Physiology in Childbearing
with Anatomy and Related Biosciences

Kaa O'Loughlin.

*This book is dedicated to the wonderful people who provide care
for mothers and babies throughout the world*

For Elsevier:

Commissioning Editor: Mary Seager
Development Editor: Catharine Steers
Project Manager: Derek Robertson
Designer: Judith Wright

Physiology in Childbearing

with Anatomy and Related Biosciences

SECOND EDITION

Edited by

Dot Stables MSc BA(Hons) MTD DN RM RN

Formerly Lecturer in Applied Biology, St Bartholomew's College of Nursing and Midwifery, City University, London, UK

Jean Rankin PhD MSc BSc(Hons) PGCE RM RGN RSCN

*Senior Lecturer (Midwifery), School of Health, Nursing and Midwifery, University of Paisley, Paisley, UK
Supervisor of Midwives – Ayrshire and Arran*

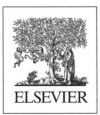

ELSEVIER

EDINBURGH LONDON NEW YORK OXFORD PHILADELPHIA ST LOUIS SYDNEY TORONTO 2005

ELSEVIER

First edition 1999
    Reprinted 2000 (twice), 2001
Second edition 2005
    Reprinted 2006, 2007

ISBN 13: 978 0 7020 2689 8
ISBN 10: 0 7020 2689 1

British Library Cataloguing in Publication Data
A catalogue record for this book is available from the British Library

Library of Congress Cataloguing in Publication Data
A catalogue record for this book is available from the Library of Congress

Note
Medical knowledge is constantly changing. Standard safety precautions must be followed, but as new research and clinical experience broaden our knowledge, changes in treatment and drug therapy may become necessary or appropriate. Readers are advised to check the most current product information provided by the manufacturer of each drug to be administered to verify the recommended dose, the method and duration of administration, and contraindications. It is the responsibility of the practitioner, relying on experience and knowledge of the patient, to determine dosages and the best treatment for each individual patient. Neither the Publisher nor the authors assumes any liability for any injury and/or damage to persons or property arising from this publication.

The Publisher

 ELSEVIER your source for books, journals and multimedia in the health sciences

www.elsevierhealth.com

Working together to grow libraries in developing countries

www.elsevier.com | www.bookaid.org | www.sabre.org

ELSEVIER   BOOK AID International   Sabre Foundation

The publisher's policy is to use paper manufactured from sustainable forests

Printed in China

Contents

Contributors

Robert Ndala MSc BSc RGN RM DMS (HSM)
Charge Midwife, Royal Berkshire Hospital, Reading, UK

Barbara V Novak MSc BA(Hons) RN RSCN RM
Lecturer in Applied Biological Sciences, St Bartholomew's School of Nursing and Midwifery, City University, London, UK

Jean Rankin PhD MSc BSc(Hons) PGCE RM RGN RSCN
Senior Lecturer (Midwifery), School of Health, Nursing and Midwifery, University of Paisley, Paisley, UK
Supervisor of Midwives – Ayrshire and Arran

Hora Soltani PhD MMedSci BSc(Midwifery)
Lecturer, Derby City General Hospital, Derby, UK

Dot Stables MSc BA(Hons) MTD DN RM RN
Formerly Lecturer in Applied Biology, St Bartholomew's College of Nursing and Midwifery, City University, London, UK

Margaret Yerby MSc RM RN ADM PGCEA
Formerly Senior Lecturer, Thames Valley University, London, UK

Preface

When the second edition of this textbook was in the planning stage it became apparent to the editor/author (Dot Stables) that the amount and depth of knowledge and its application to practice necessitated input from specialists in the different aspects of pregnancy, labour, postnatal and neonatal care. A second editor/author, Jean Rankin, was recruited and three other authors, Robert Ndala, Hora Soltani and Margaret Yerby, joined Barbara V Novak in writing about their specialist areas. This will enable students, midwifery practitioners and others caring for women during childbearing to base their decision making on detailed knowledge and understanding.

In our careers as midwives and educators the authors are aware of the increasing need to understand the physiological processes of childbearing in depth so that early recognition of pathology can prevent morbidity and mortality. We are dedicated to introducing an appreciation of the wider application of biological sciences to the practice of midwifery. Wherever possible the application of theory to practice has been discussed to demonstrate how knowledge of the biological sciences enhances the care given to mothers and babies. The aims of the second edition of this textbook remain as:

1. to provide a biology textbook for basic and post-basic students and practioners of normal and abnormal midwifery;
2. to enable an understanding of physiology and other biosciences applied to childbearing in order to ensure safe and efficient practice;
3. to foster integrated knowledge of applied biosciences and their importance for understanding humanity's place in nature;
4. to ensure the safety of mothers and babies both in the developed world and in those countries where the provision of adequate care is difficult.

We are also aware of the importance of the psychological and social aspects of reproduction and how they may affect the physiological wellbeing of childbearing women. The student should not lose sight of the integration of biology, psychology and sociology necessary to care for family health. There are many well-written books on the social and psychological implications of childbearing and the student should read the appropriate texts.

Childbearing brings about major changes in each system of the woman's body. Also an understanding of the embryological development of each system helps in an appreciation of problems arising in the neonate. For these reasons a systems approach is used throughout the textbook. Allied biosciences include anatomy, biochemistry, behavioural biology, embryology, evolution, ecology, genetics, microbiology, pharmacology and pathophysiology. Since the first edition there have been rapid advances in the field of genetics, with implications for diagnosis and treatment of diseases with a genetic basis. Therefore a new chapter has been added to consider this important field.

The book is divided into four sections. Section 1 covers preconception aspects of childbearing and includes cellular structures and functions, genetics, the anatomy and physiology of the male and female reproductive systems, fertility control and infertility. A chapter on preconception care includes wide environmental and lifestyle issues so that the practitioner can select appropriate advice for both the general public and for couples seeking specific information.

Section 2 is divided into three parts. Section 2A is concerned with the development and growth of the fetus, its placenta and membranes. The embryology is quite detailed but is hopefully presented in an easy-to-follow style. Problems of fetal health and growth are covered. Section 2B is about the physiological adaptation of the woman's body to pregnancy. Each system is described in the non-pregnant state followed by alterations brought about by pregnancy and their significance to health. Section 2C covers pathological states in pregnancy. Each disorder is discussed in depth and management in terms of diagnosis and treatment is outlined.

Section 3 is divided into two parts. Section 3A is about normal labour and includes management that arises from an understanding of physiology. There are chapters about the onset of labour, each of the three stages of labour and one devoted to the causes and management of pain in labour.

Section 3B is concerned with abnormal labour. The effects of the powers, passages and passenger on the progress of labour are considered.

Section 4 considers the mother and baby in the puerperium. It is divided into two parts. Section 4A consists of six chapters about the neonate: two chapters examine the normal neonate and adaptation to extrauterine life and four chapters explore common neonatal disorders and an outline of their management. Section 4B includes chapters on the breast and breastfeeding. The physiological changes in the puerperium and the pathological conditions that may affect women are presented. The last chapter discusses the development of mother–infant relationships in terms of biological theory.

We hope that you will find the content of this textbook as fascinating as we do and that your ability to care for mothers and babies will be enhanced by this knowledge.

Dot Stables and Jean Rankin
2005

Acknowledgements

The editors would like to thank all the contributors to this second edition as it would not have been possible without their sterling work. We are also grateful for the help of the staff of Elsevier. In particular Mary Seager and Catharine Steers, whose support made our work so much easier. We would like to mention Gordon Stables, whose unfailing support of our joint effort included providing regular meals and snacks when we editors were working together to streamline this edition.

Dot Stables believes that this book could not have been designed without the many colleagues with whom she has worked during her career in both clinical and education settings, in particular the staff of the Applied Biology Department at St Bartholomew's School of Nursing, City University, whose support allowed her to extend her knowledge of physiology and the allied biosciences, thus providing the foundation from which the chapters could be developed.

Jean Rankin would like to acknowledge Student Midwife Liz Gibson, who has been an inspiration in the face of adversity.

Section 1

PRECONCEPTION

A major aim of the book *Physiology in Childbearing* is to enable an understanding of physiology and other biosciences applied to childbearing so that safe and efficient practice is ensured. The first section of the book provides the basic knowledge to underpin the more complex content of the remaining chapters. Chapter 1 introduces basic biochemistry for those who have no previous knowledge of the subject and the content will act as a reference base. Chapter 2 examines the nature of the cell and its interactions with other cells and systems in some detail. The role of the organelles, including the nucleus and cell division, is explored. Chapter 3 is about the structure and function of the gene. It is new and has been developed because of the huge strides made in genetic theory and its practical applications in the last 5 years. Chapters 4 and 5 present the anatomy and physiology of the female and male reproductive systems. Chapters 6 and 7 examine the issues of fertility control and infertility. Chapter 8 is about preconception care and explains wide issues such as environment and lifestyle so that the practitioner can select appropriate advice both for the general public and for the couple seeking specific information.

Chapter 1

Basic biochemistry

INTRODUCTION

Organic chemistry is based on **carbon compounds** whose molecules are central to the structure and function of all living organisms (Hornby & Peach 2000). This chapter is about the chemical nature of the human body and its metabolic processes.

ENERGY

The production, storage and release of **energy** are central to the functioning of cells (Lodish et al 1999). Cells need a constant supply of energy to function and reproduce. This energy is acquired from breakdown of food molecules, in particular sugars. There are two main types of energy: **kinetic** and **potential**. Kinetic energy is the energy of movement and includes **thermal** (heat) energy. Potential or stored energy is more relevant to biological systems. Glucose stores potential energy and is broken down continuously to perform work (Alberts et al 2002, Lodish et al 1999). **Adenosine triphosphate** (ATP) is important in energy release (Ch. 23, p. 304).

Catabolic reactions (breakdown of cell products) release large quantities of energy, whereas **anabolic reactions** (such as the manufacture of proteins) are energy requiring. Cells must have a balance between energy producing and energy demanding processes (Rose 1999). All forms of energy are interchangeable and can be expressed using the same unit of measurement. The **SI unit** (International System of Units) for measuring energy is the joule (J) or kilojoule (kJ): $1\,kJ = 4.2$ calories.

THE CHEMISTRY OF LIVING ORGANISMS

Atoms

Living organisms are made up of **chemical elements**. Over 100 elements are known and each has its own symbol. Elements consist of particles called **atoms**, which are the smallest indivisible part of an element that still retains its chemical and physical properties. Atoms are constructed from

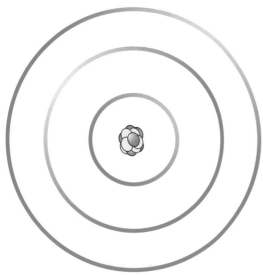

Figure 1.1   Diagrammatic representation of the structure of an atom showing the nucleus surrounded by electron orbital shells (from Hinchliff S M, Montague S E, Watson R 1996, with permission).

Table 1.1   Values for the six most common elements which make up 99% of living matter

Element	Atomic number	Number of protons	Number of neutrons	Mass number	Atomic mass
Hydrogen	1	1	0	1	1
Carbon	6	6	6	12	12
Nitrogen	7	7	7	14	14
Oxygen	8	8	8	16	16
Phosphorus	15	15	16	31	31
Calcium	20	20	20	40	40

three subatomic particles called **neutrons, protons** and **electrons** (Davis 1996). The atom has a **nucleus** made up of neutrons and protons and the very small electrons are arranged in **orbital shells** surrounding the central nucleus (Fig. 1.1).

The formation within the atom is maintained by minute electrical charges. The neutrons of the nucleus carry no charge; protons carry a positive charge, whereas electrons carry a negative charge. The number of protons is equal to the number of electrons so that most atoms are uncharged. Each element has a different number of electrons and protons, which give it its atomic number. Neutrons are heavy particles and contribute to the **mass** of the element. The number of neutrons and protons together give the element its mass number. This determines the **atomic mass** (atomic weight) of an element. Table 1.1 gives values for the six most common elements, which make up 99% of living matter.

Radioactive atoms

Variation in the number of neutrons in an atom leads to different forms of the element, called isotopes, with different mass numbers. In some isotopes the presence of extra neutrons causes them to be unstable. They will transform into a more stable configuration (break down or decay) during which they radiate energy and atomic particles. This is radioactivity and the isotopes are radioactive. Radioactive stable isotopes have been used successfully in medical diagnosis and treatment (Cooper 1992).

Molecules

Atoms are formed into **molecules** by **chemical bonds** of which there are two types: the strong, stable **covalent** bond, which is hard to disrupt, and the weaker, less stable,

non-covalent bond. The making and breaking of these bonds is associated with energy changes; the more stable the bond, the greater the thermal energy needed to disrupt it. These bonds are formed by electrons, which may be donated, received or shared by atoms. One bond is formed by one electron but some atoms have more than one electron free to form bonds. The number of available electrons is called the atom's **valency**.

Covalent bonds

When atoms are joined together by sharing electrons a molecule is formed by covalent bonds. The atoms are held closely together because electrons in their outermost shells move in orbitals that are shared by both atoms. Some atoms require more than one electron to form a bond with another atom. Bonds may be single, such as in a molecule of hydrogen gas, or double, as in a molecule of oxygen gas. Complex molecules are formed by linkage of different atoms, depending on their **valencies** (the number of electrons available to form bonds). Molecules can be represented as a molecular formula or a molecular structure (Table 1.2).

When more than two atoms form covalent bonds with a central atom, the bonds form regular structures held in shape by electrical forces. The bonds are always oriented at right angles to each other. The rigid structures formed are necessary for the structure and function of large biological molecules such as proteins and nucleic acids. The molecular mass (weight) of a substance can be calculated by adding together the mass of its component atoms. Examples are shown in Table 1.3.

The **mole** is a unit for measuring the amount of a substance and is its molecular mass expressed in grams. Concentration of a substance in a given volume of another substance is usually expressed in moles per litre: for example, a blood glucose concentration could be 4.2 millimoles per litre (mmol/L).

Non-covalent bonds

Many bonds which maintain the complex structures of large molecules are not covalent. The three-dimensional structures

Table 1.2 Examples of molecules

Atomic element	Valency	Compound	Molecular formula	Molecular structure	Bond type
H	1	Hydrogen gas	H_2	H—H	Single
O	2	Oxygen gas	O_2	O=O	Double
O	2	Water	H_2O	H H \ / O	Single
N	3	Nitrogen gas	N_2	N≡N	Triple
N	3	Ammonia	NH_3	H / H—N \ H	Single
C	4	Carbon dioxide	CO_2	O=C=O	Double
C	4	Methane	CH_4	H H \ / C / \ H H	Single
P	5	Phosphoric acid	H_3PO_4	OH | HO—P=O | OH	Single and double

Table 1.3 The molecular masses of some common chemicals

Molecular formula	Calculation	Molecular mass
H_2	1 + 1	2
O_2	16 + 16	32
H_2O	2 + 16	18
N_2	14 + 14	28
NH_3	1 + 1 + 1 + 14	17
CO_2	12 + 16 + 16	44
C_2H_5OH (ethanol)	12 + 12 + 1 + 1 + 1 1 + 1 + 16 + 1	46
$C_6H_{12}O_6$ (glucose)	$(12 \times 6) + (1 \times 12) + (16 \times 6)$	180

are stabilised by much weaker forces called non-covalent bonds. Only small amounts of energy are released in their formation. There are four main types: the **ionic bond**, the **hydrogen bond**, the **van der Waals interaction** and the **hydrophobic bond**.

Ionic bonds (electrovalent bonds)

In **ionic bonds** electrons are not shared by atoms but are donated from one atom to another, forming an **electrovalent** or ionic bond. The number of ionic bonds that can be formed is dictated by valency. Atoms of metallic elements such as sodium, calcium and iron lose electrons readily. The loss or gain of an electron is called **ionisation** and the atom becomes an **ion**. Electrons carry a negative charge so that atoms that lose an electron become positively charged **cations** such as sodium, shown by the addition of a plus sign, Na^+. The atom that receives an electron becomes negatively charged and is known as an **anion**, shown by the addition of a minus sign: for example, chlorine Cl^-. An atom or molecule that has lost or gained an electron is said to have been **polarised**.

Most ionic compounds are soluble in water because a large amount of energy is set free when ions bind tightly to water molecules. Oppositely charged ions are shielded from each other by the water and do not usually recombine. Molecules with opposite polar bonds (**dipoles**) easily form hydrogen bonds, so they attract water molecules. These polar molecules are called **hydrophilic** (water loving). Cations are attracted to anions, giving rise to compounds called **salts**. Sodium and chlorine form a very well-known salt, sodium chloride, when sodium donates an electron to chlorine:

$$Na^+ + Cl^- \rightarrow NaCl$$

In this form the salt is crystalline and consists of a rigid lattice structure but if dissolved in water the salt dissociates into free ions, which disperse in the solution. The role of fluids, solutes, acids, bases and hydrogen ion concentration (pH) in systemic function is discussed in Chapter 20.

Hydrogen bonding

Besides covalent and ionic bonds, a weak type of bond can occur between molecules. Normally a hydrogen atom forms a covalent bond with only one other atom. However, molecules containing hydrogen atoms can form an additional bond because they are attracted to each other by the weak electropositive charge left on the hydrogen atom when it is drawn towards an electronegative atom it is associating with. Hydrogen is the **donor atom** and the electronegative atom is the **acceptor atom**.

The association of oxygen and hydrogen to form water is a good example of this. Although there is no actual negative or positive charge the water molecule has become polarised. The two ends of the charge differ slightly from each other and such a molecule is a dipole. This ability of hydrogen to create weak bonds is essential for the formation of helical structures such as are found in the double helix of **deoxyribonucleic acid** (DNA) (see Ch. 3, p. 24).

The van der Waals interaction

When two atoms approach closely to each other an attractive force called a van der Waals interaction (after a Dutch physicist) is produced. Transient dipoles are created and that of one atom disturbs the electrons of the other atom, creating a second dipole. There is a weak attraction between the two dipoles. The bond formed is weaker than a hydrogen bond (Lodish et al 1999).

Both polar and non-polar molecules form this type of bond. If the van der Waals attraction between two atoms balances the repulsion between their electron clouds, the atoms stay in van der Waals contact. Distance is essential in forming this contact and each type of atom has a **van der Waals radius** at which it is in van der Waals contact with other atoms. These radii are very important in biological systems, especially when the precise shapes of two large molecules complement each other, giving many van der Waals contacts. Examples are antibody–antigen interactions (Ch. 29, p. 392) and bonds between enzymes and their substrates (Ch. 23, p. 305).

Hydrophobic interactions

Non-polar molecules contain neither ions nor dipolar bonds. They are insoluble in water and are hydrophobic (water fearing). The covalent bonds between two carbon atoms or between carbon and hydrogen atoms are the most common non-polar bonds in biological systems. That is why the hydrocarbons found in cell membranes are almost insoluble in water. A hydrophobic interaction is not a separate type of bonding force. It results from the energy needed to insert a non-polar molecule into water. The non-polar molecule cannot form hydrogen bonds and distorts the structure of water to make a cage around it. Non-polar molecules bind together comfortably using the van der Waals interaction.

CHEMICAL EQUILIBRIUM

Local environmental conditions will affect the rate at which a chemical reaction occurs and the extent to which it proceeds: concentration, temperature, pressure and so on. When two reactants come together their individual concentrations determine the formation of a product. As the concentrations decrease so does the reaction rate. Some of the products will begin to reverse the process, reforming the reactants. Eventually the forward and reverse reactions become equal. At this point a chemical mixture is said to be in **chemical equilibrium**. The presence of a specific enzyme or catalyst may speed up any reaction.

COMPOSITION OF THE HUMAN BODY

The human body is made up of about two-thirds water. The other third is composed of six main elements and traces of other elements. The chemical elements come together in various combinations to form several thousand components of living tissue (Davis 1996). Knowledge of biochemistry is essential to the understanding of physiological processes such as nutrition, respiration and metabolism. Basic substances such as **carbohydrates** (sugars), **lipids** (fats and oils) and **proteins** and their biological processes are discussed in the appropriate chapters. Other essential substances are the **nucleic acids** such as DNA. Table 1.4 lists the common elements that make up the above basic substances of the human body.

Bonds and reactions

Non-covalent bonds are not as stable as covalent bonds and that feature is essential to the working of the body. They allow complex biological compounds to change during chemical reactions without the need for large amounts of energy. Most chemical reactions in the body require the use of **enzymes** and their associated cofactors to act as **catalysts**. The types of chemical reaction found during metabolic processes are summarised in Table 1.5.

Table 1.4   Elements found in the human body

Element	Atomic symbol	Approximate weight (%)
Oxygen	O	65
Carbon	C	18
Hydrogen	H	10
Nitrogen	N	3
Calcium	Ca	2
Phosphorus	P	1
		TOTAL = 99%
Potassium	K	0.35
Sulphur	S	0.25
Sodium	Na	0.15
Chlorine	Cl	0.15
		TOTAL = 0.9%
Magnesium	Mg	trace
Iron	Fe	trace
Zinc	Zn	trace
Copper	Cu	trace
Iodine	I	trace
Manganese	Mn	trace
Chromium	Cr	trace
Molybdenum	Mo	trace
Cobalt	Co	trace
Selenium	Se	trace
		TOTAL = 0.1%

Table 1.5 Types of chemical reaction occurring during metabolism

Type	Reaction	Typical processes
Condensation	Combining molecules with the elimination of water	Formation of glycoside, ester and peptide bonds
Hydrolysis	Splitting a molecule with the addition of water	Digestion of carbohydrates, triglycerides and proteins
Dehydration	Removal of water from a molecule	Carbohydrate and fatty acid metabolism
Hydration	Incorporation of water into a molecule	Carbohydrate and fatty acid metabolism
Oxidation	Removal of hydrogen (or electrons)	Conversion of alcohols to aldehydes
Reduction	Addition of hydrogen (or electrons)	Biosynthesis of fatty acids
Carboxylation	Incorporation of carbon dioxide	Carbohydrate synthesis
Decarboxylation	Elimination of carbon dioxide	Fermentation, amine formation
Amination	Incorporation of amino group ($-NH_3$)	Amino acid biosynthesis
Deamination	Elimination of ammonia	Amino acid degradation
Methylation	Incorporation of methyl group ($-CH_3$)	Synthesis of DNA and adrenaline
Demethylation	Removal of methyl group	Amino acid degradation

MAIN POINTS

- Energy is central to the function of the cell. Kinetic energy is the energy of movement, whereas potential energy is stored in substances such as glucose which can undergo energy-releasing chemical reactions. Adenosine triphosphate is the most important substance involved in energy release.

- Living organisms are made up of atoms. The formation within the atom is maintained by minute electrical charges. Neutrons carry no charge, protons carry a positive charge and electrons a negative charge. The number of protons is equal to the number of electrons so that most atoms are uncharged.

- Variation in the number of neutrons in an atom leads to different isotopes. In some isotopes the presence of extra neutrons makes them unstable. They transform into a more stable configuration by radiating energy and atomic particles. Radioactive isotopes are used in medical diagnosis and treatment.

- Atoms join together to form compounds by using chemical bonds, of which there are two kinds – strong, stable covalent bonds and weaker less stable non-covalent bonds. The making and breaking of these chemical bonds is associated with energy changes. Stable bonds require greater thermal energy to disrupt them.

- These bonds are formed by electrons that may be donated, received or shared by atoms. The number of available electrons gives the atom's valency. When two or more atoms share electrons a molecule is formed which is held together by covalent bonds. When more than two atoms form covalent bonds with a central atom, the bonds form regular, rigid structures necessary for the function of biological molecules.

- Ionic bonds also form compounds. Electrons are not shared by atoms but are donated from one atom to another. The number of ionic bonds that can be formed is dictated by the valency. The loss or gain of an electron is called ionisation and the atom becomes an ion.

- Atoms that lose a negatively charged electron become positively charged cations. The atom that receives an electron becomes a negatively charged anion. An atom or molecule that has lost or gained an electron is polarised. Cations are attracted to anions, giving rise to salts.

- Molecules containing hydrogen atoms are attracted to each other by the weak positive charge left on the hydrogen atom when its sole electron is drawn towards the other element with which it is associating. Creation of weak bonds is essential for the formation of helical structures such as DNA.

- When two atoms approach closely to each other a van der Waals interaction is produced and transient dipoles are created. There is a weak attraction between the two dipoles. If the van der Waals attraction between two atoms balances the repulsion between their electron clouds, the atoms stay in van der Waals contact.

- Non-polar molecules contain neither ions nor dipolar bonds and are hydrophobic. They cannot form hydrogen bonds and distort the structure of water to make a cage around it. Hydrocarbons found in cell membranes are almost insoluble in water.

- Local environmental conditions affect the rate at which chemical reactions occur and the extent to which they proceed.

- Individual concentrations of reactants determine the formation of a product. As concentrations decrease, so does the reaction rate, until some of the products begin to reverse the process, reforming the reactants. When the forward and reverse reactions equalise, the mixture is in chemical equilibrium. Enzymes or catalysts may speed up reactions.

- The human body is made up of about two-thirds water and one-third of six main elements – carbon, oxygen, hydrogen, nitrogen, phosphorus, calcium and traces of other elements. Some basic substances are carbohydrates, lipids, proteins and nucleic acids.

References

Alberts B, Johnson A, Lewis J et al 2002 Molecular Biology of the Cell, 4th edn. Garland Science, Taylor & Francis Group, London.

Cooper G M 1992 Elements of Human Cancer. Jones and Bartlett, Boston.

Davis M G 1996 The Chemistry of Living Matter. In Hinchliff A S M, Montague S E, Watson R (eds) Physiology for Nursing Practice, 2nd edn. Baillière Tindall, London.

Hornby M, Peach J 2000 Foundations of Organic Chemistry. Oxford Science Publications, Oxford, UK.

Lodish H, Berk A, Zipursky L et al 1999 Molecular Cell Biology, 4th edn. W H Freeman, Basingstoke, UK.

Rose S 1999 The Chemistry of Life, 3rd edn. Penguin, Harmondsworth.

Annotated recommended reading

Alberts B, Johnson A, Lewis J et al 2002 Molecular Biology of the Cell 4th edn. Garland Science, Taylor & Francis Group, London.
This is a large, extremely well-written textbook which is worth having a look at for detailed but well-written explanations of biochemistry.

Lodish H, Berk A, Zipursky L et al 1999 Molecular Cell Biology, 4th edn. W H Freeman, Basingstoke, UK.
Parts of this textbook are very well explained, in particular the section on the molecular biology of the gene.

Rose S 1999 The Chemistry of Life, 3rd edn. Penguin, Harmondsworth.
Edition 1 of this paperback book was the author's introduction to the topic of biochemistry. Steven Rose makes the subject fascinating and easy to understand.

Hornby M, Peach J 2000 Foundations of Organic Chemistry. Oxford Science Publications, Oxford, UK.
This slim volume is suitable for the student who already understands the basic knowledge given in the chapter and would like a deeper understanding of organic chemistry.

Chapter 2

The cell – its structures and functions

PHYSICAL CHARACTERISTICS OF MAMMALIAN CELLS

All living species are made up of **cells**: small membrane-bound units filled with a concentrated aqueous solution of carefully balanced chemicals and **organelles** (Fig. 2.1). They can create copies of themselves by replication and division, thus ensuring that their **genetic lineage** is preserved and capable of competent function. Their complex structure and specialised functions, governed by complex **genetic information**, make them the fundamental units of the body. There are over 200 different cell types in the human body, assembled into tissue types such as **epithelia**, **connective tissue**, **muscle**, conducting **neural tissue** and non-conducting **neuroglia**. Most tissues consist of different cell types, functioning in harmony through coordination and communication.

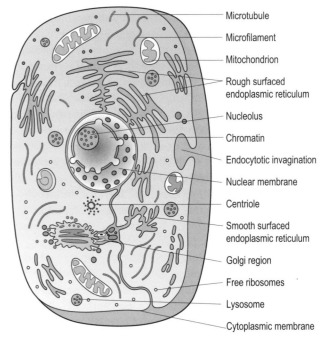

Microtubule

Microfilament

Mitochondrion

Rough surfaced endoplasmic reticulum

Nucleolus

Chromatin

Endocytotic invagination

Nuclear membrane

Centriole

Smooth surfaced endoplasmic reticulum

Golgi region

Free ribosomes

Lysosome

Cytoplasmic membrane

Figure 2.1 Diagram of the ultrastructure of a cell (from Hinchliff S M, Montague S E 1990, with permission).

Mammalian cells average 5–20 μm in diameter (Alberts et al 2002). Their microstructure cannot be determined by light microscopy but electron microscopes and electronic processing reveal structural details as small as a few nanometres. This has enabled cell biologists to reveal complex cellular ultrastructures necessary for preservation of structural and functional integrity. These are sustained, repaired or replaced when necessary by genetic expression and selective assimilation of matter from the **extracellular compartment**.

CELL SIZE AND SHAPE

Cells differentiate and modify their form and activities during their stages of development and aggregate correctly to form specific organs, systems or the whole body. In each cell biochemical control and communication are fundamental. Knowledge of the size and appearance of the cell is important. Resting **lymphocytes** are amongst the smallest of cells, their average diameter being 6 μm whereas **erythrocytes** are approximately 7.5–9.0 μm and **columnar epithelial cells** are 20 μm tall and 10 μm wide. Some cells are significantly larger than this; bone marrow **megakaryocytes** average 200 μm in diameter. Mature **ova** may be over 80 μm in diameter (Bannister et al 1995). Some neurones and skeletal muscle cells are relatively large but this may be due to their attenuated structure. These terms are discussed in later chapters.

Cellular dimensions are partly determined by **metabolic requirements** and the rate of **substrate diffusion** across the highly selective **plasma membrane** (Guyton & Hall 2000). A major advantage of cells is their capacity to permit selective but rapid diffusion of substrates over short distances of up to 50 μm. This plays a major part in sustaining the metabolic needs of active cells.

As cells increase in size their mass outstrips their surface area unless their shape changes to an irregular or elongated surface structure as in neurones. As many physiological processes such as diffusion of gases and ions and transport of nutrients depend on the surface area of the cell, an increase in mass may make maintenance of efficient metabolic processes difficult. The larger the cell, the further the cell periphery is from the nucleus and exertion of nuclear control on the **cytoplasm** and plasma membrane become problematic. In larger cells such challenges may be overcome to some extent by an increase in surface area achieved by either folding the plasma membrane and forming **microvilli**, or other surface protrusions, or flattening the entire body of the cell. This larger surface area is better designed to sustain efficient substrate transport and diffusion.

Nuclear control in larger cells can be enhanced by the presence of multiple nuclei, achieved either by a fusion of mononuclear cells as occurs in skeletal muscle or, more rarely, by multiplication of the central nucleus without cytoplasmic division. The external appearance of a cell type varies widely depending on its specific functions, interactions with other cells, external environment and the nature of the internal structures which mastermind individual cell activities.

CELL MOTILITY

Many cells display some degree of **motility** (Alberts et al 2002). This involves the movement of the cytoplasm or specific organelles from one part of the cell to another. The complexity of cell motility occurs due to an adjustment in the position of a cell, believed to be influenced and dominated by systemic environmental factors such as tissue injury. Examples of cell motility include the migration of **phagocytic** white blood cells from blood to a site of tissue injury or infection and the way that advancing tip(s) of developing axons migrate in response to growth factors along a path to their synaptic targets. Similar mechanical processes occur in **endocytosis**, **phagocytosis** and **exocytosis**.

The best example of cell migration is observed in **fibroblasts** during early embryonic development. However, the primary feature of embryonic fibroblasts is **collagen** secretion, which is essential to the development of the extracellular matrix rather than to locomotion. Fibroblasts interact with collagen by means of adhesion plaques through which they exert traction on the matrix. This process also plays a key role in the process of tissue remodelling, which is important in normal wound healing.

The exact molecular mechanisms involved in cell locomotion are unknown. However, research suggests that co-ordinated changes involve numerous molecules in different regions of the cell and that no single organelle is responsible for cell locomotion (Alberts et al 2002). Three interrelated processes are known to be essential:

1. the cell has to define its leading edge;
2. this edge adheres to the surface over which the cell is crawling; and
3. the remainder of cells drag themselves forwards by traction, using the adhesions as points for anchorage.

All three processes involve actin in different ways. The plasma membrane of the crawling cell's leading edge appears to organise the actin filaments by providing small aggregates of proteins that promote actin polymerisation (see below). Cell locomotion takes place within specific biochemical and micro-anatomic environments which modulate its speed and direction.

EPITHELIAL CELLS

Epithelial cells are derived from the three embryonic germ layers (Alberts et al 2002). Generally, epithelial cells form cell sheets which line the inner and outer body surfaces. **Ectoderm**, **endoderm** and **mesoderm** each contribute to the formation and development of epithelium:

- ectoderm contributes to the development of the epidermis, breast glandular tissue, cornea and the junctional zones of the buccal cavity and anal canal;
- endoderm forms the epithelial lining of the alimentary canal and its glands, most of the respiratory tract and the distal tract of the urogenital tract; and

• mesoderm gives rise to the epithelium-like cells lining internal cavities such as the pericardium, pleural and peritoneal cavities, the lining of the blood vessels and lymph vessels and the proximal parts of the urogenital tract.

Epithelia provide a covering for the body and its internal organs and serve as selective barriers, facilitating or preventing the transfer of substrates across the surfaces which they cover. Some epithelia protect underlying tissue from dehydration, chemical or mechanical injury, while other epithelia act as sensory surfaces, a function best illustrated by neural tissue, a modified epithelium.

Common classification of the epithelia

The polygonal, diverse shape of epithelial cells is partly determined by their cytoplasmic contents and partly by pressure and functional demands of the surrounding tissue (Bannister et al 1995). It is usual to classify the diverse epithelia according to their structural and functional characteristics.

Simple epithelia

Simple epithelia are formed by single layers of cells resting on a basal **lamina** formed of filamentous proteins and proteoglycans. They are subdivided according to the shape of their cells, which may be columnar, cuboidal, pseudostratified and squamous types. Cellular shape is largely related to cell volume. Where cells are small the volume of the cytoplasm is relatively low, denoting few organelles and low metabolic activity. Conversely, highly metabolic epithelial cells generally form secretory cells containing abundant mitochondria, endoplasmic reticulum and are tall, cuboidal or columnar. Simple epithelia are capable of special functions and help to form cilia, microvilli, secretory vacuoles or sensory features.

Stratified or squamous epithelia

Stratified or squamous epithelia consist of superficial cells, which are constantly replaced by their regenerating basal layers. These epithelia consist of flattened, interlocking, polygonal cells. Their cytoplasm may sometimes not exceed 0.1 mm thickness and their nucleus may bulge into the overlying space. As squamous epithelium is so thin, it is ideally suited to facilitating diffusion of gases and water. However, it is also engaged in active transport, a role indicated by numerous endocytic vesicles. The most critical positions for squamous epithelia are in the lining of the lung alveoli, the glomeruli and the thin segments of the loop of Henle.

Cuboidal and columnar epithelia

Cuboidal and columnar epithelia consist of regular rows of cylindrical cells. Commonly, the free surface of columnar cells has microvilli suited to the absorptive role of the small intestine, where they enhance the surface area for absorption of water and nutrients. By contrast, the columnar epithelium of the gall bladder displays a brush border, essential to concentration and storage of bile. Ciliated columnar epithelium is found in much of the respiratory tract, the lining of fallopian tubes and uterine cervix. Large cuboidal cells are found in the proximal and distal convoluted segments of nephrons, where they form a brush border which selectively reabsorbs substances from the filtrate into the renal medullary interstitium.

Transitional epithelium

The characteristic feature of transitional epithelium is its thickness, formed by an extended arrangement of 4–6 cells held together in a specific arrangement by numerous desmosomes (filamentous structures). In stretching, these cells flatten without altering their position relative to each other. Most of these epithelial cells are attached to their basal lamina by slender processes forming a basal structure where they appear cuboidal and uninucleate when relaxed. At the surface of this multilayered epithelium, cells progressively fuse to form larger, and sometimes binucleate but polyploid, cells with a plasma membrane covered by glycoprotein particles.

This cellular arrangement has two distinctive roles. It facilitates expansion and contraction, thereby stretching considerably without losing structural integrity, and provides an impermeable lining for organs that hold liquid containing toxic metabolic end-products such as urea and uric acid and high concentrations of salts such as potassium and sodium. Transitional epithelium is invaluable in forming an impermeable lining in the genitourinary tract.

Complex structures derived from epithelium

Complex organ structures derived from epithelia retain familiar cellular characteristics. For instance, the capacity of the liver or the placenta to absorb, secrete and transport substrates illustrates some of their complex physiological roles. Similarly, the diverse forms of neural tissue are functional modifications of epithelia. Most neural tissue is differentiated into conducting and non-conducting cells which provide the body with a network for processing and managing information by signal transduction.

CELLULAR ORGANISATION

A typical cell includes a single nucleus, cytoplasm and a cellular boundary known as the **plasma membrane**. The different substances making up the cell are collectively known as **protoplasm**, composed predominantly of water, electrolytes, proteins, lipids and carbohydrates, which plays a crucial role in shaping the cell and its organelles: these include the cell membrane, the nuclear membrane, the endoplasmic reticulum, Golgi apparatus, mitochondria, lysosomes and centrioles.

The plasma membrane

The cell membrane or plasma membrane is the most common feature of all cells (Alberts et al 2002). An appropriate plasma membrane is crucial to the survival and functional integrity of each cell. It encloses the cellular contents, defines its boundaries, and maintains the essential differences between the cytosol and the extracellular environment.

The lipid bilayer

The plasma membrane (Fig. 2.2) consists of a very thin lipid bilayer containing a family of protein molecules (Alberts et al 2002). This complex arrangement of lipid and specialised proteins is held together predominantly by non-covalent interactions (Ch. 1). Plasma membranes are dynamic fluid structures capable of considerable adaptation because of the ability of most of their molecules to move about within the plane of the membranes.

The lipid bilayer is composed almost entirely of fatty acids, made up of **phospholipids** and **cholesterol**. Phospholipids are small molecules constructed mainly from fatty acids and glycerol. In phospholipids, the glycerol is joined to two rather than three fatty acid chains, as in **triacylglycerols**. The third position (site) on the glycerol molecule is linked to a hydrophilic **phosphate group**, which is in turn attached to

a small hydrophilic compound such as **choline**. Each phospholipid molecule has a polar head group and two hydrophobic hydrocarbon tails consisting of fatty acids which differ in length. The differences in the length and saturation of the fatty acid tails enable the phospholipid molecules to pack against one another and construct the 'fluid' framework, ensuring plasma membrane competence. This structure gives them different physical and chemical properties to those of triacylglycerols, which are hydrophobic (Alberts et al 2002).

The lipid molecules are arranged in a continuous double layer about 5–7 nm thick (Alberts et al 2002). The hydrophobic portions of the phospholipid face each other, whereas the hydrophilic components make up the plasma membrane surface, which is in perpetual contact with the surrounding interstitial fluid. This lipid bilayer is highly permeable to lipid-soluble substances, such as oxygen, carbon dioxide and alcohol, but serves as a relatively impermeable barrier to the passage of most water-soluble molecules such as inorganic ions and glucose.

Lipid molecules are insoluble in water but dissolve readily in organic solvents. The shape and functional scope of lipid molecules results in the spontaneous formation of bilayers in aqueous solutions. When lipid molecules are surrounded by water they tend to aggregate so that their hydrophobic tails are buried in the dry, water-free interior and their hydrophilic heads are exposed to water. Lipid bilayers tend to form sealed compartments, eliminating any spaces where the hydrophobic tails would be in contact with water. This phenomenon is observed in circumstances such as damaged plasma membranes, which reseal rapidly to avoid exposure of the fatty acid tails to water.

Plasma membrane fluidity is important to the survival of the cellular infrastructure and the capacity of the membrane to sustain transport processes and enzyme activities. However, the lipid bilayer of many cell membranes is not exclusively composed of phospholipids. It can contain cholesterol, **glycolipids** and **glycoproteins**. Cholesterol molecules make the lipid bilayer more stable, less deformable and decrease its permeability to small water-soluble molecules. They also prevent the hydrocarbon chains from coming together, crystallising and damaging the functional integrity of the plasma membrane. Glycolipids and glycoproteins act as receptors for extracellular biochemical products.

The membrane proteins

Suspended in the lipid bilayer are proteins, mostly glycoproteins, which mediate many of the selective functions of the plasma membrane. These proteins fall into two groups: the **integral proteins**, which protrude through the membrane, and the **peripheral proteins**, which are attached to the inner surface of the membrane.

The transmembrane proteins   Transmembrane proteins have a unique orientation in the plasma membrane, reflecting the asymmetrical manner in which the protein is

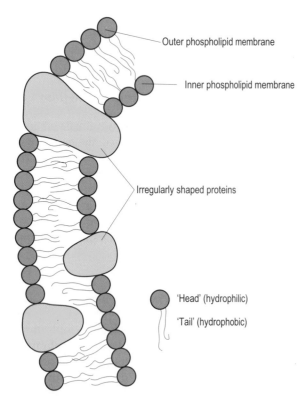

Outer phospholipid membrane

Inner phospholipid membrane

Irregularly shaped proteins

'Head' (hydrophilic)

'Tail' (hydrophobic)

Figure 2.2   Diagram of the fluid mosaic model of cell membrane structure (from Hinchliff S M, Montague S E 1990, with permission).

synthesised in the **endoplasmic reticulum** and inserted into the lipid bilayer (Guyton & Hall 2000). Membrane proteins do not flop across the lipid bilayers of the plasma membrane but rotate about an axis perpendicular to the plane of the lipid bilayer, facilitating the process of rotational diffusion. Also, many membrane proteins can move laterally within the membrane, aiding a process of lateral diffusion.

The complex role of the plasma membrane is partly attributable to the asymmetrical construction, best illustrated by the molecular lipid and protein compositions found on the outer and the inner surfaces of the membrane (Alberts et al 2002). The lipid–protein arrangements differ from one another, reflecting their different functions at the two distinctive membrane surfaces so that these epithelial cells may control the diffusion of lipids as well as protein molecules. Cells confine proteins to specific domains within a plasma membrane. For example in the epithelial cells lining the intestinal tract some of the plasma membrane transport proteins are confined to the apical surface of the cells, whereas others are confined to the basal and lateral surfaces.

Peripheral proteins   The peripheral proteins are normally attached to one of the integral proteins, usually functioning as enzymes that catalyse cellular chemical reactions. Other proteins form structural links connecting the plasma membrane to the **cytoskeleton** or to either the extracellular matrix or adjacent cells. A few proteins serve as specialised receptors for the detection and transduction of chemical signals found in the cell's environment.

The quantities and types of plasma membrane proteins vary, depending on cellular functions. For instance, the neural **myelin membrane** serves mainly as an electrical insulation for nerve cells axons, so that less than 25% of the membrane mass consists of protein. Conversely, membranes involved in energy transduction, such as the internal membranes of **mitochondria**, are composed of approximately 75% protein. Generally, plasma membrane protein content averages 50% of its total mass (Alberts et al 2002). Because lipid molecules are much smaller than protein molecules, there are many more lipid molecules in a plasma membrane than protein molecules. There may be 50 lipid molecules for each protein molecule in a membrane that is 50% protein by mass.

The selective **permeability** of the plasma membrane facilitates free passage of some gases such as oxygen, and water, but restricts the movement of larger ions such as sodium, potassium, calcium, chloride and bicarbonate to their specific protein channels, which open or close in order to regulate transmembrane ion traffic. Most integral proteins form **pores** through which water-soluble substances such as ions **diffuse** passively. The selective passage of many other substances of large molecular weight, such as glucose and amino acids, is also limited to such protein channels, most of which are ion- or substrate-specific. This contrasts with the diffusion of lipid-soluble substances, which pass directly through the lipid portion of the plasma membranes.

For instance, **steroid hormones** diffuse into the cytoplasm without passing through any form of protein channel.

Endocytosis and Exocytosis   Cells take up larger molecules by invagination of small segments of plasma membrane to create **vacuoles** or **endocytic vesicles**. These take up larger molecules and aid their transportation to other cellular regions. Extrusion of organic molecules, for example **thyroxine** and **acetylcholine**, is achieved by **exocytic vesicles**, which fuse with plasma membrane, releasing their content to the cell's exterior.

CYTOPLASM AND ITS ORGANELLES

Every living cell must communicate with its immediate environment to sustain its microstructures and functional competence. In **prokaryotic cells** (non-nucleated single cell organisms such as bacteria) communication takes place across the plasma membrane. **Eukaryotic cells** (nucleated) have developed an internal process which culminates in endocytosis and exocytosis. This elaborate internal membrane machinery is constructed by complex arrangements of cell-specific organelles contained within the cytoplasm (Bannister et al 1995).

Cytoplasm

Cytoplasm makes up approximately half of the cell volume. Due to its high protein content (20% by weight), it appears more like a gel than an aqueous solution, allowing suspension of small molecular structures, large particles and organelles. Organic and inorganic ions are dissolved in the aqueous phase of the cytoplasm and exchanged between the cell and the surrounding extracellular environment. Also dispersed in the cytoplasm are fat globules, glycogen granules, ribosomes and secretory granules. The most important organelles contained within the cytoplasm are the endoplasmic reticulum, the Golgi apparatus, the mitochondria, the lysosomes and the peroxisomes. Variations in their numbers or densities may be found in different cells, although their functions are unchanged across the cell types.

Endoplasmic reticulum

The **endoplasmic reticulum** is a network of specialised membranous structures organised into tubular or flat vesicular sacs (Fig. 2.3). These interconnect so that the entire endoplasmic reticulum forms a continuous framework within the internal cellular space. The endoplasmic reticular membrane forms a barrier between the cytosol and the reticular lumen, mediating the selective transport of molecules between these two compartments. The endoplasmic reticulum can make up as much as 50% of total cell volume.

There are two distinctive membrane types: the rough and the smooth endoplasmic reticulum. The fundamental

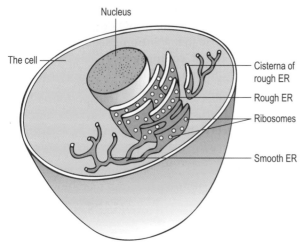

Figure 2.3   The endoplasmic reticulum. The rough endoplasmic reticulum and smooth endoplasmic reticulum with their connections are illustrated.

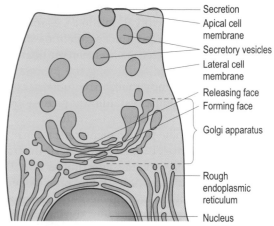

Figure 2.4   Exocytosis of secretory proteins from the Golgi apparatus (from Hinchliff S M, Montague S F, Watson R 1996, with permission).

difference between these two types of organelles is the association of ribosomes to the cytoplasmic surface of the rough endoplasmic reticulum. The rough endoplasmic reticulum is continuous with the nuclear envelope outer membrane which is also associated with **ribosomes**. By contrast, the smooth endoplasmic reticulum is ribosome-free.

The functions of rough and smooth endoplasmic reticulum differ fundamentally. Rough endoplasmic reticulum plays a central role in protein biosynthesis, including the production of all the transmembrane proteins used in the reconstruction of organelles, including its own structure! The synthesis of membrane lipids such as steroids, phospholipids and triglycerides occurs within both the rough and the smooth endoplasmic reticulum. The smooth endoplasmic reticulum of skeletal and cardiac muscle cells is known as the sarcoplasmic reticulum and acts as a reservoir for calcium, which is released into the cytoplasm to initiate contraction and taken up again to bring about muscle relaxation.

Ribosomes   There are at least two separate families of **ribosomes** in the cytoplasm (Alberts et al 2002). All ribosomes are particles or granules of no more than 25 nm in diameter, consisting of two-thirds ribonucleic acid (RNA) and one-third protein. Each ribosome is made up of a large (60S) and a small (40S) subunit which play a critical role in protein synthesis. Ribosomes are produced in the nucleus of the cell under the direction of **deoxyribonucleic acid** (DNA) and each facilitates the synthesis of one specific protein needed by that particular cell.

Membrane-bound ribosomes attached to the external surface of the rough endoplasmic reticulum and the outer nuclear membrane are involved in synthesising protein, which is then translocated into the **cisternae** of the endoplasmic reticulum. Unattached free ribosomes are involved in the synthesis of all other proteins encoded by nuclear DNA. The two types of ribosomes are structurally and functionally identical, differing only in the proteins they are synthesising at any given time.

Generally, proteins synthesised by free ribosomes are used for intracellular activities such as cytoplasmic filament formation, whereas the attached ribosomes synthesise proteins that enter the cisternae and are then transported to the Golgi apparatus. These proteins are destined for the development or construction of intra- and extracellular substrates. Protein translocation into the cisternae occurs by virtue of specific protein-conducting channels in the membrane whose opening appears to be governed by signal peptides (Alberts et al 2002).

Golgi apparatus

The **Golgi apparatus** is situated near the cell nucleus, and frequently close to the **centrosomes**. Each Golgi apparatus is adjacent to the endoplasmic reticulum and its membrane is similar in appearance to the smooth endoplasmic reticulum. The apparatus consists of four or more stacked thin, flat vesicles consisting of an entry point or *cis* face, and an exit or *trans* face. The entire Golgi apparatus functions in close association with the endoplasmic reticulum. Soluble proteins from the endoplasmic reticulum enter the Golgi apparatus where they are processed and fine-tuned to form lysosomes, secretory vesicles containing enzymes or other cytoplasmic components (Fig. 2.4).

Lysosomes

Lysosomes are vesicular organelles dispersed throughout the cytoplasm. The differentiation of lysosomes is cell-dependent, but they are usually about 250–750 nm in diameter. They are surrounded by a membranous lipid bilayer and are filled with large numbers of small granules averaging at 5–8 nm in diameter. These membranous sacs contain about 40 types of hydrolytic enzymes which are synthesised in the endoplasmic reticulum and transported through the

Golgi apparatus to the lysosomes to be stored as granules until needed. They are involved in the digestion and processing of materials entering the cells from the extracellular environment prior to its release into the cytoplasm (Alberts et al 2002).

They degrade unwanted intracellular substances such as proteins, nucleic acid, phospholipids and oligosaccharides. They also help to remove damaged structures and foreign particles such as bacteria. These digestive/hydrolytic enzymes **hydrolyse** (Ch. 1, p. 7) proteins to form amino acids, glycogen to form glucose, and obsolete parts of the cell itself such as mitochondria are degraded and removed. The degradation of the mitochondria and other organelles is initiated by its enclosure in a membrane derived from the endoplasmic reticulum. This creates an autophagosome, which fuses with local lysosomes (Alberts et al 2002). It is unclear what determines the destruction of specific organelles.

Peroxisomes

Peroxisomes are formed by the budding off of membranes from the smooth endoplasmic reticulum. Their size averages at 0.15–0.5 μm in diameter. New peroxisomes are formed by the growth and fission of existing ones. Since these organelles do not have their own genome or ribosomes, their proteins and lipids must be imported. They contain oxidases capable of catalysing many reactions, including the **oxidation** of long-chain saturated fatty acids not handled well by mitochondria. Several oxidases can combine oxygen with hydrogen ions, thereby forming **hydrogen peroxide**, also a highly oxidising substance which, in association with catalase, oxidises many substances toxic to the cell. Given their function, it is not surprising to find peroxisomes involved in cholesterol metabolism and gluconeogenesis within liver hepatocytes. In other cell types such as the myelin of the central nervous system, peroxisomes contain different enzymes which allow them to synthesise substances such as phospholipids.

Mitochondria

Mitochondria are found in the cytoplasm of most mature cells. Their distinctive structure and variable size reflect the complex nature of their function. These organelles are ellipsoid in shape with an average length of 1–2 μm and a width of 0.1–0.5 μm. However this electron microscopic picture could be misleading, because when viewed in a living cell, mitochondria change their shape, fuse, divide and move (Goodman 1998). Normally a mitochondrion doubles its mass and divides into two during each cell cycle. However, some mitochondria divide rapidly, whereas others do not divide at all.

Mitochondria have their own double-stranded circular DNA which is replicated prior to the mitochondrial division. The human mitochondrial genome consists of 16 569 nucleotide pairs (Goodman 1998). Mitochondria usually contain multiple copies of their genome. Although there are multiple mitochondria in each cell, their DNA makes up less than 1% of the total cellular DNA. Mitochondrial DNA is extremely compact, with few **intronic sequences** or untranslated regions between **coding genes** (Ch. 3). Because of asymmetric distribution of **guanines** and **cytosines**, one strand is heavier due to its guanine content and the opposing strand is lighter due to its cytosine content.

The structure of a mitochondrion   Mitochondria consist of an outer and an inner membrane, which jointly create two compartments. The outer membrane contains a major integral protein, **porin**, which forms membrane channels thought to facilitate substrate (molecular weight of less than 10 000) diffusion. The inner membrane is arranged into folds known as cristae, which increase the surface area considerably, an important feature of the function of mitochondria as power centres of the cell. This inner membrane consists of 75% protein (Goodman 1998), which may be significant in supporting the mitochondrial respiratory chain, **adenosine triphosphate** (ATP) synthesis and the transport of oxidative phosphorylation substrates in and out of the mitochondria. Mitochondria provide cells with energy by reducing oxygen and converting **adenosine diphosphate** and phosphate to ATP (Ch. 23, p. 304). Without mitochondria, cells would be unable to extract energy from nutrients and oxygen, and all cellular functions would cease (McKee & McKee 1996). Cells which are metabolically highly active usually have a large collection of mitochondria.

The **mitochondrial genome** only encodes 13 protein subunits and mitochondria must import most of their protein from the cytoplasm. These proteins are synthesised by free ribosomes, are thought to be destined for the mitochondria because they possess a mitochondrial signal peptide. This binds to a signal receptor on the mitochondrion's outer membrane and the complex moves laterally across the outer membrane until it reaches a contact site at which the outer and inner membranes are joined. The signal peptide crosses both membranes at the contact site, using the difference in the membrane potential as the energy source.

As the size and shape of the mitochondria vary considerably, their appearance varies from globular and no more than a few hundred nanometres in diameter, to elongated structures of 1 μm in diameter and up to 7 μm in length. The structural features of the mitochondria are, however, constant and arranged so that they can cope with the functional demands of cells. This is particularly evident in the cristae of the inner membrane, which project into the interior of the organelle (Fig. 2.5).

Cristae   **Cristae** may be shelflike or tubular in structure onto which the oxidative enzymes are attached. The innermost cavity of the mitochondria is filled with a matrix containing large quantities of dissolved enzymes, necessary for extraction of energy from nutrients. These enzymes function in association with oxidative enzymes and enzyme partnerships within the mitochondria to provide

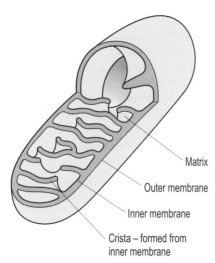

Figure 2.5   Diagram of a mitochondrion (from Hinchliff S M, Montague S E 1990, with permission).

the mechanism for oxidation of nutrients with liberation of energy and formation of carbon dioxide and water. The liberated energy is used to synthesise high-energy ATP, which is transported out of the mitochondria into the cytoplasm, as required, for the release of energy to support cellular activities. Mitochondrial self-replication is probably induced by increased cellular ATP requirements. Since mitochondria usually contain multiple copies of their own genome, its replication prior to division is one of the most important mechanisms cells have to ensure their metabolic and energy demands are met.

THE NUCLEUS

The nucleus is the ultimate control centre of the cell (Laskey 1987). As the largest structure of the cell, it measures approximately 2–10 μm in diameter. Although mainly centrally situated, its position and number can vary with cell type. For example, it is found in the periphery of **adipocytes**, at the base of epithelial and secretory cells and in the centre of the cell body in neurones. Most cells have only one nucleus although skeletal muscle cells and **osteoclasts** are examples of multinucleated cells.

Nuclei contain large quantities of DNA, which holds the genetic blueprint. The nuclear genome determines the characteristics of proteins and enzymes contained in the cytoplasm of a specific cell type. It also controls cytoplasmic activities and cellular reproduction (McKee & McKee 1996). In addition to the DNA, several other structures are essential to the normal functioning of the nucleus such as the gel-like **nucleoplasm** and the **nucleoli**: the latter are the site of **ribosomal ribonucleic acid** (rRNA) synthesis.

The genetic material, consisting chiefly of DNA, is found in a thread-like mass known as **chromatin**. Prior to cellular reproduction, chromatin shortens and coils into rod-like bodies forming (in humans) 46 recognisable **chromosomes** (Ch. 3 and below).

The outermost part of the nucleus is formed by a complex nuclear membrane composed of two lipid bilayers approximately 20–40 nm apart from each other enclosing the **perinuclear cisternae**. The outer nuclear membrane is continuous with the cell's endoplasmic reticulum. The intramembranous space of 20–40 nm serves as an extension of the internal compartments of the endoplasmic reticulum.

Several thousand **nuclear pores** penetrate the entire nuclear envelope, making it permeable to substances of low molecular weight. Large complex protein molecules surround these nuclear pores, creating central smaller pores, only 9–10 nm in diameter but large enough to permit molecules up to 44 000 in molecular weight to pass through relatively easily. Substrates of molecular weight less than 15 000 pass through the nuclear pores extremely rapidly. The selective transport of large molecules and complexes across the nuclear membrane, through the nuclear pores, occurs by a receptor-mediated process (Goodman 1998). Membrane porosity also permits the movement of messenger RNA to the cytoplasm and entry of enzymes and histones into the nucleus during DNA replication.

The nucleolus

The nucleolus is a dense structure visible within the nucleus during the cells' interphase, although its size and shape is dependent on its activity relative to the cell cycle. In cells which are actively synthesising large quantities of different proteins the nucleolus may occupy as much as 25% of the total cell volume, whereas in dormant cells the nucleolus is hardly visible. Unlike most organelles, it does not appear to have a limiting membrane. Its primary function is the production and assembly of ribosomal subunits. The nucleolus has four distinct regions Goodman (1998):

1. a fibrillar centre which contains DNA that is not being transcribed;
2. a dense fibrillar core which contains RNAs in a process of transcription;
3. a granular region where the maturing ribosomal particles are assembled; and
4. a nuclear matrix that may participate in the organisation of the nucleolus.

However, it usually contains large quantities of RNA and proteins similar to those found in the ribosomes. The nucleolus seems to become considerably enlarged when a cell is actively involved in protein synthesis, when it also increases the size and enhances the shape of the nucleus, and disappears during mitosis, when it is reassembled again in the daughter cells.

THE CYTOSKELETON

The complex network of protein filaments that extends throughout the cytoplasm is known as the **cytoskeleton**. This highly dynamic structure reorganises continuously as the cell changes shape, divides and responds to its environment (Latchman 1997). It is responsible for cellular movement such as cell crawling, muscle contraction and the many changes in cell shape that occur in the developing embryo. The cytoskeleton also provides the machinery for intracellular movement, such as the transport of organelles within the cytoplasm, and the segregation of chromosomes at mitosis. The highly diverse activities of the cytoskeleton depend on three types of protein filaments: actin filaments, microtubules and the intermediate filaments.

PLASMA MEMBRANE EXCITABILITY AND ION TRANSPORT

The hydrophobic interior of the plasma membranes acts as a barrier to the passage of most polar molecules. This barrier is crucial to the overall function of a specific cell (Goodman 1998). It allows the cell to maintain the required solutes in the cytoplasm and within each of the intracellular membrane-bound organelles at vastly different concentrations to those found in extracellular fluid. To maintain this barrier, cells use sophisticated mechanisms for transferring specific water-soluble molecules across their membranes to obtain essential nutrients, excrete metabolic waste products and regulate intracellular ion concentrations.

Specialised transmembrane proteins transport inorganic ions and small water-soluble organic molecules across the lipid bilayer. The two main classes of membrane proteins that mediate the transfer of small water-soluble molecules are called transport proteins – either **carrier proteins** or **channel proteins**. Carrier proteins are coupled to a source of energy which facilitates active transport of specific molecules across the membrane. Channel proteins form a narrow hydrophilic pore, allowing the passive movement of small inorganic ions across the lipid bilayer. This combination of passive permeability and active transport contributes significantly to the large differences in the composition of cytosol compared with extracellular fluid or the fluid within membrane-bounded organelles.

By generating ionic concentration differences across the lipid bilayer cell, membranes store **potential energy** in the form of **electrochemical gradients** which drive transport processes, convey electric signals in electrically excitable cells and generate ATP in the mitochondria. The smaller the molecule and more soluble it is in oil, the more rapidly it will diffuse across a particular lipid bilayer (Goodman 1998). Similarly, small non-polar molecules such as oxygen and carbon dioxide readily dissolve in the lipid bilayers and diffuse rapidly across them. Uncharged polar molecules also diffuse rapidly across a bilayer if they are small enough. Water and urea cross rapidly, whereas glycerol, a larger molecule, diffuses less rapidly, and the more complex glucose diffuses hardly at all without the aid of a carrier.

The lipid bilayers are impermeable to charged molecules (ions) no matter how small they are; their charge and the high degree of hydration prevent them from entering the hydrocarbon phase of the bilayer. To facilitate efficient ionic transfer, channel proteins consisting of highly selective pores form a continuous pathway across the plasma membrane to enable specific hydrophilic solutes to cross the membrane without coming into direct contact with the hydrophobic interior of the lipid bilayer. As most channel proteins are ion-species specific; their size and pore control may play a crucial role in determining ion diffusion efficiency. The advantage of channel proteins over carrier proteins is that more than 1 million ions can pass through an open channel each second, a rate 1000 times greater than the rate of transport of any known carrier protein.

Ion channels

Two important properties distinguish ion channels from single aqueous pores (Alberts et al 2002). They show ion selectivity, permitting some inorganic ions to pass but not others and, more importantly, ion channels are not continuously open but have 'gates' which open briefly, usually in response to a specific stimulus and close again once the electrogradient for a particular ion species has been reached. The main types of stimuli which cause ion channels to open are changes in **voltage** across the membrane (voltage-gated channels), **mechanical stress** (mechanically gated channels) or the binding of a **ligand** (ligand-gated channels). The ligand can be an extracellular mediator, a neurotransmitter or an intracellular mediator such as an ion or a nucleotide.

Although ion channels are responsible for the electrical excitability of muscle cells and the mediation of electrical signalling in neurones, they are not restricted to electrically excitable cells. They are present in all cell membranes, facilitating diffusion of their specific ion species and thereby maintaining the required intracellular electrochemical gradient. The most common forms of ion channels are those permeable mainly to potassium ions. This makes the plasma membrane much more permeable to potassium ions than to any other ions, a factor critical in maintaining the cell's membrane potential and the significant voltage difference across all plasma membranes.

Carrier proteins

In contrast, carrier proteins, which are responsible for selective transport of substrates across the plasma membrane, bind the specific solute and then undergo a series of conformational changes in order to transfer the solute across the plasma membrane. Each carrier protein has one or more **binding sites** for its substrate. The specialised transport process involves full saturation of the carrier sites. When all the binding sites are occupied, the rate of transport across the plasma membrane is maximal. However, solute binding can be blocked by competitive inhibitors occupying the same binding sites and which may or may not be transported by the carrier, or by non-competitive inhibitors which bind elsewhere and alter the structure of the carrier protein.

Carrier proteins are classified according to their functional capacity: some are **uniporters**; other more complex proteins are **coupled transporters**, where the transport of one solute depends on the simultaneous transfer of a second solute. This transport may be in the same direction (**symport**) or in the opposite direction (**antiport**). For example, the take-up of glucose from extracellular fluid, where its concentration is high relative to that in the cytosol, is achieved by passive transport through glucose carriers operating as uniporters, whereas intestinal and kidney epithelial cells take up glucose from the lumen of the intestine and the lumen of the nephron, respectively. In both instances the concentration of glucose is low and the epithelial cells transport glucose actively across their plasma membrane along with sodium. Carrier proteins found in human red blood cell plasma membranes function as anion carriers; they operate as antiporters in exchanging chloride for bicarbonate.

THE SODIUM–POTASSIUM PUMP

Potassium ion concentration is typically 10–20 times higher in cytoplasm than in extracellular fluid, whereas the reverse is true of sodium ions. Although ion channels play a crucial role in maintaining these differences, fine-tuning of these concentrations is achieved by the **sodium–potassium pumps** in the plasma membrane. These appear to operate as antiporters, actively pumping sodium out of the cell and pumping potassium into the cell against their steep electrochemical gradients. The sodium gradient produced by these pumps regulates cell volume through its osmotic effects, a mechanism exploited in the transportation of sugars and amino acids into cells (Fig. 2.6).

Almost one-third of the cell's energy is consumed in fuelling the sodium–potassium pumps. However, in electrically active nerve cells, which are repeatedly gaining small amounts of sodium and losing small amounts of potassium during the propagation of nerve impulses, the pump energy requirements may increase to two-thirds (Alberts et al 2002). ATP appears to supply the energy for the sodium–potassium pumps. An enzyme, sodium–potassium ATPase, consisting of a large, multipass subunit, and an associated smaller, single-pass glycoprotein, has been found in the plasma membrane.

The large subunit has binding sites for sodium and ATP on its cytoplasmic surface and a binding site for potassium on its external surface and is reversibly phosphorylated and dephosphorylated during the pumping cycle. The glycoprotein appears to be required for the intracellular transport of the large subunit to the plasma membrane. Since the sodium–potassium ATPase drives *three* positively charged ions out of the cell for every *two* it pumps in, it creates an electrical potential with the inside surface of the plasma membrane negative to the outside surface, but this effect contributes only 10% to the membrane potential.

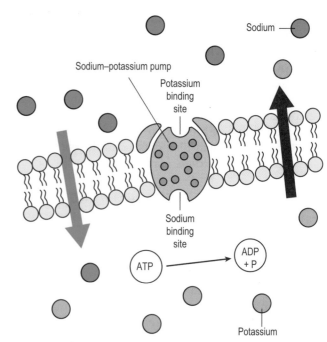

Figure 2.6   Operation of the sodium–potassium pump. Three sodium ions are moved out of the cell and two potassium ions are moved into the cell. The energy is provided by hydrolysis of one molecule of ATP.

Sodium–potassium ATPase has a further function in regulating cell volume. By controlling the solute concentration inside the cell, it regulates the osmotic forces that influence cell expansion and dehydration. Cells usually contain a high concentration of solutes, including numerous negatively charged organic molecules (fixed anions) confined to the inside of the cell. Specific cations such as sodium and potassium are required for charge balance and create a large osmotic gradient that tends to pull water into the cell. This is counteracted by an opposite osmotic gradient caused by a high concentration of inorganic ions, mainly sodium and chloride in the extracellular fluid, so that the movement of sodium contributes to intracellular hydration.

CELL DIVISION

Mitosis

Controlled cell division is vital to human reproduction, tissue growth and repair, efficient immune defence mechanisms and countless other processes (Murray & Kirschner 1991). The cycle of cell division is one of the most fundamental processes by which multicellular species replace cells damaged by wear and tear or lost during programmed cell death (apoptosis) (Latchman 1997). The body of a mature adult human being must be capable of the programmed synthesis of millions of new cells simply to maintain its physical and physiological status quo. Where ill health, trauma or planned surgery occurs, loss and replacement of new cells will increase. Where natural cell division is halted, for example in exposures to a large dose of ionising radiation, the individual is likely to die within a few days because of rapid cell destruction.

The structure of nucleotides

Cell nuclei contain large amounts of DNA. Nucleic acids are long polymers of molecules called **nucleotides**, composed of several simple chemical compounds bound together in a regular pattern. The building blocks of each molecule are phosphoric acid, a pentose sugar with five carbon atoms called deoxyribose, and four nitrogenous bases, comprising two purines (adenine and guanine) and two pyrimidines (thymine and cytosine), identified by the single letters A, G, T and C.

While details of the cell cycle may vary, certain behavioural requirements of all cells are universal. In the first instance, cells have to co-ordinate various events in the cycle. They must, for example, avoid entering mitosis or meiosis, until such time when the chromosomes have been replicated. Failure to comply with this requirement can result in cells that lack a particular chromosome, an aberration which may give rise to cancer at a later stage (Mueller & Young 1995, Goodman 1998).

Replication of DNA

In order to produce a pair of genetically identical daughter cells, nuclear DNA must be precisely replicated (Fig. 2.7) and the replicated chromosomes separated into two genetically identical cells. As the vast majority of cells also double their mass and duplicate all their cytoplasmic organelles, in each cell cycle co-ordination of the many complex cytoplasmic and nuclear processes is fundamental.

The duration of the cell cycle (Fig. 2.8) varies greatly from one cell type to another (Alberts et al 2002). However, a common standard does exist, and the cell cycle for all dividing cells consists of distinct phases: namely **interphase**, **mitosis** and **cytokinesis**. Mitosis, the critical process of nuclear division, is the most dramatic. As cells require time to grow and mature before they can divide, the standard cell cycle is fairly long, extending to 12 hours or more in fast-growing mammalian tissue. In most cells the mitotic phase takes about an hour, only a small fraction of the total cell cycle time.

- Interphase facilitates DNA replication. The vast amount of time that elapses between one mitotic phase and the next is taken up by interphase, which consists of three distinctive phases: the G1 or **gap1** phase, the S or **synthesis phase** and the G2 or **gap2** phase. During the G1 phase the cells monitor their internal environment and their size, so that when the time is appropriate decisive steps are taken that commits the cells to DNA replication, which occurs in the S or synthesis phase of the cell cycle. The subsequent G2 phase appears to provide a safety

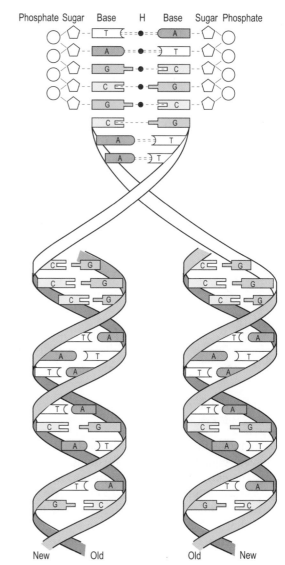

Figure 2.7 The replication of DNA showing the unwinding of the double helix and the formation of new strands with complementary base pairs (from Hinchliff S M, Montague S E 1990, with permission).

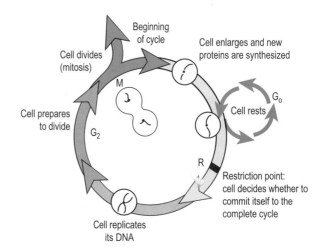

Figure 2.8 Stages of the cell cycle (reproduced with kind permission of Barbara Novak).

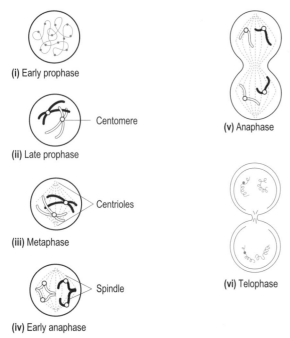

(i) Early prophase

Centomere

(ii) Late prophase

Centrioles

(iii) Metaphase

Spindle

(iv) Early anaphase

(v) Anaphase

(vi) Telophase

Figure 2.9   Stages of mitosis (from Hinchliff S M, Montague S E 1990, with permission).

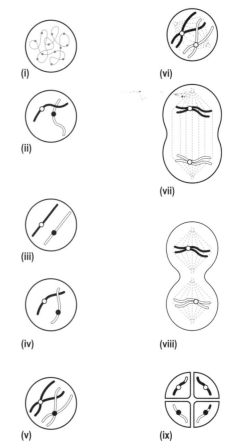

(i)

(ii)

(iii)

(iv)

(v)

(vi)

(vii)

(viii)

(ix)

Figure 2.10   The stages of meiosis. (Only one chromosome pair is shown for clarity.) (i) Interphase. (ii) Prophase I: leptotene. (iii) Zygotene. (iv) Pachytene. (v) Diplotene. (vi) Metaphase I. (vii) Anaphase I. (viii) Telophase I. (ix) Second meiotic division (from Hinchliff S M, Montague St 1990, with permission).

gap, allowing the cell to ensure that DNA replication is complete before mitosis.

- During mitosis the nuclear membrane breaks down, and the nuclear contents condense, forming visible chromosomes. The stages of mitosis are **prophase**, **metaphase**, **anaphase** and **telophase** (Fig. 2.9). During prophase, the cell's microtubules reorganise to establish the **mitotic spindle** that will eventually separate the chromosomes. The cell seems to pause briefly in metaphase as the duplicated chromosomes align on the mitotic spindle, in preparation for segregation. This segregation of the duplicated chromosomes marks the beginning of the anaphase during which the chromosomes move to the pole of the spindle where they decondense and re-establish new nuclei.

- Only at this point during telophase is the cell pinched and gradually divided by a process commonly known as cytokinesis, the critical point of the mitotic phase that terminates the end of the cell cycle.

Although the lengths of all phases of the cell cycle are variable, the greatest variation by far appears to occur in the duration of the G1 phase. One of the reasons for this variability is thought to be the cell's natural need to replicate. Thus, cells in G1, if not already committed to DNA replication, can pause in and enter a specialised resting state often referred to as the G0 phase. Cells can remain in this phase for days, weeks and even years before resuming proliferation.

In conditions that favour growth, the total protein content of a cell increases continuously throughout the cell cycle (Alberts et al 2002, Goodman 1998). Similarly, RNA synthesis continues at a steady rate, except during the mitotic phase when the chromosomes are too condensed to permit **transcription** (Ch. 3, p. 27). However, analysis of the pattern of individual protein synthesis suggests that most proteins are synthesised throughout the cell cycle. Therefore, cell growth should be considered as a steady and continuous process, interrupted briefly by the mitotic phase.

Meiosis

Meiosis, meaning diminution, is a special kind of nuclear division in which the chromosome complement is precisely halved. Meiosis involves two nuclear divisions rather then one (Fig. 2.10). With the exception of the **sex chromosomes** (different in male and female), a **diploid nucleus** contains two similar versions of each of the **autosomes** (alike in male and female). One set of these chromosomes is paternal and one set maternal in origin. These two sets of chromosomes are known as the **homologues**. In most cells these maintain a separate existence as independent chromosomes.

In contrast, a mature **haploid gamete** produced by the divisions of a diploid cell during meiosis must contain half the original number of chromosomes. This means that only one chromosome from each homologous pair is present, ensuring that either the maternal or the paternal copy of each gene but not both is present. Clearly, this specific requirement makes an extra demand on the processes governing cell division. Evidence suggests that a mechanism has evolved to accomplish the additional sorting of the chromosomes which involves the homologues recognising each other and becoming physically paired prior to lining up on the mitotic spindle. This pairing of the maternal and paternal copy of each chromosome is unique to meiosis.

It is probably only after DNA replication has been completed that the special feature of meiosis becomes evident. This suggests that, rather than separating, the sister chromatids behave as a unit, giving the impression that the earlier chromosome duplication has not occurred. The duplicated homologous pairs form a structure containing four chromatids. This close proximity allows **genetic recombination** to occur where a fragment of a maternal chromatid is exchanged for a corresponding fragment of a homologous paternal chromatid.

MAIN POINTS

- Cells are the fundamental units of life. Their morphological and functional features are governed by the genetic blueprint contained in their nuclei. Numerous physiological processes depend on the size of the surface area of the cell. Cells permit selective but rapid diffusion of substrates over short distances to ensure that metabolic needs are easily sustained.

- In larger cells there is a significant increase in surface area achieved by either folding the plasma membrane and forming microvilli or other surface protrusions or by flattening the entire cell body, generating a larger surface area for selective transport and diffusion.

- Most cells display a capacity for motility, generally involving the movement of the cytoplasm or specific organelles from one part of the cell to another. Cell motility is influenced by environmental factors such as tissue injury.

- Ectoderm, endoderm and mesoderm all contribute to the formation and development of epithelium. Epithelium provides an internal and external covering for body surfaces, protecting the underlying tissue from dehydration, and chemical or mechanical injury. Some epithelia function as sensory surfaces.

- Epithelia are classified into groups according to morphological and functional characteristics. Each epithelial cell type is identified by size, shape, cell volume and density. Where cells are small the volume of the cytoplasm is relatively low, containing few organelles, and the metabolic activity is low; large cells have more cytoplasm and organelles and the metabolic activity is high.

- Complex organs such as the liver, derived from epithelia, show a great capacity to absorb, transport and secrete substrates.

- The most common feature of cells is the plasma membrane. It is constructed of a lipid bilayer containing protein molecules and is capable of considerable adaptation because its molecular structures can move about within the membrane.

- The lipid molecule consists of a hydrophilic polar head and a hydrophobic non-polar tail. The lipid bilayer contains proteins, cholesterol, glycoproteins and glycolipids, each contributing to the structure and function of the plasma membrane. Most plasma membrane functions are carried out by membrane proteins.

- Selective permeability of the plasma membrane facilitates free passage of gases and water but restricts the movement of larger ions to their specific protein channels which can be opened or closed in order to regulate transmembrane traffic.

- The commonest form of plasma membrane ion channel is one that is permeable to potassium ions, ensuring that plasma membrane potential is maintained. The critical concentration of potassium ions may be 10–20 times higher in the cell than in the extracellular fluid, whereas the reverse is true of sodium. These ionic concentration differences are maintained by sodium–potassium pumps.

- Cytoplasm acts as a reservoir for the suspension of small molecular structures, large particles and organelles such as the endoplasmic reticulum, the Golgi apparatus, mitochondria, lysosomes and peroxisomes. The endoplasmic reticulum plays a central role in lipid and protein biosynthesis. The Golgi apparatus processes proteins for intra- and extracellular use.

- Lysosomes are filled with a granular protein aggregate which constitutes the necessary digestive enzymes. Peroxisomes contain oxidases. Several oxidases can combine intracellular oxygen with hydrogen ions, thus forming hydrogen peroxide, which is used in turn to oxidise substances that might otherwise be poisonous to the cell.

- Mitochondria vary in size and shape but their structure is constant, being mainly composed of two limiting membranes. Mitochondria generate ATP, a form of energy essential to normal cellular function. Mitochondria are self-replicating and contain their own DNA.

- The nucleus is the largest structure of the cell. Nuclei contain large quantities of DNA, which holds the cell's genetic blueprint. The nuclear genome determines the characteristics of proteins and enzymes contained in the cellular cytoplasm.

- Controlled cell division is vital to human reproduction, tissue growth, repair and other processes. To produce a pair of genetically identical daughter cells the nuclear DNA must be precisely replicated and the replicated chromosomes must be separated into two genetically identical cells.

- Meiosis leads to gamete formation where the chromosome numbers are halved. After exchanging genetic material, one of each pair of homologous chromosomes is represented in the mature gamete.

References

Alberts B, Johnson A, Lewis J et al 2002 Molecular Biology of the Cell, 4th edn. Garland Science, Taylor & Francis Group, London.

Bannister L, Berry M, Collins P et al 1995 Gray's Anatomy. Churchill Livingstone, New York.

Goodman S 1998 Medical Cell Biology. Lippincott-Raven Publishers, Philadelphia.

Guyton A, Hall J 2000 Textbook of Medical Physiology. W B Saunders, New York.

Laskey R A 1987 Basic molecular and cell biology – the cell nucleus. British Medical Journal 295:1121–1123.

Latchman D 1997 Basic Molecular and Cell Biology. BMJ Publishing Group, London.

McKee T, McKee J 1996 Biochemistry. W C Brown, London.

Mueller R, Young I 1995 Emery's Elements of Medical Genetics. Churchill Livingstone, Edinburgh.

Murray A, Kirschner M 1991 What controls the cell cycle? Scientific American 3:34–41.

Annotated recommended reading

Byrne J, Schultz S 1994 An Introduction to Membrane Transport and Bioelectricity. Raven Press, New York.
This short textbook provides a comprehensive account of the many features involved in membrane transport and outlines a detailed rationale for electroconductivity, one of the most fundamental concepts in cell physiology.

Glover D M, Gonzalez C, Raff J W et al 1993 The centrosome. Scientific American 6:32–38.
This article provides an enlightening account of some of the roles of the centrosome in cell division. The excellent use of illustrations enhances the overall quality of the evolving discussion.

Hoffman A, Thanh H 1996 Genomic imprinting. Science and Medicine 3(1):52–61.
This article offers an easy-to-understand account of how genes may play a part in marking or imprinting proteins and other intracellular molecules, which then control cell structure and function.

Karp G 2002 Cellular and Molecular Biology – Concepts and Experiments. John Wiley, New York.
This textbook offers a refreshing account of the relationship between molecular structures and functions. It details the way chemical energy may be used in running the diverse cellular activities.

Linder M 1992 G Proteins. Scientific American 7:36–43.
This article provides an account of G proteins and how these contribute to cell structure and function. As many G proteins function as signal transductors, particularly in response to stimuli such as hormones, enzymes and drugs, appreciating their normal intracellular position and function may contribute to a better understanding of their role.

Chapter **3**

Structure, organisation and regulation of genes

OVERVIEW OF MODERN GENETICS

'Life depends on the ability of cells to store, retrieve and translate the genetic instructions to make and maintain a living organism' (Alberts et al 2002). Over the last decade there have been major developments in the science of genetics. The finding that there is a genetic basis for many aspects of human disease has led to the search for treatments. The research has involved the **Human Genome Project**, the identification of the structure and function of all human genes. The study of the human genome is called **genomics**.

The completion of mapping the human genome in the year 2000 identified ethical and moral implications. The rate of development of industries based on recombinant gene technology, cloning and gene therapy has been so fast that the general public and the government have been unable to understand the implications. This has led to a sense of fear and distrust of technologies: for example, genetically modified (GM) foods. Developments will continue but the legal and moral aspects must be thought out.

Key discoveries

In 1865 a monk called **Gregor Mendel** presented a paper on the results of his experiments on garden peas. He had studied varieties of pea that differed in a single characteristic, such as tall and short plants or wrinkled and smooth seeds. He found an inheritance pattern where one of two characteristics – for example, tall plants – seemed to dominate the next generation' i.e. the **first filial (F1) generation**, and these were called **dominant** factors. The opposite characteristic – short plants – disappeared, to reappear in the 'grandchildren', the second or F2 generation. These were called **recessive factors**. Mendel proposed that each pair of characteristics was controlled by a pair of factors, one of which was inherited from each parent plant.

These factors were called **genes** by a Danish botanist, Johannsen (Mueller & Young 2001). Pure bred peas plants were **homologous** (*homo* means alike) and inherited two identical genes from their parents. The F1 generation that resulted from the breeding of a tall plant with a short plant were all tall plants. However, they inherited two different genes from their parents and were **heterozygous** (*hetero* means different). The alternative versions of genes are called *allelomorphs*, usually shortened to **alleles**.

Mendel's Laws

Out of Mendel's work, three main principles were developed:

1. *The Law of Uniformity*
   When two homozygotes with different alleles are crossed, all the offspring of the F1 generation are identical and heterozygous. Characteristics do not blend and can reappear in subsequent generations.
2. *The Law of Segregation*
   Each individual possesses two genes for a particular characteristic, only one of which can be passed on in the ovum or sperm to the next generation.
3. *The Law of Independent Assortment*
   Members of different gene pairs segregate to offspring independently of one another.

This third law is not strictly true, because if two genes are situated closely together on the same chromosome they may be linked and inherited together. Maternal and paternal chromosomes become closely apposed during meiosis and exchange segments of DNA between homologues, a phenomenon called crossing over.

Mendel's findings were ignored until 1900, but once the importance of his experiments was recognised, interest in inheritance developed. At that time thread-like structures had been seen in the nuclei of cells. These are the chromosomes and in 1903 two people independently proposed that they carried the hereditary factors known as genes. The correct number of 46 human chromosomes was identified in 1956. However, it was only in 1952 that **deoxyribonucleic acid** (DNA) was identified as the universal genetic material. In 1953 the structure of DNA was discovered by James D Watson and Francis H C Crick. Without Rosalind Franklin, who developed the skills of X-ray crystallography, their discovery might not have occurred.

COMPOSITION OF DNA

Building blocks

Cell nuclei contain large amounts of species-specific DNA. A second form of nucleic acid is **ribonucleic acid** (RNA). Nucleic acids are long polymers of molecules called **nucleotides**, composed of several simple chemical compounds bound together in a regular pattern. The building blocks of DNA are phosphoric acid, a pentose sugar with five carbon atoms called deoxyribose and four nitrogenous bases, comprising two purines (adenine and guanine) and two pyrimidines (thymine and cytosine), identified by the single letters A, G, T and C. In RNA, thymine is replaced by uracil (U).

RNA is found in the cytoplasm, particularly concentrated in the nucleolus, whereas DNA is found mainly on the 46 chromosomes, arranged in 23 pairs in somatic cells. One chromosome of each pair originates with the ovum and the other with the sperm. A cell containing two sets of chromosomes is called **diploid**. Gametes are **haploid**, i.e. there is only one of each pair. In 22 of the pairs the chromosomes are identical and these pairs are called **autosomes**. Each pair is alike and the two are called homologues. The 23rd pair is the sex chromosomes: 2 X chromosomes in females and an X and a Y chromosome in males.

The double helix

DNA molecules consist of a double helix made up of two complementary chains of nucleotides. Two sugar-phosphate strands wind around each other and the base pairs are stacked between these strands, pointing inwards to the centre of the double helix (Lodish et al 1999). The two chains are held together by hydrogen bonds between the base pairs which are easily broken, a feature necessary for DNA replication. The sugar–phosphate molecules form the backbones of the chains.

Pentose sugars

The five carbon atoms in the pentose sugar are numbered with **primes**, represented as 1′ to 5′. The carbon atoms 3′ and 5′ are on the same side of the molecule. The 5′ carbon is always linked to the phosphate molecule and the 1′ carbon to the base. The two strands run in opposite directions as indicated by their 3′ and 5′ carbon atoms and are complementary or **antiparallel** (Fig. 3.1). A purine always pairs with a pyramidine; A is paired with T by two hydrogen bonds and C is paired with G by three hydrogen bonds. The pairs stack one above the other and the structure is stabilised by two other forms of bond – hydrophobic and van der Waals interactions (Ch. 1) – between adjacent base pairs.

DNA holds the instructions for constructing, organising and maintaining a body and must be replicated accurately during mitosis. One strand or the other must be passed on to the next generation by means of ova and sperm in meiosis (Ch. 2, p. 20).

Chromosomes

Chromosomes take up different states depending on the stage of the cell cycle (Ch. 2, p. 18). When the cell is not dividing, chromosomes are extended and their chromatin is in the form of long, thin, tangled threads known as interphase chromosomes. The highly condensed chromosomes in a dividing cell are called mitotic chromosomes (Alberts et al 2002), which are much wider than the DNA double helix.

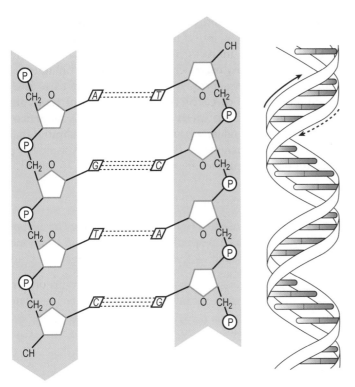

Figure 3.1 DNA double helix. A: sugar phosphate backbone and nucleotide pairing of the DNA double helix (P, phosphate; A, adenine; T, thymine; G, guanine; C, cytosine). B: representation of the DNA double helix.

If the DNA of a single human cell was stretched out it would be several metres long, yet the total length of the chromosomes placed end to end is less than 0.5 mm! DNA is packaged into chromosomes by coiling and folding (Mueller & Young 2001). Besides the double helix there is a secondary coiling around spherical molecules called histones, to form **nucleosomes**. A tertiary coiling of nucleosomes forms the chromatin fibres, which are then wound into a tight coil to make the chromosome.

Circulating lymphocytes from peripheral blood are commonly used to study chromosomes but skin or bone marrow cells can be used. Fetal cells from the chorionic villi or found in amniotic fluid (amniocytes) can be sampled. The cell samples are encouraged to divide. The process is stopped during mitosis by adding colchicines, which prevents the formation of the spindle and arrests the cells in metaphase. Hypotonic saline solution is added, which destroys the cells, releasing the chromosomes. A photograph is taken. The chromosomes images are cut out, laid out in a standard fashion and then photographed again to produce a **karyotype** (Fig. 3.2). Chromosomes are identified by their size, light and dark banding patterns and the position of the centromere.

At that moment DNA replication has taken place and the chromosomes consist of two identical strands called sister chromatids, which are joined together by a **centromere**. Centromeres consist of lengths of repetitive DNA and are responsible for the movement of the chromosomes that takes

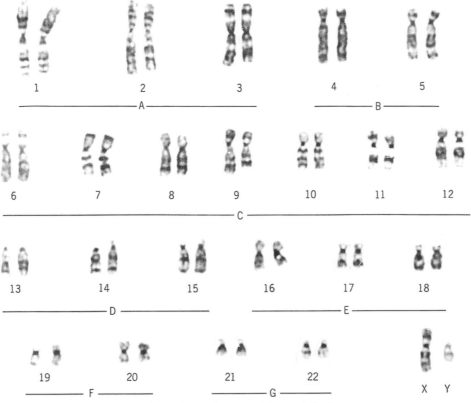

Figure 3.2 A normal karyotype (from Sweet B 1997, with permission).

place in cell division. A chromosome is divided by its centromere into short and long arms. The short arm is referred to as 'p' and the long arm 'q'. Chromosomes can be classified by the position of their centromeres. If located centrally, the chromosome is **metacentric**, if intermediate it is **submetacentric** and if found at one end the chromosome is acrocentric. Acrocentric chromosomes may have stalks with satellites attached to them which contain multiple copies of the genes for ribosomal RNA.

The tip of each chromosome arm is called the telomere, consisting of many repeats of a TTAGGG sequence, and these seal the ends of the chromosome to maintain its structural integrity. The length of these sequences is reduced each time the cell divides. This is part of normal cellular ageing and most cells can only undergo 50–60 divisions before becoming senescent.

Genes

The full complement of DNA is called the **genome**. Along the genome about 60–70% of DNA is in the form of single or low copy sequences, whereas 30–40% consists of highly repetitive sequences that appear inactive. DNA is arranged in discrete segments called genes, and there may be up to 100 000 of these in the human genome. There is a rule of genetics that says 'one gene, one protein'. However, genes often exist in families: e.g. those that code for the various types of haemoglobins (Ch. 16, p. 206) and those that code for antibodies (Ch. 29).

Genes code for polypeptides, which include enzymes, hormones, receptors or structural and regulatory proteins (Mueller & Young 2001). The alternative alleles of any gene are present at a specific place or *locus* on each of a pair of chromosomes. If both parents contribute an identical allele

for a locus, the new individual is **homozygous**. If the two alleles differ, the new individual is **heterozygous**.

Discrete single genes form about 25% of the DNA and are separated from each other by long runs of inactive, repetitive DNA sequences. It is not known why there is so much redundant DNA. The coding sequences of genes are called **exons** and the intervening non-coding sequences **introns**. Exons are usually interrupted by introns. Individual introns can be much larger than the exons and some have been found to contain a gene within a gene.

The role of the environment

Genes act in response to environmental changes. These may be internal, such as a response to fluctuations in hormone level, or external, such as the response to a meal. The full complement of genes inherited by an individual is called the *genotype*. The outward appearance of an individual, i.e. their physical, biochemical and physiological nature, is known as the *phenotype* and results from gene–environment interactions.

FROM DNA TO RNA TO PROTEIN

Proteins are the working components of the cell. DNA stores the information. RNA (Fig. 3.3) carries out instructions encoded in DNA and synthesises the proteins involved in cellular function (Lodish et al 1999).

The genetic code

Twenty different amino acids are found in proteins, so it became obvious to Watson and Crick that, as there were

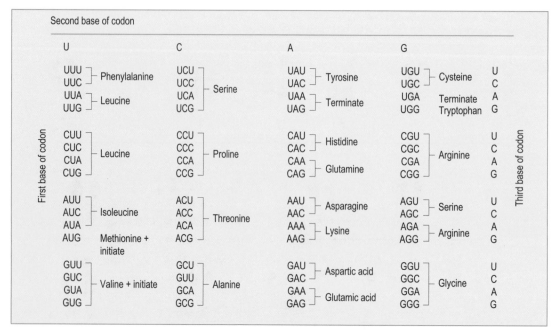

Figure 3.3   Messenger RNA (m-RNA) code words (from Hinchliff S M, Montague S E 1990, with permission).

only four bases, more than one base must be necessary to specify a particular amino acid. Even two bases wouldn't be enough, as 4^2 gives only 16 possibilities. However 4^3 bases allows 64 possibilities of codon to occur with some redundancy. A group of three nucleotides, called a **triplet codon** (Fig. 3.4), spells out each amino acid and the sequence of amino acids shape a particular protein. There are also codons at the ends of genes that signify start and stop.

The process of reading the code of DNA that results in a functional protein product involves two processes: transcription and translation.

Transcription

There are three types of RNA involved in the production of a protein:

1. messenger RNA (mRNA) copies the genetic code of a stretch of DNA in the form of a sequence of bases that codes for a sequence of amino acids;
2. transfer RNA (tRNA) carries the correct amino acids specified by the DNA to the ribosome and places them in the right order;

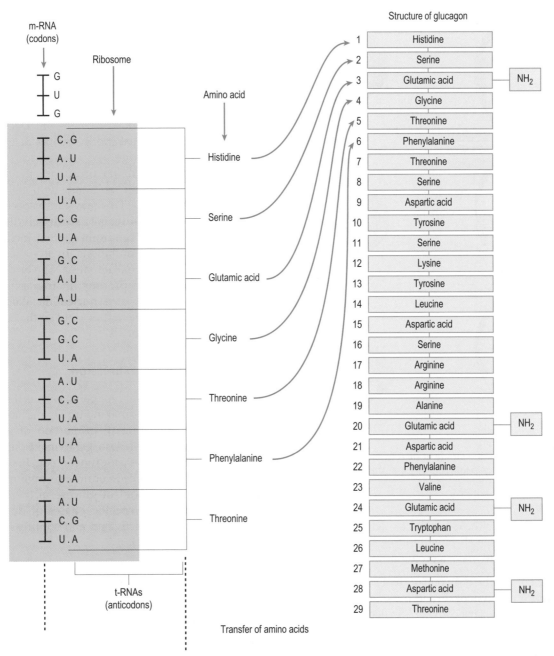

Figure 3.4   An example of protein synthesis: glucagon (from Hinchliff S M, Montague S E 1990, with permission).

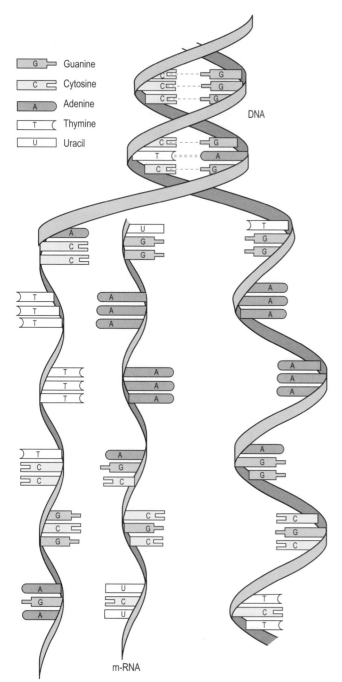

G   Guanine
C   Cytosine
A   Adenine
T   Thymine
U   Uracil

DNA

m-RNA

Figure 3.5   Transcription of a strand of DNA by messenger RNA (mRNA) (from Hinchliff S M, Montague S E 1990, with permission).

3. ribosomal RNA (rRNA) combines with proteins to make ribosomes, which have binding sites for all the molecules needed to make a protein.

In any particular gene only one of the DNA strands acts as a **template** for a polypeptide and must be copied before it can be read (Fig. 3.5). This copying is called **transcription**. It must be accurate, as mistakes may lead to an inactive product. The information stored in the gene is transmitted from the DNA to mRNA. Every base in the single-stranded mRNA is complementary to the DNA, but uracil replaces thymine. An enzyme called **RNA polymerase** tacks the bases onto the developing strand in the correct order.

Translation

Following transcription, non-coding introns are excised and the coding exons spliced together to form mature mRNA. This is transported to the ribosomes in the cytoplasm for **translation** into a specific protein (Fig. 3.6). In the cytoplasm a particular amino acid is bound to its tRNA for transporting to the ribosome, where it is linked up with others to form a polypeptide chain. The ribosome moves along the mRNA, linking up the amino acids to build the protein.

Mutations

Genes usually produce their product faithfully, but rarely a mutation or alteration in the arrangement or amount of genetic material in a cell arises, either naturally or because of the effects of environmental challenges called **mutagens**: these include radiation, chemical or physical stressors. Mutations can be minor changes in DNA or macro-mutations involving alterations such as deletions of large amounts of a chromosome.

Mutations often result in harmful or lethal defects. Point mutations cause amino acid substitutions, resulting in faulty protein products. This may cause specific functional defects such as **cystic fibrosis** or **sickle cell disease**. Macro-mutations may cause syndromes, often including mental retardation. Nonsense mutations involve the creation of a stop codon in an abnormal situation. The broken gene does not code for a protein product. In frameshift mutations, additions or deletions of a nucleotide alter the reading frame of the DNA to the left or right so that triplet codons do not code for amino acids.

Regulation of gene expression

Every cell in the body (except gametes) has the full complement of genes. The cells making up organs have specialised functions and only a small proportion of genes will be active in a particular cell. Also, genes make only the amount of their product necessary for functioning. Imagine a person whose pancreas produced continuous amounts of insulin, regardless of the amount of glucose in the blood! Genes may only function at specific phases of development in an organism and are activated and suppressed as needed (Mueller & Young 2001).

PATTERNS OF INHERITANCE

Dominant genes

Specific genes may be inherited as **dominant**, **recessive** or **sex-linked**. A dominant allele manifests its effects in

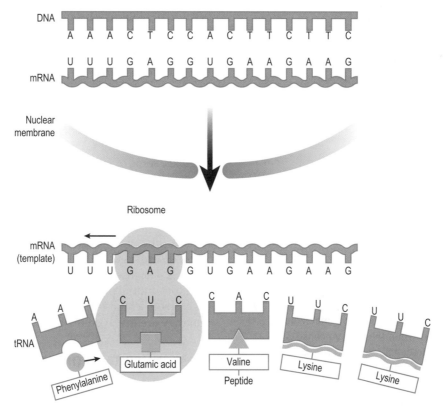

Figure 3.6   Representation of the way in which genetic information is translated into protein.

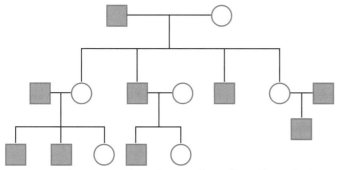

Figure 3.7   An autosomal dominant pedigree (from Sweet B 1997, with permission).

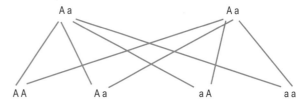

Figure 3.8   In an autosomal recessive disorder, the disease is only manifest if both members of a pair of chromosomes are abnormal. If both parents are carriers of the abnormal gene (a), then there is a one in four chance that a child will have the disease (from Sweet B 1997, with permission).

heterozygotes, as only one copy is needed to affect the phenotype. Except in cases of new mutation, every child with that particular phenotype receives a copy of one allele from a similar parent. Most genes work normally but, if the gene codes for an abnormality where one parent is affected, a child will have a 1 in 2 chance of inheriting the gene and being affected (Fig. 3.7).

Recessive genes

A recessive allele only affects the phenotype in homozygotes. People with one copy of the allele are carriers. If the gene codes for an abnormality, the children of two carriers will have 1 in 4 chance of having an affected child or a normal

child and a 1 in 2 chance of a child carrying the disorder (Fig. 3.8).

Sex-linked genes

The X chromosome carries a large number of genes involved in development and function. Males only have one X chromosome and are **hemizygous** for X chromosome genes. If there is an abnormal X chromosome gene, boys will be affected by an X-linked disorder. Females are usually heterozygous for X chromosome and will not be affected because of the opposing normal allele (Fig. 3.9). They will be asymptomatic carriers. However, in the rare case of homozygosity females will be affected. This occurs in a girl born to an affected man and a carrier woman. In females

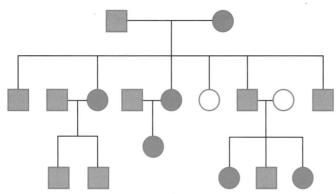

Figure 3.9 An X-linked pedigree (from Sweet B 1997, with permission).

Box 3.1 Lyonisation

In females one or other of the X chromosomes is randomly inactivated in cells early in embryonic life. Inactivation occurs at around 15 days when the embryo consists of about 5000 cells. Their descendants retain the same activated X chromosome, so that half the cells of a female will contain one activated X chromosome and half the other. All daughter cells of a particular cell line contain the same inactivated X chromosome. This effect is called *lyonisation*, after its discoverer Dr Mary Lyon. Each female is a mosaic of half paternal and maternal X chromosomes. Abnormal X chromosomes appear to be preferentially inactivated (Mueller & Young 2001, Bainbridge 2003).

In females or males with more than one X chromosome, any inactivated X chromosome can be seen during interphase as a dark mass of chromatin called sex chromatin or a Barr body. Looking for Barr bodies was used as a method of sex determination by taking a buccal smear, but this method is now obsolete as chromosomal abnormalities can be complex.

---

only one X chromosome is functional in each cell and the other is randomly activated in the early embryo. This is called lyonisation (Box 3.1).

Genomic imprinting

It has recently been discovered that genes on homologous chromosomes are not expressed equally. Different clinical features can arise depending on whether a gene was inherited from the mother or father. This is **genomic imprinting**, affecting only a small proportion of the genome. **Prader–Willi syndrome** is characterised by short stature, obesity, small gonads and learning difficulty. In 55% of those affected there is deletion of the proximal portion of the long arm of chromosome 15. A further 15% involves a submicroscopic deletion. The chromosome deleted is almost always on the paternal homologue. The remaining cases occur

because of maternal disomy – two maternal and no paternal chromosome 15 (Mueller & Young 2001).

Mitochondrial DNA

Each mitochondrion has its own circular double-stranded DNA, called mitochondrial DNA (mDNA), inherited only from mothers. Sperm mitochondria are situated in their necks and do not enter the embryo. Mitochondrial DNA codes for 37 genes, some of which are important in cellular respiration. It has a higher rate of spontaneous mutation than nuclear DNA and accumulations of mistakes may be responsible for some of the physical effects of ageing. Mitochondrial inheritance may cause rare disorders which affect males and females but are transmitted only through their mothers. These disorders usually combine muscular and neurological features. The diseases involving muscle weakness are known as mitochondrial myopathies. Mitochondria are important in tissues with a high-energy requirement, so it is not surprising that they are involved in abnormalities of these systems.

SOME INHERITED CONDITIONS

Most inherited disorders are due to nuclear gene mutations, either dominant (Table 3.1), recessive (Table 3.2) or sex-linked (Table 3.3). Some may be due to a mutation in mitochondrial DNA (Table 3.4). Slight differences in a protein brought about by a genetic mutation may cause devastating diseases such as sickle cell disease or cystic fibrosis. Whole chromosomes may be involved. About 50% of spontaneous abortions result from chromosomal defects during oogenesis. Some genes are **pleiotropic**, underpinning multiple functions, and an abnormality may affect multiple systems. In the recessive disorder phenylketonuria low tyrosine levels lead to lack of pigment in hair, skin and eyes because of reduced melanin production.

CHROMOSOMAL DEFECTS

Chromosomal defects may be present in 6% of all pregnancies and cause up to 50% of spontaneous abortions. Numerical or structural changes may affect the autosomes or sex chromosomes. People with chromosomal defects usually have characteristic phenotypes: e.g. Down's syndrome, where the typical features may cause children to look more similar to each other than to relatives.

Numerical chromosomal defects

Many of these numerical defects arise during failure of **dysjunction**, an error in cell division where the sister chromatids fail to separate at anaphase. The resulting number of chromosomes may be too many or too few:

- **Polyploidy** means the presence of multiples of the haploid number of 23 chromosomes.

Table 3.1 Disorders of systems caused by dominant genes

System	Disorder
Nervous	Huntington's disease
	Neurofibromatosis
Bowel	Polyposis coli
Kidney	Polycystic disease
Eyes	Blindness
Ears	Deafness
Blood	Hypercholesterolaemia
Skeleton	Osteogenesis imperfecta
	Achondroplasia

Table 3.2 Some recessively inherited conditions

System	Disorder
Metabolism	Cystic fibrosis
	Phenylketonuria
Nervous	Friedreich's ataxia
Blood	Sickle cell anaemia
	Beta-thalassaemia
Ears	Congenital deafness
Eyes	Recessive blindness

Table 3.3 Some X-linked disorders

System	Disorder
Locomotor	Duchenne muscular dystrophy
Blood	Haemophilia
Brain	Fragile X syndrome
Vision	Childhood blindness

Table 3.4 Some mitochondrial disorders

System	Disorder
Vision	Chronic progressive external ophthalmoplegia
Hearing	Aminoglycoside-induced deafness
Cardiovascular	Hypertrophic cardiomyopathy with myopathy

- **Triploidy**, the presence of 69 chromosomes, may occur because the chromosomes of the second polar body fail to be ejected from the ovum or because of the entry of two sperms into the ovum. Triploidy occurs in about 2% of fertilisations, mostly lost early in development.

- **Monosomy** is when one of a chromosomes pair is missing, leaving 45 chromosomes. This is only compatible with survival if the missing chromosome is an X chromosome, resulting in Turner's syndrome.

- **Trisomy** is the presence of an extra chromosome. The usual cause is non-dysjunction, so that either the ovum or sperm carries 24 chromosomes instead of 23. At fertilisation, the zygote has 47 chromosomes. The most common condition is Down's syndrome, where there are 3 copies of chromosome 21. Non-dysjunction occurs with increasing frequency as maternal age increases.

- **Trisomy** of the sex chromosomes is quite common and XXX females (triple X) or XXY males (Klinefelter's syndrome) occur. There are also XYY males. There may be tetrasomy (4 copies) of the X chromosome or even pentasomy (5 copies). Mental retardation is associated with increases in sex chromosomes. The greater the number of X chromosomes, the more severe is the mental retardation.

- **Mosaicism** results when the zygote develops into an individual with two genotypes or cell lines. The condition arises due to non-dysjunction during early mitosis. The defects seen in full monosomic or trisomic disorders are less serious in mosaicism.

Structural chromosomal defects

Environmental factors may induce breaks in chromosomes, resulting in structural rearrangements called macromutations. Two of these, inversion and translocation, may be transmitted from parent to child.

- **Translocation** is the transfer of a piece of one chromosome to another non-homologous chromosome. This may be a reciprocal translocation where two non-homologous chromosomes exchange pieces. If the translocation is balanced, the individual receives the normal complement of chromosomal material and there will be no abnormality. However, if the translocation results in extra chromosomal material, abnormality will occur. About 4% of people with Down's syndrome receive their third chromosome 21 translocated to another chromosome, often chromosome 14 or 15.

- **Deletion** is the loss of part of a chromosome. Loss of the termination of chromosome 5 causes cri du chat syndrome where affected infants have a weak, cat-like cry, microcephaly, heart defects and mental retardation.

- **Duplication** is where a section of a chromosome is repeated, either within a chromosome, attached to another chromosome or as a separate fragment. These are less harmful, as there is no loss of chromosome material.

- **Inversion** occurs if a segment of a chromosome breaks free and becomes reattached in reverse position. Paracentric inversion involves just one arm of the chromosome, whereas pericentric inversion involves both arms and the centromere.

- **Isochromosome** – The centromere divides horizontally instead of longitudinally and this occurs most often in the X chromosome. Loss of the short arm of the X chromosome is associated with features of Turner's syndrome.

APPLICATION TO PRACTICE

The Human Genome Project

The Human Genome Project involved mapping all the human genes to their chromosomes. It began in Utah under the auspices of the US Department of Energy (DOE) who were interested in finding out the mutation rates of DNA in response to exposure to radiation and chemicals. The project began in 1991 and France, the UK and Japan soon joined, followed by many other countries. The short-term hope of the project is to enable better diagnosis and counselling for families with genetic disease. In the longer term, the aim is to develop preventative strategies and treatments of genetic disorders. The project was completed in 2000.

Detection of abnormality

Following the production of a karyotype, chromosomes can be identified by their size, banding patterns and the position of the centromere. Gross chromosomal defects can be seen (Fig. 3.10). Single gene defects where the identity of the gene is known can be found by using gene probes, commercially available synthetic sections of DNA, which are attracted to the appropriate gene and can even identify single base changes.

DNA technologies

Those wishing to learn more about the techniques are referred to either Mueller & Young (2001) or Jorde et al (2003). Techniques include the use of enzymes called restriction endonucleases, which cut DNA at a specific point, polymerase chain reaction (PCR) and the Southern Blot Technique. DNA technology can be split into two main areas:

DNA cloning (producing identical copies) and DNA analysis. There are two types of DNA cloning: in-vivo (in-life) cell-based mechanisms of DNA replication and cell-free or in-vitro (in-glass) methods. Possible applications include medical cures, increased food production, crime detection, lessening of pollution and better energy production (Mueller & Young 2001, Jorde et al 2003).

THERAPEUTIC APPLICATIONS OF RECOMBINANT DNA TECHNOLOGY

The medical applications of the new technology include the manufacture of hormones and enzymes; the production of human insulin is already in use. Uses also include preimplantation genetic screening for disease and the sex of the embryo, fetal screening, screening of adults and targeted gene replacement as therapy. Stem cell therapy can be added to this list.

Victor McKusick, the man behind the Human Genome Project, began a catalogue of all known human genetic conditions. In 1998 the 12th edition contained over 8500 conditions. An on-line version has been created known as Online Mendelian Inheritance in Man (OMIM) which can be accessed by the Internet (McKusick 2002). At the beginning of 2000 there were 11 084 entries. Non-therapeutic uses such as selecting attributes for a child or, as has recently been in the news, cloning of a person may cause ethical and moral problems as the techniques come into use.

Population screening

The issue of confidentiality and privacy and who accesses medical data about an individual is of supreme importance. If techniques for screening populations are used, how much information could be asked for by employers, providers of insurance, possible life partners and others? Could a person be penalised for possessing a particular genetic defect which has yet to show its effect: for instance, Huntington's disease?

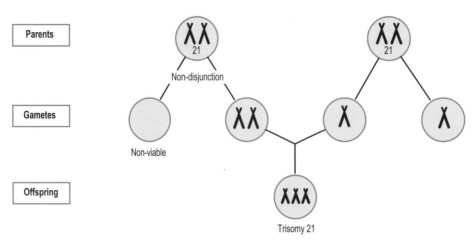

Figure 3.10 Non-dysjunction of chromosome 21 leading to Down's syndrome (from Hinchliff S M, Montague S E, Watson R 1996, with permission).

These questions must be addressed now. If carrier detection becomes available, it must be voluntary and there must be adequate counselling services in the event of a positive result.

Gene therapy

Therapeutic uses of rDNA techniques include gene therapy or 'the replacement of a deficient gene product or correction of an abnormal gene' (Mueller & Young 2001). When the gene enters the new cell it may change the way the cell works or the chemicals that the cell secretes. Advances in molecular biology leading to the identification of many abnormal human genes and their products have led to the possibilities of treatments for some important diseases.

These recent developments promise a new type of medicine but have also brought moral and ethical dilemmas. Anxieties about eugenics (Horgan 1993) raise questions about the application of genetic engineering to diagnosis and treatment of genetic diseases. Recently (2003) their have been concerns about the development of leukaemia in children undergoing gene therapy. This has led to the halting of programmes in some countries. Regulatory bodies have been set up to oversee the technical, therapeutic and safety aspects of gene therapy. Whereas *somatic cell therapy*, which affects only the individual, is acceptable, *germ cell therapy*, in which the changes could be transmitted to future generations, is currently considered morally and ethically unacceptable.

Important considerations

Before gene therapy trials can take place there are a number of technical aspects to overcome (Mueller & Young 2001):

1. At the present time gene therapy is only possible in vitro, not in vivo. For instance, in order to treat bone marrow it would have to be removed, altered and returned to the patient by transfusion.
2. The gene involved must have been cloned. This means not only the structural gene but the sequences involved in its expression and regulation.
3. The specific targets – cell, tissue and organ – must be identified and accessible.
4. There must be an efficient vector system to carry the gene into the target cells.
5. There should be no harmful effects, such as malignancy, on the target cells.

METHODS OF GENE THERAPY

These can be divided into two groups: viral and non-viral.

Viral

- Retroviruses are RNA viruses which can insert themselves into target cells where their RNA is transformed into DNA and inserted into the cellular genome. They

must be rendered inactive prior to use so that they cannot produce infection. The main problem with their use is that only very small stretches of DNA can be introduced.

- Adenoviruses are especially suitable for targeting the respiratory tract. They are more stable than retroviruses. They do not integrate into the genome, so there is no risk of mutagenesis, but their effect is likely to be transient. They contain genes involved in the production of cancer (oncogenes), so there could be a danger of provoking malignancy.
- Other viruses such as the herpes virus, influenza virus and other RNA viruses could produce large quantities of the gene product but are likely to have the same problems as already discussed. Viruses elicit an immune response which limits their repeated use.

Non-viral agents

These methods are likely to be safer but differ in their ability to produce sufficient gene product to be useful. They include:

- direct injection of naked DNA
- liposome-mediated DNA transfer – DNA packaged in a lipid bilayer surrounding an aqueous vesicle
- receptor-mediated endocytosis where specific receptors on the cell surface are targeted.

Stem cell therapy

At fertilisation the single cell and its early offspring are totipotent and can form any tissue in the body. After 4 days these totipotent cells begin to specialise (Lodish et al 1999). The embryo-forming cells can become any tissue type but are not capable of developing a placenta and membranes. These *stem cells* could theoretically be used to treat human diseases such as diabetes, liver failure, Parkinson's disease and Alzheimer's disease. Stem cells become dedicated to producing tissue with a specific function: for instance, blood stem cells are located in the bone marrow and may also circulate in the bloodstream in small numbers. They continually replenish red cells, white cells and platelets. There are various sources of stem cell lines to use therapeutically: the embryonic inner cell mass, embryonic tissue retrieved after a termination of pregnancy, cord blood and some adult somatic cell lines.

Embryonic cells

Obtaining these cells means in-vitro fertilisation and artificial growing of human embryos. There are ethical problems with developing embryos to harvest cells and in the USA President G W Bush has banned any funding for research requiring the creation and destruction of human embryos (Ezzell 2002). Taking cells from an aborted fetus may also be ethically unsound.

Adult cells

Recent research into adult cells suggests there be some multipotent cells that, even though they appear to be specialised, may have the ability to produce other types of cells. Some stem cells found in bone marrow have been able to produce liver cells. However, Ezzell (2002) mentions that when such cells were transplanted in mice, they did not form new cell lines but fused with recipient cells to create giant cells with more than the usual number of chromosomes. Such abnormal cells may not have the ability to change tissue type and could lead to cancer.

Umbilical cord blood

Allogenic (tissues of two unalike individuals) stem cell transplantation has revolutionised the outcome for a wide range of malignant and non-malignant haematological conditions (Lennard & Jackson 2000). Infusion of cord blood, very rich in highly proliferative stem cells, has been used with success in children and young adults with some haematological and immunological disorders. The best results were from HLA-matched siblings, with a success rate of 63%. The results have been less good with unmatched donor/recipient pairs, only 30% of recipients being alive after 1 year. An advantage of cord blood over other tissue is reduced incidence of graft versus host reaction. There are a four cord blood banks in the UK.

In-utero transplantation

Stem cell transplantation in utero may treat genetic disorders. The immature fetal immune system will tolerate novel cells, ending the need for a matched donor. Trials are underway for severe combined immunodeficiency (SCID), alpha- and beta-thalassaemia and sickle cell disease (Mueller & Young 2001).

Cystic fibrosis In-utero fetal gene therapy has been successful in mice with cystic fibrosis, so the possibility of treatment for the human fetus is real. However, because there is a risk of inadvertent germ cell therapy, it is considered unacceptable at present. Trials are being carried out in the USA and the UK treating cystic fibrosis patients using a liposome–gene complex or an adenovirus vector sprayed into the nasal passages. The presence of the introduced gene appears to cause no harm but also there is no evidence of its effectiveness.

Somatic cell nuclear transfer

Somatic cell nuclear transfer (SCNT) involves placing a somatic cell next to an ovum emptied of its nucleus. The two cells fuse together and the resultant cell may be totipotent. If the newly created ovum were allowed to grow, cells from the inner cell mass would give rise to pluripotent stem cell lines. The donor cell could be from the individual needing treatment, which would solve the problem of tissue rejection. An ethical problem arises because the totipotent cell is a clone of the donor somatic cell.

Conclusion

The moral and ethical issues accompanying gene technologies are of major importance to the future of human health and medical treatment. It is essential that countries develop safeguards to ensure that safety, privacy and confidentiality are not at risk. On a national and global scale how can we ensure that any developments are available to the maximum number of affected people? Biochemistry and its associated disciplines have real power to change the world. It is important to consider how this occurs and in whose interests the changes are made.

MAIN POINTS

- The genetic basis for health and disease has led to the search for preventative, palliative and curative treatments. The development of industries based on recombinant gene technology has been so fast the general public and governments have not been able to keep up with the implications.

- Gregor Mendel proposed that each pair of characteristics in his pea plants was controlled by a pair of factors, one inherited from each parent plant. He developed three main laws – the Law of Uniformity, the Law of Segregation and the Law of Independent Assortment.

- The correct number of 46 human chromosomes was identified in 1956. A cell containing two sets of chromosomes is referred to as diploid. One chromosome of each pair originates with the ovum and the other with the sperm. Gametes contain 23 single chromosomes are called haploid.

- In the 22 pairs of autosomes the chromosomes are identical. The 23rd pair is the sex chromosomes. The DNA molecule consists of a double helix made up of two complementary chains of nucleotides packaged into discrete chromosomes by coiling and folding. Chromosomal images can be photographed to produce a karyotype.

- The genome is arranged in genes which carry the code for polypeptides. Discrete single genes called exons are separated from each other by long runs of non-coding repetitive DNA sequences called introns. The coding sequences of most genes are interrupted by introns. The genotype is the full complement of genes of individuals. The phenotype is their outward appearance and results from an interaction between genes and environment.

- A triplet codon spells out each amino acid in the specific order for a particular protein. The process of reading the code of DNA involves transcription and translation. Genes must make only the amount of their product necessary for functioning and are regulated by being activated and suppressed as needed.

- Genes may be dominant, recessive or sex-linked. A dominant allele affects heterozygotes, whereas a recessive allele only affects homozygotes. Males only have one X chromosome and are hemizygous. In female cells one X chromosome is deactivated at random, an effect called lyonisation. In genomic imprinting different clinical features arise depending on whether a gene was inherited from the mother or father.

- Mitochondrial DNA is inherited only from our mothers. Mitochondrial inheritance may cause rare disorders usually combining muscular and neurological features. These affect males and females but are transmitted only through their mothers.

- Slight differences in a protein brought about by a genetic mutation may lead to devastating diseases such as sickle cell disease or cystic fibrosis. Numerical and structural defects may affect the autosomes or sex chromosomes. Chromosome numbers may be too many or too few.

- Environmental factors may induce breaks in chromosomes, resulting in inversions and translocations which may be transmitted from parent to child.

- The Human Genome Project aims to achieve better diagnosis and counselling for families with genetic disease and to develop new preventative strategies and treatments of genetic disorders.

- Developments in gene technology highlight moral dilemmas and raise questions about the application of genetic engineering to diagnosis and treatment of genetic diseases. Regulatory bodies have been set up to oversee the technical, therapeutic and safety aspects of gene therapy.

- Fetal transplantation of pluripotent stem cells may treat genetic disorders because the fetal immune system will tolerate foreign cells. Infusion of cord blood has been used with success in some haematological and immunological disorders. Somatic cell nuclear transfer (SCNT) could give rise to pluripotent stem cell lines.

- Cystic fibrosis patients have been treated using a liposome–gene complex or an adenovirus vector sprayed into the nasal passages. The introduced gene appears to be harmless but there is little evidence of its effectiveness. The moral and ethical issues accompanying gene technologies are of major importance to medical treatment. Countries must develop safeguards to ensure that safety, privacy and confidentiality are not at risk.

References

Alberts B, Johnson A, Lewis J et al 2002 Molecular Biology of the Cell, 4th edn. Garland Science, Taylor & Francis Group, London.

Bainbridge D 2003 The X in Sex. Harvard University Press, Cambridge, Massachusetts.

Ezzell C 2002 The Child Within. Scientific American 286(6):16.

Horgan J 1993 Eugenics revisited. Scientific American June 1993:90–100.

Jorde L, Carey J, Bamshad M J, White R 2003 Medical Genetics, 3rd edn. Mosby, St Louis.

Lennard A L, Jackson G H 2000 Stem cell transplantation. British Medical Journal 32:433–437.

Lodish H, Berk A, Zipursky L et al 1999 Molecular Cell Biology. W H Freeman, London.

McKusick V 2002 Online Mendelian Inheritance in Man (OMIM), URL: http://www3.ncbi.nih.gov/omim/

Mueller R F, Young I D 2001 Emery's Elements of Medical Genetics, 11th edn. Churchill Livingstone, Edinburgh.

Annotated recommended reading

Bainbridge D 2003 The X in Sex. Harvard University Press, Cambridge, Massachusetts.
This is a highly readable book on the X chromosome, including lyonisation and its effects on women.

Jones S 1996 In the Blood, God, Genes and Destiny. Harper Collins, London.
Steve Jones writes clearly and entertainingly about the topic of genetics and its benefits and limitations. This book takes a measured look at the role of the science of genetics in a social world.

Jorde L, Carey J, Bamshad M J, White R 2003 Medical Genetics, 3rd edn. Mosby.

Mueller R F, Young I D 2001 Emery's Elements of Medical Genetics, 11th edn. Churchill Livingstone, Edinburgh.
Students looking for a book on the subject of genetics will find either of these two books excellent, with clearly written text and good diagrams.

Chapter 4

The female reproductive system

INTRODUCTION

The male and female reproductive systems ensure the future of the species by producing the **gametes**, i.e. **spermatozoa** and **oocytes**. Sex is not strictly necessary and single-celled animals reproduce asexually. However, there is great benefit in producing unique combinations of genes by reshuffling genes from two parents. This ensures the genetic variability needed to provide adaptation to changing environments (Alberts et al 2002). Female mammals also provide optimum conditions for fertilisation and fetal development. Nourishment and protection is ensured until the offspring is able to survive indepenently. Finally, expulsion from the mother's body at the correct gestation must occur and lactation initiated.

SEXUAL DIFFERENTIATION

In the early embryo there is no anatomical evidence of sexual difference internally or externally prior to the 7th week of development. Two pairs of genital ducts are present, the **paramesonephric** or **Müllerian** ducts with the potential to develop into female genitalia and the **mesonephric** or **Wolffian ducts** with the potential to develop into male genitalia. A Y chromosome gene called **SRY** (sex determining region Y gene) is expressed in male embryos (Jones 2003). Under its influence testes and functioning Sertoli cells are formed in the presence of testosterone (Ch. 5, p. 56).

If the genetic make-up of the embryo is XX, ovaries will form and the female ducts develop into female genitalia. The ducts not required to develop degenerate. This influence on the indifferent tissues leads to **homologous structures**, i.e. structures differentiating in male and female developed from the same origin (Moore & Persaud 1998). Examples include testis and ovary, penis and clitoris. Rarely, the tissues develop in such a way as to make instant recognition of the sex of the baby difficult or impossible without genetic testing.

THE FEMALE REPRODUCTIVE TRACT ANATOMY

The soft tissues forming the female internal genitalia are situated in the pelvic cavity. Although the organs are separate structures, they form a continuous tract. The organs are: vulva, vagina, uterus and cervix, uterine tube and ovary. Figure 4.1 is a diagram of the whole female reproductive tract.

The vulva

Figure 4.2 shows the external organs constituting the vulva, each of which will be described in turn.

The labia majora

These are two folds containing sebaceous and sweat glands embedded in adipose and connective tissue. They are covered

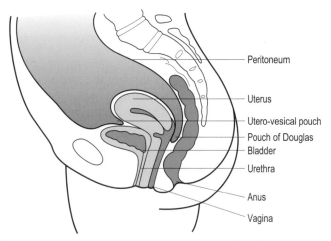

Figure 4.1 The pelvic organs in sagittal section (from Sweet B 1997, with permission).

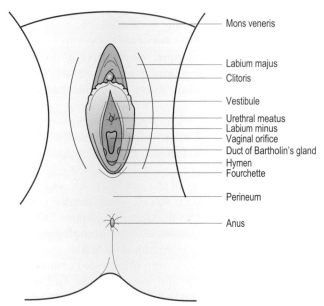

Figure 4.2 The external genitalia (from Sweet B 1997, with permission).

with skin and form the lateral boundaries of the vulval cleft. They are homologues of the scrotum. They unite anteriorly to form the **mons veneris**, an adipose pad over the symphysis pubis. Hair covers the mons veneris and terminates in a horizontal upper border. Posteriorly, the labia majora unite to form the posterior commissure. Hair grows on the outer surface of the labia majora but not on the inner surface.

The labia minora

These are two delicate folds of skin containing connective tissue, some sebaceous glands but no adipose tissue. On the medial aspect keratinised skin epithelium changes to squamous epithelium with many sebaceous glands. Anteriorly, the labia minora split into two parts. One passes over the clitoris to form its **prepuce** and the other beneath the clitoris to form a homologue of the frenulum in the male. Posteriorly, the two labia minora unite to form the fourchette. The size of the labia minora varies between women but this is of no significance.

The clitoris

This is the homologue of the male penis. It is composed of erectile tissue and can enlarge and stiffen during sexual excitement. Only the glans and prepuce are normally visible but the corpus can be palpated as a cord-like structure along the lower surface of the symphysis pubis.

The vestibule

This is the cleft between the labia minora onto which opens:

- the urethral meatus;
- the vaginal orifice.

Bartholin's glands

Bartholin's glands are two pea-sized glands embedded in connective tissue that are connected to the vestibule by ducts that are 2 cm long. These glands are homologues of Cowper's glands in the male. The ducts are lined with columnar epithelium, which produces a mucoid secretion onto the vestibule for lubrication during coitus.

Blood supply

The vulva is very vascular, receiving its arterial supply from the internal pudendal arteries which are branches of the internal iliac arteries and the external pudendal arteries which are branches of the femoral arteries. Venous drainage is usually by corresponding veins which accompany the arteries but from the clitoris a plexus of veins joins the vaginal and vesical venous plexi.

Lymphatic drainage

Lymphatic vessels form an interconnecting meshwork through the labia minora, prepuce, fourchette and vaginal introitus. These drain into the superficial and deep femoral nodes, inguinal nodes and the internal iliac nodes.

Nerve supply

Branches of the pudendal nerve and the perineal nerve supply the vulval structures.

The vagina

The vagina is a fibromuscular sheath and a potential canal extending from the vulva to the uterus. The walls are normally in apposition. The widest diameter is anteroposterior in the lower one-third and transverse in the upper two-thirds of the vagina. This is important to remember when inserting vaginal speculae. It runs upwards and backwards from the vestibule at 85° to the horizontal, which is parallel to the plane of the pelvic brim when the woman is standing erect. The vagina is surrounded and supported by the pelvic floor muscles.

The posterior wall ends blindly to form the **vault** of the vagina and is 9 cm long. The cervix projects into the anterior wall of the vagina, shortening it to 7 cm in length. This cervical projection divides the vault of the vagina into four **fornices**: shallow anterior and lateral fornices and a more capacious posterior fornix.

The entrance to the vagina is partially covered by the membranous **hymen** which has one or two uneven perforations to allow flow of the menses. This membrane varies in elasticity and is usually torn at the first coitus and more so at the first birth. Imperforate hymen is a possible cause of failure to menstruate. Once ruptured, remnants are left called **carunculae myrtiformes**. The walls of the vagina fall into transverse folds or **rugae** to allow for distension. These spread out from two longitudinal columns which run sagittally in the anterior and posterior walls.

Layers of the vagina

- Stratified squamous non-keratinized epithelium 10–30 cells deep rests on a basement membrane to form the inner lining. This is continuous with the epithelium of the infravaginal cervix. The cells are divided into three layers, all derived from the basement membrane and changing as they near the surface. These are the **parabasal cells**, **intermediate cells** and **superficial cells**.

- A layer of vascular connective tissue contains elastic tissue, nerves, lymphatics and blood vessels.

- An involuntary muscle coat whose inner muscle fibres are more oblique than circular while the outer are longitudinal. The vagina varies in size functionally, mainly as a function of muscle tone and contraction in the above muscle layer, which is under voluntary control.

- Fascia or loose connective tissue surrounds the vagina.

The entire epithelium shows cyclical changes with the ovarian and menstrual cycles. There is further development and differentiation during pregnancy in response to **circulating oestrogens**, **progesterone** and **androgens**. The vaginal epithelium does not secrete mucus but secretions seep between the cells to moisten the vagina. Superficial cells and some intermediate cells contain glycogen. Superficial cells are continuously exfoliated and release their glycogen, which is metabolised by **Döderlein's bacillus**, producing lactic acid as a waste product. This results in a normal vaginal acid medium of 4.5, preventing pathogenic organisms from invading. The cells can also absorb drugs, in particular oestrogen.

Relations

The lower half of the anterior wall is in contact with the urethra to which it is tightly bound. The upper half is in close contact with the base of the bladder. The lower third of the posterior wall is separated from the anal canal by the perineal body, the middle third is in apposition with the rectum and the upper third with a pouch of peritoneum – the pouch of Douglas. Laterally, the upper third of the vagina is supported by pelvic connective tissue, the middle third by the **levatores ani** and the lower third by the **bulbocavernosus** (see pelvic floor).

Blood supply

Arterial supply is from the vaginal and uterine arteries, both branches of the internal iliac artery. Venous drainage is by rich venous plexi in the muscular layer. These communicate with pudendal, vesical and haemorrhoidal plexi and then to the internal iliac vein.

Lymphatic drainage

Vessels from the lower one-third of the vagina drain to inferior gluteal nodes and the upper two-thirds drain to internal iliac, obturator and sacral nodes.

Nerve supply

Nerve supply to voluntary vaginal muscle is via the pudendal nerve.

Vaginal functions

- Escape of menstrual blood flow.
- Coitus with entry of the male penis.
- Birth of the fetus, placenta and membranes.

The non-pregnant uterus

The uterus develops from fusion of the two embryonic Müllerian ducts (Johnson & Everitt 2000). It is a thick-walled, muscular, hollow, pear-shaped organ flattened in its antero-posterior diameter. Its lower third forms the cervix, which projects into the vault of the vagina through its anterior wall. The uterus lies in the pelvic cavity in an anteverted and anteflexed position. Its normal measurements are shown in Table 4.1

Structure

The uterus (Fig. 4.3) consists of the body, which is 5 cm long, the narrow **isthmus** 0.5 cm long and the cervix 2.5 cm long. The fundus is the area above and between the **uterine tubes** and the junction between each uterine tube and the uterus is called the **cornu** (plural cornua). A constriction at the upper end of the isthmus is called the **anatomical internal os** whilst where the endometrium meets the columnar cervical epithelium is called the **histological internal os**. The cavity has a triangular shape when viewed in coronal section and a capacity of about 10 ml.

Although the cervix is continuous with and part of the uterus, it differs in structure and function from the body of the uterus and some aspects of cervical anatomy and physiology are described separately. The cervix is barrel-shaped and penetrated by the cervical canal. It is 2.5 cm long and separated from the body of the uterus by the isthmus. It is divided into two equal parts.

1. The **supravaginal cervix** lies above the vaginal vault and is surrounded by pelvic fascia, the **parametrium**, except posteriorly where it is in apposition to the **pouch of Douglas**.

2. The cone-shaped **infravaginal cervix** projects into the vagina and is covered by stratified squamous epithelium. This is continuous with the vaginal epithelium and joins the columnar epithelium of the cervical canal at the external os, a site called the **squamo-columnar junction** which is an important site of cellular change (see Box 4.1).

Lining of the body (corpus) The mucous lining or **endometrium** builds up from a layer of basal cells. It consists of **stroma**, which means the connective tissue component of an organ (Abercrombie et al 1992) covered by a layer of ciliated cuboid cells. This layer dips down into the stroma to form mucus-secreting tubular glands opening into the uterine cavity (Fig. 4.4). The thickness varies depending on the phase of the menstrual cycle and is thinnest at the isthmus.

Lining of the cervix The spindle-shaped cervical canal connects the cavity of the uterus at the internal os with the vagina at the external os. The canal is lined by columnar mucus-secreting epithelium thrown into anterior and posterior folds from which circular folds radiate like branches from the trunk of a tree. This appearance has led to it being called the arbor vitae (tree of life). The epithelium dips into the stroma in a complex system of crypts and tunnels separated by ridges of stroma, which consists of 80% collagen, 10% muscle fibre and 10% blood vessels. Compound racemose

Table 4.1 Measurements of the non-pregnant uterus

Dimension	Measurement
Length, including cervix	7.5 cm
Breadth	5.0 cm
Depth	2.5 cm
Average thickness of walls	1.5 cm
Weight	60 g

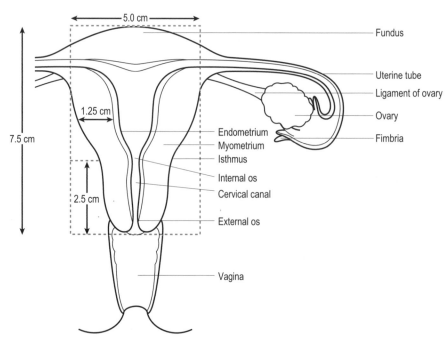

Figure 4.3 The uterus and the left uterine tube and ovary (from Sweet B 1997, with permission).

The squamocolumnar junction is between the columnar epithelium of the cervical canal and the squamous epithelium, continuous with the vaginal epithelium. This may be an abrupt transformation but sometimes the two tissue types merge in a **transformation zone**, which is the usual site for cervical carcinoma to arise. The position of this junction is determined by the amount of stroma, which is influenced by the level of the hormones oestrogen and progesterone.

Oestrogen softens the cervical collagen by binding water to the molecules. This increases the volume of stroma, which causes the clefts and tunnels to unfold. The squamocolumnar junction is displaced downwards and out of the cervical canal, an event called **eversion**. Exposure of the columnar epithelium causes the tissues to **hypertrophy** (squamous metaplasia), leading to the development of the transformation zone.

The cervix is readily accessed and the squamous epithelium has been studied widely. In some women the cervical epithelium seems unstable and cells with **nuclear dyskaryosis** (abnormal appearance of the nucleus) and **cellular dysplasia** (abnormal cell growth) are likely to lead to cervical carcinoma. These abnormalities are due to infection with the **human papillomavirus** (HPV) types 16, 18 and 6. HPV can be a cause of genital warts. Evidence from epidemiology has indicated that up to 30% of sexually active women have been affected by HPV by age 30.

Early recognition of these precancerous changes allows surgical treatment to be successful so that screening women on a regular basis can be life-saving. The technique is called **cervical exfoliative cytology** and is offered to antenatal patients who have not been recently screened. A specially shaped spatula such as an Ayres spatula is used to obtain cells from both outside and inside the cervical canal.

The cells are examined under the microscope and reported as:

1. unsatisfactory – insufficient cells or incorrect processing of the slide;
2. inflammatory or inconclusive – cells distorted by other infections such as Monilia;
3. normal;
4. mild dyskaryosis (CIN 1) (CIN means cervical intraepithelial neoplasia);
5. moderate dyskaryosis (CIN 2);
6. severe dyskaryosis (CIN 3).

Over 90% of smears will be reported as normal. Categories 1, 2 and 4 need a repeat smear after 3–4 months following treatment for infection if necessary. Categories 5 and 6 need direct vision examination by colposcopy followed by a tissue biopsy. The extent of surgical treatment will depend on the results of the biopsy and whether the woman wishes to have more children. It will vary from destruction of the abnormal cells by laser or cryosurgery to cone biopsy to hysterectomy. More serious and likely to lead to death of the woman is invasive carcinoma of the cervix, where the cancer has spread beyond the epithelial tissues.

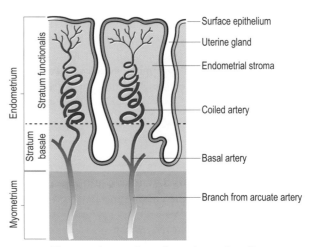

Figure 4.4   The vascular supply to the endometrium (from Hinchliff S M, Montague S E 1990, with permission).

glands secrete cervical mucus that varies in quality and quantity under the influence of the sex hormones.

Muscle layer   The muscle layer or **myometrium** is made up of bundles of smooth muscle fibres. The outer longitudinal layer and inner circular layer are not well developed in the non-pregnant uterus so that the most fibres run obliquely and interlace to surround blood vessels and lymphatic vessels. The proportion of muscle begins to diminish in the isthmus, being replaced by connective tissue. As mentioned above, the cervix has only 10% muscle content.

Peritoneal layer   The peritoneal layer is a double serosal layer known as the perimetrium. It covers the anterior and posterior surfaces but is absent from the narrow lateral surfaces. It is reflected off the uterus onto the superior surface of the bladder at the level of the anatomical internal os, an important point for understanding the technique of lower segment Caesarean section.

Relations

- Anterior – uterovesical pouch and bladder.
- Posterior – pouch of Douglas and rectum.
- Lateral – broad ligaments, uterine tubes and ovaries.
- Superior – intestines.
- Inferior – vagina.

Supports

The structures supporting the uterus are shown in Fig. 4.5.

Four pairs of ligaments support the uterus: three pairs support its position in relation to the vagina (cardinal, pubocervical and uterosacral ligaments), whereas one pair of ligaments maintains uterine anteversion and anteflexion (the round ligaments) (Table 4.2).

The broad ligaments are not true ligaments but thickened folds of peritoneum running from the uterus to the side walls of the pelvis.

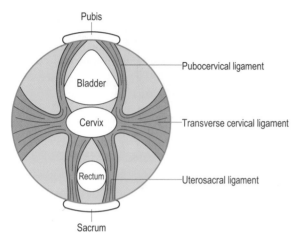

Figure 4.5   The uterine supports seen from above (from Sweet B 1997, with permission).

Table 4.2   Ligaments supporting the uterus

Ligament	Origin	Insertion
Cardinal ligaments	Cervix	Side walls of pelvis
Pubocervical ligaments	Cervix	Under bladder to the pubic bones
Uterosacral ligaments	Cervix	Sacrum
Round ligaments	Cornua	Via inguinal canal to labia majora

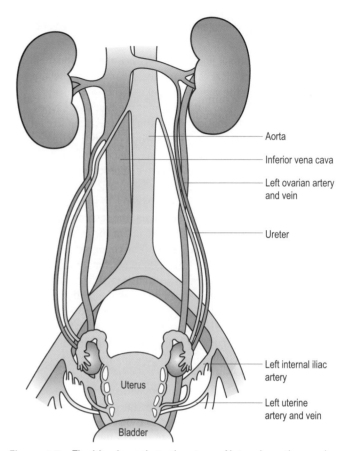

Figure 4.7   The blood supply to the uterus. Note where the ovarian vein terminates (from Sweet B 1997, with permission).

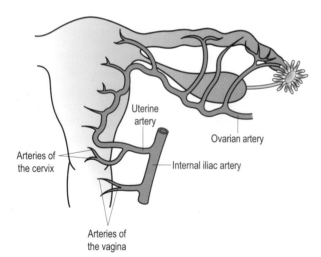

Figure 4.6   The blood supply to the uterus and its appendages as below (from Sweet B 1997, with permission).

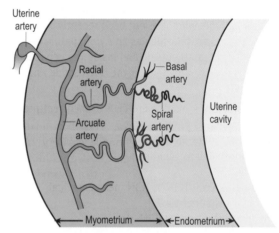

Figure 4.8   The arterial supply to the uterine endometrium. (Reproduced with permission from Studd 1989.)

Blood supply

The blood supply to the uterus is complex and rich and is contributed to by both **ovarian** and **uterine** arteries (Fig. 4.6). The uterine artery, which is a branch of the internal iliac artery, enters at the level of the internal os and sends a small branch downwards to join the vaginal arteries in supplying the cervix and vault of the vagina (Fig. 4.7). The main branch of the uterine artery turns upwards and takes a tortuous path to anastomose with the ovarian artery, which enters along the broad ligament to supply the ovaries and uterine tubes. Anterior and posterior divisions anastomose with the opposite side of the uterus. Branches leaving these vessels at right angles supply blood to the myometrium; they enter the endometrium as the **basal arteries** (Fig. 4.8).

Venous drainage is by the uterine and ovarian veins after the blood has been collected into **pampiniform plexuses** (tendril-like), some of which communicate with veins from the bladder.

Lymphatic drainage

Good lymphatic drainage of the uterus protects against uterine infection, especially following birth. There are three communicating networks of vessels and small nodes at the level of the endometrium, myometrium and subperitoneal layers of the uterus. The lymph is collected into major ducts and taken to lumbar and sacral nodes centrally and inguinal, internal and external iliac nodes laterally.

Nerve supply

The body of the uterus is supplied by autonomic supply nerves originating in thoracic 11 and 12 and lumbar 1 vertebrae. Sensation from the body of the uterus is perceived as pain in response to stretch, infection and contraction. The cervix is innervated by the sacral plexus from sacral 2, 3 and 4 vertebrae nerves which pass through the **transcervical** or **Lee–Frankenhäuser nerve plexi**. Pain sensation from the cervix is felt in response to rapid dilatation.

Functions of the uterus

- To receive the fertilised ovum.
- To nurture and protect the developing embryo and fetus.
- To expel the fetus and placenta.

The uterine tubes (fallopian tubes or oviducts)

The **uterine tubes** develop from the right and left Müllerian ducts in the embryo. They are two small, muscular, hollow tubes 10 cm long. Each tube extends from a uterine cornu, travels to the side walls of the pelvis, turning downwards and backwards before reaching them. The tubes lie within the broad ligament and communicate with the uterus at their medial end and the ovaries at their lateral end. Note that there is a direct pathway between the vagina and the peritoneal cavity, risking entry of ascending infection to the peritoneal cavity.

Structure

Each uterine tube is divided into four sections:

1. The interstitial part is the narrowest part of the tube. Its lumen is only 1 mm in diameter and it runs within the uterine wall.

2. The isthmus is a straight, narrow, thick section extending 2.5 cm laterally from the uterine wall.

3. The ampulla is the longest and widest section. It extends 5 cm from the isthmus to the side walls of the pelvis. Its lumen is tortuous, relatively thin and distensible.

4. The infundibulum or fimbriated portion is trumpet-shaped and ends in fimbriae or finger-like processes. It is the lateral 2.5 cm of the tube which turns downwards and backwards. Although the fimbria have little or no contact with the ovary, they become very active during ovulation and sweep the ovarian surface.

The three layers of the uterine tubes

1. There is an inner epithelial layer of cuboid cells arranged in plicae (folds), most pronounced in the ampulla. The complexity of the folds and the diameter of the lumen increase from the interstitial portion to the infundibular portion. Many of the cuboid cells are ciliated, whereas others are goblet cells and secrete mucus.

2. Involuntary muscle fibres in two layers, inner circular and outer longitudinal, continuous with the fibres make up the middle wall of the tube in the body of the uterus. These undergo peristaltic contractions during ovulation.

3. There is an outer covering of peritoneum on the superior anterior and posterior surfaces but it is absent on the inferior surface.

Relations

- Anterior, posterior and superior – the peritoneal cavity and intestines.
- Lateral – the side walls of the pelvis.
- Inferior – the broad ligaments and ovaries.
- Medial – the uterus.

Supports

The uterine tubes are held in position by their attachment to the uterus and the broad ligaments.

Blood supply, lymphatic drainage and nerve supply

These are shared with the ovaries and are described below.

Functions

- The mucus, cilia and peristaltic movements of the uterine tubes move the ovum towards the uterus.
- Fertilisation normally takes place in the ampulla.
- The mucus secreted by the uterine tubes may provide nourishment for the ovum.

The ovary

The pair of ovaries develops from the embryonic **gonadal ridges**. Undifferentiated primitive germ cells that begin life on the wall of the yolk sac migrate into the gonadal ridges using amoebic movements at about 4 weeks of embryological development (Moore & Persaud 1998). In the female the ovary is recognisable as such slightly later than the male testis, at about 10 weeks of development.

The mature ovary consists of **interstitial tissue** and **follicles** (Fig. 4.9). The ovaries are small almond-shaped glands measuring 3 cm × 2 cm × 1 cm and weighing just 6 g. They have a dull, pinkish grey, uneven external appearance. They lie in a shallow peritoneal fossa adjacent to the lateral pelvic wall, outside the posterior layer of the broad ligaments and inside the peritoneum. The long axis of each ovary is in the vertical plane but the position is influenced by movements of the uterus and broad ligament. If the uterus is retroverted they may lie in the uterorectal pouch or pouch of Douglas and cause pain during coitus. The uterine tubes arch over the ovaries.

Macroscopic structure

- The **medulla** is the inner part of the ovary which is directly attached to the broad ligament by the mesovarium. It consists of fibrous tissue containing blood vessels, lymphatics and nerves carried by the infundibulopelvic ligament.
- The **cortex** is the functional part of the ovary and consists of highly vascular stroma in which ovarian follicles are embedded.
- The **tunica albuginea** is a tough fibrous capsule forming the outer part of the cortex.
- The **germinal layer** consists of cuboidal cells developed from modified peritoneum and is continuous with the broad ligament. It forms an outer covering for the ovary.

Microscopic structure – the follicles

Tiny sac-like structures, called **ovarian follicles**, at different stages of maturation are embedded in the ovarian cortex.

These stages of maturation, shown in Fig. 4.9, are brought about by neurohormonal changes. The **primordial follicle** contains an immature egg or oocyte encased in a single layer of squamous-like follicle cells. These cells stay in a state of arrested development at the first meiotic prophase and will not complete their development until they are prepared for ovulation. This could be as long as 50 years (Johnson & Everitt 2000).

Over 2 million primordial follicles, consisting of the ovum surrounded by a single layer of flattened cells, are present in the fetal ovary prior to birth and no mitosis occurs after birth (Johnson & Everitt 2000). By the menarche only 200 000 remain, more than 80% having regressed. Only 300–400 will be shed at ovulation. It is not understood why these cells behave in this unusual way.

Development of the mature follicle Each day a few primordial follicles begin to develop but the mechanism behind this development or how particular follicles are selected is unknown (Johnson & Everitt 2000). Interactions between the oocyte and the follicular cells lead to oocyte growth. When a primordial follicle begins to develop, it passes through three stages:

1. First it becomes a **primary follicle** or **preantral follicle** and is surrounded by two or more layers of cuboidal **granulosa cells**.
2. Then it becomes a **secondary follicle** or **antral follicle** (the Graafian follicle). An outer layer of cells known as the **thecal layer** develops from the interstitial cells of the stroma.
3. Finally it becomes a **preovulatory follicle**.

Under the influence of hormones the granulosa and theca cells proliferate and differentiate and the oocyte increases in

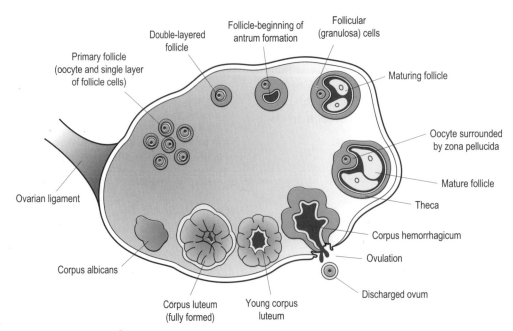

Figure 4.9 Diagrammatic section of an ovary showing stages of follicular maturation. (Reproduced with permission from Blackburn 2003.)

size by a factor of 300. The granulosa cells divide to become several layers thick, and gap junctions, which allow easy transfer of molecules between cells, develop. Secretion of fluid droplets leads to the formation of a single fluid-filled space called the **antrum**, which separates the granulosa cells into distinct layers. A dense layer called the cumulus surrounds the oocyte, while a thin outer layer lines the theca.

As the follicle continues to grow, the mature oocyte surrounded by a dense mass of granulosa cells, called the **cumulus oophorus**, becomes suspended in fluid called the **liquor folliculi**. It is attached to a stalk of granulosa cells, which connects the two layers. It then breaks away and floats freely in the fluid. The follicle bulges out from the surface of the ovary. The ovum is next to the outer wall and the stroma overlying it becomes thin. The theca cells differentiate into the **theca interna**, a highly vascularised glandular layer, and the **theca externa**, which is the dense, fibrous outer capsule of the follicle (McNabb 1997a). Glycoproteins secreted from the cell surface of the oocyte form a transparent layer called the **zona pellucida**.

Each month from the menarche to the menopause about 12 growing follicles emerge from the primordial follicles. One or occasionally more of the ripe follicles matures, ruptures and the oocyte escapes. After ovulation the ruptured follicle is transformed into a structure called the **corpus luteum** (yellow body) which, in the absence of a pregnancy, will degenerate in about 6 months into a **corpus albicans** (white body).

Relations

- Anterior – the broad ligaments.
- Posterior – the intestines.
- Lateral – the infundibulopelvic ligaments and the side walls of the pelvis.
- Superior – the uterine tubes.
- Medial – the uterus and ovarian ligament.

Supports

The ovary is held suspended in position:

- to the uterus by the ovarian ligament;
- to the posterior surface of the broad ligament by the mesovarium, which is modified peritoneum carrying blood vessels and nerves;
- to the side walls of the pelvis by the suspensory or infundibulopelvic ligament, another modified peritoneal structure.

Blood supply

The long slender ovarian arteries arise high up on the aorta, immediately below the renal arteries, demonstrating the joint development of the renal and reproductive systems (Moore & Persaud 1998). Each of the two ovarian arteries crosses over the pelvic brim laterally and enters the broad ligament where branches supply the uterine tube and the ovary. They then anastamose with the uterine artery, forming the uterine blood supply. The right ovarian vein drains directly into the inferior vena cava, whereas the left ovarian vein joins the left renal vein which then joins the inferior vena cava.

Lymphatic drainage

Lymphatic drainage is into the lumbar glands.

Nerve supply

The nerve supply of the ovary is well developed via the ovarian plexus. Sympathetic fibres and sensory nerves from the ovary run with the arteries to be relayed in the 10th thoracic segment of the spinal cord. The ovaries, like the testes, are extremely sensitive organs if handled or squeezed.

Functions of the ovary

1. To produce ova.
2. To produce the female steroid hormones oestrogen and progesterone.

CYCLICAL CONTROL OF REPRODUCTION

The ovarian cycle

In each **menstrual cycle** stromal cells surrounding the developing follicle take on an endocrine function. Developmental changes are much more complex than those that occur during spermatogenesis and the sequence of events is still being researched. The formation of receptors on follicle cells is in response to cyclical alterations in circulating hormones from the pituitary gland and the ovary itself (see below) and occurs in the late preantral and antral phases. There may also be involvement of local intraovarian regulators such as **epidermal growth factor** (EGF). The ovum is prepared for ovulation, fertilisation and implantation. At the same time changes occur within the woman's body, both in reproductive and non-reproductive tissues, to prepare for pregnancy and lactation. These also depend on the cyclical presence of specific hormone receptors on cells (McNabb 1997b).

Ovulation

The ovarian capsule stretches until it bursts, the follicle ruptures and the ovum with its surrounding tissues and liquor is flushed into the abdominal cavity. There it is picked up by the fimbria of the uterine tubes, which waft the ovum into the ampulla of the tube where it awaits fertilisation. Some women feel a pain at this time called **mittelschmerz**. The follicle now collapses to become the corpus luteum.

The lining cells of the follicle, granulosa and theca interna absorb fluid, swell and proliferate until the corpus luteum is 1–2 cm across.

Neurohormonal control of the ovarian cycle

Although the cyclical changes which occur are an integrated process, they can be discussed individually to achieve understanding of the whole process. The following aspects will be considered:

1. the hormonal function of the hypothalamic–pituitary–ovarian axis;
2. growth and development of the oocyte;
3. the menstrual cycle;
4. changes in other tissues.

The hormonal function of the hypothalamic–pituitary–ovarian axis

The average ovarian cycle lasts 28 days with ovulation on day 14. However, the cycle shows considerable variation, both from cycle to cycle in an individual woman and between women. The cycle is known to be responsive to stress, disease, allergies, physical activity and also to nutritional deficiencies (Bradley & Bennett 1995). It is usually the duration of the follicular phase leading up to ovulation that is variable.

The hypothalamus   The control of the rhythmicity of the ovarian cycle and thus the menstrual cycle is via the **hypothalamus** and **anterior pituitary gland** (Fig. 4.10). Hormonal interactions between the hypothalamus and the pituitary gland occur by vascular and neuronal pathways (Johnson & Everitt 2000). The larger anterior lobe or **adenohypophysis** has no direct neural connections with the hypothalamus, whereas the posterior lobe or **neurohypophysis** consists mainly of axons whose cell bodies are situated in the hypothalamus. The hormone **oxytocin** released by the posterior pituitary gland is important in the physiology of labour.

The anterior pituitary gland   At least five groups of hormone-producing cells are found in the anterior lobe of the pituitary. Their function is regulated by neuronal substances from the hypothalamus. Those concerned with reproduction include:

- follicle-stimulating hormone (FSH);
- luteinising hormone (LH);
- adrenocorticotrophic hormone;
- prolactin.

A detailed consideration of the many interactions involved in the process of cyclical changes can be found in Johnson & Everitt (2000). Hypothalamic **gonadotrophin-releasing hormone** (GnRH) is transferred via a portal blood system to the anterior lobe of the pituitary where it interacts with specific cell receptors to bring about the release of the gonadotrophins FSH and LH (Fig. 4.11).

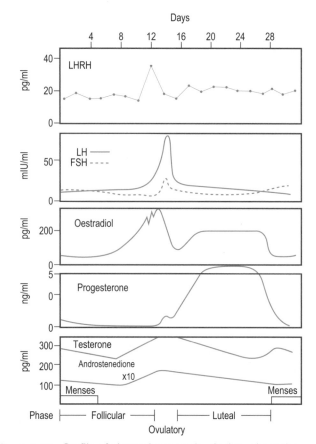

Figure 4.10   Profile of plasma hormone levels throughout the menstrual cycle. (Reproduced with permission from Berne & Levy 1993.)

The ovary   Rising plasma levels of the ovarian hormones **oestrogen** and **progesterone**, synthesised from cholesterol, can reduce the production of GnRH in a negative feedback mechanism, especially oestrogen. There are three main oestrogens: the most important is estradiol, with estrone second and estriol third in potency. If pregnancy does not occur, the corpus luteum begins to degenerate and both FSH and LH begin to rise on day 1 of the cycle and steadily increase towards the late follicular phase.

Ovulation is dependent upon a mid-cycle surge of LH and FSH, occurring 24 hours after the surge. Although plasma levels of both hormones rise, the level of LH is higher and this hormone appears to be more important in causing ovulation. Generally a single ovum is released in each cycle and the others that have begun developing regress to become **corpora atretica**.

If two follicles develop simultaneously with double ovulation, **dizygotic twinning** could occur. The frequency of double or even multiple ovulation increases with age. Black women are more likely and Asian women less likely than Caucasian women to have multiple ovulation. If there is no pregnancy, the corpus luteum begins to regress after 14 days and production of oestrogen and progesterone declines rapidly. When the plasma levels of these ovarian steroids become low enough, the anterior pituitary gland begins to produce FSH and LH again and the cycle begins again.

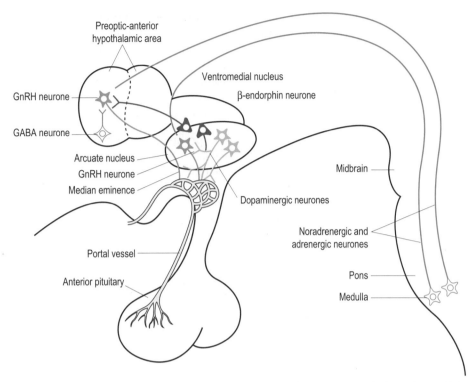

Figure 4.11   Schematic diagram to show some of the postulated neurochemical reactions which may control GnRH secretion. (Reproduced with permission from Johnson & Everitt 1995.)

Local control of growth and development of the oocyte

Within the follicle, local activities aimed at its growth and development occur. Some are carried out by theca cells, some by granulosa cells and some involve cooperation between both types of cells.

Oestrogen and progesterone   During follicular development LH stimulates the theca cells to produce the steroid hormones **androstenedione** and **testosterone**. These are transported to the granulosa cells to be converted to oestrogen, which causes proliferation of granulosa and theca cells and further growth of the follicles. The follicle that develops most rapidly may produce larger amounts of oestrogen. This may inhibit the release of FSH by negative feedback to the pituitary gland, preventing further growth of the remaining follicles. Further growth of the dominant follicle results in the surge of oestradiol that immediately precedes ovulation. Within 12 hours progesterone takes over as the dominant steroid hormone produced by the theca and granulosa cells.

Some other hormones involved locally   Research into the causes of infertility and the techniques of in-vitro fertilisation have led to the realisation that some peptide hormones, as well as the better-known steroid hormones, have major influences on follicular development. In particular, two that have been found in follicular fluid are worth mentioning – **inhibin** and **growth hormone**.

Inhibin is known to have an effect on sperm production. It has also been found in relatively high quantities in follicular fluid and may be one of the factors that determines the number of follicles released at ovulation (Herbert 1996). The rise in concentration of inhibin in follicular fluid may be a response to the surge in GnRH from the hypothalamus (Yding Andersen et al 1993).

Growth hormone may increase the intraovarian production of insulin-like growth factor 1 (IGF 1), which in turn amplifies the response of the granulosa cells to gonadotrophins (Adashi et al 1985). The GH receptor gene and GH-binding sites have been found in human granulosa cells (Carlsson et al 1992). However, GH augmentation does not improve the rate of pregnancies in women who had a poor follicular development response to treatment with gonadotrophin (Tulandi et al 1993).

Triggering of ovulation   The actions of FSH and oestrogen combine to induce the development of LH receptors on the outer layers of the granulosa cells. This coincides with the FSH and LH surge from the anterior pituitary gland brought about by GnRH from the hypothalamus, and ovulation occurs. Ovulation is facilitated by the local release of **prostaglandin E_2** (PGE_2) and the vasodilatory substances **histamine** and **bradykinin**. PGE_2 initiates breakdown of the collagen of the follicular wall, whereas the vasodilatory substances cause local inflammation. Proteolytic enzymes break down the follicular wall, allowing ovulation to occur.

The menstrual (endometrial) cycle

The changing levels and interactions between oestrogen and progesterone lead to alterations in endometrial tissues and selected tissues elsewhere, depending on the presence of hormone receptors in the tissue cells. The endometrium is itself an endocrine organ and secretes oestrogens, progesterone and prolactin; it is not totally dependent on ovarian hormones. The menstrual cycle is divided into three phases – **menstrual**, **proliferative** and **secretory** phases (Fig. 4.12). The menstrual and proliferative phases coincide with the follicular phase of the ovarian cycle and the secretory with the luteal.

Menstrual phase – days 1 to 5   As the corpus luteum degenerates, plasma progesterone, which has a shorter half-life than oestrogen, falls more rapidly, changing the balance of the two hormones in favour of oestrogen. This causes the endometrium to become unstable. Fluid is lost from the tissues, which shrink, compress the spiral arteries and cause endometrial anoxia. Autolysis begins and the upper endometrium sloughs away from the basal layer with extensive bleeding into the tissues.

Oestrogen also increases the excitability of the myometrium which further increases tissue anoxia and expels the sloughed tissue and blood. Menstrual fluid does not normally clot due to high levels of plasmin which breaks down fibrin as it forms. Blood loss is normally between 10 and 80 ml, with a mean of 35 ml and an average loss of about 0.5 mg of iron. At this point the endometrium is thin and poorly vascularised `and only the bases of the endometrial glands remain.

The proliferative phase – days 6 to 14   Rising oestrogen levels now cause rapid proliferation of stoma cells, with some oedema, and the endometrium thickens from 1 to 6 mm by ovulation. The outer epithelium remains one cell thick throughout the cycle. At the same time the glands lengthen and eventually become tortuous. The blood vessels regrow and begin to show a spiral formation. The epithelial cells and the cells of the glands begin to synthesise and store glycogen.

The secretory phase – days 15 to 28   After ovulation the corpus luteum secretes large amounts of progesterone. This acts on the oestrogen-primed endometrium to convert it to a secretory tissue. The endometrium is now highly vascular,

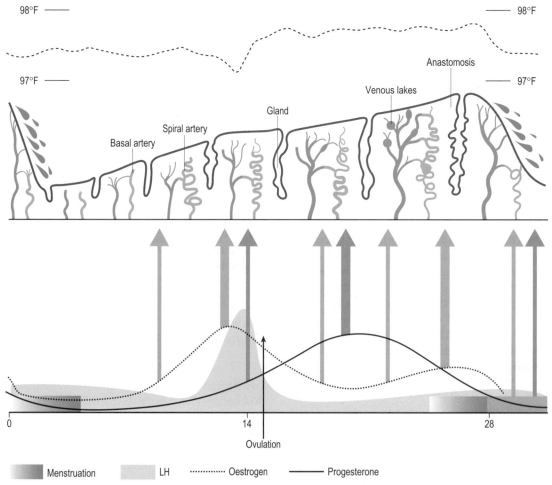

Figure 4.12   Changes in human endometrium during the menstrual cycle. (Reproduced with permission from Johnson & Everitt 1995.)

the arteries have developed pronounced spiralling and venous lakes are formed. The stroma becomes even more oedematous, the cells themselves become larger and there is a further thickening of the endometrium to 6 mm. The highly convoluted endometrial glands now secrete glycogen into their lumens. The endometrial surface becomes folded and is prepared for implantation, which normally occurs 7 days after ovulation. It is completed 14 days after ovulation at the time of the next menstrual cycle.

Non-endometrial sites of hormone action

The myometrium   Excitability of the myometrium is dependent on the balance between progesterone and oestrogen. Oestrogen increase brings about cyclical changes in the thickness of the myometrium and in muscle excitability. It stimulates spontaneous contractions, while progesterone reduces excitability. High levels of oestrogen also increase myometrial response to oxytocin.

The cervix   The mucus secreted by the cervical glands during the follicular phase is watery and turbid, while that secreted after ovulation is thicker and clearer. Mucus secreted at the time of ovulation will crystallise in a fern-like pattern if left to dry on a glass slide.

The vagina   During the follicular phase the cells of the vaginal epithelium are large and flat with an acidophilic cytoplasm. During the luteal phase they become polygonal and more basophilic. There is an increase in the glycogen content of the vagina, due partly to the secretory activity of the endometrium and partly to activity of the vaginal

epithelial cells. Lactobacilli present in the vagina metabolise the glycogen to lactic acid, lowering the pH of the vagina from 6.5 during the follicular phase to 4.5 in the luteal phase.

The uterine tubes   During the follicular phase there is an increase in the number of ciliated cells and in the frequency and coordination of the peristaltic contractions of the muscle, reaching a maximum at the time of ovulation. Subsequently, the tubes become more quiescent under the influence of progesterone.

Other actions (Johnson & Everitt 2000)   Oestrogen causes:

- development of the typical female shape;
- growth of breasts and nipples;
- development of the adult vulva, vagina and uterus;
- control of FSH production by feedback mechanism;
- maintenance of bone density;
- reduction of capillary fragility;
- increase in the ability of the cardiovascular system to withstand high blood pressures.

Progesterone causes:

- development of the secretory endometrium;
- development of alveolar breast tissue prior to menstruation;
- increase of body temperature by 0.5°C following ovulation;
- reduction of anxiety;
- interaction with aldosterone receptors to cause retention of sodium and water.

MAIN POINTS

- In the early embryo there is no evidence of sexual difference prior to the 7th week of development. If the genetic make-up of the embryo is XY, the SRY gene on the Y chromosome causes the development of the testes and male genitalia. If the genetic make-up of the embryo is XX, ovaries form and female genitalia develop.

- The continuous tract of the female internal genitalia has a direct opening to the peritoneal cavity from the external environment, necessary to allow fertilisation of the ovum, which increases the risk of pelvic infections.

- The vulva consists of the labia majora, labia minora, the clitoris and the vestibule onto which opens the urethral meatus and the vaginal orifice. The vagina is a fibromuscular sheath and a potential canal extending from the vulva to the uterus. The lining of the vagina is stratified, squamous, non-keratinized epithelium. Superficial cells are continuously exfoliated and release glycogen, which Döderlein's

bacillus metabolises to produce lactic acid to ensure an acid medium of 4.5, minimising the risk of infection.

- The endometrium of the uterine body consists of vascular connective tissue containing mucus-secreting tubular glands which open into the uterine cavity. This stroma is covered by a layer of cuboid cells which dip into it to form the glands. The thickness varies, depending on the phase of the menstrual cycle.

- The barrel-shaped cervix is divided into two equal parts: the supravaginal cervix and the cone-shaped infravaginal cervix. The spindle-shaped cervical canal is lined by columnar mucus-secreting epithelium thrown into anterior and posterior folds from which the arbor vitae radiate.

- The squamocolumnar junction is between the columnar epithelium of the cervical canal and the squamous epithelium continuous with the vaginal epithelium. In some women changes may lead to cervical carcinoma.

Early recognition by screening of precancerous changes allows surgical treatment to be life-saving.

- The myometrium is made up of bundles of smooth muscle fibres, most of which run obliquely and interlace to surround blood vessels and lymphatic vessels. The proportion of muscle diminishes in the isthmus, being replaced by connective tissue. The cervix has only 10% muscle content.

- The peritoneal layer or perimetrium covers the anterior and posterior surfaces but is absent from the narrow lateral surfaces. It is reflected off the uterus onto the superior surface of the bladder at the level of the anatomical internal os. The uterus receives the fertilised ovum, nurtures and protects the developing fetus and expels the fetus and placenta.

- The two uterine tubes communicate with the uterus at their medial end and the ovaries at their lateral end. The inner cuboid epithelial layer is arranged in plicae. Half the cells secrete mucus, while the other half are ciliated. Involuntary muscle fibres are incompletely covered by the outer layer of peritoneum. Fertilisation takes place in the ampulla.

- The ovaries lie in a shallow peritoneal fossa next to the lateral pelvic wall, outside the broad ligaments and inside the peritoneum. They consist of a medulla, cortex, tunica albuginea and germinal layer. The ovaries produce ova and the female hormones oestrogens and progesterone.

- The mature ovum consists of the haploid cell with its 23 chromosomes floating in liquor folliculi surrounded by the zona pellucida and the follicular cells of the corona radiata. The ovarian capsule stretches until it bursts and the ovum with its surrounding tissues and liquor is flushed into the abdominal cavity to be picked up by the fimbria of the uterine tube.

- The average ovarian cycle lasts 28 days with ovulation on day 14. The control of the rhythmicity of the ovarian cycle and menstrual cycle is via the hypothalamus and anterior pituitary gland. The development of the dominant follicle with its oocyte to maturity and the subsequent ovulation are complex processes involving local as well as distant steroid and peptide hormonal changes.

- The interactions between oestrogen and progesterone lead to alterations in endometrial tissues. The menstrual and proliferative phases of the menstrual cycle coincide with the follicular phase of the ovarian cycle and the secretory phase with the luteal phase.

- Steroid hormones also affect the myometrium, the cervix, the vagina, the uterine tubes and development of secondary sexual characteristics.

References

Abercrombie M, Hickman M, Johnson M L, Thain M 1992 Dictionary of Biology. Penguin Books, Harmondsworth.

Adashi E Y, Resnick C E, D'Ercole A J et al 1985 Insulin-like growth factors as intra-ovarian regulators of granulosa cell growth and function. Endocrine Review 6:400–420.

Alberts B, Bray D, Johnson A et al 2002 Essential Cell Biology. Garland Publishing, New York.

Bradley S G, Bennett N 1995 Preparation for Pregnancy. Argyll Publishing, Argyll, Scotland.

Carlsson G, Bergh C, Bentham J et al 1992 Expression of functional growth hormone receptors in human granulosa cells. Human Reproduction 76:1205–1209.

Herbert R A 1996 Reproduction. In Hinchliff S M, Montague S E, Watson R (eds) Physiology for Nursing Practice, 2nd edn. Baillière Tindall, London, pp 679–734.

Johnson M H, Everitt B J 2000 Essential Reproduction, 5th edn. Blackwell Science, Oxford.

Jones S 2003 Y: The Descent of Men. Little, Brown, London.

McNabb M 1997a Male and female reproduction – early development. In Sweet B R, Tiran D (eds) Mayes Midwifery, 12th edn. Baillière Tindall, London, pp 48–56.

McNabb M 1997b Neurohormonal regulation of female reproduction. In Sweet B R, Tiran D (eds) Mayes Midwifery, 12th edn. Baillière Tindall, London, pp 57–72.

Moore K L, Persaud T V N 1998 Before We Are Born, 5th edn. WB Saunders, Philadelphia.

Tulandi T, Falcone T, Guyda H et al 1993 Effects of synthetic growth hormone-releasing factor in women treated with gonadotrophin. Human Reproduction 8:525–527.

Yding Andersen C, Westergaard L G, Figenschau Y et al 1993 Endocrine composition of follicular fluid comparing human chorionic gonadotrophin to a gonadotrophin-releasing hormone agonist for ovulation induction. Human Reproduction 8:840–843.

Annotated recommended reading

Bainbridge D 2003 The X in Sex. Harvard University Press, Boston, Massachusetts.
This is a highly readable, entertaining account of all you need to know about the X chromosome.

Johnson M H, Everitt B J 2000 Essential Reproduction, 5th edn. Blackwell Science, Oxford.
All the major areas of reproduction are covered in this book. In particular, sexual differentiation and regulation of gonadal function are clearly described.

McNabb M 1997b Neurohormonal regulation of female reproduction. In Sweet B R, Tiran D (eds) Mayes Midwifery, 12th edn. Baillière Tindall, London, pp 57–72.
This chapter provides an easily readable account of the regulation of female hormone production.

Chapter 5

The male reproductive system

CHAPTER CONTENTS

INTRODUCTION

An understanding of the anatomy and physiology of the male reproductive system is essential knowledge for the extended role of the midwife. Many aspects of fertility, infertility and preconception care depend on the general and sexual health of both partners.

THE MALE REPRODUCTIVE SYSTEM – ANATOMY

The male genitalia are mainly outside the body cavity, a situation necessary for both production and transfer of **spermatozoa**. The organs to be described below are the scrotum, testis, rete and epididymis, ductus deferens, seminal vesicles, prostate gland, bulbourethral glands and penis with the urethra (Fig. 5.1). Unlike the female urinary system where the urethral orifice is separate to the vagina, the male genital and urinary systems share a common outlet through the urethra.

The scrotum and testes

Embryonic development

To recap, SRY gene activity on the Y chromosome converts what is known as an indifferent gonad to a testis. In the absence of this factor the gonad develops into an ovary (Jones 2003). It is a very efficient process and there are very few true **hermaphrodites** who have both testicular and ovarian tissue. Once the gonad is established, the developmental SRY gene is permanently switched off. The **Sertoli cells** (see below) of the **testes** also secrete **müllerian inhibiting hormone** (MIH), which remains active until puberty, when there is a rapid decline in production. The **Leydig cells** (see below) of the testes produce **testosterone** from about 13–15 weeks (Johnson & Everitt 2000).

In the embryo the testes develop high up on the lumbar region of the abdominal cavity (Johnson & Everitt 2000). In the last few months of fetal life they begin to descend through the abdominal cavity, over the pelvic brim and

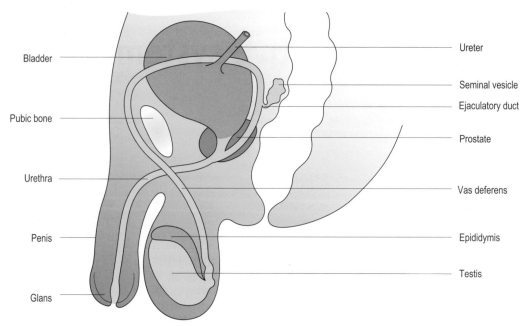

Figure 5.1   The male reproductive system (from Sweet B 1997, with permission).

down the inguinal canal into the scrotal sac outside the body cavity. This descent occurs under the influence of the male hormone testosterone and is completed in 98% of baby boys by birth.

The mature testis

At maturity each testis measures 4 cm long and 2 cm in diameter and is surrounded by two coats: the outer coat is the **tunica vaginalis** and is derived from peritoneum; the inner coat is a thick fibrous capsule, the **tunica albuginea**. One testis sits in each pocket of the **scrotal sac**. The scrotum is a thin-walled sac covered with hairy rugose skin well supplied with sebaceous glands. The scrotal skin is highly vascularised and has a large surface area (Marieb 2000).

The temperature of the testes is maintained at 2–3°C below that of the body core to facilitate spermatogenesis. The position of the scrotum in relation to the body can be adjusted by a spinal reflex in order to regulate testicular temperature. In a cold environment contraction of the scrotal muscle, the **dartos muscle**, wrinkles the scrotal skin and reduces the size of the sac, whereas the **cremaster muscle**, skeletal muscle arising from the internal oblique muscle, contracts and lifts the testes nearer to the body. Relaxation of these muscles will allow the testes to be held away from the body to facilitate cooling.

Structure   Each testis is divided into 200–300 wedge-shaped **lobules** by thin fibrous partitions that are extensions of the tunica albuginea (Fig. 5.2). Each lobule contains up to four **seminiferous tubules**, which are highly coiled loops. About 80% of the testis by weight consists of seminiferous tubules in which spermatozoa (sperm) develop. The seminiferous tubules of each lobule converge to form a straight tubule or

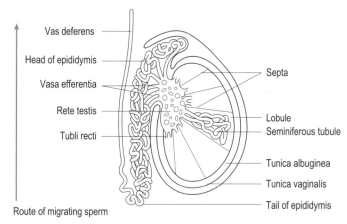

Figure 5.2   The testis (from Hinchliff S M, Montague S E 1990, with permission).

tubulus rectus that conveys the sperm into the **rete testis**, a tubular network on the posterior aspect of the testis. From here sperm enter the **epididymis**, which is in close apposition to the external surface of the testis. Macrophages that phagocytose dead sperm are found in the lumen of the epididymis. Interstitial tissue is packed around the seminiferous tubules and contains blood vessels and endocrine cells, called Leydig cells, which secrete testosterone.

Blood supply   The testes are supplied by the testicular arteries that arise from the abdominal aorta. The testicular veins form a network around the testicular artery, called a pampiniform plexus (tendril-like). This absorbs heat from the artery before the blood enters the testis.

Lymphatic drainage   Lymph drainage is by the inguinal nodes.

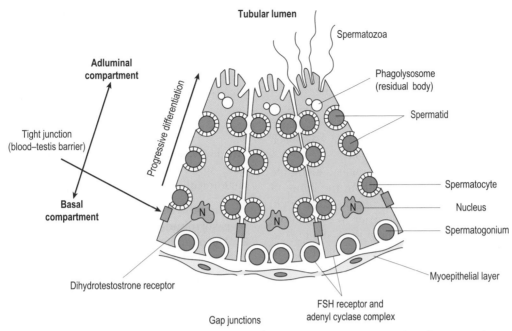

Figure 5.3   Sertoli cells with developing germ cells. (Reproduced with permission from Tepperman & Tepperman 1987.)

Nerve supply   There is an innervation by the autonomic system – both sympathetic and parasympathetic. There is also a rich sensory nerve supply, resulting in much pain and nausea if the testes are struck. The nerve fibres run with the blood vessels and lymphatics in the fibrous connective tissue sheath called the spermatic cord.

Function of the testes

- To produce spermatozoa.
- To produce the hormones testosterone and inhibin.

Spermatogenesis (the production of spermatozoa)   Each testis consists of two separate compartments: the cells that produce sperm and those that produce the hormones. There is an actual physical barrier consisting of cellular barriers which limit free exchange of water-soluble materials. This barrier develops at puberty and is formed of multiple layers of gap and tight junction complexes which surround each Sertoli cell. This is sometimes called the **blood–testis barrier** (Johnson & Everitt 2000). Its functions are:

1. to prevent sperm from entering the systemic and lymphatic circulations where they could set up antisperm antibodies, leading to infertility;
2. to maintain distinct chemical environments on either side of the barrier to facilitate sperm health and development.

Seminiferous tubules contain two types of cell: germ cells and Sertoli cells (Fig. 5.3). Primary germ cells are dormant in the testis from the fetal period of life and begin to increase in number at puberty. The production of sperm in the seminiferous tubules of the testes has three phases:

1. mitotic proliferation, which produces large numbers of cells;
2. meiotic division, which generates diversity and halves the chromosome number;
3. cytodifferentiation, which packages the chromosomes for effective delivery.

In a functioning testis, germ cells will be present at various stages of development, all originating from **spermatogonia**. Spermatogonia divide by mitosis continuously, to ensure a constant supply of cells maturing towards spermatozoa. After undergoing several mitotic divisions, they mature, become larger and are known as **primary spermatocytes**, which are diploid cells. Although nuclear division (**karyokinesis**) occurs, cytoplasmic division is incomplete and spermatogonia are linked by cytoplasmic bridges to form a **syncytium**. This syncytium persists throughout the meiotic phase and individual cells are only released as mature sperm (Johnson & Everitt 2000).

Primary spermatocytes undergo the first meiotic division to form two secondary spermatocytes, which have only 23 chromosomes – one of each pair. Half will receive the X chromosome of the male cell genotype and half will receive the Y chromosome. Secondary meiosis results in four haploid cells called **spermatids**.

Spermatids are found in close association with Sertoli cells, which are polymorphic cells attached to a basement membrane but extending into the lumen of the seminiferous tubule. They provide nutrition and support to the sperm and are sometimes called 'nurse cells'. Here the spermatids are transformed from fairly basic cells into highly specialised sperm.

As a sperm matures excess protoplasm is lost and the chromatin of the nucleus condenses to become its head. One centriole develops into the tail, which is composed of a central filament of 2 microfibrils surrounded by a circle of

9 fibrils. Mitochondria aggregate into the neck region and the Golgi apparatus helps to form the acrosome cap which develops over the head of the sperm and contains enzymes called **hyaluronidases** and **proteases**.

The process takes about 70 days and several hundred million sperm per day (300 and 600 sperm per gram of testis per second) are produced continuously from puberty. As men age, the seminal tubules undergo involution and, by 70 years, extensive atrophy may be present. Germ cells may have been reduced in number but the Sertoli cells remain.

When sperm are fully formed they are pushed along the duct system to the epididymis by the cilia in the lining of the tubuli recti and the smooth muscle in the tubal wall. Here they mature and become motile prior to ejaculation. The columnar epithelium of the epididymis is thought to secrete hormones, enzymes and nutrients to enable sperm maturation. Sperm can be stored in the epididymis for as long as 42 days, which has implications for pre-conception advice on the environmental effects present for at least 2 months before the ejaculation event which results in fertilisation of an ovum.

The duct system

The epididymis

The **epididymis** is a comma-shaped tightly coiled tube about 6 metres long. The head of the comma which caps the superior aspect of the testis receives sperm from the efferent ductules of the testis. Here the sperm become more motile and fertile. However, they do not actively swim until ejaculated into the vagina. During ejaculation, the smooth muscle in the wall of the epididymis contracts strongly, expelling sperm from the tail portion into the ductus deferens.

The vas (ductus) deferens

This muscular tube runs upwards from the epididymis, through the **inguinal canal** into the pelvic cavity. It can be felt easily as it passes over the pubic bone. Its terminus expands to form the ampulla and joins with the duct from the **seminal vesicle** to form the short **ejaculatory duct**. The two ejaculatory ducts pass into the **prostate gland** and empty into the **urethra**. The wall of the **vas deferens** is composed of an outer layer of loose connective tissue and three layers of smooth muscle which can undergo rapid peristaltic contractions during ejaculation to pass the sperm forward.

This movement is facilitated by the autonomic nerve supply. The cells of the mucosal layer are pseudostratified epithelium arranged in longitudinal ridges. In the extra-abdominal portion, the ductus is accompanied by the testicular artery, the pampiniform plexus of veins, a nerve plexus, lymphatic vessels and the cremaster muscle. The whole complex is called the spermatic cord.

If no ejaculation occurs, the sperm in the epididymis degenerate and phagocytic cells in the epithelial layer remove them. Male sterilisation involves ligating and cutting the vas deferens, an operation called vasectomy. Fertility may remain for 6–8 weeks because of the presence of viable sperm above the sectioned segment. Although the operation prevents the presence of sperm in the ejaculate, ejaculation still occurs because of the presence of fluids from the accessory glands.

The urethra

This is the terminal portion of the duct system and serves both urinary and reproductive systems. It is divided anatomically into three three regions:

1. The prostatic urethra, which exits from the bladder and is surrounded by the prostate gland.
2. The membranous urethra, which passes through the urogenital diaphragm.
3. The spongy urethra (penile), which passes through the penis to exit at the external urethral meatus. The spongy urethra is 15 cm long and is 75% of the total urethral length.

Accessory glands

These include the paired seminal vesicles, the bulbourethral glands and the single prostate gland. They provide a transport medium and nutrients and the bulk of the ejaculate.

The seminal vesicles

The **seminal vesicles** lie behind the prostate gland and are finger-shaped and sized, i.e. 5–7 cm long (Marieb 2000). They have a capacity of $3 \, cm^3$. They secrete an alkaline, sticky yellowish fluid containing fructose, globulin, ascorbic acid and prostaglandins which accounts for 60% of the semen. Sperm and seminal fluid mix in the ejaculatory duct and enter the urethra together during ejaculation.

The prostate gland

The **prostate gland** is situated around the bladder neck and first part of the urethra. It is about 3 cm in diameter in the normal adult and may involute or hypertrophy after middle age, resulting in urological problems. It produces a thin, acidic, milky fluid and contains enzymes, calcium and citrates. This fluid may act to stimulate motility in the sperm.

Semen **Semen** is a milky white sticky fluid mixture of sperm and accessory gland secretions which forms the transport medium and provides nutrients and chemicals that activate the sperm. The **prostaglandins** in semen are thought to decrease the viscosity of the cervical mucus and to cause reverse peristalsis in the uterus, facilitating movement of the sperm up the female reproductive tract. It is relatively alkaline with a pH of 7.2–7.6 which helps to neutralise the acid medium of the vagina to protect the sperm and maintain their motility.

Semen also contains a bacteriostatic chemical called **seminal plasmin** and clotting factors, including **fibrinogen**, which coagulate the semen shortly after it has been ejaculated. Once established in the vault of the vagina, the **fibrinolysin** also contained in the semen causes it to liquefy so that the sperm can swim freely into the female duct system. The average ejaculate is found to be about 3–6 ml and contains 60–200 million sperm of which at least 60–80% should be normal and 50% motile after 1 h at 37°C

The bulbourethral (Cowper's) glands

These are tiny pea-sized glands situated inferiorly to the prostate. They secrete thick clear mucus that drains into the spongy urethra, acting as a lubricant prior to ejaculation.

The penis

The **penis** is the organ of copulation which normally hangs flaccidly from the **perineum** in front of the scrotum. It has an attached root and a free shaft that ends in an enlarged tip – the **glans penis**. Internally it has three long columns of erectile tissue (Fig. 5.4), consisting of two dorsal **corpora cavernosa** side by side and one **corpus spongeosum** containing the urethra. The erectile tissue is a spongy network of connective tissue and smooth muscle full of vascular spaces.

The root of the penis is broad and firmly fixed to the pubic rami by the proximal ends of the corpora cavernosa, known as the **crura**. Each crus is surrounded by an ischiocavernosus muscle. The terminal glans penis is perforated by the urethral meatus and is very well supplied by sensory nerve endings. It is the main erogenous zone in the male. In the resting state the glans penis is covered by a folded cylinder of skin known as the **prepuce** or foreskin.

HORMONAL CONTROL OF MALE REPRODUCTIVE FUNCTION

Control is by hormones from the hypothalamus, anterior pituitary lobe and testis. Gonadotrophin-releasing hormone (GnRH) from the hypothalamus influences the anterior pituitary to produce the same hormones as in the female – follicle-stimulating hormone (FSH) and luteinising hormone (LH). In the male, plasma levels of LH are usually three times higher than FSH.

Actions of LH

LH acts on the interstitial tissue to cause synthesis and release of testosterone, and plasma testosterone levels are directly related to plasma LH levels. Testosterone is a steroid molecule synthesised from cholesterol. It binds loosely to

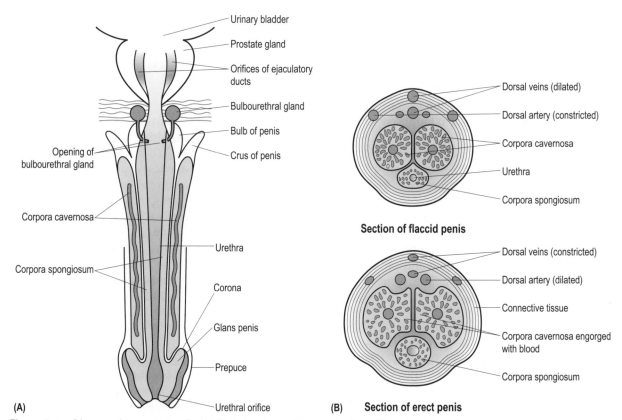

Figure 5.4   Diagram demonstrates A: detailed structure of the penis, B: section of erect penis.

Table 5.1 Functions of testosterone

Action	Functions
Before birth	Masculinisation of the reproductive tract and external genitalia Promotion of testicular descent
Sex specific tissues	Growth and maturation at puberty Maintenance of reproductive tract throughout adult life Essential for spermatogenesis
Other reproductive effects	Increased libido and sex drive Control of gonadotrophic hormones secretion
Secondary sexual characteristics	Development of male distribution of body and facial hair Deepening of the voice due to thickening of the vocal cords and enlargement of the larynx
Other effects	Anabolic effect on protein production Growth of the long bones at puberty and fusion of epiphyses Increased secretion from sebaceous glands Possible role in aggressive behaviour

plasma proteins to be taken to its target organs. The functions of testosterone are shown in Table 5.1.

Inhibin is a non-steroidal factor which has been isolated in the testis and may inhibit FSH secretion. It is possibly produced by the Sertoli cells and acts by a negative feedback loop.

Actions of FSH

FSH seems to act on the later stages of sperm maturation and cannot initiate spermatogenesis in the absence of LH.

The role of prostaglandins in reproduction

The group of chemical messengers known as the prostaglandins have been found to be active in multiple sites in the body and are involved in many physiological processes. Some have been found to act on smooth muscle: for example, in both bronchodilation and bronchoconstriction. Prostaglandins also promote pain and inflammation and modulate platelet aggregation. The common drug aspirin is a prostaglandin inhibitor and this is why it has many pharmaceutical uses.

Prostaglandins are fatty acid derivatives that are produced wherever they occur in the body from arachidonic acid; they produce their effect locally. After they have acted local enzymes rapidly inactivate them so that they do not gain access to the circulatory system. They were first identified in semen and were thought to be produced by the prostate gland, hence the name.

In the reproductive system prostaglandins:

- increase uterine activity during menstruation;
- play a role in ovulation by influencing follicular rupture;
- promote sperm transport by causing smooth muscle contraction in male and female reproductive tracts;
- mediate the renal vasodilation of pregnancy;
- are involved in preparing the cervix for labour by softening it;
- are probably the final mediator in the regulation of uterine contractions.

THE PHYSIOLOGY OF SEXUAL INTERCOURSE

Stated simply, this is the process by which male and female gametes are brought together. In mammals fertilisation occurs internally so that sperm must be deposited inside the female body. In evolutionary terms the behaviour must be pleasurable so that male and female are willing to take part. In humans there is an enormous psychological and social input to sexual behaviour and arousal includes both cognitive and emotional aspects, equally as important as the physiological context (Haeberle 1983). Classical studies of human sexual response were made by Masters & Johnson (1966), who described the response by both sexes as having the four phases of their sexual cycle, which are **excitement**, **plateau**, **orgasm** and **resolution**. This is known as their 'EPOR' model (Johnson & Everitt 2000).

The male response

In the male two stages can be described – erection and ejaculation.

Erection

Erection is brought about by a spinal reflex triggered by local stimulation of sensitive mechanoreceptors in the tip of the penis (Fig. 5.5). When the man is sexually excited, increased parasympathetic and decreased sympathetic activity cause the arterioles in the erectile tissue of the corpora cavernosa and the corpus spongeosum to dilate and engorge. Normally there is no parasympathetic control over blood vessels and it is the variation in sympathetic stimulation that causes vasodilation or vasoconstriction in blood vessels. Erection is the major instance in which both branches of the autonomic nervous system control blood vessels and vasodilation is accomplished much more rapidly than usual.

Ejaculation

Ejaculation is also controlled by a spinal reflex with a patterned sequence of events following the efferent nerve messages. Sympathetic nerve impulses cause sequential contractions of smooth muscle in the prostate, epididymis, ductus deferens, ejaculatory duct and seminal vesicles.

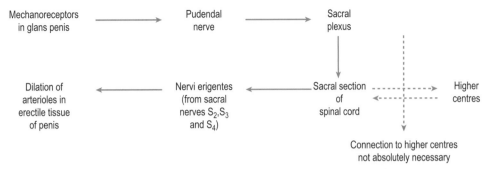

Figure 5.5   The nervous pathways (simplified) involved in the erection reflex. (Hinchliff S M, Montague S E 1990, with permission.)

This causes **emission** when the genital ducts and accessory glands empty their contents into the posterior urethra. This is followed by the expulsion phase of ejaculation when the semen is expelled from the penis by a series of rapid muscle contractions. The filling of the urethra with semen triggers nerve impulses that activate skeletal muscles at the base of the penis to contract at about 0.8 s intervals and expel the semen forcibly.

During ejaculation the sphincter at the base of the bladder is closed so that spermatozoa do not enter the bladder and urine cannot be voided. **Orgasm** occurs, which is a feeling of intense pleasure accompanied by involuntary rhythmic action of the pelvic muscles and generalised contraction of skeletal muscle throughout the body. This is followed by resolution, with physical and psychological relaxation. Loss of erection follows due to vasoconstriction of the penile arterioles and venous drainage: this varies, depending on circumstances, from a few minutes to several hours. There is now an absolute latent or refractory period during which further erection cannot occur.

The female response

In the female there is erection of the **clitoris** and the erectile tissue in the **labia minora**. **Nipples** also have erectile tissue and respond to sexual excitement. Lubrication from **Bartholin's glands** facilitates intromission. Orgasm may occur following movement of the penis in and out of the vagina. During the plateau phase vasocongestion of the outer third of the vagina occurs which tightens the introitus

around the penis. The uterus is raised upwards lifting the cervix and enlarging the upper two-thirds of the vagina. This is called ballooning and increases the space for deposition of the ejaculate.

If orgasm occurs, the same pelvic muscle contractions as in the male occur, mostly in the outer third engorged section of the vagina. This region is sometimes called the **orgasmic platform**. The uterus may contract, beginning at the fundus. During resolution, vasocongestion and the cardiac and respiratory changes return to normal. The descriptions of orgasm given by men and women are similar but orgasm appears not to occur with the same regularity in females.

Stimulation of the clitoris can enhance the pleasure and contribute to female orgasm but 10–20% of women appear never to achieve orgasm. Cross-cultural studies suggest that orgasm in women may not be reflex but learned. In societies where women are expected to enjoy sex, orgasm is much commoner (Johnson & Everitt 2000). Although orgasm is not necessary for fertilisation, contractions of the uterus may aspirate semen and help the sperm on their journey.

Cardiovascular and respiratory changes

In both sexes there are changes in the cardiovascular and respiratory systems. There is a marked increase in heart rate to between 100 and 170 beats/min, systolic blood pressure may increase by 30–80 mmHg and diastolic by 20–40 mmHg. Respiration may double to 40/min and flushing of the chest, neck and face occurs.

MAIN POINTS

- In the embryo the testes develop high up on the posterior wall of the abdominal cavity, descending into the scrotal sac in the last few months of fetal life. This maintains testicular temperature at 2–3°C below that of the body core, which facilitates spermatogenesis. The male genital and urinary systems share a common outlet through the urethra.

- The testes produce spermatozoa and the hormones testosterone and inhibin. There is a physical barrier surrounding each Sertoli cell between the tissues that produce sperm

and those that produce hormones. This prevents sperm from entering the systemic and lymphatic circulations and maintains environments which facilitate the health and development of sperm.

- Seminiferous tubules contain two types of cell – germ cells and Sertoli cells. Primary germ cells are dormant in the testis from the fetal period of life and begin to increase in number at puberty. Germ cells all originate from spermatogonia, which divide by mitosis continuously.

- After undergoing several mitotic divisions, sperm mature to become diploid primary spermatocytes. Although nuclear division occurs, cytoplasmic division is incomplete and spermatogonia are linked by cytoplasmic bridges to form a syncytium. Individual cells are only released as mature sperm.

- Primary spermatocytes undergo the first meiotic division to form two secondary haploid spermatocytes: half receive the X chromosome of the male cell genotype and half the Y chromosome. Secondary meiosis results in four haploid spermatids found in close association with Sertoli cells, which provide nutrition and support.

- The process of sperm maturation takes about 70 days and several hundred million a day are produced continuously from puberty. As men age, the seminal tubules undergo involution and there may be extensive atrophy by 70 years. Germ cells are reduced in number but Sertoli cells remain.

- When sperm are fully formed they are pushed along the duct system to the epididymis where they mature and become motile prior to ejaculation. Sperm can be stored in the epididymis for 42 days.

- Interstitial tissue packed around the seminiferous tubules contains blood vessels and Leydig cells which secrete testosterone.

- The accessory glands of the male reproductive system, including the seminal vesicles, bulbourethral glands and the prostate gland – provide a transport medium and nutrients and the bulk of the ejaculate. Semen is both a transport medium and a provider of nutrients and chemicals that activate the sperm. The average ejaculate is about 3–6 ml and contains 60–200 million sperm.

- The penis has three long columns of erectile tissue internally – two dorsal corpora cavernosa side by side and one corpus spongeosum containing the urethra. The glans penis, perforated by the urethral meatus, is very well supplied by sensory nerve endings.

- Control of the male reproductive system is via the hypothalamus, anterior pituitary and testis. Gonadotrophin-releasing hormone influences the anterior pituitary to produce FSH and LH. LH acts on the interstitial tissue to cause synthesis and release of testosterone. Inhibin may inhibit FSH secretion and prevent sperm manufacture by acting as a negative feedback loop.

- In the reproductive system prostaglandins increase uterine activity during menstruation, influencing follicular rupture and promotion of sperm transport by causing smooth muscle contraction in the male and female reproductive tracts.

- Sexual activity in humans is more than a physiological response. Psychological and social factors are important in developing the relationship between partners. Research has found that there are similar stages in the male and female physiological sexual response, although the psychosocial attitudes differ between the sexes.

References

Haeberle E J 1983 The Sex Atlas. Sheridan Press, London.
Johnson M H, Everitt B J 2000 Essential Reproduction, 5th edn. Blackwell Science, Oxford.
Jones S 2003 Y: The Descent of Men. Little, Brown, London.

Marieb E N 2000 Human Anatomy and Physiology, 5th edn. Benjamin/Cummings, Redwood City, California.
Masters W, Johnson V 1966 Human Sexual Response. J and A Churchill, London.

Annotated recommended reading

Jones S 2003 Y: The Descent of Men. Little, Brown, London.
This book is both learned and humorous and contains much information on all levels from molecular to social about being male.

Johnson M H, Everitt B J 2000 Essential Reproduction, 5th edn. Blackwell Science, Oxford.
All the major areas of reproduction are covered in this book. In particular, sexual differentiation and regulation of gonadal function are clearly described.

Chapter 6

Fertility control

INTRODUCTION

Throughout women's lives, from puberty to the menopause, fertility control is of prime concern. Many young women are unsure whether they could become pregnant at the first sexual encounter and if they need to take precautions against pregnancy. If they are sexually active, pregnancy will result. Yet the human species is not as fertile as some mammals. A **fecundity rate** of 20% has been quoted (Evers 2002); i.e. there is a 1:5 chance of conceiving at the most fertile time.

At birth the female ovary contains immature ova which remain in limbo until puberty. Under hormonal influence one ovum matures at each ovarian cycle. If more follicles ripen in a cycle, the potential of several ova is lost as partially ripened follicles, including their ova, die. Men produce an almost infinite supply of spermatozoa continuously. Few men take control of their own fertility but should do so as this would help prevent unwanted pregnancies. Reproduction and contraception constitute a significant health issue.

WORLD POPULATION

The rate of fertility and the steady rise in world population throughout the 1950s to the 1990s (Fig. 6.1) is directly related to health, environment and poverty. The development of many medical interventions and the greater prosperity of the developed countries have brought about a lower death rate. The trend to have 2.9 children instead of the 6.9 in the 1950s with the lowering death rate has meant that we have an ageing population in Western society with a growth rate declining to 0.1%, whereas population growth in many underdeveloped countries is currently 97%.

Despite the graph showing a decline in population in the 21st century, this is misleading and the world population is still expected to increase. It is difficult to predict trends in this area as infertility is increasing and must be compared to the fertility rate at that time (Speidel 2000). Many of the world's population are young and have still to have their families and there is concern that unless something can be

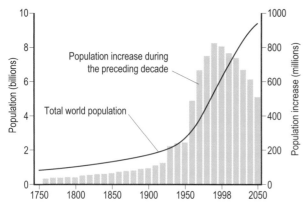

Figure 6.1 The rate of fertility and rise in world population related to health, environment and poverty.

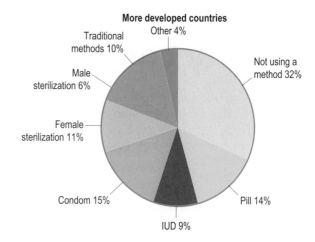

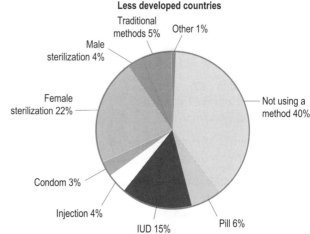

Figure 6.2 Contraception use among married women in the late 1990s.

done to slow down this increase in humanity, famine, infections and wars may intervene.

Contraception and the future

Contraception should be able to curb population growth and the destruction of the environment but people must be assured firstly that their present children will survive. Two further concepts involving the status of women and how to empower their ability to make decisions about their fertility have been considered. These are the equal right of girls and women to education and the involvement of women in paid employment (Dasgupta 1995). Obviously, population problems differ and some Western countries such as Britain have an ageing population as the number of children born drops.

Various countries are involved in contraceptive trials to combat overpopulation. China has conducted trials into a 'male pill' and the Indian National Institute of Immunology has been testing a female immunocontraceptive (vaccine) targeting human chorionic gonadotrophin. Such methods need to be cheap, easily accessible to rural as well as urban dwellers and be acceptable to both partners and to the culture in which they live.

Contraception worldwide

Worldwide, the contraceptive effect of breastfeeding probably has as much impact as all the other forms of contraception put together. However, as education increases in underdeveloped countries, so also will the use of contraception. In the year 2030 it is estimated that 60% of the world's population will live in urban communities. This will mean environmental change, population change and planning for resources. This planning must include birth control to prevent over-population and starvation. Urban women tend to have fewer children than women living in rural communities, which may in part be associated with improved education and health resources. However, surveys by the Population Reference Bureau state that a quarter of births worldwide are still unplanned. Figure 6.2 shows

contraceptive use among married women in the late 1990s (Nash & De Souza 2002).

THE EFFECTIVENESS OF CONTRACEPTION

Contraception has probably been an issue ever since the link was made between sexual behaviour and pregnancy. It certainly occupied the minds of the ancient Egyptians, Greeks and Romans. However, in modern times contraception has been openly discussed, used and become legal in most countries only during the last 50 years. There are religious, moral and cultural issues to be considered and therefore it is unlikely that one method would ever become universal.

The ideal contraceptive would be 100% effective, painless, easy to use independently of the user's memory, cheap and accessible and without medical control. Great strides have been made in the development of contraceptive methods but there has been anxiety about the safety of some methods. However, the death rate from childbearing-related problems has been very high in the past and risk must be measured against the physical, social and psychological effects of unwanted or too frequent pregnancies.

Table 6.1 Methods and their failure rates per hundred woman years (HWY). The variations in numbers indicate the commitment and skill with which the method is used

Method	Failure rate per HWY
The combined oestrogen with progestogen pill	0.1–7
The progestogen-only pill	0.5–7
Injectable progestogen	0–1
Female barrier methods	2–15
The male condom	2–15
The female condom	not yet known
The intrauterine device	0.3–4
Spermicidal preparations (used alone)	14–25
The contraceptive sponge	9–25
Symptothermal method (temperature + cervical mucus)	1–4
Coitus interruptus	25
Male sterilisation	0–0.2
Female sterilisation	0–0.2

Calculating effectiveness

A mathematical concept used to assess the effectiveness of contraceptive methods is the calculation of the **failure rate per hundred woman years (HWY)**: i.e. the number of pregnancies if 100 women used the method for 1 year (Table 6.1), also known as the **Pearl Index** (Bromwich & Parsons 1990). In a perfect world this would be truly representative of a method's effectiveness but it is complicated by factors such as changes in fertility with age, motivation to use the method correctly every time and the infertility of about 10% who will not know it whilst they are using contraception. It is difficult to differentiate between failure of the method and failure of the user to comply with instructions. Failure often occurs in the early months following commencement of any method; developing skills in using the method make it more reliable.

PHYSIOLOGICAL APPLICATION OF CONTRACEPTION

The stages of reproduction of male and female gametes (Fig. 6.3) offer choices of sites for the development of effective methods of contraception (Fig. 6.4).

Prevention of gamete production – ovum

Combined oral contraception (COC)

All the ova available to the woman for reproduction are already present in her ovary at birth. Therefore it is not a matter of preventing ovum production but of preventing their maturation and ovulation by suppressing follicle-stimulating hormone (FSH) and luteinising hormone (LH) at the pituitary

level. This, in turn, will prevent the feedback mechanisms between the hypothalamus and the pituitary gland (Rivera et al 1999).

The concept of hormonal control of fertility began in the late 1940s when it was realised that the roots of the wild Mexican yam contained a chemical from which **steroid hormones** could be produced. Unfortunately, natural hormones are expensive to produce and when taken orally are inactivated by the digestive processes. The word **combined** is used because the preparations include oestrogens and progestagens. The synthetic oestrogen **is ethinylestradiol** or **mestranol**. The synthetic progestogens used are various, including **norethisterone**, **levonorgestrel** and **gestodene**.

The oestrogen component inhibits FSH release and stops the maturation of the follicle, while the progestogen inhibits the release of LH, preventing ovulation. The dose of oestrogen is constant amongst all preparations: a maximum of 30–35 μg. The dose of progestagen is more variable and progestagens add to the contraceptive effect by causing thickening of the cervical mucus (Billings et al 1972), making the endometrium unsuitable for implantation and reducing the motility of the uterine tubes (Franey 1999).

Since the COC became available in the 1960s it has been beset by media scares, and research has some evidence suggesting that the higher-dose pills created thrombotic problems in some women. Studies published in 1968 showed a link between the use of COCs and thrombosis. This was thought to be due to the high level of ethinylestradiol in the early pills. However, it has since been realised that a family history of thrombosis or an anti-clotting disorder, obesity and cigarette smoking greatly increase the risk of thromboembolism in pill users.

The synthetic oestrogen thought to cause the side effects has been greatly reduced in many pills manufactured today. Recently, doses of 15 μg ethenylestradiol and 16 μg gestodene with 4 free pill days per month have been effective in inhibiting ovulation. A follow-up of 23 000 women which included women on the higher-dose pills found no excessive deaths over a 10-year period. There appeared to be an 80% reduction in ovarian cancer and a 30% reduction in hip fracture at 75 when taken into the forties. Venous thrombosis occurred in 2:100 000 women years of usage (Kubba et al 2000).

Benefits of the combined pill

- Couples with sexual difficulties because of a fear of pregnancy are relieved of that fear and are able to relax and enjoy a better sex life.
- The COC enables freedom in the sexual act, couples being enabled a natural flow of coitus.
- The pill can be used to combat irregular, painful or heavy periods often found in younger women. For some women, this may be of value in preventing anaemia.
- Some men find that using a condom is so embarrassing and distasteful they may lose their erection or ejaculate prematurely.

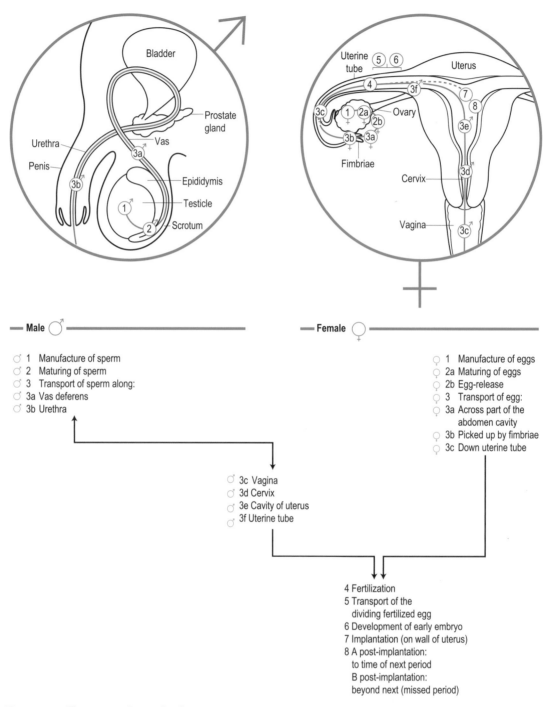

Figure 6.3   The stages of reproduction.

- The combined pill may offer protection against ovarian cancer, possibly due to the cessation of ovulation and quiescence of the ovary. A similar protection against cancer of the endometrium has been noticed.
- The pill protects against some forms of pelvic infection by altering cervical mucus and, because it prevents ovulation and tubal infection (salpingitis), it reduces the risk of ectopic pregnancy (Bromwich & Parsons 1990).

Side effects of the combined pill   For some women the pill may be dangerous and it is better to offer them alternative forms of contraception. Side effects can be divided into those related to oestrogen and those related to progestogen, although it is not always possible to be simplistic as the two hormones interact (Bromwich & Parsons 1990). Oestrogen side effects are less severe and less frequent in low-dose preparations. Headaches, dizziness, nausea and water

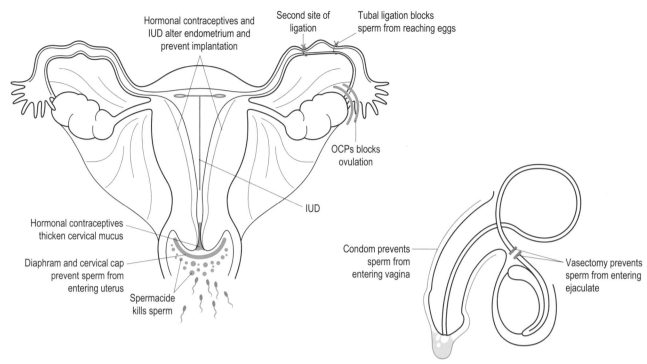

Figure 6.4   Mechanisms by which contraceptives work.

retention are reported and there may be a rise in blood pressure. Most serious is the increased risk of blood clotting.

Progestogens may predispose women to long-term weight gain, tiredness, depression and reduced libido. The progestogen content in the presence of oestrogen may predispose to arterial thrombosis rather than venous thrombosis. Any reported side effect should be considered as soon as possible by a medical practitioner so that the treatment can be reviewed and contraception usage changed.

- **Thrombosis** – Some of the side effects occur because the altered physiology of taking the combined pill mimics that of pregnancy. The risk of arterial or venous thrombosis occurs because of increased clotting factors, platelet aggregation and serum lipids. The risk is probably low in slim women under 35 who are normotensive, do not smoke and have no personal or family history of thrombosis. The consequences of thrombosis include deep vein thrombosis, pulmonary embolism and cerebral ischaemia. However, the effects of an unwanted pregnancy on physical health are far more severe.

- **Cancer** – The link between taking the pill and cancer is mixed. Research indicates that women taking the pill have a reduced incidence of ovarian and endometrial cancer but women taking oral contraceptives lose the protection that barrier methods give to the cervix. While there may have been an increase in breast cancer since the 1960s which may be related to taking oestrogenic compounds, it is possibly due to earlier diagnosis, postponement of the first pregnancy and increased fat

consumption, all known risk factors for breast cancer. However, the World Health Organisation (WHO) has found a link between women on the COC and cervical cancer linked to women carrying the human papillomavirus (HPV): 99% of women diagnosed with cancer of the cervix are HPV-positive and one-third were in their twenties (Dyer 2002).

- **Hypertension** – The risk increases with age and is more likely in those who smoke.

- **Migraine** – Some women find their migraines improve while they take the pill and some find there is deterioration. However, it is serious if women experience focal migraine with transient weakness, numbness of part of the body or loss of part of the visual field, symptoms which may indicate reduced blood flow to the brain.

- **Jaundice** – The pill is metabolised by the liver and affects liver function. Most women have a change in bile composition, which may lead to the formation of gallstones. This may be due to an acceleration of the problem rather than being the sole cause. A few women may develop jaundice and intense itching of the skin and even fewer women may develop liver tumours.

- **Effect on pregnancy** – Large-scale studies fail to find a link between taking the pill in early pregnancy and congenital abnormality (Franey 1999). However, in the past, women were given diethylstilbestrol (DES) in pregnancy and their teenage daughters developed clear cell carcinoma. Although no such link has been seen with other oestrogenic compounds, it is safer to discontinue taking the pill once pregnancy has been confirmed. Women who have taken the pill have no increase in absolute infertility but may take longer to become pregnant, with 98% of women resuming normal periods within 3 months of discontinuing the pill.

- **Effect on lactation** – Oestrogen suppresses the hormone prolactin secreted by the anterior pituitary gland. Prolactin acts on the alveoli of the breast to stimulate milk production. The result will be diminished milk production and a shorter duration of lactation (see 'The progestagen-only pill' section below).

- **Drug interactions** – Synthetic oestrogens taken orally are well absorbed by the intestinal tract. Unlike natural oestrogens which are rapidly broken down by the liver, synthetic compounds take longer to be metabolised and degraded (Rang et al 1999). The combined pill is probably effective up to 36 h. Other medication may interfere with the contraceptive action of the combined pill. Broad-spectrum antibiotics such as ampicillin may impair intestinal absorption, while most anticonvulsant drugs increase liver enzyme production and hasten drug breakdown (British National Formulary 2003). Vomiting and diarrhoea may prevent absorption and the pill should be considered non-effective for that cycle. Women with malabsorption disorders such as those with an iliostomy should not be prescribed the oral combined pill.

Contraindications Because of the above side effects, those involved in advising women about contraception or in prescribing the pill to women may be guided by the following contraindications, although these must be considered in the context of each woman's needs. Contraindications against prescribing the combined contraceptive pill include:

- a history of thromboembolic conditions or abnormal clotting factors;
- hypertension;
- familial hyperlipidaemia;
- valvular heart disease;
- diabetes mellitus with complications;
- oestrogen-dependent malignancy;
- gross obesity;
- smokers over the age of 35;
- current liver disease;
- a history of idiopathic jaundice of pregnancy;
- puerperal psychosis;
- during lactation.

Prevention of gamete production – sperm

Testosterone

Men typically generate 1000 sperm a minute. The hormones involved are hypothalamic **gonadotrophin-releasing hormone** (GnRH), which controls pituitary production of LH and FSH. LH stimulates the testes to produce testosterone, which together with FSH induces sperm production. The WHO is currently interested in injectable testosterone, which could act as a negative-feedback mechanism to reduce the production of GnRH. However, there are problems of high levels of circulating androgens, namely irritability, increased risk of cholesterol production with risk of vascular disease and acne (Franey 1999). Adding a synthetic form of progesterone (progestogen) may allow a lower dose of testosterone to be given without reducing the contraceptive effect. Researchers (Anderson et al 2002) report on the use of implants containing both progestogens and testosterone and, although spermatogenesis was suppressed, this was variable. This is promising, but requires more research before it becomes acceptable.

Gossypol

Other drugs have been considered, the most famous of these being gossypol discovered in the 1980s. People in a certain part of China who cooked their food in cotton seed oil were infertile. There are two major problems with the compound. First, the reduction in sperm production is not always reversible and, secondly, some men experience a fall in serum potassium, which could endanger their lives. Also many drugs that are successful in preventing sperm production have proved toxic to the spermatogonia in the testes, leading to irreversible sterility (Franey 1999). Senior (2001) discusses a non-hormonal contraceptive for men. The sperm tail contains a calcium channel which, when absent, renders the male infertile. Potentially, men could have a patch or injectable substance to immobilise this calcium channel, which would effectively produce a reversible male contraceptive. This has been tested in mice.

Prevention of fertilisation

The progestogen-only pill (POP)

Progestogens thicken cervical mucus and prevent sperm penetration. The endometrium is also made inhospitable to a possible embryo embedding. Uterine tube contractions become less coordinated, so that sperm that have managed to penetrate the cervical mucus find it impossible to journey up the uterine tubes. Ovulation may be suppressed in 50% of women but this is not the main mode of action.

The POP is taken continuously without breaks and should be taken at the same time each day to maintain mucus and endometrial changes which inhibit implantation (Rivera et al 1999). This may be why the progestogen-only pill appears less effective than the combined pill. Also there may be some women for whom the dosage of progestogen is insufficient to produce effective contraception. Drugs used are similar preparations to those in the COC (Rang et al 1999). One study suggests that women on desogestrel 75 μg tended to have heavier more frequent bleeding or alternately amenorrhea more than women on levonorgestrel 30 μg but there were more pregnancies in the levonorgestrel group which may be dose related (Collaborative Study Group on POP 1998).

Benefits of the progestogen–only pill

- Cervical mucus thickens after a few hours, so that contraceptive protection is achieved after 48 h. There is protection against some bacterial pathogens, so that the risk of pelvic inflammatory disease is lessened.
- Milk production is not diminished and little hormone seems to cross into breast milk.
- The very small doses of progestogen used in the pill are unlikely to have an effect on blood vessels and clotting, so this pill is considered a safe option for women who cannot be prescribed the combined pill (BNF 2003).
- Cigarette smokers are likely to develop blood vessel changes. Although stopping smoking is the best option, this pill will not add to the risk.
- Women over the age of 35 have reduced fertility and high motivation to prevent pregnancy. The progestogen-only pill is often prescribed for perimenopausal women.
- Hypertension may indicate the use of the progestogen-only pill. All oestrogen pills are likely to raise blood pressure, which may lead to heart disease.

Side effects of the progestogen–only pill   This form of contraception has been taken by limited numbers of people compared to the combined pill and there have been far fewer studies. Nevertheless the progestogen only pill has been prescribed for as long as the combined pill and there have been sufficient studies to indicate that no significant problems occur.

- *Bleeding* – Alteration in menstrual bleeding patterns is the commonest side effect. The endometrium grows irregularly because progestogens alone are insufficient to balance growth of the lining of the uterus. This usually settles down after the first 3 months but some women find the bleeding troublesome and discontinue the medication.

- *Glucose homeostasis* – Progestogen-only pills may alter the way that glucose is handled in women who have diabetes although the effect is not as strong as that produced by the combined pill.

- *Effects on pregnancy* – Besides the risks of any pregnancy there is an extra risk of becoming pregnant whilst taking the progestogen-only pill. The motility of the uterine tubes is reduced so that the embryo cannot reach the uterine cavity before it begins to increase in size, causing an ectopic pregnancy, a rare but dangerous complication (Bromwich & Parsons 1990).

Long-acting progestogen injections

The two preparations available in Britain are Depo-Provera and Monistat. These act similarly to the progestogen-only pill but with a more profound effect on the ovary. The endometrium immediately becomes thinner and theoretically prevents implantation (Rivera 1999). Depo-Provera is a long-acting injectable progestogen, given every 12 weeks, which contains medroxyprogesterone acetate. Menstrual disturbances occur and there may be a delay in fertility return (BNF 2003). There are some reports that bone mineral density is lower than average with long-term use (Banks et al 2001).

Side effects of long-acting progestogen injections

- Heavy, irregular bleeding may occur, although some women have no bleeding at all.
- Delayed return of fertility.
- The drugs need to be repeated every 12 weeks.

Benefits of long-acting progestogen injections   At present, in some countries, these drugs are only licensed to be used when other forms of contraception are not possible. There has been controversy in the treatment of women with learning difficulties, who are thought not able to cope with pregnancy and child rearing. The concept of informed consent must be a prime consideration. Worldwide, these drugs have been controversial when used in developing countries. It should be noted that:

- progestogens increase the stability of red cells and women with sickle cell disease may benefit;
- women who cannot take oral preparations where absorption is poor or the large intestine has been removed may benefit from an injectable preparation;
- the risk of repeated pregnancies may outweigh the side effects of the progestogen injection.

Emergency contraception (the morning-after pill)

It is not certain how the morning-after pill works but it may disrupt sperm motility in the uterus and change the uterine environment, thus preventing implantation, or it may prevent ovulation by stopping the LH surge. It may work in a variety of ways, depending on the phase of the cycle and the woman's own hormone basis (Rivera 1999). However, it does not cause an abortion. The Family Planning Association (FPA) won a case in February 2002 against the Society for the Unborn Child (FPA web site).

Emergency contraception may be given orally up to 72 h following unprotected intercourse at any time in the menstrual cycle. The pill contains levonorgestrel 750 μg; two doses are given 12 h apart but no longer than 16 h (BNF 2003). Controversially, this pill may be given without prescription to those over 16 years of age. Pharmacists are at the front line of counselling these women and giving morning-after pill without a medical practitioner's intervention.

Progestogen implants

The contraceptive preparation levonorgestrel 38 mg is contained in small silicone rods which are inserted under the skin of the upper arm, allowing slow release of the preparation. Norplant and Implanon are trade names for these preparations. A study in China followed 130 women using Norplant 2 for 4 years and found that irregular menstruation was the prime cause for giving up its use. Only one patient conceived in this study (Qin et al 2001). Norplant has since been discontinued although some women may have the system in place until 2004 (BNF 2003).

Implanon is the latest implant system using one rod containing 68 mg of etonogestrel. Ovulation is stopped a day after insertion and it will continue as an effective contraceptive for 3 years. Again, this implant causes irregular bleeding, which may be partly due to its effect on the endometrium (Rivera et al 1999). Once inserted, this contraceptive device can be forgotten, is not affected by antibiotics and does not have to be metabolised by the liver as it is not a systemic preparation. Some patients experience skin irritation and may have to discontinue its use (BNF 2003).

Barrier methods of contraception

The aim of these methods is to prevent sperm that are deposited in the vagina from ascending the cervix and reaching the ovum. This type of method has a long history and has been reasonably successful: for example, Egyptian women placed pessaries coated in honey into their vaginas and honey is known to kill both spermatozoa and bacteria. Similar acidic preparations have been used.

The female diaphragm

The female diaphragm is made of rubber, and when inserted into the vagina covers the cervix. It must be fitted to the individual and any loss or gain in weight of more than 7 lb (3 kg) necessitates refitting. Cervical and vault caps which adhere to the cervix by suction are less-commonly used. Diaphragms are normally used with the addition of a spermicidal preparation and should be left in situ long enough for the sperm to be killed (see Figs 6.5 and 6.6).

Benefits of the diaphragm   The diaphragm is an efficient alternative to hormonal contraception and women can take responsibility for avoidance of pregnancy. It may also be protective against some sexually transmitted diseases.

Side effects of the diaphragm   Despite its simplicity, there are a few problems with the diaphragm. Some women may be allergic to the rubber or to the spermicide and those with a degree of uterine prolapse may find the diaphragm uncomfortable and difficult to maintain in place. The diaphragm predisposes to vaginal candidiasis, especially in diabetic women, and some women may develop recurrent cystitis. Using the diaphragm may be distasteful to women who object to its messiness and the need to handle their bodies or to remember to insert it prior to coitus.

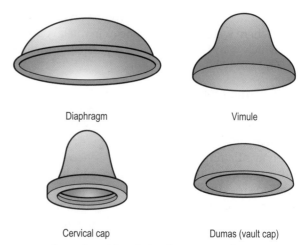

Figure 6.5   Examples of female barrier methods. (Reproduced with permission from Cowper & Young 1989.)

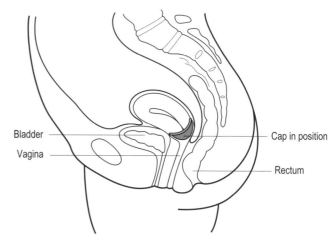

Figure 6.6   Diaphragm cap in position. (Reproduced with permission from Cowper & Young 1989.)

The contraceptive sponge

This consists of a one-size sponge impregnated by spermicide. One side has an indentation and the other side has a ribbon for removal of the sponge. It is moistened with water and inserted high into the vagina with its indented side against the cervix. It must be left in situ for at least 6 h after intercourse and can be left for 24 h. It can be purchased in a chemists shop without prescription. In the early 1980s it was thought to be ideal for modern young women as it needed no contact with professionals and its failure rate given by the manufacturer seemed reasonable – between 9 and 11 HWY. However, research by Bounds & Guillebaud (1984) using well-motivated young women suggested the true rate was nearer to 25 HWY. This method may be more suitable to women who are spacing their families and would not be too concerned if they became pregnant or to perimenopausal women whose fertility is low. It is less successful when used by women who have had children. Some researchers have suggested that the spermicide can effectively prevent chlamydial infection.

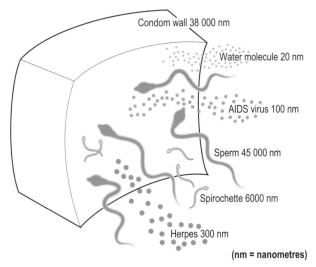

Figure 6.7   The condom barrier.

The male condom

These tubular devices have been made from various materials (Fig. 6.7). Historically, sheep's intestines were used but currently condoms are made from rubber. They must be placed on the erect penis prior to sexual contact, as there may be sperm in the fluid released from the tip of the penis following arousal. After coitus, the penis must be removed from the vagina before the erection is lost and no further genital contact must occur. They are cheap, easily purchased and successful. If a spermicide is used with the condom it increases its efficiency but interrupts spontaneity. Condoms are also barriers to various organisms and help in the prevention of the spread of sexual diseases.

The female condom

These were introduced under the trade name of Femidom and are made of polyurethane, which is tougher and finer than rubber. The device lines the vagina with an inner rim that fits into the vaginal fornices and an outer rim around the vulva. They are lubricated to aid penile insertion. They may provide an efficient barrier to sexually transmitted disease and should be as efficient as the diaphragm or condom.

Spermicidal preparations

These chemical preparations come in the form of foaming tablets, aerosols, films, creams, pessaries and jellies. While they are efficient at killing sperm, hundreds of millions of sperm may be released per ejaculate, so they should not be used alone. Spermicides may reduce the incidence of sexually transmitted organisms such as the gonococcus and spirochaete of syphilis and also viruses. This is because they do not differentiate between the sperm and single-celled microorganisms, killing them all. Also, some microorganisms hitch a ride into the female genital tract through

the channels in the cervical mucus made by the sperm. The commonest spermicidal agent, nonoxynol-9, attaches itself to the spermatozoa and prevents them taking in oxygen. It also destroys the surface tension of the outer membrane so that the sperm bursts.

Intrauterine device (IUD)

Intrauterine devices for the purpose of contraception began in the 1950s with the development of the plastics industry. Many different shapes have been tried but they must be small enough to insert through the cervix yet large enough to fill the small uterine cavity. This involves a device that can be reduced in diameter during insertion and will recoil to its effective shape once in the uterus. In the past, IUDs big enough to prevent pregnancy have caused problems of discomfort, bleeding and rejection so that the so-called 'third-generation' devices have been developed (Fig. 6.8).

These devices are smaller and the plastic holds substances that will prevent pregnancy. The most successful substances have been copper and progesterone. A comparison was made between women using the Nova-T (copper) and levonorgestrel (progestogen) IUD (LNG IUD). There were fewer pregnancies in the LNG IUD but more spotting in the earlier days of use than with the Nova-T. It was important to counsel women of this and that it improved over time. Fertility returned following removal of both IUDs. The LNG IUD was considered an effective contraceptive that could also be used for the treatment for menorrhagia (Andersson 2001).

IUDs work by reducing the likelihood of the sperm being able to swim through the uterine cavity. They also alter the contractability of the uterine tubes, reducing the chances that a fertilised ovum will reach the uterine cavity but increasing the risk of ectopic pregnancy (Andersson 2001). Finally they prevent a fertilised ovum from embedding in the uterus. This last fact is unacceptable to some people, who see it as a form of early abortion.

Advantages of the IUD   The advantage of these devices is that once inserted they can be forgotten about except for periodic checking that they are still in situ by the woman feeling for the nylon cords in the vagina. This could be a disadvantage for some!

Disadvantages of the IUD

- **Menstrual disorders** – Some women have an increase in duration of blood loss. This is not a straightforward lengthening of the menstrual phase of the cycle but an annoying light loss, beginning 2 or 3 days before true bleeding commences and a similar tailing off at the end of the period. The only IUD without this effect is the progesterone-containing type (Andersson 2001).

- **Infection** – Although the increased risk is only 1 or 2%, pelvic infections are dangerous and lead to heavy, irregular

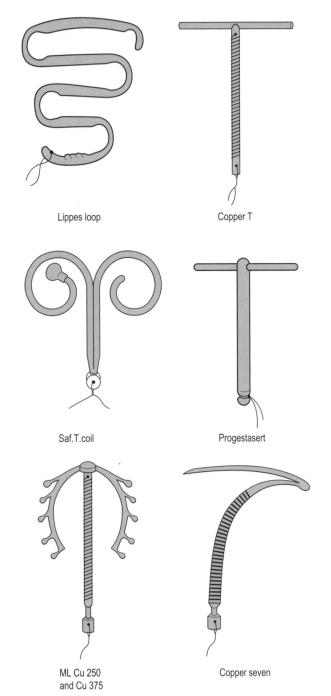

Lippes loop Copper T

Saf.T.coil Progestasert

ML Cu 250
and Cu 375 Copper seven

Figure 6.8 Intrauterine devices. (Reproduced with permission from Cowper & Young 1989.)

menstrual bleeding, infertility, miscarriage and ectopic pregnancy. This increased tendency to pelvic infection is the most important problem that may occur (Herzer 2001). This is not related to promiscuity, as some of the organisms are commonly found in the bowel. Women in steady partnerships are equally at risk. There is no barrier to bacteria and these organisms accompany the sperm through the cervical mucus and ascend to cause infection.

- **Failure** – Although the IUD is a very efficient type of contraceptive, it can fail. IUDs fail because they have become displaced or expelled from the uterus, so that about two people per 100 would become pregnant per year.

- **Fetal abnormalities** – Although no damage has been seen to a baby conceived with an IUD in situ, miscarriage is commoner, occurring in about 50% of pregnancies, and ectopic pregnancy may occur. If the IUD remains in situ and the pregnancy continues, premature onset of labour may occur.

Natural methods

Preventing ejaculation into the vagina

Various techniques of preventing ejaculation into the vagina are practised. Withdrawing the penis from the vagina at climax, termed coitus interruptus, avoiding ejaculation or coitus reservatus and coitus intracrura where the penis is placed between the thighs of the woman are all still used as contraceptive techniques. The more unusual coitus saxonicus, where hard pressure to the male perineum just prior to ejaculation results in retrograde ejaculation into the bladder, is a difficult but effective technique. Anal intercourse is also used by some couples. These methods are easy to use and do not need medical supervision so that, despite their relatively high failure rate, they will continue to be used.

Timing, temperature and cervical mucus

For some people physiological methods of contraception are the only acceptable methods (Cowper 1997). There is a very brief window in each ovulatory cycle when the ovum is available for fertilisation. If intercourse is avoided at that time, it is reasonable to assume that a pregnancy will not occur. In women with a regular menstrual cycle the calendar or timing method has been used.

Ovulation may occur irregularly so methods of pinpointing it have been discovered. These rely on changes brought about by the secretion of progesterone. The first is the change in cervical mucus and the second is the rise in core temperature (Fig. 6.9). A combination of the last two, the symptothermal method, is quite successful for highly motivated women. Chemical methods of testing urine have been developed which can be carried out in the home. These are based on the detection of rising LH in the urine by using a test strip which changes colour.

Sterilisation

Fertilisation occurs in the ampulla of the uterine tube and the zygote then travels down the tube to the uterus. The aim of female sterilisation is to remove sections of the uterine tubes to prevent the sperm reaching the ovum (Fig. 6.10). Spermatozoa travel up the vas deferens towards the urethra to be ejaculated into the vagina. The aim of male sterilisation or vasectomy is to remove a section of the vas deferens to prevent the sperm entering the ejaculatory fluid

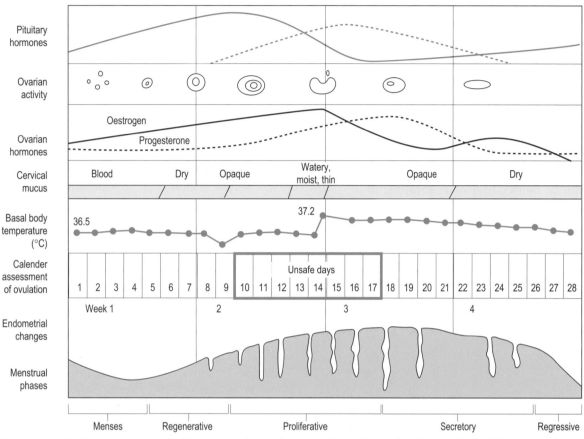

Figure 6.9   Physiological changes in the menstrual cycle in conjunction with physiological methods of birth control. (Reproduced with permission from Cowper & Young 1989.)

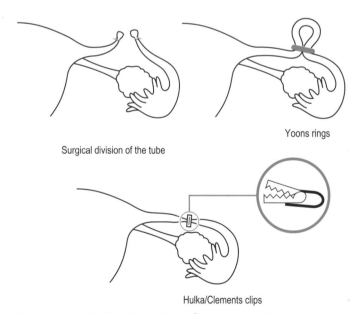

Surgical division of the tube

Yoons rings

Hulka/Clements clips

Figure 6.10   Sterilisation methods. (Reproduced with permission from Cowper & Young 1989.)

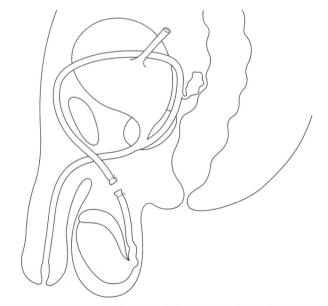

Figure 6.11   Ligation of the vas deferens (from Sweet B 1997, with permission).

(Fig. 6.11). The application of clips has been tried to increase the chances of reversal. In an American survey of 10847 women between 15 and 44 years of age, 41% had been sterilized; the incidence rose as age increased (Moore 1999).

These are not difficult operations but must be considered permanent as reversal may be difficult, involving micro-surgery. Despite this, recanalisation of the ducts occurs in up to 2 in 1000 men or women, resulting in a pregnancy.

Following vasectomy, it may take up to 20 ejaculations to clear sperm from the ducts and ejaculate should be tested until two clear specimens are obtained. In certain parts of the world where it would be difficult to carry out these tests, 20 condoms are given to the man who is told that when these have been used he can begin unprotected intercourse. There may be a short-term risk of infection or haematoma, but despite multiple studies no statistical link with long-term health problems has been made.

Prevention of embedding or development of a conceptus

Intrauterine device (IUD)

The insertion of an IUD following unprotected intercourse may prevent implantation of the conceptus, particularly when the client presents after more than 72 h. The morning-after pill could still be used in these circumstances, but, if not available, an IUD could be inserted (Rodrigues et al 2002).

Abortion

For some women abortion may be the only answer to an unwanted or dangerous pregnancy. As failure occurs in most of contraceptive methods, there is always likely to be a demand. The 1967 Abortion Act requires that two doctors state that they have formed the opinion that one of four circumstances applies to this pregnancy:

1. continuing the pregnancy would involve risk to the life of the pregnant woman greater than if the pregnancy were terminated;

2. continuing the pregnancy would involve risk of injury to the physical or mental health of the pregnant woman greater than if the pregnancy were terminated;

3. continuing the pregnancy would involve risk of injury to the physical or mental health of the existing child or children of the family of the pregnant woman greater than if the pregnancy were terminated;

4. there is substantial risk that if the child were born it would suffer from such physical or mental abnormalities as to be seriously handicapped.

Menstrual extraction or suction emptying of the uterus following an endometrial scrape can be performed when the period is 10–14 days late. This is not as popular now as it used to be because of discomfort. Dilatation of cervix and curettage of endometrium (D & C) can be used followed by vacuum aspiration of the products of conception up to 12 weeks from the last menstrual period. After 12 weeks, prostaglandin induction of uterine contractions is used to expel the fetus. These contractions are painful and the placenta may be retained in the uterus, necessitating a trip to theatre and a D & C.

Future advances

Vaccines – immunocontraceptives

Vaccines that give contraceptive protection for up to 1 year may be available in 10–15 years. Antibody production could be raised against GnRH in men, but, as this would prevent testosterone production, replacement therapy would be necessary. Female vaccines currently being developed target human chorionic gonadotrophin (hCG). Anti-sperm antibodies could also be a possibility.

As yet, there is no perfect contraceptive method that could be used globally. Also, there are some countries where, for social, cultural or religious reasons, contraception is either forbidden or frowned upon. It is not just an academic problem, as the ability of countries to produce food or avoid war is compromised by growing populations. Perhaps the saddest result of uncontrolled population growth is the effect on children's health. For this reason it is important to maintain the research into ever simpler and acceptable contraception and to support people in their chosen optimum spacing of their children.

MAIN POINTS

- The growth of the human population is occurring rapidly and the world population is now over 6 billion (2003). The changes are not brought about totally by a surfeit of births. In some countries improving health is reducing the number of children dying and preventing early adult deaths.

- Various countries are involved in contraceptive trials to combat overpopulation. China is conducting trials into a 'male pill' and the Indian National Institute of Immunology has been testing a female immunocontraceptive vaccine targeting hCG.

- There are religious, moral and cultural issues to be considered and it is unlikely that one method of contraception could become universal.

- The calculation of the failure rate per hundred woman years (HWY) is used to assess the effectiveness of contraceptive methods.

- All the ova available to the woman are present in her ovary at birth. It is not a matter of preventing ovum production but of preventing their maturation and ovulation. This is the basis for the combined oral contraceptive.

Risks of taking the contraceptive pill include its oestrogen content, cigarette smoking, obesity, a sedentary way of life and a family history of thrombosis.

- Progestagen adds to the contraceptive effect by thickening cervical mucus, making the endometrium unsuitable for implantation and by reducing uterine tubes motility.

- Other medication that the woman may be taking may interfere with the contraceptive action of the combined pill. Vomiting and diarrhoea may prevent absorption and the pill should be considered non-effective for that cycle. Women with malabsorption disorders should not be prescribed the oral combined pill.

- The WHO is interested in injectable testosterone to prevent sperm production but the side effects of high levels of circulating androgens include irritability, increased risk of cholesterol production with risk of vascular disease and acne. Adding a synthetic form of progesterone seems to allow a lower dose of testosterone to be given without reducing the contraceptive effect.

- Other drugs that might suppress sperm production such as gossypol have been considered. Many drugs that are successful in preventing sperm production have led to irreversible sterility.

- Milk production is not diminished when women take progestogen only and little hormone seems to cross into breast milk. Alteration in menstrual bleeding patterns, changes in the way that glucose is handled in women who have diabetes and ectopic pregnancy may occur. Methods of progestogen delivery by subcutaneous implant and by release from an intrauterine device have been tried.

- Barrier contraception methods include the diaphragm, contraceptive sponge, the male condom, the female condom and spermicidal preparations. Some of these methods may prevent the spread of sexually transmitted disease. Other methods include preventing ejaculation taking place in the vagina, timing, temperature and cervical mucus testing, control of coital frequency, male and female sterilisation and insertion of an IUD.

- Modern methods of postcoital contraception interrupt implantation or even ovulation depending on the time in the menstrual cycle. They include IUD insertion, taking 4 tablets of the combined pill and anti-progesterone pills such as RU486.

- Not all requests for terminations of pregnancy are due to lack of prevention. As failure occurs in most methods, there will always be a demand. The 1967 Abortion Act legalises abortion by requiring two doctors to agree that one of four circumstances applies to the pregnancy.

- Menstrual extraction can be performed when the period is 10–14 days late. D & C can be used followed by vacuum aspiration of the products of conception up to 12 weeks from the last menstrual period. After 12 weeks prostaglandin induction of uterine contractions is used to expel the fetus.

- There is no perfect contraceptive method that could be used globally. Also, there are some countries where for social, cultural or religious reasons contraception is either forbidden or frowned upon. Possibly the saddest result of uncontrolled population growth is the effect on children's health.

References

Anderson R A, Kinniburgh D, Baird D T 2002 Suppression of spermatogenesis by etonogestrel implants with depot testosterone: potential for long lasting male contraception. Journal of Clinical Endocrinology Metabolism 87(8):3640–3649.

Andersson K 2001 The Levenorgesterel intrauterine system: more than a contraceptive. European Journal Contraceptive Reproductive Health Care Jan 6, Suppl 1:15–22.

Banks E, Berrington A, Casebonne D 2001 Overview of the relationship between use of progestogen-only contraceptive and bone mineral density. British Journal of Obstetrics and Gynaecology 108(12):1214–1221.

Billings E L, Billings J J, Brown J B, Burger H G 1972 Symptoms and hormonal changes accompanying ovulation. Lancet I:282–284.

Bounds W, Guillebaud J 1984 Randomised comparison of the use-effectiveness and patient acceptability of the Collatex (Today) contraceptive sponge and the diaphragm. British Journal of Family Planning 10:69–75.

British National Formulary (BNF) 2003 Contraceptives 7.3 (46) September. British Medical Association and Royal Pharmaceutical Society of Great Britain.

Bromwich P, Parsons T 1990 Contraception, the Facts. Oxford University Press, Oxford.

Collaborative Study Group on the Desogesterol containing Progestogen only Pill 1998 A double blind study comparing the contraceptive efficacy, acceptability and safety of two progesterone-only pills containing desogestrel 75 µg/day or levonorgestrel 30 µg/day. European Journal Contraception Reproductive Health Care 3(4):169–178.

Cowper A 1997 Family planning. In Sweet B R, Tiran D (eds) Mayes Midwifery, 12th edn. Baillière Tindall, London, pp 748–761.

Dasgupta P S 1995 Population, poverty and the local environment. Scientific American February:26–31.

Dyer O 2002 WHO links long term pill use to cervical cancer. British Medical Journal 324:808.

Evers L H 2002 Female subfertility. Lancet 9327:151–159.

Franey J 1999 Family planning. In Bennett V R, Brown L K (eds) Myles Textbook for Midwives. Churchill Livingstone, Edinburgh.

Herzer C M 2001 Toxic shock syndrome: broadening the differential diagnosis. Journal of the American Board of Family Practitioners 14(2):131–136.

Kubba A, Guillebaud J, Anderson RA, MacGregor EA 2000 Contraception. Lancet 356(9245):1913–1919.

Moore M 1999 Most US couples who seek sterilization do so for contraception fewer than 25% seek reversal. Family Planning Perspectives 31(2):102–103.

Nash J G, De Souza R M 2002 Making the link: population, health, environment. Population Reference Bureau PRB Web Site: http://www.prb.org.

Qin L H, Goldberg J M, Hao G 2001 A 4 year follow-up study of women with Norplant-2 contraceptive implant. Contraception 64(5):301–303.

Rang H P, Dale M M, Ritter J M 1999 Pharmacology, 4th edn. Churchill Livingstone, Edinburgh.

Rivera R, Yacobson I, Grimes D 1999 The mechanism and action of hormonal contraceptives and intrauterine contraceptive devices. American Journal of Obstetrics and Gynecology 181(5):1263–1269.

Rodrigues I, Grou F, Joly J 2002 Effectivness of the emergency contraceptive pills between 72 and 120 hours after unprotected sexual intercourse. American Journal of Obstetrics and Gynecology 186(1):167–168.

Senior K 2001 Non-hormonal male contraceptive on the horizon? Lancet 358(1244).

Speidel J J 2000 Environment and health: 1. Population, consumption and human health. Canadian Medical Association Journal 163(5):552–554.

Annotated recommended reading

British National Formulary 2003 Contraceptives 7.3 (46).
This is always a good reference book held in the ward area so it can be used as an immediate check on drug interactions and appropriate dosage. A specific section in the appendix covers drugs in pregnancy and breastfeeding.

Family Planning Association 2002 Website, http://fpa.org.uk.
This website is useful for anyone: students, midwives and their clients. It covers all aspects of family planning and abortion.

Franey J 1999 Family planning. In Bennett V R, Brown L K (eds) Myles Textbook for Midwives, 13th edn, Ch. 32.
This is a good chapter giving a comprehensive view of family planning with some good diagrams and further references.

Chapter 7

Infertility

INTRODUCTION

Considering the size of the world's population, the fertility of human beings is quite low compared with other mammals. Fertility in Western couples appears to be declining at present but there may be a trend to smaller families. Infertility could occur because many women pursue their careers before having a family and are older at their first pregnancy. There may be environmental problems in the workplace or social hazards such as smoking or alcohol (Hruska et al 2000). In the 1950s and 1960s if a couple did not produce a child they accepted that nothing could be done. After the widely publicised birth of Louise Brown, the first 'test tube' baby in 1978, couples realised that they could be helped to conceive. As more couples seek advice, midwives will come into contact with families who have a problem in conceiving and will need to understand infertility and its treatment (Sidebotham 2001).

DEFINING INFERTILITY

The World Health Organisation defined subfertility as failure to achieve a pregnancy after 1 year of unprotected intercourse (Johnson & Everitt 2000). For couples who do not conceive the desire to have a baby may be all consuming. There may be a sense of failure every month menstruation commences (Bryan 2000). The couple may blame each other and this could cause marital/partnership disharmony. In some couples it has led to suicide (Fishel et al 2000). It may be difficult to seek help, as the couple must recognise that a problem exists and a third party has to be brought into their intimate lives.

Infertility affects as many as 1 in 6 couples, some 14% of the population, but 80% can be assisted by modern reproductive technology using their own gametes and a further 10–15% can be helped by using donated gametes (Fishel et al 2000). Possibly 0.4% live births in the UK result from assisted reproduction (Ledger 2001). The apparent increase in the incidence of infertility may depend on the fact that many couples are delaying their first pregnancy and fertility

Table 7.1   Causes of infertility

Male	Female
Defective spermatogenesis	**Defective ovulation**
● Endocrine disorders – dysfunction of the hypothalamus, pituitary, adrenal glands or thyroid gland	● Endocrine disorders – dysfunction of the hypothalamus, pituitary, adrenal glands or thyroid gland
● Systemic disease such as diabetes mellitus	● Systemic disease such as renal disease
● Testicular disorders – trauma or environmental	● Ovarian disorders – hormonal or cystic disorders such as Stein–Leventhal syndrome or ovarian endometriosis
Defective sperm transport	**Defective transport**
● Obstruction or absence of seminal ducts	● Ovum because of tubal obstruction or fimbrial adhesions
● Impaired secretions from accessory glands	● Sperm because of thick cervical mucus or loss of tubal patency
Ineffective sperm delivery	**Defective implantation**
● Impotence due to psychosexual problems	● Due to hormone imbalance, congenital anomalies, fibroids or infection
● Drug-induced problems either prescription or recreational drugs	
● Physical anomalies	

declines increasingly after 30 years old. The mother's age at her first delivery averages 28.9 years (Office of National Statistics 2000).

THE CAUSES OF MALE AND FEMALE INFERTILITY

Causes of infertility (Table 7.1) can be divided into one-third women's factors, one-third men's factors and the remaining one-third a combination of male and female problems (Sidebotham 2001). Table 7.2 indicates the causes of subfertility, expressed as a percentage (Johnson & Everitt 2000).

About 75% of all disorders involve (Johnson & Everitt 2000):

● female genital tract problems, such as blocked or damaged tubes;
● disorders of ovulation;
● male disorders of poor sperm production, either quantity or quality.

INVESTIGATIONS FOR INFERTILITY

For both men and women it is important to rule out any past or present systemic disease as a cause of infertility before proceeding to a detailed examination of the reproductive systems. General health is important: for example, hypertensive men treated with calcium channel blockers have been shown to have poor sperm motility, inhibiting their ability to reach and fertilise the ovum (Enders 1997).

Frequency and behavioural aspects of coitus and any reproductive history of both partners should be discussed (Corson 2001). Vaginismus, where the pelvic muscles surrounding the lower part of the vagina go into spasm at penetration or in anticipation of sexual intercourse, occurs in

Table 7.2   Subfertility in UK couples expressed as a percentage

Cause	Approx. percentage frequency
Endometriosis	12
Tubal damage	14
Ovulatory problems	22
Sperm defects	24
Unexplained	28

5% of infertile women. The cause may be psychosocial; the woman fears painful intercourse and coitus is impossible (Hefner 2001). The causes of infertility listed in Table 7.1 indicate that investigations should ensure that:

1. adequate numbers of sperm are deposited around the cervix (postcoital test);
2. the endometrium is in an appropriate state to receive the fertilised ovum (endometrial biopsy);
3. the fallopian tubes are patent (laparoscopy, salpingography);
4. ovulation occurs (endometrial biopsy, hormonal assays);
5. the woman is psychologically prepared for pregnancy.

The appropriateness of some investigative techniques for infertile couples is questionable and the WHO (2000) guidelines are not always followed. A particular specialist may prefer one test to another. An abnormal test may suggest that a particular problem exists, but only when that abnormality has been treated and pregnancy ensues can it be identified as the cause. As treatment for infertility develops, it may be found inappropriate to test every couple in an automated fashion.

MALE INFERTILITY

Semen analysis and sperm deposition

Some men find it difficult to accept the investigations for semen analysis. Specimens of semen are obtained into a clean dry glass jar by coitus interruptus or by masturbation following 2 days of abstinence from coitus and examined in the laboratory within 1 h of collection. The alternative to this is a postcoital test, which also assesses the reaction of the sperm on the cervical mucus and could give an indication of the sperm's ability to fertilise the ovum. Semen analysis is more accurate when performed alone and ideally an average of three specimens at 2- to 3-week intervals allows calculation of a semen value. Normal values for semen are given as (Johnson & Everitt 2000):

- volume 2–6 ml;
- sperm concentration (no per ml) $50–150 \times 10^6$;
- total sperm count more than $100–700 \times 10^6$;
- motility – more than 60% should be moving steadily;
- morphology – less than 30% should appear abnormal on examination;
- viscosity after liquefaction – low;
- cellular debris, leucocytes and immature sperm cells – low but variable.

Postcoital test

A specimen of cervical mucus taken at the fertile part of the woman's cycle and within 6 h of intercourse is examined. This test can be used to ascertain the following:

- the quality of the cervical mucus;
- the sperm's ability to penetrate cervical mucus;
- the effectiveness of intercourse;
- the presence of immunological problems.

Defective spermatogenesis

There is inconclusive evidence suggesting that sperm counts have dropped in the past 50 years by 50%. Absence of sperm (azoospermia), which may be due to defective spermatogenesis or damage to the transport ducts, is usually untreatable. Defective spermatogenesis may follow abnormal development of the testes due to poor development of the Sertoli cells which nourish sperm at puberty. This may be genetic in origin. Late or non-descent of the testes may also have a genetic background and is now treated early in the baby's first year of life by surgery. Biopsy of the testes and epididymis will show whether sperm are being produced.

Two techniques are available: microsurgical epididymal sperm aspiration (MESA) and extraction of individual sperm cells from testicular tissue or testicular sperm extraction (TESA). Chromosomal studies will indicate whether the problem is the presence of Klinefelter's syndrome (XXY karyotype) (Bittles & Matson 2000). While it is possible to assist couples with a genetic disorder, preimplantation chromosomal analysis of the conceptus is necessary to prevent abnormal fetuses being implanted.

Infection, such as mumps with its complication of orchiditis, may damage the male tubular system. *Chlamydia trachomatis* is often asymptomatic and is associated with unexplained male infertility, and certain uropathogenic organisms were found to affect sperm motility when bacterial counts were high. A reduced sperm count (oligospermia) may be caused by deficient spermatogenesis or by raised testicular temperature. Varicoceles, varicose veins of the scrotum, cause a raised testicular temperature but surgical correction can be made (Cockett et al 1998). Sperm production may be improved by eating healthily and by reducing alcohol intake and smoking.

Blood tests for hormone levels sometimes indicate possibilities for treatment. Reduced follicle-stimulating hormone (FSH) may respond to clomifene, while high levels of prolactin may respond to bromocriptine. Treatment with testosterone does not appear to stimulate sperm production. Some authorities recommend that fructose, zinc and acid phosphatase levels in seminal fluid should be measured when the sperm count is reduced. Low levels of fructose and zinc or high levels of acid phosphatase suggest a low-grade vesiculoprostatitis. Antibiotic treatment of prostatic infection may improve sperm count and motility.

Poor sperm delivery

A sperm penetration test can be carried out by introducing fresh sperm into a sample of cervical mucus on a glass slide to determine whether sperm function or mucus hostility is the problem. Crossed hostility tests can indicate whether the woman is producing antisperm antibodies against her partner's sperm. Passive immunity to the husband's sperm can be improved by the injection of his purified lymphocytes but some authorities doubt whether the condition exists (Bittles & Matson 2000). Other causes of infertility include impotence and retrograde ejaculation into the bladder. Artificial insemination by the husband's semen (AIH) may be useful in these cases or intracytoplasmic sperm injection (ICSI) (see below).

FEMALE INFERTILITY

Following general health questions, a pelvic examination will rule out gross abnormalities of the genital tract such as imperforate hymen and partial or incomplete absence of the vagina or uterus. This was found in some of the young women whose mothers had been treated with synthetic oestrogens to prevent miscarriage (Bentley 2000). A pelvic examination could also elicit ovarian tumours, tubal problems and size and shape of the uterus.

Ovulation

Ovulation problems may occur because of hypothalamic, pituitary or ovarian dysfunction (Hefner 2001):

- hypothalamic dysfunction may be caused by weight loss, low body mass index, strenuous exercise as in dancers and athletes, stress and travel/night duty which unbalance 'body clock' mechanisms;
- pituitary dysfunction may be caused by hyperprolactin-aemia, an antagonist to oestrogen, hypothyroidism;
- ovarian dysfunction may be due to polycystic ovarian syndrome, premature ovarian failure.

Tests to establish whether ovulation is occurring relate to the physiological changes accompanying ovulation. Some can be carried out in the woman's home, whereas others require hospital involvement. At ovulation, cervical mucus should become clear, copious and stretchy and show a fern-ing pattern when dried on a glass slide. Basal body temperature drops slightly and then should rise about 0.3°C. Ovulation predictor kits are available which work by measuring levels of luteinising hormone (LH). More detailed assays using venepuncture examine the changing relationships of the four hormones oestrogen, progesterone, FSH and LH throughout the cycle. Ultrasound scanning can detect a ripening Graafian follicle and a thickening endometrium.

Stimulation of ovulation

Depending on the results of investigations and where in the cyclical events the failure of ovulation originates, various drug treatments may be successful in stimulating ovulation (BNF 2003):

- Clomifene citrate (Clomid) will stimulate FSH production;
- Human chorionic gonadotrophin (hCG) is identical to LH and can be used to trigger ovulation, often in conjunction with clomifene;
- Human menopausal gonadotrophin (HMG or Pergonal) or FSH (Metrodin) may be used if clomifene has failed or in cases of polycystic ovarian syndrome (PCOS);
- Bromocriptine (Parlodel) can be used to inhibit pituitary prolactin release in hyperprolactinaemia.

The process of ovulation induction produces many ripe ova for harvesting which may then be used for in-vitro fertilisation (IVF) or stored for future use as embryos or ova. Artificial stimulation of the ovary may be repeated four to six times but Dickey et al (2002) suggested, 'pregnancy rates remained constant over four cycles, and then fell significantly for diagnoses other than ovulatory failure'. There was a slight risk of ovarian cancer with prolonged use of ovulation-stimulating drugs (Dickey et al 2002). It is important to treat underlying causes of infertility such as PCOS and endometriosis. It may be necessary to surgically remove ovarian cysts if present.

Polycystic ovarian syndrome

PCOS is the commonest cause of anovulatory infertility (Hopkinson et al 1998). Gynaecologists often see women who have suffered from this problem for years before attending the infertility clinic. The syndrome may be caused by subclinical insulin resistance, yet only 5–10% of women present with the syndrome in their reproductive years (Hopkinson et al 1998). Clinically, these women have irregular menstruation, may be hirsute, overweight, suffer from acne and have endocrine abnormalities. Testosterone and LH may be raised and there may be insulin resistance. These hormone imbalances affect the ovary, thickening the thecal layer, stopping ovulation and creating the menstrual abnormalities. Not all women with PCOS have every symptom, and when presenting with infertility the relevant problem must be treated to enable pregnancy to occur.

Tubal patency

Fertilisation takes place in the outer third of the fallopian tube and the zygote takes 4 days to reach the uterine cavity. The normal acidity of the vagina inhibits bacterial growth, and monthly shedding of the endometrium may reduce the risk of chronic infection (Profet 1995), which is a common cause of loss of tubal patency. Generally, organisms ascend through the cervix and uterus to affect the fallopian tubes (salpingitis), the ovaries and the pelvic peritoneum, causing pelvic inflammatory disease (PID). Pelvic adhesions may distort the fallopian tubes. Alternatively, the endothelial folds lining the tubes may be functionally damaged and blocked, with reduced or absent ciliated cells or peristaltic movements. The tubal lumen varies in width at the isthmus and the narrowest part of the uterine tube may be only $100\,\mu m$ to 1 mm wide, the width of a pencil lead.

The commonest organisms implicated in PID are those causing chlamydial infection and gonorrhoea. Women presenting with infertility and diagnosed with PID may have no recollection of an infection. A chlamydial serology screen is useful and a raised titre of more than 1:256 is indicative of tubal damage (Cahill & Wardle 2002). Current and past infections can be treated, if necessary, in both partners. According to a study undertaken in Leeds, the incidence of bacterial vaginosis (BV) is higher in women suffering from tubal infertility (Wilson et al 2002). To investigate and diagnose tubal patency, a hysterosalpingography can be carried out by injecting a radio-opaque contrast medium through the cervix and monitoring its passage through the uterus and fallopian tubes using X-rays. A laparoscopy can also examine the pelvic organs and check on tubal function and general pelvic structures.

Endometriosis

This is a condition where endometrial tissue which is reactive with the hormonal changes of menstruation is found outside the uterus causing dysmenorrhoea, pelvic pain, hormonal disturbances and fatigue (Prentice 2001). Llewellyn-Jones (1990) reported that 40% of patients with endometriosis were infertile and 10% of women attending infertility clinics had endometriosis. These figures are now debated (Burns & Schenken 1999). Unless tubal occlusion is present, the relationship between infertility and endometriosis needs clarification. There is no evidence that mild or moderate endometriosis affects fertility but women do present with endometriosis and subfertility.

REPRODUCTIVE TECHNOLOGIES

Treatment for infertility

Infertility treatment would be impossible without the ability of the embryologist to manipulate ova and sperm outside the body. Table 7.3 outlines the abbreviations and processes used in assisted conception.

Sperm and ova donation

The donation of ova and sperm is essential in the treatment of infertility for some couples. Donors are carefully selected for health and family history of disease under the age of 35. The National Gamete and Donation Trust was launched in 2000 to increase awareness of the need for ova and sperm

Table 7.3 Terminologies for assisted conception techniques

Term	Explanation
AIH	Artificial insemination by husband treats problems with sperm delivery, antisperm antibodies and where semen has been stored prior to chemotherapy or radiotherapy
AID	Artificial insemination by donor to prevent risk of transmission of an hereditary disease or rhesus incompatibility, where sperm are totally abnormal on semen analysis
ART	Assisted reproductive technology
IVF	In-vitro fertilisation: conception takes place outside the body
GIFT	Gamete intrafallopian transfer: sperm and ova are inserted into the uterine tube for conception to take place in a natural way
ZIFT	Zygote intrafallopian transfer: fertilised ovum replaced into the uterine tube following conception in vitro
ICSI	Intracytoplasmic sperm injection: sperm is manipulated via a pipette into the ova and then implanted into the uterus
MESA	Microsurgical epididymal sperm aspiration: the extraction of sperm from the epididymis
TESA	The aspiration of sperm from the testes
PGD	Preimplantation genetic diagnosis

donation (Klein & Sauer 2002). Sexually transmitted diseases are excluded and the semen is frozen and stored for at least 3 months to ensure that repeated tests for donor HIV are negative. Donors are matched to the physical and mental characteristics of the couple.

The Human Fertilisation and Embryology Authority (HFEA) maintain a register of donors so that any child born following sperm or ovum donation has access to details about their biological parentage but, at present, not the identity of this parentage. It is not clear whether access to the donor will be allowed in the future. Confidentiality is a major consideration for most donors (Grice 2002).

Assisted conception techniques have resulted in public concern and the report of the Warnock Committee of Enquiry into Human Fertilisation and Embryology (HMSO 1984) led to the Human Fertilisation and Embryology Act 1990. The HFEA was set up by the act to regulate research or treatment involving the creation, keeping and use of human embryos and the storage and donation of human eggs and sperm (HMSO 1990). This is achieved by a licensing system; all clinics must be licensed and data maintained for analysis.

Principles of in-vitro fertilisation

In-vitro fertilisation assists in conception by using laboratory techniques to assist sperm and egg to unite and produce an embryo which is then inserted into the uterus. Steinberg (1990) discusses four phases in the technique of IVF:

- superovulation;
- egg recovery;
- fertilisation;
- embryo transfer.

Superovulation involves using drugs to stimulate development of multiple ova. The investigations necessary to ensure that the phase of egg recovery results in mature ova involve frequent blood tests for estradiol levels and ultrasound scans for follicle tracking. At least six eggs are usually recovered by various methods, including laparoscopy. The ova are placed in a Petri dish in what is thought to be an optimum environment for fertilisation, and donor sperm are added.

The embryos that begin to develop are assessed for quality and at 24 h embryonic cleavage is noted. About 48 h after the two-cell stage, the embryo is transferred to the uterus. Usually two embryos are implanted into the uterus and the remainder are cryopreserved. The HFEA stipulates no more than three embryos and recent reports suggest that two is ideal (Alvero 2002). The woman receives hormones to prepare the endometrial lining for pregnancy. It is possible to observe the ova until the blastocyst stage (about 5 days) which would permit the insertion of one embryo. However, the later the implantation into the uterus the more risk there is for embryo survival. The delay in implanting the embryo would assist in preimplantation genetic diagnosis, which is not a routine procedure in IVF.

Intracytoplasmic sperm injection (ICSI)

Multiple ova are collected, as in the technique for IVF. Sperm are put into a solution that slows down motility to make them easier to work with. Each egg is sucked into a holding pipette. A microneedle, the diameter of which is 7 times smaller than a human hair, is used to inject a sperm directly into the centre of each ovum and then the technique continues exactly as for IVF and embryo transfer (ET). The sperm are collected by electroejaculation technology.

The transfer of genetic disease during ISCI has been a concern, as the natural selection of healthy sperm is bypassed by artificial techniques (Tindall 2003). Why the sperm have been immotile or abnormal should be considered as should the fact that ageing ova may have aneuploidy (Ch. 3), which leads to early pregnancy loss. Infertility may be nature's way of preventing abnormality. Preimplantation genetic diagnosis (PGD) involves polymerase chain reaction (PCR) to define abnormal DNA in the embryo by biopsy of the polar body, blastomere or blastocyst (Bagness & Yerby 2004).

Surrogacy

When infertility treatment with IVF or ICSI fails, the only alternative may be surrogacy. This is accepted more in the USA than in the UK. In Queensland, Australia it is illegal. The HFEA may need to lay down some guidance to clarify issues. In the USA surrogate mothers are paid for their services, but in the UK this is banned. Surrogacy has implications on family values and the child's future belief in its adoptive parents such as whether children should be told about their surrogate mother. There are many unanswered questions.

Statistics and conclusions

Assisted reproductive technology (ART) has revolutionised the treatment of infertility and has given many childless couples the healthy baby they desire. This treatment has costs, including monitory, social and psychological aspects, if IVF fails (Bergart 2000). HFEA figures for 2000/2001 showed a success rate of 25.1% if aged less than 38 and slightly lower at 21.8% for all ages. There were 23 737 patients treated, with 4621 singleton births, 1579 twin births and 109 triplet births. This means that 3 out of 4 patients' treatment failed (HFEA website).

Babies born following IVF treatment have problems. Preterm birth and its consequent small for dates and high mortality is common in multiple births. There appears to be a higher risk of bleeding, hypertension and diabetes. There is also concern regarding ICSI and genetic abnormality. Tindall (2003) cites an Australian study suggesting that any infant born of any form of ART has double the risk of an abnormality. Despite these facts, couples that are desperate for a baby are determined to surmount all odds and may be slightly 'blinkered' to the pitfalls and what lies ahead for them when embarking on infertility treatment.

MAIN POINTS

- The World Health Organisation defined subfertility as failure to achieve a pregnancy after 1 year of unprotected intercourse. The implications are that 1 in 6 couples will be rated as infertile: 80% of these couples can be helped by reproductive technology and a further 10–15% by donated gametes.

- The apparent increase in the incidence of infertility may be because many couples delay first pregnancy and fertility declines after age 30. The average mother's age at first birth is 28.9 years. Causes of infertility involve one-third woman's factors, one-third men's factors and the remaining one-third a combination of male and female problems.

- For both men and women, past or present systemic disease must be ruled out as a cause of infertility before proceeding to examination of the reproductive systems. A discussion of frequency and behavioural aspects of coitus is necessary.

- Fresh specimens of semen for analysis are obtained following 2 days of abstinence from coitus. The environmental effect on diminishing sperm counts is a worrying problem. Heavy alcohol use causes testicular atrophy, but has not been proven to cause low sperm counts. Sperm production may be improved by eating a healthy diet and by reducing alcohol intake and smoking.

- Blood hormone levels may indicate possibilities for treatment of oligospermia. Reduced FSH may respond to clomifene. High levels of prolactin may respond to bromocriptine. Direct treatment with testosterone appears to be of little use.

- Tests for establishing the cause of infertility in women include a pelvic examination, tests to establish whether ovulation is occurring, examination of cervical mucus and basal body temperature changes. Detailed blood assays examine the changes of hormone levels during the menstrual cycle. Ultrasound scanning can detect a ripening Graafian follicle and a thickening endometrium. Depending on the test results, various drug treatments may be successful in stimulating ovulation.

- Malformation, infection of the uterus or poor endocrine control of endometrial development may cause infertility. A hysterosalpingotomy can be carried out, preferably just prior to ovulation. Laparoscopy allows examination of the pelvic organs and checking of tubal function.

- Clinically, women with polycystic ovarian syndrome suffer from irregular menstruation, may be hirsute, overweight, suffer from acne and have endocrine abnormalities.

Testosterone and LH may be raised, and there may be insulin resistance.

- A common cause of loss of tubal patency is ascending infection, which, with pelvic adhesions, distort the fallopian tubes. The endothelial folds lining the tubes may be damaged with reduced or absent ciliated cells or peristaltic movements.

- About 40% of patients with endometriosis have involuntary infertility and 10% of women attending infertility clinics have endometriosis. However, this does not imply a direct causal factor unless tubal occlusion is present.

- IVF treatment consists of a series of steps: superovulation, egg recovery, fertilisation and embryo transfer. The HFEA keep statistics and registers of all IVF treatment and donors, and regulates any research or treatment involving the creation, keeping and use of human embryos and the storage and donation of human eggs and sperm.

References

Alvero R 2002 Assisted Reproductive Technologies: toward improving implantation rates and reducing high order multiple gestations. Obstetrical and Gynaecological Survey 57(8):519–529.

Bagness C, Yerby M 2004 Genetics. In Henderson C, MacDonald S (eds) Mayes Midwifery, 13th edn. Baillière Tindall, London.

Bentley G R 2000 Environmental pollutants and fertility. In Reproductive possibilities for infertile couples: present and future. In Bentley G R, Mascie-Taylor C G N (eds) Infertility in the Modern World. Cambridge University Press, Cambridge.

Bergart A 2000 The experience of women in unsuccessful infertility treatment: what do patients need when medical intervention fails? Social Work in Health Care 39(4):45–69.

Bittles A H, Matson P L 2000 Genetic influences on human infertility. In Reproductive possibilities for infertile couples: present and future. In Bentley G R, Mascie-Taylor C G N (eds) Infertility in the Modern World. Cambridge University Press, Cambridge.

BNF (British National Formulary) 2003 (46) September. British Medical Association and Royal Pharmaceutical Society of Great Britain.

Bryan A 2000 The psychological effects of infertility and the implications for midwifery practice. Midirs Midwifery Digest 10(1):8–12.

Burns W, Schenken R 1999 Pathophysiology of endometriosis-associated infertility. Clinical Obstetrics and Gynaecology 42(3):586–604.

Cahill D, Wardle P 2002 Management of infertility. British Medical Journal 325:28–32.

Cockett A T, Takihara H, Iwamura M, Koshiba K 1998 Pathophysiology of clinical varicoceles in infertile men. International Journal of Urology 5(2):113–115.

Corson S L 2001 Evaluation of the subfertile couple: the fine points. International Journal of Fertility and Women's Medicine 46(6):309–314.

Dickey R, Taylor S, Lu P et al 2002 Effect of diagnosis, age, sperm quality, and number of preovulatory follicles on the outcome of multiple cycles of clomiphene citrate intrauterine insemination. Fertility and Sterility 78(5):1088–1095.

Enders G 1997 Clinical approaches to male infertility with a case report of possible Nifedipine-induced sperm dysfunction. The Journal of the American Board of Family Practice 10(2):131–136.

Fishel S, Dowell K, Thornton S 2000 Reproductive possibilities for infertile couples: present and future, Ch. 2, p. 17. In Bentley G R, Mascie-Taylor C G N (eds) Infertility in the Modern World. Cambridge University Press, Cambridge.

Grice E 2002 Donating life. Telegraph Magazine April 13:36–40.

Hefner L 2001 Human Reproduction at a Glance. Sexual Dysfunction. Blackwell Science, Oxford.

HMSO 1984 Warnock M (Chair), Report of the Committee of Enquiry into Human Fertilisation and Embryology, London.

HMSO 1990 Human Fertilisation and Embryology Act 1990. Paul Freeman.

HFEA Website: www.hfea.org.uk.

Hopkinson Z, Satter N, Flemming R, Greer I 1998 Fortnightly review: polycystic ovarian syndrome: the metabolic syndrome comes to gynaecology. British Journal of Medicine 317(7154):329–332.

Hruska K, Furth P, Seifer D et al 2000 Environmental factors in Infertility. Clinical Obstetrics and Gynaecology 43(4):821–829.

Johnson M H, Everitt B J 2000 Essential Reproduction, 5th edn. Blackwell Science, Oxford.

Klein J, Sauer M 2002 Oocyte donation. Best practice research. Clinical Obstetrics and Gynaecology 3:277–291.

Ledger W L 2001 Assisted conception: what does the future hold? Current Opinion in Gynaecology 3(3):305–307.

Llewellyn-Jones D 1990 Fundamentals of Obstetrics and Gynaecology: Vol. 2, Gynaecology, 5th edn. Faber and Faber, London.

Office of National Statistics 2000 Health Statistics Quarterly 7.

Prentice A 2001 Endometriosis. British Medical Journal 323(7304):93–95.

Profet W 1995 On the costs and benefits of menstruation. Quarterly Review of Biology 68:335–386. Cited in Nesse R M, Williams G C 1995 Evolution and Healing. Weidenfield and Nicholson, London.

Sidebotham M 2001 Assisted conception: an issue for midwives. Practising Midwife 4(11):10–12.

Steinberg D L 1990 The depersonalisation of women through the administration of 'in vitro fertilisation'. In McNeil M, Varcoe I, Yearley (eds) The New Reproductive Technologies. Macmillan, Basingstoke, pp 74–122.

Tindall G 2003 Mixed blessings: ethical issues in assisted conception. Journal of the Royal Society of Medicine 96:4–35.

Wilson J D, Ralph S G, Rutherford A J 2002 Rates of bacterial vaginosis in women undergoing in vitro fertilisation for different types of infertility. British Journal of Obstetrics and Gynaecology 109(6):714–717.

World Health Organisation 2000 Laboratory recommendations. World Health Organisation, Geneva. http://www.who.org/

Annotated recommended reading

Bryan A 2000 The psychological effects of infertility and the implications for midwifery practice. Midirs Midwifery Digest 10(1):8–12.
This article will help midwives to understand infertility and its effect on women.

Caldwell J 1999 Paths to lower fertility. British Medical Journal 319(7215):985–987.
This paper discusses fertility and its relationship to world trends.

Hruska K, Furth P, Seifer D et al 2000 Environmental factors in infertility. Clinical Obstetrics and Gynaecology 43(4):821–829.
This paper gives an overview of environmental effects on fertility, including smoking, alcohol and occupational exposure.

Chapter **8**

Preconception matters

INTRODUCTION

Preconception care is an important part of maternal and fetal health care. It is a preventative approach through which factors that could potentially affect pregnancy outcome are identified and a prospective strategy developed to reduce or eliminate the risks made evident by family or medical history and/or specific tests. This is the background for the development of preconception counselling and of groups such as Foresight (an association for the promotion of preconception care). To minimise potential risks, it is ideal to have preconception clinics either through family doctors or family planning centres. Almost half of pregnancies are unplanned, and these women may be at greater risk, which is a great challenge to the effectiveness of such services. Systematic approaches to raise public awareness of the importance of preconception counselling need exploring. This chapter focuses on the evidence for its effectiveness, the components of programmes and the influence of lifestyle and environment on the physiology of childbearing. The implications of radiation, toxic waste and drug ingestion are also discussed.

PREPREGNANCY CARE

By the time most women realise they are pregnant, 1 or 2 weeks after missing their first period, many embryonic organs have been developing, and this is the most vulnerable stage of embryogenesis. Embryogenesis is completed by the eighth week of pregnancy and few women attend for their first antenatal visit that early in pregnancy. It is then too late for early preventative strategies such as folic acid intake for elimination of neural tube defects. Ethical considerations limit the conduction of randomised trials to investigate efficacy of preconception counselling. Nevertheless, there is evidence from retrospective, prospective and case control studies to indicate that preconception counselling improves pregnancy outcome.

There has been a progressive reduction of prenatal mortality in the last century. There should be greater emphasis on prepregnancy care and counselling to reduce these low rates further (Smith 1992). Research suggests that pregnancy outcome is improved markedly when couples are screened and advised prior to conception (Ward 1995). The mother's diet and possibly the father's also, immediately prior to and at the time of conception, may influence the developing embryo. There is evidence from animal studies that spermatogenesis is influenced by diet (Wynn & Wynn 1991).

Aims of prepregnancy care

Few couples currently seek prepregnancy advice and limited services are available to promote and provide preconception care. To be effective, preconception care should be embraced in the health education of schoolchildren, continued to adult life and special programmes established targeted at groups most in need, such as people in lower social class, smokers or obese women. The aims of prepregnancy care according to Chamberlain (1992) are:

- to bring the woman and her partner to pregnancy in the best possible health;
- to provide the means of ensuring that preventable factors are attended to before pregnancy starts – for example, rubella inoculation;
- to give advice about the effects of pre-existing disease and its treatment on the pregnancy and unborn child;
- to consider the likelihood and effects of any recurrence of events from previous pregnancies and deliveries.

Concepts in prepregnancy care

Preconception care is particularly effective in women who have chronic medical disorders such as diabetes or epilepsy. The pathological effects of hyperglycaemia and the importance of blood glucose regulation in reproduction are well-known; therefore timely advice and care for such women is essential. Preconception counselling significantly reduces malformations and neonatal morbidity and is cost-effective in the care of diabetic women, as they are less likely to require hospitalisation. Recommendations for practice are summarised below:

1. preconception care and counselling has shown to be effective in improving pregnancy outcome;
2. few couples seek advice from health professionals on preconception matters;
3. health education programmes including preconception matters should be offered as early as school age to raise awareness;
4. targeted programmes for people in lower social class or people with know high-risk factors (e.g. smokers or obese) should be considered;
5. preconception is particularly effective/cost-effective in women with chronic disease.

THE HEALTHY GAMETE

Bradley & Bennett (1995) describe the importance of preconceptual health care:

> In a biological sense the life process begins about 100 days before conception when the sperm and the ovum begin their maturation process. During these processes both ova and sperm are extremely vulnerable to nutritional disturbances, toxins and radiation.

Genetic, microbial, biochemical, dietary and environmental factors play a major role in affecting fertility and fetal outcome (Ward 1995). Although these categories are interwoven, each will be explored in regard to the health of spermatozoa and ova.

In terms of outcome there is no clear demarcation between the health of the gametes immediately prior to conception and the developing embryo. In both instances cells are developing rapidly and are vulnerable to disruption. Even when pregnancies are planned, it is unlikely that a couple will consider the importance of those 100 days of gamete formation. The continuously produced sperm is seemingly most at risk of environmental insult. In the female fetus the primary oocytes have already undergone their first reduction division early in the first trimester and no further ova will be generated after the 5th month of gestation (McCloy 1989). In this arrested stage of development they are relatively resistant to mutagenic damage. Sensitivity increases just prior to ovulation and the mutation rate from radiation may rise sharply.

Following fertilisation, the zygote becomes resistant to genetic injury while undergoing cleavage but after 16 days intense organogenesis begins. Sensitivity is high but so few cells are present that either the fetus will be affected and aborted spontaneously or not affected and normal. This may account for a considerable proportion of pregnancy losses within the first 6 weeks.

GENERAL HEALTH CARE

Prepregnancy counselling should begin with a thorough review of the medical, obstetrical, social and family histories. The history of both man and woman is taken and known personal or familial health problems discussed. A gynaecological examination of the woman and screening of blood and urine and in some cases hair, stool and semen analysis would be carried out. Any infections could be treated, dietary problems discussed and possible work and lifestyle hazards considered.

Long-term health problems such as diabetes mellitus need stabilising prior to conception. In conditions such as epilepsy, which are treated with known teratogenic drugs, a discussion of the risks and possible alteration of treatment may be necessary. Social factors such as the age of the prospective parents, especially the mother, are important as the frequency of reproductive problems, including chromosome abnormalities, increases with maternal age.

Social history

The impact of maternal age on pregnancy outcome at both end of the reproductive age is important. Teenagers are more likely to be anaemic, or at risk of having growth restricted infants, preterm labour and higher infant mortality. Most teenage pregnancies are unplanned; therefore, they rarely present for preconception care. Early pregnancy counselling could still be helpful. Pregnancies in later life (after 35) are also more likely to be at risk of obstetric complications. However, for physically fit women the risks are lower than previously reported. Some pregnancy outcomes have been shown to be strongly related to the socioeconomic and health status of the mothers, particularly in this age group; these are hypertension, diabetes, abruption, preterm delivery, stillbirth and placenta praevia.

Hair mineral analysis

Hair analysis for mineral content – which involves taking a sample of scalp hair and using equipment that can measure contaminants present at levels of 0.1 parts per million or less – is still regarded as fringe research by some practitioners, but studies confirm its usefulness. Both excess of toxic minerals and shortage of essential minerals may cause reproductive problems (Barnes 1995). Some toxins are eliminated from blood and stored in body tissues. Hair grows slowly and will show traces of whatever has passed into the follicle in the previous 6–8 weeks. Hair analysis can therefore be a useful addition to blood and urine tests to screen for minerals (Bradley & Bennett 1995). The group Foresight includes testing for the following minerals and gives advice depending on the findings:

- Essential minerals – calcium, magnesium, potassium, iron, chromium, cobalt, copper, manganese, nickel, selenium and zinc.
- Toxic minerals – aluminium, cadmium, mercury and lead. The last two are discussed below.

Either supplementation of essential minerals or removal of toxic minerals by such methods as chelating may be offered.

Inherited disorders

Some couples may be anxious to discuss the possibility of inherited conditions where genetic mutations have led to abnormalities serious enough to be a health or even life threat to the child. Such couples may need referring to genetic counsellors so that an accurate family tree can be obtained and the genetic risk calculated.

Nutrition and weight

The importance of nutrition before and during pregnancy is increasingly recognised in modern health care. Dallison & Lobstein (1995) state that, 'over recent years there has been increasing evidence about the importance of nutrition to a satisfactory birth.' Establishing a balanced diet and a healthy lifestyle prior to pregnancy increases the chance of a successful pregnancy outcome. Prepregnancy weight is positively related to infant birth weight. In developed countries it is rare to find overt malnutrition except in people with eating disorders such as anorexia nervosa.

Poor nutrition

Ethically it is not acceptable to experiment on the effects of food restriction on the human fetus. However, retrospective studies during famine provide some information. The Dutch famine of 1944–45 showed that there was more early pregnancy perinatal mortality in undernourished women and that fertility can be reduced by sudden falls in energy intake (Barker 1992). Perhaps, as a protective measure, nature ensures that women who are too thin or too fat have difficulty in achieving ovulation and fertilisation. There may be a difference in an acute energy deprivation in comparison to a chronic nutritional deprivation as a study of Gambian women showed an ability to reproduce with reasonable pregnancy outcome despite an habitually low energy intake (Poppit et al 1993). Healthy eating is discussed in Chapter 23, p. 311.

Obesity

Obesity is a growing problem in industrialised societies. Up to one in two adult Britons is overweight and one in seven obese. The increase in obesity in Great Britain is probably due to a decrease in physical activity as despite the increase in types of available food British people eat less than their grandparents but exercise less. Obesity is associated with increased risk of complications such as gestational diabetes and pre-eclampsia, thrombophlebitis, post-term pregnancy, Caesarean delivery, macrosomia and instrumental deliveries (Wolfe 1998). Obese women are prone to further development of obesity after pregnancy, particularly central type of obesity (Soltani & Fraser 2000). This is the pathological type which leads to higher risk of metabolic disorders such as diabetes and cardiovascular disease.

It is not advisable to diet during pregnancy, therefore it is very important to adjust maternal diet and weight prior to conception. Prepregnancy weight influences pregnancy outcome. Being undernourished is associated with fetal abnormality and low birth weight, while being obese brings the risk of complications of pregnancy mentioned above. A guide to ascertaining the optimum weight for a woman is the Quetelet index or body mass index. This is obtained by using the formula weight in kilograms divided by height in metres squared. The following range is used for a guide:

Less than 20 = underweight
20–24.9 = desirable weight
25–29.9 = overweight
30 and over = obesity
35 and over = severe obesity

Specific nutrient abnormalities

Suboptimal dietary deficiencies are common, especially in areas of high unemployment and poverty. More people are vegetarian but may not have the correct knowledge of nutrient content, and suboptimal nutrition may occur. A further complication is in the high level of prepared and processed foods that make up a large part of the modern diet. Processing may destroy essential nutrients, whereas chemical additives such as preservatives, artificial colouring and flavouring are added to increase the shelf life of food and to increase its attractiveness. The effects of artificial fertiliser and pesticides used to increase crop production are considered in the section on environmental issues. The increase in food allergy and the possibility of sensitisation of the fetus in utero is a growing concern.

The importance of nutrition in male fertility has rarely been investigated. Protein, energy and possibly zinc deficiencies may be linked to reduced spermatogenesis (Wharton 1992). There is mounting evidence implicating specific dietary deficiencies of affecting the process of organogenesis in the embryo, mainly related to folic acid and zinc.

Although the mechanism is not clear, studies showed that supplementation with folate/folic acid around conception can prevent neural tube defect (NTD) in the fetus (Schorah & Smithells 1991). However, 95% of pregnancies resulting in NTD are first occurrence. It is therefore advised that women planning a pregnancy should take 0.4 mg folic acid as a daily supplement from when they try to conceive until the 12th week in pregnancy (DOH 1993). Women are encouraged to eat more folate-rich foods (e.g. green beans, peas and dark green leaf vegetables) and avoid overcooking them.

Maternal zinc status is also essential in fetal development. The degree to which maternal zinc deficiency can lead to teratogenic effects in humans is unclear but there is limited evidence that severe maternal zinc deficiency may lead to fetal abnormality (Soltan & Jenkins 1982).

Excessive intake of fat-soluble vitamins is harmful. High doses of vitamin A have been shown to lead to congenital abnormalities of the eyes, brain and skeleton in animal studies. An epidemiological study in Spain (Martinez-Frias & Salvador 1990) showed an increased risk of birth defects in babies of mothers who had taken high levels of vitamin A (6000–167 000 µg) during the first 2 months of pregnancy. Although its role in causing human abnormalities is not confirmed, in the UK it is advised that women who might become pregnant should avoid vitamin A supplements unless suggested by a doctor or antenatal clinic. Women who are pregnant or might become pregnant are also advised against eating liver or liver products because of its high vitamin A content (National Dairy Council 1994).

Infection

During successful preconception care, any maternal infection should be investigated and treated. Appropriate advice should be given to prevent infection, as it can adversely affect the pregnancy outcome. Commonly, urinary or genital infections may lead to preterm labour or miscarriage (Wynn & Wynn 1991).

Systemic infections may cause reproductive problems such as infertility and congenital defects (see Ch. 15). Vaccination may be available, as in rubella, or advice on how to minimise the risk of infection during pregnancy when no vaccine is available. Rubella acquired in the first trimester of pregnancy is associated with a 90% increase in the risk of congenital malformations (Best et al 2002). Preventative policies have led to a major reduction in the incidence of congenital rubella syndrome. However, two cases of infants born to mothers who recently arrived in UK have been reported (Mehta & Thomas 2002). Therefore, prepregnancy or early pregnancy investigation of rash, particularly in a high-risk group such as recent immigrants, is important. In a preconception clinic, women should be screened for rubella antibodies and immunised if necessary. Following immunisation, pregnancy should be avoided for at least 3 months.

Toxoplasmosis – caused by the parasite *Toxoplasma gondii*, which is found in soil and vegetation and is able to multiply in refrigerator temperatures (4–6°C or above) – and *Listeria monocytogenes* can cause miscarriage, stillbirth or fetal abnormalities. Women planning a pregnancy or already pregnant should be advised on handling cat litter trays to avoid toxoplasmosis and to cook meat thoroughly. To avoid listeriosis they should be advised on hygienic food handling and avoid eating soft, ripened cheeses such as Brie and blue-vein types. Cooked chilled meals and ready-to-eat poultry should be reheated until piping hot prior to consumption. At the preconception clinic women could be screened for other infections such as sexually transmitted diseases. Most bacteria are too large to cross the placenta but viruses and the spirochaete of syphilis can penetrate the placental membrane to infect the fetus.

Drugs

Drugs are naturally occurring or synthesised chemicals that alter biological systems by affecting the functioning of cells, tissues and organs. Drugs may affect reproductive health at different times in the life cycle. They may damage sperm or ova and may have an adverse effect on nutrient absorption so that essential nutrients are absent at crucial times during embryonic development. They often have a wider range of effects than medically optimal and may be teratogenic, interfering in normal growth and development. The placenta is not a complete barrier against all chemicals.

Many people are exposed to drugs used to treat medical conditions. These may be essential for treatment and difficult to withdraw or reduce. Sometimes they can be substituted by less toxic drugs or stopped altogether during pregnancy. Women of childbearing age should only take medicines under medical supervision and medical practitioners should be alert to the teratogenic side effects of drugs.

People may purchase drugs for minor problems such as pain and indigestion without their doctor's knowledge. The doctor may then prescribe drugs that exacerbate the effects of the over-the-counter drugs. The public should be informed about the danger of taking drugs in pregnancy.

Women are usually advised to discontinue the use of hormonal contraceptives at least 3 months prior to the time they wish to get pregnant. This allows the body to readjust its hormonal system and resume physiological menstrual cycle as well as regulating the level of minerals and vitamins which may be affected by the contraceptive pill. Mineral and vitamin levels may also be affected by intrauterine devices, especially if they contain copper which can interfere with absorption of zinc and cause zinc deficiency.

Drugs may be taken for recreational reasons because of their mood-altering abilities. It is sometimes difficult to ascertain whether they are being taken and to help people to stop taking them. Such substances include alcohol, tobacco and caffeine as well as addictive drugs such as cocaine and its derivative crack, marijuana and heroin. With appropriate referral systems, preconception counselling would be most effective for habitual drug user women, as drug abuse is associated with malnutrition, alcohol abuse, smoking and higher risk of sexually transmitted diseases.

Smoking

The dangers of smoking for general health and during pregnancy are well documented. Tobacco smoking with its pharmaceutical and psychoactive effects originated at least 5000 years ago (Tuormaa 1995). Many chemicals are known to be harmful to the smoker and to cross the placenta to damage the fetus; polycyclic aromatic hydrocarbons, carbon monoxide, cyanide, lead and cadmium are inhaled in cigarette smoke. The influence of smoking can be explained partly by differences in nutrient intake (Haste et al 1991). The effects of smoking on reproduction are summarised below:

- male and female infertility;
- reduced length of gestation;
- low birth weight;
- spontaneous abortions;
- preterm labour;
- increased perinatal mortality (stillbirths + deaths in the 1st week);
- fetal malformations;
- attention deficit hyperactivity disorder (ADHD) and learning difficulties when school age reached;
- reduced immunocompetence.

Fertility

Besides experiencing infertility, women who smoke often undergo an early menopause (Jick et al 1977). In men, smoking reduces testosterone levels (Wynn & Wynn 1991),

reduces the number and motility of sperm and increases the number of abnormal sperm (Evans et al 1981). Alcohol is a direct testicular toxin, causing atrophy of seminiferous tubules and on Leydig cells. A reduction in the synthesis of testosterone occurs and similar effects on sperm are seen as those in tobacco smoking.

Reduced fetal growth

One of the most frequent adverse effects of smoking during pregnancy is reduced fetal growth, which is dose dependent. Conter et al (1995) carried out a longitudinal study of 12 987 babies – 10 238 from non-smoking mothers, 2276 from mothers smoking 1–9 cigarettes/day and 473 from mothers smoking more than 9 cigarettes/day. Their results confirmed the association of smoking during pregnancy with lower birth weight. However, the reduction of birth weight was overcome by 6 months of age. They suggested that the birth weight deficit is probably not permanent when smoking during pregnancy is not associated with other unfavourable variables such as lower socioeconomic class.

Harmful effects on babies

Once the baby is born, being in contact with these chemicals through passive smoking continues to have harmful effects on the child. There is an increased risk of sudden infant death syndrome (SIDS) associated with maternal smoking during pregnancy and evidence that household exposure to tobacco smoke has an independent additive effect (Blair et al 1996).

Fetal malformations

Tuormaa (1995), summarising findings from multiple studies, stated:

> As maternal smoking reduces both the rate of cell replication and protein synthesis, it is speculated that maternal smoking may cause most of its damage during the first weeks of gestation when the rates of embryonic and fetal cell replication are the most active, leading to various congenital malformations.

Conditions associated with smoking include hare lip and cleft palate, nervous system abnormalities and congenital heart defects. Smoking is probably the most dangerous avoidable risk taken by people and it is essential that men and women thinking about starting a family should stop smoking both for the child's sake and for their own safety (Tuormaa 1995).

ENVIRONMENTAL ISSUES

With advancing technology and scientific progress, almost everybody is exposed to novel environmental substances, some of which are of concern during pregnancy; it should be emphasised that when harmful prenatal exposure is likely, the woman (the couple) planning a pregnancy should avoid exposure before conception and during pregnancy.

Toxins

Toxins, which can be natural or manufactured, form part of the ecological system in which humans live and reproduce. Natural toxins have evolved alongside humans and a degree of mutual tolerance exists. Manufactured toxins have been developed since the beginning of the industrial revolution and there has been insufficient time for tolerance to develop. These substances cause concern to the public and to scientific researchers, leading to the setting up of international pressure groups such as Greenpeace.

Natural toxins

Many natural toxins were developed by plants as a defence against being eaten. Examples include the tannins and alkaloids found in oak acorns. Acorns eaten during famines may have caused almost as many deaths as the famines themselves. Some plants make cyanide as part of their defence system. These include apples and apricots and, although the flesh is nutritious, the seeds in quantity are poisonous. Cassava, the staple diet in some cultures, also contains cyanide but this can be neutralised by special preparation and cooking.

Randerson (2003) reports Huffman's work on primate self-medication that sifaka lemurs living in Madagascar eat small doses of tannin when they are pregnant but not at other times. Veterinary surgeons use tannin to prevent miscarriage in some animals. Tannins kill intestinal parasites and increase milk production. Low levels taste good and may act as a mild central nervous system stimulant. Finally, tannin may aid digestion by promoting production of the proteolytic enzyme trypsin. Other primates have been found to use plants as medicine.

Defence systems   Animals, including humans, have developed defence systems against plant toxins. The first line of defence is avoidance mediated by sight, smell and taste. People avoid eating mouldy or rotten food as a defence against the toxins produced by bacteria and fungi. Profet (1992), an American researcher into evolutionary aspects of reproduction, has developed a theory to explain why 80% of pregnant women suffer from nausea and morning sickness during the early weeks of pregnancy. She believes an aversion to bitter-tasting foods protects against possible teratogenic effects of naturally occurring toxins.

Some hidden toxins are ingested and the next line of defence is to expel them by vomiting and diarrhoea. People are reluctant to eat foods that have affected them in that way and often develop lifetime avoidance. Stomach acids and enzymes play a part in neutralising some toxins. There are two other cellular defence mechanisms: cells in the epithelial lining of the stomach secrete a thin layer of protective mucus to prevent toxin absorption but, should the toxin breech this mucus layer and damage cells, they are quickly replaced by the high turnover of epithelial tissue.

The liver is the main organ responsible for the detoxification of ingested substances. Toxins absorbed by the gastrointestinal tract are taken via the portal vein directly to the liver where a wide range of enzymes can render them harmless. The detoxified substances are then excreted via the kidneys.

Low levels of toxin   Plants generally produce levels of toxin insufficient to have major effects on humans. The potato produces diazepam but not enough to produce relaxation. Continuous bombardment of low levels but multiple types of toxin would occur in a typical 'stone-age' diet. Although many toxins are potentially damaging, some increase liver enzyme production. Reducing exposure to everyday toxins may reduce the preparedness of liver enzyme systems to a sudden toxic overload (Johns 1990). Also, cooking and food preparation can make some toxic substances safe to eat. Pomo Indians of California detoxify acorns by cooking bread made from acorn meal in red clay that binds tannin to make the food safe (Nesse & Williams 1995).

Manufactured toxins

The development of the chemical industry has resulted in contamination of the environment by vast quantities of synthetic pollutants such as DDT, polychlorinated biphenyls (PCBs) and polycyclic aromatic hydrocarbons (PAHs) (Colborn et al 1996). The effect of environmental toxins on the formation of the gametes must be researched. Although much of the data is new and unconfirmed, implications for changes in lifestyle may become apparent. A small study in Canada carried out on herring gulls suggested that air pollution from coal fires and other fossil fuels which release PAHs may trigger inheritable genetic defects. However, the effect is difficult to separate from other forms of pollution such as drinking contaminated water or eating contaminated fish (Cohen 2002).

Scientists in America, including Theo Colborn (1996), suspected that pesticides such as DDT and other chemical pollutants such as PCBs were disrupting sexual development by mimicking the effect on tissues of oestrogen, causing feminisation of male reproductive organs across species of fish, reptiles, birds and mammals. The effect was seen on younger rather than older animals. These chemicals were found in high levels in human blood and body fat as well as in human breast milk.

Colborn is still researching the role of pollutants as endocrine disruptors and, while some researchers believe there is no proven link between endocrine disruptors and human reproduction problems, she and her team believe even low levels of the chemicals have serious effects. The debate is unresolved but new chemicals called androgen disruptors which suppress the effects of testosterone are worrying scientists (Wakefield 2002). These block signals to cells to switch on key developmental genes normally switched on by testosterone. They enter our food by fungicide use and scientists found that the fungicide vinclozin stunted sexual development of rat pups in utero. Theoretically, humans could be at risk.

Human infertility

In 1992 Niels Skakkebaek at the University of Copenhagen found male reproductive problems such as reduced sperm counts with an increase in abnormal sperm and a threefold increase in the rate of testicular cancer in Denmark (Carlsen et al 1992). A review of the literature, which included 61 studies of 15 000 men in 20 countries, indicated a fall in sperm count between 1938 and 1990 of 50%.

The findings included:

1. The average male sperm count dropped 45% between the 1940s and 1990s.
2. This drop was seen to occur in younger men. The younger the man, the lower the sperm count.
3. The average volume of ejaculate had dropped by 25%.
4. The number of men with an internationally agreed extremely low sperm count of less than 20 million per ml had increased from 6% to 18%.

Skakkebaek is currently trying to find out whether the differences in testicular cancer rates between Denmark and Finland are due to differences in exposure to endocrine disruptors (Wakefield 2002).

A problem with sperm production data is the amount of variation around the world and through time. Earlier results in the 1940s and 1950s may not have been as accurate, and artificially high counts obtained. Currently, sperm counts may depend on who donates the sperm and what time of day. For instance, some data obtained from infertility clinics suggest a biased population and semen donated in the morning has a lower sperm count than that collected in the afternoon (Jones 2003). A new survey of potency involves men in four European cities: Edinburgh, Paris, Copenhagen and Turku in Finland. Jones (2003) suggests it may be a combination of physics and chemistry. Both increased testicular temperature due to modern clothing and sedentary occupations such as driving and chemical pollutants may affect sperm production.

Oestrogenic compounds

Sharpe, at the Medical Research Council's Reproductive Biology Unit in Edinburgh, found similar problems and believed that oestrogenic compounds affect fetal testes by preventing development of the full complement of Sertoli cells (Sharpe & Skakkebaek 1993). This reduces sperm counts, as the number of sperm produced depends on how many can be nurtured by Sertoli cells.

Oestrogenic mimics There are problems associated with oestrogenic compounds such as PAHs; PCBs; dioxins; phthalates used in plastics, paints and adhesives; breakdown products of alkylphenol polyethoxylates (APEs) used in detergents (nonylphenol); and organochlorine pesticides such as DDT, aldrin and dieldrin. These include:

- in men – increased incidence of prostatic cancer, undescended testicles and penile abnormalities such as hypospadias;
- in women – increased incidence of endometriosis and oestrogen-dependent breast cancer (an increase of 32% between 1980 and 1987 in America).

Leaching from plastics Soto and Sonnenschein (Soto et al 1991) investigated growth inhibition in cell cultures and were examining the role of oestrogen. They had cultures growing in various strengths of oestrogen, including an oestrogen-free culture. In these latter cultures cell division occurred at an unprecedented rate. The scientists suspected that the dishes holding the cultures must be acting as an oestrogenic source. Although the manufacturer refused to say which chemicals were used in their dishes, nonylphenol was leaching out of the plastic into the tissue culture. This oestrogen-acting compound was widely used in domestic cleaners, and many countries have banned its use. Bisphenol-A leaches from polycarbonates and there is bisphenol-A in the plastic lining of food cans. These substances are not biodegradable.

River pollution In Britain, anglers found it was difficult to sex the fish they caught. Most appeared to be female or have some female characteristics. Male fish were producing huge quantities of vitellogenin, a substance necessary for egg production that is normally produced by females in response to ovarian release of oestrogen (Sumpter & Jobling 1995). At first, Sumpter postulated that oestrogens in the urine of women taking the contraceptive pill were to blame but no trace of these were found in the water. Having read of the findings of Soto et al (1991), he believed that nonylphenol entering rivers in detergents was responsible.

Milk products

The latest theory attempts to explain the large differences in sperm counts between the Danish men and their neighbouring countries. It is possible that drugs used to encourage massive milk production in cattle have contaminated milk and dairy produce. Men taking large amounts of dairy produce such as those in Denmark may have much lower sperm counts than men eating less dairy produce (Jones 2003).

Unto the third generation

Environmental factors are probably as important in gametogenesis and fetal development. The more rapidly developing cells will be most affected. The effect must be considered over three generations. The ova of today's childbearing woman were developed while she was still in her mother's uterus as were the numbers of Sertoli cells present in the testicles of today's prospective fathers. Around the world 100 000 synthetic chemicals are on sale. Some banned in developed countries such as DDT are still used in Third World countries. Worldwide use of pesticides is increasing annually so the problem is likely to be with us for years ahead.

Heavy metals

Lead

Lead has been known to be toxic to the fetus for at least 100 years. The United Kingdom Lead Regulations (HMSO 1985a) legislate for 'a woman of reproductive capacity to be withdrawn from work which exposes her to a specific blood level of lead (40 micrograms per 100 ml) and for pregnant women to be suspended from any work involving exposure to lead' (McCloy 1989). Lead is stored in the bones and may enter the fetus along with calcium mobilised from bone to supply fetal skeletal needs. Exposure to lead in early life affects mental development.

Mercury

Organic mercury was shown to be exceedingly toxic when methyl mercury was discharged into the Minamata Bay area of Japan. The mercury entered the food chain in fish and Nelson (1971) reported that 6% of all births resulted in children with severe neurological abnormalities resembling cerebral palsy.

Pathogen pollution

Another threat is the release of pathogenic organisms into drinking water or the food chain. A current problem is that of the trend to keep cats indoors with the use of a toilet tray. Owners throw cat excrement down their toilet where it, plus its load of *Toxoplasma gondii*, goes into the sewage system. In 1995 the biggest outbreak of toxoplasmosis in humans was traced to the municipal water supply in British Columbia. In California this resulted in a plague affecting sea otters which died (Syufy 2003).

A second example is that of the food poisoning bacterium *E. coli* O157. Reilly of the Scottish Centre for Infection and Environmental Health (Glasgow) believes a percentage of people have contracted the infection from animal manure near camp sites. He believes that animals should be removed from camp sites and venues for pop festivals at least 3 weeks before the use of the field (Randerson 2002).

Radiation

Radiation can be divided into ionising radiation, such as is emitted by X-rays and nuclear medicine, and by atomic weapons testing, and non-ionising radiation, emitted as ultraviolet and infrared rays and by microwaves. Visual display units are now widely used in both the home and the workplace and release low levels of mixed wavelength radiation.

Ionising radiation

Ionising radiation damages DNA by transferring its energy into living cells (Moore & Persaud 1998). Atoms lose electrons and develop an electric charge. These charged particles penetrate the body and damage molecules, producing free radicals and oxidising agents which break and destroy DNA. An intense dose can kill cells during their actively dividing state.

Diagnostic X-ray Because of the known dangers of radiation, X-ray examinations of the abdomen, pelvis or hips of women should only be made during the 10 days following a menstrual period to avoid irradiating an early embryo. Modern shorter wavelength X-rays are safer (Moore & Persaud 1998) and radiology during pregnancy has been reduced because of the development of ultrasound. Shielding the gonads of both men and women whenever possible during diagnostic X-rays helps to prevent possible damage to ovum and sperm.

Natural radiation Humans are exposed to low-level natural background radiation. This low-level radiation, stemming mainly from natural γ-radiation from uranium in the ground, may be more dangerous than originally thought. High doses are associated with deaths from anaemia, respiratory infections, diseases of the nervous system and problems at birth.

Risks of atomic bomb and chemical weapons Radiation may damage actively maturing sperm and ovum and the rapidly dividing cells of the fetus. In August 1945, following the dropping of atomic bombs at Hiroshima and Nagasaki in Japan by Americans, fetuses were found to be very sensitive to radiation as many babies born to mothers who had survived were born dead or deformed. The critical exposure time seems to be between 8 and 15 weeks post conception (Pochin 1988). Bithell & Stewart (1975) found a link between prenatal irradiation of the fetus and childhood leukaemia. The United Kingdom Ionising Radiations Regulations (HMSO 1985b) legislated dose limits for women 'of reproductive capacity' and for the 'abdomen of a pregnant woman who is at work'.

Whereas the rapidly developing fetus is known to be at risk, the Radiation Effects Research Foundation has checked the children of Japanese bomb survivors and found no evidence of genetic damage to the gametes of those exposed. There has been no sign of damaged chromosomes amongst children conceived after the bomb had fallen (Jones 1996).

Chernobyl Scherbak (1996) called the Chernobyl nuclear accident in 1986, 'the worst technogenic environmental disaster in history.' Hot air carried fission products far more reactive than uranium and plutonium into the atmosphere. Amongst the most dangerous were iodine 131, strontium 90 and caesium 137. One-third of the workers who attempted to contain the explosion have developed sexual or reproductive disorders, including impotence and sperm abnormalities with reduced fertilising capacity. There has also been an increase in the number of complicated pregnancies (Scherbak 1996). Radiation has its worst effect on the DNA of rapidly dividing cells such as spermatozoa, the ovum in late menstrual cycle and the early embryo as well as tissues that divide rapidly such as skin cells and epithelial linings.

Urquhart, a statistician, found statistical evidence for a significant increase in babies born with spina bifida, cleft palate and other abnormalities between 1986 and 1989 in five regions of England, mainly in the north and west of the country. Other regions were not affected and there was a similar pattern for infant deaths (Edwards 2002).

Non-ionising radiation (electromagnetic fields)

Non-ionising rays include ultraviolet, infrared, lasers, microwaves, radar and radiofrequency waves. There are three types of electromagnetic field (Falk 2000):

1. High-frequency electromagnetic fields (microwaves) in microwave ovens and mobile phones.
2. Low-frequency electromagnetic fields around high-voltage power lines and domestic electrical equipment. They are linked to electrical currents when the equipment is turned on.
3. Low-frequency electrical fields around domestic electrical equipment. They depend on voltage and are still emitted when the equipment is turned off as long as it is connected to a power source.

There is currently public anxiety about the incidence of leukaemia linked to electromagnetic fields produced by high-voltage power lines and transformer stations. There is little agreement on whether electromagnetic fields affect human health: some studies believe there are risks and others that the findings are negative. Some studies have revealed clusters of effects, including increased miscarriages, stillbirths and congenital defects. Interpretation of these studies is complicated by the possible effects of work stress as some of the women worked uninterrupted for long periods of time (Falk 2000).

Many people are exposed to visual display units (VDUs) at work and at home. VDUs may release low levels of radiation, including X-rays, microwaves, ultraviolet and infrared light. McCloy (1989) found no evidence to show any link between reproductive risk and VDU emissions. A conference on the health effects of electromagnetic fields held in Stockholm in 1999 found no evidence of danger to reproductive health from electromagnetic fields. The conference concluded that more research with less emotive content is needed (Falk 2000). Meanwhile, caution is advised: for instance, women should avoid standing directly in front of their microwave ovens when they are switched on.

Chemical weapons

Other agents that have devastating consequences on reproduction as well as disabling effects on developing fetus are chemical weapons. These have been used in many conflicts during the 20th century, most recently by Iraq during the Iran–Iraq war as well as terrorist attacks (Evison et al 2002).

MAIN POINTS

- By the time women present themselves for antenatal care organogenesis is mostly complete and advice on healthy living may be too late. Research suggests that pregnancy outcome is improved markedly when couples are screened and given preconception advice.

- The continuously produced sperm are most at risk of environmental insult. Ova are in a state of arrested development and are relatively resistant to mutagenic damage until just prior to ovulation. During cleavage the zygote is resistant to genetic injury but after 16 days a period of intense organogenesis begins and sensitivity is high but so few cells are present that an affected fetus will be aborted.

- Any infections should be treated, dietary problems discussed and possible work and lifestyle hazards considered. Long-term health problems should be stabilised

prior to conception. In other conditions which are treated with known teratogenic drugs, possible alteration of treatment may be necessary.

- The age of the prospective parents is important as the frequency of all reproductive problems, including the incidence of chromosome abnormalities, increases with maternal age. Some couples may be anxious to discuss their risk of inherited conditions.

- In developed countries malnutrition is rare but suboptimal dietary deficiencies are common. Processing may destroy essential nutrients while chemical additives such as preservatives, artificial colouring and flavouring are added to increase the shelf life of the food.

- Prepregnancy weight is known to influence pregnancy outcome. Women who are outside the optimal weight range may develop amenorrhoea and infertility.

- Systemic infections may cause reproductive problems such as infertility and congenital defects. Specific organisms can be prevented by vaccination and advice on avoidance of infection.

- Drugs may damage sperm or ova or have an adverse effect on nutrient absorption so that essential nutrients are absent at crucial times during embryonic development. Many chemicals inhaled in cigarette smoke damage the developing fetus. The influence of smoking could be explained partly by differences in nutrient intake.

- Toxins, natural or manufactured, form part of the ecological system in which humans live and reproduce. Natural toxins have evolved alongside humans and a degree of mutual tolerance exists, including human defence systems against plant toxins.

- The development of the chemical industry has resulted in the emission release into the environment of vast quantities of synthetic chemicals which may disrupt human reproduction. The heavy metals lead and mercury are exceedingly toxic to the developing nervous system of the fetus and young child.

- Environmental factors are important in gametogenesis and fetal development. It is important to look back over three generations. The ova of today's childbearing women were developed while she was still in her own mother's uterus as were the numbers of Sertoli cells currently present in the testicles of today's prospective fathers.

- Ionising radiation damages DNA. The critical exposure time may be between 8 and 15 weeks of development. The Radiation Effects Research Foundation found no evidence to indicate genetic damage to the gametes of adults exposed to radiation. Leukaemia, lung cancer and thyroid cancer have increased amongst atomic bomb survivors.

- A conference on the health effects of electromagnetic fields found no evidence of danger to reproductive health, although they concluded that more research is needed: meanwhile, caution is advised. Women should avoid standing directly in front of their microwave ovens when they are switched on.

- Other agents that affect reproduction and have disabling effects on developing fetus are chemical weapons. These have been used in many conflicts during the 20th century, most recently by Iraq during the Iran–Iraq war as well as terrorist attacks.

References

Barker D J P (ed.) 1992 Fetal and Infant Origins of Adult Disease. BMJ Books, London.

Barnes B 1995 Hair mineral analysis, supplementation and cleansing. In Bradley S G, Bennett N (eds) Preparation for Pregnancy. Argyll Publishing, Argyll.

Best J M, O'Shea S, Tipples G et al 2002 Interpretation of rubella serology in pregnancy – pitfalls and problems. British Medical Journal 325:147–148.

Bithell J F, Stewart A M 1975 Prenatal irradiation and childhood malignancy: a review of British data from the Oxford survey. British Journal of Cancer 31:271–287.

Blair P S, Fleming P J, Bensley D et al 1996 Smoking and the sudden infant death syndrome: results from 1993–5 case-control study for confidential inquiry into stillbirths and deaths in infancy. British Medical Journal 313:195–198.

Bradley S G, Bennett N 1995 Preparation for Pregnancy. Argyll Publishing, Argyll.

Carlsen E, Giwercman A, Keiding N, Skakkebaek N 1992 Evidence for decreasing quality of semen during the past 50 years. British Medical Journal 305:609–613.

Chamberlain G 1992 ABC of Antenatal Care. British Medical Journal, London.

Cohen P 2002 Pollution triggers genetic defects. New Scientist 176(2373):8.

Colborn T, Patterson J P, Dumanoski D 1996 Our Stolen Future. Little, Brown, Boston.

Conter V, Cortinovis I, Rogari P, Riva L 1995 Weight growth in infants born to mothers who smoked during pregnancy. British Medical Journal 310:768–771.

Dallison J, Lobstein T 1995 Poor Expectations, Poverty and Undernourishment in Pregnancy. The Maternity Alliance, London.

Department of Health (DOH) 1993 Pregnancy, folic acid and you. Heywood: Health Publication Unit. In National Dairy Council, Nutrition Service, Maternal and Fetal Nutrition, fact file number 11.

Edwards R 2002 Are hundreds of British baby deaths and defects down to Chernobyl? New Scientist 174(2349):6.

Evans H J, Fletcher J, Torrance M, Hardgreave T B 1981 Sperm abnormalities and cigarette smoking. Lancet 1:627–629.

Evison D, Hinsley D, Rice P 2002 Chemical weapons. British Medical Journal 324:332–335.

Falk R 2000 Health effects of electromagnetic fields. www.niwl.se/wl2000/workshop36article_en.asp

Haste F M, Brooke O G, Anderson H R, Bland J M 1991 The effect of nutritional intake on outcome of pregnancy in smokers and non-smokers. British Journal of Nutrition 65:347–354.

HMSO 1985a Control of Lead at Work Regulations 1980: Approved Code of Practice – Control of Lead at Work. HMSO, London.

HMSO 1985b The Ionising Radiations Regulations (SI 1985 No 1333). HMSO, London.

Jick H, Porter J, Morrison A S 1977 Relation between smoking and age of natural menopause. Lancet 1:1354–1355.

Johns T 1990 With Bitter Herbs They Shall Eat It. University of Arizona Press, Tucson.

Jones S 1996 In the Blood, God, Genes and Destiny. HarperCollins, London.

Jones S 2003 Y: The Descent of Man. Little, Brown, Boston.

McCloy E C 1989 Work, environment and the fetus. Midwifery 5:53–62.

Martinez-Frias M L, Salvador J 1990 Epidemiological aspects of prenatal exposure to high doses of vitamin A in Spain. European Journal of Epidemiology 6:118–123.

Mehta N M, Thomas R M 2002 Antenatal screening for rubella – infection or immunity? British Medical Journal 325:90–91.

Moore K L, Persaud T V N 1998 Before We Are Born, 5th edn. W B Saunders, Philadelphia.

National Dairy Council 1994 Nutrition Service, Maternal and Fetal Nutrition, fact file number 11.

Nelson 1971 Hazards of mercury. Environmental Research 4:1–69.

Nesse R M, Williams G C 1995 Evolution and Healing. Weidenfield and Nicolson, London.

Pochin E E 1988 Radiation and mental retardation. British Medical Journal 297:154–156.

Poppit S D, Prentice A M, Jequier E, Schutz Y, Whitehead R G 1993 Evidence of energy sparing in Gambian women during pregnancy: a longitudinal study using whole-body calorimetry. American Journal of Clinical Nutrition 57:353–364.

Profet M 1992 Pregnancy sickness as adaptation: a deterrent to maternal ingestion of teratogens. In Barkow J, Cosmides L, Tooby J (eds) The Adapted Mind: Evolutionary Psychology and the Generation of Culture. Oxford University Press, New York, pp 327–365.

Randerson J 2002 Go easy on the manure. New Scientist 175(2361):11.

Randerson J 2003 Primates pop prenatal drug. New Scientist 177(2379):22.

Scherbak Y M 1996 Ten years of the Chernobyl era. Scientific American 1274(4):32–37.

Schorah C J, Smithells R W 1991 Maternal vitamin nutrition and malformations of the neural tube. Nutrition Research Reviews 4:33–49.

Sharpe R, Skakkebaek N 1993 Are oestrogens involved in falling sperm counts and disorders of the male reproductive tract? Lancet 341:1392–1395.

Smith N C 1992 Detection of the fetus at risk. European Journal of Clinical Nutrition 46(Suppl 1):S1–S5.

Soltan M H, Jenkins D M 1982 Maternal and fetal plasma zinc concentration and fetal abnormality. British Journal of Obstetrics and Gynaecology 89:56–58.

Soltani H, Fraser R B 2000 A longitudinal study of maternal anthropometric changes in normal weight, overweight and obese women during pregnancy and postpartum. British Journal of Nutrition 84:95–101.

Soto A, Justicia H, Wray J, Sonnenschein C 1991 p-Nonylphenol: an Estrogenic xenobiotic released from 'modified polystyrene'. Environmental Health Perspectives 92:167–173.

Sumpter J, Jobling S 1995 Vitellogenesis as a biomarker for oestrogen contamination of the aquatic environment. In The Proceedings of the Estrogens in the Environmental Conference, Environmental Health Perspectives Supplements.

Syufy F 2003 Sea otters and cat feces. http://cats.about.com/cs/parasiticdisease/a/seaotters.htm

Tuormaa T E 1995 The adverse effects of tobacco smoking on reproduction. Foresight. AB Academic Publishers, Tacoma, Washington.

Wakefield J 2002 Boys won't be boys. New Scientist 174(2349):42–45.

Ward N I 1995 Preconceptional care and pregnancy outcome. Journal of Nutritional and Environmental Medicine 5:205–208.

Wharton B A 1992 Food and biological clocks. Proceedings of the Nutrition Society 51:145–153.

Wolfe H 1998 High prepregnancy body mass index – a maternal fetal risk factor. New England Journal of Medicine 338:191.

Wynn M, Wynn A 1991 The case for preconception care of men and women. A B Academic Publishers, Oxford.

Annotated recommended reading

Colborn T, Myers J P, Dumanoski D 1996 Our Stolen Future. Little, Brown, Boston.
If you are anxious about the impact the modern chemical industry has on human reproductive health this is a good starting point.

Falk R 2000 Health effects of electromagnetic fields. www.niwl.se/wl2000/workshop36article_en.asp
This summary of a workshop on electromagnetic fields and their effect on health provides an overview of the current research areas on issues affecting reproductive and general health.

Nesse R M, Williams G C 1995 Evolution and Healing. Weidenfield and Nicolson, London.
Evolutionary medicine is a relatively new concept in health care. This book is written by two early researchers and gives a good introduction to an alternative way of thinking about health and disease.

Schettler T, Solomon G, Valenti M, Huddle A 2000 Generations at risk: reproductive health and the environment. MIT Press, Boston.
This book is recommended to interested readers. It is a source book on human exposure to toxic chemicals that can have reproduction and development effects.

Wakefield J 2002 Boys won't be boys. New Scientist 174(2349):42–45.
This article provides a sensible and easy-to-understand update on the research into environmental pollution and problems of human reproduction.

Section 2A

PREGNANCY – THE FETUS

SECTION CONTENTS

The care of the childbearing woman includes complex screening tests for fetal wellbeing. The midwife must have knowledge and experience of these procedures in order to inform her clients. This section is concerned with the development and growth of the fetus, placenta and membranes. The topic is presented in some detail because developments in the treatment of infertility and in the detection and management of fetal abnormalities are expanding rapidly. The writing style has been made as easy to follow as possible and the diagrams should clarify three-dimensional concepts. Chapter 9 discusses general points about embryological development, Chapters 10 and 11 look in detail at the development of individual systems, and Chapter 12 examines that important fetal organ, the placenta and membranes and the nature of amniotic fluid.

Chapter 13 explores fetal growth and development while Chapter 14 discusses some common fetal problems. Finally, the very important topic of the causes, diagnosis and management of common congenital defects is discussed in Chapter 15.

Chapter **9**

General embryology

INTRODUCTION

This section of the book is about the **developmental processes** that take the human from one fertilised cell to a fetus ready to be born. The general principles of embryology are outlined in this chapter. Chapter 10 covers the development of the skeletal system and Chapter 11 discusses the development of the internal organs. Chapter 12 examines the structure and function of the placenta and amniotic fluid. Chapters 13 and 14 discuss fetal growth and fetal problems. Chapter 15 examines the congenital abnormalities arising when the processes go wrong.

EMBRYOLOGY

Human embryology involves the study of human development. Discoveries about development of the human embryo are gained from research into the development of other species because of the problem of unethical experimentation on humans (The Human Fertilisation and Embryology Act 1990). Although there are more than 10 million species of animals, there are surprising similarities in the basic machinery of development (Alberts et al 2002).

The study of embryology enables us to understand the causes of the congenital abnormalities present in about 6% of live births; half of these are detectable at birth and most of the others are detected during the first year of life (Fitzgerald & Fitzgerald 1994). Malformations vary from minor to major in their effects on the wellbeing of the individual. At least half of all conceptuses are malformed but are usually aborted spontaneously (Moore & Persaud 1998).

GAMETOGENESIS

Following fertilisation of an ovum by a sperm, the resulting zygote regains its full complement of 46 chromosomes. **Gametogenesis** is the formation of the ova and spermatozoa. The primary spermatocyte and primary oocyte are diploid cells, having 46 chromosomes. **Meiosis** consists of two cell divisions, resulting in the reduction of the number

Normal gametogenesis

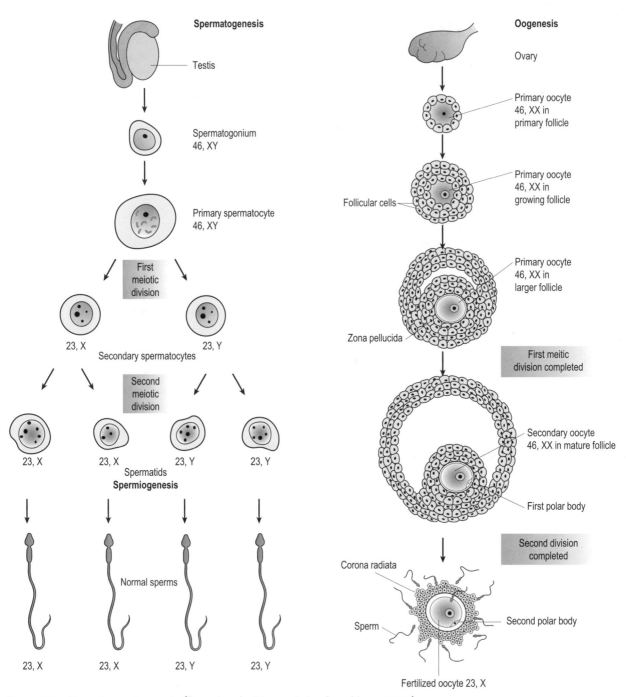

Figure 9.1   Normal gametogenesis. (Reproduced with permission from Moore 1989.)

of chromosomes to the **haploid** 23 found in the mature sperm and ovum (Fig. 9.1).

Meiosis allows the independent assortment of maternal and paternal chromosomes with their genes amongst the gametes and crossing over between homologues of segments of the maternal and paternal chromosomes. This recombination of genetic material ensures that each gamete is a mixture of maternal and paternal genes. At fertilisation a zygote which has received a mixture of genes from its mother and father is produced.

Oogenesis

Primary oocytes are present in a woman's ovaries before birth. **Oogenesis**, the process of transforming oocytes into ova, begins before a woman's birth but is not completed

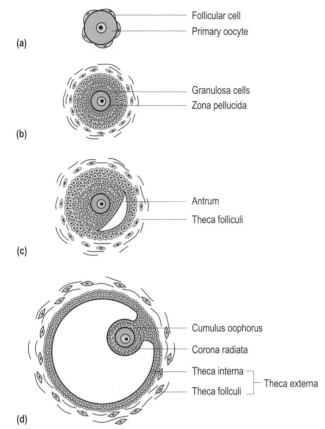

Figure 9.2   The stages of development in the follicle: (a) primordial follicle, (b) primary follicle, (c) secondary follicle, (d) Graafian follicle (from Hinchliff S M, Montague S E 1990, with permission).

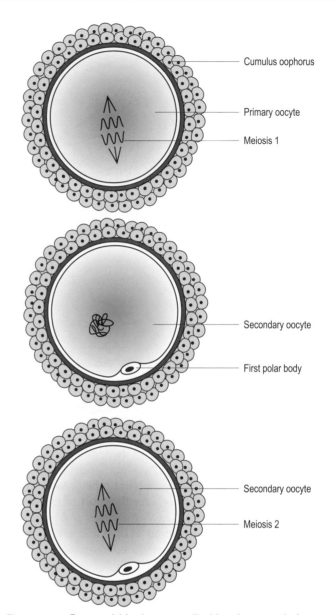

Figure 9.3   Events within the zona pellucida prior to ovulation (from Fitzgerald M J T, Fitzgerald M 1994, with permission).

until after puberty. By the time a girl is born her **primary oocytes** have undergone the prophase of the first meiotic division (meiosis 1). Just before ovulation a surge in pituitary hormones FSH and LH results in maturation of the ovum (Fig. 9.2) and the first meiotic division is completed (Fig. 9.3) (Larsen 2001).

The process results in the formation of a **secondary oocyte**, which receives most of the cytoplasm, and a non-functional cell called the first **polar body**. The secondary oocyte receives 23 chromosomes, including an X chromosome, and the first polar body receives the other 23 chromosomes but degenerates. At ovulation the secondary oocyte begins the second meiotic division but becomes arrested in metaphase of secondary meiosis (Fig. 9.4). If penetrated by a sperm, this division completes and one mature ovum with a second polar body results, which also degenerates (Larsen 2001).

Spermatogenesis

Spermatozoa are produced in the seminiferous tubules of the testes (Ch. 5, p. 53). **Primary spermatocytes** begin to increase in number from puberty. In a functioning testis germ cells will be present at various stages of development,

all originating from **spermatogonia** which divide by mitosis continuously to ensure a constant supply of cells. After undergoing several mitotic divisions, spermatogonia mature, grow larger and become **primary spermatocytes**, diploid cells that still contain 46 chromosomes.

These undergo the first meiotic division to form two **secondary spermatocytes**, which have only 23 chromosomes. Half will receive the X chromosome of the male cell genotype and half will receive the Y chromosome. Secondary meiosis results in four haploid **spermatids** found in close association with Sertoli cells, which provide nutrition and support to the sperm. The spermatids are transformed into highly specialised **spermatozoa** (Fig. 9.5).

As a sperm matures, excess protoplasm is lost and the nuclear chromatin condenses to become the head of the sperm. One centriole develops into the **tail**, which is

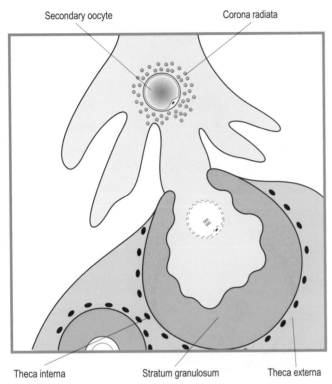

Figure 9.4   Ovulation (from Fitzgerald M J T, Fitzgerald M 1994, with permission).

composed of a central filament of two microfibrils surrounded by a circle of nine fibrils. Mitochondria aggregate in the neck region and the Golgi apparatus helps to form the **acrosome cap**, which develops over the head of the sperm and contains enzymes called hyaluronidases and proteases (Fig. 9.6). The process takes about 70 days and several hundred million sperm a day are produced continuously from puberty. As men become older, the seminal tubules undergo involution and by 70 years extensive atrophy may be present.

Gamete size

The oocyte is a very large cell, just visible to the unaided eye and usually only one is released at ovulation. It contains all the material necessary for early embryonic growth and development following fertilisation. In sharp contrast, the mature sperm has lost most of its cytoplasm, is very small and millions of them are released during ejaculation. About 1000 sperms will reach the ovum (oocyte) and these will all be needed to allow just one to enter. When one sperm enters a secondary oocyte a diploid zygote is formed, the first cell of a unique human being.

FERTILISATION

Capacitation

Freshly ejaculated sperm are unable to fertilise an oocyte and undergo a process of maturation called **capacitation**. While travelling through the female genital tract, usually in the uterus or uterine tubes, glycoproteins are removed from the surface of the acrosome. When a capacitated sperm meets the corona radiata of the oocyte the acrosome develops perforations in it. This is known as the **acrosome reaction**.

The acrosome reaction

Binding of a sperm to the zona pellucida of the oocyte is species specific. Lytic (digestive) enzymes such as **hyaluronidase** are released around the oocyte and it takes the enzymes from many sperm to create a passageway for one sperm to enter. These enzymes disperse the corona radiata follicular cells, allowing the head of one sperm to make contact with the zona pellucida. Other enzymes such as **acrosin**, which produce an opening in the zona pellucida, are now released. The sperm cell membrane fuses with the oocyte cell membrane and the sperm nucleus passes into the oocyte (Fig. 9.7). This occurs in the ampulla of the uterine tube.

Blocks to polyspermy

Two mechanisms prevent **polyspermy** (the entry of multiple sperm) immediately following entry of the first sperm, ensuring that the fertilised oocyte contains only 46 chromosomes.

Fast block

The oocyte plasma membrane electrical resting potential is normally negatively charged at −70 millivolts (mV), with which sperm can readily fuse. Immediately after sperm entry, sodium channels open in the cell membrane and extra positively charged sodium ions are allowed into the oocyte cytoplasm. This rises to a positive charge of +20 mV and more sperm are prevented from entering the oocyte. This reaction is brief and resting potential soon returns to −70 mV.

Slow block (cortical reaction)

The brief depolarisation has two other effects. First, it allows **subcortical granules** lying just under the oocyte plasma membrane to rupture and release chemicals which bind water into the cytoplasm. The oocyte swells and detaches any remaining sperm in contact with it. Secondly, the secondary oocyte is activated to complete the second meiotic division and expel the second polar body and the ovum is now mature (Larsen 2001). Its nucleus is now called the **female pronucleus**. Once the head of the sperm enters the cytoplasm of the ovum its head enlarges to form the **male pronucleus**. The male and female pronuclei fuse and paternal and maternal chromosomes intermingle.

Mitochondrial deoxyribonucleic acid (MtDNA)

The energy-producing mitochondria (Ch. 3, p. 30) are all inherited from the ovum because sperm mitochondria used

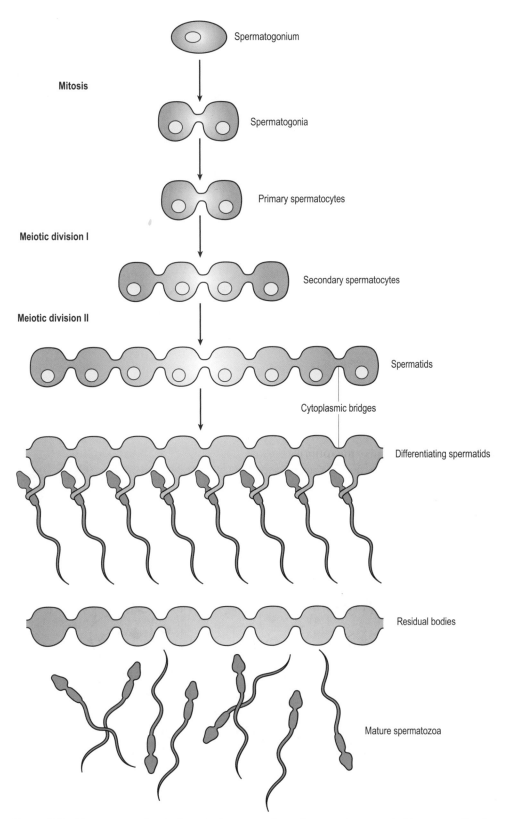

Figure 9.5   The progeny of a single maturing spermatogonium remain connected to one another by cytoplasmic bridges throughout their differentiation into mature sperm. (Reproduced with permission from Alberts et al 1994.)

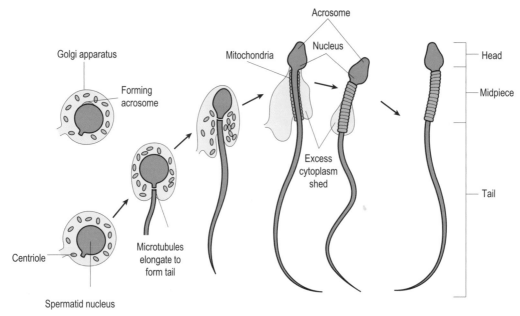

Figure 9.6 Sperm formation. (Reproduced with permission from Chiras 1991.)

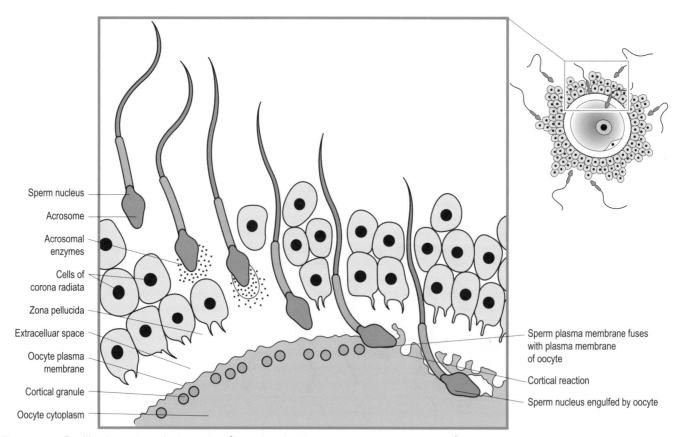

Figure 9.7 Fertilisation and cortical reaction. (Reproduced with permission from Chiras 1991.)

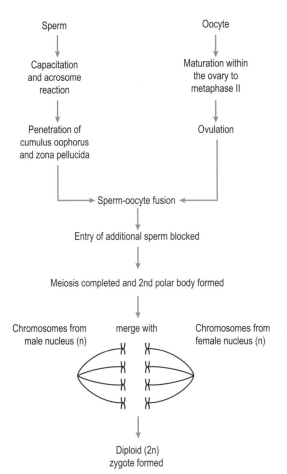

Figure 9.8   Events in the female reproductive tract leading up to fertilisation (from Hinchliff S M, Montague S M, Watson R 1996, with permission).

in motility are shed with the tail and do not enter the oocyte. In humans MtDNA is circular and very compact, being one of the smallest known in the animal kingdom.

Results of fertilisation (Fig. 9.8)

- The number of chromosomes is restored to the diploid 23 pairs or 46 chromosomes.
- The new individual inherits a unique set of genes from its parents.
- Sex determination occurs depending on which type of sperm fertilises the ovum.
- Initiation of cleavage stimulates the zygote to begin mitotic cell division.

THE EMBRYO

Terminology

The term **conceptus** refers to the products of fertilisation and comprises the embryo with its supporting tissues or adnexae. The developmental process is divided into discrete sections of time. The **preimplantation period** is the

time between fertilisation and implantation and lasts about 6 days. The conceptus is called an **embryo** from implantation until the end of the 8th week after fertilisation when it becomes known as a **fetus**. The size of embryos is expressed as the crown–rump length from the crown of the head until the terminal part of the caudal end. In the fetus, the standing length from crown to heel is used.

General concepts used in embryology

It is important to understand the general concepts of embryology and some detail about the development of specific systems and the processes involved. How does one cell develop into millions of cells and hundreds of variations? What instructions does the cell use and what processes carry out the instructions? There are three important concepts towards understanding embryology:

1. a programme of simple instructions can generate complex forms;
2. most developmental processes depend upon an interaction of genetic and environmental factors;
3. each system in the body has its own developmental pattern (Moore & Persaud 1998).

PROGRAMMING THE EMBRYO

The information to make an embryo is located in the DNA of the zygote. The sperm and ovum each contribute 23 chromosomes but the ovum contributes all the organelles and MtDNA. Regulatory genes control development by influencing where and when proteins are made (Wolpert et al 2002). Development involves various processes (Wolpert et al 2002):

- pattern formation;
- differentiation;
- morphogenesis;
- development of the germ layers;
- growth.

Pattern formation

Cells in the embryo seem to 'know' where and when to change shape and position and cell movements are part of the embryo's developmental programme. Wolpert (1991) describes this as a set of instructions, not for describing the final form but for creating shapes. A parallel can be made with knitting. The knitting pattern is the code or instruction manual but does not resemble the finished article. In order to translate the words into a garment the knitter must interpret the code and apply energy, order, control and a variety of stitches.

Cellular processes include:

- somatic cell division where the daughter cells receive identical genetic information;
- cell differentiation to make up the different tissues of the embryo;

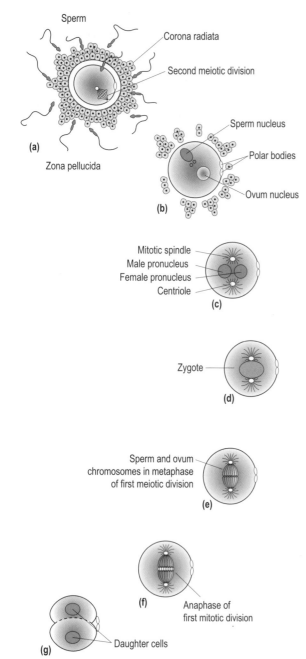

(a)

Sperm

Corona radiata

Second meiotic division

Zona pellucida

(b)

Sperm nucleus

Polar bodies

Ovum nucleus

(c)

Mitotic spindle
Male pronucleus
Female pronucleus
Centriole

(d)

Zygote

(e)

Sperm and ovum
chromosomes in metaphase
of first meiotic division

(f)

Anaphase of
first mitotic division

(g)

Daughter cells

Figure 9.9 The zygote prepares for division. (Reproduced with permission from Chiras 1991.)

- induction – cell interaction where one type of cells influences another;
- the migration of cells;
- programmed cell death to remove redundant cells.

Early cell division

Cleavage

Early in pregnancy, growth and development are very similar in any human embryo. The exact days when embryonic features develop can be given. Days of development are counted from fertilisation, not from the last menstrual period. Within 24 hours the large zygote undergoes mitosis and splits into smaller cells, each with the full complement of maternal and paternal chromosomes. This is called **cleavage**. The daughter cells are called **blastomeres** (Fig. 9.9) (Larsen 2001).

There is synthesis of new DNA but no increase in the amount of cytoplasm so that the size of the blastomeres diminishes progressively. The fertilised ovum continues its journey down the uterine tube and by the fourth day after fertilisation there are between 16 and 20 cells. The conceptus is known as the **morula** (Fig. 9.10). The cells are still **totipotent** and could contribute to any part of the embryo. If the cells are separated, multiple identical individuals could develop (clones). The formation of identical fetuses may occur in humans when hundreds of cells are present.

Differentiation

In the early embryo there is little cellular difference except their shape and the cells are not specialised. Humans have about 350 different cell types, whereas a simpler animal may have only 10–20 cell types (Wolpert 1991). Cells carry out a variety of functions, from carrying oxygen to making and secreting hormones.

Essential proteins

There are many molecular similarities between species. About 50% of genes have **homologues** (same structures) between the species (Alberts et al 2002). Recognisable versions of human genes were already present in a common ancestor of many species. Animals appear to have a set of key proteins from which to construct their bodies. Proteins are like children's building blocks. The embryo builds up different tissue types by combining proteins. There are two classes of important proteins: **transmembrane proteins** needed for cell adhesion and **cell signalling** and **gene regulatory proteins**. The development of multicellular organisms is led by cell–cell interactions and by differential gene expression. What type of cell develops depends on which path it takes as it migrates. These pathways represent gene activity and are selected depending on extracellular signals (Alberts et al 2002).

Cell–cell interactions

A handful of evolutionary cell–cell signals are used by many organisms to cause cells to differentiate to form a complex multicellular individual. All these signals are genetically controlled:

- sister cells may differ as a result of asymmetrical cell division;
- cells born alike may compete with each other and inhibit the development of those next to each other (lateral inhibition);
- a group of similar cells may be exposed to different signals called morphogens from cells outside the group.

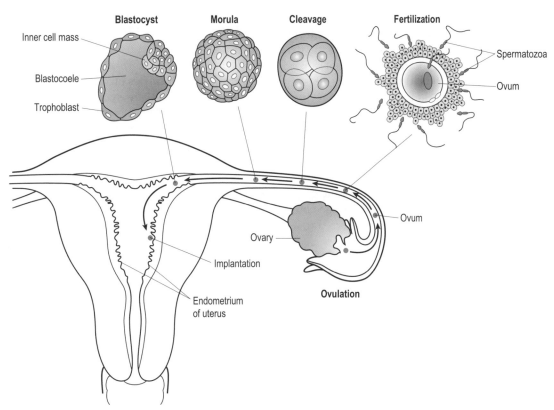

Figure 9.10   Fertilisation and early embryonic development. (Reproduced with permission from Chiras 1991.)

Morphogenesis

Regulatory genes

Cells in different parts of the embryo change shape and function to carry out their developing roles. Genes in the cell nuclei interact with environmental factors to bring about this huge variety in cell types that make up tissues and organs. All vertebrates have a similar basic **body plan** with a segmented vertebral column and the brain at the anterior end. These structures mark the **anteroposterior axis**.

The vertebrate body also has a distinct **dorsoventral axis** (back to belly) with the mouth on the ventral side. These two axes define the left–right sides of an animal with the internal organs such as the heart and liver being asymmetrically arranged. Each vertebrate has a different strategy for setting up the axes with the formation of **signalling centres** which are localised parts of an embryo influencing how nearby cells develop (Wolpert et al 2002).

Something in the embryonic environment turns on **developmental genes**, which control how cells divide, multiply and move around in the embryo. Regulatory genes control patterning in the embryo by a cascade of gene products. The most important discovery was of a discrete portion of DNA with a specific order of genes called the **homeobox** (Alberts et al 2002). These genes are present in virtually all animals.

The homeobox   Genes control **segmentation** in the developing embryo so that the correct positioning of organs is brought about. Much of the research has been carried out on the fruit fly *Drosophila* but the presence of the homeobox is likely to indicate similar functions in human embryos. A number of **homeotic** (alike) genes are active in specific positions controlling patterning in the developing nervous system (Wolpert 1991). These genes are referred to as **HOM genes** in invertebrates and **Hox genes** in vertebrates such as humans (McGinnis & Kuziora 1994) and are responsible for cell patterning locally. Different homeobox genes are switched on in the order they are positioned on the Hox complex to produce different protein products (Albert et al 2002, Wolpert et al 2002). These subdivide the embryo into discrete **homeodomains** prior to differentiation into specific tissue types, organs and systems.

Morphogens   Homeobox genes may be switched on sequentially by **chemical gradients**. Cytoplasm with special genetic properties is located at the ends of the zygote, setting up gradients called **morphogens** which, when they reach specific concentrations, activate other genes. Nusslein-Volhard (1996) writes about *Drosophila*, 'Cells in a developing field respond to a special substance – a morphogen – the concentration of which gradually increases in a certain direction, forming a gradient'.

Induction

Hans Spemann won the only Nobel Prize awarded for embryology for discovering what organises the embryo's development. He demonstrated that a nervous system will only develop if future muscle and adjacent cells move from the outside of the embryo to a situation underneath the outer layer. These migrated cells produce a signal that causes the overlying sheet of cells to develop into a nervous system. This cellular movement is said to **induce** the development of the nervous system. These influencing tissues are called **inductors** or **organisers**. The inductor needs to be near but not necessarily in contact with the tissue to be induced. Primary organisers establish the basic body plan and then a chain of secondary inductions occurs. It is generally accepted that some signal passes from inductor to induced tissue. There needs to be a sufficiently large community of cells for induction to occur. This is referred to as the **community effect**.

Cell communication

Cells communicate with each other in different ways. In some tissues the inductor may be a **diffusible molecule** passing directly from one tissue to another. In other tissues the message is mediated by an **extracellular matrix** (ECM) secreted by the inductor and with which the reacting tissue comes into contact. The ECM is a network of mesodermal cells which provides **pathways** for cells to crawl along and their chemical products appear and disappear in the ECM. Some tissues react to **direct physical contact** between the inducing and reacting tissues (Moore & Persaud 1998) and cells receive cues from their neighbours about where they should be and how they should behave. **Tissue-specific proteins** create cell recognition and accumulation. The originators of a group of cells may specify where it travels to in the embryo and the tissue it forms.

Programmed cell death

Programmed cell death or **apoptosis** (Greek for shedding leaves) plays a major part in the final pattern of cells, especially in the formation of body cavities (Wolpert et al 2002). Cells in some tissues are overproduced and those not needed commit suicide (Alberts et al 2002). Cell death is a normal feature of development of the nervous system, limbs, skeleton and heart as the following examples explain:

- In limb formation, cell death helps to achieve the final shape of the limb: for instance, the disappearance of webbing between the fingers.
- In the developing brain and nervous system over 50% too many axons arrive at target cells. The first to arrive make the best connections and send signals back in the form of nerve growth factor (NGF), which sustains neurones. There is no room for late arrivals, which cannot obtain nourishment and die.
- Too many cells are made in the development of tubes such as blood vessels, and the tube is hollowed out by cell death.

DEVELOPMENT OF THE EMBRYO

The blastocyst

The group of cells carries on cleaving for the first 4 days. The first three cleavages are synchronous, but later cleavages are asymmetrical. There is also **polarisation**, with internal cells differing from external cells. The inner cells divide less frequently and remain large and round, whereas the outer cells in contact with the zona pellucida become flattened. At this point the cells lose their totipotency and begin to **differentiate**. They are destined to become specific parts of the embryo. On the 5th day the zygote 'hatches' as the zona pellucida is digested by uterine secretions. Fluid accumulates in the space between the peripheral and central cells of the morula and it becomes the hollow **blastocyst**. The inner cell mass of the blastocyst is the **embryoblast** and will become the embryo and the flattened outer layer of cells is called the **trophoblast** which will form the placenta (Larsen 2001).

Implantation

On the 6th day the part of the blastocyst where the embryo has begun to develop, the embryoblast, begins to implant into the endometrium, most commonly on the posterior wall of the uterus. Where the trophoblastic cells make contact with the endometrium they undergo rapid DNA synthesis and become cuboid in shape to form the cytotrophoblast. The daughter cells shed their plasma membranes to form a mass of protoplasm filled with nuclei and organelles called a **syncytium**. The mass of tissue is called the **syncytiotrophoblast** (Fig. 9.11), which produces enzymes that attack the endometrium and hormones that allow the pregnancy to continue (Larsen 2001).

The effects of enzymatic erosion

As the enzymes erode the endometrium, the uterine glands release their content to nourish the embryo and the blastocyst begins to enlarge. Nutrition is also provided by the stroma cells which undergo changes known as the **decidual reaction** and become swollen with glycogen and lipid. The change commences at the implantation site and spreads within a few days throughout the whole endometrium except the lining of the cervix. The endometrium is now known as the **decidua**.

At the implantation site new blood capillaries fed by branches of the spiral arteries and drained by the endometrial veins develop and dilate (Fig. 9.12). The conceptus is completely embedded in the compact layer of the endometrium by the 12th day and is covered by the overlying uterine epithelium. Erosion of these sinuses results in maternal blood entering the syncytiotrophoblast to collect in a labyrinth of little pockets called lacunae. Human chorionic gonadotrophin (hCG) is secreted into the lacunae by the trophoblast, enters the maternal circulation and maintains the ovarian corpus luteum. This ensures the continued production of oestrogen

7 days

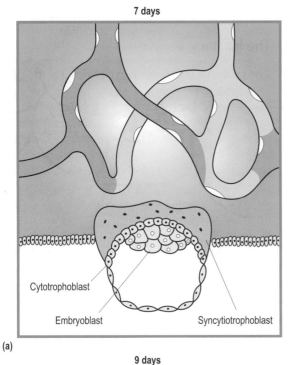

Cytotrophoblast

Embryoblast   Syncytiotrophoblast

(a)

8 days Endometrial capillaries

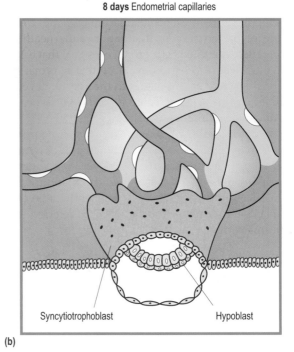

Syncytiotrophoblast   Hypoblast

(b)

9 days

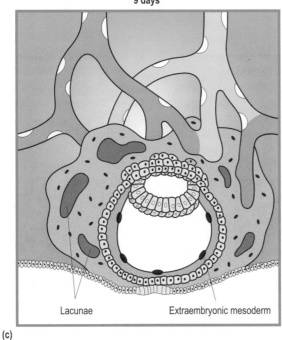

Lacunae   Extraembryonic mesoderm

(c)

Figure 9.11a–c   The implanting conceptus on days 7–9 after fertilisation. Arrows indicate direction of blood flow in endometrial capillary bed. (Uterine glands are not represented.) (From Fitzgerald M J T, Fitzgerald M 1994, with permission.)

and progesterone for maintenance of the pregnancy until the placenta produces sufficient of the two hormones at 12 weeks.

DEVELOPMENT OF THE GERM LAYERS

The bilaminar embryonic disc

The following descriptions should be studied with the accompanying diagrams, remembering that they are two-dimensional sections through a three-dimensional embryo. By the 2nd week of development the cells are well organised and the inner cell mass forms a flattened disc consisting of two layers. The inner layer or **epiblast** is composed of tall columnar epithelium and the outer layer or **hypoblast** is composed of low cuboidal epithelium. Together they are known as the **bilaminar embryonic disc** (Figs 9.13 and 9.14).

The margins of the epiblast create a thin epithelial layer, the **amnion**, and the epiblast and amnion form the amniotic sac. This sac grows more rapidly than the embryo and comes to surround the embryo. The cell margins of the

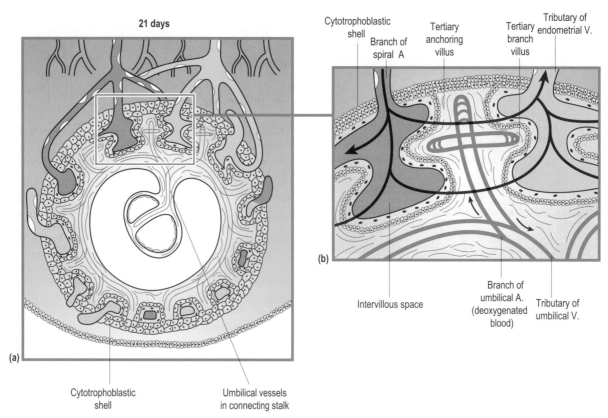

Figure 9.12a&b   Chorionic vesicle at 21 days. (b) Enlargement of upper part of (a) showing the circulation of embryonic and maternal blood (from Fitzgerald M J T, Fitzgerald M 1994, with permission).

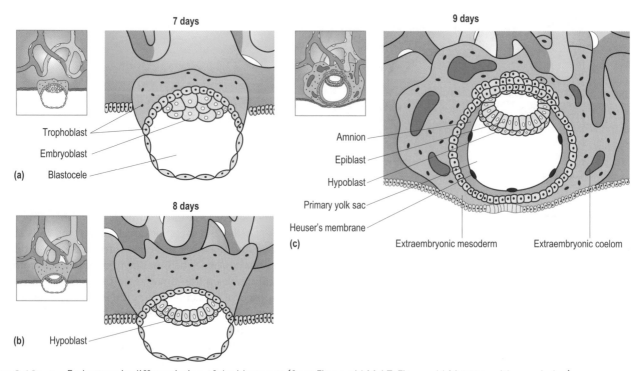

Figure 9.13a–c   Early steps in differentiation of the blastocyst (from Fitzgerald M J T, Fitzgerald M 1994, with permission).

hypoblast also divide rapidly to form branched cells that line the cavity of the blastocyst. This lining is called the **extra-embryonic mesoderm**. Spaces develop within the mesoderm and coalesce to become the **extraembryonic coelom** (coelom means cavity).

This cavity splits the mesoderm into a **visceral layer**, which is included in the **yolk sac**, and a **parietal layer**, which contributes to the **chorion** together with the tropho-blast. The visceral inner cells become flattened and form an epithelium called **Heuser's membrane** which encloses the cavity of the primary yolk sac. The visceral and parietal extraembryonic mesoderms are linked by a **connecting stalk**

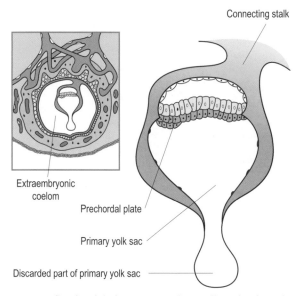

Figure 9.14   Prechordal plate; connecting stalk; reduction of primary yolk sac (from Fitzgerald M J T, Fitzgerald M 1994, with permission).

that develops into the **umbilical cord**. Towards the end of the 2nd week the flattened disc becomes ovoid. The cranial (front) part of the hypoblast thickens to form the **prechordal plate** (Larsen 2001).

The trilaminar embryo

There is an immense amount of cellular activity during **embryogenesis** and **organogenesis**. Cells migrate through the embryo, differentiating into specific cell types to form organs and systems (Larsen 2001). The formation of the **primitive streak**, **gastrulation** and formation of the **noto-chord** are important in creating the body plan (Figs 9.15 and 9.16). They will be described separately although they occur simultaneously and are interlinked in the embryo.

The primitive streak

At the beginning of the 3rd week a thick linear band of embryonic epiblast appears caudally (towards the rear) in the dorsal aspect of the embryonic disc. This primitive streak results from cells of the epiblast heaping up and migrating to the centre of the embryonic disc. It is the site of enormous cell activity when the first wave of migration forms the middle third layer of the embryo and the basic body plan is laid down with a cranial end and a caudal end. The primitive streak elongates by adding cells to its caudal end and the cranial end enlarges to form a **primitive node** (Fig. 9.17).

The primitive streak continues to form mesodermal cells until the end of the 4th week by which time it has retreated to the caudal end of the embryo. Rarely it persists and gives rise to a multi-tissued tumour called a **sacral teratoma**. Embryonic mesodermal cells migrate in three directions

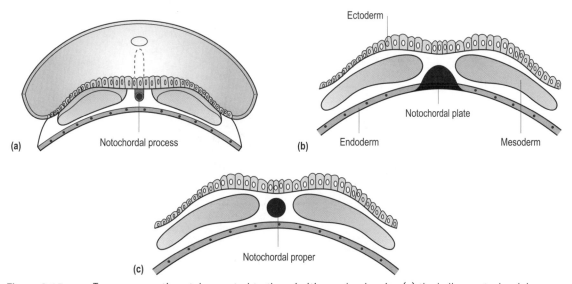

Figure 9.15a–c   Transverse sections taken rostral to the primitive node, showing (a) the hollow notochordal process; (b) the notochordal plate fused with the endoderm; (c) the notochord proper (from Fitzgerald M J T, Fitzgerald M 1994, with permission).

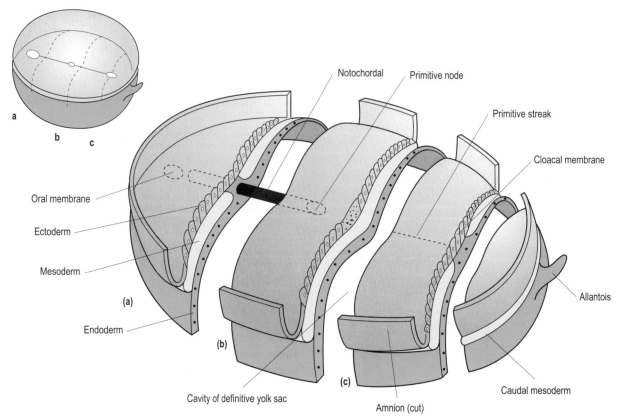

Figure 9.16   Stereosections of the trilaminar embryonic disc, viewed obliquely from above (from Fitzgerald M J T, Fitzgerald M 1994, with permission).

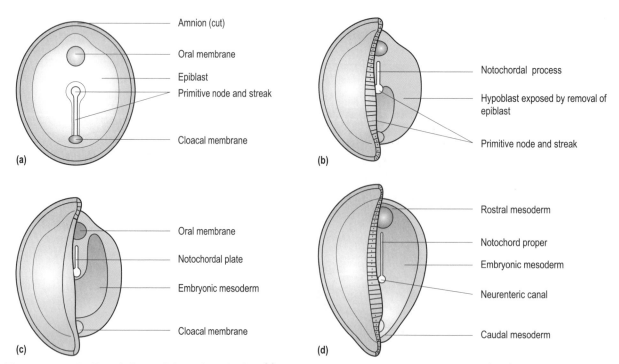

Figure 9.17a–d   Dorsal views of the embryonic disc. (a) represents the floor of the amniotic sac. In (b–d), the epiblast has been removed from the right side, to show migration of the embryonic mesoderm over the surface of the hypoblast (from Fitzgerald M J T, Fitzgerald M 1994, with permission).

from the primitive streak: laterally to the margins of the embryonic disc, cranially alongside the notochord and caudally around the **cloacal membrane** (see below).

Gastrulation

Wolpert (1991) wrote 'it is not birth, marriage or death, but gastrulation which is truly the important event in your life'. **Gastrulation** is a process of invagination by which the inner cell mass becomes the trilaminar embryo. It begins in the 1st week with the formation of the hypoblast, continues during the 2nd week with the formation of the epiblast and is completed during the 3rd week. It ends when the three primary germ layers of **ectoderm**, **mesoderm** and **endoderm** are in situ and the embryo is a trilaminar disc. It may help to visualise a simple hollow three-layered animal such as a sea urchin: the inner layer or lining is epithelium, surrounded by muscle and covered by skin. A human being is a complex elaboration of those three layers.

Epiblastic cells dip through the primitive streak and spread laterally beneath it. Wolpert (1991) wrote, 'movements occur simultaneously over many parts of the embryo with sheets of cells streaming past each other, contracting and expanding.' Some of the cells displace the underlying hypoblast to form the embryonic endoderm, while the remainder form the embryonic mesoderm or **mesenchyme**. Epiblastic cells that do not migrate remain on the surface to form embryonic ectoderm. The endoderm migrates inside the wall of the primary yolk sac to become the secondary yolk sac. A finger-like projection of the yolk sac, the **allantois**, becomes pinched off and extends into the connecting stalk.

Development of body cavities   Late in the 2nd week fluid-filled spaces appear in the cranial half of the embryonic mesoderm. These coalesce during the 3rd week to form the 'U'-shaped **embryonic coelom**. The bend of the U at the cranial end of the embryonic coelom is the **pericardial coelom**. This is divided by the **septum transversum** from the caudal two arms of the U which form the **pericardioperitoneal canals** (pleural canals) leading to two branches of the **peritoneal coelom**. Three body cavities develop – a **pericardial cavity** around the heart, two smaller **pleural canals** and a large **peritoneal cavity**. The septum transversum is incorporated into the **diaphragm**.

Formation of the notochord

The notochordal process grows out cranially from the primitive knot beneath the ectoderm until it reaches the prechordal plate. Where the prechordal plate is firmly attached to the ectoderm and remains bilaminar it forms the **oropharyngeal membrane** or future site of the mouth. Caudal to the primitive streak is a circular area which also remains bilaminar called the **cloacal membrane** or future site of the anus and urogenital orifices. The notochord, a rigid cellular rod stretched out along the embryo, develops from the notochordal process. Mesodermal cells gather around it to form the **vertebral column** and it is almost completely formed by the end of the 3rd week. It degenerates and disappears once it is surrounded by the vertebral bodies.

Organogenesis

From 3 weeks the embryo enters the vulnerable stage of organogenesis, which is completed by 8 weeks (Fig. 9.18). Organs are made up of cell types that originate from different sources and obey different instructions. From about day 20 until day 30 the dorsal surface of the embryo develops a segmented appearance with the appearance of **paired somites** which are clumps of embryonic tissue (Wolpert et al 2002). From the somites develop the vertebral column, and the segmentally innervated muscles of the trunk. The somites are still visible at 6 weeks but have differentiated by 8 weeks.

Differentiation of the germ layers

Figure 9.19 summarises the tissues and organs developing from the three layers.

Ectoderm

- Tissues derived from **neuroectoderm** include the central and peripheral nervous systems, the retina of the eye and the posterior lobe of the pituitary gland.
- Tissues derived from **surface ectoderm** include the outer layer of the skin called the epidermis with its hair follicles and cutaneous glands, including the breasts, the lens of the eye, the special sense cells of the inner ear, the anterior lobe of the pituitary gland and the enamel of the teeth.

Neurulation   Development of the human brain and nervous system is known as **neurulation** (Figs 9.20–9.25). The notochord induces its overlying ectoderm to thicken and form a neural plate. These cells are known as the neuroectoderm and differ from the remaining surface ectoderm. A flat sheet of cells on the upper surface of the embryo folds up into a tube which will develop into the brain and spinal cord. On about day 18 the neural plate develops a midline neural groove with lateral neural folds. At the beginning of the 4th week the folds come together to form the neural tube.

Fusion of the folds begins at the level of the 4th pair of somites and proceeds simultaneously in cranial and caudal directions. Cells near to the crests of the neural folds escape from the neural tube during closure and come to lie on either side of the neural tube, forming the neural crest. The two ends of the neural tube are open and termed **neuropores**. The cranial neuropore closes about day 25 and the caudal neuropore about day 27. The neural tube becomes the brain and spinal

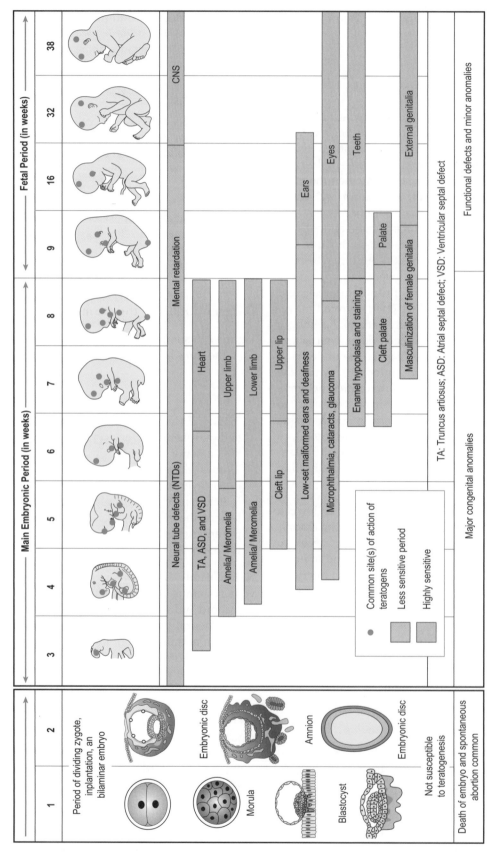

Figure 9.18 Schematic illustration of critical periods in human prenatal development, showing periods of sensitivity to teratogens. (Reproduced with permission from Moore 1989.)

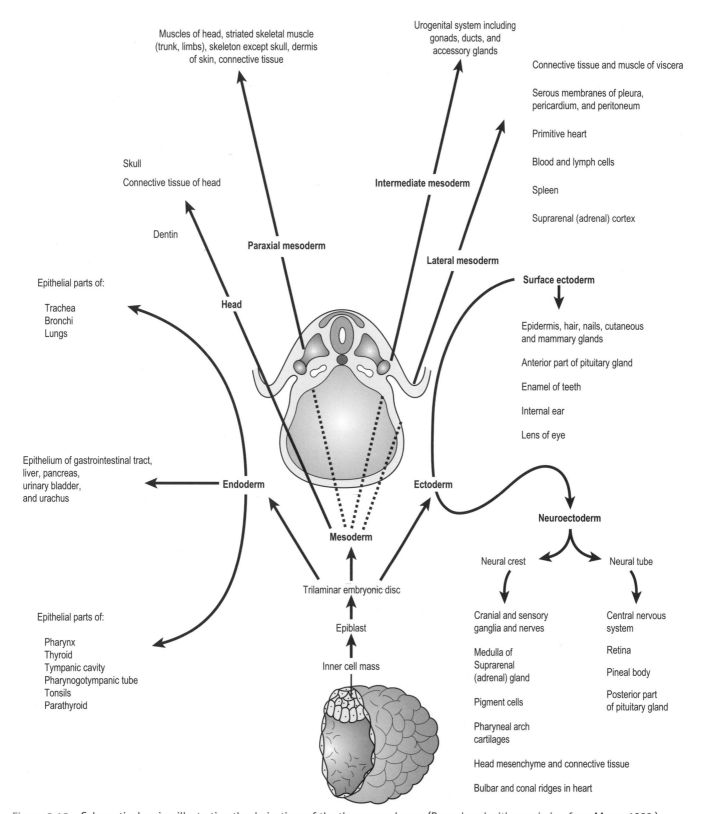

Muscles of head, striated skeletal muscle
(trunk, limbs), skeleton except skull, dermis
of skin, connective tissue

Urogenital system including
gonads, ducts, and
accessory glands

Connective tissue and muscle of viscera

Serous membranes of pleura,
pericardium, and peritoneum

Primitive heart

Blood and lymph cells

Spleen

Suprarenal (adrenal) cortex

Skull

Connective tissue of head

Intermediate mesoderm

Dentin

Paraxial mesoderm

Lateral mesoderm

Surface ectoderm

Epithelial parts of:

Trachea
Bronchi
Lungs

Head

Epidermis, hair, nails, cutaneous
and mammary glands

Anterior part of pituitary gland

Enamel of teeth

Internal ear

Lens of eye

Epithelium of gastrointestinal tract,
liver, pancreas,
urinary bladder,
and urachus

Endoderm

Ectoderm

Neuroectoderm

Mesoderm

Neural crest

Neural tube

Trilaminar embryonic disc

Epiblast

Cranial and sensory
ganglia and nerves

Central nervous
system

Inner cell mass

Retina

Medulla of
Suprarenal
(adrenal) gland

Pineal body

Epithelial parts of:

Pharynx
Thyroid
Tympanic cavity
Pharynogotympanic tube
Tonsils
Parathyroid

Pigment cells

Posterior part
of pituitary gland

Pharyneal arch
cartilages

Head mesenchyme and connective tissue

Bulbar and conal ridges in heart

Figure 9.19   Schematic drawing illustrating the derivatives of the three germ layers. (Reproduced with permission from Moore 1989.)

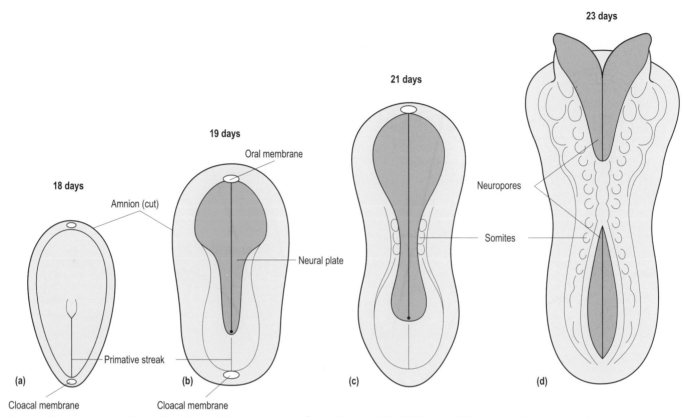

Figure 9.20a–d   Dorsal views of the floor of the amniotic sac (from Fitzgerald M J T, Fitzgerald M 1994, with permission).

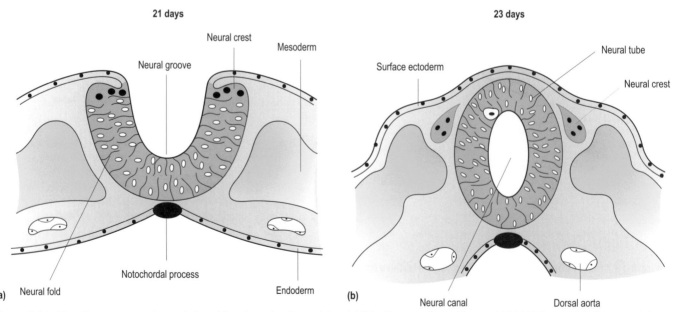

Figure 9.21a&b   Transverse sections of the mid-region of embryos (c) and (d) in Fig. 9.20 (from Fitzgerald M J T, Fitzgerald M 1994, with permission).

19 days

Pericardioperitoneal canal

Amnion (cut)   Septum transversum

(b)

C

D

Oral membrane

Brain plate

Pericardial coelom

(a)

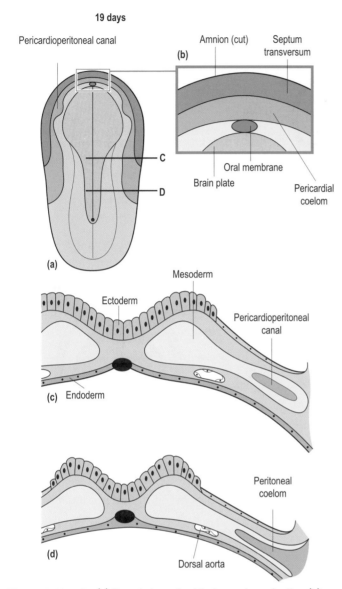

Mesoderm

Ectoderm

Pericardioperitoneal canal

(c) Endoderm

Peritoneal coelom

(d)

Dorsal aorta

Figure 9.22a–d   (a) Dorsal view of a 19-day embryonic disc. (b) Enlargement from the rostral part of (a). (c,d) Transverse sections at the levels indicated in (a) (from Fitzgerald M J T, Fitzgerald M 1994, with permission).

18 days

Ectoderm

Amnion (cut)

Notochordal process

(a)   Endoderm

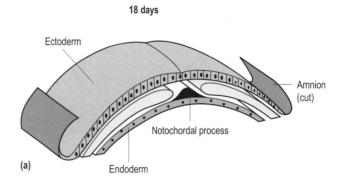

Surface ectoderm

Somites

Intermediate mesoderm

Notochord

Embryonic coelom

Endoderm

(b)

Splanchnic mesoderm

Somatic mesoderm

Lateral plate

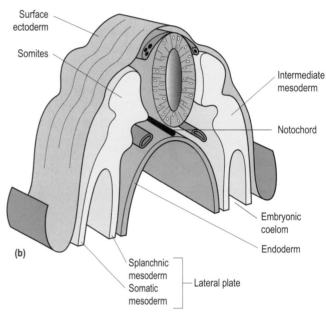

Figure 9.23a&b   Early differentiation of the embryonic mesoderm (from Fitzgerald M J T, Fitzgerald M 1994, with permission).

cord and the neural canal within the tube becomes the ventricular system of the brain and the central canal of the spinal cord. This early closure of the neural tube has implications for the causation and prevention of open neural tube defects.

Mesoderm

The mesoderm nearest the midline axis of the embryo is called **paraxial mesoderm** and undergoes segmentation to form somites. Next to the somites and not undergoing segmentation is the **intermediate mesoderm** and outside that is the **lateral plate**. The lateral plate is divided into

somatic mesoderm that lies just beneath the body wall and **splanchnic mesoderm** lying next to the endoderm of the yolk sac. Tissues derived from mesoderm are:

- from the paraxial mesoderm cranial to the somites: part of the skull and the muscles of the face and jaws;
- from the somites: the vertebral column and the skeletal musculature of the trunk and the connective tissue or dermis of the skin;
- from the intermediate mesoderm: the kidneys and ureters, the gonads, the ductus deferens and the uterus and fallopian tubes;
- from the somatic mesoderm: the limb skeleton and muscles, the sternum and the anterior part of the ribs;
- from the splanchnic mesoderm: the cardiovascular system and blood, the spleen and the smooth muscle of the gastrointestinal tract.

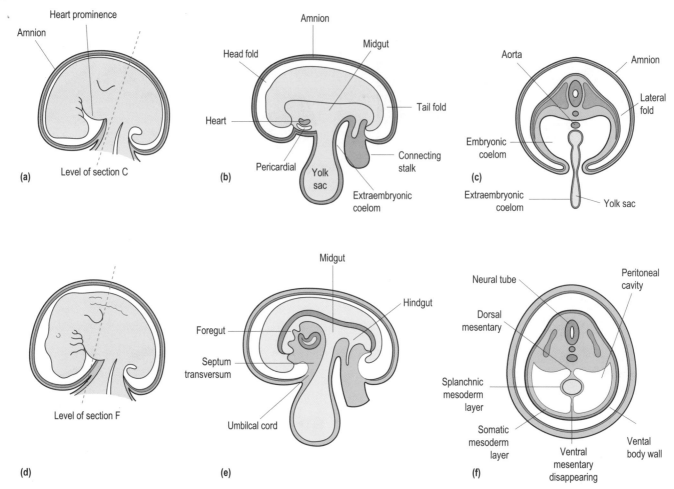

Figure 9.24 Drawings illustrating embryonic folding and its effects on the intraembryonic coelom and other structures. (Reproduced with permission from Moore 1989.)

Endoderm

• Tissues derived from endoderm include the epithelial linings of the alimentary tract and its glands, the liver and pancreas, the epithelial lining of the lower respiratory tract and of the bladder and urethra.

Folding of the embryo

Folding of cell sheets forms the basis of the early development of organs and folding of the embryo changes its shape and the relationships of the organs (Figs 9.24 and 9.25). Neurulation is a good example. A flat sheet of cells on the upper surface of the embryo folds up into a tube which develops into the brain and spinal cord. Events in the longitudinal and transverse planes are described separately.

Longitudinal folding

Longitudinal folding brings about flexion and development of the head and tail folds (Figs 9.26 and 9.27) and an

hourglass constriction of the yolk sac. There is partial extrusion of the yolk sac, the portion retained within the embryo being the gut. The portion of the yolk sac extruded from the embryo is called the **vitelline duct** which remains attached to the gut at the **vitellointestinal communication** and eventually disappears. When flexion is completed the brain overhangs the developing heart and the heart is ventral to the foregut. The midgut faces into the vitelline duct and the hindgut extends from the vitellointestinal communication to the cloacal membrane.

Transverse folding

The lateral margins of the embryonic disc form the lateral body folds which turn the embryo from a flattened disc into a cylinder. The peritoneal coelom on each side initially opened out into the extraembryonic coelom. Transverse folding directs these openings ventrally and, with the constriction of the yolk sac, the two openings communicate across the midline to form the peritoneal cavity.

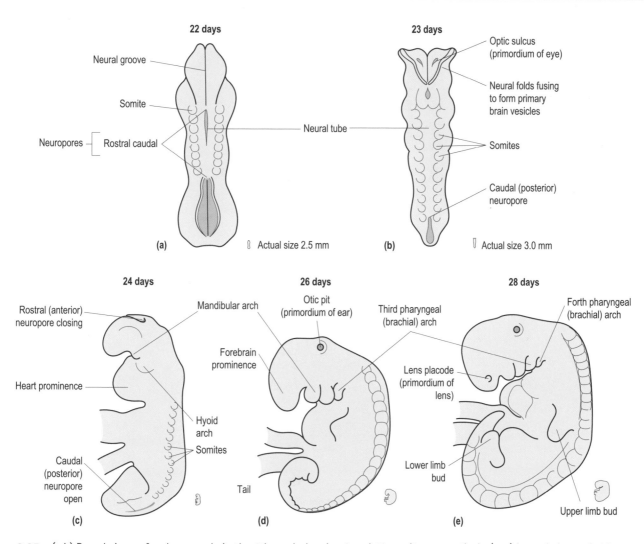

Figure 9.25   (a,b) Dorsal views of embryos early in the 4th week showing 8 and 12 somites respectively. (c–e) Lateral views of older embryos showing 16, 27 and 33 somites respectively. The rostral neuropore is normally closed by 25–26 days and the caudal neuropore by the end of the 4th week. (Reproduced with permission from Moore 1989.)

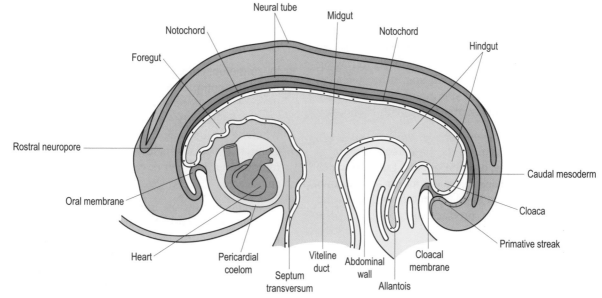

Figure 9.26   Longitudinal section of a 25-day embryo (from Fitzgerald M J T, Fitzgerald M 1994, with permission).

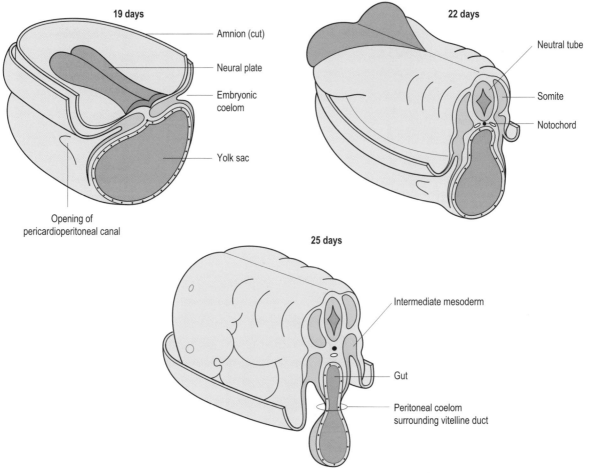

Figure 9.27   Schematic transverse sections depicting formation of the lateral body folds (from Fitzgerald M J T, Fitzgerald M 1994, with permission).

MAIN POINTS

- Gametogenesis allows the independent assortment of maternal and paternal chromosomes amongst the gametes. The oocyte contains all the material necessary for growth and development of the embryo following fertilisation. Millions of very small sperm are released during ejaculation. When one sperm enters a secondary oocyte the first cell of a new human being with 46 chromosomes is formed.

- When a capacitated sperm meets the corona radiata of the oocyte the acrosome reaction occurs. Lytic enzymes disperse the follicular cells of the corona radiata, allowing the head of the sperm to make contact with the zona pellucida. Other enzymes produce an opening in the zona pellucida.

- One sperm cell membrane fuses with the oocyte cell membrane and its nucleus passes into the oocyte. The ability of the oocyte to fuse with the sperm is lost immediately following entry of the first sperm to prevent polyspermy. Mitochondria and other organelles are inherited from the ovum.

- During embryology a programme of simple instructions generates complex forms. Most developmental processes depend upon interaction of genetic and environmental factors. Each body system has its developmental pattern whereby embryonic cells change shape and position. Cellular processes include somatic cell division, cell differentiation, induction, cell migration and programmed cell death.

- Cleavage occurs as the very large zygote splits into smaller cells called blastomeres through the process of mitosis. By the 4th day after fertilisation there are between 16 and 20 cells and the conceptus is known as the morula. The cells at this stage are totipotent and if separated there is the potential for identical individuals.

- Regulation of the complex development of the embryo is by a cascade of gene products. Homeobox genes switched on sequentially by chemical gradients produce their protein products which control segmentation in the developing embryo so that the correct positioning of organs is brought about.

- During early development some embryonic tissues influence the development of adjacent tissues. These influencing tissues are called inductors or organisers.

- The group of cells carries on cleaving during the next 4 days. There is also polarisation, with internal cells differing from external cells. The inner cells divide less frequently and remain large and round, whereas the outer cells in contact with the zona pellucida become flattened.

- On the 5th day the zygote 'hatches' as the zona pellucida is digested by uterine secretions. Fluid accumulates in the space between the peripheral and central cells of the morula and the conceptus becomes a blastocyst. The inner embryoblast becomes the embryo and the flattened outer trophoblast forms the placenta.

- On the 6th day the blastocyst begins to implant into the endometrium. Where trophoblastic cells touch the endometrium they become cuboid, forming the cytotrophoblast. Daughter cells form a syncytium which produces enzymes that attack the endometrium and hormones such as hCG which maintains the maternal corpus luteum and continued production of oestrogen and progesterone until the placenta produces them at 12 weeks. At the implantation site new blood capillaries develop.

- During embryogenesis and organogenesis cells migrate throughout the embryo to differentiate into specific cell types forming organs. Formation of the primitive streak, gastrulation and formation of the notochord are important in creating the body plan. From day 20 until day 30 the dorsal surface of the embryo develops paired somites from which the vertebral column and the segmentally innervated muscles of the trunk originate.

- Tissues derived from neuroectoderm include the central and peripheral nervous systems, the retina of the eye and the posterior lobe of the pituitary gland. Tissues derived from surface ectoderm include the epidermis with its hair follicles and cutaneous glands, the breasts, the lens of the eye, the special sense cells of the inner ear, the anterior lobe of the pituitary gland and tooth enamel.

- During neurulation a flat sheet of cells on the upper surface of the embryo folds up into a tube which develops into the brain and spinal cord. The cranial neuropore closes about day 25 and the caudal neuropore about day 27. This early closure of the neural tube has implications for the causation and prevention of open neural tube defects.

- Folding of cell sheets forms the basis of the early development of organs and folding of the embryo changes its shape and the relationships of the organs. Longitudinal folding and transverse folding of the sheets of cells both occur in the early embryo.

References

Alberts B, Johnson A, Lewis J et al 2002 Molecular Biology of the Cell, 4th edn. Garland Science, Taylor & Francis Group, London.

Fitzgerald M J T, Fitzgerald M 1994 Human Embryology. Baillière Tindall, London.

Human Fertilisation and Embryology Act 1990. HMSO, London.

Larsen W J 2001 Human Embryology, 3rd edn. Churchill Livingstone, Edinburgh.

McGinnis W, Kuziora M 1994 The molecular architects of body design. Scientific American February:36–42.

Moore K L, Persaud T V N 1998 Before We Are Born, 5th edn. W B Saunders, Philadelphia.

Nusslein-Volhard C 1996 Gradients that organise embryo development. Scientific American August:38–43.

Wolpert L 1991 The Triumph of the Embryo. Oxford University Press, Oxford.

Wolpert L, Beddington R, Jessel T et al 2002 Principles of Development, 2nd edn. Oxford University Press, Oxford.

Annotated recommended reading

Larsen W J 2001 Human Embryology, 3rd edn. Churchill Livingstone, Edinburgh.
  This book examines both molecular biological and clinical aspects of embryology. Each chapter is about a specific embryological stage and the clinical applications arising out of the advancing knowledge base.

McGinnis W, Kuziora M 1994 The molecular architects of body design. Scientific American February:36–42.
  This article provides a clear overview on the conservation of control of body plan throughout the animal kingdom.

Moore K L, Persaud T V N 1998 Before We Are Born, 5th edn. W B Saunders, Philadelphia.
  This textbook clearly describes embryo development week by week and provides an excellent source for understanding the origins of congenital defects. The illustrations in this latest edition are excellent.

Nusslein-Volhard C 1996 Gradients that organise embryo development. Scientific American August:38–43.
  For anyone wishing to understand how the early embryo develops the axes that lead to final body plan this article is clear and well illustrated.

Chapter 10

Embryological systems 1 – trunk, head and limbs

INTRODUCTION

This chapter and the next explain when and how normal systems develop and are a knowledge base for the understanding of congenital abnormalities. Explanations will be kept simple as the student is not expected to be an expert.

THE TRUNK

Skeletal features

The vertebral column

There are three phases in the development of the vertebral column (Fig. 10.1): **precartilaginous**, **cartilaginous** and **bony** (Moore & Persaud 1998).

Precartilaginous phase   Precursors of the vertebrae called **sclerotomes** are derived from the **somites**. Mesenchymal cells surround the **notochord** to form the segmented **mesenchymal vertebral column**. The cranial end of each mesenchymal vertebra is thinner than the caudal end because of a relative sparseness of cells. The cells at the interface between the two tissues form an intervertebral disc and the remainder of the condensed element merges with the vertebra caudal to it to form the centrum. As this is formed from parts of two sclerotomes, it is an intersegmental structure. From the condensed upper part of the centrum a pair of **neural arches** grows and surrounds the neural tube, giving rise to pairs of costal and transverse processes.

Cartilaginous phase   **Chondrification centres** appear in the centrum and the neural arch late in the 5th week. In the 12 thoracic vertebrae the cartilaginous costal processes which will develop into the ribs become detached from their parent neural arches by the formation of synovial joints. Synovial joints also appear between the costal and transverse processes. The remaining costal processes are incorporated into the vertebrae.

Bony phase   During the 8th week ossification centres appear in the central and neural arches and in the ribs. Ossification of the whole skeleton is not completed until the 25th year.

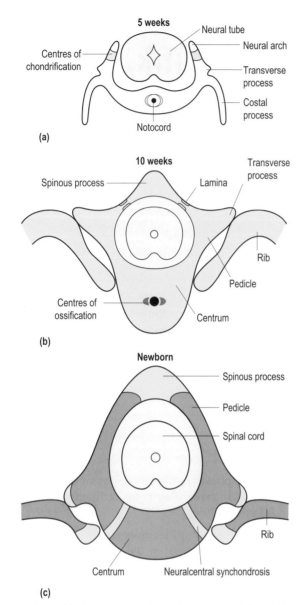

Figure 10.1   (a) Blastemal vertebra with centres of chondrification (shaded dark). (b) Cartilaginous vertebra with centres of ossification (shaded dark). (c) Bony vertebra (from Fitzgerald M J T, Fitzgerald M 1994, with permission).

Ribs and sternum

As the lateral body folds develop in the 4th week, the somatic mesoderm is penetrated from the thoracic costal processes. These induce the mesoderm to add to their tips, completing the formation of the prechondrial ribs. Two sternal bars develop in the ventral part of the somatic mesoderm which meet in the midline and unite to form a prechondrial sternum. The xiphisternum often remains bifid. The ventral ends of the seven cranial costal processes fuse with the sternum, and cartilage persists at the junction as the costal cartilages (Moore & Persaud 1998).

Soft tissues

During the 4th week the somites subdivide into three kinds of mesodermal primordia: **myotomes**, **dermatomes** and **sclerotomes** (Larsen 2001).

Myotomes

Myotomes give rise to all the muscles that link the vertebrae and skull together and the muscles of the abdominal and thoracic walls. Spinal nerves divide into **dorsal** and **ventral rami**. Dorsal rami supply the muscles with motor fibres originating in the ventral horn of the spinal cord. Ventral rami supply the muscles and their overlying dermatome with sensory fibres originating in the appropriate dorsal root ganglion. Limb muscles are not formed from myotomes.

Dermatomes

The dermatomes merge with each other and migrate to form the **dermis** layer of the skin. Each dermatome is accompanied by sensory nerve fibres derived from the level in the spinal cord that the dermatome originated. Neurologists divide the body surface into regions called dermatomes.

The skin and mammary glands

The dermis develops from the dermatomes but the **epidermis** and its appendages are derived from surface ectoderm. Surface ectoderm begins as a single cuboidal layer but becomes two-layered in the 2nd month. The superficial layer is shed, leaving the underlying germinal layer to form the structures of the skin. In the 3rd month the epidermis becomes stratified and its basal layer sends pegs down into the dermis to form the root sheath of the hair follicles. **Lanugo**, which is very fine hair, grows all over the body. True or **vellus hair** is derived from a second set of hair follicles and replaces lanugo, which is shed shortly before birth.

During the 5th month the sebaceous glands bud into the dermis from the root sheath and the sweat glands grow down from the epidermis. The sebaceous glands produce a secretion which, when mixed with peridermal cells and lanugo, becomes the vernix caseosa. The mammary glands make their appearance in the 6th week as paired strips of ectodermal thickening formed longitudinally on the ventral surface of the embryo called the mammary ridge. In humans only one pair of breasts forms from the thoracic part of the ridge and the rest of the ridge disappears.

THE SKULL

The adult skull forms from mesenchyme around the developing brain. It consists of the neurocranium, which encloses the brain, and the viscerocranium making up the bones of the face. The base of the skull or **chondrocranium** develops out of cartilage, while the **vault** bones (Ch. 24) develop from membrane (Moore & Persaud 1998). Intramembraneous ossification begins from the 4th month, separate ossification centres giving rise to the parietal bones, frontal bones, occipital bone and the squamous part of the temporal bone.

The viscerocranium

All the facial bones ossify in membrane, starting with the mandible early in the 6th week. Detailed development of the face is given later.

The teeth

Tooth buds form from thickened ectoderm called the **dental lamina**: 10 in the upper jaw and 10 in the lower jaw. These are responsible for the deciduous (milk) teeth. Later the dental lamina forms the buds of the permanent dentition. The permanent molar teeth do not have precursors in the deciduous dentition but develop from a backward extension of the dental lamina. The crowns of the teeth begin when cells called **odontoblasts** form predentine, which later calcifies to become dentine. This calcification signals cells called **ameloblasts** to lay down tooth enamel on the surface of the dentine. The central cells constitute the pulp of the tooth which is richly supplied with blood and sensory nerve endings as many of us can testify!

Deep to the level of enamel production the outer and inner enamel epithelia fuse to form the **epithelial root sheath**. Predentine and dentine are again induced to form the root of the tooth. The mesoderm of the dental sac produces a specialised form of bone called cement and the **periodontal ligament** which anchors the cement to the wall of the tooth socket. Eruption of the deciduous teeth normally occurs between 6 months and 2 years after birth.

THE BRAIN

A full description of the mature central nervous system brain is found in Chapter 26, p. 349. The neural tube cranial to the fourth pair of somites develops into the brain (Moore & Persaud 1998). The human nervous system begins to form approximately 19 days after fertilisation and is the earliest system to differentiate. The brain is a complex structure made up of separate sections with very different functions. By 19 days three expansions of the brain are present (Fig. 10.2). These primary brain vesicles (Moore & Persaud 1998) are:

- forebrain – **prosencephalon**;
- midbrain – **mesencephalon**;
- hindbrain – **rhombencephalon**.

From 4 weeks the major regions of the brain are distinct and neurons begin to differentiate from the epithelium of the neural tube. The **thalamus** and **hypothalamus** are differentiated by the 5th week (Fig. 10.3). By the end of the 8th

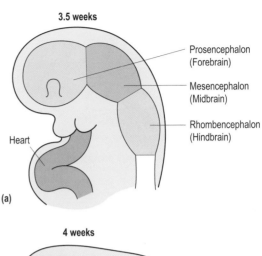

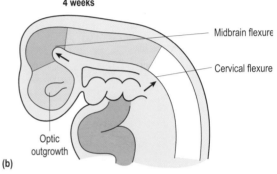

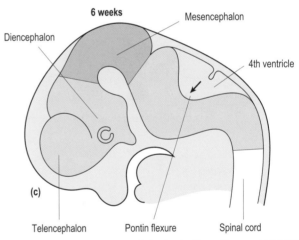

Figure 10.2   Early development of the brain (from Fitzgerald M J T, Fitzgerald M 1994, with permission).

week the head is equal to half the length of the embryo and controls the first movement of the limbs (McNabb 1997).

The changing shape of the brain

The brainstem buckles and a cervical flexure appears at the junction of the brainstem and spinal cord. A midline flexure moves the mesencephalon to the summit of the brain. The rhombencephalon folds on itself, causing the walls of the neural tube to expand into the fourth ventricle. The dorsal region of the prosencephalon expands on either side to form the cerebral hemispheres or **telencephalon**. Within the

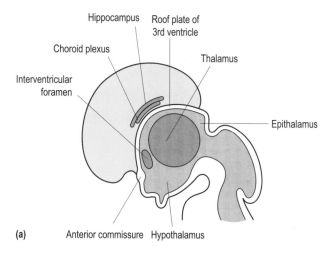

(a)

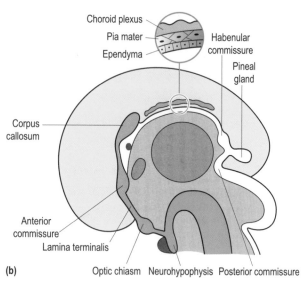

(b)

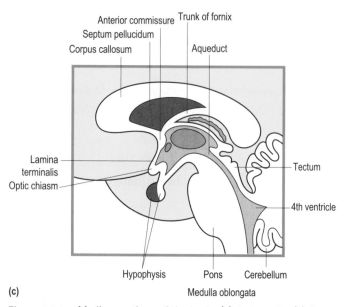

(c)

Figure 10.3   Median sections of the brain. (a) At 8 weeks. (b) At 12 weeks. (c) Postnatal (from Fitzgerald M J T, Fitzgerald M 1994, with permission).

cerebral hemispheres the neural canal dilates to form the lateral ventricles (Moore & Persaud 1998).

The remainder of the prosencephalon which straddles the midline is known as the diencephalon. The third ventricle, a cavity within the diencephalon, communicates with the fourth ventricle through the **aqueduct of Sylvius**. An outgrowth from the diencephalon becomes the two retinas and optic nerves. The cranial end of the rhombencephalon gives rise to the **pons** and the **cerebellum**, while the caudal end becomes the **medulla oblongata**.

The forebrain

Neurons migrate from the ventricular zone of the telencephalon to the surface to form the cerebral cortex. The frontal, parietal, occipital and temporal lobes are present by 12–14 weeks. Complex processes give rise to the structures within the cerebral hemispheres. Two **commissures** of nerve fibres link right and left cerebral hemispheres. The anterior commissure connects the olfactory regions and the much larger corpus callosum links matched areas of the cerebral cortex.

Other brain structures

The diencephalon gives rise to the **pineal gland**, the paired and linked thalami which contain about 30 separate nuclei (small discrete sections) and the hypothalamus. The **basal ganglia** develop immediately below the thalamus and are involved in the control of body movement.

Blood supply to the brain

The arterial blood supply develops from cranial segments of the **dorsal aortae**, comprising two **internal carotid arteries** and two **vertebral arteries**. The internal carotid arteries branch to form the **anterior**, **middle** and **posterior cerebral arteries**. Each vertebral artery gives off a branch which supplies the cerebellum and medulla oblongata before uniting with its partner to form the **basilar artery**. This gives off two pairs of arteries to the cerebellum and upper brainstem before dividing into two terminal branches that link up with the ends of the internal carotid arteries. These intercommunicating arteries at the base of the brain are known as the **circle of Willis**. The venous drainage is discussed in Chapter 24, p. 332.

THE SPINAL CORD

Following the closure of the neural tube and the formation of the somites, neural crest cells form clusters corresponding to the somites. Corresponding levels of the neural tube develop from the primitive streak during the process of secondary neurulation. At first, the neural tube is solid but becomes canalised by caudal extension of the neural canal.

Zones of the spinal cord

During the 5th week three zones can be distinguished in the side walls of the neural tube. From within outwards, these are the **ventricular**, **intermediate** and **marginal zones**.

- The ventricular zone is where neuroepithelial cells divide. After several cell divisions daughter cells move out of the ventricular zone. The first cells to move out become neurons and the last become the connective tissue cells called **neuroglia**.

- The intermediate zone is the forerunner of the grey matter of the spinal cord and is composed of **neuroblasts** that have migrated from the ventricular zone. These differentiate into neurons. **Glioblasts** enter the intermediate zone and differentiate into **astrocytes**, which provide structural support for the central nervous system (CNS), and **oligodendrocytes** which form **myelin sheaths**. Phagocytic microglial cells develop from blood monocytes and migrate from the capillary bed to the CNS during the 3rd month.

- The marginal zone is the forerunner of the white matter of the spinal cord. Small neurons invade the marginal zone and emit axons alongside the grey matter to form pathways that link the different levels of the spinal cord.

During the 6th week an accumulation of neuroblasts in the dorsolateral plate gives rise to the sensory **dorsal horn** of grey matter. The dorsal horn communicates with neural crest cells that have accumulated outside the neural tube to form **dorsal root ganglia**. Large accumulations of cells in the ventrolateral plate form the motor **ventral horn** of grey matter. Axons emerging from the ventral horn form the **ventral nerve roots**, joining with peripheral processes to form mixed spinal nerves.

During weeks 7–10 the spinal cord is formed. The neural canal shrinks to become the central canal of the spinal cord. Cells left behind in the ventricular zone develop cilia and become the lining cells of the central canal called ependymal cells. The discrete ascending and descending columns in the white matter are finalised.

Cells from the neural crest

Neural crest cells are **pluripotent** and the following cell types are thought to originate in the neural crest, many of them involved in regulation of body systems:

- the dorsal root ganglia cells;
- autonomic ganglion cells;
- the **chromaffin cells** of the adrenal medulla;
- the **Schwann cells** producing myelin sheaths;
- the **pia mater** and **arachnoid mater** around the brain and spinal cord;
- the **melanocytes** of the skin;
- the connective tissue in the wall of the heart and great vessels;

- **parafollicular cells** of the thyroid gland;
- the **glomus cells** of the carotid and aortic bodies;
- much of the craniofacial skeleton;
- the odontoblasts of the developing teeth.

STRUCTURES OF THE HEAD AND NECK

Pharyngeal apparatus

The pharyngeal (formerly known as branchial) apparatus, (Moore & Persaud 1998), consists of:

- **pharyngeal arches**;
- **pharyngeal pouches**;
- **pharyngeal grooves**;
- **pharyngeal membranes**.

Pharyngeal arches

Head and neck mesoderm originates from two sources: the paraxial mesoderm and the neural crest. The pharyngeal arches begin to develop early in the 4th week as neural crest cells migrate into the future head and neck region. During the 5th week a side view of the embryo shows five pairs of arches. These are numbered I, II, III, IV and VI in craniocaudal sequence. In mammals a fifth pair may never develop or is transient (Larsen 2001).

These mesodermal arches are remnants of the gill arches (branchia) in fishes. However, in mammals there are no gill slits and the arches are linked by mesoderm (Fig. 10.4). On the surface ectoderm there are thickenings of ectoderm called placodes; three are the nasal placode, lens placode and otic placode, whilst four contribute sensory ganglion cells to the cranial nerves. Most malformations of the head and neck happen during transformation of pharyngeal arch structures into their final form.

The structure of the pharyngeal arches

Every arch contains the following structures:

1. migrated neural crest cells surrounding a central core of mesenchyme cells;
2. unsegmented mesoderm which can form muscle and bone;
3. an artery that branches of the dorsal aorta on the same side as the arch;
4. a nerve carrying motor fibres called branchial efferents to support the striated muscles;
5. an external covering of ectoderm;
6. an internal covering of endoderm.

Pharyngeal pouches and grooves

Pockets called pharyngeal pouches develop between the pharyngeal arches from endoderm. There are four well-defined pairs and a rudimentary fifth pair. The primitive

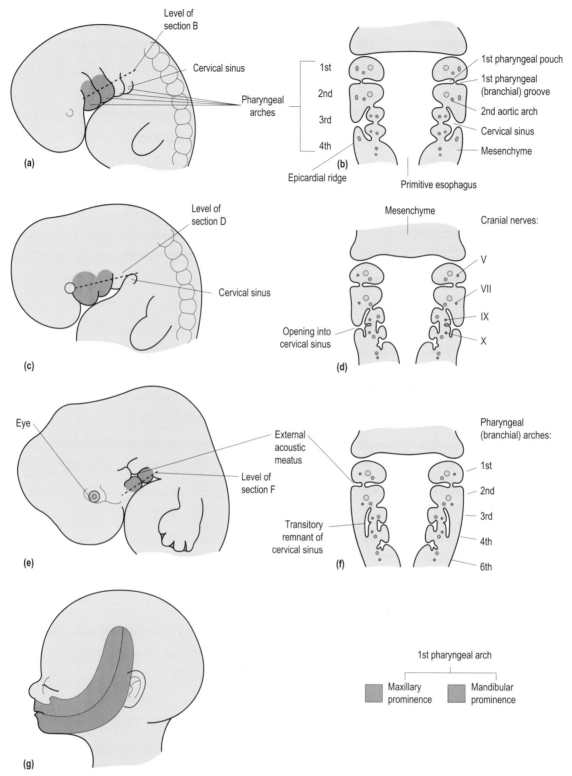

Figure 10.4   (a) Lateral view of the head, neck and thoracic regions of an embryo (about 32 days), showing the pharyngeal arches and cervical sinus. (b) Diagrammatic section through the embryo at the level shown in (a), illustrating growth of the second arch over the third and fourth arches. (c) An embryo of about 33 days. (d) Section of the embryo at the level shown in (c), illustrating early closure of the cervical sinus. (e) An embryo of about 41 days. (f) Section of the embryo at the level shown in (e), showing the transitory cystic remnant of the cervical sinus. (g) Drawing of a 20-week fetus illustrating the area of the face derived from the first pair of pharyngeal arches. (Reproduced with permission from Moore 1989.)

pharynx develops from the foregut and widens cranially. It is lined by the endoderm covering the internal surfaces of the pharyngeal arches. Externally, the pharyngeal arches are separated by pockets of ectoderm named pharyngeal grooves.

Derivatives of the pharyngeal arches

First pharyngeal arch

The first pair or **mandibular arches** are involved in the development of the face. The cartilage of this arch forms **Meckel's cartilage** which serves as a template for the development of the **mandible**. During the 6th week the mandible develops around the ventral portion of the cartilage by ossification of surrounding membrane and the cartilage mostly disappears. The dorsal end of Meckel's cartilage is incorporated into the middle ear to form the **malleus** and **incus**. From the dorsal part of each mandibular arch develop the mandibular prominence and the maxillary prominence.

Second pharyngeal arch

The second pair or **hyoid arches** have a much smaller skeletal component than the first. Their dorsal ends form the **stapes** of the middle ear and the **styloid process** of the temporal bone. The ventral ends form part of the **hyoid bone**. Most of the mesoderm migrates to form the muscles of facial expression. The sensory facial nerve supplies the muscles formed from the hyoid arches.

Third pharyngeal arch

The third pair forms the posterior part of the tongue and the lower half of the hyoid bone. The **stylopharyngeus muscle** running from the styloid process of the temporal bone to the pharynx is the only muscle formed from this arch. It is innervated by the **glossopharyngeal nerve** which also carries the sensory nerve fibres for taste at the posterior part of the tongue. The artery of this arch persists as part of the internal carotid artery.

Fourth and sixth pharyngeal arches

These form the cartilages, ligaments and muscles of the larynx. The nerve supply to the muscles is via the vagus nerve through laryngeal and pharyngeal branches. The left artery of the fourth arch contributes to the arch of the aorta, while the right one forms most of the right subclavian artery.

Derivatives of the pharyngeal pouches

Derivatives of the pharyngeal pouches are:

- first pouch – the **Eustachian tube** and the **middle ear cavity**;
- second pouch – the **tonsils**;
- third pouch – the **thymus gland** and **inferior parathyroid gland**;
- fourth pouch/fifth pouch – **superior parathyroid gland**, **parafollicular** and **C cells** of the **thyroid gland**.

The thyroid gland is the first endocrine gland to develop, arising during the 4th week from a thickening of midline endoderm in the floor of the pharynx. The median rudiment bifurcates, forming two lobes connected by an isthmus. By 7 weeks the thyroid gland reaches its final destination in the neck.

The tongue develops from five tongue buds, the first or median tongue bud develops at the end of the 4th week on the floor of the pharynx. Two distal tongue buds develop on each side of the median tongue bud and overgrow it to merge together to form the anterior or oral two-thirds of the tongue. The posterior part of the tongue develops from mesoderm in the third and fourth branchial arches.

Derivatives of the pharyngeal grooves

The first pharyngeal groove is the only one that contributes to final structures, forming the **external canal of the ear**. The others form a deep ectodermal depression called the **cervical sinus** during the 5th week. The cervical sinus is obliterated by the 7th week, giving the neck a smooth contour.

THE FACE

The development of the face is complex and it is not possible to cover every detail (Fig. 10.5). The primitive mouth begins as a slight depression of the surface ectoderm called the **stomodeum**. It is separated from the foregut by the **oropharyngeal membrane** which ruptures about day 24 to bring the digestive tract into communication with the amniotic cavity. Early in the 4th week, five prominences emerge around the stomodeum: the frontonasal prominence, two pairs of mandibular and two pairs of maxillary prominences. These merge with each other and are covered by surface ectoderm.

The mandibular prominence forms the lower jaw or mandible and the maxillary prominence gives rise to the upper jaw or **maxilla**, the zygomatic bone and the squamous portion of the temporal bone as well as the outer parts of the upper lip. Mandibular arch mesoderm forms the muscles of mastication which are inserted into the mandible. These muscles are innervated by the mandibular branch of the **trigeminal nerve**. The skin of the face and mucous membranes of the mouth are formed from mandibular arch ectoderm. They receive a somatic sensory nerve supply from the three branches of the trigeminal nerve: **ophthalmic**, **maxillary** and **mandibular**.

By the end of the 4th week bilateral thickenings of the ectoderm called **nasal placodes** appear. The formation of the nose, palate and upper lip begins early in the 5th week

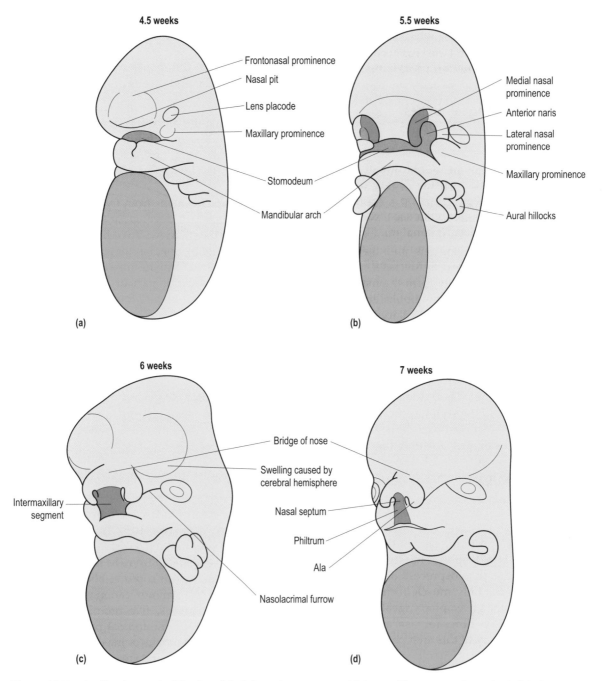

Figure 10.5a–d Development of the face. Medial nasal processes and intermaxillary segment are shaded dark (from Fitzgerald M J T, Fitzgerald M 1994, with permission).

when the two nasal placodes recede into **nasal pits** whose openings become the nostrils. A week later the frontonasal prominence extends onto both sides of the nasal pits to form the medial and lateral nasal prominences. The two medial nasal prominences merge across the midline to form the **intermaxillary segment**. During the 7th week this produces three midline structures: the lower border of the **nasal septum**, the **philtrum** of the upper lip and the **primary palate**. If these structures fail to develop cleft lip and palate result.

THE EARS

The outer and middle ear

The **pinna** (auricle) of the ear develops from six **aural hillocks**, three on the first pharyngeal arch and three on the second. It begins in the upper part of the neck and is displaced cranially during development of the mandible. The first pharyngeal cleft gives rise to the **external acoustic** meatus (outer ear canal). The middle ear cavity extends outwards from the first pharyngeal pouch during the 5th week. It makes contact with the outer ear canal and where they meet a thin layer of mesoderm forms the **tympanic membrane** (eardrum). The ear ossicles develop from the dorsal ends of the first and second pharyngeal arches.

The inner ear

At the end of the 3rd week, an **otic placode** develops on either side of the head. These sink below the surface to form the **otic vesicles** (otocysts) which develop a **vestibular sac** and a **cochlear sac**. From the vestibular sac three plate-like expansions become the **semicircular canals** and the remainder of the sac becomes the **utricle**. From the cochlear sac the coiled **cochlea** containing the **organ of Corti** arises and the remainder becomes the **saccule**. A shell of chondrified mesoderm surrounds the membranous labyrinth and ossifies to become the bony labyrinth. The **vestibulocochlear nerve** originates from neural crest cells. The inner ear, tympanic cavity and ossicles are almost full sized at birth but the outer ear is short and easily damaged by insertion of objects into the canal.

THE EYES

In the 4th week two important events happen in the development of the eyes (Fig. 10.6):

● the **optic vesicles** develop as an outgrowth of the diencephalon, remaining attached to it by the **optic stalk**;
● under the inducing influence of the optic vesicles the lenses develop as an ingrowth of a thickened patch of surface ectoderm – the **lens placode**.

As the lens vesicle sinks inwards, the optic vesicle becomes a double-walled optic cup by invagination. This creates the **optic fissure** on the under surface of the optic cup and its stalk. Before the lips of the optic fissure come together during the 6th week it is infiltrated by mesenchyme (Fig. 10.7). Within the cup the mesenchyme produces a gelatinous secretion that fills the **vitreous component** of the eye. During the 5th and 6th weeks, a shell of mesenchyme covers the outer surface of the optic cup and differentiates into the vascular **choroid coat** of the eyeball and the outer fibrous coat consisting of the **sclera** and **cornea**. The six **extraocular muscles** develop from mesoderm. The cells in the posterior wall of the lens vesicle elongate and lay down primary **lens** fibres. Secondary lens fibres are laid down later by cells migrating into the interior from the margins of the lens.

The optic cup

The outer epithelium of the optic cup accumulates **melanin pigment** and becomes the pigmented layer of the **retina**.

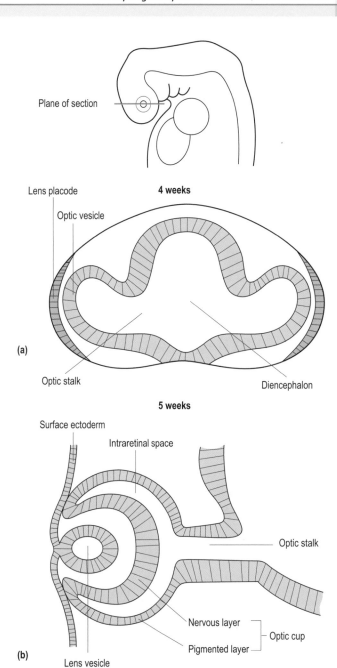

Figure 10.6   Early development of the eye (from Fitzgerald M J T, Fitzgerald M 1994, with permission).

Around the rim of the cup the outer and inner layers form the **ciliary body** and the **iris**. The ciliary muscles develop from ectomesenchymal cells in the ciliary body and the sphincter and dilator muscles of the pupil develop from the posterior epithelium of the iris. The inner epithelium of the optic cup becomes the nervous layer of the retina, differentiating into the various visual sensory cells. The axons of these neurons converge on the optic stalk and form the **optic nerve**, which is an extension of the white matter of the CNS.

The ciliary processes secrete **aqueous humour** which accumulates between the cornea and the lens. Between the iris and cornea is the anterior chamber and between the iris and the lens is the posterior chamber. Aqueous humour

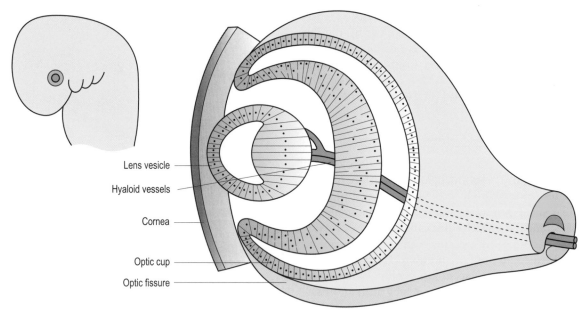

Figure 10.7   The eye at 6 weeks, showing the optic fissure (from Fitzgerald M J T, Fitzgerald M 1994, with permission).

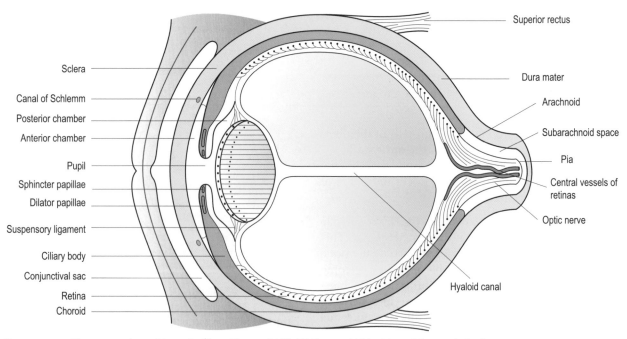

Figure 10.8   The eye at about 20 weeks (from Fitzgerald M J T, Fitzgerald M 1994, with permission).

moves from posterior to anterior chamber through the pupil and then into a small vein encircling the eye at the anterior margin of the choroid coat called the **canal of Schlemm**. The eye is more or less complete by 20 weeks (Fig. 10.8).

The eyelids and lacrimal apparatus

The eyelids develop from mesodermal folds lined by surface ectoderm that grow to meet each other in front of the cornea during the 2nd month. From the 3rd to the 6th months the eyelids are fused, allowing clinicians to esti-

mate the gestational age of a very premature baby. The **lacrimal glands** develop from the outer part of the conjunctival sac and are an exocrine gland. It is said that newborns do not produce tears but there is a continuous lacrimal secretion to protect the cornea.

THE LIMBS

When the author was studying for her BA a visiting lecturer (Lewis Wolpert) asked a question, 'How do limbs know when to stop making one bone and change to two and then

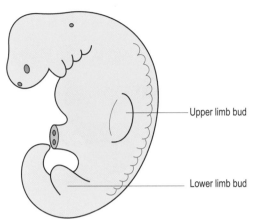

Figure 10.9   Limb buds at 4 weeks (from Fitzgerald M J T, Fitzgerald M 1994, with permission).

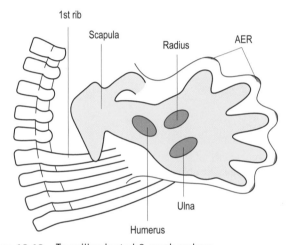

Figure 10.10   Transilluminated 6-week embryo.

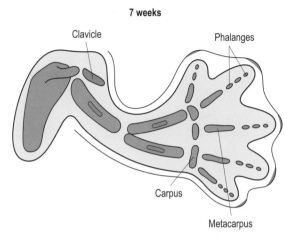

Figure 10.11   Upper limb skeleton at 7 weeks. Centres of ossification (red) have appeared in the clavicle and in three major long bones (from Fitzgerald M J T, Fitzgerald M 1994, with permission).

to form multiple bones at the wrist and ankle terminating in five digits and how do the two arms end up the same length?' These are profound questions in developmental biology – what controls the process of development from a single cell to a complete organism? Some answers are beginning to be found and are referred to in Chapter 9. This encounter fired the author's interest in embryology.

Development of the limbs

The limbs form from the somatic mesoderm of the lateral body wall (Figs 10.9–10.13). Minute upper limb buds appear in the middle of the 4th week at the level of the lower cervical somites. The lower limb buds appear 2 days later at the level of the lower lumbar somites. This is typical of the **craniocaudal development** of the fetus (Moore & Persaud 1998).

Development of the limbs is regulated by **Hox genes** (Wolpert et al 2002). Proliferation of somatic mesodermal cells is induced in each limb by the **apical ectodermal ridge** (AER), a thickening of surface ectoderm over the limb bud (Larsen 2001). This covers the whole surface at first but is later confined to the growing tip of the limb. The limb bud is filled with loose mesenchyme. Cell division in the mesenchyme is restricted to a progress zone immediately below the AER. Daughter cells separate out from this zone and add to the limb's length.

Formation of the hands and feet

During the 5th week the hands and feet develop in the form of flat limb plates. The AER breaks up into five ridges that mark the positions of the future digits. Each of these induces and maintains a progress zone which lays down a rod of mesoderm. The five rods are called **digital rays**. Webs of loose mesenchyme connect the rays but programmed cell death creates **interdigital clefts**.

Development and rotation of the limbs

The limb skeleton passes through precartilaginous, cartilaginous and ossification stages, except the clavicle, which develops from membrane. During the 5th week condensations of the limb mesenchyme form a rough skeletal plan. Later in that week chondrification centres appear and, by the end of the 6th week, the skeleton is fully cartilagineous. By the end of the 7th week ossification begins and primary ossification centres are present in the limb long bones by the 12th week (Moore & Persaud 1998). Ossification of the ankle bones begins late in fetal life but the wrist bones remain cartilaginous until after birth. At first the limbs grow out laterally from the trunk but during the 8th week the limbs rotate to bring them into the human position. Elbow and knee creases appear.

Muscles and nerves of the limbs

The skeletal muscle of the arms and legs develops from cells which migrate from the nearest somites, while tendons

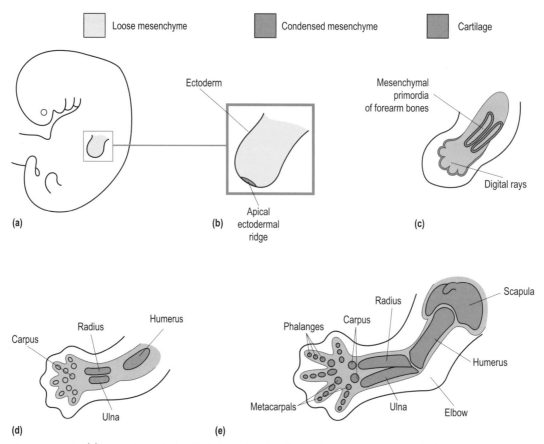

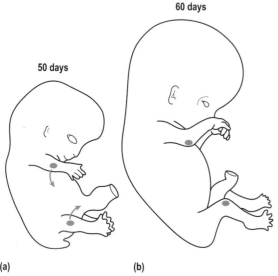

Figure 10.12 (a) An embryo at about 28 days, showing the early appearance of the limb buds. (b) Schematic drawing of a longitudinal section through an upper limb bud. The apical ectodermal ridge has an inductive influence on the mesenchyme and appears to give it the ability to form specific cartilaginous elements. (c) Similar sketch of an upper limb bud at about 33 days, showing the mesenchymal primordia of the limb bones. The digital rays are mesenchymal condensations that undergo chondrification and ossification to form the bones of the hand. (d) Upper limb at 6 weeks showing the cartilage models of the bones. (e) Later in the 6th week showing the completed cartilaginous models of the bones of the upper limb. (Reproduced with permission from Moore 1989.)

Figure 10.13 Positions of the extensor aspects (red marks) of elbow and knee (a) before and (b) after rotation of the limbs (from Fitzgerald M J T, Fitzgerald M 1994, with permission).

develop from somatic mesoderm already present in the limb buds. Spinal nerves called **ventral rami** invade the limbs in their original positions prior to rotation. They are mixed nerves carrying motor fibres from the ventral grey horn of the spinal cord and sensory fibres from dorsal root ganglia (Larsen 2001). The 31 pairs of spinal nerves are named by the first letter of the name and the number of the vertebra from above downwards:

- cervical = C1–8;
- thoracic = T1–12;
- lumbar = L1–5;
- sacral = S1–5.

There is also one coccygeal nerve. Neural crest cells surround these nerves, forming myelin sheaths (Moore & Persaud 1998). The upper limbs receive nerves from vertebrae C5 to T1 while the lower limbs are invaded by nerves from L2 to S2.

Blood supply to the limbs

The limb buds are invaded early by branches of the **intersegmental** blood vessels. A single **axial** artery is later displaced by the developing skeleton and replaced by new blood vessels. In the upper limb these are the **axillary**, **brachial** and **interosseous** arteries with the brachial artery branching into the **radial** and **ulnar** arteries to supply the forearm and hand. In the lower limb the **popliteal** and **peroneal** arteries replace the axial artery, and the **femoral** artery develops to join the popliteal artery, which branches into the anterior and posterior tibial arteries to supply the lower leg and foot.

MAIN POINTS

- Three phases lead to the development of the bony vertebral column: the precartilaginous, cartilaginous and bony phases.

- Myotomes give rise to the muscles of the head and trunk. Dermatomes merge with each other and migrate to form the dermis layer of the skin. Each dermatome is accompanied by sensory nerve fibres derived from the level in the spinal cord that the dermatome originated.

- Lanugo grows all over the body and the sebaceous glands produce a secretion which, when mixed with peridermal cells and lanugo, becomes the vernix caseosa. True or vellus hair replaces lanugo shortly before birth. Mammary glands appear in the 6th week as paired longitudinal strips of ectodermal thickening on the embryonic ventral surface.

- The adult skull is divided into the neurocranium, which encloses the brain, and the viscerocranium making up the bones of the face. Intramembraneous ossification begins in the vault of the skull from the 4th month with separate ossification centres giving rise to the parietal bones, frontal bones, occipital bone and the squamous part of the temporal bone.

- Tooth buds form from thickened ectoderm called dental lamina. These are responsible for the deciduous teeth. Later the dental lamina forms the buds of the permanent dentition. Eruption of deciduous teeth occurs between 6 months and 2 years after birth.

- The human nervous system is the earliest system to differentiate. By 19 days three primary brain vesicles of the brain are present: the forebrain or prosencephalon, the midbrain or mesencephalon and the hindbrain or rhombencephalon.

- Neurons migrate to form the cerebral cortex. Frontal, parietal, occipital and temporal lobes are present at 14 weeks. Two commissures of nerve fibres link the right and left cerebral hemispheres – the anterior commissure connects the olfactory regions and the corpus callosum links matched areas of the cerebral cortex.

- At first the neural tube is solid but it becomes canalised by caudal extension of the neural canal. During the 6th week neuroblasts in the dorsolateral plate give rise to the sensory dorsal horn of grey matter. Accumulations of cells in the ventrolateral plate form the motor ventral horn. During week 7 to week 10 the spinal cord is finalised.

- Five mesodermal pairs of pharyngeal arches develop on the future head and neck region. The first pair is involved in the development of the face. The second forms the stapes of the middle ear and the styloid process of the temporal bone, part of the hyoid bone and the muscles of facial expression. The third forms the posterior part of the tongue and the lower half of the hyoid bone. The fourth and sixth form the cartilages, ligaments and muscles of the larynx.

- Derivatives of the first pharyngeal pouches are the Eustachian tube and the middle ear cavity. The second pouch forms the tonsils. The third pouch forms the thymus gland and inferior parathyroid gland and the fourth/fifth pouches form the cells of the thyroid gland.

- The primitive mouth begins as a slight depression of the surface ectoderm called the stomodeum. It is separated from the foregut by the oropharyngeal membrane which ruptures about day 24 to bring the digestive tract into communication with the amniotic cavity.

- The pinna of the ear develops from six aural hillocks, three on the first pharyngeal arch and three on the second. The first pharyngeal cleft gives rise to the outer ear canal. The middle ear cavity extends outwards during the 5th week to make contact with the outer ear canal. Where they meet a thin layer of mesoderm forms the eardrum. Otic placodes develop on either side of the head and sink below the surface to form the semicircular canals.

- Between the 3rd and 6th weeks development of the eye takes place. The eyelids develop during the 2nd month but are fused from the 3rd to the 6th months. The exocrine lacrimal glands develop from the outer part of the conjunctival sac.

- The limbs form from the somatic mesoderm of the lateral body wall in a craniocaudal pattern. Minute upper limb buds appear in the middle of the 4th week at the level of the lower cervical somites and lower limb buds appear 2 days later at the level of the lower lumbar somites.

- During the 5th week the hands and feet develop as flat limb plates. The apical epidermal breaks up into five ridges that mark the positions of the future digits. Each lays down a rod of mesoderm called a digital ray. Webs of loose mesenchyme connect the rays but programmed cell death creates interdigital clefts. At first the limbs grow out laterally from the trunk. During the 8th week the limbs rotate to bring them into the human position.

References

Larsen W J 2001 Human Embryology, 3rd edn. Churchill Livingstone, Edinburgh.

McNabb M 1997 Embryonic and fetal developments. In Sweet B R, Tiran D (eds) Mayes Midwifery, 12th edn. Baillière Tindall, London, pp 89–105.

Moore K L, Persaud T V N 1998 Before We Are Born, 5th edn. W B Saunders, Philadelphia.

Wolpert L, Beddington R, Jessel T et al 2002 Principles of Development, 2nd edn. Oxford University Press, Oxford.

Annotated recommended reading

Larsen W J 2001 Human Embryology, 3rd edn. Churchill Livingstone, Edinburgh.
This book examines both molecular biological and clinical aspects of embryology. Each chapter is about a specific embryological stage and the clinical applications arising out of the advancing knowledge base.

Moore K L, Persaud T V N 1998 Before We Are Born, 5th edn. W B Saunders, Philadelphia.
The layout of this textbook remains excellent. It clearly describes embryo development week by week and provides an excellent source for understanding the origins of congenital defects. The illustrations in this latest edition are excellent.

Chapter 11

Embryological systems 2 – internal organs

THE CARDIOVASCULAR SYSTEM

The cardiovascular system must be in place early in the embryo before it becomes too big to receive nourishment by diffusion (McNabb 1997). From the end of the 3rd week the embryo must obtain nutrients from the maternal circulation. The cardiovascular system is able to pump blood around vessels early in the 4th week.

Blood

At about day 17 **blood islands** appear in the extraembryonic mesoderm lining the yolk sac (Larsen 2001). The central cells of these islands are the **haemacytoblasts** which become primitive nucleated red blood cells. The peripheral cells are called **angioblasts** and form a capillary endothelium around each of the blood islands (Fig. 11.1).

There are three phases of blood cell formation (Fig. 11.2):

1. The **yolk sac period** from weeks 3–12.
2. The **hepatic period** from weeks 5–36 when clones of blood-forming cells migrate to the spleen.
3. The **bone marrow period** from week 12 of fetal life and for the rest of the individual's life. During week 12 clones settle in the spleen, liver and bone marrow and produce red blood cells, while clones settling in the bone marrow, thymus and lymph nodes produce white blood cells.

All red cells contain the red pigment haemoglobin but in cells made in the yolk sac and liver the haemoglobin is fetal or HbF which takes up and releases O_2 and CO_2 more readily than adult haemoglobin. Red cells produced by the bone marrow are mature. They lose their nucleus and contain adult haemoglobin or HbA.

Development of arteries

Three parts of the embryonic arterial system develop:

1. A pair of **umbilical arteries** carry blood to the placenta.
2. **Vitelline arteries** arise from the dorsal aortas linking up with the capillary bed of the yolk sac. These eventually become the three **mesenteric arteries** supplying the gut.

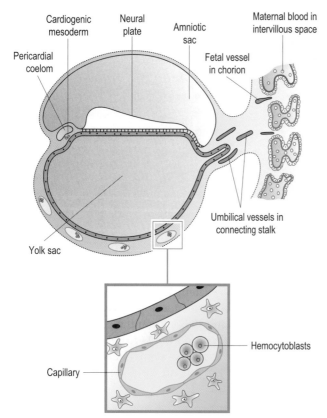

Figure 11.1 Longitudinal section of 18-day embryo, showing primitive vasculature (from Fitzgerald M J T, Fitzgerald M 1994, with permission).

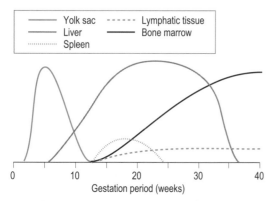

Figure 11.2 Sites and times of haemopoiesis (from Fitzgerald M J T, Fitzgerald M 1994, with permission).

3. **Intersegmental arteries** supply blood to the somites and neural tube.

As the pharyngeal arches form during the 4th and 5th weeks they are supplied by **aortic arches** arising from the aortic sac and terminating in the **dorsal aortas** running the length of the embryo (Fig. 11.3). The paired dorsal aortas soon fuse to form a single dorsal aorta (Moore & Persaud 1998). About 30 branches of the dorsal aorta, called the dorsal intersegmental arteries, carry blood to the somites and

their derivatives. Those in the neck join to form the **vertebral artery** on either side of the neck. In the thorax they become the **intercostal arteries**. Most of the abdominal branches become **lumbar arteries** but the fifth pair of lumbar intersegmental arteries remains as the **common iliac arteries**. Finally, the sacral intersegmental arteries become the **lateral sacral arteries** (Moore & Persaud 1998).

Development of veins

Three pairs of veins drain into the tubular heart of the 4 week embryo:

1. **umbilical veins** form in the body stalk but only the left one persists to carry well-oxygenated blood back to the embryo;
2. the **vitelline veins** carry blood from the yolk sac to the heart tube;
3. **common cardinal veins** return poorly oxygenated blood from the embryo.

Development of the heart

The **primordium** (primitive form) of the heart is visible at 18 days and begins to beat at 22 days. Before the head fold develops, cardiogenic mesoderm occupies the floor of the pericardial coelom and gives rise to a pair of **endothelial heart tubes** (Marieb 2000). As folding proceeds, these unite to form a single heart tube and a **primordial myocardium** develops (Fig. 11.4). A **pericardial sac** forms around the heart tube. The tubular heart elongates and forms a series of alternating dilatations and constrictions (Fig. 11.5):

- **truncus arteriosus**;
- **bulbus cordis**;
- **ventricle**;
- **atrium**;
- **sinus venosus**.

Because the bulbus cordis and the ventricle grow faster than the other regions the heart tube buckles to form a twisted U shape called the **bulboventricular loop**. The **atrioventricular canal** divides the primordial atrium and ventricle. The truncus arteriosus is continuous with the aortic sac from which the aortic arches rise. The sinus venosus receives the umbilical, vitelline and common cardinal veins mentioned above.

Blood flow through the early heart

Blood flows via veins from the yolk sac, embryo and chorionic villi to the sinus venosus and into the primitive atrium. The blood then passes through the atrioventricular canal into the primordial ventricle. The ventricle contracts and blood is pumped through the bulbus cordis and truncus arteriosus into the aortic sac and to the aortic arches. It then passes into the dorsal aortas to return to the yolk sac and placenta.

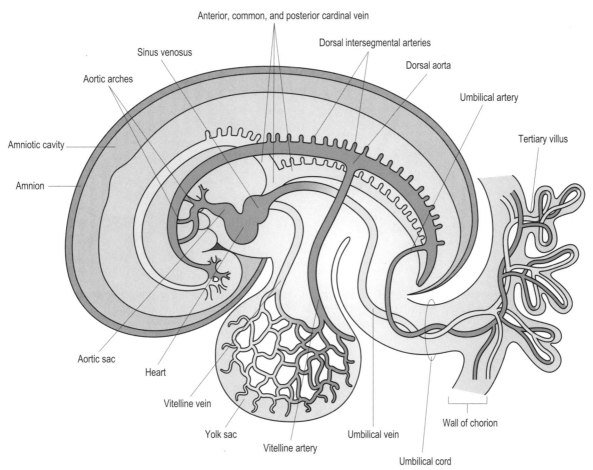

Figure 11.3   Diagram of the primitive cardiovascular system in an embryo of about 20 days, viewed from the left side. Observe the transitory stage of paired symmetric vessels. Each heart tube continues dorsally into a dorsal aorta that passes caudally. Branches of the aortae are (1) umbilical arteries, establishing connections with vessels in the chorion; (2) vitelline arteries to the yolk sac; and (3) dorsal intersegmental arteries to the body of the embryo. An umbilical vein returns blood from the chorion and divides into right and left umbilical veins within the embryo. Vessels on the yolk sac form a vascular plexus that is connected to the heart tubes by vitelline veins. The anterior cardinal veins return blood from the head region. The umbilical vein carries oxygenated blood and nutrients from the chorion (embryonic part of the placenta) to the embryo. The arteries carry poorly oxygenated blood and waste products to the chorionic villi for transfer to the maternal blood. (Reproduced with permission from Moore 1989.)

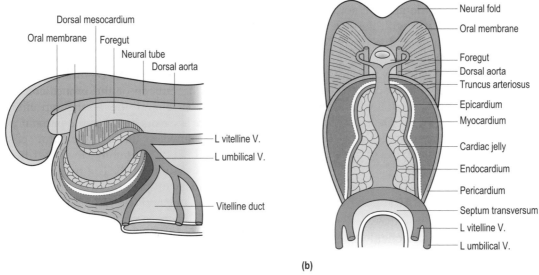

(a)   (b)

Figure 11.4   'Straight' heart tube. (a) Viewed from the left. (b) Ventral view (from Fitzgerald M J T, Fitzgerald M 1994, with permission).

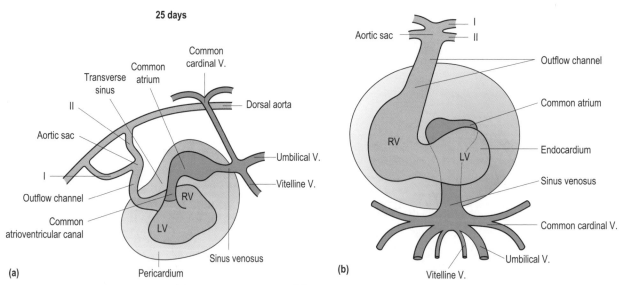

Figure 11.5   The ventricular loop. (a) Viewed from the left. (b) Ventral view. I, II, first and second aortic arches; LV, RV, presumptive left and right ventricles (from Fitzgerald M J T, Fitzgerald M 1994, with permission).

Partitioning of the heart

Partitioning of the heart begins in the middle of the 4th week. The primitive atrium is partitioned into two by the growth and fusion of two septa: the **septum primum** from the dorso-cranial wall and the **septum secundum** from the ventro-cranial wall. An opening with a flap-like valve formed by the septum secundum is left between the left and right atria to accommodate a left-to-right shunt of blood across the atrial septum. This is the **foramen ovale**, which closes at birth.

Division of the primitive ventricle begins at the end of the 4th week with the development of a ridge of tissue called the **interventricular septum**. An **interventricular foramen** closes at the end of the 7th week and the pulmonary arterial trunk taking blood to the lungs then communicates with the right ventricle and the aorta carrying blood to the body communicates with the left ventricle. After this formation of two atria and two ventricles, the fetal circulation is established.

Valves and their supporting papillary muscles and chordae tendinae and the tissue forming the conducting system of the heart begin developing at about 5 weeks and are in place by the end of organogenesis. Development of the heart and great vessels is a highly complex process, leading to the possibility of many different types of malformation.

THE LOWER RESPIRATORY TRACT

Development of the laryngotracheal tube

A median **laryngotracheal groove** appears on the floor of the primitive pharynx in the middle of the 4th week.

A septum grows into the laryngotracheal groove, converting it into the laryngotracheal tube with a laryngeal opening into the pharynx. The epithelial lining at the cranial end of this tube, the laryngeal cartilages and the vocal cords develop from the fourth and sixth pharyngeal arches. The cranial epithelium becomes the epithelial lining of the **larynx** and **trachea** and the caudal part lines the **bronchial tree**. **Tracheo-oesophageal folds** grow towards each other to form a septum that divides the cranial part of the foregut into the laryngotracheal tube and the oesophagus (Fig. 11.6).

Development of the lungs

The lung bud develops as a bulge in the caudal part of the laryngotracheal tube during the 4th week. It splits to form two bronchial buds which give rise to the **primary bronchi**. The bronchial buds invaginate the **pericardioperitoneal canals** which become the pleural cavities. The epithelium covering the outside of the bronchial buds becomes the **visceral pleura** and the epithelium lining the pericardioperitoneal canals becomes the **parietal pleura**. The connections between the two pleural cavities and the pericardial cavity containing the heart become closed off (Moore & Persaud 1998). The two primary bronchi divide into secondary or lobar bronchi; three serve the three lobes of the right lung and two serve the two lobes of the left lung (Fig. 11.7). Each secondary bronchus further subdivides into tertiary or segmental bronchi which have a cuboid epithelial lining. During the 7th month respiratory **bronchioles** become more abundant and terminate in **alveolar ducts** and **sacs**.

From 5 to 17 weeks the developing lungs are in the **pseudoglandular period**, resembling an exocrine gland. Respiration is not possible. In the **canalicular period**, from 16 to 25 weeks, air passages become patent and blood capillaries surround the future alveoli. Towards 25 weeks, respiration is possible but survival is improbable. From 24 weeks until birth, alveoli develop in the **terminal sac period** and by 28 weeks sufficient terminal sacs are present to permit survival. Budding of fresh bronchioles, alveolar ducts and alveolar sacs continues for the first 8 years of life. This is the **alveolar period** (Moore & Persaud 1998).

At first these terminal sacs are lined by **type 1 alveolar cells** which will take part in gas exchange. At the end of the 6 months, **type 2 alveolar cells** can be found. These cells secrete **surfactant** to lower the surface tension between the alveolar epithelium and inspired air. Babies born before 34 weeks may develop **respiratory distress syndrome** because of insufficient surfactant production.

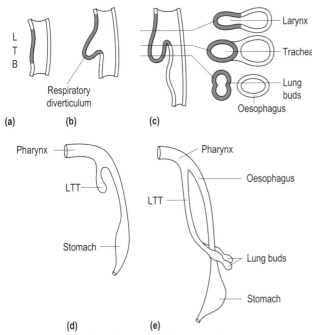

Figure 11.6   Early development of lower respiratory tract. (a) At 24 days. L, T, B, presumptive epithelial linings of larynx, trachea, bronchial tree. (b) At 25 days. (c) At 26 days. (d) At 4 weeks. (e) At 5 weeks. LTT, laryngotracheal tube (from Fitzgerald M J T, Fitzgerald M 1994, with permission).

The diaphragm

The diaphragm is quite complex in its origins with five elements contributing to its formation:

- the third to fifth somites contribute cells that form the muscles of the diaphragm;
- ventral extension of the pleural sacs forms a layer of cells for diaphragmatic connective tissue;
- oesophageal mesentery supplies connective tissue around the oesophagus and inferior vena cava;
- the septum transversum gives rise to the fibrous tissue of the central tendon;
- the pleuroperitoneal membranes contribute connective tissue surrounding the central tendon.

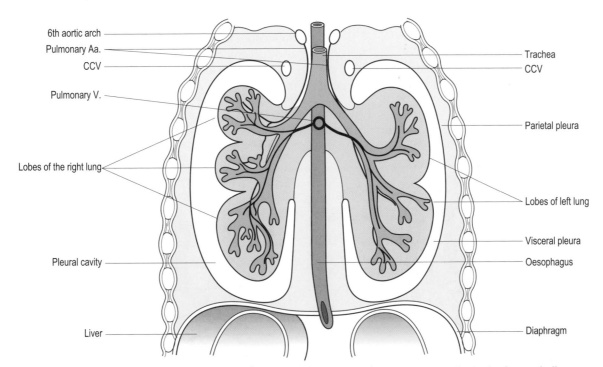

Figure 11.7   Coronal section of the posterior mediastinum at 7 weeks. CCV, common cardinal vein. Arrows indicate directions of expansion of pleural cavities and lungs. The septum transversum has been incorporated into the diaphragm (from Fitzgerald M J T, Fitzgerald M 1994, with permission).

THE ALIMENTARY TRACT

The primitive gut begins to form during the 4th week when the dorsal part of the yolk sac becomes incorporated into the embryo. The endoderm of this primitive gut gives rise to most of the epithelial lining and glands of the digestive system. By the middle of the 4th week the alimentary tract consists of **foregut**, **midgut** and **hindgut**, each with different arterial blood supply (Larsen 2001). The epithelial linings of the cranial and caudal ends of the gut, the stomodeum and anal pit, are derived from ectoderm as are the stomodeum and anal pit. The muscular and fibrous parts of the digestive tract form from splanchnic mesoderm.

The foregut

By the 5th week the foregut is visibly divided into the oesophagus, stomach and proximal duodenum (Fig. 11.8) (Larsen 2001).

The oesophagus

Although the **oesophagus** is part of the alimentary tract, it is in close proximity to the respiratory tract and is a thoracic structure. As the thoracic cavity lengthens and the heart and lungs descend into it, the oesophagus also lengthens. The upper and lower parts of the oesophagus differ in origin. Pharyngeal arch mesoderm contributes striated muscle to its upper part and the vagus nerve gives off recurrent laryngeal branches to supply this part. Splanchnic mesoderm contributes smooth muscle to its lower part and the nerve supply is autonomic from the neural crest.

The stomach

The **stomach** begins as a spindle-shaped dilatation of the caudal end of the foregut. It is attached to the dorsal wall of the abdominal cavity by the dorsal mesentery. During the 5th and 6th weeks the dorsal border elongates to form the convex **greater curvature** of the stomach while the ventral border forms the concave **lesser curvature**. The stomach now rotates clockwise on its axis through 90° taking the **dorsal mesentery** to the left. This rotation ensures that the liver becomes a right-sided organ and the spleen a left-sided organ (Larsen 2001).

The duodenum

The **duodenum** develops from the caudal part of the foregut and the cranial end of the midgut. The junction of the two parts of the duodenum is just distal to the entrance of the **common bile duct**.

The liver, gall bladder, pancreas and spleen

About day 24 the endoderm thickens directly caudal to the **septum transversum** to form the **hepatic diverticulum** or liver bud, which grows out from the duodenum (Fig. 11.9). The liver bud gives off the **gall bladder** and **biliary duct system**. The hepatic diverticulum divides into left and right hepatic buds which develop into the **lobes** of the liver. The stalk of the gall bladder becomes the **cystic duct** and the stalks of the hepatic buds become the **hepatic ducts**. The **bile duct** is formed by the union of the conjoined hepatic ducts with the cystic ducts. The hepatic buds produce a network of **hepatocytes** arranged in branching and anastomosing plates.

The **pancreas** develops as two separate structures. The smaller ventral pancreas arises from the hepatic diverticulum, which will become the bile duct, to form the uncinate process of the pancreas. The larger dorsal pancreas arises from the duodenum to form the head, body and tail. The main **pancreatic duct** enters the duodenum along with the bile duct.

The **spleen** develops from mesenchymal cells between the layers of the dorsal mesentery. It appears about the 5th

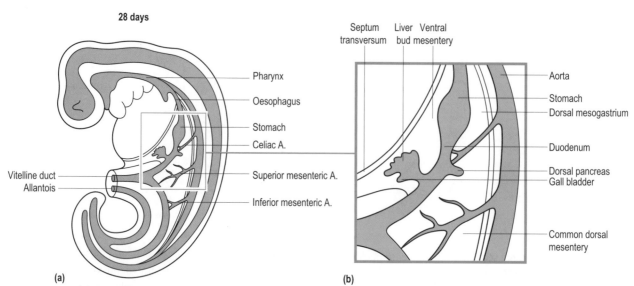

Figure 11.8 (a) Digestive system at 4 weeks. (b) Enlargement from (a) (from Fitzgerald M J T, Fitzgerald M 1994, with permission).

week on the left side of the abdomen. The spleen is seeded by **haemopoeitic cells** from the wall of the yolk sac and manufactures both fetal red and white cells in the middle trimester of pregnancy.

Development of the veins of the liver   The vitelline veins infiltrate between the hepatocytes to form the **liver sinusoids**. The **portal vein**, which drains the entire gut below the diaphragm, also develops from segments of the two vitelline veins. During the 5th week the right umbilical vein disappears, while the left one enlarges to receive returning placental blood. During the 6th to 8th weeks a large vascular shunt called the **ductus venosus** diverts oxygenated blood from the left umbilical vein to the right hepatic vein, ensuring that the highly metabolic liver receives sufficient oxygen and nutrients.

The midgut

The derivatives of the midgut are the **small intestine**, the **caecum** and **vermiform appendix**, **ascending colon** and right half or more of the **transverse colon**. During the 6th week the midgut lengthens and becomes too big for the abdominal cavity and is found in the umbilical cord (Fig. 11.10). This is called physiological herniation of the midgut (Larsen 2001).

As it enters the umbilical cord, the midgut begins to twist on itself in a counterclockwise direction when viewed from in front. This occurs because of the space taken up by the developing liver and kidneys and proximal colon. By 10 weeks the peritoneal coelom has increased sufficiently in size to allow the intestines to slide back into the abdomen.

The small intestine returns first and the colon follows to frame it. The caecum with its attached appendix enters last and enters on the right side below the liver.

The hindgut: the rectum and anal canal

The hindgut extends from the midgut to the **cloacal membrane**. The **cloaca** will form the bladder and urethra with development of the **urorectal septum**, formed by migration of cells from the **urogenital tubercle**. It is completed during the 7th week, forming the **urogenital sinus** ventrally and the **rectum** and upper **anal canal** dorsally (see Fig. 11.11 and next section). The upper half of the anal canal is lined by columnar epithelium continuous with the rectum, whereas the lower half develops from the anal pit and is lined by stratified epithelium continuous with the epidermis of the surrounding skin.

The urorectal septum fuses with the cloacal membrane by the end of the 6th week to form the **dorsal anal membrane** and the larger **urogenital membrane**. The anal membrane ruptures at the end of the 7th week to form the anal orifice. Imperforate anus occurs in 1 in 5000 births but is easily resolved if noticed early. The mesoderm of the urorectal septum persists as the **perineal body**.

THE URINARY AND GENITAL TRACTS

The urinary and genital systems are closely related embryologically and functionally. They develop from intermediate mesoderm, with the urinary system developing before the

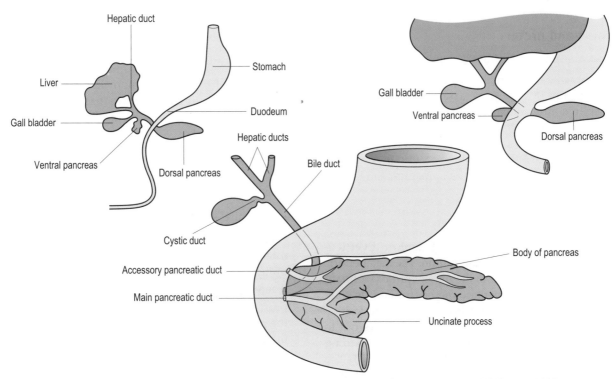

Figure 11.9   Development of duct systems of liver, gallbladder, and pancreas (from Fitzgerald M J T, Fitzgerald M 1994, with permission).

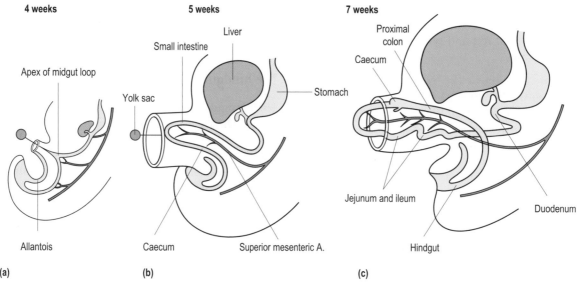

Figure 11.10 (a) Intestine at 4 weeks. (b) Entry of midgut loop into umbilical cord. Arrow indicates rotation of the midgut loop. (c) Rotation through 180° carries caecum and proximal colon to a cranial position (from Fitzgerald M J T, Fitzgerald M 1994, with permission).

genital system (Moore & Persaud 1998). During embryonic folding, the intermediate mesoderm is carried ventrally and loses its contact with the somites. A longitudinal ridge of mesoderm on either side of the primitive aorta is called the **urogenital ridge**. Part of the urogenital ridge called the **nephrogenic cord** or ridge gives rise to the urinary system and the **gonadal** or **genital ridge** gives rise to the genital system.

The kidneys and ureter

Three pairs of kidneys appear in succession during embryonic development. These are the **pronephros, mesonephros** and **metanephros** (Moore & Persaud 1998, Larsen 2001). The pronephros appears early in the 4th week but is non-functional in mammals and soon degenerates. It remains functional in some fishes. It is replaced between weeks 4 and 8 by the mesonephros, a form of kidney found in Amphibia (Fig. 11.12). Finally, the metanephros or mammalian kidney appears.

Development of the collecting system

The metanephros develops from the **metanephric diverticulum** and a mass of **metanephric mesoderm**. The metanephric diverticulum, a dorsal bud from the mesonephric (Wolffian) ducts, grows into the metanephric mesoderm and its stalk becomes the **ureter**. As this advances towards the kidney it acquires a lumen by apoptosis and its tip hollows out to become the **renal pelvis**. The ureteric bud keeps dividing to form generations of **collecting tubules** (Fig. 11.13). The first four generations enlarge and coalesce to form the **major calyces** and the next four become the **minor calyces** of the

kidney. The remaining generations form the collecting tubules (Moore & Persaud 1998).

The cells of the intermediate mesoderm surrounding the kidney multiply to form a **metanephric cap** over the renal pelvis. A cluster of metanephric cells gathers at the tip of each collecting tubule to form a **nephron**. Different growth rates within the embryo cause the kidneys to ascend into the abdomen and come into contact with the **adrenal glands** by the 8th week. The fetal kidney produces small amounts of urine from about 9 weeks and becomes more functional from about 15 weeks, with excretion of urine into the amniotic cavity. At first the developing kidneys receive their blood supply from the common iliac arteries but by the time they are in their correct position the renal arteries have developed.

The bladder and urethra

The urogenital sinus

The urogenital sinus has three parts:

- A **vesical part** above the level of entry of the mesonephric ducts expands to form the bladder and receives the two ureters.
- A narrow **pelvic part** forms the lining epithelium of the prostatic and membranous parts of the **urethra**. In females the pelvic part forms the lining of the whole of the short urethra.
- A **phallic part** extends ventrally beneath the male phallus. At first the urethra opens on the underside of the phallus behind the developing **glans** but during the 4th

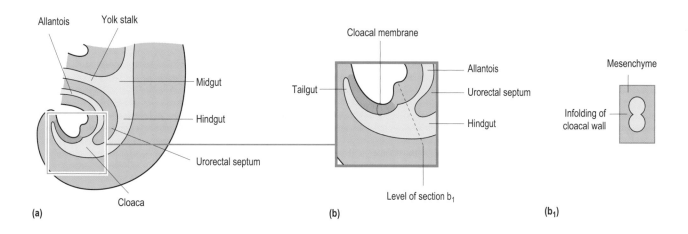

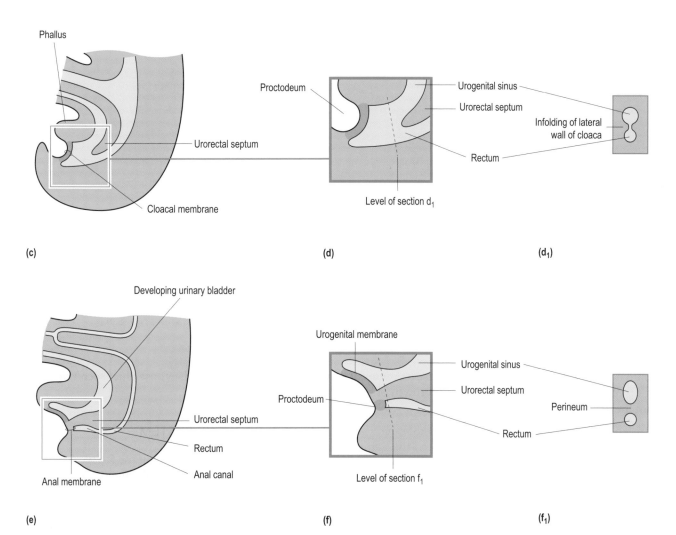

Figure 11.11 Drawings illustrating successive stages in the partitioning of the cloaca into the rectum and urogenital sinus by the urorectal septum. (a,c,e) Views from the left side at 4, 6, and 7 weeks respectively. (b,d,f) Enlargements of cloacal region. (b$_1$, d$_1$, f$_1$) Transverse sections of the cloaca at the levels shown in (b), (d) and (f), respectively. Note that the tailgut (shown in (b)) degenerates and disappears as the rectum forms from the dorsal part of the cloaca (shown in (c)). (Reproduced with permission from Moore 1989.)

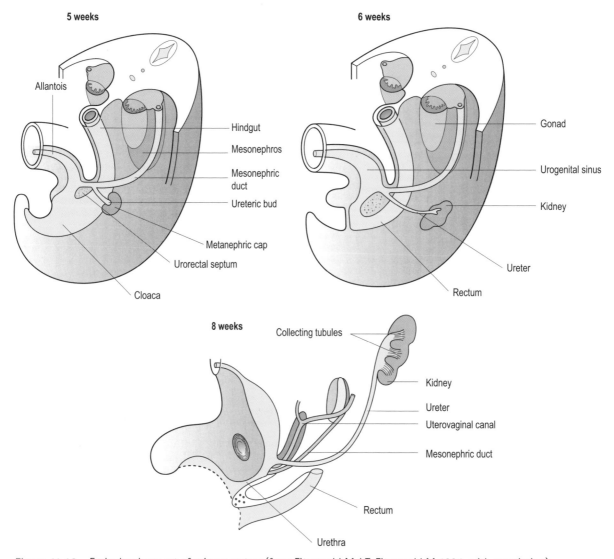

Figure 11.12   Early development of urinary system (from Fitzgerald M J T, Fitzgerald M 1994, with permission).

month a glandar urethra forms and the urethra opens at the tip of the glans. The **prepuce** is an outgrowth of skin from the glans.

Between the umbilicus and the cloacal membrane, caudal mesoderm forms a midline swelling called the genital tubercle. Migration of cells from this forms the urogenital sinus which gives rise to the bladder and urethra. As the bladder enlarges, the caudal parts of the mesonephric ducts are incorporated into its dorsal wall so that the ureters open into the urinary bladder.

The suprarenal (adrenal) glands

The cortex and the medulla of the **suprarenal glands** are formed from separate tissues. The cortex develops from mesoderm and the medulla is derived from neural crest cells. The **chromaffin cells** of the medulla are modified sympathetic ganglion cells whose chief secretion is adrenaline (epinephrine).

THE REPRODUCTIVE SYSTEM

The gonads can be identified about the 5th week and develop from three sources. The gonadal ridge on the medial side of the mesonephros includes cells from two sources, the **coelomic epithelium** and underlying **intermediate mesoderm**. The epithelium releases a chemical that attracts a third source of cells, **primordial germ cells**, which become ova or sperm. About 100 are present on the caudal surface of the yolk sac during the 4th week, migrate into the interior of the gonadal ridge and are enclosed in columns of epithelial cells called **sex cords** (Moore & Persaud 1998). At first the indifferent gonads are identical in males and females (Fig. 11.14). They differentiate into recognisable male and female forms from the 7th week (Fig. 11.15).

6 weeks

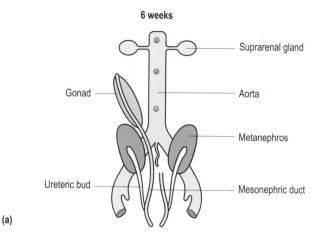

Suprarenal gland

Gonad

Aorta

Metanephros

Ureteric bud

Mesonephric duct

(a)

8 weeks

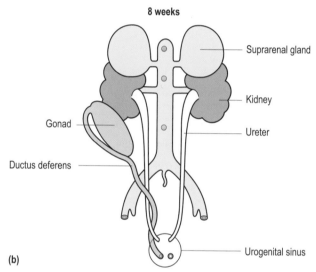

Suprarenal gland

Kidney

Gonad

Ureter

Ductus deferens

Urogenital sinus

(b)

Figure 11.13   Renal ascent. (a) At 6 weeks. (b) At 8 weeks (from Fitzgerald M J T, Fitzgerald M 1994, with permission).

Testes and the male genital tract

In the presence of SRY (sex-determining region Y) gene at about day 50 intermediate mesoderm forms the **tunica albuginea**. The sex cords become **testicular cords** and the primordial germ cells become **prospermatogonia**. The testicular cords are gathered into lobules separated by testicular septa derived from the tunica albuginea. The inner ends of the cords are linked together in a network called the rete testis. Two sets of endocrine cells form in the lobules:

1. Sertoli cells are the most numerous type of cell in the early testis. Their earliest function is to produce a **Müllerian duct inhibitory factor** which enters the fetal circulation and causes regression of the paramesonephric ducts during the 9th week.

2. Leydig cells arise in the stroma between the lobules and secrete **testosterone** into the fetal circulation. This

hormone ensures the survival and growth of the **Wolffian ducts** and the formation of the epididymis, ductus deferens, seminal vesicle and the ejaculatory duct.

The testes descend gradually from their original site in the lumbar region into the pelvis and out into the scrotal sac, usually by term. They are accompanied by a pocket of peritoneum called the **processus vaginalis**, which becomes the **tunica vaginalis** on completion of descent. The testes are accompanied by the ductus deferens, testicular blood vessels, nerves and lymphatics which constitute the two spermatic cords. In females the Wolffian ducts disappear by programmed cell death without any ovarian influence. Remnants are found in the broad ligament and may form **parovarian cysts**.

Ovary and the female genital duct

In the absence of SRY no tunica albuginea forms. The sex cords accumulate in the outer cortex of the gonadal ridge and this becomes filled with **primordial follicles** consisting of an oocyte derived from the primordial germ cells, an inner shell of follicular cells derived from cell-cord epithelium and an outer shell, the theca, derived from intermediate mesoderm. The number of primordial follicles reaches a maximum of 6–7 million in the 15th week. Programmed cell death reduces this number drastically so that 2 years after birth only 1 million remain and at puberty only 300 000 are present. The ovary descends from the abdominal lumbar region into the true pelvis after the 12th week.

The upper and middle sections of the Mullerian ducts form the epithelial lining of the **Fallopian tubes** and the lower segments fuse into one during the 9th week to become the **uterovaginal canal** which eventually forms the epithelial lining of the uterus. The muscle walls of the Fallopian tubes and the myometrium of the uterus are formed from splanchnic mesoderm.

The vagina

If the Müllerian system develops, a small tubercle called the Müllerian eminence gives rise to the **vaginal plate**. This lengthens along the dorsal wall of the urogenital sinus. The lumen of the vagina is formed by canalisation from below upwards. The lumen extends around the cervix to form the fornices. The hymen is left as a partition between the vagina and the vestibule.

The external genitalia

Early in the 3rd month it is not possible to see a sexual difference. Externally, the phallic urethra is an open urethral groove flanked by paired inner urogenital folds and outer genital swellings derived from mesenchyme.

● In males the matching pairs under the influence of testosterone come together. The urogenital folds unite

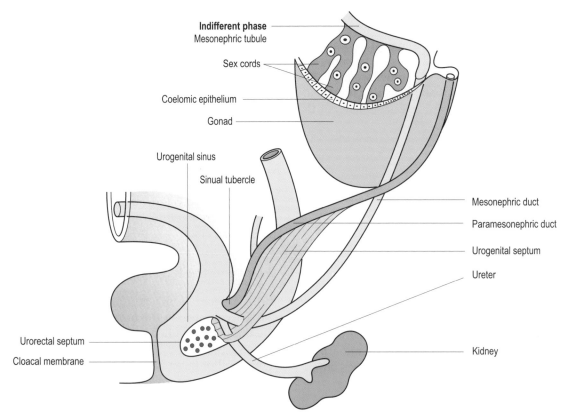

Figure 11.14   Indifferent gonad and genital ducts at 4 weeks (from Fitzgerald M J T, Fitzgerald M 1994, with permission).

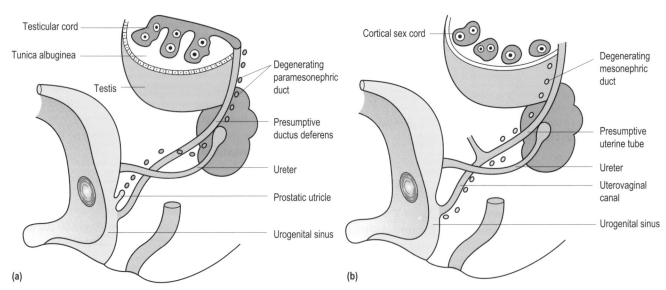

Figure 11.15   Early sexual differentiation. (a) Male. (b) Female (from Fitzgerald M J T, Fitzgerald M 1994, with permission).

below the urethral groove to complete the spongy urethra and the genital swellings form the two halves of the scrotum. A line of union at the junction of the two halves of the scrotum is called the scrotal raphe and the line of union of the urogenital folds is marked by the urethral raphe.

● In females they stay apart and there is growth in situ of the urogenital folds and genital swellings. The phallus forms the clitoris with a small glans at its tip. The urethral groove and the phallic part of the urogenital sinus remain open as the vestibule and the urogenital folds become the labia minora while the genital swellings become the labia majora.

ESTIMATION OF EMBRYONIC AGE

By 8 weeks the embryo is recognisably human although the head is rounder and very large in proportion to the body.

The rest of pregnancy is concerned mainly with growth and maturation. The usual calculations of embryonic age are made by ascertaining the date of the first day of the last menstrual period (LMP). However, it is unusual to know the exact day of fertilisation and there are other ways of estimating the age of an embryo if spontaneously or therapeutically aborted. External features and measurements of the embryo are useful and careful ultrasound scanning can confirm the age of a viable embryo in utero. At 4 weeks after fertilisation (6 weeks from the first day of the LMP) the embryo and its sac measure 5 mm long. A week later discrete embryonic features can be visualised and crown–rump measurements can be made.

MAIN POINTS

- The cardiovascular system is in place in the embryo from the end of the 3rd week and its nutrients are obtained from the maternal circulation. Blood is pumped around vessels by a heart early in the 4th week. Early in the 3rd week blood islands appear in the extraembryonic mesoderm lining the yolk sac. The heart is derived from mesoderm by a highly complex process.

- Three sets of arteries develop: two umbilical arteries carry blood to the placenta, vitelline arteries arising from the dorsal aortas become the three mesenteric arteries supplying the gut and intersegmental arteries supply blood to the somites and neural tube.

- Veins link to the arteries in capillary beds: two umbilical veins form in the body stalk to link with the arteries in the placental capillary bed, a large pair of yolk sac veins become the vitelline veins to the yolk sac capillary bed and the two main common cardinal veins from the fetus.

- A median laryngotracheal groove appears on the floor of the primitive pharynx in the middle of the 4th week. A septum converts it into the laryngotracheal tube with a laryngeal opening into the pharynx. Tracheo-oesophageal folds form a septum dividing the cranial part of the foregut into the laryngotracheal tube and the oesophagus.

- The lung bud splits to form two bronchial buds. These divide into secondary bronchi serving the three lobes of the right lung and the two lobes of the left lung. Each secondary bronchus subdivides into tertiary or segmental bronchi. During the 7th month respiratory bronchioles terminate in alveolar ducts and sacs lined by type 1 alveolar cells. At the end of the 6th month type 2 alveolar cells which secrete surfactant appear.

- The primitive gut begins to form during the 4th week when the dorsal part of the yolk sac becomes incorporated into the embryo during folding. By the middle of the 4th week the alimentary tract consists of foregut, midgut and hindgut.

- The stomach begins as a spindle-shaped dilatation of the caudal end of the foregut. During the 5th and 6th weeks the dorsal border elongates to form the greater curvature of the stomach while the ventral border forms the lesser curvature.

- On day 24 the hepatic diverticulum or liver bud grows out from the duodenum and gives off the gall bladder and biliary duct system. Left and right hepatic buds develop into the lobes of the liver. The gall bladder stalk becomes the cystic duct and the stalks of the hepatic buds become the hepatic ducts. The bile duct is formed by the union of hepatic and cystic ducts.

- The pancreas develops as two separate structures. The smaller ventral pancreas arises from the hepatic diverticulum to form the uncinate process of the pancreas. The larger dorsal pancreas arises from the duodenum to form the head, body and tail.

- The spleen appears about the 5th week and develops from mesenchymal cells between the layers of the dorsal mesogastrium. It is seeded by haemopoeitic cells from the wall of the yolk sac and manufactures both red and white cells in the middle trimester of pregnancy.

- Derived from the midgut are the small intestine, the caecum and vermiform appendix, ascending colon and right half of the transverse colon. During the 6th week the midgut lengthens and is too big for the abdominal cavity and is found in the umbilical cord – the physiological herniation of the midgut. The small intestine returns first and the colon follows to frame it.

- The cloaca forms the bladder and urethra with development of the urorectal septum. The urorectal septum fuses with the cloacal membrane forming the dorsal anal membrane and the urogenital membrane. The anal membrane ruptures at the end of the 7th week to form the anal orifice.

- The urogenital ridge gives rise to the nephrogenic cord or ridge, primordium of the urinary system. The part giving rise to the genital system is called the gonadal or genital ridge. Three pairs of kidneys appear in succession during embryonic development; the last is the metanephros or permanent mammalian kidney.

- The gonadal ridge includes cells from two sources, the coelomic epithelium and underlying intermediate mesoderm. The epithelium releases a chemical that attracts the primordial germ cells which will form the ova or sperm. The gonads are identical in males and females up to the 7th week. Two pairs of genital ducts are present; the Wolffian ducts are forerunners of the male genital tract and the Müllerian ducts are forerunners of the female genital tract. In the absence of a trigger all embryos become female. The SRY factor influences the gonads to become testes.

- Early in the 3rd month the phallic urethra is an open urethral groove flanked by paired inner urogenital folds and outer genital swellings. In males testosterone influences the matching pairs to come together to complete the spongy urethra and the genital swellings form the two halves of the scrotum. In females the urethral groove and the phallic part of the urogenital sinus remain open and the urogenital folds become the labia minora while the genital swellings become the labia majora. The phallus forms the clitoris with a small glans at its tip.

- By 8 weeks the embryo is recognisably human. The rest of fetal intrauterine time is concerned mainly with growth and maturation.

References

Larsen W J 2001 Human Embryology, 3rd edn. Churchill Livingstone, Edinburgh.

Marieb E N 2000 Human Anatomy and Physiology, 5th edn. Benjamin/Cummings, California.

McNabb M 1997 Embryonic and fetal developments. In Sweet B R, Tiran D (eds) Mayes Midwifery, 12th edn. Baillière Tindall, London, pp 89–105.

Moore K L, Persaud T V N 1998 Before We Are Born, 5th edn. W B Saunders, Philadelphia.

Annotated recommended reading

Larsen W J 2001 Human Embryology, 3rd edn. Churchill Livingstone, Edinburgh.
This book examines both molecular biological and clinical aspects of embryology. Each chapter is about a specific embryological stage and the clinical applications arising out of the advancing knowledge base.

Moore K L, Persaud T V N 1998 Before We Are Born, 5th edn. W B Saunders, Philadelphia.
The layout of this textbook remains excellent. It clearly describes embryo development week by week and provides an excellent source for understanding the origins of congenital defects. The illustrations in this latest edition are excellent.

Chapter **12**

The placenta, membranes and amniotic fluid

INTRODUCTION

The embryo obtains nutrients and oxygen and disposes of waste products via its mother's circulation through the highly complex organ called the placenta. In evolutionary terms this organ has developed to ensure that the fetus is well protected during its early development but occasionally problems and malfunctions arise. By understanding the development and function of the placenta, treatments that can save some babies' lives may be possible.

IMPLANTATION

The embryo obtains nutrients and oxygen and disposes of waste products via its mother's circulation through the **placenta** which is derived from embryonic trophoblast cells and a few inner cell mass mesodermal cells. The initial trophoblastic cells, called collectively the **cytotrophoblast**, give rise to the **syncytiotrophoblast** (trophoblast without cells) that has undergone nuclear division without forming daughter cells. This structure invades the uterine lining, allowing the embryo to embed, a process completed by the 10th day when a plug of clotted blood and cellular debris closes over its point of entry. The syncytiotrophoblast at the embryonic pole of the zygote forms a thick multinucleated layer.

Maternal endometrial capillaries surrounding the embryo swell to form **sinusoids** which are eroded by the invasive syncytiotrophoblast. Small spaces called **lacunae** appear in the syncytiotrophoblast and become filled with a mixture of blood from the sinusoids and secretions from eroded endometrial glands. This fluid is the **embryotroph** and passes to the embryonic disc by diffusion (Moore & Persaud 1998). The lacunae fuse to form the **intervillous spaces** of the placenta through which maternal blood begins to flow.

In normal pregnancy decidual and myometrial arteries undergo changes to convert them to **uteroplacental arteries**. Two types of **migratory cytotrophoblast** (MC) cause this:

1. Endovascular MC invades spiral arterioles on the decidua and myometrium and replaces arterial endothelium,

destroying muscle and elastic tissues in the tunica media. The tissues are replaced by maternal fibrinoid. The migration takes place in two waves: 6–10 weeks into the decidua and 14–16 weeks into the myometrium.

2. Interstitial (stromal) MC destroys the ends of decidual blood vessels, promoting blood flow into the lacunae. The maternal arteries are functionally denervated so that they are completely dilated and unresponsive to circulatory pressor substances or autonomic neural control. Local prostacyclin maintains vasodilation of uterine radial arteries.

Soon mesodermal tissue from the developing embryo migrates through the primitive streak and joins trophoblast extensions to form the connecting stalk. This mesoderm gives rise to the umbilical blood vessels and the structure becomes the umbilical cord. By the end of the second week trophoblastic cells have formed finger-like projections called **primary chorionic villi** all around the embryo. The embryo, its yolk sac and early amniotic sac are suspended in the **chorionic sac**, which consists of a layer of mesoderm nearest the embryo, the cytotrophoblast and the syncytiotrophoblast nearest the endometrium. The **amniotic sac** is nearest to the uterine wall and is divided from the chorion by a fluid-filled cavity, the **extraembryonic coelom**.

DEVELOPMENT OF THE CHORIONIC VILLI

Early in the 3rd week a core of loose connective tissue developed from embryonic mesenchyme invades each primary chorionic villus to form the **secondary chorionic villi**. Some of the mesenchymal cells in the core differentiate into fetal blood capillaries, forming mature **tertiary chorionic villi**. By 15–20 days there is a functioning **arteriocapillaryvenous network** which becomes connected to the embryonic heart vessels. By the end of the 3rd week fetal blood circulates through the chorionic villi and an exchange of substances between maternal and fetal circulations begins (Figs 12.1 and 12.2).

Formation of the cytotrophoblastic shell

At the same time the cytotrophoblastic cells proliferate and extend through the syncytiotrophoblast to from a **cytotrophoblastic shell**. This attaches the chorionic sac to the maternal endometrium by specialised chorionic villi called **stem** or **anchoring villi**. From the sides of the stem villi **branch villi** grow through which the main exchange of materials between maternal and fetal circulations occurs.

Until about 20 weeks the placental membrane (Fig. 12.3) consists of four layers of tissue separating the two circulations – syncytiotrophoblast, cytotrophoblast, connective tissue of the mesenchymous core and the endothelium of the fetal capillary (Moore & Persaud 1998). Maternal and fetal bloods do not mingle unless there is damage to the villi (Bennett & Brown 1999). As pregnancy advances, this

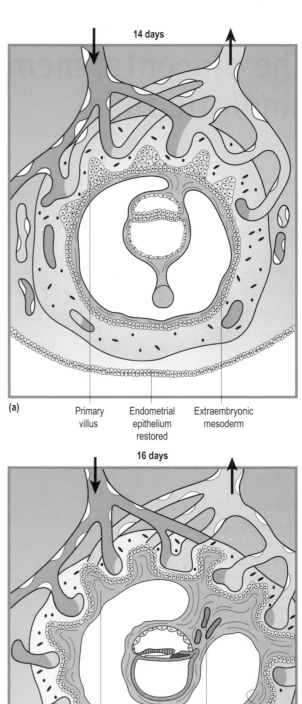

(a)   Primary   Endometrial   Extraembryonic
      villus   epithelium   mesoderm
                  restored

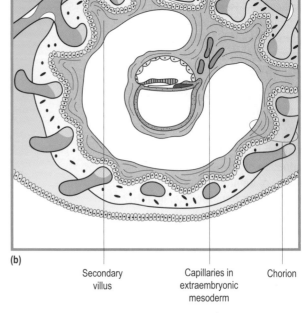

(b)   Secondary   Capillaries in   Chorion
      villus   extraembryonic
                             mesoderm

Figure 12.1   Formation of chorionic vesicle (from Fitzgerald M J T, Fitzgerald M 1994, with permission).

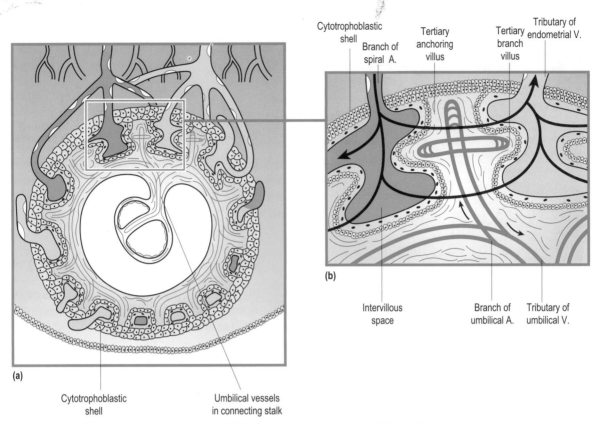

Figure 12.2   Chorionic vesicle at 21 days. (b) Enlargement of upper part of (a) showing the circulation of embryonic and maternal blood. (From Fitzgerald M J T, Fitzgerald M 1994, with permission.)

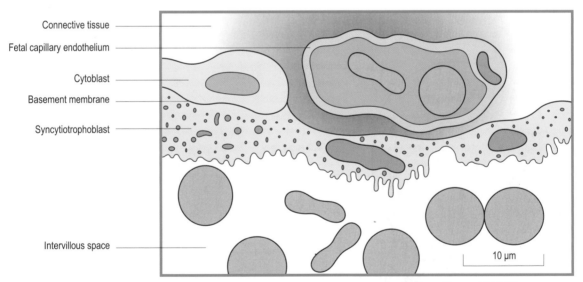

Figure 12.3   Structure of the placental membrane. All erythrocytes are coloured grey (from Fitzgerald M J T, Fitzgerald M 1994, with permission).

placental membrane becomes thinner and many fetal capillaries lie very close to the syncytiotrophoblast.

Later placental development

Once the conceptus has implanted, the decidual reaction spreads outwards from the embedding site and the endometrium is called the decidua because it is shed at the end of pregnancy. Three regions of the decidua are described, based on their relation to the implantation site:

- the **decidua basalis** lies beneath the conceptus, forming the maternal component of the placenta;
- the **decidua capsularis** overlies the conceptus;
- the **decidua vera** or **parietalis** is the name of the remaining uterine lining.

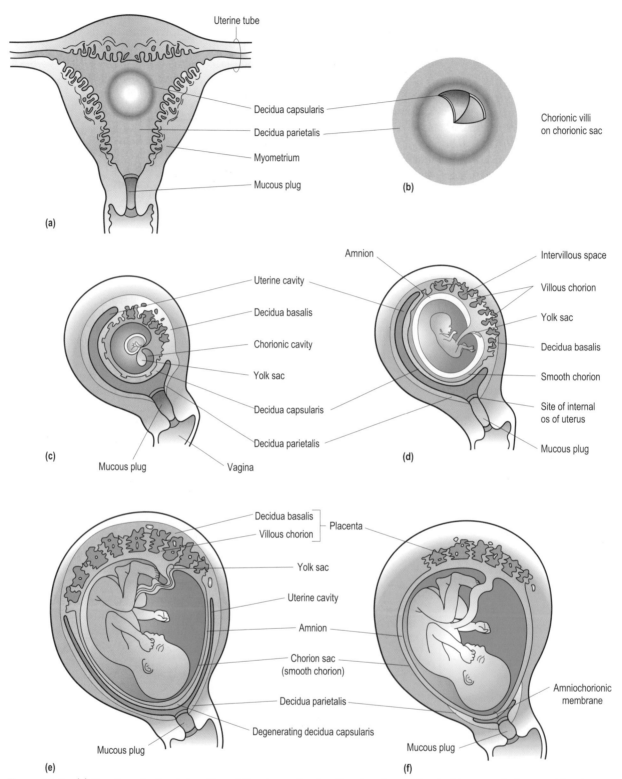

Figure 12.4   (a) Drawing of a frontal section of the uterus showing the elevation of the decidua capsularis caused by the expanding chorionic sac of an implanted 4-week embryo. (b) Enlarged drawing of the implantation site shown in (a); the chorionic villi have been exposed by cutting an opening in the decidua capsularis. (c–f) Drawings of sagittal sections of the gravid uterus from the fourth to the twenty-second weeks, showing the changing relations of the fetal membranes to the decidua. In (f) the amnion and chorion are fused with each other and the decidua parietalis, thus obliterating the uterine cavity. Note that the chorionic villi persist only where the chorion is associated with the decidua basalis; here they have formed the villous chorion (from Moore K, Persand T V N 1998, with permission).

As the conceptus grows the decidua capsularis bulges into the uterine cavity and eventually fuses with the decidua vera, obliterating the uterine cavity. By 22 weeks the decidua capsularis has degenerated and disappeared (Fig. 12.4).

The entire surface of the chorionic sac is covered by chorionic villi until the 8th week. As the sac grows the chorionic villi associated with the decidua capsularis become compressed, reducing their blood supply and they degenerate leaving a bare area, the **chorion laeve** (smooth), which becomes the **chorionic membrane**. The chorionic villi of the decidua basalis increase, branch and enlarge rapidly to form the **chorion frondosum**, the fetal part of the placenta. By 16 weeks the placenta reaches its full thickness and no new lobes or stem villi develop. Circumferential growth continues with branching of villi. The size and number of maternal capillaries increases, as does the surface area for gas exchange. Cellular proliferation stops at about 35 weeks but cellular hypertrophy continues until term.

THE MATURE PLACENTA

Appearance

The placenta is a flattened discoid organ about 20 cm in diameter. It is about 2.5 cm thick at the centre and thins out towards its circumference, where it is continuous with the chorion. It is about one-sixth of the baby's weight at term. There are two distinct surfaces (Fig. 12.5): the **maternal surface** attached to the maternal decidua and the **fetal surface** covered with amnion into which the umbilical cord inserts. At delivery the maternal surface is dark red because it contains maternal blood. Part of the decidual basalis will have been separated with it during delivery. The surface is formed of about 20 **cotyledons** (lobes) separated by **sulci** (grooves). The decidua dips down into these sulci to form **septa**. The lobes are made up of **lobules**, each containing a tertiary villus and its branches.

Because of the presence of the amnion the fetal surface is a shiny greyish white. From the insertion of the umbilical

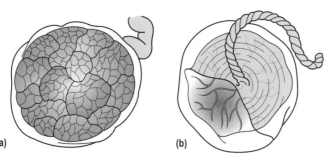

(a)   **(b)**

Figure 12.5   The placenta. (a) The maternal surface, showing cotyledons. (b) The fetal surface (from Sweet B 1997, with permission).

cord, branches of the single umbilical vein and two arteries spread out and dip down into the tissue. The amnion can be peeled off the surface, leaving the chorionic plate from which the placenta has developed. This is the portion continuous with the chorion.

The membranes

The amnion and chorion grow until about 28 weeks of gestation and then increase their size by stretching. They resist rupture as the fetus grows mainly due to the strength of the amnion. Rupture of the membranes in labour is probably brought about by increased intrauterine pressure from amniotic fluid as contractions reduce the intrauterine space and fluid cannot be compressed. The amnion and chorion are not fused and contain up to 200 ml of amniotic fluid between them.

The outer chorion adheres closely to the decidua but the amnion moves over it aided by mucus. This may lead to rupture of the amnion, with the formation of amniotic bands which may constrict or amputate fetal limbs (Blackburn 2003). The chorion is a thick, opaque, friable membrane continuous with the edge of the placenta. At term it varies from about 0.02 to 0.2 mm thick and consists of four layers of tissue (Fig. 12.6) which atrophy as pregnancy advances. The cells of the chorion laeve are metabolically active, producing enzymes that can reduce the level of locally produced progesterone and a protein that can bind progesterone. The chorion also produces prostaglandins, oxytocin and platelet-activating factor, stimulators of uterine myometrial activity (McNabb 1997a).

The inner amnion is derived from the inner cell mass. It is tough, smooth and translucent and lines the chorion and the surface of the placenta, continuing over the outer surface of the umbilical cord. At term it is about 0.02–0.5 mm thick and consists of five layers (Fig. 12.6). It is lined by non-ciliated cuboid epithelial cells which possibly help in the formation and regulation of amniotic fluid (Bennett & Brown 1999). The amnion also produces prostaglandins, in particular PGE_2 which may help to initiate the onset of labour (Germain et al 1994).

The umbilical cord

The umbilical cord or **funis** is usually attached to the centre of the placental fetal surface. It is 1–2 cm in diameter and varies in length from 30 to 90 cm with an average of 50 cm. There are normally two **umbilical arteries** and one **umbilical vein** in the umbilical cord surrounded by a mucoid connective tissue called **Wharton's jelly**. The umbilical vein is longer than the arteries which spiral around it. The vessels are longer than the cord and non-significant loops of vessel called **false knots** may be seen. Rarely a **true knot** may be present and the blood vessels may become occluded, causing fetal distress, especially during labour.

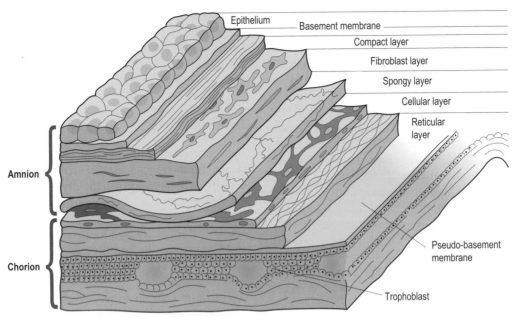

Figure 12.6   Layers of the human amnion and chorion. (Reproduced with permission from Blackburn & Loper 1992.)

The yolk sac and allantois

By 9 weeks the **yolk sac** has shrunk to a pear-shaped remnant about 5 mm in diameter. Once its functions in producing blood cells during weeks 3–5 are completed, it becomes detached from the gut and remains present in the umbilical cord (Coad & Dunstall 2001). The **allantois** degenerates, forming the **urachus** (median umbilical ligament) that connects the umbilicus to the urinary bladder. In 2% of adults the urachus persists as a diverticulum of the ileum and is known as a **Meckel's diverticulum**.

THE PLACENTAL CIRCULATION

The placental villi form a huge surface area for substance exchange between maternal and fetal circulations. Maternal blood enters the intervillous space in spurts via 80–100 endometrial spiral arteries. It flows slowly over the surface of the villi and substance exchange occurs in both directions. The maternal blood reaches the floor of the **intervillous space** where it drains into the endometrial veins (Figs 12.7–12.9). Anything interfering with the uteroplacental circulation will result in fetal hypoxia and may interfere with growth or cause death. An analogy can be made to the placental circulation as if you are taking a shower. If you stand under the shower, your body is the tertiary villus, the shower head delivering water is the spiral arteriole delivering blood and the shower drainage is the endometrial vein.

Deoxygenated blood leaves the fetus and passes into the two umbilical arteries which take it to the placenta. Here the blood vessels form the extensive arterio–capillary–venous system within the chorionic villi where fetal blood is brought very close to maternal blood. Oxygenated fetal blood then converges in thin-walled veins to enter the umbilical vein, which returns it to the fetus. The fetal circulation is described in detail in Chapter 48.

ANATOMICAL VARIATIONS OF THE PLACENTA

Placentae may be abnormally shaped and it is important to examine the placenta and seek medical aid if it appears incomplete.

Succenturiate lobe

Sometimes a separate placental lobe is linked by blood vessels to the main placenta. Failure to deliver this succenturiate lobe may lead to infection and haemorrhage. Each placenta must be examined to ensure there is no hole in the membranes with blood vessels leading away from it (Fig. 12.10).

Battledore placenta

The umbilical cord is inserted into the edge of the placenta, giving it the appearance of a battledore, the bat used in a medieval game similar to badminton.

Velamentous insertion of the umbilical cord

The umbilical cord insertion is into the membranes outside the placental boundary. Rarely the umbilical cross the internal os, a condition called vasa praevia. If these

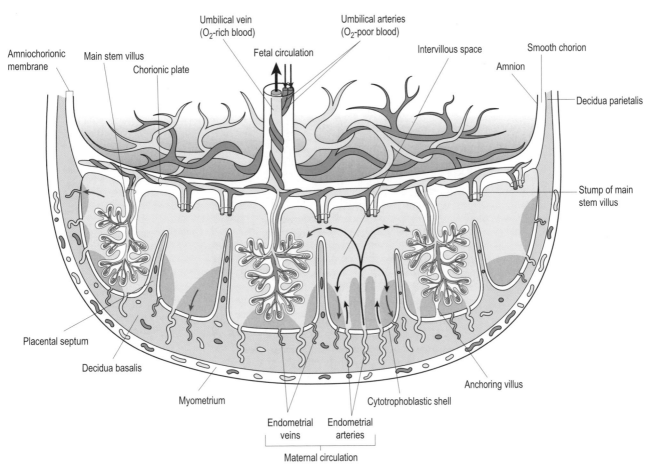

Figure 12.7 Schematic drawing of a transverse section through a full-term placenta, showing (1) the relation of the villous chorion (fetal part of placenta) to the decidua basalis (maternal part of placenta); (2) the fetal placental circulation; and (3) the maternal placental circulation. Maternal blood flows into the intervillous spaces in funnel-shaped spurts from the spiral arteries, and exchanges occur with the fetal blood as the maternal blood flows around the branch villi. It is through the branch villi that the main exchange of material between the mother and embryo/fetus occurs. The inflowing arterial blood pushes venous blood out of the intervillous space into the endometrial veins, which are scattered over the entire surface of the decidua basalis. Note that the umbilical arteries carry poorly oxygenated fetal blood (shown in dark grey) to the placenta and that the umbilical vein carries oxygenated blood (shown in light grey) to the fetus. Note that the cotyledons are separated from each other by placental septa, projections of the decidua basalis. Each cotyledon consists of two or more main stem villi and their many branches. In this drawing, only one stem villus is shown in each cotyledon, but the stumps of those that have been removed are indicated. (Reproduced with permission from Moore 1989.)

vessels rupture during labour, the fetus may have a massive haemorrhage.

Circumvallate placenta

An opaque thickened ring is seen on the fetal surface of the placenta which forms because of doubling back of the membranes (Fig. 12.11). The membranes may leave the placenta nearer to the centre than normal. It is associated with an increased risk of growth retardation (Coad & Dunstall 2001).

Bipartite (tripartite) placenta

A placenta may be divided into two (or three) fairly equal lobes.

Infarcts

Infarcts are patches on the maternal surface of the placenta caused by localised death of placental tissue that result from an interruption of blood supply. They are red when newly formed and degenerate into white fibrous patches. Any placenta may contain them but they are more common on the placentae of women with hypertension of pregnancy.

Calcification

Small gritty, greyish white patches may be found on the surface of the placenta, especially if the pregnancy is post term. These are deposits of lime salts and are of no significance.

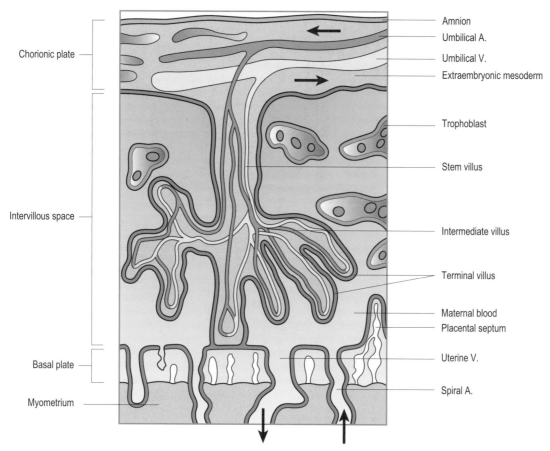

Figure 12.8   Diagrammatic section through the placenta. The arteries carry deoxygenated blood; the veins carry oxygenated blood. Arrows indicate directions of blood flow (from Fitzgerald M J T, Fitzgerald M 1994, with permission).

The major placental pathologies of **abruptio placentae** and **placenta praevia** are discussed in Chapter 31, p. 409.

FUNCTIONS OF THE PLACENTA

The key function of the placenta is **transport of nutrients** to the fetus and **waste products** away from the fetus. The placenta has other functions, including **production of hormones** and **transfer** during metabolism. It also **protects** the fetus against environmental hazards such as toxins and infective agents and has an **immunological role** in preventing fetal rejection. These functions are energy consuming and the placenta utilises about one-third of the nutrients devoted to the fetoplacental unit (Chard 2000).

Endocrine function

Although the maternal part of the placenta and the decidua secrete the hormones **prolactin**, **relaxin** and **prostaglandins**, decidual production of these hormones probably influences pregnancy most. **Pregnancy-associated placental protein A** (PAPP-A) is produced by the decidua as well as by

placental trophoblast. These decidual hormones target the fetoplacental unit and bind to the fetal membranes and trophoblast.

The fetoplacental hormones alter maternal metabolic processes to benefit the fetus. They can be divided into two groups – **steroid hormones** and **protein hormones**. Steroid hormones such as **oestriol** are made by sending a series of molecules backwards and forwards between fetus and placenta until the final hormone structure is reached. Steroid hormones are found in higher concentrations in fetal blood than in maternal blood.

The placenta produces specific protein hormones in substantial amounts and produces small quantities of every protein produced by the adult body (Chard 2000). The manufacture of protein hormones does not appear to need fetal input but may be linked directly to the amount of active trophoblastic tissue. They are found only in maternal blood and are implicated in changing maternal physiology. There does not appear to be a feedback mechanism controlling their production. The syncytiotrophoblast produces its own **luteinising hormone releasing hormone** (LHRH) which controls **human chorionic gonadotrophin** production in the same cell.

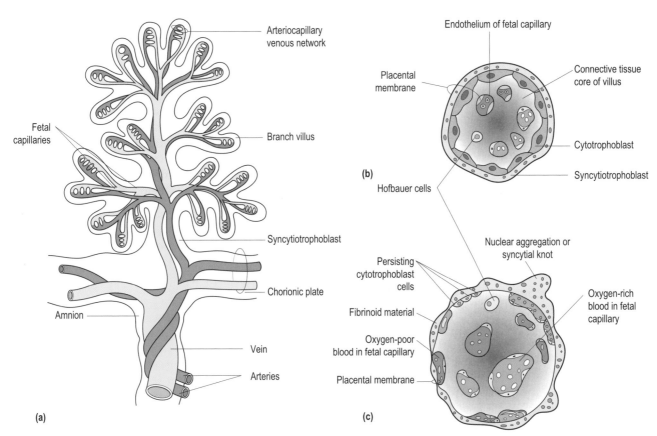

Figure 12.9 (a) Drawing of a stem chorionic villus showing its arteriocapillary venous system. The arteries carry poorly oxygenated fetal blood and waste products from the fetus, whereas the vein carries oxygenated blood and nutrients to the fetus. (b,c) Drawings of sections through a branch villus at 10 weeks and full term, respectively. The placental membrane, composed of extrafetal tissues, separates the maternal blood in the intervillous space from the fetal blood in the capillaries in the villi. Note that the placental membrane becomes very thin at full term. Hofbauer cells are thought to be phagocytic. (Reproduced with permission from Moore 1989.)

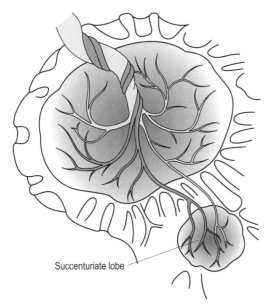

Figure 12.10 Succenturiate placenta (from Sweet B 1997, with permission).

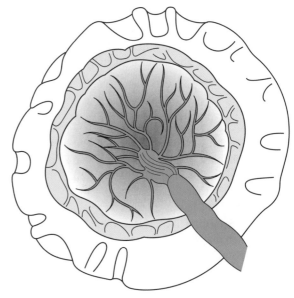

Figure 12.11 Circumvallate placenta (from Sweet B 1997, with permission).

The protein hormones

The main placental protein hormones are:

- human chorionic gonadotrophin (hCG);
- human placental lactogen (hPL);
- Schwangerschaftsprotein 1 (SP₁);
- pregnancy-associated protein A (PAPP-A);
- pregnancy-associated protein B (PAPP-B);
- placental protein 5 (PP5).

The above hormones are analogous to some anterior pituitary hormones (see Box 12.1): For example, hCG has a similar structure to LH and hPL is similar to prolactin and growth hormone.

The steroid hormones – oestrogens

Three oestrogens are important: **estrone**, **estradiol** and **estriol**. In the non-pregnant woman estriol is derived from estradiol and estrone, whereas in pregnancy estriol is synthesised by the fetoplacental unit. The fetal liver and suprarenal glands are important in estriol production and estriol is a direct measure of fetal wellbeing. **Pregnenolone sulphate**,

---

Box 12.1 Placental protein hormones

Human chorionic gonadotrophin

Human chorionic gonadotrophin (hCG) is a glycoprotein consisting of two subunits α (alpha) and β (beta), joined by a disulphide bond. The smaller α subunit contains 92 amino acids. The larger β subunit contains 147 amino acids and is probably the biologically active one. In early pregnancy there is a rapid increase in hCG production, the urinary excretion rate doubling every 36–48 hours (Klopper 1991). The curve flattens out at about 9 weeks and declines. The lower level is maintained until just before term when there is another rise. The plasma concentration is measured in international units (IU)/ml and rises from 7 to 100 IU/ml. Pregnancy tests kits contain antibodies which bind to the β subunit to show a positive pregnancy test. It can be detected in maternal blood 9 days after fertilisation.

The hCG influences the maternal ovary to produce the extra oestrogen and progesterone necessary for the maintenance of pregnancy. It appears to control placental production of progesterone, the amount of hCG determining the level of progesterone production. However, scientists have found no association between insufficient hCG production and spontaneous abortion. The fall in hCG levels found in miscarriages occurs after the death of the conceptus. An early pregnancy placental abnormality called hydatidiform mole produces large amounts of hCG (Ch. 31).

Human placental lactogen

Human placental lactogen (hPL) is produced by the syncytiotrophoblast. It consists of 190 amino acids, of which 163 are found in **human growth hormone**. It is the only placental protein that does not contain carbohydrate. Maternal blood hPL level rises from a value of 0.3 μg/ml at 10 weeks to 5.4 μg/ml at 36 weeks. There is then a fall until delivery which may correspond to a fall in functioning placental tissue. Maternal plasma hPL levels have been used to check placental function.

In pregnancy hPL probably acts as a growth promoter affecting carbohydrate metabolism. It causes the mobilisation of free fatty acids and antagonises the action of insulin. Pregnant women must manufacture more insulin and, where the insulin reserve is poor, carbohydrate metabolism may be compromised, especially in diabetic women. For this reason hPL is called diabetogenic.

Schwangerschaftsprotein 1

SP₁ is another high-carbohydrate glycoprotein present in large amounts. It can be detected in early pregnancy and is easily measured in late pregnancy. Like hPL, there is a steady rise until 36 weeks, followed by a steady decline until delivery. The hormone has no use as a test of placental function because of large subject-to-subject variation. The role of this hormone is unknown but it may affect immunosuppression, preventing rejection of the placenta as a foreign protein.

Pregnancy-associated plasma proteins A and B

A series of **pregnancy-associated plasma proteins** (PAPPs) were discovered in the early 1970s. Of these, **PAPP-A** and **PAPP-B** are produced by the trophoblast. PAPP-A is a large glycoprotein detectable in maternal plasma early in pregnancy with a rising concentration as pregnancy progresses. The values continue to rise until the onset of labour. It is probably involved in the prevention of rejection of the fetoplacental unit by the cellular lymphocyte component of the maternal immune system. PAPP-B is the largest placental glycoprotein and rises throughout pregnancy, with the steepest part of its curve occurring after 30 weeks. It has been used to ascertain the progress of the placenta in such diseases as pre-eclampsia and diabetes mellitus.

Placental protein 5

This hormone is a small glycoprotein which has different properties from the others. It is found in the stroma of the chorionic villi as well as in the syncytiotrophoblast. In studies it has been found to inhibit the proteolytic activity of trypsin and may inhibit protease activity in the placenta.

the precursor of all fetoplacental steroids, is converted to oestrogens by enzymes in the placenta. The steps are:

1. acetate to cholesterol;
2. cholesterol to pregnenolone;
3. pregnenolone to dehydroepiandosterone;
4. 16-hydroxylation to 16-hydroxydehydroepiandosterone;
5. 16-hydroxydehydroepiandosterone to estriol.

Oestrogen levels in normal pregnancy   Most tissues and organs are affected by oestrogens in pregnancy. Oestrogens are growth stimulators and cause hypertrophy and hyperplasia of uterine muscle as well as growth and development of the breasts. In a normal pregnancy maternal serum levels of all three hormones rise but the curve for plasma estriol is the most useful, showing a steep rise from about 34 to 36 weeks. This late surge may not occur if pregnancy pathology affects the fetus, when the curve may flatten out or even fall away. Serial assays of estriol have been useful in monitoring fetal wellbeing.

Estriol estimations and fetal wellbeing   Previously, urinary estriol assays were used because blood levels were not as clearly defined, but new tests have allowed accurate estimations of plasma estriol and maternal blood is now taken. The unit of measurement is nmol/L. The overlap between physiological and pathological levels is large and the best use is in serial estimations in a pregnancy known to be at risk rather than as a single screening device.

The steroid hormones – progesterone

Progesterone is produced by the syncytiotrophoblast: some hormone is sent to the maternal circulation and some to the fetus. The likely pathway of progesterone production by the placenta is from cholesterol through pregnenolone to progesterone. Progesterone is broken down into the inactive substance pregnanediol and excreted via urine.

Progesterone levels in normal and abnormal pregnancy It used to be thought that progesterone levels were indicative of fetal wellbeing and that a low level caused spontaneous abortion. However, treatment with progesterone was unsuccessful and the low level of progesterone follows rather than causes fetal compromise. Some sources have found a slight drop in maternal progesterone levels at the 9th week when placental production is taking over from ovarian production, with a sharp rise from the 10th week onwards. There is no agreement on what constitutes a normal level, as it fluctuates throughout pregnancy, but the average is from 275 nmol/L at 32 weeks to 450 nmol/L at term (Klopper 1991). Much progesterone is stored in body fat and may act as a buffer against transient low production.

The function of progesterone in pregnancy Ovarian progesterone plays a part in ovum transport and implantation. It is involved in endometrial development in the second part of the menstrual cycle and the decidual reaction is caused by progesterone secretion for 48 h followed by superimposed oestrogen. Progesterone has a sedative effect on uterine muscle contractability. With relaxin it may alter membrane potential in myometrial cells to reduce contractile impulses. Progesterone relaxes all smooth muscle during pregnancy, leading to many of the minor disorders of pregnancy. It competes with aldosterone for binding sites in the kidney, leading to urinary sodium loss. Aldosterone secretion is increased to counteract this effect. There is little evidence that a fall in progesterone level initiates the onset of labour.

Transfer of substances

The fetus is completely dependent on the mother for respiration, nutrition, excretion and protection, and the placenta acts as the fetal lungs, alimentary tract, kidneys and endocrine system. The placenta continues to grow throughout pregnancy, weighing about 300 g at 28 weeks of gestation and about 900 g at term. During the latter half of pregnancy, fetal growth is extremely rapid, whereas that of the placenta slows or even ceases. The placenta keeps pace with fetal needs by increase in blood flow on both maternal and fetal sides (Chard 2000).

New villi are formed until term when their surface area exposed to the maternal circulation is about 11 m². By late pregnancy there is thinning of the syncytium in small areas known as **vasculosyncytial membranes**. There are fewer microvilli and the syncytium is closely applied to the capillary basement membrane and has a large number of **intracellular vesicles**, possibly enabling the transfer of macromolecules such as immunoglobulins.

Mechanisms of transfer

Substances such as gases, nutrients, waste materials and drugs are transported across the placental membrane by the usual cellular membrane transport systems (Fig. 12.12):

- simple diffusion of lipid-soluble substances;
- water pores transfer water-soluble substances;
- facilitated diffusion of substances such as glucose by carrier proteins;
- active transport mechanisms against a concentration gradient of ions such as calcium and phosphate, of amino acids and of some vitamins;
- endocytosis (pinocytosis) of macromolecules.

Transport across the placenta increases during the course of gestation, as the placenta increases in size and becomes modified in structure. The rate of transfer is influenced by increased maternal and fetal blood flow and increased fetal demands. It is also influenced by maternal nutritional status, exercise and disease. Glucose transfer increases in diabetes mellitus due to maternal hyperglycaemia. Hypertension decreases nutrient transfer because of the reduced placental blood flow and alcoholism impairs placental uptake of glucose and amino acids.

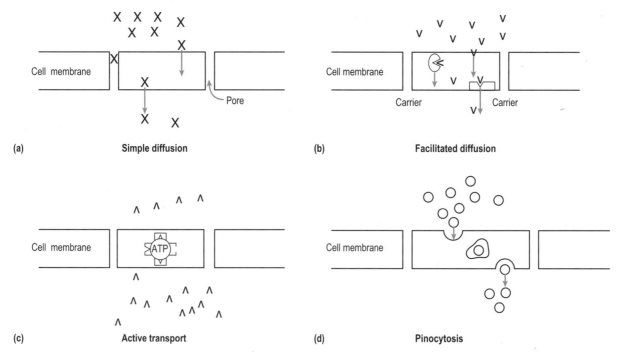

Figure 12.12   Mechanisms of placenta transfer. (Reproduced with permission from Blackburn & Loper 1992.)

Respiration

The major respiratory gases oxygen and carbon dioxide are moved between mother and fetus by simple transfer down a partial pressure concentration gradient. This is made more complex by maternal and fetal differences in haemoglobin concentration and type. If there is any disorganisation of blood flow by maternal or fetal disease, respiratory exchange may be compromised.

Fetal oxygen supply   Most oxygen in maternal and fetal blood is bound to haemoglobin in the form of **oxyhaemoglobin** (HbO$_2$). A gram of haemoglobin can carry 1.34 ml of oxygen at full saturation. A litre of maternal blood contains about 115 g Hb and can carry 154 ml of oxygen. A litre of fetal blood contains about 165 g Hb and can carry 221 ml oxygen (Stacey 1991).

Maternal blood arrives in the intervillous spaces of the placenta saturated with oxygen at a high partial pressure. Fetal blood arrives in the placenta with a low partial pressure and low oxygen content. Oxygen diffuses readily down the partial pressure gradient from mother to fetus. Maternal blood is not as good a source of oxygen as atmospheric air but fetal blood contains more Hb in order to maximise O$_2$ uptake. The diffusion gradient is enhanced by the increased affinity for oxygen of fetal haemoglobin (HbF), which combines more readily with oxygen than adult haemoglobin (HbA). Fetal systemic Po$_2$ is much lower than adult systemic Po$_2$ and parts of the fetal vascular tree are extremely sensitive to oxygen. This is important after the onset of respiration when a rise in Po$_2$ leads to closure of the ductus arteriosus and constriction of the umbilical vessels.

Carbon dioxide   Most of the metabolic processes of the fetus are aerobic and depend on a constant oxygen supply, and the fetus produces carbon dioxide for excretion. The much higher lipid solubility of carbon dioxide over oxygen results in a much more rapid transfer of the gas across cell membranes.

Nutrition

The fetus needs **amino acids** for cell building, **glucose** for energy, **calcium** and **phosphorus** for bones and teeth, and **iron** and **other minerals** for the formation of blood. Simple forms of nutrients such as amino acids, glucose and **fatty acids** pass from maternal to fetal blood through the walls of the villi. The placenta selects the substances required by the fetus and will deplete maternal supplies if necessary. Water, electrolytes and water-soluble vitamins cross the placenta (Bennett & Brown 1999).

Carbohydrate transfer   Glucose is a principal substrate for the production of energy which the fetoplacental unit utilises for the synthesis of macromolecules not obtained from the mother. The main form of transport for glucose is facilitated diffusion via a carrier protein molecule. Some glycogen is stored in the placenta and may act as an energy store for its own needs. The healthy placenta has a capacity for glucose transfer that far exceeds fetal needs. The transfer is affected by maternal blood glucose levels and by insulin.

Amino acid transfer   Fetal proteins are synthesised from amino acids obtained via carrier systems from the maternal circulation. The fetus accumulates amino acids against a concentration gradient and the placenta contains more amino acids than either maternal or fetal circulations (Stacey 1991).

Lipid transfer The fetus synthesises fatty acids from carbohydrate and short-chain organic acids, compensating for their absence in the diet of strict vegetarians. However, it is probable that the fetus obtains and stores fatty acids from the mother by passive transfer. Cholesterol also crosses the placenta.

Vitamin transfer As **vitamins** cannot be synthesised in the body, the fetus is dependent on its mother for supply. Vitamins differ in their molecular structure, which affects their transfer. The lipid-soluble vitamins A, D and E pass from maternal to fetal blood down a concentration gradient. Water-soluble vitamins such as vitamin C appear to be transferred to the fetus against a gradient and cannot be passed back to maternal circulation.

Trace element transfer Small amounts of crucial trace elements, including iron, zinc and copper, are transferred to the fetus.

Water and electrolyte transfer Water balance is achieved by diffusional gradients brought about by hydrostatic pressure and colloid osmotic pressure. Solutes such as sodium, potassium, calcium and phosphate are also freely transferred between maternal and fetal circulations. The fine balance maintained between maternal and fetal fluid components can be disturbed by the administration of hypotonic intravenous solutions such as 5% dextrose to the mother, especially if it contains the **antidiuretic oxytocin**. Transfer of water to the fetus occurs, resulting in **fetal hyponatraemia**.

Excretion

Besides carbon dioxide, discussed above, the placenta also passes other metabolic by-products as urea, uric acid and bilirubin to the maternal circulation to be excreted.

Protection

The placental membrane is a barrier against most bacteria, which are too large to penetrate it. However, the organisms causing syphilis and tuberculosis cross the barrier to form **transplacental infection**. Rubella virus also crosses freely. Drugs with a small molecular structure may cross to the fetus and some may cause congenital abnormalities. Other drugs such as antibiotics may be beneficial: for example, in the treatment of syphilis. Towards the end of pregnancy there is a transfer by pinocytosis of immunoglobulin G (IgG), conferring passive immunity for the first 3 months of extrauterine life.

Immunological role

The trophoblast appears to have immunological properties that make it inert so that maternal antibodies do not reject the fetus as foreign tissue (see Ch. 29).

AMNIOTIC FLUID

Production of amniotic fluid

Amniotic fluid is an alkaline clear, pale straw coloured fluid consisting of about 98% water with organic and inorganic substances in solution.

Sources of amniotic fluid

- Before keratinisation of the fetal skin there is free exchange of fluid and solutes between the fetus and amniotic cavity.
- Amniotic fluid may be secreted by the amniotic membrane cells which are separated by intracellular channels, leading to the amniotic cavity. Between 4 and 8 weeks of gestation amniotic fluid increases to about 20 ml. The expanded amnion reaches and lines the chorion.
- From the 11th week the fetus excretes urine into the amniotic cavity (Lind et al 1972). Amniotic fluid volume increases to 400 ml at 20 weeks, 800 ml at 36 weeks and declines slightly until term.
- Fluid is also secreted by the fetal respiratory tract.
- Although some water and solutes cross a transmembrane pathway from maternal blood to placenta and membranes into the amniotic cavity, this is not a significant amount.
- Diffusion from maternal interstitial fluid across the amniochorionic membrane from the surrounding decidua is probably the main source of the amniotic fluid (Moore & Persaud 1998).

Circulation of amniotic fluid

Amniotic fluid is in a constant state of circulation and renewal and the water content changes every 43 h (Moore & Persaud 1998). The fetal gastrointestinal tract is a major pathway for its removal. It is swallowed by the fetus and absorbed into its bloodstream; large amounts diffuse across the placenta into maternal circulation and some is excreted by the fetus into the amniotic sac. In the second half of pregnancy the chief sources of amniotic fluid are the fetal kidneys, which contribute 700 ml/day and fetal lungs, which contribute 350 ml/day (Fig. 12.13).

Content of amniotic fluid

During the first half of pregnancy the fetal skin is not a barrier to fluid and is a site for water and solute transfer. The composition of amniotic fluid in early pregnancy is similar to fetal tissue fluid (Moore & Persaud 1998). After keratinisation of

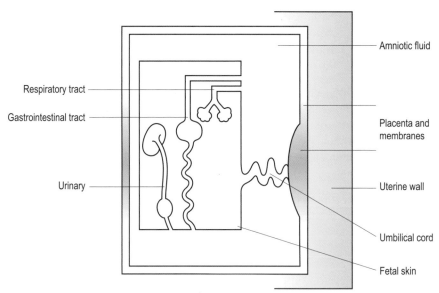

Figure 12.13 Pathways of amniotic fluid production and exhange. (Reproduced with permission from Wallenburg 1977.)

fetal skin at 17 weeks, the continuity between the fetal amniotic fluid and extracellular fluid is lost and the pattern of content and flow changes. Diffusible solutes such as sodium and urea can no longer be equilibrated with fetal or maternal plasma (Hytten 1991). In the latter half of pregnancy osmolality decreases to about 90% of maternal plasma and the composition resembles dilute urine (Blackburn 2003).

Mature amniotic fluid contains electrolytes, proteins and protein derivatives such as urea and creatinine, carbohydrates, lipids, hormones, enzymes, desquamated fetal cells, vernix and lanugo. Sodium and chloride content decreases and urea, uric acid and creatinine increases as fetal kidney function matures. Increasing amounts of phospholipids from the lungs appear as the fetal lung matures.

Regulation of amniotic fluid quantity

Decidual prolactin and **prostaglandins** (PGE$_2$) from the amnion and umbilical cord may aid regulation of amniotic fluid volume (McNabb 1997b). Concentration of prolactin in amniotic fluid is up to 10 times that of maternal circulation, increasing sharply in the second trimester and declining to a lower plateau by 34 weeks. Prolactin may regulate the volume of amniotic fluid by controlling electrolyte exchange across the chorioamniotic membrane. PGE$_2$ may regulate amniotic fluid by removing it into the maternal circulation to counterbalance the large volume of fetal urine output in the second half of pregnancy.

Functions of amniotic fluid

Amniotic fluid provides the following (Bennett & Brown 1999):

- space for fetal growth and movement;
- an equal pressure on the fetus to protect it from injury;
- a constant temperature for the fetus;
- small amounts of nutrients;
- prevention of placental and cord compression during labour;
- an aid to cervical effacement and dilatation.

Clinical implications: abnormalities of quantity

Moore & Persaud (1998) relate abnormalities of the fetus to abnormalities of amniotic fluid quantity. In fetal conditions such as renal agenesis or urethral obstruction, where there is obstruction to the flow of urine, the volume of amniotic fluid is very low (**oligohydramnios**). In conditions where the fetus cannot swallow, such as oesophageal atresia or anencephaly, there is an excess of amniotic fluid (**polyhydramnios**).

Polyhydramnios

One of the commonest anomalies found on ultrasound examination is polyhydramnios, which affects up to 1.5% of all pregnancies. Queenan (1996) defines polyhydramnios as 'a pathological accumulation of amniotic fluid volumes greater than 2000 ml clinically detectable in the third trimester of pregnancy (which) may or may not be associated with other problems.' Polyhydramnios may be chronic and acute:

- Chronic polyhydramnios is more common and is gradual in onset from about the 30th week of pregnancy.
- Acute polyhydramnios is rare, occurs at about 20 weeks and comes on rapidly. It is associated with monovular twins and occasionally with severe fetal abnormality.

Diagnosis   Polyhydramnios can be suspected clinically if:

- the uterus is larger than expected for gestational age;
- there is easy ballottement of the fetus;
- fetal parts are difficult to find;

Box 12.2 The causes of polyhydramnios

Fetal causes – number of fetuses	Multiple pregnancy
Fetal causes – anomalies	Central nervous system anomalies – anencephaly, hydrocephaly, spina bifida
	Gastrointestinal anomalies – oesophageal atresia, small bowel atresias, diaphragmatic hernia
	Cardiac anomalies
	Haematological abnormalities – α-thalassaemia, fetomaternal haemorrhage
	Fetal tumours
	Skeletal malformations – achondroplasia, osteogenesis imperfecta
	Chromosomal/genetic abnormalities
	Intrauterine infections – Rubella, syphilis, toxoplasmosis
Maternal causes	Diabetes mellitus
	Rhesus isoimmunisation
Placental causes	Placental chorioangioma
	Circumvallate placenta syndrome
Idiopathic causes	

Box 12.3 The causes of oligohydramnios

Post-term pregnancy	
Intrauterine growth retardation	
Premature rupture of membranes	
Fetal renal anomalies	Renal agenesis (Potter's syndrome)
	Urethral obstruction
	Prune belly syndrome
	Multicystic, dysplastic kidneys
Fetal non-renal anomalies	Triploidy
	Thyroid gland agenesis
	Skeletal dysplasia
	Congenital heart block
Chronic abruptio placentae	
Following medical procedures	Amniocentesis
	Chorionic villus sampling

- the fetal heart is muffled;
- maternal symptoms include breathlessness, vulval varicosities, oedema and gastric problems.

Ultrasonography is now the technique chosen to diagnose polyhydramnios and, if suspected clinically, should be confirmed by ultrasound (Moore & Persaud 1998).

Causes In 65% of cases of polyhydramnios the cause is unknown. Fetal causes are associated with 18%, maternal causes with 15% and placental causes with less than 1% of cases (Box 12.2).

Complications Polyhydramnios is associated with an increase in maternal and fetal mortality. Maternal complications include pregnancy-induced hypertension and respiratory discomfort. Fetal mortality is associated with conditions incompatible with life and fetal morbidity with minor abnormalities and preterm birth. Obstetric complications include unstable lie, malpresentation, cord presentation and prolapse, preterm labour, premature rupture of membranes (PROM), placental abruption and postpartum haemorrhage.

Management Diagnostic tests include:

- ultrasound examination to detect fetal and placental abnormalities and to confirm gestational age;
- studies of **fetal karyotype** to rule out chromosomal or genetic abnormalities (Barnhard et al 1995);
- fetal swallowing studies;

- TORCH screening for intrauterine infection;
- maternal antibody screening and diabetic screening.

Maternal comfort will be improved if the woman rests in bed in an upright position to relieve dyspnoea. She may require antacids to relieve heartburn and nausea. Amniotic fluid decompression of no more than 500 ml at a time (Abdel-Fattah et al 1999) may be carried out as needed if it is necessary to conserve the pregnancy. This will relieve maternal discomfort and reduce intrauterine pressure with its increased risk of preterm labour. Risks include infection and provoked onset of labour.

Oligohydramnios

Oligohydramnios is an abnormally small amount of amniotic fluid, less than 500 ml at term. In some cases much less than this is present (Rankin 1996). Oligohydramnios may affect 4% of pregnancies.

Diagnosis The condition may be suspected on abdominal examination if the following findings are present:

- the uterus appears smaller than expected for gestational age;
- the mother may have noticed a reduction in fetal movements;
- the uterus feels compact and fetal parts are easily felt.

Ultrasound examination confirms the absence of normal amniotic fluid pockets.

Causes Decreased amniotic fluid is a serious sign of severe fetal growth retardation, usually associated with maternal disease such as hypertension or chronic renal disease. Causes of oligohydramnios are outlined in Box 12.3.

Complications Prognosis is poor because of the complications of **premature rupture of membranes** (PROM) and fetal abnormalities. **Pulmonary hypoplasia** affects 60% of fetuses deprived of amniotic fluid for several weeks. It is generally lethal, with small anatomically immature lungs, poor surfactant levels and pulmonary hypertension. Oligohydramnios is often associated with **amnion nodosum**. Yellow-grey nodules consisting of desquamated fetal epidermal cells, hair and vernix are found in and on the amnion and on the fetal surface of the placenta, probably pressed into the amnion because of its close application to the fetus.

Management Management depends on the length of gestation, the maturity of the fetus, fetal and maternal health and the relative risks to the fetus of conservative management or delivery. The means of delivery depends on achieving maximum safety for mother and fetus. **Amnioinfusion**, where saline solution is infused into the amniotic cavity transabdominally or by a transcervical catheter, has been used in labour to prevent fetal distress and reduce the incidence of caesarean section. This invasive procedure can be performed either antenatally or during labour to:

- improve ultrasound imaging in oligohydramnios with suspected fetal abnormality;
- facilitate rapid fetal karyotyping;
- replace fluid in conservative management of PROM;
- prevent the development of fetal lung hypoplasia;
- decrease cord compression and reduce fetal distress during labour;
- reduce recurrent variable decelerations;
- dilute meconium (Telfer 1997).

Hofmeyr (1995) found no difference in outcomes between two groups of women, one who received prophylactic amnioinfusion and one where treatment was related to the onset of signs of fetal danger. He concluded that there was no advantage to be gained by prophylactic amnioinfusion over therapeutic amnioinfusion when signs were present. A meta-analysis of randomised controlled trials to evaluate the use of intrapartum amnioinfusion in pregnancies complicated by oligohydramnios concluded that intrapartum amnioinfusion improved neonatal outcome and lowered the rate of caesarean sections without increasing endometrial infection rates (Pitt et al 2000).

Diagnostic uses of amniotic fluid

Biophysical profile

Biophysical profile is a non-invasive test of fetal wellbeing using ultrasound imaging. Five variables are measured (Telfer 1997):

- fetal heart rate;
- fetal tone;
- somatic movements;
- breathing movements;
- amniotic fluid volume.

The variables are scored individually and added together to give a total. It can be an accurate predictor of fetal danger and imminent death but in a meta-analysis of 2839 pregnancies, when compared with conventional monitoring (e.g. cardiotocography), biophysical profile showed no effects, beneficial or deleterious, on pregnancy outcome in high-risk pregnancies (Alfirevic & Neilson 1997).

Amniocentesis

Cellular and biochemical components of amniotic fluid change with gestational age and provide useful indicators of fetal wellbeing and maturity (Blackburn 2003). Although the procedure is considered safe when warranted by fetal risk, there are possible complications of spontaneous abortion, infection, haematoma, haemorrhage, leakage of amniotic fluid or preterm labour. Amniotic fluid can be obtained by amniocentesis to gain knowledge about the fetus:

- cells can be used for chromosomal and genetic studies;
- α-fetoprotein can be used to assess the likelihood of neural tube defects or as part of the triple test for Down's syndrome;
- creatinine levels increase as the fetus matures;
- bilirubin estimates can monitor fetal red cell haemolysis in rhesus incompatibility;
- the ratio of the phospholipids lecithin and sphingomyelin can be used to assess fetal lung maturity;
- enzyme studies of cultured cells can help diagnose over 50% of inborn errors of metabolism.

MAIN POINTS

- The placenta is derived from the extraembryonic trophoblast cells with a few mesodermal cells from the inner cell mass. The cytotrophoblast gives rise to the syncytiotrophoblast, which invades the uterine lining to allow embedding. Lacunae fuse to form the intervillous spaces, which become filled with a mixture of blood and secretions from the eroded endometrial glands.

- In pregnancy decidual and myometrial arteries become dilated and unresponsive to circulatory pressor substances

or autonomic neural control. By the end of the 3rd week fetal blood circulates through the capillaries of the chorionic villi.

- About the 8th week of pregnancy the chorionic villi of the decidua capsularis degenerate and form the chorion laeve, which becomes the chorionic membrane. The chorionic villi of the decidua basalis branch to form the fetal part of the placenta. The outer chorion and inner amnion form the fetal sac.

- The placenta produces protein hormones and steroid hormones. Protein hormones include hCG, hPL, SP_1, PAPP-A and PAPP-B. The steroid hormones are mainly oestrogens and progesterone. The hormones alter maternal metabolic processes to benefit the fetus.

- The hormone hCG stimulates ovarian production of extra oestrogen and progesterone to maintain pregnancy. The hormone hPL probably promotes growth, mobilising free fatty acids and antagonising the action of insulin. A pregnant woman must manufacture more insulin in pregnancy, which is why hPL is diabetogenic.

- The levels of the hormones SP_1, PAPP-A and PAPP-B rise as pregnancy progresses. SP_1 and PAPP-A may be important in the immunosuppressive mechanism preventing rejection of the placenta and fetus.

- The fetal liver and suprarenal glands are important to the production of estriol. Plasma estriol levels rise steeply from about 34 to 36 weeks.

- Progesterone produced by the syncytiotrophoblast is sent to both the maternal circulation and the fetus. Progesterone relaxes smooth muscle during pregnancy and is responsible for some minor disorders of pregnancy. There is little evidence that a fall in progesterone production influences the onset of labour.

- Fetal growth depends on sufficient placental transfer of nutrients and oxygen. Transport across the placenta increases during the course of gestation as the placenta increases in size. Transfer across the placental membrane can be modified by maternal nutritional status, exercise and disease.

- Oxygen and carbon dioxide cross the syncytiotrophoblast and fetal capillary epithelium by simple transfer down a partial pressure concentration gradient. Nutrients, trace elements and vitamins pass from maternal to fetal blood through the walls of the villi. The placenta excretes urea, uric acid and bilirubin via the maternal circulation.

- Water balance is achieved by diffusional gradients brought about by hydrostatic pressure and colloid osmotic pressure. Solutes such as sodium, potassium, calcium and phosphate are freely transferred between maternal and fetal circulations.

- Most bacteria are too large to penetrate the placental membrane but those causing syphilis and tuberculosis do so, as does the rubella virus. Drugs of small molecular structure cross the placental barrier and may cause congenital abnormalities. Others such as antibiotics may be beneficial.

- Mature amniotic fluid contains electrolytes, proteins, urea and creatinine, carbohydrates, lipids, hormones, enzymes, desquamated fetal cells, vernix and lanugo. Sodium and chloride content decreases and urea, uric acid and creatinine increases as fetal kidney function matures. There are increasing amounts of phospholipids from the lungs as they mature.

- Amniotic fluid is in a constant state of circulation and renewal. The fetal gastrointestinal tract is a major pathway for its removal. Decidual prolactin and prostaglandins from the amnion and umbilical cord may regulate amniotic fluid volume.

- Amniotic fluid provides space for fetal growth and movement and protects the fetus from injury. A constant temperature is maintained. Intact membranes prevent placental and cord compression during labour and act as an aid to cervical effacement and dilatation.

- Polyhydramnios affects up to 1.5% of all pregnancies. Chronic polyhydramnios is more common. Causes include multiple pregnancy, fetal anomalies, diabetes mellitus and placental abnormalities. Acute polyhydramnios is rare and is associated with monovular twins and severe fetal abnormality.

- Obstetric complications include unstable lie, malpresentation, cord presentation and prolapse, preterm labour, premature rupture of membranes, placental abruption and postpartum haemorrhage. Diagnostic tests include ultrasound examination, fetal karyotype, fetal swallowing studies, TORCH screening for intrauterine infection, maternal antibody screening and diabetic screening.

- Maternal comfort will be improved with bed rest in an upright position to relieve dyspnoea. Antacids will relieve heartburn and nausea. Amniotic fluid may be removed to conserve the pregnancy.

- Causes of oligohydramnios include post-term pregnancy, intrauterine growth retardation, fetal renal anomalies and chronic abruptio placentae. Fetal complications include pulmonary hypoplasia, which is generally lethal. Amnioinfusion has been used in labour as a means of preventing fetal distress and reducing the need for caesarean section.

- Biophysical profiling can be an accurate predictor of fetal danger and imminent death. In comparison to cardiotocography, biophysical profile results may have no effect on pregnancy outcome.

- Cellular and biochemical components of amniotic fluid change with gestational age and provide useful indicators of fetal wellbeing and maturity. Although amniocentesis is considered safe when warranted by fetal risk, there are complications of spontaneous abortion, infection, haematoma, haemorrhage, leakage of amniotic fluid and preterm labour.

References

Abdel-Fattah S A, Carroll S G, Kyle P M, Soothill P W 1999 Amnioreduction: How much to drain? Fetal Diagnosis and Therapy 14(5):279–282.

Alfirevic Z, Neilson J P 1997 Biophysical profile for fetal assessment in high risk pregnancies. Cochrane Review: In The Cochrane Library, Issue 2. Update Software 2003, Oxford.

Barnhard Y, Bar-Hava I, Divon M Y 1995 Is polyhydramnios in an ultrasonographically normal fetus an indication for genetic evaluation? American Journal of Obstetrics and Gynecology 173(5):1523–1527.

Bennett V R, Brown L K 1999 The placenta. In Bennett V R, Brown L K (eds) Myles Textbook for Midwives, 12th edn. Churchill Livingstone, Edinburgh, pp 43–50.

Blackburn S T 2003 Maternal, fetal and neonatal physiology – a clinical perspective. W B Saunders, Philadelphia.

Chard T 2000 The placenta as patient. Yearbook of Obstetrics and Gynaecology 8:61–73.

Coad J, Dunstall M 2001 Anatomy and Physiology for Midwives. Mosby, St Louis.

Germain A M, Smith J, Casey M L et al 1994 Human fetal membrane contribution to the prevention of parturition: uterotonin degradation. Journal of Clinical Endocrinology and Metabolism 78(2):463–470.

Hofmeyr G J 1995 Prophylactic versus therapeutic amnioinfusion for oligohydramnios in labour. Cochrane Review: In the Cochrane Library, Issue 2. Update Software 2003, Oxford.

Hytten F 1991 Weight gain in pregnancy. In Hytten F, Chamberlain G (eds) Clinical Physiology in Obstetrics. Blackwell Scientific, Oxford.

Klopper A 1991 Placental metabolism. In Hytten F, Chamberlain G (eds) Clinical Physiology in Obstetrics. Blackwell Scientific, Oxford.

Lind T, Kendall A, Hytten F E 1972 The role of the fetus in the formation of amniotic fluid. Journal of Obstetrics and Gynaecology of the British Commonwealth 79:289; cited in Hytten F E 1991 Weight gain in pregnancy. In Hytten F E, Chamberlain G (eds) Clinical Physiology in Obstetrics. Blackwell Scientific, Oxford.

McNabb M 1997a Embryonic and fetal developments. In Sweet B R, Tiran D (eds) Mayes Midwifery, 12th edn. Baillière Tindall, London.

McNabb M 1997b Implantation and development of the placenta. In Sweet B R, Tiran D (eds) Mayes Midwifery, 12th edn. Baillière Tindall, London.

Moore K L, Persaud T V N 1998 Before We Are Born, 5th edn. W B Saunders, Philadelphia.

Pitt C, Sanchez-Ramos L, Kaunitz A M et al 2000 Obstetrics and Gynaecology 96(5)part 2:861–866.

Queenan J T 1996 Polyhydramnios. Contemporary Obstetrics and Gynaecology 41(5):11–16.

Rankin S 1996 Disorders of the pregnancy. In Bennett V R, Brown L K (eds) Myles Textbook for Midwives, 12th edn. Churchill Livingstone, Edinburgh.

Stacey T E 1991 Placental transfer. In Hytten F, Chamberlain G (eds) Clinical Physiology in Obstetrics, 2nd edn. Blackwell Scientific, Oxford, pp 415–437.

Telfer F M 1997 Antenatal investigations of maternal and fetal wellbeing. In Sweet B R, Tiran D (eds) Mayes Midwifery, 12th edn. Baillière Tindall, London.

Annotated recommended reading

Alfirevic Z, Neilson J P 1997 Biophysical profile for fetal assessment in high risk pregnancies. Cochrane Review: In The Cochrane Library, Issue 2. Update Software 2003, Oxford.
This review on the Cochrane database provide an excellent start to studying a particular subject in depth.

Chard T 2000 The placenta as patient. Yearbook of Obstetrics and Gynaecology 8:61–73.
This paper provides a highly readable account of previous and recent knowledge about the physiology and pathology of the placenta. There are many good references cited within the work.

Hofmeyr G J 1995 Prophylactic versus therapeutic amnioinfusion for intrapartum oligohydramnios. Cochrane Review: In The Cochrane Library, Issue 2. Update Software 2003, Oxford.
This review on the Cochrane database provide an excellent start to studying a particular subject in depth.

Moore K L, Persaud T V N 1998 Before We Are Born, 5th edn. W B Saunders, Philadelphia.
The layout of this textbook remains excellent. It clearly describes the formation of the placenta and amniotic fluid. The illustrations in this latest edition are excellent.

Chapter 13

Fetal growth and development

INTRODUCTION

The general organising principles of embryology, the development of systems and the structure and function of the placenta have been discussed in previous chapters. During the development of the zygote into a recognisable human form, the baby is referred to as an embryo. From the beginning of the 9th week of intrauterine life most of the organs are in place even though they may be non-functional. This fetal period is primarily concerned with an increase in size and maturation of the systems.

THE FETAL PERIOD

Care must be taken to avoid confusion when calculating fetal age. Fetal age has traditionally been calculated from the 1st day of the **last menstrual period** (LMP). Following the use of ultrasound scanning (US), it has become more common to calculate fetal age by using the estimated day of fertilisation. The date of birth is about 266 days or 38 weeks after fertilisation and about 280 days or 40 weeks from the first day of the LMP. Tanner (1978) stated that it is usual to use **postfertilisation age** when describing organ differentiation and development and this method will be used throughout this chapter.

Fetal growth

Moore & Persaud (1998) remind us that the fetal period from the 9th week following ovulation to the delivery is characterised by 'rapid body growth and differentiation of tissues and organ systems' that appeared in the embryonic period. Wolpert et al (2002) define growth as 'an increase in the mass or overall size of a tissue or organism'. Cell death is important in determining overall growth rate.

Tissues may grow by:

- **cell proliferation** or hypertrophy (increased cell numbers);
- **cell enlargement** without division or hyperplasia (increased cell size);

- **accretion of extracellular material** such as bone matrix or even water.

During cleavage and blastula formation there is little growth, cells becoming smaller with each cleavage division. There is then a remarkable rate of growth during weeks 9–24. From 24 weeks, growth slows and remains constant until just before term when it slows again. In early pregnancy growth is mainly by **hyperplasia**. This is followed by a period of simultaneous hyperplasia and **hypertrophy** (Bogin 2001). After 34 weeks, growth is mainly by hypertrophy (Blackburn 2003). Few new nerve cells or new muscle cells appear after 30 weeks. **Growth** and **maturation** of the systems is directly linked to the ability of the fetus to survive outside the uterus, a concept known as **viability**.

Control of cell growth and proliferation

Cells divide by going through a fixed sequence of events during the cell cycle (Ch. 2, p. 18). **Growth factors** and other **signalling proteins** play a key role in controlling cell growth and proliferation. Cells must receive these signals not only to divide but also to survive. Without them they commit **apoptosis** (cell suicide), brought about by activation of an internal cell death programme (Wolpert et al 2002). However, the mechanisms underlying embryonic cell division are poorly understood.

The fetal genome has the greatest effect on fetal growth but maternal and fetal factors may alter the inherited pattern (Johnson & Everitt 2000) (Box 13.1).

KEY EVENTS IN THE FETAL STAGE OF DEVELOPMENT

The details of developmental stages are adapted from Moore & Persaud (1998) and are given in Table 13.1. Note that there is no line of week or measure when a fetus can be said to be viable. Dimensional variations increase with age, making the judgement of gestational age less accurate (Figs 13.1 and 13.2). It is still unlikely that a fetus of less than 22 weeks or weighing less than 500 g could survive.

Fetal size

Before birth it is usual to measure the fetus in the form of sitting height or **crown–rump length**. Table 13.2 is based on post-fertilisation age and is derived from Moore & Persaud (1998).

ESTIMATION OF FETAL AGE AND ASSESSMENT OF FETAL GROWTH

Growth curves

If a series of measurements is taken, these can be plotted on a graph and used to calculate growth. Growth can be viewed as a motion through time (Bogin 2001) and, if measurements are taken and plotted at regular intervals of time, a steady curve called a **distance curve** (Fig. 13.3) results. It is more usual to plot a distance curve when monitoring fetal growth. In order to show how the rate of growth alters over time, the speed or velocity of growth is measured and

---

Box 13.1 Maternal control of fetal size

As mentioned above, maternal factors may alter the inherited pattern of fetal growth. Tanner (1978) stated that 'there is considerable evidence that, beginning at 34 to 36 weeks, the growth of the fetus slows down owing to the influence of the uterus, whose available space is by then becoming fully occupied'. He also wrote that twins begin to slow in growth earlier, when their combined weight is that of a 36-week fetus. This slowing down allows a genetically large child growing in the uterus of a small mother to be safely delivered.

A genetic explanation

Haig (1993) suggested a genetic mechanism for control of fetal size. He hypothesised that how big a baby grows is determined by a conflict between maternal and paternal genes. A gene present on chromosome 11 called **IGF2** (insulin-like growth factor 2) is responsible for the regulation of fetal size. The gene inherited from the father

makes a growth factor which helps the fetus to grow while the maternal gene is programmed to be non-functional and to inhibit the effect of the father's gene.

In humans evidence for this is seen in the genetic condition **Beckwith–Wiedemann syndrome** where babies are born very large and with enlargement of various tissues in the body. The gene for this syndrome is on C11 and in affected tissues two paternal genes were found to be present instead of one from each parent. This would double the amount of the protein enhancing fetal growth produced.

Evidence for maternal control of fetal growth is also found in the size of foals from horse crosses between a large shire horse and a smaller Shetland pony. If the mother is a shire horse the newborn foal is similar in size to a normal shire foal, but if the mother is a Shetland pony the newborn is much smaller. During growth after birth both foals achieve a similar size, midway between shires and Shetlands (Wolpert et al 2002). Intrauterine growth retardation is discussed in Chapter 14.

Table 13.1 Fetal development based on weeks from fertilisation

Weeks	Developmental feature
9	The fetal head measures half the fetal crown–rump length
10	Intestinal coils have all re-entered the body cavity
12	Fetal length has more than doubled The upper limbs have attained their relative length in comparison to the fetal trunk but the lower limbs remain short The mature forms of the external genitalia appear There is a decrease of red blood cell formation by the liver and onset in the spleen The formation and excretion of urine begins The beginning of fetal muscle movements occurs The eyelids fuse
13–16	This is a period of very rapid growth
16	By now the head is smaller in comparison to the trunk and the lower limbs have reached their correct proportions The skeleton can be seen clearly on X-ray films The face has become more human with the eyes facing anteriorly rather than laterally The external ears have moved to their positions on the sides of the head
17–20	Growth slows down Fetal movements are felt by the mother The skin becomes covered with vernix caseosa, protecting it from the amniotic fluid Lanugo which has developed over the whole body by the 20th week may help to hold the vernix on the skin Head and eyebrow hair become visible The highly metabolic brown fat is formed during this period
21–25	Surfactant production in the lungs begins Towards the end of this time there is a chance of survival if the baby is born The skin lacks subcutaneous fat and is wrinkled The skin appears red because of blood capillaries just under the surface The fetus now has periods of sleep and activity and responds to sound
26–29	The lungs are capable of breathing air and allowing gas exchange The nervous system can control rhythmic breathing movements and body temperature. Intrauterine respiratory movements are made The eyes reopen Head and lanugo hair is well developed White subcutaneous fat is laid down under the skin At 28 weeks erythropoeisis ends in the spleen and begins in the bone marrow
30–34	The pupillary light reflex is present The quantity of body fat increases to 8% of total body weight The skin is opaque and smooth From 32 weeks most fetuses will survive Lanugo disappears from the face The fetus begins to store iron
35–38	A fetus of 35 weeks will have a firm grasp Most fetuses become plump At 36 weeks the head and abdominal circumferences are equal. Later the abdominal circumference becomes greater. Growth slows as term approaches By 38 weeks the body fat content has to be about 16% of body weight Breast tissue is present in both sexes The testes are in the scrotum in male infants The nails reach the tips of the fingers Lanugo disappears from the body

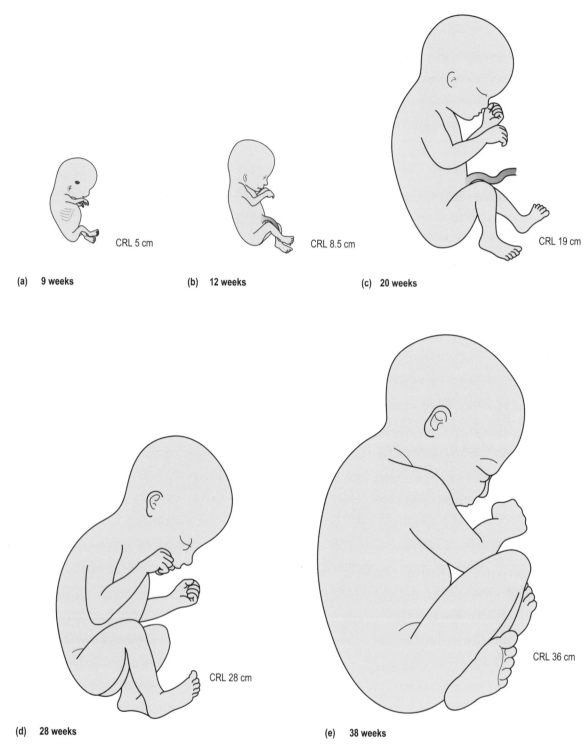

CRL 5 cm

(a) **9 weeks**

CRL 8.5 cm

(b) **12 weeks**

CRL 19 cm

(c) **20 weeks**

CRL 28 cm

(d) **28 weeks**

CRL 36 cm

(e) **38 weeks**

Figure 13.1   Drawings of fetuses at various stages of development. CRL, crown–rump length. (Reproduced with permission from Moore 1989.)

plotted. This generates a **velocity curve**, showing how the rate of growth alters (Fig. 13.4).

Maternal weight and fetal growth

Maternal weight gain has traditionally been used to assess fetal wellbeing in pregnancy and continued weight gain is thought to be a favourable sign of maternal adaptation and fetal growth and wellbeing (Thomson 1996). However, weight gain varies widely: from weight loss to a gain of 23 kg and more (Hytten 1991). Many factors affect maternal weight gain, including the presence of oedema, maternal metabolic rate, dietary intake, gastrointestinal problems, smoking and the size of the fetus.

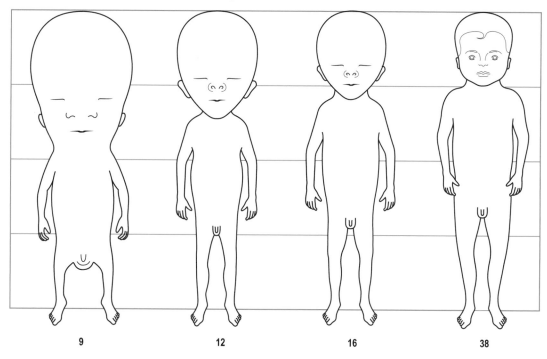

9   12   16   38

Fertilization (conception) age in weeks

Figure 13.2   The changing proportions of the body during the fetal period. At 9 weeks the head is about half the crown–rump length of the fetus. By 36 weeks, the circumferences of the head and the abdomen are approximately equal. After this, the circumference of the abdomen may be greater. All stages are drawn to the same total height. (Reproduced with permission from Moore 1989.)

Table 13.2   The average size of the fetus related to weeks of gestation

Age in weeks	Crown–rump length in mm	Weight in grams
10	61	14
12	87	45
14	120	110
16	140	250
18	160	320
20	190	460
22	210	630
24	230	820
26	250	1000
28	270	1300
30	280	1700
32	300	2100
36	340	2900
38	360	3400

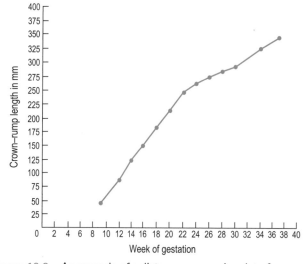

Figure 13.3   An example of a distance curve using data from fetal crown–rump measurements.

Attempts to control maternal weight gain in order to reduce the size of the fetus and make delivery easier have been made but were unsuccessful and had little effect on fetal size. The only components of weight gain available for manipulation are maternal fat and extracellular fluid and Hytten (1990) does not believe that either obesity or oedema can be influenced by regular weighing. An average weight gain appears to be about 12 kg and should be 2 kg in the first 20 weeks and 0.5 kg thereafter until term (Thomson 1996). It can be broken down into its components, as shown in Table 13.3.

Hytten (1990) reviewed the literature on weight gain in pregnancy. Poor weight gain was associated with **intrauterine growth retardation** (IUGR) but was not a very sensitive indicator. Weight gain may have been normal when a baby with IUGR is delivered. Daily fluctuations in a woman's

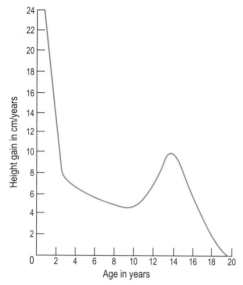

Figure 13.4   An example of velocity curve demonstrating the growth of body from birth to age 18.

Table 13.3   Distribution of maternal weight gain in pregnancy

Component of weight gain	Gain in grams
The fetus	3400
The placenta	600
The amniotic fluid	600
The uterus	900
The breasts	500
Fat stores	3500
Blood volume	1500
Extracellular fluid	1000
Total	12000

weight can be up to 1% of the total body weight and there are better ways of assessing the fetus.

Uterine **fundal height** is the most common method used to assess fetal growth. Fundal height measurements are made in centimetres from the upper border of the symphysis pubis to the top of the fundus of the uterus. Care must be taken to allow for any deviation of the uterus to one side of the abdomen. Errors may occur if a woman is too thin or obese or has too much or too little abdominal muscle tone. Breech presentation and transverse lie will also result in error. Fundal height can be plotted against a standard curve.

Ultrasound

The gestational age is calculated from the mother's LMP or taken from an early first or second trimester scan. Plotting of later measurements must be charted accurately to avoid wrong diagnosis. The rate of success of US in detecting IUGR may be as high as 95%. Measurements taken by ultrasound scan are plotted against a normal curve. Linear and non-linear measurements can be used (Proud 1996).

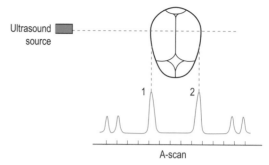

Figure 13.5   An A-scan sonogram; 1 and 2 indicate the parietal eminence (from Sweet B 1997, with permission).

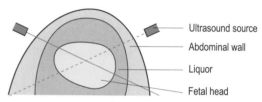

Figure 13.6   A diagram showing the abdominal wall and the fetal head (from Sweet B 1997, with permission).

Linear measurements

Crown–rump length is used to estimate gestational age in the first trimester. The measurement between the two parietal eminences is called the **biparietal diameter** or BPD (Fig. 13.5). This can be assessed once the correct position of the fetal head is located (Fig. 13.6). This is a useful estimate of gestation in the second trimester but becomes less accurate later in pregnancy. Femur length is also useful in assessing gestational age.

Non-linear measurements

Measurement of the head circumference (HC) is preferred in the third trimester when moulding of the head may alter the BPD. Abdominal circumference (AC) is measured at the level of the bifurcation of the hepatic vein in the centre of the fetal liver. A reduction in AC suggests a reduction in liver size due to depletion of stores.

Ratios

- HC to AC ratio compares the status of the brain to the liver. A raised ratio because of reduced AC suggests IUGR

- Femur to AC ratio compares the length of the femur, which is minimally affected by asymmetric IUGR, to the AC. A raised ratio suggests IUGR

Doppler wave form analysis

Measuring the velocity of blood in the umbilical cord using **Doppler ultrasound** has been suggested as an additional means of assessing fetal wellbeing (Ch. 14, p. 181).

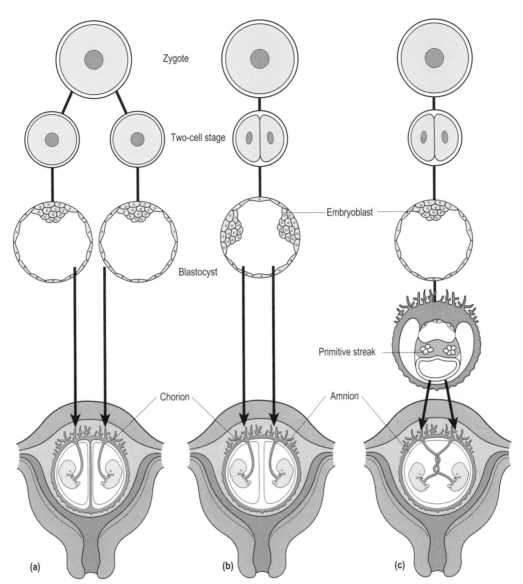

Figure 13.7   Three kinds of twins. (a) Dichorionic–diamniotic, (b) monochorionic–diamniotic, and (c) monochorionic–monoamniotic (from Fitzgerald M J T, Fitzgerald M 1994, with permission).

MULTIPLE PREGNANCIES

Multiple pregnancy (multifetal gestation) is the term used to describe the development of more than one fetus in utero at the same time. At delivery the prevalence of twins is about 1 in 100 but this has now increased due to infertility treatment and is now about 1 in 75 births (Divon & Weiner 1995).

Types of twin pregnancy

Dizygotic

About two-thirds of twin pregnancies are **dizygotic** (binovular, non-identical or fraternal twins), having developed from the fertilisation of two separate ova. This type of twinning varies between ethnic groups (Moore & Persaud 1998, Sebire et al 2000). Dizygotic twins have separate placentas, two chorions and two amnions (**dichorionic-diamniotic**) and only share the same genetic make-up as any brother or sister (Fig. 13.7). They may be the same or different sexes. The incidence of congenital malformation is only slightly greater than normal.

Monozygotic

About one-third of twinning occurs when a single fertilised ovum divides into two separate fetuses. These are **monozygotic** (uniovular or identical) twins. About one-third of monozygotic twins are **dichorionic** and two-thirds share one placenta and chorion. In 95% of these each baby has its own amnion (**monochorionic-diamniotic**). In about 5% of twins the babies share one amnion (**monochorionic-monoamniotic**) and about 1% of monoamniotic twins are **conjoined** or **Siamese twins** (Sebire et al 2000).

They are identical in their genetic make-up, having developed from the one fertilised ovum and the twins are always of the same sex, except in very rare abnormalities of the sex chromosomes (Fig. 13.7). There is a connection between the two fetal circulations via the placenta. The high incidence of errors of development and of congenital malformations may be linked to the abnormality that caused the twinning.

The incidence of multiple pregnancies

Since the advent of the treatment of infertility by stimulation of ovulation multiple births have become much more common. In naturally occurring pregnancies twins occur about once in 90 pregnancies, triplets about once in 90^2 pregnancies, quadruplets once in 90^3 pregnancies and quintuplets once in 90^4 pregnancies (Moore & Persaud 1998). The incidence of multiple pregnancy varies naturally around the world. It is higher in black people and lower in Asian peoples. The differences in twinning rates result from variations in dizygotic twinning and the incidence of monozygotic twins is constant at 3.5 per 1000 across all nationalities. Factors influencing the frequency of dizygotic twinning are:

- maternal age – the incidence increases up to 35 years of age;
- maternal parity;
- conception soon after discontinuing oral contraceptives – if oral contraceptives have been used for more than 6 months and conception occurs within a month of discontinuation, the chances of a twin pregnancy doubles.

The development of ultrasound scanning techniques has shown that the incidence of twin pregnancy at conception in humans may be double the number of eventual twin births. Half may never be recognised as twin pregnancy because of the death of one embryo in early pregnancy. The embryo may be reabsorbed (**vanishing twin syndrome**) or rarely may remain in between the membranes of the second twin as a **fetus papyraceous** (paper fetus). The earlier the ultrasound scan is performed, the higher the probability of only one baby being born (Divon & Weiner 1995).

Triplets and higher-order pregnancies

The introduction of drugs such as **clomifene** which stimulate ovulation has led to an increase in pregnancies where five to eight fetuses are conceived (Duncan & Denbow 2001). The incidence of multiple pregnancies following clomifene is between 6.8% and 17% and, if **gonadotrophins** have been used, the rate increases to between 18% and 53%. In the United Kingdom assisted pregnancy has led to an increase in the number of multiple births, and triplet births have more than doubled since 1989.

The implications for maternity and neonatal care of these **high-risk pregnancies** are a cause for concern (Spillman 1997). The outcome of such pregnancies can be poor and some centres have advocated **multifetal reduction** to ensure survival of fewer fetuses. This is carried out between 9 and 12 weeks when an intracardiac injection of potassium chloride is given under ultrasound guidance. This ensures the survival of the two or three remaining fetuses, but the procedure may lead to loss of all the fetuses.

When the figures on fetal survival in triplet, quadruplet and quintuplet pregnancies are contrasted with the risk associated with selective feticide, it is difficult to support a decision to reduce fetal numbers if there are four fetuses or less. More than 50% of women in whom three or more fetal sacs were found on ultrasound scan had a spontaneous reduction of fetal number before 12 weeks of pregnancy (Dickey et al 2002). This was commoner in spontaneous multiple ovulations than in induced ovulations.

Skrablin et al (2000) compared triplet pregnancies with quadruplet and quintuplet pregnancies in 64 women. They found that, although birth weight was significantly lower in pregnancies with four or five fetuses than in triplet pregnancies, survival rates were the same. As the spontaneous loss rate in triplets and higher-order births was similar to the pregnancy loss rate following multifetal reduction they advocate conservative management in specialist centres, especially in triplet pregnancies. Leondires et al (2000) found no significant differences in perinatal mortality, gestational age at delivery and healthy survival of triplets between pregnancies where all fetuses were allowed to develop and those in which fetal reduction was carried out.

Diagnosis of twin pregnancy

It is apparent that the earlier the diagnosis of twins is made, the more successful the outcome. Perinatal losses may be much larger when the diagnosis is made after 28 weeks. Since the development of routine ultrasound scanning, the incidence of undiagnosed twins at delivery is rare. However, not all midwives work in countries where access to scanning is easy or possible, therefore it is important to be able to diagnose a multiple pregnancy by clinical examination. A family history of twinning should alert the professional carer to the possibility. However, vigilance in all pregnancies should be equal.

Abdominal examination

Inspection This method is unlikely to diagnose twins before 20 weeks of pregnancy but the uterus may appear larger than expected for the gestational age. The uterus may look large and broad and fetal movements may be very obvious over the whole uterus.

Palpation The fundal height may be greater than expected for the period of gestation. The presence of two fetal poles in the fundus may help to identify a twin pregnancy. Location of three poles suggests the presence at least a twin pregnancy. Multiple fetal limbs may also be present. A later clue is the apparent smallness of the fetal head in relation to the size of the uterus. Lateral palpation may find two fetal backs or the presence of fetal limbs on both sides of the uterus.

Auscultation   It is said by some that hearing two fetal hearts simultaneously with a difference of 10 beats per minute is diagnostic of twins. Practically, this is difficult to achieve as the fetal heart of a singleton fetus can be heard over a wide area.

Ultrasound

Ultrasound diagnosis of a multiple pregnancy can be made as early as 5 weeks following the last menstrual period. However it may not be possible to confirm a twin pregnancy until after 12 weeks because of the likelihood of vanishing twin syndrome (Divon & Weiner 1995). Ultrasound diagnosis should be made to ascertain the number of placentas present and types of membranes present. Diagnosis of monoamniotic twins is essential because of the higher risk of abnormalities so that management can be planned (Sebire et al 2000).

Complications of pregnancy

Sebire et al (2001) analysed more than 400 000 pregnancies in the United Kingdom in their attempt to 'provide estimates of risk for common obstetric problems in multiple pregnancies compared to singleton pregnancies'. They found that the incidence of certain obstetric complications were more frequent in multiple births than in singleton births. These included pre-eclampsia, antepartum haemorrhage, anaemia, delivery by caesarean section, preterm delivery, low birth weight, stillbirth, admission of the babies to neonatal intensive care unit, postpartum haemorrhage and maternal infections. For most of the complications the incidence increased with the number of fetuses present.

Fetal problems

Loss of pregnancy   Abortion is more commonly associated with multiple pregnancies. This may be due to fetal abnormality in early pregnancy or to overdistension of the uterus in later pregnancy.

Single fetal demise   Single fetal demise may occur. Before 14 weeks this will probably cause no problems for the survivor. Later there may be transfer of **thromboplastin** released from the tissues of the dead twin, which may cause arterial occlusion, brain damage and renal cortical necrosis. A serious maternal problem is the onset of disseminated intravascular coagulation (DIC) about 3 weeks after fetal death.

Fetal abnormality   Congenital malformation is more likely to occur in twin pregnancies. Although the incidence was about the same in monozygotic and dizygotic twins,

abnormalities in dizygotic twins tended to be minor while those in monozygotic twins were multiple and lethal. The most common abnormalities are cleft lip and palate, central nervous system defects and cardiac defects. In monozygotic twins abnormalities also include conjoined twins and **fetal acardia**.

Monoamniotic twins   When monoamniotic twins are present the perinatal mortality is as high as 50%, mainly because of entanglement of the umbilical cords. Other causes of fetal loss are **twin-to-twin transfusion syndrome**, congenital abnormalities and preterm birth (Sebire et al 2000). Ultrasound scanning should be carried out at regular intervals to diagnose any problems and allow planning for management (Divon & Weiner 1995). It is best to deliver the babies by caesarean section to avoid increasing cord entanglement during vaginal birth.

Conjoined twins   The joining of twins by a bridge of tissue affects about 1% of monozygotic twin pregnancies (Fig. 13.8). This means that 1 in 900 of twin pregnancies and 1 in 40 000 to 1 in 100 000 live births are affected. In pairs of **conjoined twins** 70% will be female and the cause is unknown. Partial or complete duplication of just the upper or lower part of the body may occur and associated malformations are usually present (Table 13.4) (Craven & Ward 1996). There are two possibilities of causation: first, and more likely, possibility is incomplete separation of the embryonic cell mass at the embryonic plate/primitive streak stage 14–17 days after ovulation. The second possibility is partial fusion of two separate centres of embryonic growth, which probably happens before the 14 days (Craven & Ward 1996).

A diagnosis can be made by ultrasound and suspicion should be raised in the following cases:

1. monoamniotic twins;
2. twins that face each other;
3. the heads are at the same level and in the same plane;
4. the thoracic cages are in close proximity;
5. both fetal heads are hyperextended;
6. there is no change in the fetal positions on a later scan.

Once the diagnosis is confirmed, delivery by caesarean section should be planned. The outcome for conjoined twins is poor. About one-third of conjoined twins are stillborn and another third die within 24 hours of delivery (Craven & Ward 1996). Surgical separation of conjoined twins is the only means by which independent lives can be achieved. The presence of shared organs may make it impossible to save both babies. However, Spitz & Kiely (2000) state that there has been improvement in survival following surgery because of advances in diagnosis, meticulous anaesthesia and improved surgical techniques.

Acardiac twinning   This is a malformation that occurs in about 1% of monozygotic twins where one twin has no heart structures and the circulation for both is maintained by the heart of the second twin. The acardiac twin is non-viable

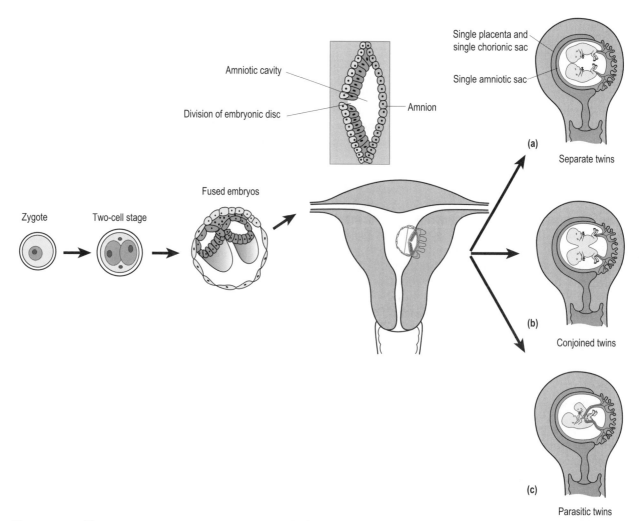

Figure 13.8   Diagrams showing how some monozygotic (MZ) twins develop. This method of development is very uncommon. Division of the embryonic disc results in two embryos within one amniotic sac. (a) Complete division of the embryonic disc gives rise to twins. Such twins rarely survive because their umbilical cords are often so entangled that interruption of the blood supply to the fetuses occurs. (b,c) Incomplete division of the disc results in various types of conjoined twins. (Reproduced with permission from Moore 1989.)

Table 13.4   Classification of conjoined twins by the site of union

Name	Percentage of occurrence	Description
Thoracopagus	40	Joined at the chest
Omphalopagus	35	Joined at the anterior abdominal wall
Pygopagus	18	Joined at the buttocks
Ischiopagus	6	Joined at the ischium
Craniopagus	2	Joined at the head

and circulatory overload may lead to heart failure in the normal twin; the mortality rate for the normal twin is 35%. Some obstetricians have successfully terminated the acardiac fetus and others have treated the normal twin for congestive cardiac failure by giving the mother drugs (Craven & Ward 1996).

Twin–twin transfusion syndrome   Twin–twin transfusion syndrome (TTTS) affects between 15% and 35% of monozygotic twins. Vascular communications in the placenta occur between the fetuses, causing a circulatory imbalance. This results in **hypovolaemia**, **oliguria** and **oligohydramnios** in the donor twin who may suffer from 'stuck twin' phenomenon and growth retardation. If anaemia is severe, the donor may develop **hydrops fetalis** and heart failure. **Hypervolaemia**, **polyuria** and **polyhydramnios** occur in the recipient who often **develops circulatory overload** and **congestive cardiac failure**. Fetal loss occurs and survivors are very ill and risk long-term morbidity (Van Gemert et al 2001). Prenatal diagnosis is made when the following conditions are present:

- same sex twins;
- a thin membrane between the twins showing diamniotic-monochorionic membranes;
- a 20% difference in estimated fetal weight of the twins;

- a discrepancy in the amniotic fluid surrounding the fetuses;
- fetal hydrops in one or both twins.

Attempts to deal with the problem antenatally may reduce the mortality rate to 40%. These include bed rest and preterm delivery, **serial amniocentesis**, occlusion of the vascular anastomoses by **laser coagulation** and **septostomy** (creating a hole between the two chorionic membranes). Researchers differ in their appraisal of which method of treatment is more successful. Johnson et al (2001) favour septostomy, while Van Gemert et al (2001) prefer laser abla-tion. Serial amniocentesis may provoke preterm labour, with loss of both babies, but individual women may need different treatments depending on the severity of the fetal conditions (Johnson et al 2001).

Polyhydramnios Polyhydramnios is associated in particu-lar with monozygotic twins and with fetal abnormality. Acute polyhydramnios occurs in mid pregnancy and usu-ally leads to abortion. The author remembers one unusual evening when she was recently qualified as a midwife. Two women, both with monozygotic twins and acute polyhy-dramnios, were being cared for in the same room. Both women delivered identical twin boys within half an hour of each other. All four boys were under 300 g and all died.

Intrauterine growth retardation Most twins show dis-cordant growth, with one twin being larger than the other. The smaller twin is more at risk of perinatal complications. Discordant growth occurs because one twin obtains less nourishment from the maternal circulation. This is a feature of placental mass and occurs more commonly in dizygotic twins. Genetic syndromes and TTTS may also result in dis-cordant growth. If preterm delivery of the twins is antici-pated, to safeguard the smaller twin weekly injections of **betamethasone** may be given to the mother to hasten fetal lung maturity.

Maternal problems

Detailed accounts of the following maternal problems are given in other chapters.

Exacerbation of minor disorders The presence of more than one fetus in utero means a higher level of pregnancy hormones and more pressure from the growing uterus. This will tend to cause an exacerbation of all minor disorders of pregnancy: in particular, morning sickness, nausea and heartburn may be more troublesome.

Anaemia The rate of anaemia in multiple pregnancy is about double that of singleton pregnancies. **Iron deficiency** and **folic acid deficiency** occur commonly in multiple pregnancy. Early in pregnancy iron is utilised in the growth of tissues, in particular the expansion of the plasma volume with formation of extra red blood cells. After the 28th week fetal demands deplete the remaining iron stores.

Table 13.5 Fetal presentations by percentage	
Fetal presentation	Per cent
Vertex-vertex	39.6
Vertex-breech	27.7
Vertex-transverse	7.2
Breech-breech	9.0
Breech-vertex	6.9
Breech-transverse	3.6
Other combinations	6.9

Pregnancy-induced hypertension Hypertension is more common in women with multiple pregnancy. Both hyper-tension and oedema may develop because of the extra increase in blood volume. With rest, the hypertension usu-ally improves and pregnancy can be allowed to continue. A more worrying occurrence is the onset of pre-eclampsia with proteinuria, vasoconstriction and reduced blood volume.

Antepartum haemorrhage There is a significant increase in **antepartum haemorrhage** in multiple pregnancies (Sebire et al 2001). **Placenta praevia** may occur because of the large placental site and **abruptio placentae** because of polyhydramnios, with risk of sudden decrease in uterine size if the membranes rupture early.

Complications of labour

Fetal malpresentations

At the commencement of labour, Farooqui et al (1973) found fetal presentations to be as shown in Table 13.5. After deliv-ery of the first twin the lie, presentation and position of the second twin may change and must be checked and the fetal heart listened to before proceeding with the delivery.

Locked twins

Locked twins occur in 1 in 1000 twin labours. Typically, the babies will have presented in a breech-vertex pattern with the head of the first breech twin obstructed by the head of the second or vertex twin. Other types of locked twins are rarer. If diagnosed before the onset of labour, a situation that should be checked in every breech-vertex combination, an elective caesarean section should be carried out.

If the body of the first baby has already been born, an attempt to manipulate the babies to free the head should be made. It may be successful, as the babies are usually small; otherwise, an emergency caesarean section should be carried out. With one of the sets of twins the author has observed vaginal manipulation was successful and both babies sur-vived with good Apgar scores. Unfortunately, in the second set of twins, vaginal manipulation was unsuccessful and both babies died during the caesarean section. It is pleasant to report that the 40-year-old woman who lost her babies went on to have a beautiful little girl born by caesarean section within a year.

Umbilical cord problems

Problems affecting the umbilical cord are more common in multiple pregnancies. These include:

- the presence of a single umbilical artery;
- cord prolapse;
- velamentous insertion of the cord;
- vasa praevia;
- umbilical cord entanglement in monoamniotic twins.

Preterm onset of labour

Labour may begin spontaneously before term or may be induced for maternal or fetal complications. It is unusual for a twin pregnancy to go beyond term. If this happens labour is usually induced. Previously it was thought that bed rest from 24 to 34 weeks decreases preterm onset of labour and perinatal mortality and morbidity in twins. However, Crowther (2000) reviewed six trials of hospitalisation for bed rest in uncomplicated multiple pregnancies involving 600 women and 1400 babies and found no evidence that bed rest could prevent preterm birth or perinatal mortality. If labour threatens, a tocolytic drug such as ritodrine or salbutamol may be given in an attempt to stop the uterine activity. The rationale is that it prevents pressure on the cervix and also increases utero-placental circulation.

Mode of delivery

Many obstetricians believe that indications for an elective caesarean section should include breech presentation or transverse lie of the first twin. However, in 75% of twin pregnancies, the first twin presents by the vertex and there is no contraindication to vaginal delivery. The second twin should deliver easily as long as the lie is longitudinal. If the lie of the second twin is oblique or transverse, most can be easily converted to longitudinal by external cephalic version. Labour may be prolonged by poor uterine action because of overdistension of the uterine muscle. This can be remedied by oxytocin infusion. Epidural analgesia is the first choice, as it does not affect the fetuses and allows any unforeseen manipulative manoeuvres such as external cephalic version or breech extraction to be made.

Postpartum haemorrhage

Poor uterine tone and the presence of a large placental site predispose women giving birth to more than one fetus to postpartum haemorrhage, a life-threatening condition if the woman's haemoglobin level is low. Prevention of haemorrhage should be a priority. An intravenous infusion of oxytocin should be in situ and intramuscular Syntometrine 1 ampoule or intravenous ergometrine 500 μg administered.

Undiagnosed twins

If the head of the baby appears small in contrast to the known size of the uterus before delivery, if the uterus still looks large after the delivery of the baby or the baby itself appears small a second twin should be suspected and the uterus quickly palpated. If an oxytocic drug has already been given, delivery of the second twin needs to take place quickly as its life may be in danger. The second baby is likely to be asphyxiated and will need active resuscitation.

Postnatal care of mother and babies

Care of the babies

Following the birth, once the babies are breathing well, care will depend on the size and maturity of the babies. If the babies are **premature** or **light for dates**, appropriate care will be needed. Some twins may not need any special care other than helping the mother to care for them. The babies may be breastfed if the mother wishes.

Care of the mother

Involution of the uterus may be painful because of the increased muscle bulk (Grant 1996). Analgesia should be offered. If the mother decides to breastfeed both babies, a high-protein, high-calorie diet will be needed. Anaemia should be treated and postnatal exercises geared at improving muscle tone of the abdominal wall and pelvic floor encouraged.

Management of pregnancy with a high fetal number

In the late 1990s a woman conceived eight babies. She had refused selective termination of babies. In the end she lost all her babies at 20 weeks of pregnancy. More recently, a woman in the USA delivered seven babies, all of whom survived. The more fetuses in the uterus, the earlier labour is likely to commence. Complications are more likely to occur and despite an improvement in mortality and morbidity over the last few years, they remain high. Caesarean section is the commonest mode of delivery and, if the babies are delivered in a centre of excellence, survival is quite good. It never ceases to amaze the author that the Dionne quintuplet identical girls were born vaginally in their parent's home in Canada and survived. Sextuplets have survived and grown into healthy children in Britain.

MAIN POINTS

- Following the use of ultrasound scanning, it is more common to calculate the age of the fetus using the estimated day of fertilisation. Maximum growth rate occurs between 16 and 24 weeks with both hyperplasia and hypertrophy. Growth then slows until term.

- How big a baby grows may be determined by maternal and paternal genes. There is a pattern of developmental stages clearly seen from the 9th week until delivery.

- Continued maternal weight gain is thought to be a favourable sign of growth but is affected by many factors. Poor weight gain is associated with intrauterine growth retardation. Fundal height can be used to assess fetal growth and a series of measurements can be plotted on a graph.

- About two-thirds of twin pregnancies are dizygotic. Dizygotic twins share the same genetic make-up as any brother or sister. The incidence of congenital malformation is only slightly greater than normal. Ethnic origin, maternal age, parity and conception soon after discontinuing oral contraception influence the frequency of dizygotic twinning.

- About one-third of monozygotic twins are dichorionic and two-thirds share one placenta and chorion. In 95% of these each baby has its own amnion and in 5% the babies are monoamniotic. About 1% of these are conjoined. Monozygotic twins are identical in their genetic make-up. There is a higher incidence of congenital abnormalities. The incidence of monozygotic twins is 3.5 per 1000 across all nationalities.

- The outcome of higher-order multiple pregnancies can be poor and some centres have advocated multifetal reduction to ensure survival of two or three fetuses, but the procedure itself may lead to the loss of all the fetuses. Conservative management in specialist centres is advocated.

- The earlier the diagnosis of twins is made, the more successful the outcome and perinatal losses may be much larger when the diagnosis is made after 28 weeks. In developing countries with no access to scanning, midwives must diagnose multiple pregnancies by clinical examination.

- Obstetric complications include abortion, pre-eclampsia, antepartum haemorrhage, anaemia, delivery by caesarean section, preterm delivery, low birth weight, stillbirth, admission of the babies to neonatal intensive care unit, postpartum haemorrhage and maternal infections. For most complications the incidence increased with the number of fetuses present.

- Congenital malformation is more likely to occur in twin pregnancies. Abnormalities in dizygotic twins tend to be minor while those in monozygotic twins are multiple and lethal. The most common abnormalities are cleft lip and palate, central nervous system defects and cardiac defects.

- When monoamniotic twins are present the perinatal mortality is as high as 50%, mainly because of entanglement of the umbilical cords, twin-to-twin transfusion syndrome, congenital abnormalities, conjoined twins and preterm birth. It is best to deliver the babies by caesarean section to avoid increasing cord entanglement during vaginal birth.

- The outcome for conjoined twins is poor. About one-third are stillborn and another third die within 24 hours of delivery. The presence of shared organs may make it impossible to save both babies. In acardiac twinning, circulatory overload may lead to heart failure in the normal twin.

- Twin-to-twin transfusion syndrome affects between 15% and 35% of monozygotic twins. Attempts to deal with the problem antenatally include serial amniocentesis, occlusion of the vascular anastamoses by laser coagulation and septostomy.

- Most twins show discordant growth because one twin obtains less nourishment from the maternal circulation. Genetic syndromes and twin-to-twin transfusion syndrome may also result in discordant growth. The smaller twin is more at risk of perinatal complications.

- Maternal complications of multiple pregnancies include minor disorders of pregnancy, iron and folic acid deficiency, pregnancy-induced hypertension, pre-eclampsia and antepartum haemorrhage. At the commencement of labour, fetal malpresentations may be present.

- If locked twins are diagnosed before the onset of labour, an elective caesarean section should be carried out. If the body of the first baby has already been born, an attempt to manipulate the babies to free the head should be made. It may be successful as the babies are usually small.

- Labour may begin before term or be induced for maternal or fetal complications. A recent review found no evidence that bed rest prevented preterm onset of labour or perinatal mortality and morbidity.

- In 75% of twin pregnancies the first twin presents by the vertex and there is no contraindication to vaginal delivery. Labour may be prolonged by poor uterine action because of overdistension of the uterine muscle. The presence of a large placental site predisposes to postpartum haemorrhage. Following the birth, care will depend on the size and maturity of the babies.

- If the mother decides to breastfeed both babies, a high-protein, high-calorie diet will be needed. Anaemia should be treated and postnatal exercises geared at improving muscle tone of the abdominal wall and pelvic floor encouraged.

- The more fetuses that are in the uterus, the earlier labour is likely to commence. All the complications mentioned above are more likely to occur and, despite an improvement in mortality and morbidity over the last few years, they remain high. Caesarean section is the commonest mode of delivery and, if the babies are delivered in a centre of excellence, survival is quite good.

References

Blackburn S T 2003 Maternal, Fetal and Neonatal Physiology, a Clinical Perspective. W B Saunders, Philadelphia.

Bogin B 2001 Patterns of Human Growth. Cambridge University Press, Cambridge.

Craven C, Ward K 1996 Placental causes of fetal malformation. Clinical Obstetrics and Gynecology 39(3):588–606.

Crowther C A 2000 Hospitalisation and bed rest for multiple pregnancies. Cochrane Review: In the Cochrane Library, Issue 3. Update Software 2003, Oxford.

Dickey R P, Taylor S N, Lu P Y et al 2002 Spontaneous reduction of multiple pregnancy: incidence and effects on outcome. American Journal of Obstetrics and Gynecology 186(1):77–83.

Divon M Y, Weiner Z 1995 Ultrasound in twin pregnancy. Seminars in Perinatology 10(5):404–412.

Duncan K R, Denbow M L 2001 Multiple pregnancy. Current Obstetrics and Gynaecology 11(4):211–217.

Farooqui M O, Grossman J H, Shannon R A 1973 A review of twin pregnancy and perinatal mortality. Obstetric and Gynaecological Survey 28:144–153.

Grant B 1996 Multiple pregnancies. In Bennett V R, Brown L K (eds) Myles Textbook for Midwives, 12th edn. Churchill Livingstone, Edinburgh.

Haig D 1993 Genetic conflicts in human pregnancy. Quarterly Review of Biology 68(4):495–519.

Hytten F 1990 Is it important or even useful to measure weight gain in pregnancy? Midwifery 6:28–32.

Hytten F 1991 Weight gain in pregnancy. In Hytten F, Chamberlain G (eds) Clinical Physiology in Obstetrics, 2nd edn. Blackwell Scientific, Oxford.

Johnson M H, Everitt B J 2000 Essential Reproduction, 5th edn. Blackwell Science, Oxford.

Johnson J R, Rossi K Q, O'Shaughnessy R W 2001 Amnioreduction versus septostomy in twin–twin transfusion syndrome. American Journal of Obstetrics and Gynecology 185(5):1004–1047.

Leondires M P, Ernst S D, Miller B T et al 2000 Triplets: outcomes of expectant management versus multifetal reduction for 127 pregnancies. American Journal of Obstetrics and Gynecology 183(2):454–459.

Moore K L, Persaud T V N 1998 Before We Are Born – Essentials of Embryology and Birth Defects, 5th edn. W B Saunders, Philadelphia.

Proud J 1996 Specialised antenatal investigations. In Bennett V R, Brown L K (eds) Myles Textbook for Midwives, 12th edn. Churchill Livingstone, Edinburgh.

Sebire N J, Souka H, Skentou L et al 2000 First trimester diagnosis of monoamniotic twin pregnancies. Ultrasound in Obstetrics and Gynecology 16(3):223–225.

Sebire N J, Jolly M, Harris J et al 2001 Risk of obstetric complications in multiple pregnancies: an analysis of more than 400,000 pregnancies in the UK. Prenatal and Perinatal Medicine 6(2):89–94.

Skrablin S, Kuvacic I, Pavacic D et al 2000 Maternal and neonatal outcome in quadruplet and quintuplet versus triplet gestations. European Journal of Obstetrics and Gynecology and Reproductive Biology 88(2):147–152.

Spillman J 1997 Multiple pregnancy. In Sweet B R, Tiran D (eds) Mayes Midwifery, 12th edn. Baillière Tindall, London.

Spitz L, Kiely E 2000 Success rate for surgery of conjoined twins. Lancet (Correspondence) 356:1765.

Tanner J M 1978 Foetus into Man. Open Books, London.

Thomson V 1996 Psychological and physiological changes of pregnancy. In Bennett V R, Brown L K (eds) Myles Textbook for Midwives, 12th edn. Churchill Livingstone, Edinburgh.

Van Gemert M J C, Umur A, Jijssen J G P, Ross M G 2001 Twin–twin transfusion syndrome: etiology, severity and rational management. Current Opinion in Obstetrics and Gynecology 13:193–206.

Wolpert L, Beddington R, Jessell T et al 2002 Principles of Development, 2nd edn. Oxford University Press, Oxford.

Annotated recommended reading

Craven C, Ward K 1996 Placental causes of fetal malformation. Clinical Obstetrics and Gynecology 39(3):588–606.
This excellent paper is informative about the relationship between the placenta and developmental abnormalities of fetal structure, including problems in twins such as acardia, conjoined twins and twin–twin transfusion syndrome.

Divon M Y, Weiner 1995 Ultrasound in twin pregnancy. Seminars in Perinatology 10(5):404–412.
The authors have evaluated the role of ultrasound in the management of twin pregnancies and focus on both its uses in detecting fetal growth and perinatal complications in twins. They also include a discussion on determining the types of placentation and membranes.

Duncan K R, Denbow M L 2001 Multiple pregnancy. Current Obstetrics and Gynaecology 11(4):211–217.
This paper discusses the management of multiple pregnancies and how clinical expertise along with serial ultrasonic and biophysical monitoring produces good results.

Moore K L, Persaud T V N 1998 Before We Are Born – Essentials of Embryology and Birth Defects, 5th edn. W B Saunders, Philadelphia.
Chapter 7 discusses the fetal period from the 9th week until birth. The illustrations, both diagrams and photographs, and tables make this an excellent visual guide to developmental stages.

Van Gemert M J C, Umur A, Jijssen J G P, Ross M G 2001 Twin–twin transfusion syndrome: etiology, severity and rational management. Current Opinion in Obstetrics and Gynecology 13:193–206.
The authors present a detailed review of the causes and management of twin–twin transfusion syndrome, including amnioreduction and laser therapy of anastomoses. They conclude that with optimal treatment in all centres survival rate could be as high as 85%.

Chapter **14**

Common fetal problems

INTRODUCTION

This chapter covers a variety of topics concerning fetal danger. Although there is a blurred line between concepts applied to the fetus and the neonate, this chapter is concerned with the fetus. Some fetal problems such as rhesus isoimmunisation are discussed in relation to the neonate in Chapters 48–53.

INTRAUTERINE GROWTH RETARDATION

Before discussing intrauterine growth retardation (IUGR), it is useful to understand some definitions:

- **A low birth weight baby** (LBW) is a baby who weighs 2500 g or less at birth.
- **A very low birth weight baby** (VLBW) is a baby who weighs 1500 g or less at birth.
- **A light for dates** or **small for gestational age** (SGA) baby describes a baby whose birth weight is below the 10th centile for its gestational age but is not necessarily growth restricted.
- **A large for gestational age** (LGA) is a baby whose birth weight is above the 90th centile for gestational age.
- **A preterm infant** is a baby born before 37 completed weeks of pregnancy irrespective of the birth weight. A preterm infant may also be SGA or LGA.

There are two categories of fetus which appear SGA:

1. The fetus shows early departure from normal limits of growth that continues until delivery. The fetus is small because of conditions such as chromosomal abnormality or intrauterine infection.

2. The fetus shows arrest of previously normal growth where the growth failure is caused by a factor outside the fetus such as maternal disease or placental pathology.

   The term IUGR should be used only for the second category where growth is known to be arrested (Enkin et al 2000). Wrong classification of IUGR does not allow for fetuses that are small and healthy. This may lead to inappropriate interference in the course of the pregnancy.

Complications of IUGR

In the antepartum and intrapartum periods there is an increase in the number of stillbirths, oligohydramnios and fetal distress. Neonatal complications including meconium aspiration syndrome, persistent fetal circulation, hypoglycaemia, hypocalcaemia, hyperviscosity syndrome and poor temperature control will be discussed in Section 4A of the book.

Factors adversely affecting fetal growth

Fetal growth depends on interacting factors such as genetic determinants, maternal health and nutrition, availability of growth substrates, and an effective maternal blood supply to the placenta (Blackburn 2003). The essential substrates are oxygen, glucose and amino acids. Any decrease in substrate availability due to pathological conditions affecting mother, placenta or fetus will result in poor growth.

Maternal conditions most frequently associated with poor fetal growth are:

- hypertension;
- chronic renal disease;
- diabetes mellitus with vascular lesions;
- sickle cell anaemia;
- severe cardiac disease;
- severe malnutrition;
- smoking;
- alcohol ingestion.

The commonest fetoplacental problems are:

- chromosomal abnormalities;
- intrauterine infections;
- multiple pregnancy;
- small placental size and inadequate changes in uterine spiral arteries;
- placental infarcts;
- placenta praevia.

The commonest socioeconomic factors are maternal smoking and a history of a previous growth-retarded fetus. The commonest medical condition involved with IUGR is hypertensive disease (Ch. 32). Smoking is discussed below.

Maternal malnutrition

Maternal influences associated with IUGR include malnutrition and low weight gain in pregnancy (Ott 2001). However, low birth weight due to malnutrition is more likely to occur in developing countries. Babies born in the Dutch famine of 1944–45 had a reduced birth weight in proportion to their length. Severe protein calorie malnutrition, especially during the second half of pregnancy, will reduce birth weight. Low maternal weight gain in the second and third trimesters is associated with IUGR and it has been seen in American women who have had gastric bypass operations for gross obesity (Arias 1993).

Smoking

Smoking is a prime cause of IUGR (Ott 2001, Robinson et al 2000). Tobacco smoking induces fetal hypoxia by vasoconstriction due to the effect of nicotine on adrenergic neurons which decreases placental blood flow and leads to placental underperfusion. This reduces fetal nutrition, leading to growth retardation. Maternal smoking may reduce term weight by 10–15 g for every cigarette smoked per day (Ott 2001). The increase in carboxyhaemoglobin causes a sustained reduction of oxygen to the fetus, which has a more prolonged effect on growth (Longo 1977). The combined effect of nicotine and carboxyhaemoglobin is associated with preterm labour and exacerbates the low birth weight. Birth weight reduction is between 120 and 430 g.

Alcohol consumption

Fetal alcohol syndrome (FAS) was first recognised in America and more recently in Great Britain. Alcohol has a low molecular weight and crosses the placental barrier. It is a known teratogen and fetal damage has been associated with any drinking, from slight social drinking to heavy intake. It is not possible to state how much alcohol causes the abnormalities associated with FAS, so it is wise to abstain from drinking alcohol during pregnancy. In a few women alcohol-induced malnutrition will add to the fetal problems.

The characteristic features of FAS (not all are present in a particular infant):

- deficient overall growth;
- facial abnormalities – small eyes with inner epicanthic folds; poorly formed nasal bridge, giving the nose a retrousse appearance; poor or absent vertical groove in a narrow top lip; ears that are large and simple in formation; and cleft palate;
- musculoskeletal abnormalities – congenital hip lesions and thoracic cage abnormalities;
- genitourinary abnormalities – undescended testes, male urethral abnormalities, hypoplastic labia in females and kidney abnormalities;
- cardiac abnormalities are common – mainly atrial or ventricular septal defects;
- poor coordination of movement and learning difficulties;
- alcohol withdrawal symptoms.

Placental insufficiency

In **placental insufficiency** the placenta is usually small with a reduction in the number of stem and villous capillaries

(Robinson et al 2000). The muscle layer of the spiral arteries is intact because of incomplete penetration by the trophoblastic cells. Blood flow to the fetus is restricted, limiting the availability of nutrients. These placental changes may be an isolated pathology or may be found in maternal conditions, particularly hypertension. The extent of the placental changes is related to the severity of the maternal disease.

Multiple pregnancy

Poor fetal growth occurs in about 21% of twins, mainly due to abnormal placentation.

Genetic factors and chromosomal aberrations

The prevalence of genetic and chromosomal disorders amongst babies with IUGR is higher than normal, with an incidence of congenital abnormalities between 5 and 27% as compared with an incidence of 0.1–4% in babies with normal growth (Ott 2001). It is particularly common in babies with trisomies such as Down's syndrome. The majority of these babies have symmetric growth retardation.

Diagnosis and management of IUGR

The first step in managing IUGR is to identify those women at risk, then to differentiate the small healthy babies from those with genuine IUGR (Robinson et al 2000). Monitoring at-risk fetuses allows management decisions to be made. Using a combination of the clinical and ultrasound methods outlined in the section on assessing fetal growth, a diagnosis should be possible in 95% of cases.

Umbilical artery Doppler velocimetry

Assessment of flow patterns and velocities in fetal vessels has become a significant method for assessing fetal growth in utero. Doppler velocimetry used in conjunction with either estimated fetal weight or abdominal circumference improves accuracy of antenatal diagnosis of IUGR (Ott 2001). Soregaroli et al (2002) found a correlation between umbilical Doppler velocimetry abnormalities and an increased incidence of perinatal complications. The more abnormal the umbilical arterial blood flow, the more risk to the fetus.

Measuring fetal subcutaneous fat

Ultrasonographic measurement of subcutaneous fat in the fetal abdomen may be of value in predicting IUGR (Gardeil et al 2000). This developed from measuring the fetal abdominal circumference and measuring skinfold thickness in neonates. In their research group of 137 women there was a correlation between babies with less than 5 mm of subcutaneous fat at 38 weeks and a low height/weight ratio (**ponderal index**) at birth. There were more instances of neonatal morbidity in those babies than in the control group with a subcutaneous abdominal fat measurement of more than 5 mm.

Other tests of placental function

Neither serial estriol estimation nor human placental lactogen (hPL) assays are of value in assessing placental function and fetal wellbeing and are of historical interest only. While fundal height measurements may not detect all cases of IUGR, it is a method that allows the referral of women to a consultant unit for ultrasonic screening. Monitoring daily fetal movements has also been shown to be of no value as a screening technique (Enkin et al 2000).

Contraction stress testing

Continuous **cardiotocography** recording fetal heart rate and uterine activity is monitored in response to an **oxytocin challenge**. It has no benefits and is time consuming and potentially dangerous for the fetus. Its use is contraindicated in at-risk pregnancies such as antepartum haemorrhage, placenta praevia and preterm labour. A similar test using **nipple stimulation** to induce contractions has proved to be so dangerous that its use has been discontinued (Enkin et al 2000).

Non-stress cardiotocography

Antepartum cardiotocography has been used to detect the at-risk fetus using such variables as **baseline heart rate**, **beat-to-beat variability** and **accelerations of the fetal heart**. Readings can be divided into **reactive**, with good baseline variability, and **non-reactive**, if there is an inadequate baseline with loss of variability or accelerations in response to fetal movement. Interpreting the printouts is difficult and intervention has been carried out too early, increasing morbidity and mortality (Enkin et al 2000). Doppler assessment combined with non-stress cardiotocography plays an important part in diagnosing and managing IUGR (Ott 2001).

Fetal biophysical profile

The method is derived from research into serial ultrasound examinations and antenatal cardiotocography (non-stress test). Five fetal physiological variables are combined to try and reduce the incidence of false-positive diagnoses: these are movement, tone, reactivity, breathing movements and amniotic fluid volume. In the small number of studies reported, **biophysical profile** was a better predictive test than the non-stress test in identifying babies with a low 5-min Apgar score. However, its use did not result in an improvement in outcome for the baby. A meta-analysis by Hofmeyr (1995) found no effect, beneficial or otherwise on the outcome of pregnancy. A modified biophysical profile with non-stress test and fluid volume only is a useful standard for fetal monitoring. Measurement of the amount of liquor amnii (amniotic fluid) will indicate oligohydramnios, a late sign of fetal malnutrition. Serial estimations of the amount of amniotic fluid can indicate the need to expedite delivery.

Delivery of the baby

Once fetal lung maturity is achieved and, preferably after 34 weeks postfertilisation age, the baby should be delivered. Excluding congenital malformations, intrapartum asphyxia is a major cause of morbidity and mortality. The increased incidence of low 5-min Apgar scores and later neurological deficits is a major worry. Every method to avoid asphyxia should be used:

- direct fetal monitoring by scalp electrode should be utilised to monitor fetal condition
- care should be taken with analgesia and an epidural anaesthetic may be best
- the second stage of labour should be short and a low forceps delivery used if necessary
- a paediatrician should be present at the delivery.

Most of these babies now survive the neonatal period but they remain smaller than their age cohorts for several years after their birth. A major concern is that chronic intrauterine malnutrition may lead to a permanent decrease in brain cell number. Poor fetal growth has been studied in context of the early onset of fetal diseases (Robinson et al 2000). Small size at birth and low ponderal index are linked to coronary heart disease, high blood pressure and diabetes in adult life (Barker 1998).

RHESUS ISOIMMUNISATION AND ABO INCOMPATIBILITY

Rhesus isoimmunisation

The reader should ensure they understand blood group inheritance before reading on. The fetus inherits a gene for the **rhesus factor** from each parent and as rhesus D is a dominant gene if either or both genes for rhesus are inherited the baby will be rhesus positive (Rh+). Only if the baby inherits two recessive d genes will the blood group be rhesus negative (Rh−) (Fig. 14.1).

If the mother is Rh− and the fetus Rh+, **haemolysis** of fetal red cells may occur (Fig. 14.2). This rarely affects the first baby as there are no spontaneous anti-D antibodies present in a woman prior to her first pregnancy unless fetal red blood cells have crossed the placental barrier during that pregnancy or she has been accidentally transfused with Rh+ blood.

During pregnancy and labour there is normally no mixing of maternal and fetal circulation. When the placenta separates, the chorionic villi tear and there is a risk of a **fetomaternal transfusion**; usually between 0.5 ml and 5 ml of fetal blood enters the maternal circulation. If the fetus is Rh+ the production of antibodies will be stimulated and memory cells will mount a secondary response should the

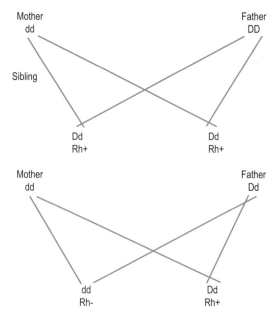

Figure 14.1 Inheritance of the rhesus factor (from Sweet B 1997, with permission).

mother become pregnant with a second Rh+ baby. This process is called **isoimmunisation**.

Spontaneous or therapeutic abortion, amniocentesis, antepartum haemorrhage or external cephalic version may lead to fetomaternal transfusion and antibody formation. The problem arises in subsequent pregnancies because anti-D antibodies cross the placenta and haemolyse fetal red cells. Some protection occurs if the mother and fetus are ABO incompatible, as the naturally occurring anti-A or anti-B will destroy fetal red cells before the maternal immune system responds to the rhesus factor.

Prevention of maternal isoimmunisation

In the past **haemolytic disease of the newborn** led to fetal or neonatal death but this is now largely a preventable event if three conditions are met:

1. Rhesus-positive blood should never be used in a transfusion if a woman's blood group is unknown.

2. Unnecessary risk of fetomaternal transfusion should be avoided, for example by placental location prior to amniocentesis. Abdominal palpation in women with an antepartum haemorrhage should be kept to a minimum.

3. If there has been a risk of fetomaternal transfusion, anti-D immunoglobulin (rhesus D antibodies) must be administered to the mother within 72 h, which confers passive immunity for about 3 months. The antibodies will coat and destroy any fetal red cells in the maternal circulation.

The dose of **anti-D immunoglobulin** is normally 250 IU (international units) before 20 weeks of pregnancy and 500 IU after 20 weeks. Occasionally the fetomaternal haemorrhage

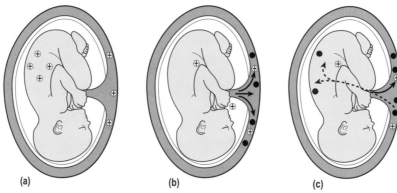

Figure 14.2   Antibody formation. (a) Transfer of rhesus antigen (+) to the maternal circulation. (b) Antibody formation (•) in the rhesus-negative mother. (c) Transfer of rhesus antibody to the fetus (from Sweet B 1997, with permission).

is so large that one dose of anti-D immunoglobulin is insufficient to prevent isoimmunisation. The number of fetal red cells in the maternal blood is estimated by means of a Kleihauer test and, if a second dose is needed, the laboratory will inform the doctor.

Antenatal management

Every pregnant woman has her blood tested for ABO and rhesus types early in pregnancy. Besides the information being readily available should a blood transfusion be necessary, any rhesus-negative woman will be screened for rhesus antibodies. If the test is negative her blood will be retested later, usually at 28 and 34 weeks of pregnancy.

Anti-D prophylaxis   Because some fetomaternal bleeds are undetected in pregnancy, some authorities recommend the use of antepartum rhesus D immunoglobulin prophylaxis. Some women still do not receive anti-D, including those who attend accident and emergency departments with bleeding in early pregnancy. Women are still being sensitised to RhD antigen because of the two above instances (Benbow & Wray 1998). Wickham (2001) suggested that more research is needed into the midwife's role if a policy of routine administration were to be adopted.

Care at delivery

When a mother is rhesus negative, the umbilical cord is clamped immediately to minimise the amount of placental blood with possible maternal antibodies entering the baby's circulation and cord blood is taken for testing by using a syringe and needle into a placental vein to avoid the risk of contamination by maternal blood and Wharton's jelly, which would make interpreting the test results difficult. The needle is removed prior to transferring the blood to a bottle to avoid haemolysis. Cord blood is tested for ABO and rhesus type; **direct Coombes' test**, looking for maternal antibodies on fetal red cells; and a haemoglobin estimation to check for haemolysis. If the mother has rhesus antibodies, the cord blood is also tested for serum bilirubin level.

Management if rhesus antibodies are present during pregnancy

If antibodies are detected, the titre will be checked. Although titre does not relate directly to the fetal condition, it indicates the necessity of carrying out an amniotic fluid test. The amount of **bilirubin** excreted from the breakdown of red cells can be measured against a **Liley chart** which relates the level to the week of gestation and allows judgement to be made about future management. However, the value of this measure should be weighed against the risk of provoking a fetomaternal bleed by performing an amniocentesis. It is usual to delay this examination until after 26 weeks when the fetus is viable (Bennett & Brown 1999). The possible outcomes are:

- The pregnancy is allowed to continue and bilirubin level is estimated at intervals. If the titre is rising it may be necessary to deliver the fetus.

- If the fetus is considered mature enough to survive and it is considered to be dangerous to continue the pregnancy, the baby is delivered in a consultant unit when all facilities, such as the pathology laboratory and paediatrician, are available.

- The fetus may be given an intrauterine transfusion of group O rhesus-negative packed cells to prolong life if it is considered too immature to survive.

Rhesus haemolytic disease

All babies whose mothers have Rh antibodies should be transferred to a neonatal intensive care unit until the results of the tests on the cord blood are known. Depending on the percentage of red blood cells destroyed, this disease has varying degrees of severity:

1. **Congenital haemolytic anaemia** occurs if haemolysis is minimal. There will be a slow-onset anaemia, enlargement of the liver and spleen but jaundice will not be severe. If the baby's haemoglobin level is low a small blood transfusion of packed cells can be given.

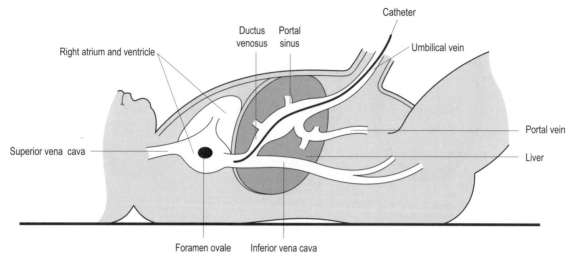

Figure 14.3 The umbilical vein and its connections in the neonate. The position of the umbilical venous catheter is shown. Note how easy it would be to push it accidentally into the right atrium. (Reproduced with permission from Wallis & Harvey 1979.)

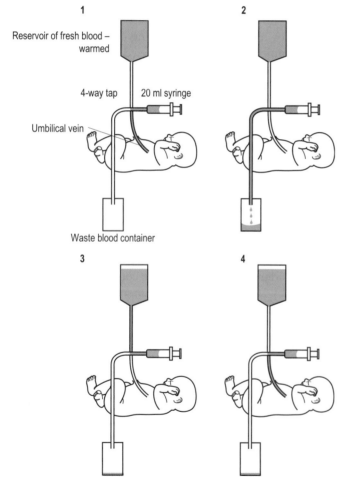

Figure 14.4 Exchange transfusion. 1. Blood is drawn out into a syringe via an umbilical vein catheter. 2. This blood is discarded into a waste container. 3. Blood warmed to body temperature is drawn into this syringe. The blood is crossmatched for compatibility with blood from the baby's mother. 4. This blood is injected slowly. The process is repeated until the twice the baby's blood volume has been exchanged. (Reproduced with permission from Wallis & Harvey 1979.)

2. **In icterus gravis neonatorum** (severe jaundice of the newborn) haemolysis has occurred in the fetus and the baby is born with a low haemoglobin level. Because the placenta transfers bilirubin to the mother for excretion, the baby is usually not jaundiced at birth. After delivery when the baby's liver must cope with the excessive bilirubin, jaundice rapidly develops. Treatment includes restoring the haemoglobin level, reducing the bilirubin level and removing maternal antibodies.

3. In **hydrops fetalis** severe intrauterine anaemia results in congestive cardiac failure. The baby and placenta are pale and oedematous and the baby may be stillborn. If the baby is alive an immediate transfusion of packed cells will allow tissue oxygenation. Bilirubin and maternal antibodies are removed by an exchange transfusion (Figs 14.3 and 14.4) when the baby's condition is stable.

ABO incompatibility

In this condition the mother is blood group O and the baby is group A or B. The baby cannot be group AB as it inherits an O gene from its mother. The mother's blood contains unprovoked anti-A and anti-B antibodies even in the first pregnancy so the first child may be affected. Immunoglobulin M (IgM) antibodies (Ch. 29, p. 393) are too large to cross over the placenta, but IgG antibodies may cross over the placenta and haemolyse fetal red cells. Although jaundice appears in the first 24 hours it is usually mild. Treatment will depend on the rate of rise of bilirubin level in the blood.

MATERNAL INFECTION IN PREGNANCY

Microbes are small organisms that live in and on the human body. They can be divided into five major classes: **bacteria**, **viruses**, **algae**, **fungi** and **protozoa**. Some are helpful **commensal organisms** like the **lactobacillus** that increases the acidity of the vagina. However many are **pathogens**, entering the body and causing infection. Over time, the immune system develops defence systems against pathogens. Systemic infections may cause reproductive problems such as infertility and congenital defects and some infections are specific to the genitourinary tract. In the vagina other organisms may be present in non-invasive numbers. These include yeasts, streptococci and sometimes *Escherichia coli* (*E. coli*). Some organisms that specifically cause genital tract disease will be outlined first, followed by some systemic disorders that may damage the fetus.

Suppression of cell-mediated immunity

Despite the alterations in the maternal immune system in pregnancy, most women are not **immunocompromised**. However, the suppression of cell-mediated immunity means that some infections are more likely to be more severe in pregnancy, especially viruses and the **opportunistic pathogens** associated with HIV such as *Pneumocystis carinii* and *Toxoplasma gondii*. The viruses include poliomyelitis and influenza. Pregnancy may also cause reactivation of latent cytomegalovirus (CMV) and herpes.

Sexually transmitted diseases

The control of **sexually transmitted diseases** (STDs) constitutes a difficult public health problem. Each year worldwide there may be 300 million new cases in adults. In men they may cause few problems, but in women **pelvic inflammatory disease** (PID) and decreased fertility are frequently seen. The diseases may also have an adverse effect on the fetus. Pregnant women may pass the STD to the fetus, resulting in birth defects or stillbirth (Moodley & Sturm 2000). About one-third of cases in developed countries affect teenagers because young people are more likely to have more than one sexual partner.

Many STDs have no symptoms or vague non-specific symptoms. The social stigma attached to these diseases means that people are less inclined to seek treatment, yet untreated, these diseases have long-term serious health consequences (Madigan et al 1999). The presence of a second disease often complicates treatment: For example, an asymptomatic chlamydial infection may remain after successful treatment for gonorrhoea has been completed. This trend is worrying as most STDs with the exception of HIV infection are treatable. An overview of the more common diseases follows.

Gonorrhoea

This infectious disease is still one of the most widespread of human diseases and symptoms are different in males and females. In women the initial symptoms are a mild vaginitis and this may even go unnoticed while in men the organism

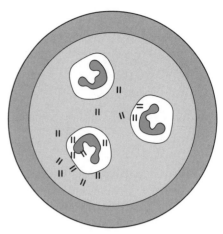

Figure 14.5   *Neisseria gonorrhoeae* in pus cells (from Sweet B 1997, with permission).

causes a painful infection of the urethral canal. The organism can also cause a severe eye infection in neonates.

The causative organism, *Neisseria gonorrhoeae* (Fig. 14.5), is easily killed outside of the body and the disease is transmitted by intimate bodily contact. Severe complications include PID and damage to heart valves and joint tissues. Most cases still respond to the antibiotic penicillin but **penicillin-resistant** strains of the organism are evolving. Despite the ease with which gonorrhoea can be treated, there are three major factors for the high level of infection:

1. there are at least 16 types of the organism, causing difficulty in development of immunity and likelihood of reinfection;
2. oral contraceptives mimic the pregnant state, with reduced vaginal glycogen production and reduction in Döderlein's bacillus, allowing the gonococcus to access the female reproductive tract;
3. symptoms may go unrecognised in women who may act as a reservoir for infection of men.

Syphilis

Syphilis is more serious than gonorrhoea but better controlled as penicillin is very effective against the causative spirochaete *Treponema pallidum* (Fig. 14.6). The organism enters the body through a break in the skin or mucous membrane. In men infection is usually on the penis, while in women it may be hidden in the vagina or on the cervix. In about 10% of cases the infection is extragenital, usually in the oral region. The disease can be transmitted across the placenta to the fetus to cause congenital syphilis.

The organism multiplies within 2–6 weeks at the site of entry to form a primary lesion or **chancre**, which soon heals. It then spreads to other tissues and a **generalised skin rash** develops – the secondary stage. About 25% of people undergo a spontaneous cure, 25% remain symptomless although the organism stays in their bodies and about 50% of infected people will develop the tertiary stage with

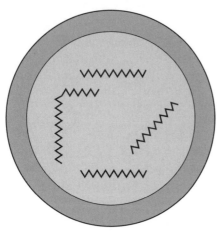

Figure 14.6 *Treponema pallidum* (from Sweet B 1997, with permission).

possible fatal involvement of the cardiovascular and/or central nervous systems. Because the symptoms are noticeable in both sexes, sufferers usually seek treatment. In Great Britain pregnant women are screened for the presence of syphilis and offered treatment to prevent or treat infection in the fetus.

Chlamydia

The incidence of infection with the intracellular organism *Chlamydia trachomatis* probably greatly outnumbers infections with the two organisms already discussed. One strain causes severe eye infections but separate strains of the organism cause venereal disease. Contamination of the neonate during birth may cause severe conjunctivitis and respiratory disease. Chlamydia can cause **non-gonococcal urethritis** (NGU) in males and cervicitis and PID in females.

Asymptomatic chlamydial infection is common in sexually active men and women and can result in infertility in both sexes. In men testicular swelling and prostate inflammation can occur. In women fallopian tubes may be damaged or blocked by destruction of the epithelial lining cells, leading to adhesions. If chlamydial infection is diagnosed in pregnancy, **tetracycline**, which would normally be used, cannot be given because of the effects on fetal bones and teeth. **Erythromycin** is a good alternative (Moodley & Sturm 2000). Chlamydia is often present in people infected with the gonococcus and treatment to eradicate both organisms is given. Factors common to all STDs are:

1. the pathogens are not shed in enormous numbers except during sexual activity;
2. many of the organisms are sensitive to drying;
3. the organisms have lost their ability to survive outside the body.

Group B streptococcus

One in three women in Great Britain may have vaginal carriage of **group B streptococcus** (GBS) at some time during their pregnancy. Maternal infection is asymptomatic but the organism has become the commonest cause of overwhelming sepsis in neonates (Enkin et al 2000).The prevalence is between 0.6 and 3.7 per 1000 live births and the mortality rate of infected babies may be as high as 50%. Screening and treatment of these women is difficult because of recurrence of infection but intrapartum antibiotic treatment of women carrying GBS appears to reduce the risk of neonatal infection (Smaill 2003).

Acquired immune deficiency syndrome

Currently 22 million people have died from acquired immune deficiency syndrome (AIDS) and 42 million people are thought to be infected with the **human immunodeficiency virus** (HIV), most of them living in developing countries (Wilson 2003), especially in sub-Saharan Africa. More than 1.5 million are children under the age of 15 (Brocklehurst & Volmink 2002).

The HIV is a **retrovirus** carrying its genetic information as **ribonucleic acid** (RNA), unlike most organisms which contain **deoxyribonucleic acid** (DNA). Cells of the immune system (Ch. 29, p. 387) containing **CD4 molecules** – which include T lymphocytes, monocytes and macrophages – are its targets. On entering a cell the viral genetic message is converted from RNA to DNA and inserted into the host DNA.

This disease is not strictly sexually transmitted. As the retrovirus is transferred by blood from one person to another, skin or mucous membrane lesions must be present during sexual activity for infection to occur. This disease is almost always fatal and there is as yet no cure or effective treatment. Promiscuity is a key factor in the spread of the disease, as is blood contamination of needles shared by drug addicts or used (in certain countries) in mass vaccinations. Medically, HIV transmission has involved blood transfusion or blood products such as **factor VIII** used to treat **haemophilia**. Infection from mother to fetus may occur during pregnancy, at birth or through breast milk (Enkin et al 2000).

Recent controversy Much controversy continues about the risks to the heterosexual population. The Department of Health (2001) reported over 3500 new cases of HIV infection in the UK in the year 2000. The four major routes of infection were 39% homosexual, 49% heterosexual, 2.6% intravenous drug users and 2.5% mother to child. As other routes are declining, heterosexual exposure seems to be increasing. Africa is currently the primary source of exposure for UK-diagnosed heterosexual infection, accounting for two-thirds of cases.

Reducing the risk of transmission The world is becoming a 'global village' and as travel becomes easier it is probably not wise to exclude any mode of transmission from any country. Those caring for a multicultural society need to be aware of the risk factors of viral transmission through contamination with blood and body fluids. The following recommendations are valid:

1. Avoid mouth contact with penis, vagina and rectum.

2. Avoid sexual activities that may result in tears in the linings of the rectum, vagina and penis.

3. Avoid sexual activity with individuals from high-risk groups. These include male and female prostitutes, homosexual or bisexual individuals and intravenous drug users.

4. If a person has unprotected sexual intercourse with a member of a high-risk group, a blood test should be taken to ascertain whether infection has occurred. If the test is positive future sexual partners should be protected by the use of a condom.

The effect on mothers and babies   Women who are HIV positive may pass the virus across the placenta to affect their unborn child or the baby may be infected by contact with maternal blood during birth. A third way of transmission is through breastfeeding. This transmission from mother to child is called **vertical transmission** (transmission from person to person is called **horizontal transmission**). As HIV may not be obvious at birth but may present with recurrent infections and failure to thrive months or years later, it is difficult to assess the risk for mother–baby transmission. Studies suggest that there is a risk of transmission during breastfeeding and it may be best in developed countries to advise women not to breastfeed. Most cases occur in developing countries so the risk has to be offset by the benefits of breastfeeding when mothers have no access to artificial milk or to hygienic homes.

Attempts to reduce the risk of mother to baby vertical transmission seem promising. **Zidovudine** given to mothers from 35 weeks of pregnancy and their babies until they are 3 days old appears to be protective. One large trial has shown that a single dose of **nevirapine** given to mothers at the onset of labour and to babies within 72 h of birth may be more effective than zidovudine. It may be possible to use nevirapine for longer periods in breastfeeding populations (Brocklehurst & Volmink 2002). However, most cases occur in countries where such drugs are unaffordable.

The search for a cure   T cells stimulate production of antibodies by B lymphocytes. As the T-cell population is reduced over a few years, production of antibodies falls, the immune system becomes crippled and the person becomes ill with opportunistic infections. The mutation rate of HIV has resulted in so many different variants that no **vaccine** against the whole virus can be developed. Trials of vaccines against **viral subunits** are underway but this common method of triggering antibody response has so far proved futile.

Scientists working on vaccines realised they had concentrated on antibody stimulation and ignored the cellular component of immunity (Ch. 29, p. 387). **Cytotoxic lymphocytes** (CTLs) kill cells that have foreign protein attached to their surfaces (Clayton 2003). CTLs may account for a group of Nairobi prostitutes who have no virus or HIV antibodies in their blood although they are at high risk. These women's immune systems seem to be very efficient at provoking a strong CTL response. Researchers are trying to find a way of provoking a strong CTL response in people with a normal CTL response.

Until a successful vaccine is developed, a way to minimise the risk of sexual transmission is needed. In many parts of the developing world men refuse to use condoms and Stone (2003) believes that what is needed is a method of protection that women have control over. He discusses attempts to manufacture **microbicides** to destroy causative organisms in situ. These could be gels, foams, creams and impregnated sponges placed in the vagina (or anus) prior to intercourse.

There are several promising agents under development which could be available in 5–6 years. Stone (2003) says that even if these were only 60% effective, 3.7 million cases of HIV infection could be prevented in the first 3 years! The WHO and governments have seen the value of this research, which could be as cheap as 25p per dose. Two problems need addressing: first such products may also kill sperm; secondly, it is more difficult to protect anal epithelium, which is more fragile than vaginal epithelium. Also, the microbicide may dissipate through the lower gut rather than being contained in situ, as in the vagina, making it difficult to achieve an effective dose.

TORCH organisms and the risk in pregnancy

TORCH is a word derived from the first letters of a series of infections that can cross the placenta to affect the fetus. These are **Toxoplasmosis**, **Others**, **Rubella**, **Cytomegalovirus** and **Herpes**. Most of these infections will cause congenital abnormality if acquired in the first trimester and neonatal infection, often affecting the lung, liver, spleen and brain, if acquired late in pregnancy.

Rubella

In 1941 Gregg in Australia described an association between maternal rubella (German measles) and **congenital cataracts**. Rubella infection during the first few weeks of pregnancy inhibits cell division in the embryonic eyes, ears, heart and brain. After the 3rd month the commonest defect is congenital deafness. An infant born with congenital rubella is highly infectious and must be isolated (Bennett & Brown 1999). The virus may remain in the body for up to a year. Rubella vaccination of girls has been carried out in this country and pregnant women are screened so that women who are not immune can be offered vaccination in the postnatal period. Those working with women and their babies should also be screened and offered vaccination if needed.

Varicella

Varicella (chickenpox) is a childhood illness transmitted by respiratory droplets. If it occurs in pregnancy a woman may develop **adult respiratory distress syndrome** (ARDS) with a mortality rate of up to 35%. Preterm labour and delivery are more common, as is **herpes zoster** (shingles).

Varicella syndrome with developmental abnormalities may occur in the fetus if maternal infection occurred in the first trimester. This includes low birth weight, eye lesions, undeveloped limbs, skin scars and psychomotor retardation. Infection in the third trimester may result in neonatal infection with **pneumonitis, hepatitis** and **disseminated intravascular coagulation** (DIC). Hyperimmune varicella zoster immune globulin (VZIG) can be offered to susceptible pregnant women who have been in contact with chickenpox or shingles. Ultrasound monitoring of the fetus for limb and other external abnormalities is advised. Prophylactic aciclovir can be given to susceptible women.

Cytomegalovirus

Infection with this virus belonging to the double-stranded DNA herpesvirus is transmitted by contact with infected blood, saliva, urine or by sexual contact (ACOG 2000). It is often asymptomatic. If the primary infection occurs during pregnancy, cytomegalovirus (CMV) may cause abortion, preterm labour, intrauterine growth retardation or fetal death. The greatest risk to the fetus is within the first 20 weeks of pregnancy. The virus may damage the fetal liver and nervous system and microcephaly may be present. Neonatal infections are seen in two-thirds of infants born by vaginal delivery.

Toxoplasmosis

The causative organism is a protozoon, *Toxoplasma gondii*, found in dog and cat faeces and in uncooked meat. It may also be acquired by insect contamination of food (ACOG 2000). Infection is usually asymptomatic and occurs in 1 in 500 pregnant women. About 36% of their babies will be affected. **Microcephaly, hydrocephalus** and **hepatosplenomegaly** (enlarged liver and spleen) may occur. Screening in pregnancy with treatment by **spiramycin** could be offered. Umbilical cord blood may be tested to see if the fetus is infected. Some women may consider termination of pregnancy.

Herpes simplex

Genital infection with the organisms type 1 or type 2 *herpes simplex virus* (HSV-1 and HSV-2) may lead to serious neonatal infection, more commonly due to HSV-2 and less so to HSV-1 (Moodley & Sturm 2000). An infected baby may develop localised lesions, encephalitis or generalised herpes infection including septicaemia, pneumonitis, liver dysfunction and coagulopathy (Garland & Jones 2001). The problem is difficult as many women have been infected but shown no clinical signs. The first diagnosis may be at made on appearance of neonatal infection. The diagnosis of HSV infection is established by clinical signs in conjunction with viral isolation (Moodley & Sturm 2000).

If the woman gives a history of infection the mode of delivery should be discussed with her. In the past caesarean section (CS) has been used to prevent exposure of the baby to the virus. Trials of **aciclovir** for suppressing viral shedding have been inconclusive. Although aciclovir has been used in the neonate there have been no trials to judge its usefulness. A large number of surveys have shown that CS does not protect completely against neonatal infection, as intrauterine transplacental infection may have occurred (Moodley & Sturm 2000), nor has there been an increase in neonatal infections in places where abdominal deliveries are no longer performed.

The method of delivery may be based on the clinical appearance of the genital tract at the onset of labour (Randolph et al 1993). If no active lesions are present a vaginal delivery may be carried out. Use of techniques likely to break the skin of the fetus such as scalp electrodes should be avoided. Even overt lesions from a repeat flare up are not necessarily a reason for surgical delivery as they may not be shedding virus.

However, if the woman has acquired a new infection or infection with a different serotype there is a high risk of viral transmission and delivery by CS should be considered. If infection occurs within 6 weeks before delivery, CS is safer for the fetus (Moodley & Sturm 2000). There are two possible future strategies. The search for a vaccine has had no success because many people are infected asymptomatically and because the organism rapidly establishes a latent infection. Viral subunit vaccines have been tried but are only successful if a person is seronegative for both HSV-1 and HSV-2. Mass screening is too expensive in countries where the incidence of neonatal infection is low.

Listeriosis

The foodborne pathogen *Listeria monocytogenes* is a bacterium found throughout the environment and may cause abortion, fetal disease or death. Cook-chill produce in particular has been implicated in the transmission of infection. Diagnosis in women or neonates is by culturing the organism from blood and/or cerebrospinal fluid and it is susceptible to penicillin and erythromycin. Health education on safe preparation of food would help to reduce the incidence of infection.

Hepatitis B (serum hepatitis)

The hepatitis B virus (HBV) is highly infectious and can be transmitted by blood, sexual intercourse and by vertical transmission to the fetus. Virus particles are found in the blood and body fluids of infected people. Long-term infection can lead to chronic hepatitis, cirrhosis of the liver and liver cancer. It is more commonly carried in people from Asia, sub-Saharan Africa, the Caribbean, Central and South America and Alaska and immigrants from these regions have a 1 in 10 risk of carrying the virus against a background rate in the UK of 0.1%. The risk factors for HIV infection are shared by HBV.

Antenatal screening of all pregnant women is recommended so that the baby can be treated and anyone involved in the delivery can take sensible precautions. As in many viruses, the structure includes a **central core** carrying the genetic material, an **outer envelope** and an **outer surface**. This gives rise to three sites that can stimulate antibody production: the surface antigen **HBs Ag** (formerly Australia antigen), the envelope antigen **Hbe Ag** and the core antigen **HBc Ag**. The presence of Hbe Ag indicates that the disease is highly infectious and these women have a 25% probability of transmitting the virus to their babies. If women are Hbe Ag positive or have had a late pregnancy infection their babies are given hepatitis B vaccine, the first dose within 24 h of birth and repeated at 1 month and 6 months of age. This will protect the babies against the long-term dangers.

MAIN POINTS

- Optimal birth weight depends on an interaction between fetal growth potential and the intrauterine environment. Growth potential varies between races and individuals, creating a problem of diagnosis of intrauterine growth retardation. The classification of IUGR does not allow for small but healthy fetuses and may lead to inappropriate interference in pregnancy.

- In IUGR there is an increase in the number of stillbirths, oligohydramnios and fetal distress. Complications in the neonatal period include meconium aspiration syndrome, persistent fetal circulation, hypoglycaemia, hypocalcaemia, hyperviscosity syndrome and poor temperature control.

- Fetal growth depends on interacting factors such as genetic determinants, maternal health and nutrition, availability of growth substrates, fetal growth hormones and sufficient maternal blood supply to the placenta.

- Associated maternal conditions are hypertension, chronic renal disease, diabetes mellitus, sickle cell anaemia, severe cardiac disease, smoking and alcohol ingestion. Placental problems include small placental size, inadequate changes in the spiral arteries and placental infarcts. Fetal causes include chromosomal abnormalities, infections and multiple pregnancy.

- Maternal influences associated with asymmetrical fetal growth include malnutrition and low weight gain in pregnancy. Tobacco smoking decreases placental blood flow, causing fetal growth retardation. Alcohol crosses the placental barrier and causes fetal alcohol syndrome. Genetic and chromosomal disorders amongst babies with symmetric IUGR are common.

- A combination of clinical and ultrasound methods make a diagnosis of IUGR possible in 95% of cases. Umbilical Doppler velocimetry with either estimated fetal weight or abdominal circumference may improve accuracy of antenatal diagnosis of IUGR. Ultrasonographic measurement of fetal abdominal subcutaneous fat may be a useful predictor.

- Tests such as serial estriol estimation, serial hPL assays and daily fetal movement monitoring have little value. Fundal height measurements select women for ultrasonic screening.

- Serial measurements of the amount of liquor amnii may demonstrate oligohydramnios, a late sign of fetal malnutrition and the need to expedite delivery. Fetal biophysical profile may be a better predictive test than the non-stress test in identifying babies with a low 5-min Apgar score.

- Once fetal lung maturity is achieved, the baby can be delivered. IUGR babies remain smaller than their age cohorts for several years. Some studies have reported increased incidence of minimal brain dysfunction and speech defects; others have found no difference.

- Rhesus haemolysis of fetal red cells rarely affects the first baby as there are no spontaneous maternal anti-D antibodies present prior to a first pregnancy. Antibody formation may occur because of abortion, antepartum haemorrhage or obstetric manoeuvres such as amniocentesis. If a fetomaternal transfusion is likely, anti-D immunoglobulin must be administered to the mother within 72 h.

- Rhesus-negative women are screened for rhesus antibodies. If there is a high titre a direct test on the amniotic fluid is performed. The amount of bilirubin allows judgement to be made about management of the pregnancy. Some authorities recommend the use of antepartum rhesus D immunoglobulin prophylaxis.

- At delivery, cord blood is taken for testing from all babies of rhesus-negative women for ABO and rhesus type, direct Coombes' test and haemoglobin estimation. If the mother has rhesus antibodies, cord blood is also tested for serum bilirubin level.

- In ABO incompatibility the mother has unprovoked anti-A and anti-B antibodies in the first pregnancy so the first child may be affected. Jaundice appears in the first 24 h but is usually mild.

- Systemic infections may cause infertility and congenital defects in the babies of pregnant women. Despite the suppression of cell-mediated immunity in pregnancy, most women are not immunocompromised. However, some infections such as poliomyelitis and influenza are likely to be more severe in pregnancy. Pregnancy leads to reactivation of latent cytomegaloviruses and herpes.

- If untreated, sexually transmitted diseases can have long-term serious health consequences and pregnant women may pass the infection on to the fetus, resulting in birth defects or stillbirth.

- Severe complications of gonorrhoea include pelvic inflammatory disease and damage to heart valves and joint tissues. The organism can cause severe neonatal ophthalmia. Most cases respond to penicillin but penicillin-resistant strains of the organism are evolving.

- Syphilis is more serious than gonorrhoea but better controlled, as penicillin is very effective against the causative organism. The disease can be transmitted across the placenta to the fetus to cause congenital syphilis.

- Contamination of the baby with *Chlamydia trachomatis* during birth may cause severe conjunctivitis and respiratory distress. Chlamydial infection responds to tetracycline or erythromycin.

- Infection with group B streptococcus is most often responsible for overwhelming neonatal sepsis with a high mortality rate. Screening and treatment of women is difficult because of the recurring infection but giving antibiotics to labouring women may be useful.

- The transmission of the HIV virus is associated with sexual activity where skin or mucous membrane integrity is broken. Women who are HIV positive may pass the virus across the placenta to the fetus or the baby may be infected by contact with maternal blood during birth. A third way of transmission is through breastfeeding.

- TORCH infections will cause congenital abnormality, if acquired in the first trimester, and neonatal infection, often affecting the lung, liver, spleen and brain, if acquired late in pregnancy.

- *Listeria monocytogenes* is a foodborne pathogen which may cause abortion, fetal disease or death.

- The hepatitis B virus is transmitted by blood, sexual intercourse and by vertical transmission to the fetus. Long-term infection can lead to chronic hepatitis, cirrhosis of the liver and liver cancer. Antenatal screening of pregnant women ensures that the baby can be treated.

- Maternal genital infection with the type 1 or type 2 *herpes simplex virus* may lead to serious neonatal infection. Many infected women show no clinical signs. Trials of antiviral agents have been inconclusive. Delivery by caesarean section does not protect completely against neonatal infection because of transplacental infection. There are two alternative strategies for the future: a vaccine or mass screening.

References

ACOG 2000 Practice bulletin No 20. Perinatal Viral and Parasitic Infections 26(3):1–12.

Arias F 1993 Practical Guide to High Risk Pregnancy and Delivery. Mosby Year Book, Chicago.

Barker D J P 1998 Mothers, babies and health in later life. Harcourt Brace, Edinburgh.

Benbow A, Wray J 1998 Recommendations for the use of anti-D immunoglobulin for RhD prophylaxis. British Journal of Midwifery 6(3):84–86.

Blackburn S T 2003 Maternal, Fetal and Neonatal Physiology – A Clinical Perspective. W B Saunders, Philadelphia.

Bennett V R, Brown L K (eds) 1999 Myles Textbook for Midwives, 13th edn. Churchill Livingstone, Edinburgh.

Brocklehurst P, Volmink J 2002 Antiretrovirals for reducing the risk of mother-to-child transmission of HIV infection. Cochrane Review: In The Cochrane Library, Issue 1. Update Software 2003, Oxford.

Clayton J 2003 Beating the odds. New Scientist 177(2381):34–37.

Department of Health 2001 First national strategy for sexual health and HIV services published: new information campaign and targeted chlamydia screening. Press Release 2001/0354. Department of Health, London.

Enkin M, Keirse M J N C, Neilson J et al 2000 A Guide to Effective Care in Pregnancy and Childbirth, 3rd edn. Oxford University Press, Oxford, pp 79–92.

Gardeil F, Greene R, Stuart B, Turner M J 2000 Sonographic measurement of subcutaneous fat in the fetal abdomen: a new predictor of growth restriction? Contemporary Reviews in Obstetrics and Gynecology March.

Garland S, Jones C 2001 Herpes simplex virus in pregnancy. Obstetrics and Gynaecology 3(2):108–111.

Hofmeyr G J 1995 Prophylactic versus therapeutic amnioinfusion for intrapartum oligohydramnios. Cochrane Review: In The Cochrane Library, Issue 1. Update Software 2003, Oxford.

Kelly J, Mathews K A, O'Conor M 1984 Smoking during pregnancy, effects on mother and the fetus. British Journal of Obstetrics and Gynaecology 95:111–117.

Longo L D 1977 The biological effects of carbon monoxide on the pregnant woman, fetus and newborn infant. American Journal of Obstetrics and Gynecology 129:69–103.

Madigan J, Martinko J M, Parker J 1999 Brock's Biology of Micro-organisms. Prentice Hall, New Jersey.

Moodley P, Sturm W 2000 Sexually transmitted infections, adverse pregnancy outcome and neonatal infection. Seminars in Neonatology 5(3):255–269.

Ott W J 2001 The ultrasonic diagnosis and evaluation of intrauterine growth restriction. Ultrasound Reviews in Obstetrics and Gynecology 1:205–215.

Randolph A G, Washington E, Prober C G 1993 Caesarean delivery for women presenting with genital herpes lesions. Efficacy, risks and costs. Journal of the American Medical Association 270:77–82.

Robinson J S, Moore V M, Owens J A, McMillen I C 2000 Origins of fetal growth restriction. European Journal of Obstetrics and Gynecology and Reproductive Biology 92:13–19.

Smaill F 2003 Intrapartum antibiotics for Group B streptococcal colonisation. Cochrane Review: In The Cochrane Library, Issue 1. Update Software 2003, Oxford.

Soregaroli M, Bonera R, Danti L et al 2002 Prognostic role of umbilical artery Doppler velocimetry in growth-restricted fetuses. The Journal of Maternal-Fetal Medicine 11:199–203.

Stone A 2003 Protect and survive. New Scientist 177(2381):42–44.

Wickham S 2001 Routine antenatal anti-D: an overview of the evidence. MIDIRS Midwifery Digest 11(2):201–203.

Wilson C 2003 World without AIDS. New Scientist 177(2381):38–41.

Annotated recommended reading

Barker D J P 1998 Mothers, babies and health in later life. Harcourt Brace, Edinburgh.
This book is an eye-opener for anybody who wishes to find out about the long-term effects of fetal disadvantage. It is well written and opens up a new field of preventative medicine.

Moodley P, Sturm W 2000 Sexually transmitted infections, adverse pregnancy outcome and neonatal infection. Seminars in Neonatology 5(3):255–269.
This paper provides an excellent overview of the effects of sexually transmitted diseases on mothers and their babies.

Ott W J 2001 The ultrasonic diagnosis and evaluation of intrauterine growth restriction. Ultrasound Reviews in Obstetrics and Gynecology 1:205–215.
The author provides not only an excellent report on his own research but also a good overview of methods of monitoring growth restriction in the fetus.

Wickham S 2001 Routine antenatal anti-D: an overview of the evidence. MIDIRS Midwifery Digest 11(2):201–203.
This is an informative review of research into the use of antenatal anti-D prophylaxis. It discusses the changing role of the midwife when new technology or treatments are introduced.

Clayton J 2003 Beating the odds. New Scientist 177(2381):34–37.

Wilson C 2003 World without AIDS. New Scientist 177(2381):38–41.

Stone A 2003 Protect and survive. New Scientist 177(2381):42–44.
These three linked articles are easily accessible and contain the latest information and ideas related to combating the AIDS epidemic.

Chapter 15

Congenital defects

INTRODUCTION

Congenital defects which are present at birth may be visible, involve obvious changes in organs or be hidden such as changes in protein molecules, for example haemoglobin or cell receptors. O'Shea (1995) outlines the terminology used to describe congenital defects as follows:

- a **defect** is a primary aberration in the zygote and is programmed to lead to abnormal development regardless of environmental influences
- **disruption** refers to destruction of normally developing tissue by some outside influence such as drug-related defects
- **deformation** is the term used for alterations in the development of normal tissues and organs by physical forces, such as occurs in oligohydramnios
- **dysplasia** describes abnormal differentiation or organisation of tissues.

Congenital defects account for most severe illness during infancy and childhood and 25% of childhood deaths. A defect is present in about 2% of liveborn infants but most are minor and of no functional significance. Other major problems are incompatible with life and result in early abortion. Recent research shows that some of the diseases that afflict older people such as heart disease, hypertension or diabetes occur because of structural or functional changes in the fetus (Barker 1992).

GENERAL CAUSES OF CONGENITAL DEFECTS

There are four main groups of causes of congenital defects (O'Shea 1995):

- genetic/chromosomal abnormalities;
- environmental teratogen;
- multifactorial disorders caused by the interaction of environment and genes;
- idiopathic defects with no known cause, the largest group.

Genes

An introduction to genetics including causation of fetal abnormalities is found in Chapter 3 and the role of genes in embryogenesis is presented in Chapter 8. Many fetal anomalies are caused by genetic and chromosomal defects. Mutations may occur in the DNA of either protein-coding genes or homeobox regulatory genes.

Teratogens

Teratology is the study of the causes, mechanisms and patterns of abnormal (fetal) development (Moore & Persaud 1998). From the 3rd to the 8th weeks, during organogenesis, the embryo is vulnerable to developmental disruption by environmental factors (Ch. 8, p. 85). **Teratogens** reach the fetus by crossing the placenta and cause **DNA mutations**. Malformations of a particular structure are usually caused only during the sensitive period of its development (Larsen 2001). The earlier teratogens are present, the more generalised the effect. If they occur during the first 17 days when the three germ layers are being formed (Ch. 9), they are usually fatal. During the rest of the embryonic period survival with major defects is likely. Following completion of organogenesis at 8 weeks their effects are greatly reduced, except in the brain where cell differentiation still continues. Some teratogens interfere with cell division by affecting **nucleic acid synthesis**, while others interfere with **cell migration** or with the **synthesis of cell products**.

Environmental and genetic interaction

The rate of new mutations can be increased by environmental factors such as microbial, biochemical, dietary factors, smoking, alcohol ingestion, radiation and many chemicals (Ward 1995). These may interfere with embryonic development at very precise times during organogenesis. Some factors such as the rubella virus are easily associated but other, vague issues such as atmospheric pollutants are more difficult to ascertain. These interactions are discussed in Chapter 8, p. 85.

Drugs

Medical drugs may be dispensed by practitioners or may be bought over the counter from a chemist. Drugs may damage gametes or have an adverse effect on nutrient absorption so that essential nutrients are absent at crucial times (Table 15.1).

Thalidomide, a drug taken for morning sickness in the early 1960s, caused major **limb reduction deformities** as well as other problems. The effects of taking thalidomide in early pregnancy (Fig. 15.1) are still being seen in South America where the drug is prescribed for leprosy. While care is taken in avoiding prescribing the drug to pregnant women, people may offer friends and relatives their drugs. Inevitably, some who take drugs in this way will be pregnant.

Table 15.1   Drugs known to cause fetal defects (British National Formulary 2003)

Drug	Effect
Thalidomide	Limb deformities, heart defects
Warfarin	Limb defects, central nervous system defects, retarded growth
Corticosteroids	Cleft palate and congenital cataract
Anticonvulsants such as phenytoin	Lip and palate deformities, mental retardation
Androgens	Masculinisation in female fetus
Oestrogens	Testicular atrophy in male
Diethylstilbestrol	Vaginal and cervical cancer at puberty
Cytotoxic drugs (especially folic acid antagonists)	Neural tube defects, cleft palate
Tetracycline	Staining of bones and teeth, thin tooth enamel, impaired bone growth

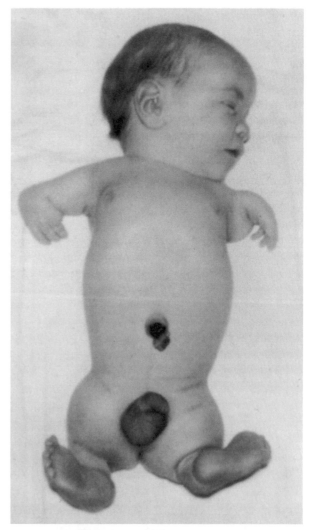

Figure 15.1   Newborn male infant showing typical malformed limbs (meromelia – limb reduction) caused by thalidomide ingested by his mother during the critical period of limb development. (Reproduced with permission from Moore 1963.)

A drug's effect may be delayed and not show itself for a generation (Colborn et al 1996).

PRENATAL SCREENING FOR CONGENITAL DEFECTS

In an ideal world congenital defects could be prevented. However, most women are seen for the first time when their pregnancy is already underway. Education of people and the offer of a **preconception service** (Ch. 8, p. 81) will help to reduce the number of abnormal embryos conceived. Early diagnosis is essential wherever possible so that a couple can be offered the choice to terminate the pregnancy. Many defects can now be detected in specific populations. Techniques include ultrasonography, chorionic villus sampling, amniocentesis and maternal serum screening.

Abramsky & Chapple (1994) consider the 'human side' of prenatal screening and late pregnancy diagnosis of fetal abnormality. They are concerned that medical technology has raced ahead with little consideration given to the ethical, legal and emotional dilemmas raised by an increased ability to detect fetal defects. Couples may not want to terminate the pregnancy and early diagnosis offers them a chance to plan for treatment of the baby after birth. Larsen (2001) discusses three techniques that have 'begun to revolutionise the diagnosis of embryonic and fetal malformations and genetic disease'. These are ultrasonography, amniocentesis and chorionic villus sampling.

Ultrasonography

Most women are offered an **ultrasound scan** (USS) in pregnancy. The embryonic sac can be seen as early as 6 weeks following conception. Ultrasound screening is probably best carried out at 18–20 weeks gestation so that an accurate fetal age can be confirmed, multiple pregnancy detected and congenital defects diagnosed. The indications for USS are controversial but many obstetricians feel the advantages of routine scanning far outweigh the disadvantages. Proud (1999) lists the advantages and disadvantages and the author adds a few more.

Advantages
- It is a non-invasive technique.
- The mother requires minimal preparation.
- It provides instant information.
- Movements of the fetus can be seen.
- Parents feel pleased to have seen their baby's image.
- It can support clinical findings.

Disadvantages
- There may be long-term dangers to the fetus.
- Clinical expertise may decline and there may be over-reliance on the ultrasound findings.
- Some practitioners have an impersonal approach compared to the midwife's examination.

- It is an expensive form of investigation with little proof of effectiveness.

Neilson (1998) updated an earlier review and found that:

routine ultrasound in early pregnancy appears to enable better gestational age assessment, earlier detection of multiple pregnancies and earlier detection of clinically unsuspected fetal malformation at a time when termination of pregnancy is possible. However the benefits of other substantive outcomes are less clear.

How ultrasound works

Ultrasound imaging depends on the differences in structure between organs. Sound at a very high pitch (frequency of 3–10 MHz) is produced by a **transducer**. Because of its frequency, high-pitched sound travels in a **narrow beam**. These sound waves pass into the body until they reach a tissue and are reflected back. The sound echoes are detected **electronically** and transmitted onto the screen as a dot. The more dense the tissue, the stronger the echo and the whiter the visual display. Weaker echoes produce various shades of grey. Fluid-filled areas reflect no echoes, resulting in a black area.

Various types of display modes are used, each with its own advantages. **M-mode** ultrasonography shows changes in position of a structure with time. **B-mode** ultrasonography shows the anatomy of a two-dimensional plane of scanning and can be carried out in real time. **Doppler ultrasonography** produces flow information and is used to study patterns of blood flow in the heart and vessels. A recent development due to miniaturisation has been **endosonography**, whereby an endoscope can be inserted into the vagina to bring it closer to the fetus and receive a higher-resolution image. **Real-time B-mode** ultrasonography is the type most often used to examine the fetus (Larsen 2001). Common defects diagnosed by ultrasound include:

- anencephaly, microcephaly and hydrocephaly;
- neural tube defects (NTDs);
- gastrointestinal defects such as atresias and omphalocele;
- renal agenesis and polycystic kidneys;
- body defects associated with chromosomal defects.

Obtaining fetal tissue for genetic testing

All invasive techniques carry a risk of infection, haemorrhage and fetal loss. The risks must be weighed against the likelihood of abnormality being present in the fetus. Cells obtained by **amniocentesis** or **chorionic villus sampling** can be used for **karyotyping** for chromosomal errors such as Down syndrome, **genetic analysis** using gene probes as in cystic fibrosis and **sexing the embryo** if there is a family history of X-linked disorders such as Duchenne muscular dystrophy. **Enzyme assay** for detection of an inborn error of metabolism is available in over 50% of disorders.

Amniocentesis

A sample of amniotic fluid is withdrawn from the amniotic cavity through a transabdominal needle using ultrasound to avoid the placenta. This procedure is usually carried out at 14–16 weeks when sufficient liquor amnii is present. It can be carried out between 9 and 13 weeks of pregnancy but is difficult because of the small amount of liquor amnii and it may not provide sufficient cells to study. A further problem lies in the culturing of **desquamated cells**, which may have to be cultured for up to 3 weeks before the chromosomes can be counted. There is a 1 in 200 chance that amniocentesis may cause a miscarriage and the long waiting period before results are available is distressing to the parents.

Chorionic villus sampling

Chorionic villus sampling (CVS) involves obtaining a small amount of tissue (10–40 mg) from the chorion frondosum by using a cannula or biopsy forceps under ultrasound guidance. CVS can be performed either transabdominally or transvaginally and can be carried out as early as 6 weeks. The cells are healthy and actively dividing so that results of karyotyping can be obtained quickly. However, maternal tissue may be mistaken for fetal tissue, leading to incorrect diagnoses and sex determination. At worst the decision to abort a normal fetus could occur (Larsen 2001). Also, the spontaneous abortion rate following chorionic villus sampling is higher than that following amniocentesis.

Cordocentesis

A needle is guided to the base of the umbilical cord using ultrasound visualisation and a sample of fetal blood withdrawn. The blood can be used to screen for blood disorders such as haemophilia and haemoglobinopathies, karyotyping for chromosome analysis, DNA analysis, testing for inborn errors of metabolism and assessment of anaemia in rhesus isoimmunisation.

Fetoscopy

An endoscope is inserted transabdominally and the fetus visualised directly. It is rarely performed and has been superseded by other procedures. Fetal skin biopsy and fetal liver biopsy have been carried out in this way but there is a fetal loss of up to 5% and preterm labour of up to 10%.

Maternal serum screening

This is carried out to search for the small amounts of **maternal serum α-fetoprotein** (MSAFP) present. Normal values of MSAFP are highest in early pregnancy, decreasing as pregnancy advances. Multiple pregnancy, fetal death, open fetal defects such as **spina bifida** or **exomphalos** and **Turner's syndrome** associated with a **cystic hygroma** are associated with raised levels of MSAFP. Low MSAFP levels are associated with Down syndrome if found with a low level of unconjugated estriol and a high level of human chorionic gonadotrophin (hCG). Following the finding of an abnormal level of MSAFP, the fetus can be examined by ultrasound and/or amniocentesis is carried out to check the AFP level.

Comparison of amniocentesis and CVS

Alfirevic et al (1998) compared chorionic villus sampling with amniocentesis for prenatal diagnosis. They found that there were multiple problems with CVS, probably because CVS is more technically demanding for both obstetricians and cytogeneticists. The problems included:

- more sampling failures;
- multiple instrument insertions;
- repeated procedures;
- laboratory failures;
- maternal contamination;
- abnormal karyotypes;
- false-positive and false-negative results;
- higher pregnancy loss because of spontaneous abortion;
- increased stillbirths and neonatal deaths.

They concluded that 'second trimester amniocentesis is safer than CVS and the benefits of earlier diagnosis by CVS must be set against its greater risks'. In a separate review, Alfirevic (1998) compared a technique of early amniocentesis (before 14 weeks) with CVS. He found that technical difficulties occurred more often with CVS but laboratory failure was more common in early amniocentesis. Pregnancy loss was more common in the women allocated to the early amniocentesis group, with an increase in preterm deliveries. However, the numbers involved in the trials were too small to be reliable.

Fetal blood cells leak through the placenta into the maternal circulation. It may be possible in the future to use such cells 'to provide safe and reliable tests for genetic defects such as Down syndrome'. However it may be 10 years before the isolating of fetal cells from maternal blood becomes routine enough to provide a screening test.

EXAMPLES OF SOME DISORDERS

The following common disorders are representative of the major factors in the causation of congenital defects. Some of the implications for society brought about by modern technology are introduced. Horgan (1993) warned of the problems that arise when genetic testing followed by termination of affected pregnancies is taken to the extremes of **eugenics**. Rennie (1994) similarly wrote about the effects of population screening for genetic diseases. The disorders to be discussed are:

- chromosomal disorder – Down syndrome (Fig. 15.2);
- dominant genetic disorder – Huntington's disease;

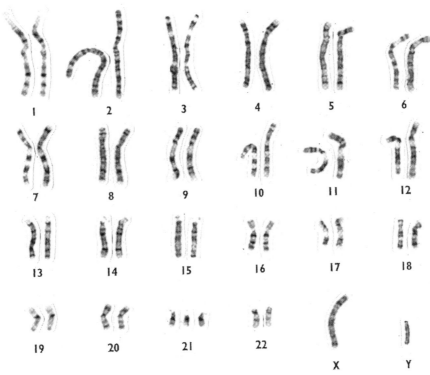

Figure 15.2   A branded karyotype of Down syndrome (trisomy 21) (from Kelnar C, Harvey D, Simpson C 1995, with permission).

- recessive genetic disorder – cystic fibrosis;
- X-linked genetic disorder – Duchenne muscular dystrophy;
- genetic predisposition with environmental trigger – neural tube defects (NTDs);
- Environmental disorder – rubella and other infections are discussed in Chapter 14.

Down syndrome

The natural incidence of Down syndrome or trisomy 21 is about 1 in 800 births but increases with maternal age (Fig. 15.3) when the incidence can be as high as 1 in 40. Many more are conceived and, even without action, three-quarters may be aborted spontaneously. About 95% are caused by non-dysjunction but translocation 14/21 (Ch. 3) may occur in any age of woman and is likely to be inherited.

The features of Down syndrome are easily recognised and include (Fig. 15.4):

- A small head with flattened occiput and a broad flat nose.
- A small mouth cavity with thick gum margins and protruding tongue.
- Epicanthic folds.
- Brushfield's spots, which are white flecks seen in the iris.
- Short hands with incurving little fingers.
- A single palmar crease.
- A wide deviation of the great toe with a plantar crease between the first and second toes.
- Dry skin.

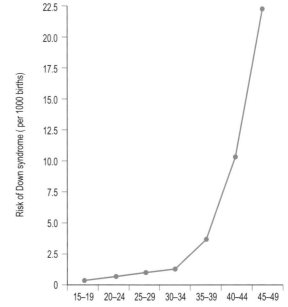

Figure 15.3   The risk of Down syndrome at different maternal ages (from Kelnar C, Harvey D, Simpson C 1995, with permission).

- Hypotonic muscles.
- Other features include heart defects, increased incidence of duodenal atresia, reduced intelligence, inadequate immune system and a tendency to develop leukaemia. By the age of 40 many Down syndrome people have developed Alzheimer's disease.

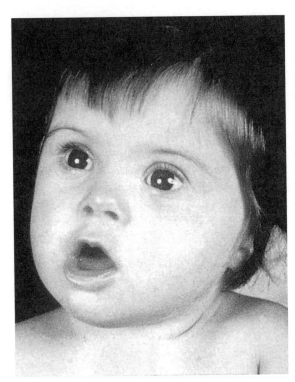

Figure 15.4   Down syndrome (from Sweet B 1997, with permission).

Detection of trisomy 21

There is controversy about the lack of inter-hospital agreement and availability of the safest and most cost-effective screening tests for Down syndrome (Hartley 2001, Brennand & Cameron 2001). There is also discussion about whether testing in the first or second trimester is better. Many positive fetuses identified in the first trimester would be spontaneously aborted. A combination of biochemical tests on maternal serum and ultrasound findings linked to maternal age could indicate the presence of an affected fetus. According to Hartley (2001) there is no continuity in which tests are offered to pregnant women and many are offered a weak combination. The best tests must be offered by all health authorities. If screening reveals a high risk, karyotyping of the fetal chromosomes is carried out. The biochemical indicators are:

- low maternal serum α-fetoprotein (AFP);
- high free beta subunit human chorionic gonadotrophin (β-hCG);
- low unconjugated estriol (uE3);
- inhibin A;
- low PAPP-A.

The first four of these form a quadrupal test that is only available privately in 2002.

Ultrasonography

- The main ultrasound marker is nuchal translucency where an increased skin-fold thickness at the back of the neck

is a recognised clinical feature (Brennand & Cameron 2001).

- Although increased nuchal translucency thickness is associated with chromosomal defects, it is not a clear indicator of Down syndrome. Other ultrasound markers such as duodenal atresia and cardiac septal defects can avoid false-positive tests.

Huntington's disease

Huntington's disease (HD), caused by a dominant gene, occurs in about 1 in 2000 births. The gene was found in 1983 on the terminal band of the short arm of chromosome 4. It affects the **basal ganglia** and **cerebral cortex**, resulting in involuntary movement called **chorea**, which begin in the arms and face and eventually affect the whole body. **Dementia** follows with impaired memory and judgement. It affects all races and the average age of onset is 40 years.

Onset is earlier if the gene is inherited on the paternal chromosome rather than the maternal but the mode is not understood. The disease tends to commence earlier in succeeding generations (Mueller & Young 2001). There is no treatment for halting or even delaying symptoms. Death occurs from cerebral degeneration after 15–20 years. The onset of HD is delayed until an affected person has already had their own children and might even have grandchildren. Genetic presymptomatic testing and testing of children are just two of the ethical issues that follow the identification of any gene.

Cystic fibrosis

Cystic fibrosis (CF) is a recessive inherited disease of the **exocrine glands** with production of thick mucus that obstructs the gastrointestinal tract and the lungs. Although the disease mainly affects white populations, slightly different mutations of the gene occur in black and other populations. The gene is located in the middle of the long arm of chromosome 7 and codes for a transmembrane regulator protein. Its full name is the **cystic fibrosis transmembrane regulator** (CFTR). The CFTR protein controls the entry of sodium and chloride ions into the cells so that both cells and their secretions lack water. The resulting thick mucus obstructs and dilates the ducts of the pancreas and the lungs, destroying the structure and the function of the organs. In the lung secondary bacterial infection is common and there is progressive involvement of the bronchial tree, beginning in the alveolar ducts and resulting in large cystic dilations of all bronchi.

Genetic markers allow the prenatal diagnosis of CF and carriers can be detected in over 70% of families with a history of CF. More than 900 individual mutations have now been found on or near this gene, not all of which cause severe disease. One in particular, present in about 1 in 20 people, is called **5T**. It only causes cystic fibrosis in the presence of a

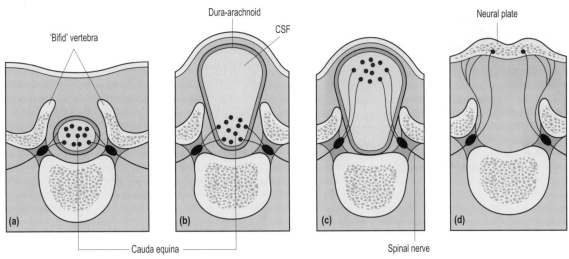

Figure 15.5 Variants of spina bifida. (a) Spina bifida occulta. (b) Meningocele. (c) Meningomyelocele. (d) Myelocele (from Hinchliff S M, Montague S E 1990, with permission).

second, rarer mutation called **R117H**. This has led to problems of interpretation in the USA and many women have been offered unnecessary terminations of pregnancy (Concar 2003). This demonstrates that before national screening, protocols must be in place and the implications fully understood by all practitioners. The United Kingdom is at present considering national screening for carriers.

With early diagnosis and active treatment, life expectancy has increased from death in childhood until 30 years. The financial cost of treatment for a person with CF is great and there is the likely need for a heart–lung transplant. CF is a disease where the treatment with a genetically engineered product may be possible. The gene for the CFTR proteins could be attached to a retrovirus for administration to the lungs by a nebulizer. However, the research is still at the experimental stage.

Duchenne muscular dystrophy

Duchenne muscular dystrophy (DMD) is the commonest muscular dystrophy. It occurs only in boys and is an X-linked disorder. The abnormal gene is carried on the short arm of the X chromosome and may be a deletion. This is a severe disorder and sufferers die before they have children. The normal allele at the site codes for a muscle protein called **dystrophin** which is absent in boys with DMD.

Muscle bulk diminishes and connective tissue and fat replace muscle fibres. DMD begins at about the age of 3 with slow motor development, progressive weakness and muscle wasting. Muscle weakness begins in the pelvic girdle and the boys develop a waddling gait. There is hypertrophy of the calf muscles in 80% of cases (McCance & Huether 2002). Muscular weakness affects pulmonary function and cardiac involvement occurs in over 90% of children. Boys are usually confined to a wheelchair by 12 years of age and die of respiratory or cardiac failure before the age of 20.

Fetal diagnosis is possible but not as routine screening. Women with an affected son are offered screening in subsequent pregnancies.

Neural tube defects

Most major defects of the brain are the result of defective closure of the anterior neuropore neural canal during the 4th week from conception. The result may be anencephaly with absence of the forebrain and covering skull. Most of the embryonic brain is exposed and extruding from the skull. Life following birth is not possible. Failure of closure of the caudal neuropore at the end of the 4th week results in congenital defects of the spinal cord such as spina bifida (Fig. 15.5).

Severe NTDs involve the tissues lying over the spinal cord – the meninges, vertebral arch, muscles and skin (Moore & Persaud 1998). Spina bifida occulta may have no external signs and no clinical symptoms. The defect usually involves the vertebrae L5 or S1. The severe types of spina bifida involve protrusion of the spinal cord and meninges through defects in several vertebral arches. This happens only 2 weeks after the woman misses her menstrual period and long before most women present for antenatal care. Once the woman is receiving care, detection of NTD and counselling concerning the termination of pregnancy is offered.

Terminology

- If the protruding sac contains only meninges and cerebrospinal fluid, it is called **spina bifida cystica**.

- If the spinal cord and nerve roots are included in the sac (75% of fetuses), it is called **spina bifida with meningomyelocele** (Fig. 15.6). Meningomyeloceles may

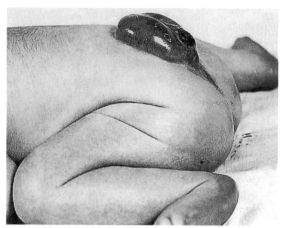

Figure 15.6   Meningomyelocele. The 'frog leg' posture is characteristic of combined femoral and sciatic nerve paralysis, with preservation of hip flexion by the ilio psoas muscle (from Hinchliff S M, Montague S E 1990, with permission).

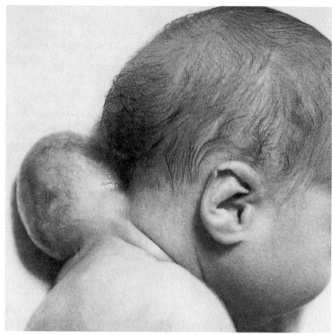

Figure 15.8   Cervical meningocele (from Kelnar C, Harvey D, Simpson C 1995, with permission).

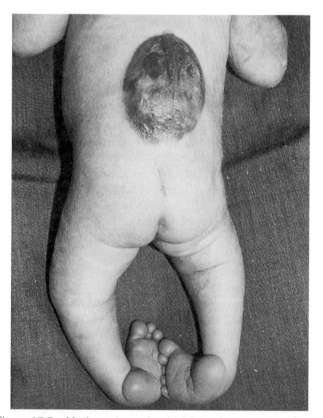

Figure 15.7   Myelomeningocele with bilateral severe talipes (from Kelnar C, Harvey D, Simpson C 1995, with permission).

be covered with skin or with a thin, easily ruptured membrane and may be associated with talipes (Fig. 15.7).

● When the spinal cord is only a flattened mass of nervous tissue, the condition is called **myeloschisis**.

● A **meningocele** may be found at the cervical part of the spine (Fig. 15.8).

It would be much better if the occurrence of NTDs could be prevented. There was suspicion that **folic acid deficiency** (Hibbard & Smithells 1965) was somehow implicated in the causation of NTDs. Two intervention studies (Smithells et al 1980, Laurence et al 1981), where folate had been given to women who had had a previous pregnancy resulting in a fetus with an NTD, suggested that supplementation might prevent recurrence. This led to a randomised double-blind trial being conducted at 33 centres in seven countries. The results were so clear that the research group recommended that folic acid supplementation should be given to all women who were likely to bear children.

MAIN POINTS

- Congenital defects account for most severe illness during infancy and childhood and 25% of childhood deaths. Some diseases that afflict older people such as heart disease may occur because of structural or functional changes in the fetus. During organogenesis the embryo is vulnerable to disruption of development by environmental processes.

- Teratogens lead to genetic mutations. Drugs may damage sperm or ova or may affect embryonic nutrient absorption, making essential nutrients absent at crucial times. They may be teratogenic and interfere in normal development.

- Screening for congenital defects may involve ultrasonography, amniocentesis and chorionic villus sampling. Fetal tissue can be used for karyotyping for chromosomal errors, embryonic sexing if there is a history of X-linked disorders and enzyme assay for detecting inborn errors of metabolism.

- The incidence of trisomy 21 increases with maternal age and can reach as high as 1 in 40. The risk of a mother carrying a Down syndrome baby can be estimated by using a combination of maternal serum biochemical tests and ultrasound findings. Fetal karyotyping for chromosomal abnormality is carried out if the fetus is at high risk.

- The onset of Huntington's disease (HD) is earlier if the gene is inherited on the paternal chromosome rather than the maternal chromosome. As the onset of HD is delayed until an affected person has already had children, genetic presymptomatic testing and testing of children are ethical issues.

- Cystic fibrosis mainly affects white populations but different mutations of the gene occur in other populations. The gene codes for the cystic fibrosis transmembrane regulator (CFTR), which controls the entry of sodium and chloride ions into cells. The CFTR gene could be attached to a retrovirus for administration to the lungs by a nebulizer but research is still experimental.

- The X-linked disorder Duchenne muscular dystrophy is so severe that sufferers die before they have children. Fetal diagnosis is possible and women who have borne an affected son can be offered screening for subsequent pregnancies.

- Most major defects of the brain are the result of defective closure of the anterior neuropore during the 4th week from conception. The result may be anencephaly or spina bifida. Diet, in particular folic acid deficiency, may be implicated in their cause.

References

Abramsky L, Chapple J (eds) 1994 Prenatal Diagnosis: The Human Side. Chapman and Hall, London.

Alfirevic Z 1998 Early amniocentesis versus transabdominal chorionic villus sampling for prenatal amniocentesis. Cochrane Review: In The Cochrane Library, Issue 2. Update Software 2003, Oxford.

Alfirevic Z, Gosden C, Neilson J P 1998 Chorionic villus sampling compared with amniocentesis for prenatal diagnosis. Cochrane Review: In The Cochrane Library, Issue 2. Update Software 2003, Oxford.

Barker D J P (ed.) 1992 Fetal and Infant Origins of Adult Disease. BMJ Books, London.

Brennand J E, Cameron A D 2001 Current methods of screening for Down's syndrome. The Obstetrician and Gynaecologist 3(4):191–197.

British National Formulary 2003 BNF 46. British Medical Association and Royal Pharmaceutical Society of Great Britain.

Colborn T, Myers J P, Dumanski D 1996 Our Stolen Future. Little Brown, Boston.

Concar C 2003 Test blunders risk needless abortions. New Scientist 178(2393):4–6.

Hartley J 2001 NHS Downs test is flawed. Reprinted in MIDIRS Midwifery Digest 12(1):62.

Hibbard E D, Smithells R W 1965 Folic acid metabolism and human embryopathy. Lancet i:1254.

Horgan J 1993 Eugenics revisited. Scientific American June:90–100.

Larsen W J 2001 Human Embryology, 3rd edn. Churchill Livingstone, Edinburgh.

Laurence K M, James N, Miller M H et al 1981 Double-blind randomised controlled trial of folate treatment before conception to prevent recurrence of neural-tube defects. British Medical Journal 282:1509–1511.

McCance K L, Huether S E 2002 Pathophysiology. The Biologic Basis for Disease in Adults and Children, 3rd edn. Mosby, St Louis.

Moore K L, Persaud T V N 1998 Before We Are Born, 5th edn. W B Saunders, Philadelphia.

Mueller R F, Young I D 2001 Emery's Elements of Medical Genetics. Churchill Livingstone, Edinburgh.

Neilson J P 1998 Ultrasound for fetal assessment in early pregnancy. Cochrane Review: In The Cochrane Library, Issue 2. Update Software 2003, Oxford.

O'Shea P A 1995 Congenital defects and their causes. In Coustan D R, Haning R V, Singer D B (eds) Human Reproduction Development. Little Brown, Boston.

Proud J 1999 Specialised antenatal investigations. In Bennett V R, Brown L K (eds) Myles Textbook for Midwives, 13th edn. Churchill Livingstone, Edinburgh.

Rennie J 1994 Grading the gene tests. Scientific American June:66–74.

Smithells R W, Shephard S, Schorah C J et al 1980 Possible prevention of neural-tube defects by periconceptional vitamin supplementation. Lancet 1:339–340.

Ward N 1995 Preconceptional care and pregnancy outcome. Journal of Nutritional and Environmental Medicine 5:2205–2208.

Annotated recommended reading

Larsen W J 2001 Human Embryology, 3rd edn. Churchill Livingstone, Edinburgh.
This book examines both molecular biological and clinical aspects of embryology. Each chapter is about a specific embryological stage and the clinical applications arising out of the advancing knowledge base.

Moore K L, Persaud T V N 1998 Before We Are Born, 5th edn. W B Saunders, Philadelphia.
This textbook clearly describes embryo development week by week and provides an excellent source for understanding the origins of congenital defects. The illustrations are excellent.

Alfirevic Z 1998 Early amniocentesis versus transabdominal chorionic villus sampling for prenatal amniocentesis. Cochrane Review: In The Cochrane Library, Issue 2. Update Software 2003, Oxford.
The Cochrane reviews are carefully constructed and written in an unbiased manner. This makes them useful to practitioners who are involved in decision making and carrying out policies.

Brennand J E, Cameron A D 2001 Current methods of screening for Down's syndrome. The Obstetrician and Gynaecologist 3(4):191–197.
This paper gives an extremely good overview of the current availability of first and second trimester screening tests for Down's syndrome.

Neilson J P 1998 Ultrasound for fetal assessment in early pregnancy. Cochrane Review: In The Cochrane Library, Issue 2. Update Software 2003, Oxford.
The Cochrane reviews are carefully constructed and written in an unbiased manner. This makes them useful to practitioners who are involved in decision making and carrying out policies.

Section 2B

PREGNANCY – THE MOTHER

Women who are pregnant develop an altered physiology to compensate for the needs of the developing baby and Section 2B is about those physiological adaptations. In anticipation of those students who enter midwifery by the direct route, each system is first described in the non-pregnant state, then the adaptations brought about by pregnancy are discussed and finally their significance to health is discussed. Related systems have been grouped as far as possible. The chapters also provide revision for those qualified nurses who enter the midwifery profession. The haematological system (Ch. 16) and the cardiovascular system (Ch. 17) are integral to the support of the growing fetus. Three other systems involved in gas exchange, acid–base control (pH) and fluid balance are the respiratory system (Ch. 18), the renal system (Ch. 19) and fluid balance (Ch. 20). Chapters 21–23 examine the organs of the digestive tract and nutrition while Chapters 24 and 25 explore the musculoskeletal system. The relationship between the nervous, endocrine and immune systems provides much knowledge about human health. The relatively new science of psychoneuroimmunology is gaining ground. However, to foster understanding, each system is given its own space in Chapters 26–29.

Chapter 16

The haematological system – physiology of the blood

CHAPTER CONTENTS

BLOOD AS A TISSUE

In small-cell organisms, diffusion of substances is sufficient to maintain the metabolic needs of the cell. However, multicellular organisms need more advanced mechanisms other than diffusion to enable the transport of substances. During evolution of multicellular organisms this has been achieved through the cardiovascular system and the circulation of blood.

Blood is a fluid connective tissue, which communicates between internal cells and the body surface, and between the various specialised tissues and organs. In an adult human, blood will normally comprise 6–8% of body weight: this is 5–6 litres in a man and 4–5 litres in a woman.

If a sample of blood is placed in a test tube and prevented from clotting, the heavier cellular elements settle and the plasma rises to the top. The **haematocrit**, or packed cell volume fraction, essentially represents the percentage of total blood volume occupied by erythrocytes. White cells and platelets form only 1%, settle on top of the red cells and can be seen between the two main layers as a thin cream-coloured layer called the **buffy coat**. The haematocrit averages 45% and the plasma averages 55% of the total volume. Table 16.1 details the specific properties of blood.

FUNCTIONS OF BLOOD

Blood has three general functions.

1. **Transportation:** blood transports oxygen from the lungs to the cells and transports carbon dioxide from the cells

Table 16.1   Specific properties of blood

Property	Value
Specific gravity (relative to water)	1.026
Viscosity (relative to water)	1.5–1.75 (cells contribute equally to viscosity)
pH	7.35–7.45
H^+ concentration	35–45 nmol/L

to the lungs, nutrients from the gastrointestinal tract, hormones from endocrine glands and heat and waste products away from the cells.

2. **Regulation:** blood is involved in the regulation of acid–base balance, body temperature and water content of cells.

3. **Protection:** clotting factors in blood protect against excessive loss from the cardiovascular system. White blood cells protect against disease by producing antibodies and performing phagocytosis. In addition, blood also contains interferons and complement proteins that help protect against disease.

CONSTITUENTS OF BLOOD

Blood has a characteristic constituency of living cells suspended in a plasma matrix. It is a sticky, viscous, dark red, opaque fluid consisting of 55% plasma and 45% cells. More than 99% of the cellular component consists of erythrocytes (red blood cells or RBCs). White cells and platelets are present in small quantities. Blood also contains many chemicals in suspension. If blood is exposed to the air it solidifies into a clot and exudes a clear fluid called serum.

PLASMA

Plasma is the liquid portion of the blood which acts as the transport medium of substances being carried in the blood. Water comprises approximately 90% of the plasma volume, with the remainder containing protein 8%, inorganic ions 0.9% and organic substances 1.1%. The characteristic straw colour of plasma is produced by bilirubin, the waste product of haemoglobin breakdown. Table 16.2 outlines the constituents and function of plasma.

Serum is blood plasma without fibrinogen and other clotting factors. Protein molecules are too large to pass into

the interstitial fluid at the capillary beds; therefore, there is a higher protein content in plasma than in interstitial fluid (i.e. 8% compared with 2%). Most of the protein that does pass into interstitial fluid is taken up by the lymphatic system and returned to the blood. The main plasma proteins are presented in Table 16.3.

The functions of plasma proteins are to:

- Prevent fluid loss from blood to tissues by exerting colloid osmotic (**oncotic**) pressure. This is mainly due to the presence of the protein albumin. If plasma protein levels fall due to either reduced production or loss from the blood vessels then osmotic pressure is also reduced. Fluids will then move into the tissues (oedema) and body cavities. This may occur in diseases of the liver and kidneys, burns, inflammation and allergic disorders.

- Transport bound substances to prevent them from being metabolised until they reach their target tissue: for instance, albumin binds bilirubin. Some substances can displace others and compete for binding sites. An example of this is the displacement of bilirubin from albumin by aspirin or sulphonamides.

- Aid in clotting and fibrinolytic activities.

- Assist in prevention of infection – γ-globulins (also known as immunoglobulins – see Ch. 29, p. 393) function as specific antibodies for specific protein antigens such as microbial agents and pollen.

- Help regulate acid–base balance by acting in buffering systems.

- Act as a protein reserve that forms part of the amino acid pool.

- Contribute about 50% to the total viscosity of blood.

Other proteins found in the blood in small quantities are hormones, enzymes and most of the clotting factors. There is also a series of plasma proteins called **complement** that assist in the inflammatory and immune mechanisms. Albumin is the smallest of the plasma proteins with a molecular mass of 69 000 and is just too large to pass through the capillary walls in normal circumstances. If the glomerular capillaries in the kidney are damaged, albumin can be lost from the blood in large quantities.

Table 16.2   Outline of blood constituents and function

Constituent	Function
Water	Transport medium of nutrients, wastes, gases Heat distributor
Plasma protein – albumin	Transports many substances Large contribution to colloid oncotic pressure
Plasma protein globulins – α and β	Transports substances, involved in clotting
Plasma protein globulins – γ	Antibodies
Plasma protein – fibrinogen	Inactive precursor for fibrin
Electrolytes	Osmotic distribution of fluid between compartments

Table 16.3   Plasma proteins

Name	Origin	% of total
Albumin	Synthesised in the liver	60
Fibrinogen	Synthesised in the liver	4
Globulins (α) and (β)	Synthesised in the liver	36
Globulin (γ)	Synthesised in the immune system	Trace

THE CELLULAR COMPONENTS OF BLOOD

Three major cell types are present in blood, each having a very different function: red cells (**erythrocytes**), white cells (**leucocytes**) and platelets (**thrombocytes**) (Table 16.4).

Under normal circumstances, the proportions of these cells remain constant within narrow limits. However, the body may adjust these levels to maintain health. A simple routine test can measure the cellular content of blood. This is normally carried out on most people at some point in their life, either as part of health screening or to diagnose illness.

Haemopoiesis is the term used for blood cell formation. Embryonic blood cells appear in the bloodstream as early as the 3rd week of development. All blood cell types are descended from a single type of bone marrow cell called a pluripotent stem cell or **haemocytoblast**, which is an undifferentiated cell capable of giving rise to the precursor of any of the blood cell types. These include the red cells and megakaryocytes (leading to platelets). The pluripotent stem cells branch to form myeloid stem cells, which leads to the production of granulocytes and monocytes in the bone marrow. Lymphoid stem cells leave the bone marrow to reside in the lymphoid tissues and produce lymphocytes. Each person has about 1500 g of red bone marrow in the body. Two-thirds of the production is white cells and one-third is red cells (Fig. 16.1).

Red blood cells

The major function of erythrocytes or red blood cells (RBCs) is the carriage of oxygen, picked up in the lungs, to all the cells of the body. Erythrocytes contain large amounts of the protein haemoglobin with which oxygen and, to a lesser extent, carbon dioxide reversibly combine. The shape and size of the red cells are significant for this function. Erythrocyctes are biconcave discs (circular and flattened, thinner in the middle than round the edge) and are 7.5 micrometres (μm) in diameter. This provides a high surface-to-volume ratio well suited to the exchange of gases, and allows the volume of the cell to readily alter with the osmotic shifts of water between cell and plasma. The plasma membrane is strong and conveniently pliant, which allows the cells to become deformed as they squeeze through torturous and narrow capillary vessels whose diameter may be smaller than the RBC.

Erythrocytes are normally measured per cubic mm (mm^3, which is the same as a μl of blood) and average 5 million. This value may also be reported as 5.0×10^{12}/L. Women have a range of $4.3–5.2$/mm^3 and men have a higher range of $5.1–5.8$/mm^3 (Table 16.5). RBCs are the main cellular contributor to blood viscosity. Therefore any increase in this range will also raise the viscosity of blood, which may occur in circumstances such as a slower flow of blood or a move to an area of high altitude. Any subsequent decrease, such as is seen in normal pregnancy, will lower viscosity and blood will flow more rapidly.

Table 16.4   Outline of the cellular constituents of blood

Constituent	Function
Erythrocytes (red cells)	Oxygen and carbon dioxide transport
Leucocytes (white cells)	Defence against micro-organisms
Platelets	Haemostasis

Table 16.5   Red cell laboratory values

Parameter	Value
Red cell count	$5.1–5.8 \times 10^{12}$/L (males) $4.3–5.2 \times 10^{12}$/L (females)
Haemoglobin	13–18 g/dl (males) 12–16 g/dl (females) 14–20 g/dl (infants)
Mean cell haemoglobin concentration (MCHC)	32 g/dl
Mean cell volume (MCV)	85 femtolitres (fl) – 1000 million millionth/litre

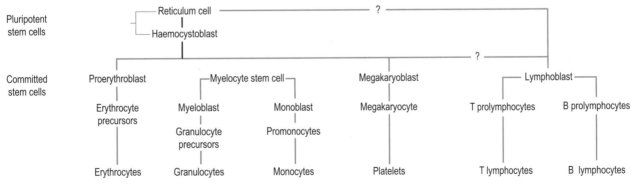

Figure 16.1   Summary of the major stages of haemopoiesis (from Hinchliff S M, Montague S E 1990, with permission).

Erythrocytes are completely dedicated to the transport of oxygen and carbon dioxide. Haemoglobin (Hb) is the oxygen-carrying capacity of the erythrocytes and is measured in grams per 100 ml of blood (g/100 ml). The normal range of values is 14–20 g/dl in infants, 12–16 g/dl in females and 13–18 g/dl in males. Haemoglobin also picks up about 20% of carbon dioxide (CO_2) returning from the tissues to form carbaminohaemoglobin, but most of the CO_2 is in solution in the blood.

Haemoglobin

Haemoglobin is a red-coloured pigment found in red cells. Each red cell contains 30 pg (picograms) of haemoglobin. This is reported as the mean cell haemoglobin or MCH. Another measure reported is the mean cell concentration of haemoglobin (MCHC), which is 32 g/dl. Haemoglobin is made up of the protein **globin** bound to the red **haem** pigment. Globin is rather complex. It consists of four polypeptide chains – two alpha (α) and two beta (β) – each bound to a ring-like haem group (Fig. 16.2). Each haem contains one iron (Fe^{2+}) ion that can combine reversibly with one oxygen molecule to form the bright red **oxyhaemoglobin** (HbO_2). The iron–oxygen interaction is very weak and the two can be easily separated without any damage. Once the oxygen has been released in the tissues, it becomes darker red and is known as **deoxyhaemoglobin**.

Each haemoglobin molecule can carry four molecules of oxygen. These are picked up one at a time and each binding changes the configuration of globin and increases the affinity of the haemoglobin molecule for oxygen. The affinity for the fourth molecule of oxygen is 20 times that of the first affinity. This aspect of oxygen uptake will be examined in greater detail when respiration is considered.

The pigment haem is made up of ring-shaped organic molecules called **pyrrole rings**. Four of these join together to from a larger ring and the nitrogen atom of each pyrrole ring holds a ferrous iron atom centrally. The globin proteins consist of long chains of amino acids. There are four types of globin chain, each with slight differences in amino acids: α (alpha), β (beta), δ (delta) and γ (gamma). They can be varied in pairs to form different types of haemoglobin, three of which are found normally:

HbA	– the major adult haemoglobin	2α	2β
HbA$_2$	– the minor adult haemoglobin	2α	2δ
HbF	– fetal haemoglobin	2α	2γ

At birth HbF makes up two-thirds of haemoglobin content and HbA one-third. From the age of 5 the adult ratio is established, i.e. HbA is greater than 95%, HbA$_2$ is less than 3.5% and HbF is less than 1.5%. Other fetal haemoglobins have substitutions for the β chains which can persist and may be life-saving in thalassaemia. Abnormal β chains are made in sickle cell disorders.

Formation of erythrocytes

Mature red blood cells develop from haemocytoblasts within the erythroid tissue in the bone marrow. After 3–5 days the cells pass into the circulation as cells called **reticulocytes** because they still contain rough endoplasmic reticulum and clumped ribosomes. This disappears when the cell is mature, which normally takes 4 days. Three or four mitotic cell divisions are involved so that each haemocytoblast gives rise to 8 or 16 red cells. There is a gradual build-up of haemoglobin made at the ribosomes which appears in the cell. Other organelles and the nucleus are extruded from the cell. There is a reduction in cell size and a change in cell shape. Reticulocytes normally comprise less than 2% of the red cells in the blood of an adult. The formation of erythrocytes is called **erythropoiesis** and the dietary substances required are summarised in Table 16.6.

The life span of red cells

About 1% of erythrocytes are replaced each day. Production is stimulated by the hormone **erythropoietin**, which originates in the kidney. This is a glycoprotein produced when the kidney cells are hypoxic: for example, during haemorrhage, haemolytic crises, at altitude and following exercise. Erythropoietin can only stimulate committed cells and there will be an increase in reticulocytes in the blood if the need is drastic. Red blood cells live about 120 days and are finally ingested and destroyed by macrophages, mainly in the spleen. As the cells circulate, their plasma membrane

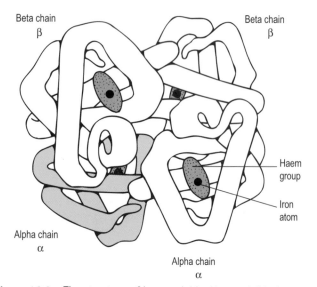

Beta chain
β

Beta chain
β

Haem group

Iron atom

Alpha chain
α

Alpha chain
α

Figure 16.2 The structure of haemoglobin. Haemoglobin is a protein with four subunits (2 α polypeptides and 2 β polypeptides). Each subunit contains a haem group with an iron atom. (From Jones et al, with permission.)

becomes progressively more damaged until it ruptures. Having no nucleus, they have no mechanism of self-repair. They are fragmented to produce protein and haem, which is mostly reclaimed in the body stores for reuse. The remainder of the haem portion is degraded and bilirubin is excreted as bile (Fig. 16.3).

Very defective cells such as those found in sickle-cell disease may be haemolysed in the circulation. The haemoglobin, which has a molecular mass of 68 000 and is small enough to be excreted in the urine, is released into the plasma. Special plasma proteins called **haptoglobins** bind to free haemoglobin to form larger molecules and prevent it from being excreted. If this mechanism becomes saturated, haemoglobin will appear in the urine (**haemoglobinuria**).

Table 16.6 Dietary substances needed for erythropoiesis

Substance	Utilisation
Protein	Synthesis of the globin part of haemoglobin and for cellular proteins
Iron	Contained in the haem portion of haemoglobin
Vitamin B$_{12}$ (hydroxycobalamin)	Needed for DNA synthesis
Folic acid	Needed for DNA synthesis
Vitamic C (ascorbic acid)	Facilitates absorption of iron

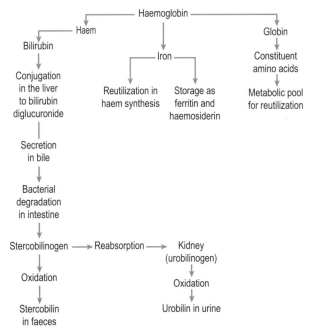

Figure 16.3 A summary of haemoglobin breakdown (from Hinchcliff S M, Montague S E 1990, with permission).

IRON METABOLISM

Absorption

A typical British mixed diet usually contains about 14 mg of iron daily but normally only 1–2 mg (5–10%) is absorbed (Letsky 1998). The composition of the diet determines how much iron is available for absorption. There are two distinct forms for absorption: iron attached to haem and inorganic iron. Iron attached to haem is found in the haemoglobin and myoglobin protein found in animal products. It is absorbed much more efficiently than non-haem iron and is not affected by factors affecting the absorption of non-haem iron. In most foods, iron is present in its ferric form and has to be converted to ferrous iron in order to be absorbed.

Absorption is enhanced if reducing agents that can aid this conversion are available. Hydrochloric acid found in the gastric juice performs this function, as can ascorbic acid (vitamin C). In grain foods iron forms a complex with phytates and only small amounts of soluble iron are available. The iron in eggs is bound to phosphates in the yolk and is poorly absorbed. The amount of iron absorbed depends on the rate of red cell production, the extent of iron stores, the content of the diet and whether or not iron supplements are given. Intestinal absorption of iron is facilitated when there is erythroid hyperplasia, rapid turnover of iron and a high concentration of unsaturated transferrin, as occurs in pregnancy.

Serum iron, transferrin and total iron–binding capacity

Non-pregnant women have a serum iron content of 13–27 μmol/L but this shows immense individual variability and fluctuates hour to hour. The process for the changes is not fully understood (Letsky 1998). A low concentration of serum iron usually indicates iron deficiency anaemia. The **total iron-binding capacity** (TIBC) is 45–72 μmol/L. A low concentration of TIBC is associated with iron deficiency anaemia. **Transferrin** is the protein that specifically binds iron and is usually between 1.2 and 2 g/L. TIBC is usually one-third saturated with iron. Transferrin rises to 4.7 g/L by the second trimester and TIBC increases to 90 μmol/L. This is also seen in women taking oestrogen-containing oral contraceptives. Oestrogen probably causes the change. TIBC returns to normal within 3 weeks of delivery.

Serum ferritin

Ferritin is a glycoprotein with a high molecular mass and is found in cells where it holds two-thirds of the iron store. It is also in small amounts in the plasma in a wide range of 15–300 μg/L. It is stable, not affected by iron ingestion and is a good indicator of iron stores, especially in the lower range as in iron deficiency anaemia in pregnancy.

Marrow iron

Occasionally it is useful to examine bone marrow to assess iron stores. Marrow is taken by aspiration from the iliac crest. A stainable iron/protein complex called **haemosiderin**, which is similar to ferritin, may be seen. No stainable iron will be seen if the serum ferritin has fallen below $40 \mu g/L$. In the absence of iron supplementation, no stainable iron is seen in 80% of women at term. The developing erythrocytes can also be examined for iron deficiency signs. The presence of infection, especially urinary tract infection, can block the incorporation of iron into haemoglobin as the microbes may utilise iron in their own metabolic processes.

FOLATE METABOLISM

Folate is a vitamin found widely distributed in nature. It is found in leafy green vegetables such as spinach and in mushrooms and oranges. Liver is a good source. Folic acid is destroyed by prolonged boiling or by the addition of bicarbonate of soda to the cooking water. Some drugs act as folic acid antagonists and prevent its absorption. A typical Western diet contains $500–800 \mu g$ daily and normal daily needs are $100–200 \mu g$. This excess intake partly compensates for the loss in cooking.

Folates are absorbed in the duodenum and jejunum and then stored in the liver. Deficiency is more likely to be seen in the winter months when the foods containing folic acid may be difficult to obtain. It is more common in certain socially and economically deprived groups. It was identified and synthesised in the 1940s. The metabolism of folic acid is the basis for cellular use of folate and it is essential for cell growth and division (Letsky 1998). Tissue that is active in reproduction and growth is more dependent on the efficient turnover and supply of folate coenzymes and during pregnancy folate metabolism is increased.

BLOOD GROUPS

Red blood cells, like all cells, have **glycoproteins** in their plasma membranes which are genetically coded for and therefore inherited. These can act as **antigens** (see Ch. 29), provoking an immune reaction if incompatible blood enters the circulation. The red cells are agglutinated and destroyed. There are over 400 different antigens found on the surface of red cells. Some of these antigens cause a more vigorous reaction than others and the two most commonly problematic are those of the ABO system and the rhesus (Rh) system.

The ABO system

The ABO blood groups are based on the presence of two red cell antigens (known as **agglutinogens**) called type A and type B. These types are co-dominant (i.e. neither gene masks the presence of the other so that both proteins are expressed). A person inheriting both antigens will have blood group AB. If neither antigen is inherited, then blood group O arises. Therefore four blood groups are possible depending on the surface antigens present on the red cells: i.e. A, B, AB and O.

A unique factor associated with the ABO system is the presence of preformed antibodies (known as **agglutinins**) in the plasma within 2 months of birth with no previous sensitisation event. A baby cannot have antibodies against any antigen carried on its own red cells or the cells would be destroyed. Therefore a baby who has neither the A nor B antigen on its red cells will have both anti-A and anti-B antibodies in the serum while a baby with the blood group AB will have neither antibody present in the serum. Those with blood group A will have anti-B antibodies and those with blood group B will have anti-A antibodies.

The rhesus system (Rh)

There are eight types of Rh antigens but only three are common. These are called the C, D and E agglutinogens. A gene codes for each type and there are two alleles to each gene, giving CDE/cde as the full range of alleles. Rhesus D is by far the most clinically important antigen. The word rhesus is used because agglutinogen D was originally identified in rhesus monkeys.

About 85% of people in the Western world are rhesus positive (Rh+), which means they have the Rh agglutinogen on their red cells, and 15% are rhesus negative (Rh−) and do not have the agglutinogen on their red cells. In Japan 99.7% of people are Rh+ and only 0.3% are Rh−. Unlike the ABO system, there are no spontaneously occurring anti-Rh antibodies and these are only formed if there is a sensitisation event with the presence of Rh+ red blood cells in the circulation of an Rh− person. There is a problem associated with the rhesus factor in pregnancy, discussed in Chapter 14.

WHITE CELLS

These cells are the **leucocytes** and can be referred to as WBCs. Taking all the types together, the average number of WBCs in the circulation is 4000–11 000 per cubic mm which can also be reported as $4–11 \times 10^9/L$. They account for only 1% of the blood's cellular content. An increase in WBCs is called **leucocytosis** and a decrease is **leucopenia**. Those white cells present in the blood represent only a small part of the body's total white cell content as the majority of the cells are in the tissues.

The reason for the wide variation in the normal count is that cells enter and leave the circulation constantly in response to physiological factors such as exercise. The newborn baby has approximately double the white cell count of an adult, which decreases to reach adult levels by about 5–10 years of age. These cells are part of the immune defence system (see Ch. 29) and are protective against bacteria, viruses, parasites, toxins and tumour cells. Some white cells undergo **diapedesis**, which means that the cells can slip out of capillaries with an amoebic action in response to positive **chemotaxis** (chemical call).

Types of white cell

Granulocytes (polymorphonuclear leucocytes) contain granules which have a lobed nucleus and substances that can fight infection in their cytoplasm. They are 10–14 micrometres (μm) in diameter. Granulocytes can be further divided into three groups, categorised by the size of their granules and the way they take up Wright's stain. All these granulocytes are phagocytic.

Neutrophils contain granules of varying sizes that stain violet because they take up both acidic red dyes and basic blue dyes. Neutrophils have the most lobular nuclei and are the most common types of granulocytes, accounting for more than 50% of all white cells. Neutrophils are chemically attracted to sites of inflammation and will ingest and destroy bacteria and some fungi.

Eosinophils have large granules which are stained red by acidic dyes. The nucleus usually has two lobes. Eosinophils make up about 1–4% of the white cell population. The most important role of this type of cell is to attack parasitic worms such as tapeworms and round worms. When such a worm enters the body the eosinophils surround it and release enzymes from their granules onto the parasite's surface to digest it from the outside. Eosinophils are also involved in dealing with allergy attacks by destroying antigen/antibody complexes.

Basophils have large granules that take up a basic dye and stain blue-black. The nucleus usually has two or three lobes. These are the rarest of the white cells, accounting for only 0.5% of the population. Their large granules contain histamine, which is an inflammatory substance that acts as a vasodilator and draws other white blood cells to the site of inflammation. Cells similar to basophils that are present in connective tissue are called **mast cells**. Both type of cells release histamine when they bind to immunoglobulin E (IgE). The immune system is discussed in full in Chapter 29, p. 387.

The production of granulocytes

Granulocytes arise from myeloid precursor cells in the red bone marrow, a process that takes about 14 days. This time can be reduced considerably if cells are urgently required, such as when infection is present. There is also a pool of granulocyte cells in the bone marrow where there can be 50 cells for every granulocyte in the circulation. During **granulopoiesis**, there is progressive condensation and lobulation of the nucleus. Granules develop in the cell cytoplasm and there is loss of organelles such as mitochondria.

Within 7 h of reaching the circulation, half of the granulocytes will have left to meet tissue needs and will not return to the blood. The normal survival of these cells in the tissues is about 4–5 days. Dead cells are eliminated from the body in faeces and respiratory secretions. Dead neutrophils form the pus at infection sites.

Agranulocytes

These include lymphocytes and monocytes and do not contain visible cytoplasmic granules.

Lymphocytes

Lymphocytes are produced in the bone marrow and immature cells migrate to the thymus and other lymphoid tissue to divide again and mature. These are round cells with large round nuclei and are the second most common type of leucocyte. Even though a large numbers of lymphocytes exist in the body, only a small number are found in the circulation. The majority of lymphocytes are often present in lymphoid tissue and are involved in immune reactions.

Monocytes

Monocytes are large cells that are produced in the bone marrow. Mature cells spend about 30 h in the blood and then migrate to the tissues where they develop into macrophages. Macrophages are also phagocytic although they respond more slowly than the neutrophils. They are also greatly involved in regulating the immune response by activating B and T lymphocytes (see Ch. 29, p. 394).

PLATELETS

Platelets are small non-nuclear cellular elements produced in the bone marrow. They are colourless discoid bodies and have a diameter of only 2–4 μm. There are about $150–400 \times 10^9$/L.

Production of platelets (**thrombopoiesis**) occurs in the bone marrow. They are formed inside the cytoplasm of large cells called megakaryocytes and bud off from the cell surface. Each megakaryocyte takes about 10 days to mature and produces about 4000 platelets (Fig. 16.4). At any time two-thirds of the body's platelets are in the circulation and one-third in the spleen. The life span of a platelet is 7–10 days and they are destroyed by macrophages, mainly in the spleen but also in the liver.

Platelets are complex and have many functions other than being involved in the clotting process of blood. They are able to phagocytose small particles such as viruses and immune complexes. They store and transport **histamine** and **serotonin** which are released when platelets are damaged. This affects the tone of smooth muscle in blood vessel walls. Platelets probably supply the endothelial cells of the blood vessels with nutrition and these cells atrophy in platelet deficiency. They secrete **platelet-derived growth**

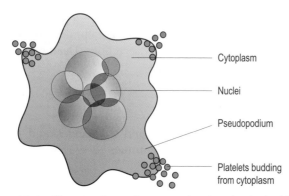

Figure 16.4 Diagram of megakaryocyte showing platelet budding (from Hinchliff S M, Montague S E 1990, with permission).

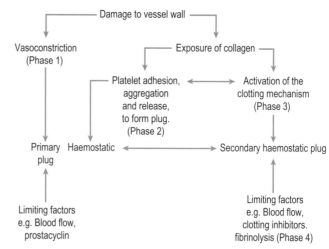

Figure 16.5 An outline of the events of haemostasis (from Hinchliff S M, Montague S E 1990, with permission).

factor (PDGF) which stimulates proliferation of smooth muscle walls to help healing after injury.

HAEMOSTASIS

If the endothelium of blood vessels is smooth and uninterrupted, blood flow is maintained. However, if a blood vessel is damaged a series of reactions occurs in order to maintain haemostasis and minimise blood loss. The mechanism is fast, localised and carefully controlled. Many blood coagulation factors normally present in plasma are involved. Some substances involved in the blood clotting process are released from platelets and injured tissues. Haemostasis involves three phases: vascular spasm, platelet plug formation and coagulation of blood (Fig. 16.5).

Vascular spasm

Vasoconstriction after injury is brought about by direct injury to vascular smooth muscle; compression of the vessel by extravasated blood; chemicals released by endothelial cells; and platelets and reflexes triggered by pain receptors. A strongly constricted artery can significantly reduce blood loss for up to 30 min. This allows time for platelet plug formation and blood clotting to occur. A blunt injury crushes tissue and is more efficient at causing vascular spasm than a sharp cut.

Formation of a platelet plug

Normally platelets do not stick to each other or to the endothelial lining of blood vessels. Damage or disruption of the endothelium exposes underlying collagen fibres. This causes platelets to swell, form spiky processes and stick to the exposed area. Once the platelets have adhered to the endothelium, lipids in the platelet plasma membrane release a short-lived prostaglandin derivative called thromboxane A_2. Degranulation of platelets occurs and other chemicals are released. These are serotonin, which enhances vascular spasm, and adenosine diphosphate, which attracts

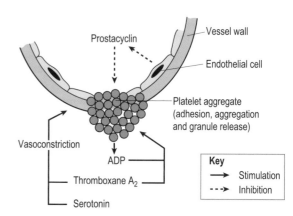

Figure 16.6 Summary of events in the formation of a platelet plug (from Hinchliff S M, Montague S E 1990, with permission).

more platelets. Within 1 min a platelet plug forms (Fig. 16.6). Prostacyclin (PG_{I2}) limits the process by confining platelet aggregation to the immediate area of damage.

Coagulation

There are three critical events in coagulation of blood:

1. Prothrombin activator is formed.
2. This converts the plasma protein prothrombin to thrombin.
3. Thrombin causes fibrinogen molecules to form a fibrin mesh. This traps blood cells and seals the hole in the blood vessel.

Over 30 different substances affect the process. There are factors that enhance clot formation, called **procoagulants** (see Table 16.7), and those that inhibit clot formation, called **anticoagulants**. Most of the clotting factors or procoagulants are plasma proteins synthesised in the liver – except factors III and IV. Many need the presence of vitamin K – factors II, VII, IX and X. The factors are released into the

Table 16.7   Procoagulant factors

Number	Name	Function
I	Fibrinogen	Converted to fibrin mesh
II	Prothrombin	Converted to thrombin which converts fibrinogen to fibrin
III	Thromboplastin	Catalyses thrombin formation
IV	Calcium ions	Needed at all stages
V	Platelet accelerator	Affects both intrinsic and extrinsic methods
VI	No substance	
VII	Serum prothrombin conversion accelerator (SPCA)	Entrinsic pathway conversion
VIII	Antihaemophilic factor	Intrinsic mechanism Absence = haemophilia A
IX	Plasma thromboplastin component (PTC, Christmas factor)	Intrinsic mechanism Absence = haemophilia B
X	Stuart-Power factor	Both extrinsic and intrinsic pathways
XI	Plasma thromboplastin antecedent (PTA)	Intrinsic mechanism Absence = haemophilia C
XII	Hageman factor	Intrinsic mechanism
XIII	Fibrin stabilizing factor (FSF)	Cross links fibrin to make it insoluble

blood where they remain inert until the clotting cascade is triggered.

Clotting may be initiated by either of two pathways. These are the intrinsic and extrinsic pathways, and in the body both pathways are usually triggered by the same tissue-damaging events. The intrinsic pathway only initiates clotting of blood outside the body, whereas the extrinsic pathway initiates clotting of blood that has escaped into the tissues. Clot formation is normally complete within 3–6 min. The extrinsic pathway involves fewer steps and is more rapid than the intrinsic pathway. In severe trauma the extrinsic mechanism can clot blood within 15 s.

Clot retraction and fibrinolysis

After 30–60 min a platelet-induced process called **clot retraction** occurs. A contractile protein, **actomyosin**, works in the same way as it does in muscle cells. Serum is squeezed out, the clot is compacted and the torn edges of the blood vessel are drawn together. This is the beginning of healing. PGDF released by degranulation of the platelets stimulates smooth muscle and fibroblasts to divide and rebuild the muscle wall.

Unnecessary clots are removed by fibrinolysis. If this did not occur the blood vessels would become occluded. Yet another of the plasma proteins, **plasminogen**, is activated to produce plasmin which is a protein-digesting enzyme.

Large amounts of plasminogen may be incorporated into a big clot but remain inactive, producing plasmin only as necessary. Plasminogen activators are released from endothelial cells when clot is present. Factor VII and thrombin are also potent plasminogen activators.

Factors limiting clot growth or formation

- Rapid removal of coagulation factors.
- Inhibitors of activated clotting factors.

Any tendency to clot in rapidly moving blood is usually unsuccessful because any activated clotting factors are diluted and washed away. **Heparin** is a natural anticoagulant normally contained in the granules of the leucocytes – mast cells and basophils. Endothelial cells also produce heparin. Small amounts released into the plasma normally prevent inappropriate blood coagulation.

MATERNAL PHYSIOLOGICAL ADAPTATIONS TO PREGNANCY

Blood volume and composition

Total blood volume is a combination of plasma volume and red cell volume. The average increase in total blood volume during pregnancy is between 30 and 50% with an increase above 50% in multiple pregnancies. Plasma volume and total red cell mass are under separate control and bear no fixed relation to one another (Letsky 1998). The increase in blood volume relates to an increase in cardiac output and is noted as early as the 6th week of pregnancy. Most increase takes place before 32–34 weeks and thereafter there is relatively little change. The increase in blood volume may be due to a hormonal mechanism. Plasma volume increases by about 50% while red cell mass increases by 18% (Letsky 1998). This difference results in hypervolaemia, haemodilution and a fall in Hb level often referred to as **physiological anaemia** (Figs 16.7 and 16.8).

Plasma volume

The aetiology of plasma expansion is poorly understood. The increase in plasma volume is directly related to the birth weight of the baby. Women with multiple pregnancy have an increase greater than women with a singleton pregnancy and the amount increases with the number of fetuses in the uterus. Multigravid women have a further increase of plasma volume, which is mirrored by the greater weight of their babies (Letsky 1998).

The benefits of the hypervolaemia are to fulfil the extra demands on the circulation in pregnancy. For instance, the basal metabolic rate increases by 20% in pregnancy with the production of more heat. Blood flow to the skin is increased

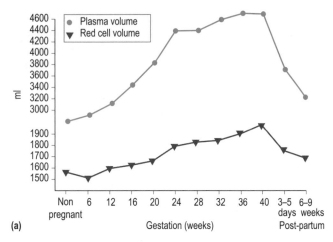

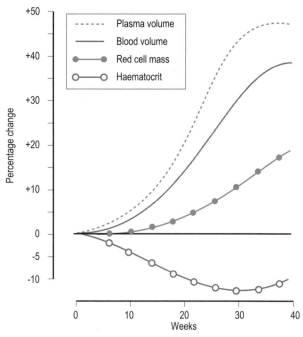

Figure 16.7a   Mean total plasma and red cell volume during normal pregnancy. (Reproduced with permission from Lund & Donovan 1967.)

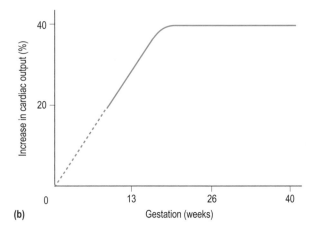

Figure 16.7b   Changes in cardiac output throughout pregnancy. (Reproduced with permission from Hytten & Chamberlain 1991.)

Figure 16.8   Changes in plasma volume, blood volume, red cell mass and haematocrit during normal pregnancy levels. (Reproduced with permission from Rosso 1990.)

and this allows heat to be lost. The increased blood volume also helps to maintain blood pressure when blood may be sequestered in the lower part of the body in the third trimester. This helps to safeguard the woman against haemorrhage at delivery. The decrease in viscosity with increase in cardiac force leads to a decreased resistance to blood flow, which is essential for placental perfusion.

Red cells

In previous research the increase in red cell content of the blood in a normal pregnancy has been difficult to ascertain because many of the women had been given iron supplements. It is estimated that the increase is about 18% in women not supplemented with iron and 30% for those given iron medication (Letsky 1998). The red cell mass should increase as oxygen needs of the body increase. Therefore an increase in red cell mass of 18% should be adequate to meet the 15% increase in oxygen requirements in pregnancy. The nature of

the increase in red cell production is not fully understood but there is a three-fold increase in erythropoietin in plasma in the second trimester. This increase is thought to be related to progesterone, prolactin and human placental lactogen (hPL), rather than by hypoxaemia (Blackburn 2003). There is also a slight rise in the production of HbF, which reaches a peak at 20 weeks and returns to normal 8 weeks after delivery (Letsky 1998).

Changes in red cell values in pregnancy

- The red cell count increase is less than the plasma increase, resulting in a reduction in red cell count from the normal $4.2–4.5 \times 10^{12}$/L in early pregnancy to $3.6–3.8 \times 10^{12}$/L by term.

- The haemoglobin level falls about 2 g/dl from a normal level of 13 g/dl to about 11 g/dl. The haematocrit falls in parallel with the fall in red cell count.

- Mean cell haemoglobin concentration (MCHC) – the average concentration of haemoglobin in each red cell – changes little in a normal pregnancy. There is a slight progressive fall in some women who are not given iron therapy.

- Mean cell volume (MCV) – is a more sensitive haematological measure of iron status in pregnancy. In normal pregnancy with sufficient iron present there is an increase in red cell size. In pregnancy complicated by iron deficiency an early sign is a reduction of cell size.

Table 16.8   The distribution of the extra iron in pregnancy

Tissue usage	Requirements (mg)
Expansion of the red cell mass	570
Fetus	270–370
Placenta	35–100
Blood loss at delivery	100–250
Breastfeeding (6 months)	100–180
Loss from skin, faeces, urine	270

Iron requirements during pregnancy

In order to meet the expansion in red cell mass and the needs of the fetus and placenta, extra iron is needed in pregnancy. The total requirements are calculated as between 700 and 1400 mg throughout pregnancy. Table 16.8 presents an overview of the distribution of iron requirements in pregnancy. Overall, the requirement is for 4 mg/day but this rises from 2.8 mg/day in the non-pregnant woman to 6.6 mg/day in the last few weeks of pregnancy. The needs can be met only by mobilising iron stores in addition to achieving maximum absorption from dietary iron (Letsky 1998).

Set against this need is the iron saved during pregnancy and breastfeeding because of amenorrhoea, which is 250–480 mg in total. Box 16.1 provides an overview of the issues surrounding iron supplementation in pregnancy.

Folate metabolism in pregnancy

Folates together with iron have a central role in the nutrition of pregnancy. Requirements for folates are increased in pregnancy to meet the needs of the growing fetus and placenta, and for the increased maternal tissues of the growing uterus and red cell mass. The placenta transports folates actively to the fetus even if maternal folate status is deficient. Maternal folate metabolism is altered early in pregnancy before fetal demands act directly.

White cells

The total white cell count rises in pregnancy, mainly due to an increase in neutrophils (Blackburn 2003). The neutrophil count rises in the menstrual cycle at the time of the oestrogen peak and continues to rise if fertilisation of the ovum occurs. A peak is reached at 30 weeks and then a plateau is maintained until delivery. There is a further rise in labour and the count returns to normal by the 6th postnatal day. Circulating oestrogen is probably the cause of the extra neutrophil production.

There is a slight rise in eosinophils in ratio to the increased white cell count. A sharp fall in circulating eosinophils occurs during labour. These are absent at delivery and return to normal by the 3rd postnatal day. The basophil and monocyte counts appear to remain unchanged.

Although the lymphocyte count remains unchanged in pregnancy with no change in circulating T cells and B cells, there is profound depression of cell-mediated immunity. This picture is also seen in women taking oral contraceptives containing oestrogen. Oestrogen may increase the number of glycoproteins on the cell surface, leading to impaired response to stimuli. Human chorionic gonadotrophin from the placenta and prolactin from the anterior pituitary are known to suppress lymphocyte function. There is no apparent impairment to the production of immunoglobulins or to humoral-mediated immunity. The depression of cell-mediated immunity is essential to the survival of the fetus but may increase susceptibility to viral infections such as rubella, influenza, poliomyelitis and influenza. Worldwide, the increased susceptibility in immune women to malaria leads to an infected placenta with increased fetal mortality.

Haemostasis in pregnancy

The major changes occur in the haemostatic components of blood and some of these are unique to pregnancy. Adaptations lead to a hypercoagulable state during pregnancy. Adequate haemostasis depends on a complex interaction between blood vessel wall, platelets, coagulation factors and fibrinolysis. Haemostasis in health has three main functions – to keep the circulating blood inside the vascular tree, to maintain the fluidity of blood and to arrest bleeding following injury to vessels (Letsky 1998).

The following changes are seen in pregnancy:

- Platelet count decreases slightly in relation to the haemodilution. No change in function has been reported.

- There are increased levels of coagulation factors VII, VIII and X and a marked increase in plasma fibrinogen from as early as the 3rd month of gestation. Plasma fibrinogen levels may double in late pregnancy and labour due to increased synthesis. Factor VII may increase 10-fold (also seen in women taking oestrogen/progesterone contraceptives) and the activity of factor VIII doubles (Letsky 1998).

- These changes are consistent with a continuous low-grade coagulation activity with fibrin deposition in the intervillous space of the placenta and in the walls of the spiral arteries supplying the placenta (Blackburn 2003). As pregnancy progresses, a fibrin matrix replaces the smooth muscle and elastic lamina of the spiral arteries. This allows expansion of the lumen to accommodate an increase in blood volume and decrease the pressure of arterial blood flowing to the placenta. This hypercoagulability is advantageous following placental separation to help in control of blood loss and to prevent haemorrhage. Following delivery, a fibrin mesh very rapidly covers the placental site. The fibrinogen used represents up to 10% of the total circulating fibrinogen.

- Fibrinolytic activity decreases during pregnancy, remains low in labour and delivery and returns to normal as

Box 16.1 Iron supplementation in pregnancy

Iron supplementation in pregnancy is a controversial issue. Those who favour supplementation recommend prophylactic iron supplements to all women from as early as 16 weeks of pregnancy onwards while others prefer supplementation only if there is an established iron deficit.

In evolutionary terms, women are adapted to the needs for iron in pregnancy but humans have changed their diet since the beginning of the agricultural revolution about 10 000 years ago. Previously people ate a high-protein diet based on fishing and hunting but changed to a mixed diet with grains and a much lower intake of fish and meat. Women at high risk of iron deficiency due to dietary factors are adolescents consuming a low-calorie diet, vegetarians and vegans (Hercberg et al 2001). In modern times, Western women now have fewer pregnancies that are often spaced out over time. This should prevent the continuous depletion of iron from the stores made by repeated pregnancies.

Iron requirements in pregnancy are significantly higher than in the non-pregnant state (Bothwell 2001). Although iron requirements are reduced in the first trimester due to the absence of menstruation, they rise steadily thereafter. The amount of iron that can be absorbed from an optimal diet is less than the demands of pregnancy. Letsky (1998) has no doubt that many women already enter pregnancy with insufficient iron stores to supply the increased maternal and fetal needs. In developing countries this may be due to dietary deficiency but also to chronic infection such as malaria. Iron supplementation during pregnancy will improve health status in these populations and may even be life-saving. She suggests that many authors do not accept that the physiological needs for iron in pregnancy are much higher than the dietary intake even of women with a good diet.

The current and most reliable approach to diagnosis and screening for iron deficiency anaemia during pregnancy remains serum ferritin levels. Recent findings suggest that **erythrocyte zinc protophyrin measurements** may be a more helpful test than either serum ferritin levels or haemoglobin measurements to determine which women have iron deficient erythropoiesis and may benefit from iron therapy (Harthoorn-Lasthuizen et al 2000). These findings warrant further investigation to determine the most accurate and reliable diagnosis or predictor for women at risk. Prevention and treatment of iron deficiency anaemia is essential. Women are more at risk in the third trimester when the fetus obtains iron from maternal stores by active transport across the placenta. Resulting iron

deficiency may have an adverse effect on exercise tolerance, cerebral function and fetal and neonatal development. Letsky (1998) strongly recommends that it would be safer, more practical and less expensive to give all women iron supplements from early pregnancy because of the potential health risks and treatment.

Numerous reviews of the literature have been carried out on this important issue. Enkin et al (2000) conclude that most pregnant women in developing countries show haematological changes indicating iron and folate deficiency. It remains common practice for pregnant women to routinely receive iron and folate supplementation and iron supplementation is essential when there is evidence of genuine iron deficiency (Allen 2002, Milman et al 1999). Data available provide evidence that iron supplementation restores normal (for non-pregnant women) values (Sloan et al 2002) and also appears to prevent low haemoglobin at birth or at 6 weeks postpartum (Mahomed 1999). The number of available trials is limited and there is inconclusive evidence on treatment of iron deficiency (Cuervo & Mahomed 2001). Controlled trials of iron supplementation have consistently demonstrated positive effects on maternal iron status at delivery but have not demonstrated reductions in factors associated with maternal anaemia such as increased risk of preterm delivery and infant low birth weight (Scholl & Reilly 2000).

The therapeutic approach to iron supplementation suffers from real or perceived problems of compliance (Beard 2000). Oral iron preparations themselves may cause gastrointestinal upsets such as nausea, constipation and diarrhoea and women may not comply with therapy. The interaction between iron intake and zinc absorption remains unclear. Oral preparations may reduce the bioavailability of zinc, important in pregnancy, and fetal growth may be adversely affected.

Ideally, women should have good iron stores before conception. Prevention and control of iron deficiency anaemia should involve good dietary advice, preferably before or early in pregnancy (Hercberg et al 2001). Dietary advice should also include the role of vitamin C in enhancing iron absorption and of the tannins in coffee and tea in inhibiting its absorption.

There is still a considerable amount of information to be explored about the benefits of maternal iron supplementation on the health and iron status of the mother and her child during pregnancy and postpartum. The current situation remains controversial. Women diagnosed with iron deficiency will require iron therapy during pregnancy and prophylactic iron supplements may be considered on a general or selective basis.

early as 1 h of placental delivery (Blackburn 2003). These changes help to combat the hazards of haemorrhage at delivery. However, the fact that they occur early in pregnancy and are accompanied by venous stasis predisposes women to thromboembolic episodes.

Intrapartum and immediate postpartum periods

Blood volume lost at delivery is possibly 500 ml for a single-ton pregnancy and up to a 1000 ml for a multiple pregnancy or following a caesarean section. The normal response to blood loss in non-pregnant women is a drop in blood volume compensated for by vasoconstriction. Over the next few days, the blood volume expands back to near normal values because of increased plasma volume. As a result, there is a fall in the haematocrit proportional to the blood loss. In the normal healthy pregnant woman the response to blood loss is modified because of the hypervolaemia of pregnancy.

After the acute blood loss at delivery there is no compensatory increase in blood volume, which remains relatively stable. There is a gradual fall in plasma volume primarily due to diuresis. The red cell mass increase during pregnancy gradually reduces to normal values as red cells come to the end of their life span. The haematocrit gradually increases and blood volume returns to non-pregnant levels (Letsky 1998).

MAIN POINTS

- Blood is a fluid connective tissue communicating with all body cells through the pumping action of the heart. It carries oxygen and nutrients to the cells and carbon dioxide and metabolic waste from the cells. Blood will normally comprise 6–8% of body weight which is about 5–6 litres in a man and 4–5 litres in a woman.

- The functions of blood are internal transport of substances for respiration, nutrition and excretion; maintenance of water, electrolyte and acid–base balance; metabolic regulation; protection against infection; protection from haemorrhage; and maintenance of body temperature.

- Blood consists of two components: 55% plasma and 45% cells. The plasma component consists of water, plasma proteins and electrolytes. The cellular component comprises 99% erythrocytes (red blood cells) and small quantities of leucocytes and platelets.

- Plasma proteins prevent fluid loss, transport substances around the body, are involved in clotting and fibrinolytic activities, assist in prevention of infection, help regulate acid–base balance, act as a protein reserve and contribute half of total blood viscosity. Serum is the fluid remaining if clotting factors are removed.

- Haemopoiesis is the term for blood cell formation. A pluripotent stem cell in the red bone marrow gives rise to progenitor cells for the three main types of cell, i.e. red cells, white cells and platelets. Each cell type performs a different function. Erythrocytes are involved in transport of gases to and from cells, leucocytes are involved in the defence of micro-organisms and platelets are involved in haemostasis.

- Red blood cells live about 120 days. They are finally fragmented and destroyed by macrophages in the spleen. Protein and haem are produced and enter the body stores while bilirubin is excreted in bile.

- White cells account for 1% of the blood's cellular content. Those in blood represent only a small part of the body's total white cell count as the majority of cells are in the tissues.

- Platelets are produced in the bone marrow inside the cytoplasm of megakaryocytes. In the clotting process they form a platelet plug. Platelets phagocytose small particles such as viruses and immune complexes, store and transport histamine and serotonin, supply the endothelial cells of the blood vessels with nutrition and secrete PDGF, which stimulates proliferation of smooth muscle cells to help healing.

- Blood flow depends on a smooth endothelial surface lining blood vessels. If a vessel is damaged a series of reactions occurs in order to maintain haemostasis and minimise blood loss. Haemostasis involves vascular spasm, platelet plug formation and blood coagulation.

- The ABO blood groups are based on the presence of two red cell antigens, type A and type B. The O blood group arises if neither antigen is inherited; if both are inherited, group AB results.

- Only three rhesus antigens are common, i.e. C, D and E agglutinogens. Rhesus D is by far the most clinically important antigen. About 85% of people in the Western world are Rh+ and 15% are Rh−. There are no spontaneously occurring anti-Rh antibodies. These are formed if there is a sensitisation event.

- Total blood volume is a combination of plasma volume and red cell volume. The increase in blood volume in pregnancy relates to an increase in cardiac output. In pregnancy red cell mass or total volume of red cells increases by 18% while plasma volume increases by about 50%. This difference results in hypervolaemia, haemodilution and a fall in Hb level, often referred to as physiological anaemia.

- The increase in plasma volume is related to the birth weight of the baby. Women with multiple pregnancy have greater increase in plasma volume than women with a singleton pregnancy. The decrease in viscosity with increase in cardiac force leads to a decreased resistance to blood flow, essential for placental perfusion.

- Extra iron is needed in pregnancy to meet the expansion in red cell mass and the needs of the fetus and placenta. There is no agreement on whether women need iron supplements if well nourished. Women in developing countries may enter pregnancy with their iron stores already depleted and iron supplementation can be life-saving.

- Requirements for folic acid are increased during pregnancy to meet the needs of the growing fetus and placenta, and the increased maternal tissues of the growing uterus and red cell mass.

- The total white cell count rises in pregnancy, mainly due to an increase in neutrophils. The lymphocyte count remains unchanged with no change in circulating T cells and B cells. There is depression of cell-mediated immunity, which may be essential to the survival of the fetus but may increase susceptibility to viral infections.

- Major changes occur in the haemostatic components of blood during pregnancy, leading to a hypercoagulable state. Fibrinolytic activity is decreased during pregnancy, remains low in labour and delivery and returns to normal within 1 h of delivery. These changes help to combat haemorrhage at delivery but are accompanied by venous stasis and predispose women to thromboembolic episodes.

- Blood volume lost at delivery is possibly 500 ml for a singleton pregnancy and up to a 1000 ml for a multiple pregnancy. After the acute blood loss at delivery, the blood volume does not increase as usual in haemorrhage. There is a gradual fall in plasma volume primarily due to diuresis. The red cell mass gradually reduces to non-pregnant levels as red cells come to the end of their life span.

References

Allen L H 2002 Anemia and iron deficiency: effects on pregnancy outcome. American Journal of Clinical Nutrition 71(5):1280S–1284S.

Beard J L 2000 Effectiveness and strategies of iron supplementation during pregnancy. American Journal of Clinical Nutrition 71(5):1288S–1294S.

Blackburn S T 2003 Maternal, Fetal and Neonatal Physiology. A Clinical Perspective, 3rd edn. W B Saunders, Philadelphia.

Bothwell T H 2000 Iron requirements in pregnancy and strategies to meet them. American Journal of Clinical Nutrition 72(1):257S–264S.

Cuervo L G, Mahomed K 2001 Treatments for iron deficiency anaemia in pregnancy. Cochrane Database Systematic Reviews (2), CD003094.

Enkin M, Keirse M J N C, Neilson J 2000 A Guide to Effective Care in Pregnancy, 3rd edn. Oxford University Press, Oxford, pp 39–46.

Harthoorn-Lasthuizen E J, Lindemans J, Langenhuijsen M M 2000 Erythrocyte zinc protoporphyrin testing in pregnancy. Acta Obstetrics and Gynecology Scandinavia 79(8):660–666.

Hercberg S, Preziosi P, Galan P 2001 Iron deficiency in Europe public health. Nutrition 4(2B):537–545.

Letsky E A 1998 The haematological system. In Chamberlain G, Broughton-Pipkin F (eds) Clinical Physiology in Obstetrics, 3rd edn. Blackwell Scientific, Oxford, pp 71–110.

Milman N, Bergholt T, Byg K E, Erikson L, Graudal N 1999 Iron status and iron balance during pregnancy. A critical reappraisal of iron supplementation. Acta Obstetrics and Gynecology Scandinavia 78(9):749–757.

Mahomed K 1999 Iron supplementation in pregnancy. Cochrane Database Systematic Reviews (2), CD000117.

Scholl T O, Reilly T 2000 Anemia, iron and pregnancy outcome. Journal of Nutrition 130(2S):443S–447S.

Sloan N L, Jordan E, Winikoff B 2002 Effects of iron supplementation on maternal haematological status in pregnancy. American Journal of Public Health 92(2):288–293.

Annotated recommended reading

Chamberlain G, Broughton Pipkin F (eds) 1998 Clinical Physiology in Obstetrics, 3rd edn. Blackwell Scientific, Oxford.
This text provides a detailed description of the major changes that occur in the body systems during pregnancy. There is an extensive review of the literature, extending from classical research studies to the more recent research findings.

Sherwood L 2001 Human Physiology: From Cells to Systems, 4th edn. Blackwell Science, Oxford.
This textbook presents a detailed overview of human anatomy and physiology, well illustrated with diagrams and pictures. It is relevant for undergraduates in a health-related profession.

Mahomed K 1999 Iron supplementation in pregnancy. Cochrane Review: In The Cochrane Library, Issue 2. Update Software 2003, Oxford.
This is a systematic review of many controlled trials dealing with related outcomes of iron levels in pregnancy. It highlights the controversy arising from the selective or compulsory use of iron supplementation in pregnancy.

Chapter 17

The cardiovascular system

INTRODUCTION

The cardiovascular system, consisting of the heart and blood vessels, is designed to meet the crucial homeostatic needs of the cells and tissues by maintaining an adequate blood supply during varying physiological circumstances. For instance, blood can be preferentially directed to individual systems as required. Flow increases to the muscles during exercise and to the gastrointestinal system following food intake. Centres in the brain control the system as a whole, although local events and reflexes may modify the end result. There are three main roles for the cardiovascular system:

1. delivery of nutrients and oxygen;
2. removal of metabolic waste and carbon dioxide;
3. dissipation of heat from active tissues and redistribution of heat around the body.

CIRCULATORY PATHWAYS

Blood flows through a network of blood vessels that extend between the heart and peripheral tissues. The circulation of blood can be subdivided into two distinct circuits, that both begin and end in the heart. The **pulmonary circulation** takes deoxygenated blood from the right side of the heart to the lungs and returns oxygenated blood from the lungs to the left side of the heart. The **systemic circulation** takes oxygenated blood from the left side of the heart to all the tissues and returns deoxygenated blood to the right side of the heart. Exchange of nutrients and metabolic waste products takes place in the systemic circulation. In a normal adult at rest the amount of blood circulated through the heart is 5 litres per min (L/min), which is the same as the amount of blood in the circulation.

The force required to move blood around the body comes from the heart, which is essentially two separate pumps: the left side supplies the systemic circulation and the right side supplies the pulmonary circulation. As a general principle, veins carry blood **to** the heart: oxygenated in the pulmonary circulatory system and deoxygenated in the systemic veins (Fig. 17.1). Arteries carry blood **away** from

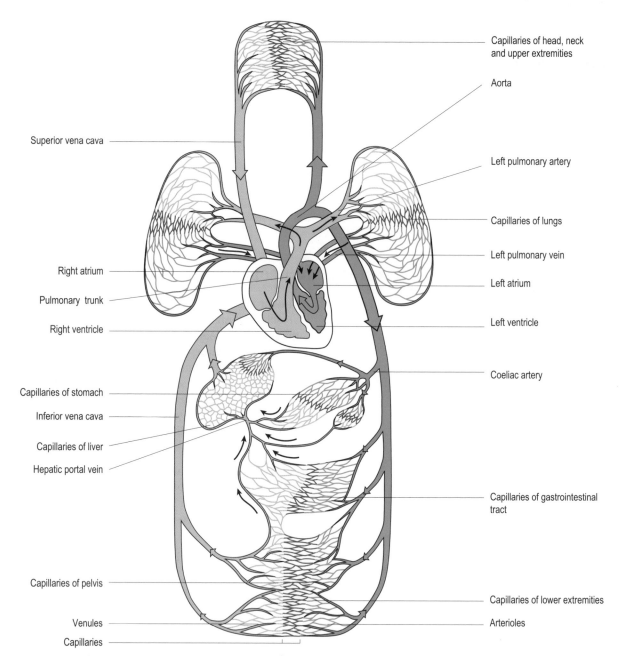

Figure 17.1   A general plan of the circulatory system (from Hinchliff S M, Montague S E, Watson R 1996, with permission).

the heart: deoxygenated in the pulmonary circulatory system and oxygenated in the systemic circulation.

ANATOMY OF THE HEART

Description

The heart lies in the mediastinum of the thoracic cavity between the two lungs enclosed in their pleural sacs. It is positioned with two-thirds of its mass to the left of the body's midline. It is shaped like a blunt cone with its apex pointing downwards and to the left. The heart covers about 12–14 cm from the second to the fifth intercostal space and its base, which points upwards towards the right shoulder,

is about 9 cm wide. The heart of an adult normally weighs about 300 g.

Layers

The myocardium, endocardium and pericardium make up the three layers of the heart.

The **myocardium** or contractile wall of the heart consists mainly of cardiac muscle. Connective tissue forms a dense fibrous network which reinforces the myocardium and anchors the muscle fibres. This fibrous network limits the spread of electrical action potentials to specific pathways.

The inner lining or **endocardium** consists of squamous epithelium resting on connective tissue. This also covers the

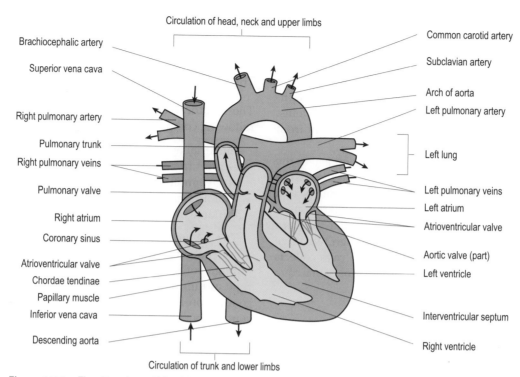

Figure 17.2 The direction of blood flow within the heart (from Hinchliff S M, Montague S E, Watson R 1996, with permission).

valves and the tendons that hold them in place. It is continuous with the endothelial lining of the blood vessels entering the heart.

The heart is enclosed in a fibroserous sac called the **pericardium**, which protects it and anchors it to the large blood vessels, diaphragm and sternal wall. It has two layers – an outer fibrous layer and an inner serous pericardium. The serous pericardium is also composed of two layers – the outer parietal layer and the inner visceral layer next to the myocardium called the **epicardium**. Between the visceral and parietal layers of the serous pericardium is the **pericardial cavity**, which is filled with **pericardial fluid**. This provides a friction-free area within which the heart can pump.

Chambers and valves

There are four **chambers** in the heart: two superior atria and two inferior ventricles. The right ventricle forms most of the anterior surface of the heart while the left and largest ventricle forms the apex and the inferior posterior aspect of the heart. These chambers are separated by valves and septa: the interatrial septum and the interventricular septum. The valves are attached to papillary muscles by the **chordae tendinae**, which anchor them in the closed position. The valves direct and control the flow of blood through the heart by opening as the associated chamber contracts and closing as the chamber relaxes. The valves ensure a one-way flow of blood through the heart (Fig. 17.2).

The atrioventricular valves

The **tricuspid** valve separates the right atrium from the right ventricle. The **mitral** or **bicuspid** valve separates the left atrium from the left ventricle.

The semilunar valves

The **pulmonary** valve separates the right ventricle from the pulmonary artery. The **aortic** valve separates the left ventricle and the aorta.

The coronary circulation

Oxygen is carried to the cardiac muscle by the right and left coronary arteries, which originate from the aorta just beyond the aortic valve. The right coronary artery supplies the right atrium, right ventricle and portions of the left ventricle. The left coronary artery divides near its origin into:

- the left anterior descending branch, supplying the anterior part of the left ventricle and a small part of the right ventricle
- the circumflex branch, which supplies blood to the left atrium and upper left ventricle.

Blood returns from the left side of the heart to the right atrium via the coronary sinus and blood returns from the right side of the heart via small anterior cardiac veins.

Pulmonary and systemic circulation

The **pulmonary circulation** takes deoxygenated blood from the right atrium to the lungs via the pulmonary trunk, which divides into two pulmonary arteries, one directed to each lung. The arteries further subdivide until the capillary level where they unite into venules and then veins. Oxygenated blood is then returned to the left atrium from the lungs via four pulmonary veins.

In the **systemic circulation**, oxygenated blood leaves the left ventricle via the aorta and is diverted to all the tissues and cells around the body through smaller arteries and arterioles. At tissue level the blood reaches capillaries, merging with venules to form veins. These veins unite to return deoxygenated blood to the right atrium through two large veins called the vena cavae: the inferior vena cava collects blood from the lower body and the superior vena cava collects blood from the upper body.

PHYSIOLOGY OF THE HEART

Cardiac muscle combines properties of both skeletal and smooth muscle (see Ch. 25). It is striated like skeletal muscle but individual muscle cell membranes have very low electrical resistance. Structures called **intercalated discs** (Fig. 17.3) allow action potentials to pass easily from one cardiac muscle cell to another so that the muscle mass can function as a whole. Intercalated discs contain anchoring units called **desmosomes** to hold the fibres together. Gap junctions between the muscle cells allow easy movement of ions to facilitate the spread of action potentials. The action potential is prolonged, allowing the electrical impulse to travel over the whole atrial and ventricular mass so that the cardiac muscle contracts as a unit. There is then a prolonged refractory period where relaxation phase occurs and no further contraction can begin. This is when the heart chambers refill with blood.

Both atria contract together, propelling blood into each ventricle. Both ventricles then contract together, propelling blood into the pulmonary and systemic circulations. As the atria contract, the ventricles are relaxed so they can fill up with blood. As the ventricles contract, the atria are relaxed and fill up with blood ready for the next cycle.

The electrical conducting system (nodal system)

The electrical conducting system of the heart has the following components:

- sinoatrial node (SA);
- atrioventricular node (AV);
- atrioventricular bundle of His;
- left and right branch bundles;
- Purkinje fibres.

The **SA node**, located in the right atrium, initiates the action potential that causes contraction. It then spreads through both atria and enters the **AV node** at the base of the right atrium. This plus the **bundle of His** provide the only conduction link to the ventricles. There is a 0.1 s delay in conduction, allowing the atria to complete contracting and emptying their blood into the ventricles. The wave now spreads via the left and right branch bundles, which lie on either side of the interventricular septum, to the **Purkinje fibres** and the ventricular muscle. The spread is simultaneous and there is coordinated contraction.

The cardiac cycle

The cardiac cycle is taken from the end of one contraction to the end of the next (Fig. 17.4). It produces two distinct sounds in a single beat, 'lub-dup'. The first heart sound is produced by the closure of the atrioventricular valves at the beginning of ventricular contraction or **systole**. The second sound is produced by the closure of the semilunar valves at the beginning of ventricular relaxation or **diastole**. The **heart rate** (HR) is the number of cycles or beats per minute (bpm). At an average heart rate of 72 bpm, each cardiac cycle lasts approximately 0.8 s with approx. 0.4 s being in systole and 0.4 s in diastole.

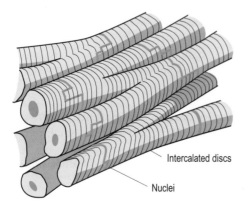

Figure 17.3 The structure of cardiac muscle showing the intercalated discs (from Hinchliff S M, Montague S E, Watson R 1996, with permission).

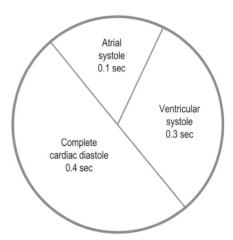

Total period of 1 cycle = 0.8 sec

Figure 17.4 The cardiac cycle.

CONTROL OF THE HEART RATE

Intrinsic control

The intrinsic conduction system of the heart allows the heart muscle to beat on its own with no external control. The heart's electrical conduction system has **autorhythmicity**. The SA node acts as a pacemaker and in the absence of any nervous or hormonal influences initiates a rate of 100 bpm. Other parts of the conducting system also have autorhythmicity. The unopposed AV node can initiate a rate of 40–60 bpm and the rest of the system will initiate a rate of 15–40 bpm.

Extrinsic control

The heart rate can also be externally influenced by the autonomic nervous system, hormones such as adrenaline (epinephrine), stretching the atria, temperature and drugs.

Nervous control

In the medulla oblongata the **cardiovascular centre (CVC)** receives input from baroreceptors, chemoreceptors and higher centres in the brain such as the cortex and hypothalamus (Fig. 17.5). The CVC can be subdivided into the **cardiac centre**, affecting heart function, and the **vasomotor centre**, affecting blood vessels, but these probably function interactively. Both sympathetic fibres (from the CVC) and parasympathetic fibres (from the vagus nerve) innervate the SA node. Sympathetic activity causes the heart rate to increase and parasympathetic activity causes the heart rate to decrease (Fig. 17.6). This parasympathetic influence, dominant at rest, is sometimes known as the **vagal brake**. This explains why a normal resting heart rate averages 70 bpm compared with the unopposed SA node rate of 100 bpm.

Hormonal control

Adrenaline (epinephrine) stimulates β_1 receptors in cardiac muscle and causes the heart rate to increase in response to stress. The hormones noradrenaline (norepinephrine) and thyroid hormone also enhance the effect of the sympathetic nervous system to increase heart rate.

Stretch

Stretching of the atrial walls can be caused by increased venous return or increased blood volume. Atrial stretching can increase the heart rate by 10–15%. This is the **Bainbridge reflex** and occurs because the stretch receptors in the atrial walls send impulses to stimulate sympathetic output.

Stroke volume

Excess blood also stretches the ventricles (**ventricular end-diastolic volume** (VEDV)). The more the ventricles are stretched before contraction, the greater the force of contraction and the greater the amount of blood leaving the heart. This is **Starling's law of the heart**. The amount of blood leaving each ventricle during one contraction is called the **stroke volume** (SV) and is normally 70 ml. A ventricle does not empty completely when it contracts. The blood left in the ventricle at the end of systole is the **ventricular end-systolic volume** (VESV). Typical values for an adult at rest are SV = 70 ml, VEDV = 135 ml and VESV = 65 ml and can be represented by the following equation:

$$SV = VEDV - VESV \qquad (17.1)$$

In health, adding the atrial contents to the remaining blood in the ventricle brings about the extra VEDV of the next cycle. This increases the contraction force, causing the ventricle to

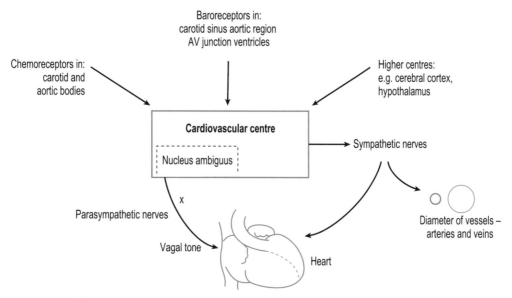

Figure 17.5   Diagrammatic representation of afferent and efferent pathways associated with the cardiovascular control centre (from Hinchliff S M, Montague S E 1990, with permission).

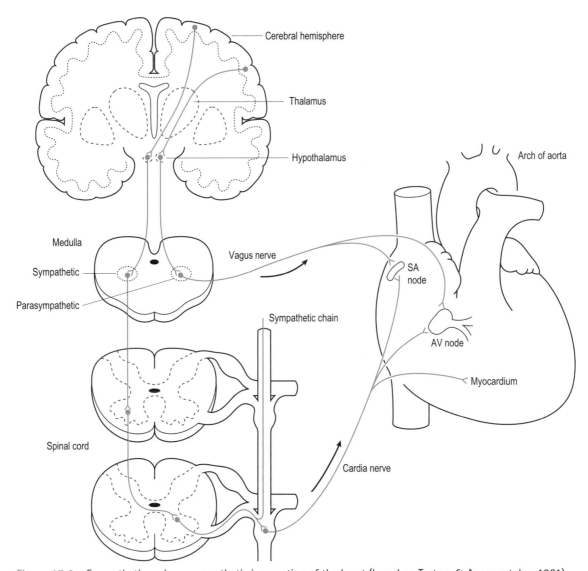

Figure 17.6   Sympathetic and parasympathetic innervation of the heart (based on Tortora & Anagnostakos 1981).

empty more completely and thus maintaining SV at a constant level.

Cardiac output

The volume of blood pumped by each ventricle per minute is called cardiac output (CO), usually expressed in L/min. It is also the volume of blood flowing through either the systemic or pulmonary circuit per minute (Vander et al 2000). The CO is determined by multiplying the heart rate, the number of beats per minute, by the stroke volume, the blood ejected by each ventricle with each beat:

$$CO = HR \times SV \qquad (17.2)$$

Thus if each ventricle has a rate of 72 bpm and ejects 70 ml of blood with each beat, from Eqn (17.2) the cardiac output is:

$$CO = 72\,\text{bpm} \times 0.07\,\text{L/beat} = 5.0\,\text{L/min}$$

These are approximate values for a healthy adult at rest. Since the total blood volume is also approximately 5 litres,

this means that essentially all the blood is pumped around the circuit once each minute. Cardiac output may reach 35 L/min in well-trained athletes during periods of strenuous exercise (i.e. total blood volume pumped around the circuit seven times a minute). Sedentary individuals can reach cardiac outputs of 20–25 L/min. The difference between the cardiac output at rest and the *potential* cardiac output is called the **cardiac reserve**.

In response to being stretched the atria secrete a hormone called **atrial natriuretic factor** (ANF) or **atrial natriuretic peptide** (ANP). This is a potent diuretic that causes the kidney to excrete excess sodium and water, resulting in a decrease of blood volume and blood pressure.

Other influences (Fig. 17.7)

- Alterations in core body temperature influence heart rate: there will be an increase in heart rate with an increase in temperature, whereas lowering of core body temperature

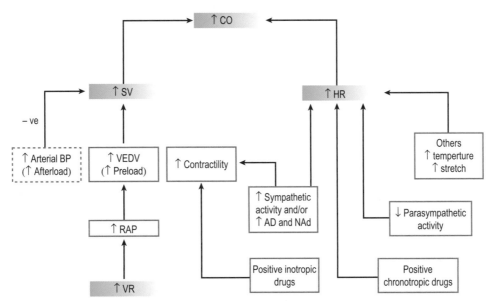

Figure 17.7   Main factors that can alter cardiac output. An increased arterial blood pressure (i.e. an increased afterload) causes a decrease in stroke volume and consequently a decrease in cardiac output. CO, cardiac output; SV, stroke volume; HR, heart rate; VEDV, ventricular end-diastolic volume; RAP, right atrial pressure; VR, venous return; Ad, adrenaline; NAd, noradrenaline (from Hinchliff S M, Montague S E 1990, with permission).

will decrease the heart rate. This latter is seen in people with hypothermia. The changes in body temperature alter the rate of electrical discharge.

- Drugs such as isoprenaline or adrenaline (epinephrine) can increase the heart rate. Drugs acting as β-adrenergic blockers such as propranolol will decrease the heart rate.
- A raised arterial blood pressure may decrease SV because the ventricles must exert force against a greater load. A normal heart will self-adjust to counter this by increasing the force of ventricular contraction. If the blood pressure is chronically raised, the left ventricle will hypertrophy and fail.

THE VASCULAR SYSTEM

The vascular system delivers blood to all tissues as needed and returns blood to the heart (Figs 17.8 and 17.9). To achieve this the system must be able to adapt to local needs. A change from pulsatile arterial blood flow to a steady capillary flow is necessary to allow the effective exchange of nutrients and waste to occur at the capillary beds.

In the systemic circulation, blood leaves the left side of the heart via the **aorta**, which subdivides into smaller arteries. The smallest are **arterioles**, branching into **capillaries** where the exchange of gases, nutrients and metabolic wastes occurs. Capillaries unite to form **venules** and these unite to form larger veins. Finally, the two largest veins, the **inferior vena cava** returning blood from the lower part of the body and the **superior vena cava** returning blood from the upper part of the body, enter the right atrium of the heart.

In the pulmonary circulation a single pulmonary artery leaves the right ventricle and divides into two branches, which deliver deoxygenated blood returning from the tissues to each lung for oxygenation. The division into smaller arteries, arterioles, capillaries, venules and veins is the same as in the systemic circulation. Four pulmonary veins deliver oxygenated blood back to the left atrium.

Structure of blood vessels

The structure of the blood vessels varies depending on their specific functions but the walls of the blood vessels, with the exception of the capillaries, contain the same three layers of tissue (Fig. 17.10):

1. **Tunica intima** is the innermost layer, called the endothelium, which is a single layer of extremely flattened epithelial cells. A basement membrane and some connective and elastic tissue support this layer, which is only found in capillaries.
2. **Tunica media** is the middle layer and consists mainly of smooth muscle and elastic tissue. This is the layer that gives rise to the variation throughout the vascular system.
3. **Tunica adventitia** is the outer layer and is composed of fibrous connective tissue, collagen and fibroblasts.

The arterial system

Elastic arteries (conducting arteries)

Large arteries contain more elastic tissue and can passively expand and recoil to accommodate changes in blood

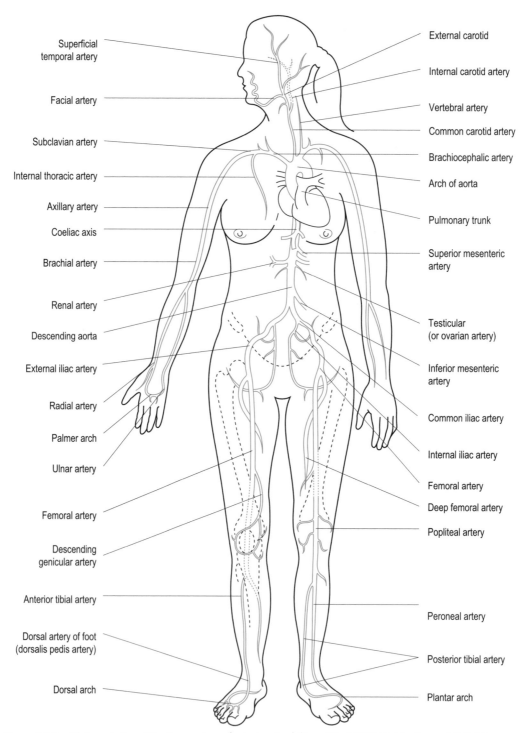

Superficial temporal artery

Facial artery

Subclavian artery

Internal thoracic artery

Axillary artery

Coeliac axis

Brachial artery

Renal artery

Descending aorta

External iliac artery

Radial artery

Palmer arch

Ulnar artery

Femoral artery

Descending genicular artery

Anterior tibial artery

Dorsal artery of foot (dorsalis pedis artery)

Dorsal arch

External carotid

Internal carotid artery

Vertebral artery

Common carotid artery

Brachiocephalic artery

Arch of aorta

Pulmonary trunk

Superior mesenteric artery

Testicular (or ovarian artery)

Inferior mesenteric artery

Common iliac artery

Internal iliac artery

Femoral artery

Deep femoral artery

Popliteal artery

Peroneal artery

Posterior tibial artery

Plantar arch

Figure 17.8 Major arteries of the human body (anterior view) (from Hinchliff S M, Montague S E 1990, with permission).

volume. This allows blood to be kept under a continuous pressure rather than starting and stopping with the pulsatile heart beat. When the heart contracts, blood is forced into the aorta and distends these vessels. When the heart rests, the large arteries return to their normal diameters. They have large diameters – that of the aorta is about 2.5 cm.

Muscular arteries (distributing arteries)

These medium-sized arteries distribute blood to all tissues. They have an average diameter of about 0.4 cm and still remain distensible so that resistance to flow is low. As they branch further and become smaller, the amount of elastic tissue decreases and the smooth muscle component increases.

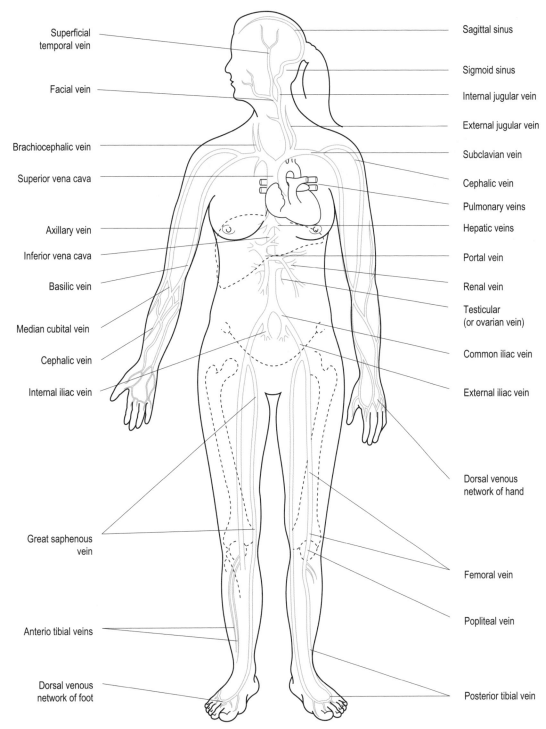

Superficial temporal vein

Facial vein

Brachiocephalic vein

Superior vena cava

Axillary vein

Inferior vena cava

Basilic vein

Median cubital vein

Cephalic vein

Internal iliac vein

Great saphenous vein

Anterio tibial veins

Dorsal venous network of foot

Sagittal sinus

Sigmoid sinus

Internal jugular vein

External jugular vein

Subclavian vein

Cephalic vein

Pulmonary veins

Hepatic veins

Portal vein

Renal vein

Testicular (or ovarian vein)

Common iliac vein

External iliac vein

Dorsal venous network of hand

Femoral vein

Popliteal vein

Posterior tibial vein

Figure 17.9   Major veins of the human body (anterior view) (from Hinchliff S M, Montague S E 1990, with permission).

Arterioles

Arterioles are the smallest arteries, less than 0.3 cm in diameter, with a thicker wall mainly composed of muscle tissue in concentric layers. The total resistance to blood flow is mainly determined by the diameter of the arterioles, which also determines the distribution of blood flow to different tissues. The **precapillary sphincters** are specialised regions near the junction between the terminal arterioles and the capillaries. They consist of smooth muscle fibres arranged in a circular manner around the vessels, which control the amount of blood flowing into a capillary bed. This action may also play a part in the formation of tissue fluid (see below).

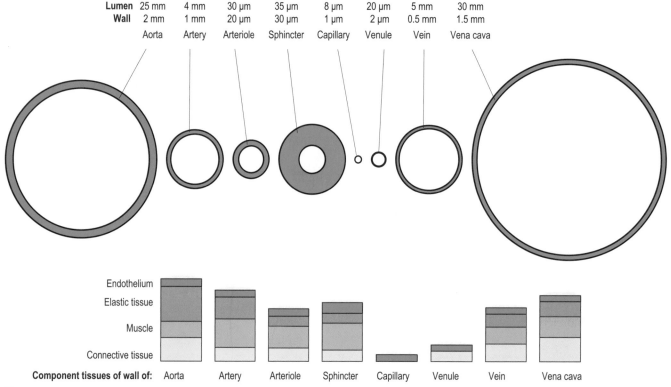

Figure 17.10 The variations in size and components of the walls of the various blood vessels in the circulatory system (from Hinchliff S M, Montague S E 1990, with permission).

Capillaries

Capillaries form a dense network of very narrow short vessels. Red blood cells pass through them in single file and may have to fold to negotiate their lumen. They are the exchange vessels where gases, nutrients and metabolic waste products pass between individual cells and the vascular system. Approximately 50 million capillaries are present in the body but at rest only 25% may be patent. Some modified, wider capillaries are known as **sinusoids**. They are found mainly in the liver, bone marrow, lymphoid tissues and endocrine organs and are lined by phagocytic white cells. Blood flows slowly through sinusoids to allow modification of its content: for instance, in the liver when nutrients are extracted.

The microcirculation

Each cell must have access to a capillary supply if it is to remain healthy. Substances need to travel a very short distance to enable adequate **diffusion**. Different tissues have varying amounts of capillaries, depending on their metabolic needs. There may also be **arteriovenous shunts**, connections between the arteries and veins that bypass the capillaries. Blood can flow rapidly through the shunts but this mechanism does not allow exchange of nutrients and gases. They facilitate dissipation of heat from the body via the skin if needed.

The venous system

Veins return blood from the capillary beds to the heart passively along a pressure gradient. As the veins become fewer and larger, resistance to flow decreases. Vein walls have the same three layers as arteries but they are thinner and more distensible than arteries. Some veins, such as those in the legs, have folds in the endothelium which act as valves to ensure that blood flows in one direction towards the heart. These valves may be damaged if overstretched by high pressures, for instance in pregnancy, and this may lead to oedema and varicose veins. The larger part of the circulating blood, about 60%, is contained in the venous system. Veins are sometimes known as capacity vessels and can change their capacity by altering the diameters of the vessels.

THE PHYSIOLOGY OF CIRCULATION

Blood vessel diameter

Changes in blood vessel diameter regulate blood pressure and blood flow to the tissues. Altering the degree of smooth muscle contraction in the tunica media changes the blood vessel diameter. Increasing contraction of the circular muscle fibres reduces blood vessel diameter (**vasoconstriction**). When the muscle relaxes, the diameter increases (**vasodilation**). The smooth muscle of the blood vessel walls is normally in a state of contraction known as **vasomotor tone**. Control of the smooth muscle involves nervous and chemical factors.

Nervous control

Sympathetic nerve fibres from the vasomotor centre innervate the smooth muscle in the tunica media. These nerve endings are more densely distributed in the arterioles, precapillary sphincters and venules. Sympathetic nerve discharge increases muscle contraction, causing vasoconstriction. A decrease in the frequency of nerve impulses brings about vasodilation. Vasoconstriction from increased sympathetic activity increases total vascular resistance, increases venomotor tone and reduces venous capacity and venous return.

Chemical control

Vascular smooth muscle is influenced by hormones and locally produced metabolites. Adrenaline (epinephrine) and noradrenaline (norepinephrine) cause vasoconstriction. Angiotensin II, formed by the action of renin (produced by the kidney) on angiotensinogen, is also a potent vasoconstrictor. Histamine and plasma kinins are released from inflamed local tissues and cause vasodilation of small vessels. Local prostaglandins may also be involved in vasodilation.

Endothelial mediated regulation

The endothelium produces a factor, **endothelial-derived relaxing factor** (EDRF), which causes relaxation of vascular smooth muscle and vasodilation. One form of EDRF is **nitric oxide** (NO), which is a free radical. It acts as a chemical messenger, carrying signals from cell to cell. Nitric oxide is released from the endothelial cells and diffuses into the muscle wall of the blood vessel. This chemical local control is extremely important when there is a localised increase in metabolism. Local chemicals largely mediate control of circulation to the brain and the heart. A major factor is the level of oxygen in the blood. The blood flow to the skin is mainly under sympathetic nervous control.

BLOOD PRESSURE

There are a few facts about the nature of a fluid that may help the reader to understand the concepts involved in blood pressure.

Fluid pressure

Hydrostatic pressure is the force a liquid exerts against the walls of its container. In the vascular system this is the pressure the blood exerts on the blood vessel walls, which is called **blood pressure** (BP). Pressure will also vary with the height of the liquid column. This is related to gravity. When

a person is standing up the venous pressure in the feet is greater than that in the head. A third factor that influences hydrostatic pressure is the distensibility of the container. Pressure is less in a distensible container compared to a rigid container. The heart generates a head of pressure that is highest in the aorta and falls throughout the vascular system along the path to the tissues.

Fluid flow

The flow of a fluid through a vessel is determined by the pressure difference between the two ends of the vessel and the resistance to flow. **Resistance to flow** is a measure of the ease with which a fluid flows through a tube. In the vascular system this is described as vascular resistance but for practical purposes most resistance is generated in the small peripheral vessels. This is referred to as **peripheral resistance** (PR). It is affected by:

- **Viscosity**, which is the thickness of a fluid. In blood, viscosity is affected by the ratio of red cells and plasma proteins to plasma fluid. Viscosity increases when there is an increase in cell content or a reduction in plasma fluid, such as in dehydration. An increase in plasma fluid will decrease viscosity. The greater the viscosity, the more force is required to move the fluid along the vessel.
- **Blood vessel length** – the longer the blood vessel, the greater the resistance to flow.
- **Arteriolar diameter** – small changes in diameter can lead to large changes in PR. The smaller the diameter, the greater the resistance. This is because particles in the fluid are more likely to collide with the vessel walls.
- **The lining** also affects flow. A smooth lining in a blood vessel will create a smooth **laminar** flow whilst a rough lining will cause a **turbulent** flow.

Blood pressure is the force exerted on the wall of a blood vessel by the blood it contains. It is measured in millimetres of mercury (mmHg). There is a typical value for different parts of the vascular tree, i.e. for arterial blood pressure, capillary blood pressure, venous blood pressure and so on. These gradients facilitate blood flow around the systems. The pressure in the systemic circulation falls during the blood's journey from the aorta to the right atrium. Pressures in the pulmonary circulation are lower than in the systemic circulation but there is still a falling gradient from right ventricle to left atrium.

Venous return

Blood pressure in the capillary beds is very low so a mechanism is needed to ensure blood return to the right atrium. Blood pressure in the venules is greater than the pressure in the right atrium but gravity opposes venous return when a person is upright and blood may pool in the feet and legs. In contrast, blood returning from the head is aided by gravity when in the upright position and dizziness may occur due to a temporary reduction in brain blood supply if a person stands up too quickly. If venous return to the heart is impeded, cardiac output will fall.

There are several mechanisms to ensure adequate blood flow:

- Increasing **venomotor tone** will reduce the capacity of the venous system.
- The **skeletal muscle pump** – contractions of the skeletal muscles, especially in the limbs, squeezes the veins and pushes the blood towards the heart. Venous valves prevent backflow most effectively when a person is walking. Standing still means the muscle pump cannot act and venous return is not as good. People may faint if they stand still for long periods.
- The **respiratory pump** – as a person breathes in, pressure in the thorax and the right atrium is lowered, which increases the pressure gradient and assists venous return.

The arterial blood pressure is of most value clinically because it ensures an adequate blood supply to the tissues. The main parameter affecting blood pressure is the relationship between cardiac output and peripheral resistance. This can be represented by the following simple equation:

$$BP = CO \times PR \qquad (17.3)$$

Arterial blood pressure

Arterial blood pressure changes throughout the cardiac cycle. Contraction of the ventricles during systole ejects blood into the aorta and raises the arterial pressure. This is the **systolic pressure** and is determined by the stroke volume and the force of the contraction. Systolic pressure will be raised if the arterial walls are stiffer because the vessels cannot distend to accommodate the extra blood. As the heart relaxes during diastole, blood leaves the main arteries and the blood pressure falls. This is the **diastolic pressure**, which is affected by peripheral resistance. Diastolic pressure therefore depends on the level of systolic pressure, the elasticity of the arteries and the viscosity of blood. If the heart rate is slow, diastolic pressure will fall as there is more time for extra blood to flow out of the artery. An increase in heart rate will raise the diastolic pressure.

Pulse pressure and mean arterial pressure

Each ventricular contraction initiates a pulse of pressure through the arteries. The difference between the systolic and diastolic pressure is called the **pulse pressure**. A typical blood pressure would be 120/70 mmHg, giving a pulse pressure of 50 mmHg, i.e. 120 − 70 = 50 mmHg. The main factors influencing pulse pressure are stroke volume and the rigidity of the arteries.

An average or mean value for arterial pressure is useful as it represents the pressure driving the blood through the arteries. **Mean arterial pressure** (MAP) is more useful as a guide to tissue perfusion than the usual systolic/diastolic BP reading. It is estimated by:

Mean arterial pressure (MAP) = Diastolic pressure
+ One-third of the pulse pressure   (17.4)

For example, using Eqn (17.4), a blood pressure of 120/70 mmHg gives:

MAP = 70 + (⅓ of 50) = 87 mmHg

The regulation of blood pressure

Neural, chemical and renal controls act to modify blood pressure by influencing cardiac output, peripheral resistance and/or blood volume.

Neural system

The neural system can either alter blood distribution or maintain adequate systemic blood pressure. The system operates by spinal reflex. The vasomotor centre sends sympathetic nerve impulses via vasomotor efferent fibres to the muscular walls of the arterial system and acts mainly on the arterioles. The more impulses from these neurons, the more constricted are the arterioles. The vasomotor centre activity is modified by baroreceptors and chemoreceptors.

Baroreceptors are situated in the tunica adventitia of the internal carotid artery (especially in the carotid sinus), the transverse section of the aortic arch and the largest vessels in the neck and thorax. These provide a short-term feedback mechanism responding to changes in posture and in activity levels. Nerve fibres run from the baroreceptors via the glossopharyngeal cranial nerve (IX) and the vagal nerve (X). The nerve endings respond to stretching of the arterial wall. The normal action of these nerves on the CVC is inhibitory. They slow the heart rate and decrease the force of ventricular contraction as well as causing arterial vasodilation.

Chemoreceptors are situated in the aortic arch and carotid bodies. They respond to a fall in blood oxygen or an increase in blood acidity. The main effect is on the respiratory system but in severe hypoxia they stimulate sympathetic activity, which increases heart rate and blood pressure. Brain centres such as the cortex and the hypothalamus also affect blood pressure.

Chemical control

Hormones from the adrenal medulla, namely adrenaline (epinephrine) and noradrenaline (norepinephrine), act to increase sympathetic activity (the flight or fight response). Antidiuretic hormone (from the posterior pituitary) is released into the circulation to retain fluid during pain and low blood pressure. Some drugs such as morphine, alcohol and nicotine will also increase the blood volume by preventing renal excretion of fluid.

The renal system

The kidneys respond to altered blood volume by altering the amount of urine excreted via the **renin–angiotensin mechanism** (see Chs 19 and 20). A reduction in blood pressure and kidney blood flow results in the excretion of renin by the kidney juxtaglomerular apparatus. Renin acts on angiotensinogen to release angiotensin I, which is then converted to angiotensin II by enzymes. Angiotensin II is a powerful vasoconstrictor and also triggers the release of aldosterone from the adrenal cortex to cause retention of sodium and increased excretion of potassium. Water is retained passively by the increased amount of sodium. Blood volume has a direct effect on blood pressure: the higher the volume, the higher the blood pressure.

Blood pressure values

Blood pressure is highly variable both between individuals and within an individual. It is difficult to quote a normal blood pressure for a population but it is possible to find a typical value for an individual. Both physiological and genetic factors and a range of external influences can affect blood pressure. It is therefore of more value to consider a normal range. Normal adult blood pressure is considered to be between 100/60 mmHg and 150/90 mmHg. Maturation and growth, as well as age, sex and race, can influence blood pressure. Blood pressure readings from 250 000 healthy people presented in Table 17.1 illustrate the range.

THE FORMATION OF TISSUE FLUID

In the tissues, blood contained in the capillaries is separated from both the interstitial fluid and intracellular fluid of the cells. Capillary walls consist of a single layer of endothelial cells resting on a basement membrane. Slit-like spaces are present between the cells. These are known as pores and represent only a small proportion of the total surface area of the capillary wall. Water and solutes diffuse to and from the blood and interstitial fluid. Although there is a high rate of substance diffusion between the two compartments, the fluid content of the plasma and the interstitial fluid changes very little. The volume of fluid moving out of the capillaries is equal to the amount returned. The hydrostatic pressure on each side of the capillary wall and the osmotic pressure of protein in the plasma and tissue fluid help to ensure this equilibrium (Fig. 17.11).

Table 17.1 Blood pressure values (Durkin 1979)

Age in years	BP systolic	BP diastolic
Newborn	80	46
10	103	70
20	120	80
40	126	84
60	135	89

Hydrostatic pressure

Hydrostatic pressure is the force of water pushing against the cell membrane. In the vascular system it is generated by the blood pressure. In the capillaries a hydrostatic pressure of 25 mmHg is sufficient to push water across the capillary membrane into the extracellular space. It is partly balanced by **osmotic pressure**. The excess water moves into the lymph system.

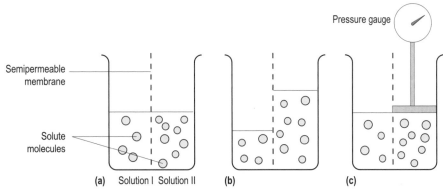

Figure 17.11 In (a) two solutions of equal volume but differing concentrations are separated by a semipermeable membrane. Solution I is less concentrated than solution II. Soluble molecules are too large to pass through the pores in the semipermeable membrane, but solvent molecules can pass through freely. In (b) solvent has moved across the semipermeable membrane from solution I to solution II, until the concentration of the two solutions is equal. This movement of solvent is called osmosis. Osmotic pressure is the pressure required to stop the movement of solvent by osmosis (c). The greater the difference in concentration between the solutions on either side of the semipermeable membrane, the greater is the pressure required to halt the osmotic movement of solvent across the membrane (from Hinchliff S M, Montague S E 1990, with permission).

Blood pressure falls from the arteriolar end of the capillary to the venous end. Fluid, with its dissolved solutes, will also cross the capillary wall. It is forced out at the arteriolar end and returns in the blood at the venous end. Capillary hydrostatic pressure (HP_C) is higher at the arteriolar end (about 25–35 mmHg) than at the venous end (10–15 mmHg). Hydrostatic pressure in the interstitial space (HP_{if}) has usually been rated as 0 mmHg because there is very little fluid present. This is because most of it is drawn into the lymphatic system. This pressure may have a negative value of about −6 mmHg (Marieb 2000). The net hydrostatic pressure is $HP_C − HP_{if}$.

Osmotic pressure

Osmosis is the movement of water down a concentration gradient across a semipermeable membrane. The water moves from high water content to lower water content. Osmosis is directly related to hydrostatic pressure and solute concentration but not to particle size. Osmotic pressure is

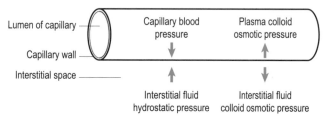

Figure 17.12 Forces affecting fluid movement across the capillary wall (from Hinchliff S M, Montague S E 1990, with permission).

created by the presence of large non-diffusable substances in a fluid. In blood this is provided by plasma proteins (mainly albumin molecules), which apply osmotic pressure if the water concentration surrounding them is lower than the water concentration on the opposite side of the capillary membrane (Fig. 17.12). Capillary osmotic pressure (OP_C) is about 25 mmHg while interstitial fluid, which contains few proteins, has a much lower pressure at OP_{if} 0.1–5 mmHg. The net osmotic pressure is $OP_C − OP_{if}$.

Fluid will leave the capillary where the net hydrostatic pressure is greater than the net osmotic pressure. Hydrostatic forces dominate at the arteriolar end at about 35 mmHg while net osmotic pressure is about 25 mmHg (+10 mmHg). Osmotic pressure dominates at the venous end of the capillary with a net hydrostatic pressure of 13 mmHg and a net osmotic pressure of 23 mmHg (−10 mmHg). Therefore, fluid is forced out of the circulation at the arteriolar end of the capillary beds and forced back in at the venous end (Fig. 17.13).

About 1.5 ml/min is lost from the circulation, picked up from interstitial fluid by the lymphatic system. This fluid, with any lost protein, is returned to the vascular system. The opening of precapillary sphincters will increase capillary pressure and force fluid into the tissues. Their closure will decrease capillary pressure, ensuring that osmotic force draws fluid back into the capillary. In the pulmonary circulation the same mechanism applies but the pressures are much lower.

Diffusion

Movement of substances always occurs along a concentration gradient, from high to low concentration. Oxygen and

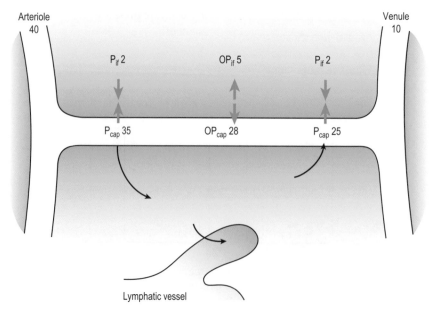

Figure 17.13 Diagram summarising the forces contributing to the formation and reabsorption of tissue fluid in the systemic circulation (all figures refer to pressures in mmHg). NB: P_{cap} is the only pressure for which magnitude alters. P_{cap}, capillary blood pressure; P_{if}, interstitial fluid pressure; OP_{cap}, plasma colloid osmotic pressure; OP_{if}, interstitial fluid colloid osmotic pressure (from Hinchliff S M, Montague S E 1990, with permission).

nutrients will pass from blood to the interstitial fluid and then to cells. Carbon dioxide and waste products of metabolism will flow from the cells into the capillary blood to be eliminated from the body.

MATERNAL ADAPTATIONS TO PREGNANCY

During pregnancy, dramatic changes occur in the cardiovascular system. These changes are necessary to meet the extra maternal and fetal demands imposed by pregnancy (Blackburn 2003). The uteroplacental circulation allows the exchange of gases, nutrients and waste products between mother and fetus. The fetal requirements place an increased load on the cardiovascular system, added to by the increased circulating blood mass, placental circulatory system and gradual increase in body weight. Under normal circumstances these changes are tolerated well but if cardiovascular disease exists the changes could be dangerous for the mother and fetus. On the other hand, no change occurring could compromise fetal health, as there may be a possible link between low blood volume and poor fetal growth (see Ch. 13).

Haemodynamic changes

An important part of the maternal cardiovascular adaptation to pregnancy is accomplished in early pregnancy. The timing of these and other changes in maternal physiology remains an enigma as to why they are initiated early in pregnancy before there is any physiological need for them (Duvekot & Peeters 1998). Current evidence suggests that the hormonal and immunological alterations act together very early to begin the process of haemodynamic adaptation. The most important haemodynamic changes in the maternal circulation during pregnancy are the increase in blood volume and cardiac output, and the decrease in peripheral vascular resistance. Other changes occur in the position and size of the heart, heart rate, stroke volume and distribution of blood flow (de Swiet 1998).

Size and position of the heart

As pregnancy progresses, the heart is pushed upwards by the elevation of the diaphragm and rotated forward so that the apex is moved upwards and laterally, appearing in the fourth rather than the fifth intercostal space (de Swiet 1998). The heart volume increases from 70 to 80 ml (about 12%) between early and late pregnancy. There is little increase in wall thickness and the increased venous filling increases the heart size rather than muscle hypertrophy.

The increase in atrial size related to the increase in venous return has been associated with more production of ANP in pregnancy. ANP has a diuretic effect and this helps to cope with the increased blood volume of pregnancy. Normal and anatomical and physiological changes may characteristically alter some heart sounds. Systolic or diastolic murmurs can be detected from as early as 12–20 weeks and may mimic pathology. Systolic murmurs are common because of the increased cardiovascular load (Blackburn 2003). In non-pregnant women, a diastolic murmur would indicate disease but in pregnant women it may not be significant because of increased blood flow through the tricuspid or mitral valves. During pregnancy there is an enhanced myocardial performance with a slight increase in myometrial contractility, probably due to lengthening of the myocardial muscle fibres (Gilson et al 1997).

Cardiac output

One of the most significant changes in cardiac output is the rapid increase early in the first trimester of pregnancy. The increase is not solely to supply uterine blood flow, as the early increase occurs before the uterus has enlarged significantly. The increased cardiac output is achieved both by an increase in heart rate and an increased stroke volume. An initial average increase in heart rate of 15 bpm occurs as early as 4 weeks following conception. This results in the myocardium requiring an increase in oxygen, which could be significant in women with heart or lung disease. This is followed by a small increase in stroke volume that occurs progressively during the first and second trimesters to about 30% above the non-pregnant rate. It is the prime instigator of cardiac output after 20 weeks (Blackburn 2003).

There is agreement that the increase in CO peaks by the end of the second trimester and then levels out. Over recent years research findings have raised some doubt as to whether these levels are now maintained in late pregnancy or decline as found in earlier studies (de Swiet 1998). Findings from studies using modern techniques have found that levels do not decline in late pregnancy until delivery (Mabie et al 1994) or small variable adjustments may be found in late pregnancy (Easterling et al 1990). There is an even greater increase in CO associated with multiple pregnancy.

The growing uterus provides the primary influence on changes in cardiac output in selected maternal positions. In the supine position the uterine mass compresses the inferior vena cava, leading to decreased venous return and 20–30% decrease in CO. This syndrome, referred to as **supine hypotension**, is associated with increased heart rate in response to the decreased output. There is somewhat less compression of the vena cava in the sitting position and the most favourable position for venous return is the lateral recumbent position.

Total blood volume

The increase in total blood volume, due to a rise in plasma volume and red cell volume occurring simultaneously, probably explains the increase in CO. Uterine blood rises from 100 ml/min at end of first trimester to 500 ml/min at term. Again, this does not parallel the early changes in CO.

Red cell mass or total volume of red cells increases by 18%, while plasma volume increases about 50%. The difference results in haemodilution of pregnancy and a fall in Hb level, often referred to as physiological anaemia.

Arterial blood pressure

The slight decrease in systolic blood pressure accompanied by the greater decrease in diastolic blood pressure leads to an increase in pulse pressure (Blackburn 2003). This is probably due to hormonal vasodilation. It is important to accurately measure BP using the correct size of cuff and standardised technique, e.g. the cuff must be level with the left atrium. Recording a woman's BP when she is lying in a supine position may have a considerable effect by resulting in a profound fall in BP (supine hypotension).

In normal healthy women, a general pattern in blood pressure recordings is noted during pregnancy. There is relatively little change in systolic pressure but there is a marked fall in diastolic pressure, which is lowest at mid-pregnancy and rises thereafter to approximately non-pregnant levels at term. Therefore, there is a raise in pulse pressure for most of pregnancy. At the beginning of labour blood pressure rises slightly and uterine contractions are associated with a rise in mean BP of 10 mmHg, which mirrors the rise in CO in labour.

Age and parity can affect blood pressure. As parity increases, regardless of age, both the systolic and diastolic blood pressures decrease with the greatest difference being between the first and second pregnancy. As age increases (after 35 years of age), systolic blood pressure remains unchanged but diastolic BP increases.

Systemic vascular resistance

Changes in cardiac output during pregnancy are accomplished without an increase in arterial pressure. This is because of the marked decrease in systemic vascular resistance (SVR), especially due to general relaxation of peripheral vascular tone in early pregnancy (Blackburn 2003). SVR (mean arterial pressure divided by cardiac output) decreases by 5 weeks, usually reaches its lowest level by 16–34 weeks and then progressively increases to term. The later change is presumed to be due both to the establishment of new vascular beds such as the low-resistance uteroplacental circulation and to a decreased peripheral vascular resistance.

Pulmonary arterial pressure

During pregnancy the pulmonary artery pressure remains unaltered, implying a large decrease in pulmonary vascular resistance, which mirrors the gestational pattern in cardiac output (Duvekot & Peeters 1998). The pulmonary circulation has a great capacity for high rates of blood flow without pressure changes and cardiac output may increase four to six times in pregnancy before pulmonary arterial pressure

becomes elevated. Reductions in pulmonary resistance are achieved by pulmonary arteriolar vasodilation capillary recruitment and possibly by arteriovenous shunting.

Venous pressure

Venous pressure increases markedly in the femoral veins in pregnancy and there is no similar rise in right atrial pressure. This indicates venous obstruction between the two points (de Swiet 1998). In pregnancy this is brought about by:

- simple mechanical pressure by the weight of the uterus on the iliac veins and on the inferior vena cava;
- pressure of the fetal head on the iliac veins;
- hydrodynamic obstruction due to the outflow of blood at relatively high pressure from the uterus.

The rate of blood flow in the leg veins is much reduced. This contributes to a risk of varicosities developing in the leg veins and vulva as well as haemorrhoids in susceptible women. Another side effect is the development of gravitational oedema.

Regional distribution of increased blood flow

The uterus

The increased circulation of pregnancy mainly targets the uterus. Estimating blood flow to the placental site has been attempted but this has been difficult to measure due to inaccessibility of the uterus and the complex blood supply. It is generally believed that the uterine vascular bed is widely dilated so that oxygen consumption is dealt with by increases in extraction rather than by increases in blood flow. This is a feature of the changes in the uterine blood vessels. Both steroid hormones and the renin–angiotensin system may contribute to the uterine blood flow of pregnancy.

The kidneys

Renal blood flow rises in early pregnancy to about 400 ml/min above non-pregnant levels; this may fall towards the end of pregnancy (see Ch. 19, p. 262).

The skin

Blood flow to the skin, particularly that of the hands and feet, is greatly increased in pregnancy. Women feel warm and often complain about the heat. Temperature is increased in both the fingers and toes.

Peripheral vasodilation

Increased blood supply to the hands may cause increased fingernail growth. The hair does change character although the rate of hair growth does not appear to be increased. In non-pregnant women, 85% of hairs are actively growing and the remainder is in the resting stage prior to falling out.

During pregnancy there are 95% of hairs in the growing stage. Therefore by the end of pregnancy the woman has more overaged hairs that fall out after delivery, leading to the common anxiety of hair coming out 'in handfuls' in the puerperium (de Swiet 1998). Increased blood supply to the nasal mucous membrane increases nasal congestion. Nose bleeds may occur as does increased snoring.

The liver

The research into increased blood flow through the liver is not clear but it is likely because of the increased metabolic rate during pregnancy (see Ch. 23, p. 311).

The breasts

Mammary blood flow is probably increased (see Ch. 54, p. 689).

Control of cardiovascular changes

Control of cardiovascular changes is partly hormonal, with increased circulating levels of oestrogen, progesterone and prostaglandins, and partly mechanical, with changes of growth and development of organs necessitating increased blood supply. Vasodilation of peripheral blood vessels is the primary haemodynamic alteration followed by increases in circulating blood volume and cardiac output. Findings from a literature review suggest that generalised vasodilation of pregnancy is unlikely to be induced by prostaglandins or that the hormones of pregnancy are the primary stimulus for vasodilation (Duvekot & Peeters 1998). They postulate that an EDRF such as nitric oxide may be the cause of the vasodilation. An increase in physical activity levels has an impact on the cardiovascular system. Box 17.1 provides an overview of the issues related to exercise during pregnancy.

Box 17.1 Exercise and the cardiovascular system

In recent years there has been a dramatic increase in the number of women who want to begin or continue with an active lifestyle during pregnancy. This has stemmed from the widespread promotion and encouragement of healthy individuals to adopt active lifestyles to gain the psychological, physical and health benefits of regular physical activity (Griffiths 1996).

Pregnancy involves anatomical and profound physiological changes unique to pregnancy. This raises important fundamental questions, including the ways in which pregnancy alters a woman's ability to exercise and to what extent exercise influences the course of pregnancy and development of the fetus. Many research studies have investigated the additional impact that exercise has on the changes normally occurring in the body during pregnancy. However, available data are insufficient to infer important risks or benefits for the mother or infant (Kramer 2002). The remaining gaps in the existing knowledge mainly focus on concerns related to safety aspects for the woman and her fetus (Stevenson 1997a). It is also important to ascertain how the impact of exercise undertaken by serious training on a regular basis differs from the more gentle exercises performed by most pregnant women.

All types of exercise place increased demands on the cardiorespiratory function, which continues to be an area of interest for researchers. Other areas of interest related to exercise in pregnancy include:

- the redistribution of weight;
- the hormone changes of pregnancy;
- pregnancy and birth outcomes;
- hyperthermia and fetal normality;
- hypoxia and the fetus.

The ability to increase cardiac output in response to exercise progressively decreases as pregnancy progresses. The theoretical redistribution of weight may affect venous return and blood may be redirected to the exercising skeletal muscles and to the skin for heat dissipation. Many women spontaneously reduce their level of physical activity. This may be due to the increased amount and distribution of weight gained, which alters the normal balance of the body and shifts the centre of gravity upwards and forwards. As a result, the pelvis tilts forward and down to keep the trunk upright. Spinal changes may be characterised by further developing of lumbar lordosis to help bear the weight of the growing fetus. Evidence suggests that pregnancy does not make much difference to exertion during non-weightbearing exercise. During weightbearing exercises, the increased cost of exercise, e.g. in oxygen consumption, is proportional to the increase in body weight (de Swiet 1998). Sufficient calories should be taken to supply the needs of the pregnancy as well as the exercise.

Uterine blood flow is reduced by exercise and this may be counteracted by an increased oxygen extraction in fit women. Evidence based on animal and human studies suggests that the fetus may experience transient hypoxia resulting in a reduction in the fetal heart rate (FHR) during maternal exercise. The range of FHR in the healthy fetus is normally between 120 and 160 beats/min (bpm) and any reduction below 110 bpm is usually associated with fetal distress. Findings from numerous studies suggest that FHR changes during maternal exercise are transient and do not interfere with normal fetal development and growth. However, there is need for further research in this area, since a reduction in heart rate is assumed to reflect fetal distress.

Box 1.1 *Continued*

Exercise can improve circulation, posture and attitude to nutrition as well as reduce complaints of constipation and varicose veins. Women who exercise regularly are reported to gain psychological benefits both during and following pregnancy (Rankin 2002). On the basis of the current state of research, physical exercise and sport can be recommended during pregnancy so long as women are aware of the contraindications and follow guidelines for safe exercise.

Exercise should be safe and undertaken under guidance from a trained person and should aim to maintain rather than improve fitness. The advice given should be appropriate to the needs of the individual woman (Stevenson 1997b). The American College of Obstetrics and Gynecology (ACOG 1994) guidelines for exercise during pregnancy include the following advice:

- women, starting exercise, should begin at a very low intensity and gradually increase activity levels;
- women already exercising can continue with their existing exercise levels and amend as pregnancy progresses.

Include

- an initial short warm up of muscles and cool down of muscles following exercise to gradually return the body to the non exercising levels;
- gentle stretching of muscles because of connective tissue laxity;
- liberal liquids to prevent dehydration and overheating.

Avoid

- perfoming in hot, humid conditions;
- activities such as jumping, ballistic movements or rapid directional changes.

In general, there appears to be no contraindication to exercise in the healthy woman (ACOG 2002). Review of controlled trials indicates that regular aerobic exercise during pregnancy appears to improve (or maintain) physical fitness and body image (Kramer 2002). There is no doubt that benefits of regular exercise will help to prepare women physically and psychologically for the challenges of pregnancy, childbirth and transition to parenthood (Rankin 2002).

MAIN POINTS

- The cardiovascular system has three main roles: delivery of nutrients and oxygen; removal of metabolic waste and carbon dioxide; and distribution of heat around the body. Blood flows in two distinct circuits: the pulmonary circulation and the systemic circulation. The systemic circulation is much larger than the pulmonary circulation and the force generated by the left side of the heart is much greater than that of the right side.

- The myocardium (middle and contractile layer), endocardium (inner layer) and pericardium (outer layer) make up the three layers of the heart. There are four chambers in the heart, two superior atria and two inferior ventricles, separated by septa and valves. Valves direct and control the flow of blood through the heart by opening as the associated chamber contracts and closing as the chamber relaxes.

- Oxygen is carried to the cardiac muscle by the right and left coronary arteries. Blood returns from the left side of the heart to the right atrium via the coronary sinus and from the right side of the heart via small anterior cardiac veins.

- Cardiac muscle is specialised tissue. The cardiac cycle is taken from the end of one contraction to the end of the next and lasts approx. 0.8 s. Cardiac output is about 5 L/min. This can increase to 35 L/min under extreme conditions.

- The structure of blood vessels depends on their specific functions. Muscle contraction will bring about vasoconstriction and muscle relaxation causes vasodilation. The smooth muscle of the blood vessel walls is normally in a state of contraction, known as vasomotor tone.

- The flow of a fluid through a vessel is determined by the pressure difference between the two ends of the vessel and the resistance to flow. Factors affecting peripheral resistance include viscosity, blood vessel length, arteriolar diameter and the nature of the lining in a blood vessel.

- Blood pressure (mmHg) is the force exerted on the wall of a blood vessel by its contained blood. The main parameter affecting BP is the relationship between cardiac output and peripheral resistance (BP = CO × PR).

- Contraction of the ventricles during systole ejects blood into the aorta and pulmonary artery and raises the arterial pressure. This is known as the systolic pressure. During diastole (relaxation) blood leaves the main arteries and BP falls to give the diastolic pressure. MAP (diastolic + one-third pulse pressure) is a useful guide to tissue perfusion.

- Neural, chemical and renal controls modify blood pressure by influencing cardiac output, peripheral resistance and/or blood volume. Blood pressure is highly variable both between individuals and within an individual.

Physiological and genetic factors and a range of external influences can set blood pressure.

- In pregnancy, the maternal cardiovascular system changes to meet the demands of the fetus. Exchange of gases, nutrients and waste products between mother and fetus occur via the uteroplacental circulation. The most important changes are increase in blood volume, increased cardiac output and reduced peripheral resistance.

- CO increases in the first and second trimesters of pregnancy. An initial rise in heart rate of 15 bpm occurs as early as 4 weeks, followed by a small increase in stroke volume.

- There is haemodilution of pregnancy and a fall in Hb level referred to as physiological anaemia. Little change is noted in the BP systolic reading, with a marked fall in the diastolic reading over the first two trimesters (lowest at mid pregnancy) and rising in third trimester to non-pregnant levels.

- The rate of blood flow in the leg veins is much reduced, sometimes leading to varicosities in the leg veins and vulva as well as haemorrhoids of susceptible women. Gravitational oedema may occur.

- The increased circulation of pregnancy mainly targets the uterus. Renal blood flow rises in early pregnancy but this may fall towards the end of pregnancy. Blood flow to the skin, particularly that of the hands and feet is increased. Mammary blood flow is probably increased.

- Control of cardiovascular system changes is partly hormonal and partly mechanical, as changes of growth and development of organs necessitate increased blood supply.

- Adopting an active lifestyle during pregnancy raises important questions about the woman's ability to exercise and to what extent exercise influences the course of pregnancy and development of the fetus. There is belief in the value of safe exercise during pregnancy, provided that any advice given is appropriate to the needs of the individual woman.

References

American College of Obstetricians and Gynecologists (ACOG) 2002 Committee on Obstetric Practice-Opinion, Number 267: Exercise during pregnancy and the postpartum period. Obstetrics and Gynecology 99(1):171–173.

American College of Obstetricians and Gynecologists (ACOG) 1994 Exercise during pregnancy and the postpartum period – Technical Bulletin Number 189. International Federation Gynecologists Obstetricians 45(1):65–70.

Blackburn S T 2003 Maternal, Fetal and Neonatal Physiology: A Clinical Perspective, 3rd edn. W B Saunders, Philadelphia.

de Swiet M 1998 The cardiovascular system. In Chamberlain G, Broughton Pipkin F (eds) Clinical Physiology in Obstetrics, 3rd edn. Blackwell Science, Oxford.

Duvekot J J, Peeters L L H 1998 Very early changes in cardiovascular physiology. In Chamberlain G, Broughton Pipkin F (eds) Clinical Physiology in Obstetrics, 3rd edn. Blackwell Science, Oxford.

Easterling T R, Watts H, Schmucker B C et al 1990 Measurement of cardiac output in pregnancy by Doppler technique. American Journal of Perinatology 7:220–225.

Gilson G J, Samaan S, Crawford M H et al 1997 Changes in hemodynamics, ventricular remodelling, and ventricular contractility during normal pregnancy – a longitudinal study. Obstetrics and Gynecology 89(6):957–962.

Griffiths A 1996 Employee exercise programme: organisational and individual perspective. In Kerr J, Griffiths A, Cox T (eds) Workplace Health: Employee Fitness and Exercise. Taylor & Francis, Nottingham.

Kramer M S 2002 Aerobic exercise for women during pregnancy. Cochrane Review: In The Cochrane Library, Issue 2. Update Software 2002, Oxford.

Mabie W C, DiSessa T G, Crocker L G et al 1994 A longitudinal study of cardiac output in normal human pregnancy. American Journal of Obstetrics and Gynecology 170:849.

Marieb E N 2000 Human Anatomy & Physiology, 5th edn. Benjamin/Cummings, New York.

Rankin J 2002 Effects of Antenatal Exercise on Psychological Well-being, Pregnancy and Birth Outcome. Whurr Publishers, London.

Stevenson L 1997a Exercise in pregnancy. Part 1: Update on pathophysiology. Canadian Family Physician 43(1):97–104.

Stevenson L 1997b Exercise in pregnancy. Part 2: Recommendations for individuals. Canadian Family Physician 43(1):107–111.

Vander A, Sherman J, Luciano D 2000 Human Physiology: The Mechanisms of Body Function, 8th edn. McGraw-Hill, New York.

Annotated recommended reading

Marieb E N 2000 Human Anatomy & Physiology, 5th edn. Benjamin/Cummings, New York.
This textbook presents a detailed overview of human anatomy and physiology. It is well illustrated with diagrams and pictures. Attention is given to the structure and function of the individual body systems, their interrelationships and homeostasis.

Rankin J 2002 Effects of Antenatal Exercise on Psychological Well-being, Pregnancy and Birth Outcome. Whurr Publishers, London.
This text is part of a series of published research studies. It includes a review of the literature related to the physiological and psychological effects of exercise during pregnancy. A randomised controlled trial study is detailed and a section on the practical aspects of an exercise programme, guidelines and contraindications is included.

Chapter 18

Respiration

INTRODUCTION

Respiration is the process by which the body exchanges gases with the atmosphere in order to provide for the changing needs of cell metabolism. Oxygen (O_2) is taken from the atmosphere and transported around the body in the blood to the tissues. Carbon dioxide (CO_2), produced as metabolic waste by the cells, is returned to the lungs and excreted into the air. Efficient respiration depends on the interactions of respiratory, cardiovascular and central nervous system functions that alter the rate and depth of respiration as needed. An adult utilises about 250 ml of oxygen per minute and this can be dramatically increased in severe exercise.

ANATOMY OF THE RESPIRATORY SYSTEM

The respiratory system consists of the airways from the nasal passages to the pharynx and larynx as well as the bronchi, bronchioles and alveoli of the lungs (Fig. 18.1). The chest structures necessary for moving air in and out of the lungs are part of the system. It is usual to divide the respiratory system into the upper and lower airways at the level of the cricoid cartilage.

The upper airways

The **nasal cavity** is a large, irregular-shaped cavity divided into two by a septum. Bony structures, called the **turbinates**, increase the surface area of the cavity and it is lined with ciliated epithelium which warms, filters and moistens the incoming air. The air now enters the upper pharynx through two internal nares.

The **pharynx** is a common passageway for water and food as well as air. It is a funnel-shaped tube extending from the internal nares to the level of the cricoid cartilage. The auditory or **Eustachian tubes** open into the upper pharynx and the mouth opens into the central portion or oropharynx. The tonsils and adenoids, which are organs of the lymphatic system, are found in the larynx. The oropharynx divides

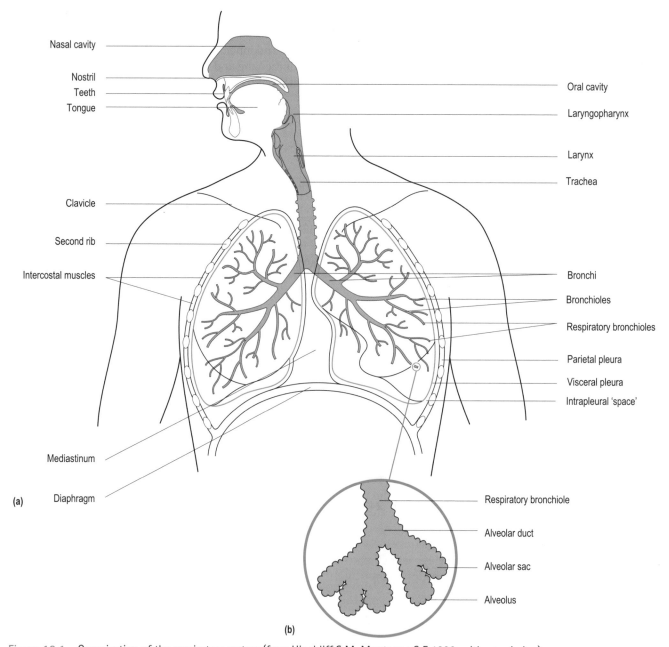

Figure 18.1   Organisation of the respiratory system (from Hinchliff S M, Montague S E 1990, with permission).

into the oesophagus, transporting food and water into the stomach, and the trachea, transporting air into the lungs.

The **larynx**, commonly called the voice box, is composed of pieces of cartilage connected by ligaments and moved by muscles. It is lined with mucous membrane continuous with the pharynx and trachea. In the larynx are the **vocal cords**, responsible for the production of sound, and between the vocal cords is the **glottis**, through which air passes. The **epiglottis** is a leaf-shaped piece of cartilage anchored to the thyroid cartilage. It moves up and down during swallowing to act as a cover for the glottis and prevent food and water from being inhaled into the larynx and lungs.

The lower respiratory tract

The lower part of the airway is also called the **bronchial tree** because of its resemblance to a trunk and branches (Fig. 18.2). The trachea is a cylindrical tube, 10–12 cm long, made up of 16–20 C-shaped cartilaginous rings joined together by fibrous and muscular tissue. This gives the trachea a firm structure to prevent the collapsing of the airway during inspiration. The posterior aspect of the cartilaginous rings is absent, facilitating the passage of food down the oesophagus, which lies immediately behind the trachea. The trachea extends from the larynx to the level of the fifth vertebra,

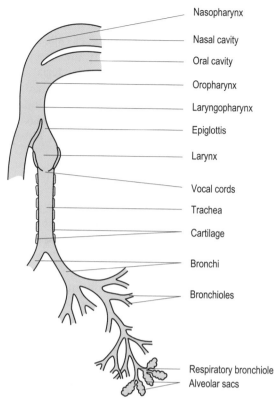

Nasopharynx
Nasal cavity
Oral cavity
Oropharynx
Laryngopharynx
Epiglottis
Larynx
Vocal cords
Trachea
Cartilage
Bronchi
Bronchioles
Respiratory bronchiole
Alveolar sacs

Figure 18.2   Organisation of the airways (from Hinchliff S M, Montague S E 1990, with permission).

where it divides into the two **primary bronchi**. The right primary bronchus is wider and shorter and more vertical than the left so that inhaled objects tend to enter the right lung rather than the left. The primary bronchi enter the lungs at the **hilum**, where the right bronchus goes on to divide into three: the right upper, middle and lower bronchi, to serve three lobes of the right lung. The left primary bronchus divides into two: the left upper and lower bronchi, to serve the two lobes of the left lung.

The lower branches of the airway, known as bronchi, still have cartilage in their structure. After this they are known as **bronchioles** and have smooth muscle in their walls. The smooth muscle is able to respond to stimuli by causing dilatation or constriction of the lumen of the bronchioles. This function is mainly under the control of the autonomic nervous system, with sympathetic impulses causing bronchodilation and parasympathetic impulses causing bronchoconstriction. There are about 8–13 divisions from the trachea to the smallest bronchi and another 3–4 before the terminal bronchioles are reached. Each terminal bronchiole divides into about 50 respiratory bronchioles. About 200 sac-like **alveoli** are supplied with air by each respiratory bronchiole.

The thoracic cage

The thoracic cage forms the cavity and contains the two conical lungs and the heart. The organs are separated from each other by the mediastinum and its contents. Each lung

is surrounded by a double-layered fluid-filled sac called the **pleura**, which also attaches them to the inner surface of the thorax. The inner, or visceral, pleura covers the outer surface of the lung and is reflected back to become the outer or parietal pleura which is attached to the inner surface of the thoracic cavity.

PHYSIOLOGY OF THE RESPIRATORY TRACT

The epithelial lining

The upper airway protects the alveolar tissues by warming, filtering and moistening the air. The structure of the epithelial lining is particularly good as a filter. It contains glands that secrete thick sticky mucus to trap particles and is ciliated to waft excess mucus and foreign particles towards the pharynx where they can be swallowed. The cilia beat about 600–1000 times per minute. Large numbers of phagocytic cells will engulf and destroy debris and bacteria trapped by the mucus.

Reflex mechanisms

Coughing is a forceful expiration reflex under the control of the respiratory centre in the medulla, which will expel irritant particles from the larynx. Air rushes out at a speed of 500 miles per hour! It is instigated by messages from a sensitive part of the airway at the bifurcation of the trachea, called the **carina**. **Sneezing** is a similar reflex, instigated by irritation of the nasal mucosa. The **swallowing reflex** is extremely important for respiration. Absence of this reflex, as is seen in unconscious or anaesthetised patients, may result in inhalation of particles of food or water into the larynx or lung. The airway may be obstructed or infection and pneumonia may occur.

Structure and function of the alveoli

The terminal bronchioles feed into respiratory bronchioles which branch into the alveolar ducts. These lead into alveolar sacs and the alveoli, where most of the gas exchange occurs (Fig. 18.3). The alveoli are expansions off the alveolar sacs, making the latter resemble bunches of grapes. Alveoli open into a common chamber called the **atrium** at the terminus of the alveolar duct. There are about 300 million alveoli in the lungs, providing an enormous area for gas exchange.

The alveolar wall (Fig. 18.4) consists of a single layer of flattened squamous epithelial cells called type I cells. The external surface of an alveolus has a few elastic fibres around the opening. There is a dense network of pulmonary capillaries surrounding each alveolus, providing a continuous encircling sheet of blood. Each capillary wall is also only one-cell thick so that the interstitial space between the alveolus and its capillary network, forming the air–blood interface, is extremely thin (i.e. 0.2 μm, compared with the 7 μm diameter of an average red blood cell). This interface is called the **respiratory** membrane and has blood flowing on one side and gas on the other. Gas exchange occurs by simple diffusion across the respiratory membrane and depends on the existence of pressure gradients between the lungs and the atmosphere. The total surface area of alveoli in contact with capillaries is roughly the size of a tennis court. This extensive area and the thinness of the barrier permit the rapid exchange of large quantities of oxygen and carbon dioxide for diffusion.

Surfactant

In addition to the type I cells forming the alveolar wall, the alveolar epithelium contains cuboidal type II alveolar cells

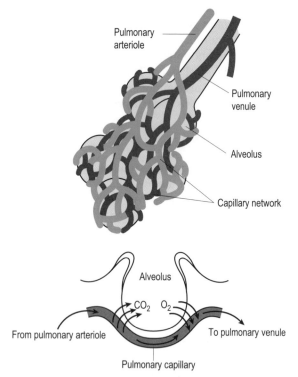

Figure 18.3   Relationship between alveoli and blood vessels. Gas exchange can occur across the vast surface area provided by the dense network of capillaries (from Hinchliff S M, Montague S E 1990, with permission).

which secrete pulmonary surfactant. This is a phospholipid that helps to keep the membrane moist and also maintains the patency of the alveolus. Macrophages called dust cells, part of the defence system of the body, are also present in the lumen of the alveoli, mopping up bacteria, dust and other inhaled particles. The alveolar surface is usually sterile. There are minute pores of Kohn present in the alveolar walls, allowing air flow between adjacent alveoli (**collateral ventilation**), which is useful if the terminal airways are blocked by disease.

Blood supply to the lungs

The lungs act to oxygenate the blood but they also need their own blood supply to maintain healthy tissue. The blood to be oxygenated reaches the lungs by branches of the pulmonary arteries, is reoxygenated in the pulmonary capillary network surrounding the alveoli and returns to the heart via the pulmonary veins. The two left and one right bronchial arteries arising from the aorta provide the blood supplying the lung tissue with oxygen. Venous return is by both bronchial veins and the pulmonary veins.

Nerve supply to the respiratory muscles

The phrenic nerve to the diaphragm (originating in cervical nerves 3, 4 and 5) and the intercostal nerves to the intercostal muscles (originating in the thoracic nerves 1–12) innervate the respiratory muscles. This is why severance of the spine above C3 results in total respiratory paralysis but, below that, diaphragmatic breathing can occur although the intercostal muscles will be paralysed.

THE PHYSIOLOGY OF PULMONARY VENTILATION (BREATHING)

There are two phases to breathing: **inspiration** or breathing in and **expiration** or breathing out. Mechanical factors and neural factors are involved in the control of respiratory rate.

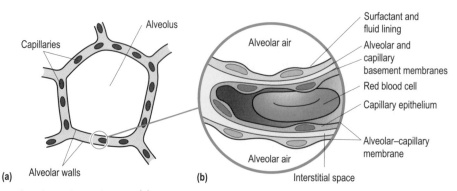

Figure 18.4   (a) Cross-section through an alveolus. (b) Higher magnification showing histology of part of the alveolar-capillary membrane. The dense network of capillaries forms an almost continuous sheet of blood in the alveolar walls, providing a very efficient arrangement for gas exchange (from Hinchliff S M, Montague S E 1990, with permission).

Atmospheric air contains about 21% oxygen and 79% nitrogen with traces of inert gases, carbon dioxide and water vapour. Alveolar air exchanges oxygen for carbon dioxide and water vapour. By the time alveolar air reaches the point of expiration it will be mixed with the atmospheric air in the dead space so that the content of expired air will be between the two extremes of atmospheric and alveolar air.

Mechanical factors

Under normal conditions and pressure gradients, oxygen passes from the alveolus into the blood and carbon dioxide from the blood into the alveolus. The movement of gases flowing from a high to a lower pressure down a gradient is said to occur by bulk flow. Air flows in and out of the lungs during breathing by bulk flow. Expansion of the thoracic cage, by contraction of the respiratory muscles during inspiration, increases lung volume and causes a temporary drop in the pressure in the alveoli. Atmospheric air flows in until pressure inside the lung is equal to the atmospheric pressure. Relaxation of the respiratory muscles causes expiration, by reducing the volume of the thoracic cage, creating a temporary rise in pressure within the lung to above atmospheric pressure.

Inspiration

The diaphragm, the most important muscle of inspiration, is a strong dome-shaped sheet of muscle separating the thoracic and abdominal cavities from each other. The diaphragm flattens when it contracts. This change in shape presses down the abdominal contents and lifts the rib cage, enlarging the thoracic cavity both from top to bottom and from front to back. Normally the external intercostal muscles, which are accessory muscles of respiration lying between the ribs, play little part in this expansion of the rib cage but do help to stabilise it. However, during any need for extra oxygen, such as in exercise and in upper airway obstruction, the upper intercostal muscles as well as other accessory muscles of respiration help to enlarge the rib cage and so enhance lung expansion.

Expiration

Under resting conditions, expiration is a passive process brought about by the relaxation and elastic recoil of the diaphragm and intercostal muscles at the end of inspiration. The elastic lung returns to its original volume as air is pushed out of the lung (the **functional residual capacity**), because the reduction in volume makes the alveolar pressure temporarily exceed atmospheric pressure. Active expiration may occur when the need for gas exchange increases under certain conditions such as during exercise or constriction of the airways.

Pulmonary ventilation

Respiratory parameters

Respiratory volumes and respiratory capacities can be described and measured using a spirograph. The measurements below are given for the average healthy adult (Marieb 2000, Sherwood 2001).

Respiratory volumes

- **Tidal volume** (TV) is the volume of air entering and leaving the lungs during a single breath. The tidal volume during normal quiet breathing averages 500 ml for both males and females.
- **Inspiratory reserve volume** (IRV) is the maximum amount of air that can be increased above the tidal volume value during the deepest inspiration. Volumes differ significantly by gender: males average 3200 ml and females average 1900 ml.
- **Expiratory reserve volume** (ERV) is the maximum amount of air that can be voluntarily expelled after a normal quiet respiratory cycle. This averages 1200 ml.
- **Residual volume** (RV) is the volume of air remaining in the lungs at the end of maximal active expiration and is typically 1200 ml in males and 1100 ml in females.

Respiratory capacities

- **Total lung capacity** (TLC) is the amount of air in the lungs at the end of a maximum inspiration. It includes TV + IRV + ERV + RV and averages 6100 ml in males and less in females (4200 ml) because of their smaller size.
- **Vital capacity** (VC) is total capacity minus RV and is typically 80% of TLC. This averages 4800 ml in males and 3100 ml in females.
- **Inspiratory capacity** (IC) is the maximum volume of air that can be inspired after a normal expiration. It is the sum of the tidal volume and the inspiratory reserve volume and averages 3600 ml for males and 2400 ml for females.
- **Functional residual capacity** (FRC) is the amount of air remaining in the lungs after a normal expiration. It is the sum of the expiratory reserve volume and the residual volume and averages 2200 ml in males and 1800 ml in females.

Minute volume

The total volume of air exchanged with the atmosphere in 1 min is called the **minute volume** or **pulmonary ventilation**. This volume depends on tidal volume and respiratory rate and varies considerably in different states of health and according to age. An average tidal volume in a resting adult is about 500 ml with a respiratory rate of 12 breaths per minute. Therefore pulmonary ventilation would be 6000 ml/min. Of this, about 150 ml of each breath is trapped in the **dead space** above the respiratory tissue and is breathed out with its composition unchanged.

Alveolar ventilation

The volume of fresh air entering the alveoli each minute is called the **alveolar ventilation**. The calculation from the parameters mentioned above is as follows:

Respiratory rate × (Tidal volume − Dead space)
= Alveolar ventilation

e.g. for values given above:

$$12 \times (500 - 150) = 4200\,\text{ml/min}$$

Shallow rapid breathing is not as efficient as slower deeper respiration because of the greater proportion of each breath wasted in the dead space.

TRANSPORT OF GASES AROUND THE BODY

Gas exchange in tissues

Gas exchange in the tissues occurs at the capillary level and the constant usage of oxygen and production of carbon dioxide by the cells creates the necessary pressure gradients, as discussed in Chapter 16. Oxygen is not very soluble in water and must therefore be carried around the blood in association with haemoglobin. Carbon dioxide is about 20 times more soluble than oxygen and readily dissolves in water to form carbonic acid. However, if all carbon dioxide was carried in solution then the acidity of the blood would be far too great to sustain life so a more complex mechanism is needed.

Transport of oxygen

About 99% of oxygen in the blood is bound to haemoglobin. There is a small quantity of oxygen dissolved in the blood, helping to determine the partial pressure of oxygen in the blood (PO_2) and maintains the pressure gradients, as the bound oxygen is not free to exert a pressure. The oxygen content of the blood is determined partly by the haemoglobin level but the hydrogen ion content of the blood also plays its part. As more oxygen is available, the PO_2 rises and haemoglobin will take it up. At a certain PO_2 when oxygen content is equal to oxygen capacity, the haemoglobin will be unable to take up any more oxygen and is said to be **fully** or **100% saturated**.

Partial pressure gradients and gas diffusion

The partial pressure gradient needed for the diffusion of oxygen is steep. For instance, the PO_2 of pulmonary blood is only 40 mmHg (5.3 kPa) while the PO_2 in the alveoli is 100 mmHg (13.3 kPa). Oxygen diffuses from the alveoli into the pulmonary capillary blood until there is equilibrium, with a PO_2 of 100 mmHg (13.3 kPa) on both sides of the respiratory membrane. Carbon dioxide moves in the opposite direction down a much less steep gradient from about 45 mmHg (6.1 kPa) to 40 mmHg (5.3 kPa) with equilibrium at 40 mmHg (5.3 kPa). Although the gradients are so different, both gases are exchanged equally well because carbon dioxide has solubility in plasma and alveolar fluid 20 times that of oxygen.

The oxygen dissociation curve

The oxygen–haemoglobin dissociation curve demonstrates the equilibrium between oxygen and haemoglobin (Fig. 18.5). The curve relates the partial pressure of oxygen to the percentage of haemoglobin that is saturated. There are two aspects of the curve that must be considered: its shape and position. The shape of the curve is sigmoid (S-shaped), indicating that at higher levels (less than 50 mmHg) the curve flattens and an increase in PO_2 produces little increase in saturation. The upper range is the PO_2 range in which oxygen binds to haemoglobin in the lungs. At low PO_2 levels the curve is steep and small changes in PO_2 result in large changes in haemoglobin saturation. In this range oxygen is released from haemoglobin and cellular activities occur. A small drop in PO_2 here allows a large amount of oxygen to be unloaded to the tissues.

Although each of the four haem groups in a haemoglobin molecule can take up a molecule of oxygen, they vary in their affinity. The first haem group in the molecule to take up oxygen does so with difficulty but also holds on to its oxygen tightly. This association changes the shape of the haemoglobin molecule so that the second and third haem

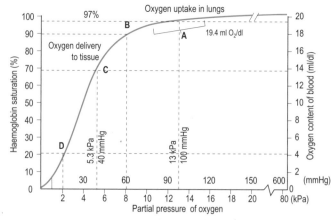

Figure 18.5 The oxygen–haemoglobin dissociation curve. This applies when pH is 7.4, PCO_2 is 40 mmHg (5.3 kPa) and blood is at 37°C. The total blood oxygen content is shown, assuming a haemoglobin concentration of 15 g/dl blood (i.e. O_2 capacity of 20 ml/dl) (from Hinchliff S M, Montague S E 1990, with permission).

molecules take up oxygen readily for a relatively small increase in PO_2 as oxygen saturation goes from 25% to 75%. This is shown on the graph as the steep part of the sigmoid curve. The fourth haem group takes up oxygen more slowly and only at high PO_2. The unloading of oxygen at the tissues is also efficient, with the unloading of one molecule facilitating the unloading of the next.

Effects of the sigmoid curve on oxygen uptake

Physiological effects of the oxygen dissociation curve include the following aspects. First, oxygen diffuses into the blood at the alveoli and by increasing the plasma PO_2, creates a pressure gradient so that oxygen can enter the red cell. Within the erythrocyte, the PO_2 rises more slowly, as the dissolved oxygen is rapidly bound to the haemoglobin molecules, so the pressure gradient is maintained. Loading to 90% saturation occurs rapidly at PO_2 of 60 mmHg (8 kPa). However, loading from 90% saturation to full saturation is slower and needs a higher erythrocyte PO_2 of 100 mmHg (13.3 kPa). Secondly, this flattened upper portion of the curve provides a safety factor in illness or at altitude as the blood leaving the lungs will still reach 90% saturation even when PO_2 remains moderate at 60 mmHg (8 kPa).

Effects of sigmoid curve on oxygen release

Blood enters the capillary circulation with a PO_2 of 100 mmHg (13.3 kPa) and is exposed to a tissue PO_2 of only 40 mmHg (5.3 kPa). This tissue pressure lies on the steep part of the oxygen dissociation curve so that up to 80% of the bound oxygen is readily released into the blood so that it can diffuse to the tissues. Below 10 mmHg (1.3 kPa) the affinity of haemoglobin for oxygen is increased so that the last molecule of oxygen associated with haemoglobin is lost with difficulty. However, this low level is very rarely reached. In working muscles, PO_2 of this low level may occur but **myoglobin**, a special oxygen-carrying molecule, can extract all the oxygen.

Factors influencing the oxygen–haemoglobin dissociation curve

The position of the curve depends on the oxygen affinity for the haemoglobin molecules. The affinity of haemoglobin for oxygen must be sufficient to oxygenate the blood during its movement through the pulmonary circulation. However it must be weak enough to allow release of the oxygen to the tissues. Several factors can influence the affinity of haemoglobin for oxygen at any given PO_2. These include factors that move the oxygen dissociation curve to the right or to the left. A shift to the right implies a lowered affinity and enhances oxygen unloading, while a shift to the left indicates that oxygen is more tightly bound to haemoglobin and unloading is inhibited.

Increase in carbon dioxide

An increase in carbon dioxide will reduce the ability of haemoglobin to bind oxygen. This reduced affinity for oxygen in the presence of increased carbon dioxide is called the **Bohr effect**. Blood entering the tissues with a PCO_2 of 46 mmHg (6.1 kPa) will release more of its oxygen than blood with a PCO_2 of 40 mmHg (5.3 kPa). This will shift the oxygen dissociation curve to the right.

Increase in hydrogen ions

The oxygen dissociation curve moves to the right when the blood becomes acidic. As acidity increases in the blood, as occurs with the addition of lactic acid to the extra carbon dioxide during anaerobic cell metabolism in exercise, oxygen release to the tissues is facilitated by the presence of extra hydrogen ions.

Increase in of 2,3-diphosphoglycerate

This substance is a product of red cell metabolism and binds reversibly to haemoglobin, reducing its affinity for oxygen. As the red cells reach the tissues 2,3-DPG is produced in more quantity and oxygen release is facilitated by moving the dissociation curve to the right.

Increase in temperature

Local elevation of temperature due to muscle cell metabolism in exercise or other actively metabolising cells will enhance the release of oxygen from the red cells. This moves the dissociation curve to the right.

The effects are reversed in the lung where the extra CO_2 is blown off and the local temperature is cooler. Haemoglobin therefore has a higher affinity for oxygen in the pulmonary capillaries, an appropriate effect!

Carbon monoxide

Carbon monoxide (CO) and oxygen compete for the same binding site on haemoglobin but the affinity of haemoglobin for CO is 240 times that of oxygen (Sherwood 2001). The product of haemoglobin with CO is carboxyhaemoglobin (HbCO). Even small amounts of CO will block the uptake of oxygen and shift the oxygen dissociation curve to the left. The amount of oxygen in the blood is reduced and the cells die from oxygen deprivation. CO is odourless, colourless and tasteless and is produced during the incomplete combustion of carbon products. If introduced into a small space it is lethal as the victim has no sense of breathlessness.

A shift in position has little effect on the saturation when the PO_2 is within normal arterial range (95–100 mmHg) due to the sigmoid shape of the curve. In the venous system (PO_2 range is around 40 mmHg) there is a right shift in the curve, leading to an increased unloading of oxygen to the tissues and improving tissue oxygenation (Blackburn 2003).

Transport of carbon dioxide

There are three ways in which carbon dioxide is carried around the blood:

1. ~5% is carried in simple solution
2. ~5% is carried in combination with the globin rather than the haem part of haemoglobin as carbamino-haemoglobin
3. ~90% is transported as hydrogen carbonate (bicarbonate) ions.

Bicarbonate ions

As the cells metabolise they constantly produce CO_2 so that the PCO_2 of intracellular fluid is always greater than that of the blood in the tissue capillaries. This creates the pressure gradient for the removal of CO_2 from the tissues into the plasma. A small quantity will dissolve in the plasma to give carbonic acid. This is a reversible reaction:

$$CO_2 + H_2O \leftrightarrow H_2CO_3 \qquad (18.1)$$

An enzyme called **carbonic anhydrase** can catalyse (speed up) this reaction. There is little of this enzyme in the plasma but the amount inside the red cell is much greater so that most of the CO_2 from the tissues diffuses through the plasma into the red cells. The rapid production of carbonic acid mops up the CO_2, keeping the red cell PCO_2 low. This ensures maintenance of the pressure gradient along which the CO_2 flows.

As is characteristic of acids, the carbonic acid in the red cell quickly ionises (dissociates) into hydrogen (H^+) and bicarbonate (HCO_3^-) ions, another reversible reaction:

$$CO_2 + H_2O \leftrightarrow H_2CO_3 \leftrightarrow H^+ + HCO_3^- \qquad (18.2)$$

The chloride shift

HCO_3^- ions can readily pass out of the red cell into the plasma, unlike the H^+ ions, so that the HCO_3^- ions, but not the H^+ ions, can pass down a concentration gradient into the plasma. HCO_3^- ions are much more soluble in blood than CO_2. This movement out of the cell of HCO_3^- ions leaves the erythrocyte with a more positive electrical charge than the plasma and creates an electrical gradient down which chloride ions (Cl^-), the main plasma anion (**anions** are negatively charged ions and **cations** are positively charged ions), can diffuse into the red cell to restore electrical neutrality. This is known as the **chloride shift**.

Hydrogen ions, carbon dioxide and the acid–base balance

Most of the accumulated H^+ ions inside the red cell become bound to the haemoglobin, as reduced Hb has an affinity for them. This action of haemoglobin acts as buffer, which neutralises the released H^+ ions to prevent any rise in acidity within the red cell. The increased affinity for the uptake of

CO_2 and H^+ ions that follows the removal of oxygen is called the **Haldane effect**. The Bohr effect and the Haldane effect work together to facilitate O_2 release and the uptake of CO_2 and H^+ ions by the red cells at tissue level. During exercise, much larger amounts of CO_2 are produced by the tissues but the increase in alveolar ventilation and in cardiac output ensure that arterial PCO_2 remains constant between 37 mmHg (4.9 kPa) and 43 mmHg (5.7 kPa).

The reactions are reversed once the blood reaches the lungs because of the reversed pressure gradients caused by the presence of atmospheric air in the alveoli. Here, CO_2 leaves the red cell to enter the plasma and crosses into the alveoli, and the freed H^+ ions combine with HCO_3^- ions to form H_2CO_3, which then separates into CO_2 and H_2O [see Eqn (18.2)], generating more CO_2 to diffuse out to the alveoli. This reaction is also catalysed by carbonic anhydrase.

As the HCO_3^- ions within the red cell are used up to generate CO_2, there is a shift inside the red cell to a positive electrical charge and plasma HCO_3^- ions and Cl^- ions now move back into the cell to restore electrical neutrality once more. This is a major pathway through which acid is removed from the body to maintain the acid–base balance: about 200 ml/min are removed from the tissues and eliminated from the lungs. Oxygen now crosses from the alveoli into the plasma and then the red cell to bind to haemoglobin.

Because of the importance of fluid and electrolyte balance and the maintenance of pH, a full discussion of the role of the respiratory system in maintaining the pH is presented in Chapter 20.

CONTROL OF VENTILATION

Breathing, like the beating of the heart, must occur in a continuous rhythmic cycle in order to provide oxygen for the cells. The control of breathing is complex. The respiratory muscles, unlike cardiac muscle with its intrinsic pacemaker, are skeletal muscles and must receive nervous stimulation from the brain to make them contract. In normal circumstances respiration is an involuntary act. The control of rhythmic breathing originates in the respiratory centre in the medulla.

Medullary respiratory centres

The dorsal respiratory group

The pace-setting nucleus within the medulla oblongata is called the **inspiratory centre** or dorsal respiratory group (DRG). There is a second nucleus called the **expiratory centre** or ventral respiratory group but its function is not well understood. Two other centres that influence the respiratory centre (higher in the brainstem in the pons) are the **pneumotaxic centre**, which sends out inhibitory impulses to the DRG to prevent overinflation of the lungs, and the **apneustic centre**, which continuously stimulates the DRG to prolong inspiration. The pneumotaxic centre normally inhibits the apneustic centre. There is also a voluntary pathway of control by the cerebral cortex with descending pathways to the respiratory centre.

The respiratory cycle

Descending neurons from the respiratory centre terminate on the motor neurons controlling the respiratory muscles. As inspiration starts, there is a rapid increase in the number of nerve impulses from the DRG travelling along the phrenic and intercostal nerves to arrive at the respiratory muscles. The force of inspiration gradually increases and thoracic expansion occurs. At the end of inspiration the DRG becomes dormant and there is a sudden reduction in the number of impulses, resulting in relaxation of the respiratory muscles and passive elastic recoil of the thoracic cage and lungs. Inspiration lasts about 2 s and expiration about 3 s. This cycle is repeated about 12–18 times in a minute but the level of ventilation is continuously adapted to changes in bodily requirements or atmospheric conditions so that adequate oxygenation is maintained.

Factors influencing the rate and depth of breathing

Multiple factors are involved in the regulation of respiration. These include neural, mechanical and chemical events and are best summarised in a diagram (see Fig. 18.6).

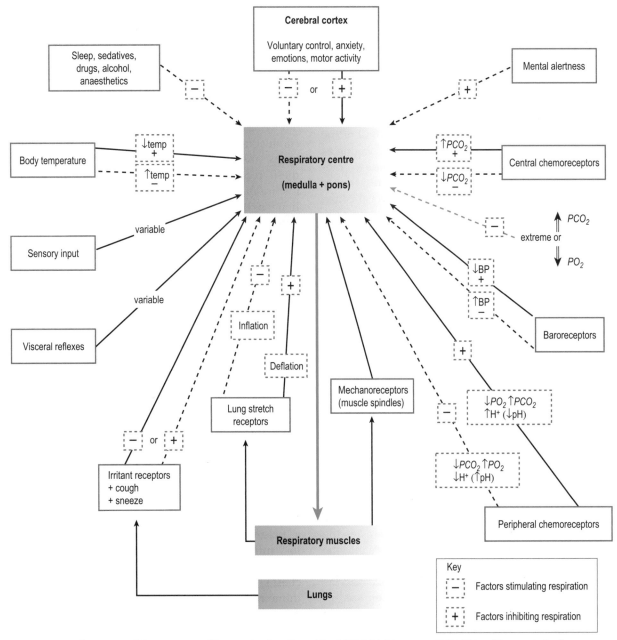

Figure 18.6   Summary of factors controlling respiration (from Hinchliff S M, Montague S E 1990, with permission).

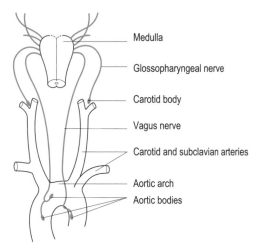

Figure 18.7 Peripheral chemoreceptor system involved in the control of breathing (from Hinchliff S M, Montague S E 1990, with permission).

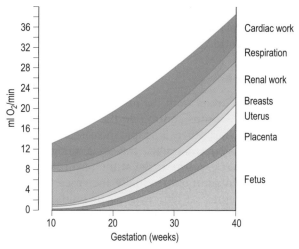

Figure 18.8 Partition of the increased oxygen consumption in pregnancy among the organs concerned. (Reproduced with permission from de Swiet 1991.)

Voluntary control of breathing

Voluntary control of the rate and rhythm of respiration, such as hyperventilation or breath holding, is limited by the chemical stimuli that such efforts induce. Complex control of the respiratory system is necessary during speech and singing as well as playing a wind musical instrument. Response to emotional states with laughing and crying also change respiratory patterns. When nerve impulses are sent to the vocal cords, simultaneous impulses are sent to the respiratory centre to control the flow of air between the vocal cords. Mental states influence respiratory rhythm: mental alertness and wakefulness have a stimulating effect and sleep, sedatives, alcohol and some anaesthetics have an inhibitory effect.

Chemoreceptor effects

Both peripheral and central chemoreceptors are able to respond to small changes in arterial PO_2 and PCO_2 to affect the rate and rhythm of respiration. **Peripheral chemoreceptors** are situated in the carotid bodies and other vascular structures around the aortic arch (Fig. 18.7). These receptors respond to chemical changes in the blood. They sense the levels of PO_2, PCO_2 and H^+ ions and relay the information to the respiratory centre.

The response to oxygen levels depends primarily on these peripheral chemoreceptors but the response to excessive levels of CO_2 (**hypercapnia**) depends on **central chemoreceptors** situated under the surface of the medulla. It is probable that with a rise in arterial PCO_2 carbon dioxide crosses the blood–brain barrier from the cerebral blood vessels into the cerebrospinal fluid (CSF). This bathes the central chemoreceptors. Once in the CSF, hydrogen ions are released [as in Eqn (18.2)] and these stimulate the central chemoreceptors, sending excitatory messages to the respiratory centre to increase the rate of respiration. A fall in PCO_2 will inhibit respiration.

The Hering–Breuer reflex

Stretch receptors are present in the visceral pleura and in the conducting passages in the lungs and are stimulated if the lungs are overinflated. Inhibitory impulses are sent by these receptors via the vagus nerve to the medullary inspiratory centre, resulting in the termination of inspiration so that expiration can occur. The stretch receptors quieten down as the lungs recoil so that inspiration can begin again. This is called the **inflation** or **Hering–Breuer** reflex.

MATERNAL ADAPTATIONS TO PREGNANCY

Pregnancy is associated with major changes in the respiratory system in lung volume and ventilation. The anatomical and functional changes during pregnancy are needed to meet the increased metabolic needs for oxygen of the maternal body and fetoplacental unit (Fig. 18.8). The changes occur very early due to hormonal and biochemical influences, even before the growing uterus impairs ventilation (de Swiet 1998).

Anatomical changes

The muscles and cartilage of the thorax relax, creating anatomical changes in the shape of the chest. These develop as pregnancy progresses and have implications for respiratory function (Fig. 18.9). The diaphragm becomes raised by a maximum of 4 cm and the transverse diameter of the chest is increased by 2 cm. The subcostal angle widens from the normal 68° to 103° in late pregnancy (de Swiet 1998). There is a change from abdominal to thoracic breathing, the main work of respiration being carried out by increased diaphragmatic movement during pregnancy. Some of these

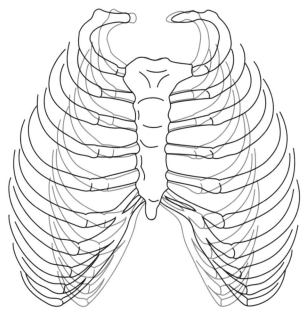

Figure 18.9 The ribcage in pregnancy and the non-pregnancy state showing the increased subcostal angle, the increased transverse diameter and the raised diaphragm in pregnancy. (Reproduced with permission from de Swiet 1991.)

changes occur in advance of the increasing size of the uterus.

Biochemical changes

Carbon dioxide

The tendency to overbreathe causes CO_2 to be washed out of the lungs so that the alveolar and arterial CO_2 concentration is lower than in the non-pregnant woman. This reduction in arterial PCO_2, from a norm of 35–40 mmHg (4.7–5.3 kPa) to a level of 30 mmHg (4 kPa), has been found in the luteal phase of each menstrual cycle before any embedding of a fertilised ovum is possible. It is the result of progesterone, which is thought to stimulate the respiratory centres directly, causing an increased sensitivity to CO_2 with a lowered threshold (Blackburn 2003). Progesterone also causes an increase in carbonic anhydrase in the red cells, which in turn facilitates CO_2 transfer, tending to decrease PCO_2 even without the presence of a change in ventilation. The resulting mild respiratory alkalosis is essential to create the gas gradients for exchange across the placenta (de Swiet 1998).

Progesterone may also contribute to the decrease in airway resistance by relaxing the smooth muscles of the bronchioles (up to 50%). This will reduce the work of breathing and facilitate a greater airway flow in pregnancy. Prostaglandins may also influence the smooth muscle in the lung tissue, with $PGF_{2\alpha}$ acting as a bronchoconstrictor and PGE_1 and PGE_2 acting as bronchodilators (Blackburn 2003). Increases have been seen in PGFs throughout pregnancy and PGEs in the last trimester but their role is not clear.

Oxygen

The increased alveolar ventilation not only causes a decrease in PCO_2 but also raises PO_2. However, this rise is only slight and has no significance on the oxygen–haemoglobin dissociation curve.

Respiratory parameters

The respiratory parameters discussed by de Swiet (1998) are summarised below.

Pregnancy causes less stress to the respiratory system than to the cardiovascular system: therefore women with respiratory disease are less likely to show deterioration in their condition than those with cardiac disease. Over the years, findings from studies both support and refute an increase in vital capacity during pregnancy. The truth may be that some, but not all, pregnant women increase or decrease their vital capacity during pregnancy and the difference may be related to body build. Where there is probably an increase, this has taken place from midpregnancy and is of the order of 100–200 ml.

Recent studies agree that inspiratory capacity increases by about 300 ml and this occurs progressively throughout pregnancy. Expiratory reserve volume reduces by 200 ml progressively from early pregnancy. Tidal volume rises throughout pregnancy from the normal 500 ml to about 700 ml, an increase of 40%. Therefore ventilation increases during pregnancy by the woman deepening her respirations and not by breathing more frequently. Minute ventilation rises by 40% in parallel with tidal volume. Oxygen consumption increases by about 16% and alveolar ventilation is increased by 50%, resulting in a physiological change to overbreathing.

Postpartum changes

The changes in the respiratory system rapidly return to normal after delivery. This is initiated by the fall in progesterone levels following delivery of the placenta and the reduction in intra-abdominal pressure following delivery of the baby. A rise in PCO_2 is seen within 48 h of delivery. Overall, anatomical changes and ventilation parameters return to normal between 1 and 3 weeks following delivery (Blackburn 2003).

CLINICAL IMPLICATIONS

Dyspnoea

As discussed above, the resting pregnant woman increases her ventilation, oxygen consumption and minute ventilation and there is a physiological change to overbreathing. The major influence leading to the overbreathing is central respiratory control but there are alterations in the lung volumes due to the anatomical changes mentioned above.

The woman may be uncomfortable with dyspnoea and giddiness and mention or complain of 'shortness of breath'. This is not always related to exercise but is more likely to be present when sitting down rather than when walking about.

Smoking

Smoking remains one of the potentially preventable factors associated with adverse pregnancy and birth outcomes and for this reason it is an important public health issue in pregnancy (Enkin et al 2000). It is probably one of the most dangerous avoidable risks taken by people and it is essential that both men and women who are thinking about starting a family should stop smoking for the health and safety of mother and baby (Tuormaa 1995). Cigarette smoking during pregnancy is common and between 1 in 5 and 1 in 3 pregnant women in developed countries report smoking.

There is strong evidence to suggest that cigarette smoking has harmful effects on the fetus in addition to the adverse health outcomes for the mother. The effects of smoking on human reproduction are discussed in Chapter 8, where the following list is addressed in detail.

Major reproductive effects of tobacco smoking on reproduction

- Male and female infertility.
- Very preterm birth.
- Low birth weight.
- Spontaneous abortions.
- Increased perinatal mortality (stillbirths + neonatal deaths in the 1st week).
- Fetal malformations.
- Reduced immunocompetence.

MAIN POINTS

- Respiration is the process by which the body exchanges gases with the atmosphere in order to provide for the changing needs of cell metabolism. Oxygen is taken from the atmosphere and transported around the body in the blood to the tissues. Carbon dioxide, produced as metabolic waste by the cells, is returned to the lungs and excreted into the air.

- The respiratory system consists of the airways from the nasal passages to the pharynx and larynx as well as the bronchi, bronchioles and alveoli of the lungs. Alveoli in the lungs provide an enormous area for gas exchange. Pulmonary surfactant helps to keep the membrane moist and also acts to maintain the patency of the alveolus.

- Inspiration and expiration are the two phases of breathing. Mechanical and neural factors are involved in the control of respiration rate. Expiration is a passive process and active expiration may occur when the need for gas exchange increases.

- Respiratory parameters include tidal volume, inspiratory reserve volume, expiratory reserve volume and residual volume. Respiratory capacities include total lung capacity, vital capacity, inspiratory capacity and functional residual capacity. Minute volume or pulmonary ventilation is the total volume of air exchanged with the atmosphere in 1 min. Alveolar ventilation is the volume of fresh air entering the alveoli each minute.

- The relationship between haemoglobin saturation and PO_2 is called the oxygen dissociation curve. Several factors can influence the affinity of haemoglobin for oxygen. An increase in carbon dioxide, hydrogen ions, 2,3-DPG and temperature move the oxygen dissociation curve to the right, enhancing oxygen unloading. An increase in carbon monoxide moves the oxygen dissociation curve to the left and inhibits oxygen transfer.

- The control of breathing involves the respiratory centre in the medulla and neural, mechanical and chemical events. Both peripheral and central chemoreceptors are able to respond to small changes in arterial PO_2 and PCO_2, affecting the rate and rhythm of respiration.

- In pregnancy, changes in the respiratory system in pregnancy are required to meet the increased requirements for oxygen and to accommodate the enlarging uterus. The changes are brought about by hormonal and biochemical influences as well as the mechanical effect of the enlarging uterus.

- Respiratory function is affected by the mechanical changes of pregnancy. The diaphragm is pushed upwards and the transverse diameter of the chest increases. Breathing changes from abdominal to thoracic, with increased diaphragmatic movement.

- Inspiratory capacity increases progressively throughout pregnancy and tidal volume increases by 40%. Ventilation during pregnancy increases by the woman deepening her respirations and not by breathing more.

- The pregnant woman may be uncomfortable with dyspnoea and giddiness perceived as shortness of breath. This is more likely to occur when sitting down.

- Smoking is a preventable factor associated with adverse pregnancy and birth outcomes. Some adverse effects on reproduction include male and female infertility, premature birth, low birth weight and increased perinatal mortality. It is an important public health issue in pregnancy.

References

Blackburn S T 2003 Maternal, Fetal and Neonatal Physiology: A Clinical Perspective, 3rd edn. W B Saunders, Philadelphia.

de Swiet M 1998 The respiratory system. In Chamberlain G, Broughton Pipkin F (eds) Clinical Physiology in Obstetrics, 3rd edn. Blackwell Science, Oxford.

Enkin M, Keirse M J N C, Neilson J et al 2000 A Guide to Effective Care in Pregnancy, 3rd edn. Oxford University Press, Oxford.

Marieb E N 2000 Human Anatomy and Physiology, 5th edn. Benjamin/Cummings, New York.

Sherwood L 2001 Human Physiology: From Cells to Systems, 4th edn. Brookes Cole, New York.

Tuormaa T E 1995 The Adverse Effects of Tobacco Smoking on Reproduction. Foresight, AB Academic Publishers, Tacoma, Washington.

Annotated recommended reading

Sherwood L 2001 Human Physiology: From Cells to Systems, 4th edn. Brookes Cole, New York.
This textbook provides an in-depth introduction to the function of human body systems and is suitable for undergraduate students in health-related studies.

Coad J, Dunstall M 2001 Anatomy and Physiology for Midwives. Mosby, Edinburgh.
This is an excellent textbook that provides an overview of the respiratory system and a detailed description of the adaptations to the respiratory system during pregnancy. The text is supported with clear illustrations and application to midwifery practice.

Chapter 19

The renal tract

CHAPTER CONTENTS

INTRODUCTION

The structure and function of the renal tract and how these change in pregnancy will be discussed within this chapter. Although the production of urine is also discussed, fluid and electrolyte balance and the regulation of acid–base balance are discussed in the following chapter in an attempt to integrate the roles of the respiratory and renal systems. This should be of value to the reader interested in the interactions between systems and may avoid turning backwards and forwards in the text to synthesise material. The role of renin and the angiotensin–aldosterone system and the control of blood pressure will be discussed in Chapter 20, p. 267.

KIDNEY FUNCTIONS

The kidneys play a major role in maintenance of homeostasis within the internal environment by their regulation of the volume and composition of the body fluids. Each day the kidneys filter several litres of fluid from the bloodstream, ensuring that toxins, metabolic wastes and excess ions are excreted from the body in urine. Other than the excretory function, the roles of the kidney are:

- regulation of the volume and chemical make-up of the blood;
- maintenance of balance between water and salts, acids and bases;
- production of the enzyme renin, which helps to regulate blood pressure, and production of the hormone erythropoietin, which stimulates red cell production in the bone marrow;
- conversion of vitamin D to its active form.

Also part of the renal system are the two ureters, which convey urine to the urinary bladder where urine is stored until it is voided through the urethra.

ANATOMY OF THE KIDNEY

The kidneys are paired, compact organs situated on either side of the vertebral column between the twelfth thoracic and the third lumbar vertebrae. They are situated behind the peritoneum and are attached to the posterior abdominal wall by adipose tissue. An adult kidney is bean-shaped with a convex lateral surface and concave medial surface. A cleft in the medial surface is called the **hilum** and leads to a space within the kidney called the **renal sinus**. The hilum is the site of entry and exit of structures that include the ureters, renal blood vessels, lymphatics and nerves. Each kidney weighs about 150 g and measures 12 cm long, 6 cm wide and 3 cm thick. The adrenal gland sits on top of the kidney.

Structure

Three layers of supporting tissue surround each kidney:

1. The **renal capsule** is closest to the kidney and is fibrous and transparent. This is a strong barrier that prevents infections in nearby regions spreading to the kidneys.
2. The **adipose capsule** is a middle layer of fatty tissue that helps hold the kidney in place and protects it from trauma.
3. The **renal fascia** is the outermost covering and is made of dense fibrous connective tissue that surrounds both kidney and adrenal gland and anchors them to surrounding structures.

Beneath the capsule lie three distinct regions: the outer **cortex**, the **medulla** and the inner **renal pelvis** (Fig. 19.1). The cortex has a light granular appearance. The medulla is darker and reddish brown with cone-shaped masses of tissue called **medullary** or **renal pyramids**. The base of each pyramid is broad and faces the renal cortex while the pointed apex (**papilla**) projects into a minor calyx. Several minor calyces open into each of two or three major calyces, which then open into the renal pelvis. The pyramids have a striped appearance because they consist of bundles of microscopic tubules. The renal columns are extensions of cortical tissue that separate the pyramids. Each medullary pyramid and its cap of cortical tissue is known as a **lobe** of the kidney. There are usually between 8 and 18 lobes in a kidney.

The renal pelvis

The renal pelvis is a flat funnel-shaped tube that is continuous with the ureter. The urine produced by the kidney flows continuously from the papillae into the calyces and down the ureter where it is then stored in the bladder. The walls of the calyces, pelvis and ureter contain smooth muscle, which contracts in peristaltic movements to propel urine towards the bladder.

Microscopic structure of the kidney

Each kidney contains over 1 million nephrons, which are the functional units of the kidney. Each nephron consists of a renal tubule and a tuft of blood vessel capillaries called the **glomerulus**. The end of the tubule, called a **Bowman's**

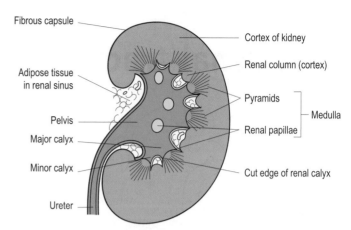

Figure 19.1   Coronal section through a kidney (from Hinchliff S M, Montague S E 1990, with permission).

capsule, is enlarged and invaginated to hold the glomerulus. The outer or parietal layer of the Bowman's capsule is composed of simple squamous epithelium and has a purely structural function. The inner or visceral layer that clings to the glomerulus is made up of branching epithelial cells called **podocytes** which form part of the filtration membrane. The branches of the podocytes end in **pedicles** or foot processes. The clefts between the pedicles form filtration slits or slit pores.

The capillary endothelium of the glomerulus is porous, which allows large quantities of solute-rich fluid to pass from the blood into the glomerular capsule. This fluid is called the **filtrate** and is processed by the renal tubules to form urine. A basement membrane divides the endothelium of the capillary from the epithelium lining the Bowman's capsule. The Bowman's capsule and its contained glomerulus is known as a **renal corpuscle** and is situated in the renal cortex. The structure comprising the capillary endothelium, basement membrane and podocytic epithelium constitutes the selective filtration barrier.

The remainder of the renal tubule is about 3 cm long and can be divided into four anatomically distinct regions: the proximal convoluted tubule, the loop of Henle, the distal convoluted tubule and collecting duct (Fig. 19.2).

The **proximal convoluted tubule** extends about 16 mm through the cortex. This region of the tubule is lined by large columnar epithelial cells, which have a brush border of microvilli on their internal surface for solute reabsorption.

The **loop of Henle** has a descending limb and an ascending limb. The thin-walled descending limb extends from the proximal convoluted tubule, dips down into the medulla and makes a U turn, moving back into the cortex by the thick-walled ascending limb. In this loop the columnar cells are flatter and contain less microvilli on their luminal (side facing into the lumen) surfaces.

The **distal convoluted tubule**, continuous with the loop of Henle, is comparatively short (about 4–8 mm) and leads into the **collecting ducts**, which fuse together as they approach the renal pelvis to form papillary ducts. These ducts open at

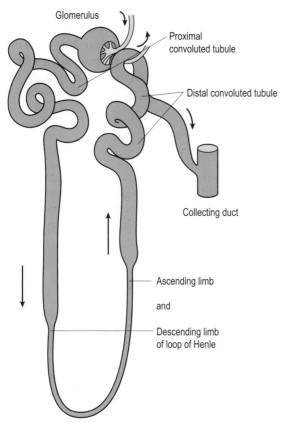

Figure 19.2   Microanatomy of nephron (from Hinchliff S M, Montague S E 1990, with permission).

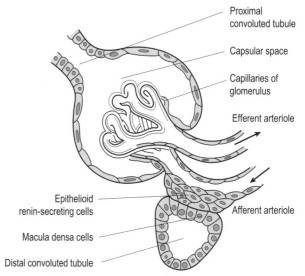

Figure 19.3   The juxtaglomerular apparatus showing the macula densa. (Redrawn from Creager 1983.)

the tips of the medullary papillae to discharge their urine into the calyces and renal pelvis. The first part of the distal tubule folds back to bring it nearer to the afferent arteriole. This forms the juxtaglomerular apparatus (see below).

Cortical and juxtamedullary nephrons

About 85% of the nephrons are called **cortical nephrons** because they are situated in the cortex (except where their loops of Henle dip into the medulla). The remaining 15% of nephrons are different in structure and are called **juxtaglomerular nephrons**. They are located near the cortex–medullary junction and their loops of Henle are found deep in the medulla. Their thin segments are more extensive than those of the cortical nephrons. The juxtamedullary nephrons have long thin-walled looping capillaries, called the **vasa recta**, running parallel with their loops of Henle.

Capillary beds of the nephron   Every nephron is closely associated with two capillary beds which form the microvasculature of the nephron. These are the glomerulus and the peritubular capillary bed. The glomerulus is unlike any other capillary bed because it is fed and drained by arterioles. Glomeruli originate from an afferent arteriole arising from interlobular arteries that permeate the renal cortex and drain into efferent arterioles. The peritubular capillary bed consists of capillaries arising from the efferent arterioles

draining the glomeruli. These capillaries cling closely to the renal tubules and empty into nearby venules. Just as the glomerular capillary bed is adapted for filtration, the peritubular bed is adapted for reabsorption. They are low-pressure porous capillaries. The additional vessels of the vasa recta play a part in reabsorption of salts.

The blood pressure within the glomerular capillary bed is very high for two reasons:

1. arterioles are high-resistance vessels;
2. the afferent arteriole has a much larger diameter than the efferent arteriole.

This high pressure forces fluids and solutes out of the glomerular blood along its entire length into the Bowman's capsule. About 99% of this filtrate is reabsorbed into the blood in the peritubular capillary beds. As blood flows into the renal circulation, it encounters high resistance, first in the afferent and then in the efferent arterioles. Renal blood pressure declines from 95 mmHg in the renal arteries to 8 mmHg in the renal veins. The resistance of the afferent arterioles protects the kidney from large fluctuations in the systemic blood pressure. Resistance in the efferent arterioles maintains the high glomerular pressure and reduces the hydrostatic pressure in the peritubular arteries to facilitate reabsorption.

The juxtaglomerular apparatus   The juxtaglomerular apparatus is a region found in each nephron where the distal convoluted tubule lies against the afferent arteriole as it supplies the glomerulus (Fig. 19.3). Where the two parts of the nephron touch, the cellular structures are modified. The afferent arteriolar wall contains juxtaglomerular (JG) cells. These are enlarged smooth muscle cells that contain granules filled with **renin**. They seem to be mechanoreceptors responding to the blood pressure in the afferent arterioles.

The **macula densa** is a group of tall, closely packed distal tubule cells that act as chemoreceptors or osmoreceptors responding to sodium chloride concentration in the distal tubule. These two types of cell are important in the regulation of filtrate formation and systemic blood pressure.

Blood supply

About 25% of cardiac output is delivered to the kidneys each minute. This is a higher blood supply than any other tissue. The two renal arteries arise high up on the abdominal aorta and enter the hilum, dividing in the renal tissue to form interlobar arteries between the pyramids. Arcuate arteries arise here and give rise to interlobular arteries, which branch to form the afferent arterioles supplying each glomerulus. Efferent arterioles emerge from the glomerulus and form a dense peritubular capillary network. Venous capillaries drain into interlobular, arcuate and interlobar veins and then into the renal veins. The renal veins drain into the inferior vena cava that lies to the right of the vertebral column. Therefore, the left renal vein must be twice as long as the right one.

Nerve supply

The kidneys are supplied by the autonomic nervous system. There is a rich supply of sympathetic fibres and a few parasympathetic fibres. These fibres supply the smooth muscle of the arterioles and the juxtaglomerular apparatus. Stimulation of these nerves causes vasoconstriction, a reduced renal blood flow, a reduced glomerular filtration rate (GFR) and the release of renin from the juxtaglomerular apparatus. The kidneys also have some sensory nerve fibres that allow the sensation of pain to be perceived. These fibres are stimulated by distension of the renal capsule in such situations as bleeding, inflammation or obstruction by renal calculi. Ischaemia may also cause pain.

RENAL FUNCTION

The production of urine

In an adult about 180 litres of plasma are filtered every day and 99% of the filtrate is reabsorbed by the nephrons. This results in the production of about 1.5 litres of urine per day. Fluid intake, diet and extrarenal fluid losses will affect the amount of urine produced (Sherwood 2001). Glomerular filtration is the first step in urine production. Prior to describing the physiology of glomerular filtration, some concepts to facilitate understanding will be briefly outlined.

Electrolytes

These substances are solutes that are electrically charged and dissociate into their constituent ions when placed in solution. Electrolytes are polarised into those carrying a positive charge (**cations**) and a negative charge (**anions**). They are located in both extracellular fluid (ECF) and intracellular fluid (ICF). In ECF, sodium is the cation (Na^+) and chloride is the main anion (Cl^-). In ICF, potassium is the cation (K^+) and protein the anion. Electrolytes are measured in milliequivalents per litre (mEq/L), which is the number of electrical charges per litre.

Diffusion

Diffusion is the movement of a solute molecule down a concentration gradient across a permeable membrane. This movement depends on the electrical potential across the membrane, the particle size, lipid solubility and water solubility.

Osmosis

Osmosis is the movement of **water** down a concentration gradient across a semipermeable membrane from a high water content to a lower one. The membrane must be more permeable to water than to the solutes and there must be a greater concentration of solutes in the destination solution for water to move easily. Osmosis is directly related to hydrostatic pressure and solute concentration but not to particle size. For example, in the plasma the protein albumin is smaller but more concentrated than the protein globulin: therefore, albumin exerts the greater osmotic force for drawing fluid back from the ECF into the intravascular compartment.

Osmolality is the concentration of molecules per weight of water, measured in milliosmoles/kilogram. **Osmolarity** is the concentration of molecules in water, measured in millosmoles/litre of water. The two terms are often used interchangeably.

Hydrostatic pressure

Hydrostatic pressure is the mechanical force of water pushing against cell membranes. In the vascular system it is generated by the blood pressure. In the capillaries a hydrostatic pressure of 25 mmHg is sufficient to push water across the capillary membrane into the extracellular space. It is partly balanced by **osmotic pressure**. The excess water moves into the lymph system.

The amount of hydrostatic pressure needed to oppose the osmotic pressure of the solution depends on the type and thickness of the plasma membrane, size of the molecules, concentration of the molecules on the gradient and solubility of the molecules. An example would be the movement of water in the glomerulus of the kidney.

Tonicity is the effective osmolality of a solution. Solutions can be **isotonic**, with the same concentration of particles as the body fluids; **hypotonic**, with less concentration of particles (will cause water to be pulled into the cells by osmosis); or

hypertonic, with more concentration of particles (will cause water to be pulled out of the cells).

Oncotic pressure is the overall osmotic effect of the plasma proteins, sometimes called colloid osmotic pressure.

pH and acid–base balance

The pH is a measure of the **hydrogen ion concentration** [H$^+$]. It is the negative logarithm of the hydrogen ions in solution on a scale of 1 to 14. This means that from one pH unit to the next there is a 10-fold change in hydrogen ion concentration. It is negative because as hydrogen decreases, the pH value increases. Low pH values with more hydrogen ions result in an acid solution and high pH values with a low hydrogen ion concentration result in an alkaline solution. A pH of 7 is neutral and most body fluids, with the exception of acid gastric juices (pH 1–3) and urine (pH 5–6), are just alkaline with a pH between 7 and 8. Many pathological conditions disturb the acid–base balance.

Glomerular filtration

Filtration is a largely passive, non-selective process in which fluids and solutes are forced through a membrane by hydrostatic pressure. The passage of water and solutes across the filtration membrane of the glomerulus is similar to that in other capillary beds, moving down a pressure gradient. However, the glomerular filtration membrane is thousands of times more permeable to water and solutes and glomerular pressure is much higher than normal capillary blood pressure. There is a high net filtration pressure (Marieb 2000).

This results in 180 litres of filtrate per day compared to the 4 L/day formed by all other capillary beds combined. Unlike other capillary beds, where water and solutes move back into the capillary as the balance of hydrostatic pressure changes, movement is one way only, from the capillary into the glomerulus. The **glomerular filtration rate** (GFR) is the volume of plasma filtered through the glomeruli in 1 min and is normally 120 ml/min.

The filtration membrane of the glomerulus lies between the blood and the interior of the glomerular capsule. As described above, it is a porous membrane made up of three layers:

1. the fenestrated capillary endothelium;
2. the podocytic visceral membrane of the glomerular capsule;
3. the intervening basement membrane.

The membrane allows free passage of water, solutes and small protein molecules (less than 3 nm in diameter) but larger molecules such as blood cells and larger protein molecules are prevented from passing through by the capillary pores. The basement membrane may also act as a selective molecular sieve. It is made up of anionic (negatively

charged) glycoproteins and therefore repels filtrate anions and prevents their passage; therefore the filtrate contains more cationic (positively charged) and uncharged molecules. The presence of the plasma proteins in the capillary provides the colloid osmotic pressure of the glomerular blood, limiting the loss of water to one-fifth of the plasma fluid.

Regulation of glomerular filtration

Intrinsic control by autoregulation The kidney can control its own blood supply over a wide range of arterial blood pressure, from 80 to 180 mmHg. This intrinsic system is called **autoregulation** and depends on alterations in the diameter of the afferent and efferent arterioles in response to a systemic blood pressure change. Factors involved in autoregulation may include:

- the myogenic mechanism – the tendency of vascular smooth muscle to contract when stretched;
- a tubuloglomerular feedback mechanism directed by the macula densa cells and solute concentration;
- the renin–angiotensin mechanism and renal vasoconstriction (see below);
- prostaglandin E$_2$ and renal vasodilation.

Extrinsic control by sympathetic nervous system stimulation When the body is stressed adrenaline (epinephrine) is released into the blood from the adrenal medulla. This causes strong constriction of the afferent arterioles and inhibits filtrate formation. Blood can be shunted to the brain and muscles at the expense of the kidneys. The JG cells are also stimulated to release renin, which activates angiotensin II to raise systemic blood pressure by generalised vasoconstriction. If there is a less intensive response, afferent and efferent arterioles are constricted to the same extent. This restricts blood flow out of the glomerulus as well as into it and GFR declines only slightly.

Tubular reabsorption and secretion

During the second stage of urine production, the filtrate is greatly modified as it moves along the tubule. Most reabsorption occurs in the proximal tubule where two-thirds of the filtrate is removed. Prior to this modification, filtrate is similar in every way to plasma, except it does not contain blood cells and large protein molecules. Figure 19.4 shows regional specialisation in reabsorption and secretion by the nephron.

Vital solutes such as glucose, amino acids and electrolytes are reabsorbed together with water. They pass from the lumen of the nephron, across the epithelial layer into the peritubular capillary network. A few substances are secreted into the filtrate from the peritubular capillaries. Mechanisms for reabsorption from the nephron may be active or passive.

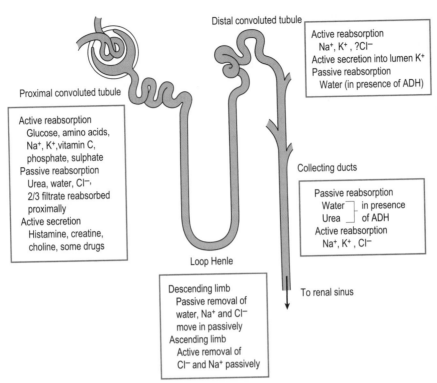

Figure 19.4 Regional specialisation in reabsorption and secretion in the nephron. Throughout the nephron, exchange of Na^+ for H^+, HCO_3 reabsorption and NH_2 secretion occur (from Hinchliff S M, Montague S E 1990, with permission).

Transport mechanisms in the nephron

Active transfer

Active transfer is the uphill movement of solutes against an unfavourable chemical or electrical gradient. Solutes move from a low to a high chemical concentration or electrical potential. Energy in the form of adenosine triphosphate (ATP) is used. Sodium is actively transported bound to a carrier protein. About 80% of energy is used in the transport of sodium ions. Substances actively reabsorbed include glucose, amino acids, lactate, vitamins and most ions. Many of these are cotransported bound to the sodium carrier complex (Marieb 2000). There is a transport maximum depending on the number of carriers available in the renal tubule. When the maximum is exceeded any surplus substance will be excreted in the urine. This is what happens when people develop glycosuria.

Passive transfer

Passive transfer is the movement of non-electrolytes and ions across cell membranes according to the chemical or electrical gradients that prevail. Solutes could be said to move downhill from an area of high to low chemical concentration or electrical potential (see Ch. 2). No energy is directly used in passive transfer. Passive transfer includes diffusion, facilitated diffusion and osmosis.

Positively charged sodium ions are moved from the tubule to the peritubular capillaries and create an electrical gradient that favours the transfer of anions such as HCO_3^- and HCl^- so that electrical neutrality is restored in the plasma and filtrate. Sodium movement also establishes a strong osmotic gradient so that water moves from the lumen of the tubule into the peritubular capillaries. This movement of water out of the tubule increases the concentration of solutes in the filtrate and they begin to follow their concentration gradients out of the tubules. This movement of solutes after the solvent is called **solvent drag**.

Non-reabsorbed substances

Substances are not reabsorbed because:

- they lack carriers;
- they are not lipid soluble and cannot diffuse through cell membranes;
- they are too large to pass through the plasma membrane pores in the tubular cells.

These include the end products of protein and nucleic acid metabolism – urea, creatinine and uric acid. Urea is a small molecule and about 45% is reabsorbed but creatinine is not reabsorbed at all. It is therefore a useful substance to measure when assessing GFR and glomerular function.

Tubular secretion

Tubular secretion is an important mechanism in clearing the blood of unwanted substances. Urine is therefore composed of both filtered and secreted substances. Secreted substances include hydrogen ions, ammonia and drug metabolites. Also secreted into the tubules are drugs such as penicillin and undesirable substances that might have been reabsorbed such as urea or excess potassium ions.

Regulation of urine concentration and volume

The role of the kidney in maintaining fluid and electrolyte balance and regulating pH is discussed in detail in the following chapter. Briefly, an important function of the kidney is to keep the solute load of the body constant by regulating urine concentration and volume. This is accomplished by a function called the **countercurrent exchange**. The term countercurrent exchange means that something flows in opposite directions through adjacent channels. In this case, the loop of Henle and its adjacent blood vessels, the vasa recta, are involved.

The descending limb of the loop of Henle is quite impermeable to solutes and permeable to water. Water passes out of the filtrate into the interstitial fluid by osmosis along the course of the descending loop and the solute load becomes concentrated. The ascending limb of the loop of Henle is impermeable to water and actively transports sodium into the surrounding interstitial fluid. The concentration of solutes in the filtrate as it enters the ascending limb is very high. Sodium is pumped out of the lumen into the interstitial fluid. The urine becomes more dilute and becomes hypotonic with respect to plasma.

The two loops are close enough to influence each other's activity. Water diffusing out of the descending limb produces the salty filtrate that the ascending limb uses to raise the osmolarity of the medullary interstitial fluid. The more salt the ascending limb extrudes, the saltier the filtrate in the descending limb becomes. This positive feedback mechanism is referred to as a **countercurrent multiplier**.

The collecting tubules add to the osmolality of the renal medulla by allowing urea to leak out into the interstitial space.

The vasa recta are freely permeable to both water and salt and provide another countercurrent exchange to regulate the content of the interstitial fluid while still maintaining the gradient established by the loop of Henle. Blood moving down the descending limb of the vasa recta gains solutes and loses water while in the ascending limb the blood loses solutes and gains water.

Formation of concentrated urine

Because water follows the osmotic gradients established by salt concentration, sodium and water balance are interrelated. Water balance is mainly regulated by antidiuretic hormone (ADH) from the posterior pituitary gland. The secretion of ADH is initiated by an increase in plasma osmolality, by a decrease in circulating blood volume and by a lowered blood pressure. If blood volume decreases, volume receptors (located in the right and left atria and thoracic vessels) and baroreceptors (located in the aorta, pulmonary arteries and carotid sinus) stimulate the release of ADH. The action of ADH is to increase the permeability of the renal tubular cells to water. Water absorption increases plasma volume and urine concentration is increased. This is called **facultative water reabsorption**. The amount of urine excreted is reduced and its concentration is increased.

The renin–angiotensin–aldosterone system

Sodium is regulated by aldosterone from the adrenal cortex. Sodium, along with its associated ions chloride and bicarbonate, regulates osmotic forces and therefore water balance. Sodium also works with potassium to maintain neurotransmission, regulate acid–base balance (via sodium bicarbonate) and participate in membrane reactions. The main anion in the ECF that neutralises the positive electrical charge of sodium is chloride. The transport of chloride is passive (following sodium) and concentrations of chloride vary inversely with concentrations of bicarbonate, which competes for sodium binding.

Concentrations of sodium are maintained within a narrow range of 136–145 mEq/L, primarily via renal tubular reabsorption. The average daily intake of sodium is 6 g but the need is only 500 mg. If sodium is taken in excess a combination of hormonal (aldosterone), neural and renal mechanisms (via the renin–angiotensin system) work together to control the balance (Fig. 19.5). Renin is produced by the juxtaglomerular apparatus in the kidney and stimulates production of the inactive blood peptide angiotensin I. This is converted into the active angiotensin II, which acts as a hormone to stimulate the secretion of aldosterone and cause vasoconstriction.

Natriuretic hormone

The atria of the heart produce antinatriuretic hormone (ANH), which promotes urinary excretion of sodium by reducing tubular reabsorption. The excretion of sodium results in a diuresis. The hormone ANH is synthesised by the atrial myocytes and secreted into circulating blood by the coronary sinus. Increased right atrial pressure stimulates this hormone release. Increased circulating blood volume causes increased pressure on the atrial myocytes and the release of hormone seems to be directly related to the degree of mechanical load.

THE LOWER URINARY TRACT

The ureters

The structural changes occurring in the lower urinary tract are important and need to be taken into account by those involved in caring for pregnant women. The two ureters are hollow muscular tubes (Fig. 19.6). Urine that is secreted into the renal pelvis drains down through the ureters to be stored

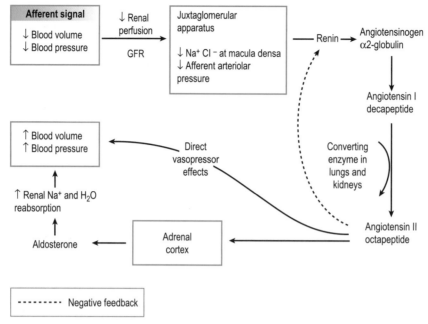

Figure 19.5 The renin-aldosterone system (from Hinchliff S M, Montague S E 1990, with permission).

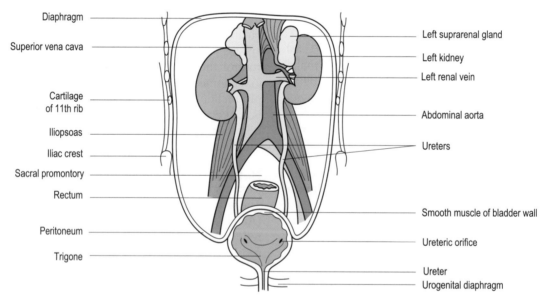

Figure 19.6 Anatomy of the lower urinary tract (from Hinchliff S M, Montague S E 1990, with permission).

in the bladder. The muscle walls of the ureter undergo peristaltic movements to propel urine towards the bladder.

Structure

The walls of the ureters are composed of the following layers:

1. a lining layer of mucous membrane in longitudinal folds;
2. a fibrous tissue layer containing elastic fibres on which the epithelium rests;
3. a smooth muscle layer consisting of three sets of fibres – a weak inner layer of longitudinal fibres, a middle layer of circular fibres and an outer well-defined longitudinal layer;
4. a coat of fibrous connective tissue.

Situation and size

The ureters lie outside and behind the peritoneum throughout their length. They extend from the renal pelvis to the posterior wall of the urinary bladder, crossing the pelvic brim anterior to the sacroiliac joints. The ureters run through the pelvic fascia and pass through special tunnels in the cardinal ligaments. They enter the posterior bladder wall in front of the cervix and run at an oblique angle for about 20 mm, which prevents the back flow of urine. They open into the cavity of the bladder at the posterior lateral angles of the **trigone**. In an adult, the ureter is about 30 cm long and 3 mm in diameter.

Blood supply, lymphatic drainage and nerve supply to the ureters

Blood supply is from the common iliac, internal iliac, uterine and vesical arteries and drainage is by corresponding veins. Lymphatic drainage is to the internal, external and common iliac nodes. The nerve supply is via aortic, renal and hypogastric plexi.

The bladder

The bladder is a hollow, distensible muscular organ acting as a reservoir for the storage of urine. It is roughly pyramidal in shape when empty and lies in the pelvis. It has a posterior base or **trigone** (resting on the vagina) and an anterior apex. The bladder lies in the pelvis when empty. The normal capacity of the bladder when full is 500 ml. It then becomes globular and expands upwards and forwards into the abdomen when full.

The trigone of the bladder is triangular in shape and each side measures 2.5 cm. The two ureteric orifices are situated on either side of the base of the trigone and the apex is formed by the internal meatus of the urethra. This region may be called the **bladder neck**.

Structure

The bladder walls are formed of the following structures:

1. A lining of transitional epithelium resting on a layer of **areolar tissue**. The lining, except for the trigone, is thrown into folds or **rugae** to allow it to distend. Over the trigone the epithelium is firmly bound to the muscle.

2. Three coats of smooth muscle (inner longitudinal, middle circular and outer longitudinal) called the **detrusor muscle**. This contracts to expel urine during micturition. Around the internal meatus the circular muscle is thickened to form the **internal sphincter** of the bladder. This thickened muscle is in a state of sustained contraction except during micturition. There is a special arrangement of muscle fibres in the trigone. The fibres, which run between the ureteric openings, form a band known as the **interureteric ridge**. The muscle fibres running from each ureteric opening to the urethral orifice are also raised into ridges.

3. The upper surface of the bladder is covered by peritoneum reflected off the uterus to form the **uterovesical pouch**. Its remaining surfaces are covered by visceral pelvic fascia.

Ligaments

There are five ligaments attached to the bladder:

- A fibrous band called the **urachus** runs from the apex of the bladder to the umbilicus.
- Two **lateral ligaments** pass from the bladder to the side walls of the pelvis.
- Two **pubovesical ligaments** attach the bladder neck anteriorly to the pubic bones. They form part of the pubocervical ligaments of the uterus.

Relations

- Anterior – the pubic bones are separated from the bladder by a space filled with fatty tissue called the **cave of Retzius**.
- Posterior – the cervix and ureters.
- Lateral – the lateral ligaments of the bladder and the side walls of the pelvis.
- Superior – the body of the uterus and the intestines lying in the uterovesical pouch.
- Inferior – the upper half of the anterior vaginal wall and the levator ani muscles.

Blood supply, lymphatic drainage and nerve supply

Blood supply is from the superior and inferior vesical arteries and drainage is by corresponding veins. Lymphatic drainage is to the external iliac and obturator nodes. The nerve supply is via sympathetic and parasympathetic fibres of the autonomic system.

The urethra

In the female the urethra is a narrow tube about 4 cm long passing from the internal meatus of the bladder to the vestibule where it opens externally. It runs embedded in the lower half of the anterior vaginal wall. The internal sphincter surrounds it as it leaves the bladder. As it passes between the levator ani muscles it is enclosed by bands of striated muscle known as the **membranous sphincter** of the urethra, which is under voluntary control.

Structure

The walls of the urethra consist of the following layers:

1. The lumen is thrown into small longitudinal folds and is lined by transitional epithelium in the upper half and squamous epithelium in the lower half. It is normally closed.
2. A layer of vascular connective tissue.
3. An inner longitudinal layer of smooth muscle.
4. An outer circular layer of smooth muscle.

Several small crypts open into the urethra at its lowest point. The two largest are **Skene's ducts** and correspond to the prostate gland in the male.

Blood supply, lymphatic drainage and nerve supply

Blood supply is from the inferior vesical and pudendal arteries and drainage is by corresponding veins. Lymphatic drainage is to the internal iliac nodes. The nerve supply to the internal sphincter is from the sympathetic system and the voluntary control of the membranous sphincter is achieved via sympathetic and parasympathetic fibres of the autonomic system.

The physiology of micturition

Micturition requires the coordination of autonomic nerves and somatic nerves. Motor and sensory sympathetic and parasympathetic nerves pass to and from the bladder but the sympathetic fibres appear to play a minor role. When the bladder contains about 300 ml of urine, stretch receptors are stimulated and sensory parasympathetic nerves convey sensations of fullness to the basal ganglia, reticular formation and cortical centres of the brain. The need to pass urine is perceived but can be voluntarily postponed until a suitable time. There is a centre for the reflex control of micturition in the second to fourth sacral segments of the spinal cord. When the bladder contains 700 ml it may become impossible to avoid micturition.

Nerve impulses from the cerebral cortex increase parasympathetic activity and decrease sympathetic activity, causing relaxation of the internal sphincter and contraction of the detrusor muscle. The external sphincter is relaxed, intra-abdominal pressure is raised and expulsion of urine occurs. Cortical control of micturition is learned in infancy and usually achieved at about 2 years of age.

MATERNAL ADAPTATIONS TO PREGNANCY

During pregnancy the renal system undergoes a variety of structural and functional changes with many of the structural changes persisting well into the postpartum period. It is important that practitioners understand these normal changes in order to be aware of the possible effects of pregnancy on women with renal disease, hypertension or following renal transplant (Baylis & Davison 1998).

The main changes of pregnancy are sodium retention and increased extracellular volume. Parameters used to assess normal renal function become altered and alterations in renal function may be difficult to assess.

The prenatal period

The maternal kidneys must act as the primary excretory organ for fetal waste besides dealing with the increased

Table 19.1 The changes in the renal tract in pregnancy

Organ	Change
Renal calyces, renal pelvis, ureters	Dilatation, elongation, increased muscle tone, decreased peristalsis
Bladder	Mucosa becomes oedematous and hyperaemic, incompetence of vesicoureteric sphincter, displacement in late pregnancy. Decreased bladder tone, bladder capacity increases to 1 litre.
Renal blood flow	Increases 35–60%
Glomerular filtration rate	Increases 40–50%
Tubular function	Increased reabsorption of solutes Increased excretion of glucose, protein, amino acids, urea, uric acid, water-soluble vitamins, calcium, hydrogen ions, phosphorus. Retention of sodium and water
Renin–angiotensin–aldosterone system	Increase in all components Resistance to pressor effects of angiotensin II

intravascular and extracellular volume and metabolic waste products (Blackburn 2003). As in many of the widespread physiological adaptations to pregnancy, renal changes are related to the effects of progesterone on smooth muscle, pressure from the enlarging uterus and cardiovascular alterations such as increased cardiac output and increased blood volume (Coad 2001). A summary of the main changes in the renal tract is presented in Table 19.1.

Structural changes – the kidneys and ureters

Kidney size Kidneys enlarge and the length may increase by 1.5 cm. This increase in size is mainly due to increased blood flow and vascular volume in addition to an increase in the interstitial space. Glomerular size increases but there is no change in the number of cells. Overall, the microscopic structure of the kidney is the same in the pregnant and non-pregnant woman.

Changes in the ureters The most striking anatomical change is dilatation of the renal calyces, renal pelvis and ureters (Fig. 19.7). These changes are accompanied with alterations in haemodynamics, glomerular filtration and tubular performance. The dilatation of the renal calyces, renal pelvis and ureters begins in the first trimester and is prominent in over 90% of women by the third trimester (Baylis & Davison 1998). The changes are mainly seen in that portion of the ureters above the pelvic brim and can be referred to as physiological hydroureter and hydronephrosis.

That portion of the ureters below the pelvic brim does not usually enlarge. This may be because the connective tissue

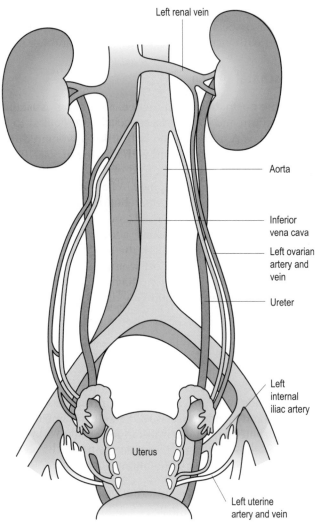

Figure 19.7   Obstruction of the right ureter at the plevic brim by an enlarged ovarian vein. Note that the ovarian vein enters the vena cava by several trunks and that the pelvic portion of the ureter is normal (from Hinchliff S M, Montague S E 1990, with permission).

surrounding the ureters hypertrophies and prevents the hormonally induced dilatation. The diameter of the lumen of the ureter increases, there is hypertrophy of the smooth muscle of the ureters, an increase in muscle tone and there is no decrease in peristalsis. The ureters elongate and become more tortuous in the latter half of pregnancy and are also displaced laterally by the growing uterus. The ureters may hold up to 25 times more urine and contain as much as 300 ml. The changes greatly increase the risk of urinary tract infection.

Physiological hydroureter   The cause of physiological hydroureter is not understood but the main factor may be the external compression of the ureters against the pelvic brim by the growing uterus. Growing blood vessels such as the iliac arteries and venous plexi may also add to the compression effect. Dilatation is more prominent in primigravidae where the firmer abdominal wall does not permit the uterus to expand anteriorly. In 85% of women the right

ureter is dilated more than the left, possibly because of dextro-rotation of the growing uterus due to the presence of the sigmoid colon in the left quadrant of the pelvis. The increased flow of urine in pregnancy may result in a small amount of dilatation.

Structural changes – the bladder

Bladder capacity doubles by term to approximately 1000 ml. Oestrogenic influences cause the trigone to become hyperplastic with hypertrophy of the bladder musculature (Blackburn 2003). The bladder mucosa becomes hyperaemic with an increase in size and tortuous route of blood vessels. The mucosa also becomes oedematous and is thus more vulnerable to trauma and infection. The decrease in bladder tone leads to incompetence of the vesicoureteric sphincters and there may be reflux of urine. This may be increased by the displacement of the bladder and of the terminal ureters.

Changes in renal physiology

Blood flow   There is a significant increase in renal blood flow in pregnancy. Blood flow increases by 35–60% by the end of the first trimester and then decreases slightly until the end of pregnancy. This is due to the increased blood volume and cardiac output as well as the decreased renal vascular resistance brought about by the relaxing effects of progesterone. There is vasodilation of the afferent and efferent glomerular capillaries.

Glomerular filtration   GFR increases 40–50% in pregnancy, with the increase beginning shortly after conception and peaking at 9–16 weeks before stabilising. The early second trimester level is maintained until term. Values for GFR may reach more than 150 ml/min. The volume of urine produced in 24 h is 25% higher during pregnancy. A greater proportion of renal blood flow is filtered and this increases the excretion of glucose, protein, amino acids, water-soluble vitamins and hydrogen ions.

No single cause has been identified for the increase in GFR in pregnancy. It is related to the increased renal blood flow. The decreased plasma oncotic pressure present because of the reduced concentration of plasma proteins due to haemodilution also increases GFR and there is involvement of hormones. Prolactin release from the pituitary gland has been found to induce changes in GFR in rats and is probably implicated in the human response to pregnancy. Prostaglandins may cause the renal vasodilation of pregnancy. Alterations in the renin–angiotensin–aldosterone system and in the role of antidiuretic hormone (see Ch. 20) accommodate the increase in blood plasma volume and thus add to renal blood flow.

Tubular function

Glucose   The rise in GFR increases the amount of fluid and solutes present within the tubules by 50–100%. Tubular reabsorption must increase to prevent the loss of sodium, chloride, glucose, potassium and water. However, tubular reabsorption rate and clearance may not accommodate the increased load and substances such as glucose and amino acids are excreted. Urinary glucose values may rise as much as 10-fold during pregnancy. There is a reduced ability of the tubules to reabsorb glucose in proportion to the amount in the filtrate (fractional reabsorption), possibly due to the changes in pregnancy steroid hormones (Baylis & Davison 1998). This leads to glycosuria commonly occurring in pregnancy. The changes are likely to be due to the increased plasma levels of oestrogen and progesterone and a similar effect is seen in some women taking the oral contraceptive pill.

Amino acids   Protein excretion increases during pregnancy and this can significantly vary on a day-to-day basis. Proteinuria is also more common during pregnancy with the extra excretion of amino acids. A value of 1+ on a protein dipstick is not abnormal and protein excretion up to 300 mg/24 h can be accepted. Protein excretion does not correlate with the severity of renal disease and may not indicate progressive deterioration of the disease. However, proteinuria associated with hypertension is serious and associated with increased risk to the woman and her fetus.

The postnatal period

During the postnatal period there is a rapid and sustained loss of sodium and a diuresis, especially on the 2nd to 5th postnatal day. A normal urine output for a woman during this time may be up to 3000 ml with voiding of 500–1000 ml at any one micturition. By the end of the 1st week urinary excretion of calcium, phosphate, vitamins, glucose and other solutes returns to normal but it may take up to 3 weeks to achieve normal fluid and electrolyte balance. Structural changes as described above may take up to 3 months to disappear although the structures will return to normal in 6–8 weeks in most women. This is important to remember when women who have had renal problems in pregnancy are assessed following delivery.

MAIN POINTS

- The kidneys play a major role in maintenance of internal homeostasis by regulating the volume and composition of the body fluids. Kidneys regulate the volume and chemical make-up of the blood, maintain balance between water and electrolytes and produce renin and erythropoietin.

- The kidneys are surrounded by three layers of supporting tissue: the renal capsule, the adipose capsule and the outermost renal fascia. Beneath the capsule lie three distinct regions: the outer cortex, the medulla and the inner renal pelvis.

- Each kidney contains over 1 million nephrons (functioning units). There are two types of nephron: superficial cortical nephrons (85%) and juxtaglomerular nephrons (15%). About 25% of cardiac output is delivered to the kidneys each minute (higher blood supply than any other tissue).

- The kidneys have a rich supply of sympathetic fibres and a few parasympathetic fibres. Stimulation of these nerves causes vasoconstriction, reduced renal blood flow, reduced glomerular filtration rate and the release of renin from the juxtaglomerular apparatus.

- In an adult about 180 litres of plasma are filtered every day and 99% of the filtrate is reabsorbed by the nephrons. As a result, 1.5 litres of urine is produced per day. Glomerular filtration is the first step in urine production.

- Filtration is a passive, non-selective process in which fluids and solutes are forced through a membrane by hydrostatic pressure. The glomerular filtration rate is the volume of plasma filtered through each glomeruli in 1 min (normally 120 ml/min). The presence of the plasma proteins (colloid osmotic pressure) limits the loss of water.

- An intrinsic system in the kidney controls blood supply over a wide range of arterial blood pressure. This autoregulation depends on alterations in the diameter of the afferent and efferent arterioles in response to a systemic blood pressure change. Extrinsic control is by sympathetic nervous system stimulation.

- During the second stage of urine production the filtrate is greatly modified as it moves along the tubule. Most reabsorption occurs in the proximal tubule where two-thirds of the filtrate is removed. Vital solutes such as glucose, amino acids and electrolytes are reabsorbed together with water.

- Transport across the nephron may be active or passive. Substances are not reabsorbed because they lack carriers, they are not lipid soluble and cannot diffuse through cell membranes or they are too large. These include the end products of protein and nucleic acid metabolism.

- Tubular secretion is an important mechanism in clearing the blood of unwanted substances. Urine is therefore composed of both filtered and secreted substances. Secreted substances include hydrogen ions, ammonia and drug metabolites.

- Water balance is mainly regulated by antidiuretic hormone. Sodium is regulated by aldosterone from the adrenal cortex. Renin is produced by the juxtaglomerular apparatus in the kidney and stimulates production of the inactive blood peptide angiotensin I. This is converted into the active angiotensin II, which acts as a hormone to stimulate the secretion of aldosterone and cause vasoconstriction.

- The two ureters are hollow muscular tubes through which the urine produced drains to the bladder for storage. The muscle walls propel urine through peristaltic movements. The bladder acts as a reservoir for urine and the normal capacity of the full bladder is 500 ml. The female urethra is about 4 cm long. Micturition requires the coordination of autonomic nerves and somatic nerves.

- The renal system undergoes structural and functional changes during pregnancy. Many of the structural changes are still present well into the postpartum period. The main changes are sodium retention and increased extracellular volume. Parameters used to assess normal renal function become altered and these alterations may be difficult to assess.

- Kidneys enlarge because of increased blood flow, and vascular volume and an increase in the interstitial space. That portion of the ureters below the pelvic brim does not usually enlarge because the connective tissue surrounding the ureters hypertrophies and prevents the hormonally induced dilatation. The ureters elongate, become more tortuous and are also displaced laterally by the growing uterus. The ureters may hold up to 25 times more urine and contain as much as 300 ml.

- Bladder capacity doubles by term to 1000 ml. Under the influence of oestrogen, the trigone becomes hyperplastic with muscle hypertrophy. The bladder mucosa becomes hyperaemic with an increase in size and tortuous route of blood vessels. The mucosa also becomes oedematous and is thus more vulnerable to trauma and infection.

- There is a 60% increase in renal blood flow by the end of the first trimester, which then decreases slightly until the end of pregnancy. GFR increases 50% in pregnancy, the rise beginning soon after conception and peaking at 9–16 weeks.

- Urinary glucose values may rise as much as 10-fold during pregnancy. The tubules have a reduced ability to reabsorb glucose in proportion to the amount in the filtrate (fractional reabsorption) and glycosuria commonly occurs in pregnancy. Proteinuria is also more common during pregnancy with the extra excretion of amino acids. Proteinuria associated with hypertension is serious.

- After birth there is a rapid and sustained loss of sodium and a diuresis, especially between the 2nd and 5th day, and it may take up to 3 weeks to achieve normal fluid and electrolyte balance.

- Structural changes may take up to 3 months to disappear although most women will return to normal in 6–8 weeks. It is important to remember this when women who have had renal problems in pregnancy are assessed following delivery.

References

Baylis C, Davison J 1998 The urinary system. In Chamberlain G, Broughton Pipkin F (eds) Clinical Physiology in Obstetrics, 3rd edn. Blackwell Science, Oxford.

Blackburn S T 2003 Maternal Fetal and Neonatal Physiology: A Clinical Perspective, 3rd edn. W B Saunders, Philadelphia.

Coad J, Dunstall M 2001 Anatomy and Physiology for Midwives. Mosby, Edinburgh.

Marieb E N 2000 Human Anatomy and Physiology, 5th edn. Benjamin/Cummings, New York.

Sherwood L 2001 Human Physiology: From Cells to Systems, 4th edn. Brookes Cole, New York.

Annotated recommended reading

Sherwood L 2001 Human Physiology: From Cells to Systems, 4th edn. Brookes Cole, New York.
This textbook provides in-depth information on the physiology of the renal system relevant for undergraduates in the health care profession.

Coad J, Dunstall M 2001 Anatomy and Physiology for Midwives. Mosby, Edinburgh.
This is an excellent textbook that provides an overview of the renal system and more detailed information on the adaptations of the renal system during pregnancy. The text provides good application to midwifery practice.

Chapter 20

Fluid, electrolyte and acid–base balance

INTRODUCTION

Cell function depends on the maintenance of a stable environment through the continuous supply of nutrients, removal of waste and homeostasis of the surrounding fluids. Therefore it is essential that the fluid, electrolyte, acid and base balances of the extracellular fluids be kept within a narrow range. For instance, changes in the composition of electrolytes can affect the electrical potentials of neurons and can move fluid from one compartment to another. Changes in pH can disrupt cellular enzyme systems. Cells also depend on a continuous supply of nutrients and the removal of metabolic wastes. Various organs are involved in coordinating this fluid balance and therefore the purpose of this chapter is to step outside of individual systems and examine the integration of systems in the control of this extremely important aspect of life. Understanding of the basic information on biochemistry provided in Chapter 1, p. 3, will be of benefit to the reader before proceeding with this chapter.

FLUID AND ELECTROLYTES

Body water content

In an adult, water accounts for about 50% of the body mass although this ratio can vary depending on age, sex, body weight and relative amount of body fat (Marieb 2000). Infants contain approximately 73% of water because of their lower bone mass and body fat. Men contain more water than women because of the extra amount of female adipose tissue and their lower muscle mass. Body fat leads to a reduction in water content as fat is the least hydrated of all body tissues so that obese people contain less water proportionate to their body weight. Older people have less water as their fat content is increased and their muscle content decreased. Also, as the kidney ages it is less able to concentrate urine so that more fluid is lost in urine. Other losses of body fluid can therefore be life threatening in the elderly. Table 20.1 provides a summary of the distribution of body fluid by weight in a 70 kg man.

Table 20.1 Distribution of body fluid by weight in a 70 kg man

Compartment	% Body weight	Volume (litres)
Intracellular fluid	40	28
Extracellular fluid interstitial	15	11
Extracellular fluid intravascular	5	3
Total body water	60	42

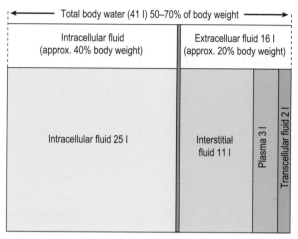

Figure 20.1 Size of the major body fluid compartments (from Hinchliff S M, Montague S E 1990, with permission).

Fluid compartments

There are three main **compartments** of the body where water can be found (Fig. 20.1). These are **intracellular fluid** (ICF), the fluid inside the cells, and **extracellular fluid** (ECF) which can be divided into **interstitial fluid**, the fluid between the cells, and **plasma**, the fluid inside the vascular system. Special types of ECF separate from interstitial fluid and plasma are lymph, transcellular fluid (secreted by cells), synovial, intestinal, cerebrospinal, sweat, urine, pleural, peritoneal, pericardial and introcular fluid. These fluids are usually considered to be part of ECF because of the similarity in composition. The sum of all of the above is the **total body water** (TBW).

Composition of body fluids

Solutes: electrolytes and non–electrolytes Water is the universal solvent and contains a variety of solutes. Broadly speaking, these can be divided into electrolytes and non-electrolytes. The **non-electrolytes** have bonds (usually covalent bonds) that prevent them dissociating into their component particles in solution and therefore do not carry electrical charges. These are mainly organic molecules such as glucose, lipids, creatinine and urea. **Electrolytes** are chemical compounds that do dissociate into ions in water. They are said to **ionise** and are charged particles capable of conducting an electric current. Electrolytes include inorganic salts, both inorganic and organic acids and bases and some proteins.

All dissolved solutes contribute to the osmotic activity of a fluid but electrolytes have the greatest osmotic power because each molecule can dissociate into at least two ions. An example is sodium chloride (NaCl):

$$NaCl \rightarrow Na^+ + Cl^- \qquad (20.1)$$

Electrolytes have the greatest ability to cause fluid shifts because water moves along osmotic gradients from areas of lesser osmolality to greater osmolality.

Differences in composition between intracellular fluids and extracellular fluids Each fluid compartment has its own pattern of electrolytes. Except for the high protein content of plasma, all extracellular compartments have a similar composition. Sodium is the most abundant ECF cation and chloride the major anion. In the ICF, potassium is the most abundant cation and the major anion is phosphate (HPO_4^{2-}).

The balance in concentrations of sodium in ECF and potassium in ICF reflects the activity of the **sodium pump** (see Ch. 2).

Movement of fluid between compartments

Water movement between plasma and interstitial fluid

The distribution of water and the movement of nutrients and waste products between the plasma in the capillary and the interstitial space occur because of changes in hydrostatic pressure and osmotic forces between the arterial and venous ends of the capillary network. The capillary membrane is semipermeable and allows interchange of fluids and solutes between the intravascular and interstitial fluid (IF) compartments.

The movement of fluid back and forth across the capillary wall is called **net filtration** (Starling's hypothesis). The major forces of filtration are within the capillary. Net filtration is the balance between forces favouring filtration, such as capillary hydrostatic pressure (blood pressure) and interstitial oncotic pressure, and forces opposing filtration, such as plasma oncotic pressure. As the plasma flows from the arterial to the venous end of the capillary, blood pressure falls, reducing the hydrostatic pressure. Oncotic pressure remains constant. At the arterial end of the capillary, hydrostatic pressure exceeds oncotic pressure and fluid is forced out into the interstitial space. At the venous end of the capillary, oncotic pressure exceeds hydrostatic pressure and fluid is drawn back into the capillary (Sherwood 2001).

Water movement between ICF and ECF

This water movement between compartments is a function of osmosis. Water moves freely across cell membranes so that the osmolality of TBW is normally at equilibrium. The ICF balance is maintained by active transport of ions out of the cell and interstitial hydrostatic pressure. However, normally, the interstitial forces are negligible because only a very small amount of plasma protein crosses the capillary membrane so that the major forces of filtration are within the capillary. Movements of respiratory gases, nutrients and wastes are unidirectional.

Water balance

Water intake must balance water loss and Table 20.2 summarises the normal daily water balance in a healthy adult.

Regulation of water intake

Regulation of water intake is by the mechanism of thirst, which is poorly understood. A thirst centre in the hypothalamus responds to either a drop in plasma volume or an increase in plasma osmolarity. It is probable that the salivary glands, which obtain their fluid from the blood, produce less saliva and the resulting dry mouth makes us drink. Thirst is quenched as soon as we have taken on board the right amount of water, even before there has been time for it to affect blood volume.

Regulation of water output

Water is lost from the body in ways that cannot be avoided. These are the **obligatory water losses** and explain why we cannot survive long without drinking. They include the insensible loss of water from the lungs and via the skin. Because of the large amount of perspiration lost daily, especially in a hot climate, humans are of necessity a riverine species. That is to say that most settlements before the advent of piped water were next to a river. Water in faeces must be added to the loss. There is an absolute minimum of 500 ml of urine per 24 hours that the kidneys must excrete even when the urine is concentrated to its maximum level possible.

Disorders of water balance

Oedema

Oedema is the accumulation of fluid within the interstitial space. It is a problem of fluid distribution and does not necessarily indicate excess intake. Oedema may be accompanied by signs of dehydration if fluid becomes sequestered (locked) within a compartment. It may be caused by factors that increase fluid flow out of the plasma or hinder its return. There are four major contributors to oedema:

1. **Increased capillary hydrostatic pressure** may occur from venous obstruction such as in thrombophlebitis, hepatic obstruction, tight clothing or prolonged standing.
2. **Reduced plasma oncotic pressure** follows the loss of plasma proteins found in renal failure, diminished production of plasma proteins found in liver disease or protein malnutrition.
3. **Increased capillary membrane permeability** is usually associated with inflammatory or immune reactions.

Table 20.2 Normal daily water losses and gains

Intake	Amount	Output	Amount (ml)
Drinking	1400–1800	Urine	1400–1800
Water in food	700–1000	Faeces	100
Water of oxidation	300–400	Skin	300–500
		Lungs	600–800
Total	2400–3200		2400–3200

Burns, crush injuries, cancer and allergy also produce this effect.

4. If the **lymphatic system is blocked** by infection or inflammation or lymphatic cancer or has had to be surgically removed in areas to prevent the spread of cancer, proteins and fluids accumulate in the interstitial spaces causing localised lymphoedema.

Clinical manifestations

Oedema may be generalised or localised. It is associated with weight gain, swelling of the tissues and puffiness. Clothing may feel tight. Movement may be limited and blood flow may be restricted. Wounds tend to heal more slowly and the risk of pressure sores and wound infections is increased. The sequestered fluid is not available for metabolic processes and dehydration may occur, for instance following burns. Hypovolaemic shock may occur. Treatment is tailored to fit the individual case and could include elevation of affected limbs, support stockings, avoiding prolonged standing, reducing salt intake and the prescribing of diuretics.

Electrolyte balance

Electrolytes include salts, acids and bases. Salts are the main electrolytes and are involved in many physiological processes. The four main electrolytes are sodium, potassium, calcium and magnesium. Salts are obtained from the food we eat and also, to a lesser extent, in our drinking water. Small amounts of salts may be released during metabolism. An example would be the release of phosphate during the breakdown of nucleic acids.

A major problem for humans is the love of salty food. This may be an acquired taste but is equally as likely to have an innate factor because of the need to replenish salts lost in perspiration. Salts are lost from the body in faeces and urine as well as in perspiration, as mentioned above. If we are depleted of salt our perspiration will be more dilute but, even so, in hot weather a good deal of salt can be lost.

The role of sodium in fluid and electrolyte balance

Salts containing sodium account for at least 90% of solutes in the ECF. Regulating the balance between sodium intake and output is a major function of the kidneys. Sodium is the most abundant cation in the ECF and is the main cause of osmotic pressure. Sodium does not cross cell membranes very easily (Ch. 2, p. 18) and is therefore ideal for controlling the ECF volume and water distribution in the body. Water follows salt so that a change in sodium content will be followed by a change in water content of a fluid compartment. Blood volume and blood pressure are linked to sodium balance and there is a hormonal regulatory effect by the hormone aldosterone, discussed more fully in Chapter 17, p. 231.

Aldosterone   Aldosterone is produced by the cortical cells of the adrenal gland and its release is mediated by the production of renin by the juxtaglomerular apparatus of the kidney, as explained in the previous chapter. The renin–angiotensin–aldosterone system is discussed fully in Chapter 19, p. 259. In brief, renin catalyses a series of reactions leading to the activation of angiotensin II, which causes aldosterone release. Normally, without the influence of aldosterone, about 75% of the sodium in the renal filtrate is reabsorbed in the proximal tubules of the nephrons of the kidneys.

If aldosterone levels are high, most of the remaining sodium is reabsorbed in the distal tubules and collecting ducts. If the permeability of the tubules has been increased by antidiuretic hormone (ADH, also known as arginine vasopressin or AVP), water will passively follow the sodium. There will be sodium and water retention. When aldosterone release is inhibited, there will be little reabsorption of sodium beyond the proximal tubules. Urinary excretion of large amounts of sodium will always result in the excretion of large amounts of water. The effect of aldosterone is to allow large amounts of sodium-free water to be excreted in times of sodium depletion. Like all hormones, aldosterone has a slow effect, taking hours or days to alter fluid compartments.

Other influences on fluid and electrolyte balance discussed in other chapters are the cardiovascular system baroreceptors, the regulation of ADH and the influence of atrial natriuretic factor. Oestrogens and glucocorticoids also play a part in enhancing tubular reabsorption of sodium.

Regulation of potassium balance

Potassium (K^+) is the main cation in ICF and is necessary for normal neuromuscular functioning and other processes such as protein synthesis. Potassium is quite toxic, especially to heart muscle. Both hyperkalaemia (excess potassium) and hypokalaemia (potassium depletion) can cause abnormalities of cardiac rhythm and even cardiac arrest. Potassium also acts as a part of the buffer system which controls the pH of body fluids. Shifts of hydrogen ions (H^+) into and out of cells is compensated by shifts of potassium (K^+) in the opposite direction to maintain cation balance.

Potassium balance is similar to sodium balance as it is maintained by renal mechanisms. However, whereas sodium loss or retention is controlled to meet the specific needs of the body, potassium loss is constant. Most potassium is reabsorbed by the proximal tubule but about 10–15% is lost in the urine despite any need changes in the body.

Tubular cell secretion of potassium   The amount of potassium secreted into the lumen of the tubule can be changed. When potassium levels in the ECF are low, potassium leaves the cells. The kidneys then conserve potassium by reducing the amount secreted into the tubule. There are three factors which alter the rate and amount of potassium secretion: the intracellular potassium content of the tubule cells, aldosterone levels and the pH of the ECF.

Tubule cell potassium   If a high potassium load is taken on, there is an increase in potassium in the ECF and then in the ICF. This triggers the tubule cell to secrete potassium into the lumen of the proximal tubule of the nephron. A low potassium intake will have the reverse effect. Low ECF potassium levels result in low ICF potassium levels and the tubule cells reduce their secretion of potassium.

Aldosterone   Aldosterone helps to regulate potassium ions as well as sodium ions. To maintain electrolyte balance, there is a one-for-one exchange of Na^+ for K^+ in the collecting tubules of the kidney and for each Na^+ absorbed, a K^+ is secreted. Therefore as plasma sodium levels rise, potassium levels fall. The adrenal cortex is also sensitive to high levels of potassium and will react by releasing aldosterone.

pH of ECF   The excretion of both K^+ and H^+ is linked to the reabsorption of sodium ions. They are cotransported with sodium and compete for places. If the pH of blood begins to fall, the secretion of H^+ ions increases and K^+ ions secretion falls.

Regulation of calcium balance

Almost all of the calcium content of the body, 99%, is found in the bones. However, ionic calcium found in the ECF is extremely important for normal blood clotting, membrane permeability and secretory behaviour (Marieb 2000). Calcium is like potassium and sodium in having a large effect on neuromuscular excitability – hypocalcaemia increases excitability and leads to muscle tetany while hypercalcaemia inhibits muscle cells and neurons and may lead to cardiac arrhythmias.

Calcium is extremely well regulated and is balanced by the interaction of two hormones: parathyroid hormone (PTH) and calcitonin. PTH is released by the parathyroid glands situated on the posterior aspect of the thyroid gland. Calcitonin is produced by the parafollicular cells of the thyroid gland.

PTH acts to release calcium into the blood from the bones. It also stimulates the small intestine to absorb calcium by causing the kidneys to transform vitamin D into its active form. Activated vitamin D is necessary for the intestinal absorption of calcium. PTH increases calcium reabsorption by the kidneys, while at the same time there is a decrease in phosphate reabsorption. Declining plasma levels of calcium stimulate the release of parathyroid hormone.

Calcitonin encourages the deposition of calcium salts in bone tissue and inhibits bone reabsorption. Although it is an antagonist of PTH, its role in calcium homeostasis is small.

Regulation of magnesium balance

Magnesium is essential as an activator of coenzymes needed in carbohydrate and protein metabolism. It is also implicated in neuromuscular functioning. About 50% of the body's magnesium is in the skeleton and the remainder is found intracellularly in heart and skeletal muscle and in the liver. Although the mechanism of magnesium balance is not well understood, the renal tubules are probably involved.

Alterations in sodium, chloride and water balance

These alterations mainly involve changes in tonicity and can be classified as isotonic, hypertonic and hypotonic (Table 20.3).

Isotonic alterations

Depletion causes contraction of the ECF volume with weight loss, dry skin and mucous membranes, decreased urinary output and symptoms of hypovolaemia: rapid heart rate, flattened neck veins and normal or decreased blood pressure. **Excesses** are usually due to overadministration of intravenous fluids, hypersecretion of aldosterone or the effect of drugs such as cortisone. There will be weight gain and a decrease in haematocrit and plasma proteins. Neck veins distend and blood pressure increases. Increased capillary hydrostatic pressure results in tissue oedema. If the excess is severe enough pulmonary oedema and heart failure may be the consequence.

Hypertonic alterations

Hypertonicity may be due to excess sodium (**hypernatraemia**) or depleted water (**dehydration**). Hypernatraemia occurs when the serum sodium concentration exceeds 147 mEq/L. This is rarely due to dietary excess. Causes include inappropriate use of hypertonic saline solution such as the administration of sodium bicarbonate to correct acidosis. Medical conditions leading to hypernatraemia include hyperaldosteronism and Cushing's syndrome with oversecretion of adrenocorticotrophic hormone (ACTH).

Dehydration occurs mainly in people who cannot take in water by themselves. Pathological causes include water loss in fever, respiratory infections, diabetes insipidus, diabetes mellitus, profuse sweating and diarrhoea. Clinical manifestations include thirst, dry skin and mucous membranes, elevated temperature, weight loss and concentrated urine except in patients who have diabetes insipidus. Isotonic salt-free solutions such as 5% dextrose can be given in both hypernatraemia and water loss until the plasma serum concentration returns to normal. Plain water cannot be given as it would increase intracellular fluid and cause cell lysis.

Hypotonic alterations

The most common causes are sodium deficit (**hyponatraemia**) and water excess (**water intoxication**). Hyponatraemia develops when plasma sodium concentration falls below 135 mEq/L. It is rarely caused by low intake and may be caused by vomiting, diarrhoea, gastrointestinal suctioning and burns. Hyperglycaemia increases ECF osmolality and pulls fluid from the plasma into the tissues.

Water excess may occur following overintake in thirsty people (**dilutional hyponatraemia**). Pathological conditions include reduced urinary output in oliguric renal failure, congestive cardiac failure and cirrhosis of the liver. Clinical manifestations include neurological symptoms such as lethargy, confusion, apprehension, nausea, headache, convulsions and coma. If symptoms are severe small doses of hypertonic saline can be given with caution. With dilutional hyponatraemias, oedema may develop. Sodium and water balances are calculated and appropriate intravenous solutions are given. Restriction of fluid may be necessary in dilutional hyponatraemias. A summary of hypertonicity and hypotonicity is presented in Box 20.1.

Table 20.3   Changes in tonicity

Tonicity	Mechanism
Isotonic (isoosmolar) imbalance	Gain or loss of ECF results in a concentration equivalent to a 0.9% NaCl solution (normal saline) with no shrinkage or swelling of cells
Hypertonic (hyperosmolar) imbalance	An imbalance with an ECF concentration greater than 0.9% salt solution due either to water loss or solute gain. Cells shrink as fluid moves out of them into the ECF
Hypotonic (hypoosmolar) imbalance	An imbalance with an ECF concentration of less than 0.9% salt solution due to either water gain or solute loss. Cells gain water from ECF and swell

Box 20.1   Summary of hypertonicity and hypotonicity

Hypertonicity		
Sodium excess	Water normal	Hypervolaemia
Sodium normal	Water deficit	Hypernatraemia
Hypotonicity		
Sodium deficit	Water normal	Hypovolaemia
Sodium normal	Water deficit	Hypervolaemia

ACID–BALANCE BALANCE

Almost all biochemical reactions in the body are influenced by the pH of their fluid environment (Ch. 1). The acid–base balance of body fluids is crucial to many biochemical reactions. There is a slight difference in pH between fluid compartments. Arterial blood pH is normally 7.4, venous blood and interstitial fluid have a pH of 7.35 while inside the cell the pH is 7.0. The fall in pH is due to the presence of acid metabolites. **Alkalosis** is present when arterial blood pH is over 7.45 and **acidosis** when arterial blood pH falls below 7.35. This could be said to be a misuse of the term, as even at pH of 7.0 a fluid is not acidic but neutral.

The structure of proteins, particularly enzymes, is affected by small changes in pH and significant alterations could disrupt metabolic processes and result in death. The pH scale may soon be replaced and the hydrogen ion concentration expressed in nanomoles per litre (nmol/L). The hydrogen ion content of arterial blood in these units is 40 nmol/L.

Chemical buffers tie up excess acids and bases as a temporary measure but cannot excrete them from the body. The lungs can dispose of carbonic acid by excreting carbon dioxide. However, it is the kidneys that dispose of the **metabolic** or **fixed acids** generated by cellular metabolism. These include phosphoric and uric acid and ketone bodies, the causes of **metabolic acidosis**. Also, only the kidneys have the power to regulate blood levels of alkaline substances. The kidneys are therefore the main regulators of acid–base status and act slowly and steadily to regulate the large acid–base imbalances that occur due to diet, metabolism or disease. Their most important mechanisms are the regulation of hydrogen ions (H^+) and the conservation or generation of bicarbonate ions.

The role of the kidney in acid–base balance

Regulation of hydrogen ion secretion

The tubule cells and the cells of the collecting ducts appear to be able to respond directly to the pH of the ECF. They then alter their H^+ secretion as needed to restore balance. The secreted ions are obtained from the dissociation of carbonic acid (H_2CO_3 (carbon dioxide + water)) within the tubule cells and for each H^+ ion secreted into the lumen, one Na^+ ion is reabsorbed into the tubule cell from the filtrate. This maintains the electrochemical balance. The rate of H^+ secretion varies directly with CO_2 levels in the ECF. The kidneys can respond to alterations in blood pH because CO_2 levels in blood are directly associated with blood pH.

Conservation of filtered bicarbonate ions

Bicarbonate ions (HCO_3^-) are an important part of the carbonate buffer system. In order to maintain the **alkaline reserve** (available bicarbonate ions) to act in the buffer system (see below) the kidneys must replenish stores of HCO_3^-

as necessary. The tubule cells are almost impermeable to bicarbonate ions and cannot reabsorb them from the filtrate. However, they can shunt bicarbonate ions generated within them into the peritubular blood. Dissociation of one molecule of carbonic acid inside the tubule cell releases one HCO_3^- ion and one H^+ ion.

There is a one-to-one exchange of bicarbonate ions depending on the numbers of H^+ ions secreted by the tubule cells. For each filtered HCO_3^- ion that is lost from the body, another one is generated from the dissociation of carbonic acid in the tubule cells. When large amounts of H^+ are secreted, equally large amounts of HCO_3^- enter the peritubular blood.

Respiratory regulation of hydrogen ions

Respiration and carbon dioxide transport have an important effect on the acid–base status (pH) of the body. The acidity of blood and body fluids is determined by hydrogen ion concentration, $[H^+]$; the hydrogen ions are the most highly reactive cations in the body. The intake and production of hydrogen ions varies according to the diet, energy output, disease and some drugs. To maintain homeostasis it is essential to both buffer these ions in body fluids and excrete them from the body via the lungs and kidneys.

These three mechanisms are brought into effect sequentially. Chemical buffers act within a fraction of a second and are the first line of defence against a change in pH. Respiratory rate is adjusted in 2–3 min. The kidneys are the most efficient regulator but it may take hours for the kidney to bring about a change in blood pH.

Excretion of hydrogen ions by the lungs

Any increase in PCO_2 and $[H^+]$ with a consequent fall in pH will be sensed by the central and peripheral chemoreceptors. Then there will be a rapid rise in alveolar ventilation, leading to a speeding up of the reaction:

$$H^+ + HCO_3^- \leftrightarrow H_2CO_3 \leftrightarrow CO_2 + H_2O \qquad (20.2)$$

This leads to the rapid excretion of excess CO_2 and H^+ ions. The reverse situation will occur with any decrease in PCO_2 and $[H^+]$, with a consequent rise in pH leading to a decrease in respiratory effort. These two mechanisms form an efficient response to short-term chemical changes in blood. The kidneys play the main role in long-term control of pH and acid–base balance.

Chemical buffer systems

Buffers are systems that minimise changes in pH. Acids are proton donors releasing free H^+ ions into a solution. Bases are proton acceptors and mop up free H^+ ions from a solution. Chemical buffers minimise the changes in pH by binding to H^+ ions when there is a fall in pH, i.e. when the fluid is becoming more acidic, and releasing H^+ ions when pH rises, i.e. when the fluid is becoming more alkaline. There are three major buffer systems in the body which work together:

1. the bicarbonate buffer system;
2. the phosphate buffer system;
3. the protein buffer system.

The bicarbonate buffer system

In a solution, strong acids dissociate into their component molecules and release H^+ ions. In a similar manner strong alkalis dissociate to release hydroxyl (OH^-) ions. The bicarbonate buffer system is important in both ECF and ICF. It is a mixture of carbonic acid (H_2CO_3) and its salt sodium bicarbonate ($NaHCO_3$) in the same solution. Carbonic acid is a weak acid that does not dissociate to release H^+ ions in neutral or acidic solutions. However, in a buffered solution in the presence of a stronger acid such as hydrochloric acid, bicarbonate ions of the salt will tie up the H^+ ions released by the stronger acid to form more carbonic acid:

$$HCl + NaHCO_3 \rightarrow H_2CO_3 + NaCl \qquad (20.3)$$

In the same manner, if a strong base such as sodium hydroxide (NaOH) is added to a buffered solution, the weak base $NaHCO_3$ will not dissociate to release hydroxyl ions (OH^-) but the carbonic acid will be forced to dissociate and release H^+ ions to mop up the OH^- ions released by the strong alkali to form water (H_2O):

$$NaOH + H_2CO_3 \rightarrow NaHCO_3 + H_2O \qquad (20.4)$$

In either Eqn (20.3) or Eqn (20.4) the result will be to drive the pH of the solution back to a biologically acceptable level. Potassium bicarbonate or magnesium bicarbonate acts as a buffer within cells where there is little sodium present. The bicarbonate ion concentration in ECF is normally about $25\,mEq/L$. The concentration of carbonic acid is about one-twentieth of the bicarbonate. It is freely available from cellular respiration and is subject to respiratory control.

The phosphate buffer system

The phosphate buffer system is almost identical to the bicarbonate buffer system with the control of H^+ ions occurring in a similar manner. Phosphate ions (HPO_4^-) replace bicarbonate ions in the equations. It is a very effective buffer in ICF and in urine, where phosphate concentrations are high.

The protein buffer system

Proteins in plasma and within the cells are the body's most plentiful and powerful source of buffers. In fact, at least three-quarters of buffering power of body fluid resides within the cells, and most of this reflects the buffering activity of intracellular proteins. Some amino acids have side groups called organic acid or **carboxyl groups** (COOH),

which can release the H^+ ion if needed. Other amino acid side chains can accept hydrogen ions. An exposed NH_2 group can bind H^+ to form NH_3 or release it as needed. This type of molecule is said to be **amphoteric**. Haemoglobin in red cells is an excellent example of a protein that acts as an intracellular buffer.

Abnormalities of acid–base balance

*   **Respiratory acidosis** is caused by any condition that impairs lung ventilation and gas exchange: rapid shallow breathing, narcotic or barbiturate overdose.
*   **Metabolic acidosis** can be caused by severe diarrhoea, untreated diabetes mellitus, starvation and excess alcohol ingestion.
*   **Respiratory alkalosis** is always caused by hyperventilation whatever the triggering factor.
*   **Metabolic alkalosis** can be caused by vomiting of acid gastric contents, diuretics that cause salt loss and severe constipation.

The effects of acidosis and alkalosis

Severe acidosis will depress the central nervous system and the person will go into a coma, shortly followed by death if not corrected. Alkalosis overexcites the CNS, resulting in muscle tetany, extreme nervousness and convulsions. Death may occur due to respiratory arrest.

Respiratory and renal compensation

If an acid–base imbalance occurs due to failure of either the lungs or kidneys, the other system will try to compensate. Changes in respiratory rate and rhythm are usually easy to observe. In metabolic acidosis the respiratory rate and depth are increased due to stimulation of the respiratory centres by high levels of hydrogen ions. The respiratory system blows off as much carbon dioxide as it can to reduce blood pH. In respiratory acidosis the respiratory rate is normally depressed and is actually the cause of the acidosis. In metabolic alkalosis respiratory compensation involves slow, shallow breathing, which allows carbon dioxide to accumulate in the blood.

MATERNAL ADAPTATIONS IN CHILDBEARING

Pregnancy

In order to meet the needs of the fetus and her own metabolic changes, a woman's body retains fluids and electrolytes. Renal processes are modified and a new balance is achieved, especially in sodium and water homeostasis (Blackburn 2003). This adaptation is achieved by the antidiuretic hormone (ADH) and the renin–angiotensin–aldosterone system.

Sodium

The increase in glomerular filtration rate (GFR) brings about an increase of up to 50% in filtered sodium. Tubular reabsorption increases so that 99% of the filtered sodium is reabsorbed. Sodium retention is highest in the last 8 weeks of pregnancy when about 60% of the retained sodium is utilised by the fetus. The rest is distributed in maternal blood and ECF.

The maintenance of sodium retention during pregnancy is influenced by multiple factors. Besides ADH and the renin–angiotensin–aldosterone system, a decrease in plasma albumin, the vasodilation effects of prostaglandins and the effects of the pregnancy hormones human placental lactogen (hPL) and oestrogen play their parts. Water accumulation is directly proportional to sodium retention.

Renin–angiotensin–aldosterone system

The increases in the components of the renin–angiotensin–aldosterone system and the decrease in response to the vasoconstrictor effects of angiotensin II are brought about by oestrogens, progesterone and prostaglandins and the alterations in sodium processing (Baylis & Davison 1998). Plasma renin activity increases by a factor of 4–10 times during the first trimester and remains elevated until delivery. Renin release is stimulated by oestrogens. Progesterone also has an effect by stimulating renal sodium loss, which causes the release of renin and aldosterone.

Angiotensinogen levels double by 8 weeks and increase 3–5 times by 20 weeks (Blackburn 2003). This is due to the effect of oestrogen on the liver, which manufactures the plasma protein. The plasma aldosterone level reaches a peak at 24 weeks of 2–5 times that in non-pregnant women. There is a second peak at 36 weeks when the aldosterone level can be 8–10 times that in the non-pregnant woman. Although angiotensin II rises during pregnancy, blood pressure actually decreases because of the decreased peripheral vascular resistance.

Water

Pregnant women accumulate about 7 L of fluid over the normal level to meet the needs of the fetus and their own altered metabolism. About 75% of the weight gain in pregnancy is due to the accumulation of fluid in the ECF. Interstitial fluid increases by about 1.5 L, beginning as early as 6 weeks and peaking at 30 weeks. This increase occurs despite decreases in plasma osmolality and colloid osmotic pressure, which would normally lower the fluid in the intravascular compartment. The vasodilation brought about by oestrogen and progesterone, which enables the vascular system to accommodate more blood volume, is probably a major cause as the increased volume is retained without

stimulating the production of ADH. Thirst and urine output remain in balance.

Antidiuretic hormone

Early in pregnancy plasma osmolality decreases, in particular the decreased solute load. ADH secretion and its effect on reabsorption of water are similar in the pregnant and non-pregnant woman. During pregnancy the osmotic threshold is reset so that ADH release occurs at the lower plasma osmolality. As mentioned above, this allows the vascular tree to accommodate more fluid volume with a lower osmolarity due to the haemodilution of pregnancy. Human chorionic gonadotrophin (hCG) may be the main influence on osmoregulation in pregnancy. Circulating hCG levels decrease the thresholds for thirst and also the secretion of ADH.

Acid–base regulation

The plasma hydrogen ion concentration decreases by 2–4 mmol/L in early pregnancy and the change is sustained until term. This makes the blood slightly more alkaline with a pH change to 7.44 from a non-pregnant value of 7.4. Plasma bicarbonate concentration also decreases. This mild alkalaemia is thought to be respiratory in origin since women normally hyperventilate in pregnancy, reducing their arterial PCO_2. Renal bicarbonate reabsorption and H^+ excretion appear to be unchanged in pregnancy. The blood changes, especially the reduction in plasma CO_2 level, place the pregnant woman at a disadvantage if she develops significant metabolic acidosis such as in diabetic ketoacidosis or acute renal failure.

Potassium and calcium excretion

There is selective retention of potassium during pregnancy, most of which is utilised by the fetus. However, urinary calcium excretion increases. This may be to combat high levels of circulating 1,25-dihydroxyvitamin D (calcitriol), which increases the absorption of calcium in the intestines. Serum calcium levels are raised and renal calcium reabsorption reduced.

The intrapartum period

During labour and delivery the renin–angiotensin–aldosterone system of both mother and fetus are altered with an elevation of the components. It is possible that this mechanism may assist uteroplacental blood flow during labour (Blackburn 2003). The result is to cause fluid retention. Labouring women may suffer from water intoxication if given too much intravenous fluid, especially if it contains oxytocin (which has an antidiuretic effect). This may produce symptoms of agitation and delirium in a few women although most women will cope with overenthusiastic fluid administration in labour (Millns 1991). Nutrition and fluid needs in labour will be discussed in Chapter 37.

A decrease in GFR and sodium excretion and an increase in vasoconstriction complicates the use of general anaesthesia. If the woman is stressed, this effect may be increased. It is important to maintain accurate fluid balance recordings in labour and after a general anaesthetic.

The postnatal period

Renal blood flow and GFR return to normal by 6 weeks following delivery. Urinary excretion of electrolytes and glucose returns to normal after 1 week. There is a diuresis with loss of sodium and water until prepregnancy levels are reached by 21 days.

MAIN POINTS

- Cell function depends of the maintenance of a stable environment. The fluid, electrolyte, acid and base balances of ECF must be kept within a narrow range. Cells depend on a continuous supply of nutrients and the removal of metabolic wastes.

- In an adult, water accounts for about 50% of the body mass although this may depend on the age, sex and weight of individuals. Water can be found in the ICF, and ECF (interstitial fluid and plasma). The sum of all of these is total body water.

- Water is the universal solvent and contains a variety of solutes, mainly divided into non-electrolytes and electrolytes. Non-electrolytes do not carry electrical charges and do not dissociate in solution. Electrolytes dissociate into ions in solution.

- Dissolved solutes all contribute to the osmotic activity of fluid but electrolytes have the greatest osmotic power because each molecule can dissociate into at least two ions. Electrolytes have the greatest ability to cause fluid shifts.

- The movement of water, nutrients and waste products across the capillary membrane is due to changes in hydrostatic pressure and osmotic forces between the arterial and venous ends of the capillary network. The movement of fluid across the capillary wall is called net filtration.

- Water intake must balance water loss. Regulation of water intake is by the mechanism of thirst. Water is lost via the lungs, skin, urine and faeces.

- Oedema is the accumulation of fluid within the interstitial space. It is a problem of fluid distribution and does not necessarily indicate excess intake. Oedema may be generalised or localised and is associated with weight gain, swelling and puffiness.

- Electrolytes include salts, acids and bases. Salts are the main electrolytes and these are obtained through ingestion of food and also, to a lesser extent, in drinking water. Regulating the balance between sodium intake and output is a major function of the kidneys.

- Baroreceptors, ADH and atrial natriuretic factor influence fluid and electrolyte balance. Oestrogens and glucocorticoids also play a part in enhancing tubular reabsorption of sodium.

- Potassium is the main cation in ICF and is necessary for normal neuromuscular functioning and other processes such as protein synthesis. It also acts as a part of the buffer system to control the pH of body fluids. Potassium balance is maintained by renal mechanisms.

- Aldosterone helps to regulate potassium ions as well as sodium ions and as plasma sodium levels rise, potassium levels fall. If the pH of blood begins to fall then the secretion of H^+ ions increases and K^+ ions secretion falls.

- Ionic calcium found in the ECF is extremely important for normal blood clotting, membrane permeability and secretory behaviour. Calcium is extremely well regulated by the interaction of parathyroid hormone and calcitonin. Calcium has a large effect on neuromuscular excitability. Hypocalcaemia increases excitability, leading to muscle tetany, while hypercalcaemia may lead to cardiac arrhythmias.

- Almost all biochemical reactions in the body are influenced by the pH of their fluid environment. There is a slight difference in pH between fluid compartments. The structure of proteins, particularly enzymes, is affected by small changes in pH and significant alterations could disrupt metabolic processes and result in death.

- Chemical buffers neutralise excess acids and bases but cannot excrete them from the body. The lungs can dispose of carbonic acid by excreting carbon dioxide but the kidneys dispose of the metabolic acids or fixed acids generated by cellular metabolism. Bicarbonate ions are important for the carbonate buffer system.

- Respiration and carbon dioxide transport have an important effect on the acid–base status of the body. The hydrogen ion concentration [H^+] determines the acidity of blood and body fluids. It is essential to buffer these ions to maintain homeostasis. Chemical buffers act in less than a second and are the first line of defence against a change in pH. There are three chemical buffer systems in the body which work together: the bicarbonate, the phosphate and the protein buffer systems.

- Respiratory acidosis is caused by any condition that impairs lung ventilation and gas exchange. Metabolic acidosis can be caused by severe diarrhoea, untreated diabetes mellitus, starvation or excess alcohol ingestion. Respiratory alkalosis is always caused by hyperventilation. Metabolic alkalosis can be caused by vomiting of acid gastric content, some diuretics or severe constipation.

- Severe acidosis will depress the CNS and lead to a comatose state, followed shortly by death if not corrected. Alkalosis overexcites the CNS, resulting in muscle tetany, extreme nervousness and convulsions. Death may occur due to respiratory arrest.

- The pregnant woman's body retains fluids and electrolytes and renal processes are modified to achieve a new balance, especially in sodium and water. Changes are due to the ADH and the renin–angiotensin–aldosterone system. Pregnant women accumulate about 7 L more water and about 75% of the weight gain due to the accumulation of ECF fluid.

- The plasma [H^+] decreases early in pregnancy and the change is sustained until term. This makes the blood slightly more alkaline. Plasma bicarbonate concentration also decreases. This mild alkalaemia may be respiratory in origin as pregnant women hyperventilate.

- There is selective retention of potassium during pregnancy, most of which is utilised by the fetus. However, urinary calcium excretion increases. Serum calcium levels are raised and renal calcium reabsorption reduced.

- During labour and delivery the renin–angiotensin–aldosterone system of mother and fetus are altered with an increase in the components. This causes fluid retention. Labouring women may suffer from water intoxication if given too much intravenous fluid, especially if it contains oxytocin (antidiuretic effect). Accurate fluid balance should be maintained in labour and following a general anaesthetic.

- Renal blood flow and GFR return to normal by 6 weeks postpartum. Urinary excretion of electrolytes and glucose returns to normal after 1 week. There is a diuresis with loss of sodium and water until prepregnancy levels are reached by 21 days.

References

Baylis C, Davison J 1998 The urinary system. In Chamberlain G, Broughton Pipkin F (eds) Clinical Physiology in Obstetrics, 3rd edn. Blackwell Science, Oxford.

Blackburn S T 2003 Maternal, Fetal and Neonatal Physiology: A Clinical Perspective, 3rd edn. W B Saunders, Philadelphia.

Marieb E N 2000 Human Anatomy and Physiology, 5th edn. Benjamin/Cummings, New York.

Millns J P 1991 Fluid balance in labour. Current Obstetrics and Gynaecology 1:35–40.

Sherwood L 2001 Human Physiology: From Cells to Systems, 4th edn. Brooks Cole, New York.

Annotated recommended reading

Chamberlain G, Broughton Pipkin F (eds) Clinical Physiology in Obstetrics, 3rd edn. Blackwell Science, Oxford.
This textbook provides a detailed description of the major changes that occur in the body systems during pregnancy. There is an extensive review of the literature, extending from classical research studies to the more recent research findings.

Sherwood L 2001 Human Physiology: From Cells to Systems, 4th edn. Brooks Cole, New York.
This is a further textbook that presents a detailed overview of the maintenance of fluid balance. Attention is given to the nature of the structure and function of body systems, their interrelationships and homeostasis.

Chapter 21

The gastrointestinal tract

INTRODUCTION

In general, the form in which we eat food is unsuitable for use by the body for growth, repair and energy production. A healthy digestive system is essential to maintaining life by converting the foods we eat into the raw materials necessary to build and fuel our body's cells. The organs of the digestive system can be divided in to two main groups: alimentary canal (*aliment = nourish*) and the accessory digestive organs, which include teeth, tongue, salivary glands, liver, gall bladder and pancreas. The alimentary canal, also called the gastrointestinal tract, will be discussed in this chapter followed by significant changes in pregnancy. The accessory organs of salivary glands, liver, gall bladder and pancreas will be discussed fully in Chapter 22 and nutrition in Chapter 23.

ANATOMY OF THE GASTROINTESTINAL TRACT

The adult gastrointestinal tract (GI tract) is a continuous, coiled, fibromuscular tube of variable diameter about 4.5 metres long, open to the external environment at both ends and extending from the mouth to the anus. It varies in structure and function throughout its length. The organs of the GI tract are the mouth, pharynx, oesophagus, stomach, small intestine and large intestine (Fig. 21.1). Readers are referred to Marieb (2000) for detailed anatomy. A brief description is given below.

The basic structure of the gastrointestinal tract is the same throughout its course. From the oesophagus to the anal canal, the walls of every organ consist of the same four basic layers (Fig. 21.2):

1. The **mucosal layer** is innermost and lines the tube. This layer is very variable along the length of the tube depending on the required function. The lumen is lined with stratified epithelial cells from which mucus-secreting cells develop. The turnover rate for the epithelial cells is high because of the amount of frictional damage. The epithelial cells are supported by a sheet of connective

tissue, called the **lamina propria**, and beneath that is a thin layer of smooth muscle called the **muscularis mucosae**. The mucosal layer also contains patches of lymphoid tissue, which defend the tract against microorganisms.

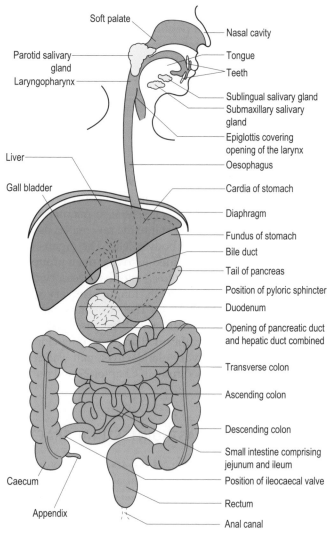

Figure 21.1   Diagrammatic representation of the gastrointestinal tract (from Hinchliff S M, Montague S E 1990, with permission).

2. The **submucosa** consists of loose connective tissue that supports blood vessels, lymphatics and nerves. The nerve fibres are called the **submucosal** or **Meissner's plexus**.

3. The **muscularis layer** is formed of smooth involuntary muscle fibres, bound together in sheets called **fasciculi**. There are two sheets: an inner circular layer and an outer longitudinal layer. In the stomach there is an additional oblique layer. Between the two layers of muscle fibres is a network of nerve fibres called the **myenteric** or **Auerbach's plexus**. The muscle fibres respond rhythmically to stimulation by the autonomic nervous system and some hormones. They respond slowly and less forcefully than striated muscle fibres and their contractions are not as finely controlled.

4. The **adventitia** or **serosa** (visceral peritoneum) is the outermost protective layer and is formed of connective tissue and squamous, serous epithelium. It is continuous with the mesentery of the abdominal cavity and supports blood vessels and nerves.

The peritoneum

Most of the digestive organs lie in the abdominopelvic cavity. All body cavities contain friction-reducing serous membranes and the peritoneum of the abdominopelvic cavity is the largest of these membranes. The visceral peritoneum covers the external surface of most of the digestive organs and is continuous with the parietal peritoneum that lines the walls of the abdominopelvic cavity. Between the two layers is the **peritoneal cavity** containing fluid secreted by the serous membranes.

The mesentery

Connecting the visceral and parietal layers of the peritoneum is a fused double layer of peritoneum called the mesentery. This supports the blood vessels, lymphatics and nerves to the digestive organs and helps support the organs. It also stores fat and is able to wall off areas of infection and inflammation to prevent the spread of peritonitis. Another fold of peritoneum, the **lesser omentum**, runs

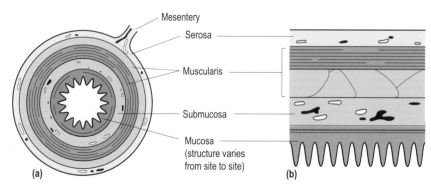

Figure 21.2   Generalised structure of the gut wall. (a) Cross-section; (b) longitudinal section (from Hinchliff S M, Montague S E 1990, with permission).

from the liver to the stomach. The **greater omentum** is a fold of peritoneum that hangs in front of the intestines and is reflected off the stomach. In most places the mesentery is attached to the posterior abdominal wall. The peritoneum surrounding the small intestine is like a fan with the small intestine attached to its outer edge.

Blood supply

Branches of the abdominal aorta serve the digestive organs and the special hepatic portal circulation. These include the hepatic, splenic and left gastric branches of the coeliac trunk supplying the liver, spleen and stomach and the superior and inferior mesenteric arteries supplying the small and large intestines. The hepatic portal circulation collects nutrient-rich venous blood from the digestive organs and takes it to the liver, as discussed in Chapter 22.

CONTROL OF THE GASTROINTESTINAL TRACT

Autonomic nervous system

Nerve fibres from the autonomic nervous system (ANS) control the function of the gastrointestinal tract. The submucosal and myenteric nerve plexi are the local tracts. In the submucosal plexus, parasympathetic nerve fibres synapse with ganglion cells present in small clusters in the submucosal tissue. Postganglionic fibres, accompanied by some sympathetic fibres, leave the ganglion cells and send impulses to the glands and smooth muscle of the tract.

In the myenteric plexus parasympathetic nerve fibres synapse with ganglion cells which lie in large clusters between the circular and longitudinal fibres of the muscularis layer. Postganglionic fibres leave the ganglion cells and send impulses to the smooth muscle. Sympathetic fibres also supply this muscle. Both plexi run the length of the gut and receive both sympathetic and parasympathetic nerve fibres. The two plexi are connected and activity in one can affect the other. Stimulation at the upper end of the gastrointestinal tract can be transmitted to more distal parts; for instance, stimulation of gastric and intestinal enzyme secretion follows entry of food into the oesophagus.

Parasympathetic activity leads to an increase in both the motility and secretory functions of the tract and to relaxation of the gut sphincters. The vagus nerve, which is the tenth cranial nerve, is the source of parasympathetic supply to the oesophagus, stomach, pancreas, bile duct, small intestine and proximal colon. The parasympathetic supply to the distal colon is via the nervi erigentes from the sacral outflow.

Sympathetic activity leads to a decrease in blood supply to the gut with a decrease in secretions and in gut motility. There is contraction of the gut sphincters. As in other parts of the body, there are two types of catecholamine receptors in the gut: α and β_2 receptors. Note that β_1 receptors are present only in cardiac muscle. Stimulation of α receptors causes contraction of the smooth muscle of the gastrointestinal tract while stimulation of the β_2 receptors causes relaxation.

Regulatory chemicals

Two chemicals produced by the tract help in neural regulation. These are substance P and serotonin:

1. **Substance P**, a small peptide of only 11 amino acids, is found in high concentrations in the gut and may be a chemical mediator. It acts like a neurotransmitter and is referred to as a regulatory peptide or neuropeptide. It is involved in the conduction of pain impulses but brings about vasodilation and contraction of non-vascular smooth muscle.
2. **Serotonin** (5-hydroxytryptamine or 5-HT) is synthesised in the myenteric plexus and may also act as an interneuronal transmitter substance.

FUNCTIONS OF THE GASTROINTESTINAL TRACT

The role of the gastrointestinal (alimentary) tract is to alter food so that it can be utilised by the body cells. Six processes can be described:

1. ingestion;
2. propulsion;
3. mastication;
4. mechanical and chemical digestion;
5. absorption;
6. elimination of non-usable residues as faeces.

Ingestion and mastication

These two processes take place in the mouth. Food is mixed with saliva, broken into small pieces by the teeth and propelled backwards into the oesophagus by the tongue. The tongue allows us to taste food. On its superior surface are numerous peg-like projections called **papillae**. These contain most of the 10 000 taste buds, which allow differentiation between the four taste modalities – sweet, sour, salty and bitter (Marieb 2000). All taste buds have the potential for recognising the four tastes, although particular ones are associated with one taste. The four tastes result in different neural firing patterns, which are interpreted in the cerebral cortex. Taste is aided by the sense of smell, which sends impulses to the brain via the olfactory nerve. This is why any inflammation and hypersecretion of the nasal mucosa, which may occur in pregnancy, will result in a loss or alteration of taste.

Saliva

The salivary glands and the production of saliva are discussed more fully in the next chapter. The three pairs of salivary glands – the parotid, submaxillary and sublingual glands – produce 1.5 L of saliva daily, consisting of 99% water and with a pH of 7.0. Saliva contains the digestive enzyme salivary **α amylase** which acts upon cooked starch to convert polysaccharides into disaccharides. It facilitates the formation of a bolus of partly broken up food ready to swallow, once lubricated by salivary mucins. Saliva is produced in response to the cerebral perception of the thought, sight or smell of food or the presence of food in the mouth.

The ingested and masticated food is propelled down the oesophagus into the stomach for digestion of the food to continue. The process is called **deglutition**. The tongue contracts and presses the bolus of food against the hard palate in the roof of the mouth. It then arches backwards and the bolus of food is propelled into the oropharynx.

THE STOMACH

Chemical breakdown of food by the secretion of enzymes begins in the stomach and is completed in the small intestine. The stomach is 25 cm long and lies in the left side of the abdominal cavity partly hidden by the diaphragm and liver. It is continuous with the oesophagus above and the duodenum below. When empty, it is J-shaped. Its mucosal layer has folds (**rugae**) which allow distension. The rugae are further folded, providing a large absorptive surface, and contain millions of deep **gastric pits** with microscopic gastric glands that produce gastric juice.

Functions of the stomach

- A reservoir for food.
- Production of the intrinsic factor.
- Gastric absorption.
- A churn to mix food.
- Secretion of mucus, hormones and gastric juice.

A reservoir for food

At rest the stomach's capacity is only 50 ml, but receptive relaxation of the stomach wall musculature can allow distension by up to 1.5 L. Under exceptional circumstances the stomach can hold 4 L of content. The pyloric sphincter prevents a too rapid transfer of food to the small intestine.

Production of the intrinsic factor

The intrinsic factor is a glycoprotein necessary for the absorption of **vitamin B_{12}** (cyanocobolamin) produced by the gastric parietal cells, which also produce gastric acid. Intrinsic factor binds to vitamin B_{12} in the terminal ileum of the small intestine to form a complex which appears to bind to receptors in the wall of the ileum and is transferred into the blood. Vitamin B_{12} is required for the maintenance of healthy myelin sheaths around the nerves and also for the formation of red blood cells in the bone marrow. Lack of

vitamin B_{12} may lead to a megaloblastic anaemia. The resulting pernicious anaemia may lead to subacute combined degeneration of the spinal cord.

Gastric absorption

Food that has reached the stomach is only partly broken down there and many of the molecules are still too large to be absorbed. There are also no carrier systems present in the gastric mucosa. Water and some drugs such as aspirin (acetylsalicylic acid), which is a weak acid, can be absorbed from the stomach. Absorption of aspirin lowers intracellular pH and may cause damage, leading to gastric irritation and bleeding.

A churn to mix food

The stomach converts food to a thick soup consistency by mixing it with gastric secretions. This also dilutes the food and makes it compatible with the extracellular fluid in the duodenum. The semiliquid, formed by waves of peristalsis of the smooth muscle in the stomach wall, is called **chyme**.

Secretion of mucus

Mucus is produced by the cells in the necks of the deep gastric glands in both the cardiac and pyloric sphincters. It adheres to the gastric mucosa to protect the stomach from being digested by the proteolytic gastric enzyme **pepsin**. The layer of mucus that protects the mucosa must be 1 mm thick.

Secretion of hormones

Enteroendocrine cells release a variety of hormones, which diffuse into blood capillaries and are returned to the GI tract to influence digestive system target organs. These include gastrin, serotonin, cholecystokinin, somatostatin and endorphins. Histamine, produced by circulating mast cells and basophils, increases gastric acid secretion by binding to histamine receptors (H_2 receptors) on the gastric parietal cells (Table 21.1).

Secretion of gastric juice

Two to three litres of gastric juice (a mixture of secretions from two types of cells present in the gastric pits but absent from the pylorus) is produced daily (Fig. 21.3). The gastric pit cells are:

1. parietal or oxyntic cells, which secrete hydrochloric acid (HCl) and the intrinsic factor;
2. chief or zygomen cells, which secrete the enzymes.

There are about a 1000 million parietal cells in the gastric pits of an adult stomach. Hydrogen ions are secreted into the lumen of the stomach against a concentration gradient, probably by an active pump mechanism in the cell membrane.

Table 21.1   Hormones that aid digestion

Hormone	Stimulus	Target organ	Effect
Gastrin	Presence of food in the stomach	Stomach	Increased gastric gland secretions, most effect on HCl production
		Small intestine	Causes contraction of intestinal muscle
		Ileocaecal valve	Relaxes valve
		Large intestine	Stimulates mass movements
Serotonin	Food in stomach	Stomach	Contraction of stomach musculature
Histamine	Food in stomach	Stomach	Release of HCl
Somatostatin	Food in stomach Sympathetic nerve stimulus	Stomach Pancreas Small intestine Gallbladder	Inhibits gastric secretion, motility, emptying Inhibits secretion Inhibits GI blood flow and intestinal absorption Inhibits contraction and bile release
Intestinal gastrin	Acidic/partly digested food in duodenum	Stomach	Stimulates gastric glands and motility
Secretin	Acidic or irritant chyme, partially digested fats and proteins	Stomach Pancreas Liver	Inhibits gastric secretion and motility during gastric phase Increases bicarbonate-rich pancreatic juice Potentiates CCK action Increases bile output
Cholecystokinin (CCK)	Fatty chyme or partially digested proteins	Liver/pancreas Gallbladder Sphincter of Oddi	Potentiates secretin's action Increases enzyme-rich output Stimulates contraction with expulsion of bile Relaxes to allow bile and pancreatic juice to enter duodenum
Gastric inhibitory peptide (GIP)	Fatty and/or glucose containing chyme	Stomach	Inhibits gastric gland secretion and motility during gastric phase

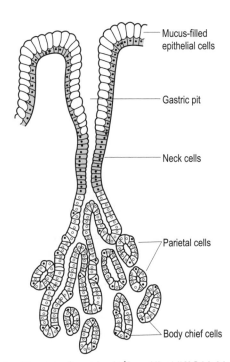

Figure 21.3   Diagram of gastric pit (from Hinchliff S M, Montague S E 1990, with permission).

CO_2 diffuses into the parietal cells from arterial blood and combines with water to form H_2CO_3 (carbonic acid). Equal numbers of hydrogen ions formed by the dissociation of H_2CO_3 into hydrogen ions (H^+), bicarbonate ions (HCO_3^-) and chloride ions (Cl^-) are secreted into the lumen of the gastric pits. This forms HCl, which is then diluted by water. Histamine or the hormone gastrin stimulates the secretion of the HCl into the lumen of the stomach.

The functions of gastric acid are:

- inactivation of salivary amylase;
- bacteriostasis;
- alteration of the molecular structure of proteins to tenderise them;
- curdling of milk;
- conversion of pepsinogen to pepsin.

Children produce an enzyme called **rennin** which acts on the milk protein casein and converts it into curds.

The chief cells produce a pepsinogen-rich secretion. When gastric pH is lower than 5.5, pepsinogen is converted into the active proteolytic enzyme pepsin by HCl, which converts proteins to polypeptides by breaking the bonds between specific amino acids. Once chyme leaves the stomach there is a change to an alkaline medium and pepsin's activity ceases.

Control of gastric juice secretion

There are both neural and hormonal aspects of control of gastric juice secretion.

Neural control

There are two phases in the neural control although the two work interdependently. The **cephalic phase** is an anticipatory conditioned reflex to the sight, smell or thought of food. This phase is mediated by the vagus nerve, which stimulates both parietal and chief cells. The **gastric phase** is mediated by stretch receptors and chemoreceptors. Stretch receptors in the stomach wall respond to distension by food. Chemoreceptors respond to the presence of protein molecules within the stomach. Impulses from these two types of receptor are sent to the submucosal plexus where they synapse with parasympathetic neurons. Excitatory impulses are then dispatched to the parietal cells.

Hormonal control

Although the neural influences described above are important, hormonal influences, especially gastrin, contribute most to the gastric phase of secretion. Throughout, the gut regulatory hormones called **peptides** are active. Many of them are also found in the central nervous system and alternative names for them are neurohormones, neuropeptides or neurotransmitters. The term **gastrin** refers to a group of similar hormones produced by **G cells** in the lateral walls of the gastric glands in the antrum of the stomach. A small amount of gastrin is produced by the duodenal mucosa, sometimes referred to as a third or **intestinal phase** of gastric juice secretion. The production of gastrin is stimulated by food in the stomach, particularly by partially digested proteins and caffeine (Tortora & Grabowski 2000).

P cells throughout the gastrointestinal tract secrete **bombesin**, the gastrin-releasing peptide. Gastrin enters the gastric circulatory capillaries and the systemic circulation and when it reaches the stomach via the bloodstream gastrin has the following actions:

- stimulates the production of gastric acid by the parietal cells by the release of histamine;
- has a minor role in stimulating the production of pepsinogen by the chief cells;
- stimulates the growth of the gastric and intestinal mucosa;
- causes enhanced contraction of the cardiac sphincter to prevent gastric reflux;
- stimulates the secretion of insulin and glucagon in the pancreas.

Control of gastric motility

Increase of gastric motility

Stomach contractions empty the stomach and also compress, knead and mix the food with gastric juice to produce chyme. Waves of peristalsis pass from the cardiac sphincter to the pylorus about three times a minute. The more liquid parts of chyme pass through the pylorus into the small intestine, while the more solid parts are sent back to the body of the stomach for further gastric mixing. The regulatory peptide **motilin**, produced by cells in the duodenum and jejunum in response to the entry of acid chyme, increases gastric motility.

Food remains in the stomach depending on its consistency and composition. Carbohydrates and liquids leave the stomach fastest followed by proteins and fats. The **enterogastric reflex** is initiated when the products of protein digestion, together with the acid, enter the duodenum, resulting in a slowing of gastric motility. Gastric emptying usually takes 4–5 h, during which the antrum, pylorus and duodenal cap contract in sequence. This is the gastric pump mechanism, which results in squirts of chyme entering the duodenum.

Inhibition of gastric motility

When glucose and fats enter the duodenum a regulatory peptide called **gastric inhibitory peptide** (GIP) is secreted by the **K cells** of the duodenal and jejunal mucosa. GIP, also known as glucose-dependent insulin-releasing peptide, decreases gastric secretion and motility and stimulates the secretion of insulin. **Vasoactive intestinal polypeptide** (VIP), produced in the D cells of the duodenum and colon, also inhibits gastric motility by acting as a smooth muscle relaxant. It also stimulates the intestinal secretion of electrolytes.

THE SMALL INTESTINE

The structure of the small intestine

The small intestine is a long coiled tube about 3–3.5 m long, that extends from the pyloric sphincter to the ileocaecal valve. Its diameter is only 2.5 cm. It is the body's main digestive organ, where food digestion is completed and absorption of nutrients and most of the water from the chyme takes place.

There are three sections of the small intestine:

1. The C-shaped duodenum lies mainly behind the peritoneum. It is about 25 cm long and surrounds the head of the pancreas.
2. The jejunum, 250 cm long, makes up about 40% of the remainder of the small intestine.
3. The ileum, 360 cm long, makes up the other 60%, joining the large intestine at the ileocaecal valve. The jejunum has thicker walls and is more vascular while the ileum has fewer folds in its lumen. Protective lymph nodes called **Peyer's patches** are present in the ileum.

The duodenum

Salivary amylase begins the digestion of cooked starch into maltose and dextrins. Pepsin begins the breakdown of proteins into polypeptides. There is no secretion of enzymes by the duodenum although it does secrete hormones. The duodenum receives the secretions of the pancreas and liver via the pancreatic duct and common bile duct (Fig. 21.4) after they join together at the ampulla of Vater, at the sphincter of Oddi. These secretions are alkaline (pH of about 8) and produce a sharp change in pH from the acidity of the stomach to the alkalinity of the duodenum. Enzymes are pH sensitive and function within a narrow range. The first few centimetres of the duodenum are called the **duodenal cap**. The tissue is protected from the acid chyme by a large number of mucus-secreting **Brunner's glands**.

Pancreatic extrinsic secretions

The exocrine function of the pancreas is achieved by secretions from **acinar cells** and plays a major role in digestion. The production of the enzymes will be discussed more fully in Chapter 22. The enzymes are secreted into the pancreatic duct and the duodenum. The three proteolytic enzymes are:

1. **Trypsinogen**, which is in an inactive form to safeguard the gut from autodigestion.
2. **Trypsin**, which is formed from trypsinogen in a reaction catalyzed by the enzyme enterokinase (enteropeptidase). Trypsin completes the breakdown of proteins to amino acids.
3. **Carboxypeptidase**, which acts on peptides.

Other enzymes are:

- pancreatic amylase, which converts starch to maltose;
- pancreatic lipase, which breaks down triglycerides to three fatty acids and glycerol;
- ribonuclease (RNAase), which breaks down RNA;
- deoxyribonuclease (DNAase), which acts on DNA to release free nucleotides.

Control of pancreatic juice secretion

The hormone **secretin** results in the secretion of the watery component, rich in bicarbonate but low in enzymes. Another hormone, **cholecystokinin** (CCK), causes the release of the enzymes. Stimulation of pancreatic juice secretion can be divided into a cephalic phase, with vagal control brought about by the sight, smell or thought of food or the presence of food in the mouth, and a gastric phase stimulated by the release of gastrin (Fig. 21.5).

CCK causes:

- stimulation of enzyme-rich pancreatic secretion;
- augmentation of the activity of secretin;
- slowing of gastric emptying and inhibition of gastric secretion;
- stimulation of the secretion of enterokinase;
- stimulation of glucagon secretion;
- stimulation of intestinal motility;
- contraction of the gall bladder with the release of bile.

Bile

Bile is produced by the liver and stored in the gall bladder. It contains no digestive enzymes but emulsifies fats so that the fat-soluble vitamins and iron can be absorbed. Its production, content and function will be discussed more fully in Chapter 22. The control of bile secretion also involves neural and hormonal factors. CCK is the major controller, causing contraction of the gall bladder and relaxation of the sphincter of Oddi. Once the gall bladder is empty, further flow of bile into the duodenum occurs directly from the liver. Vagus nerve stimulation will bring about a similar action. About 97% of bile salts are reabsorbed into the portal circulation and returned to the liver.

Intestinal juice

The process of digestion is completed by juices secreted by the duodenum and jejunum. This juice is rich in mucus, some of which comes from the Brunner's glands in the proximal duodenum. **Lieberkühn's glands** in the jejunum and ileum secrete most of the watery juice. The nutrients are absorbed into the circulating blood through small finger-like projections in the surface of the small intestine called **villi**, which are covered by a layer of mucus to prevent autodigestion.

Intestinal enzymes

These enzymes are produced by enterocytes in the villi and break down food particles into their absorbable form.

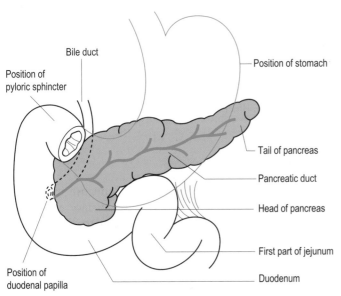

Figure 21.4 The position of the pancreas (from Hinchliff S M, Montague S E 1990, with permission).

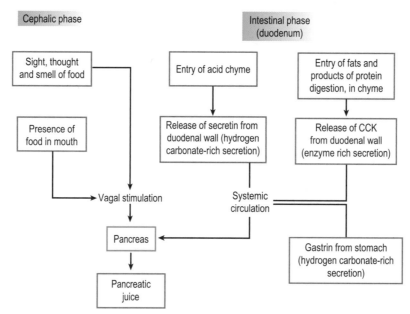

Figure 21.5   Flow chart to illustrate pancreatic juice secretion (from Hinchliff S M, Montague S E 1990, with permission).

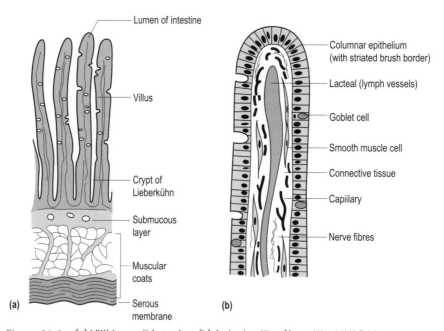

Figure 21.6   (a) Villi in small intestine. (b) A single villus (from Hinchliff S M, Montague S E 1990, with permission).

They are probably released from shed enterocytes. Proteins are broken down into amino acids, while fats are in the form of fatty acids and glycerol. Carbohydrates are broken down into monosaccharides – glucose, fructose and galactose. The enzymes are:

- aminopeptidases – act on peptides;
- dipeptidases – act on dipeptides;
- maltase – converts maltose to glucose;
- lactase – converts lactose to glucose and galactose;
- sucrase – converts sucrose into glucose and fructose.

The villi

Visible folding of the mucosa and submucosa into **plicae circularis** (circular folds) increases the surface area of the small intestine. The addition of villi and microvilli increases the surface area to 600 times that of a simple tube of the same size, giving a surface area of 200 m^2 (Hinchliff et al 1996). Between the villi are small pits called the **crypts of Lieberkühn** where the mucus-secreting glands are situated. Villi have an external covering of simple columnar epithelium continuous with the crypts (Fig. 21.6) and a central lacteal containing lymph, which empties into the local lymphatic circulation. There is a capillary blood supply linked to both hepatic and portal veins.

Two other types of cell are associated with the villi: **goblet cells** that secrete mucus are situated mainly in the crypts while **enterocytes** are tall columnar cells involved in digestion and absorption. Enterocytes have many mitochondria to provide the energy for enzyme secretion and nutrient absorption. They have a high rate of mitosis and those at the tip of the villi are replaced every 30 h.

A few smooth muscle cells are present in villi, contracting to assist lymph drainage in the central lacteals. Lymphocytes and plasma cells are situated at intervals between the enterocytes. The plasma cells secrete immunoglobulin A (IgA) to protect the gut from pathogens.

There are also cells in the intestinal wall secreting 5-HT, which may increase intestinal motility.

ABSORPTION

Eight to nine litres of water and 1 kg of nutrients daily are absorbed across the gut wall. The transport of nutrients can be either active or passive. **Active transport** requires energy and is usually against a concentration gradient. Most such substances require carrier molecules, including vitamin B_{12}, iron, sodium ions, glucose, galactose and amino acids. Water follows passively along an osmotic gradient. **Passive transport** requires no energy, depending on the direction of concentration and electrical gradients. It includes water, lipids, drugs and some electrolytes and vitamins. Some substances passively cross the gut wall membrane, with the help of carrier molecules, by **facilitated diffusion**.

Nutrients and minerals

Monosaccharides

About 500 g of monosaccharides are absorbed daily. Galactose and glucose pass into the villous capillaries and then to the hepatic portal vein. A high concentration of sodium ions on the surface of the enterocytes facilitates the active transport of these molecules. Glucose and sodium ions share the same carrier molecule. Sodium concentration in the enterocyte is low so that sodium moves into the cell along a concentration gradient accompanied by glucose. Fructose has a different carrier molecule and its transport is not influenced by sodium.

Monosaccharides are transported to the liver where galactose and fructose are converted to glucose (Fig. 21.7). Some of the glucose is converted to glycogen (**glycogenesis**) under the influence of insulin. About 100 g of glucose are stored in the liver, sufficient to maintain blood glucose levels for 24 h. Some glycogen is stored in skeletal muscle to provide energy for muscle action. The liver converts any glucose that is surplus to the body's needs into adipose tissue.

Blood glucose is maintained normally at a level of 3.5–5.5 mmol/L. When the glucose level falls, liver glycogen is broken down (**glycogenolysis**) to release glucose. This occurs under the influence of glucagon and adrenaline (epinephrine). Once glycogen stores in the liver are depleted, the liver manufactures glucose from amino acids and glycerol (**gluconeogenesis**).

When circulating glucose arrives at the tissues, the cells take it up by facilitated diffusion, under the influence of insulin. In the mitochondria of the cells glucose is oxidised to form energy in the **Krebs** or **citric acid cycle**. The glucose is converted to pyruvic acid, which, in turn, is converted to acetyl coenzyme A, usually referred to as **acetyl CoA** in a process requiring oxygen, i.e. aerobic. Acetyl CoA enters the Krebs cycle to undergo changes mediated by enzymes. The process of oxidation forms the energy-storage molecule adenosine triphosphate (ATP), along with water and carbon dioxide. If there is insufficient oxygen to convert pyruvic acid to acetyl CoA, lactic acid is formed.

Amino acids

In an adult, approximately 200 g of amino acids are absorbed daily from the ileum, of which 50 g/day are needed to maintain nitrogen balance and to provide for tissue growth and repair. The mechanism for absorption of amino acids is not fully understood but may depend on whether the amino acid is acidic, basic or neutral. Sodium appears to facilitate the absorption of amino acids.

Amino acids cannot be stored by the body and are absorbed into the blood to enter a common circulating pool from which cells can remove them as necessary (Fig. 21.8). However, the liver can interconvert amino acids by utilising the eight essential amino acids to synthesise the nonessential amino acids. The process of **deamination** in the liver breaks down any excess amino acids. The nitrogen portion is converted into urea, which enters the blood and is excreted by the kidney.

Fats

About 80 g of fat is absorbed daily, mainly in the duodenum. The contents of the micelles are discharged onto the microvilli and enter the enterocytes by passive diffusion. Short-chain fatty acids enter the capillary network and travel in the hepatic portal vein as free fatty acids. Longer-chain fatty acids are resynthesised in the enterocyte to become triglycerides coated with a layer of lipoprotein, cholesterol and phospholipid. These complexes enter the central lacteals to form **chyle**, which enters the lymphatic system and then the bloodstream. Faeces contain about 5% fat.

Bile salts, steroid hormones and cell membranes are formed from cholesterol. Cholesterol is found in the blood, mainly in combination with a protein carrier, as lipoproteins, of which there are three types:

- high-density lipoproteins (HDLs);
- low-density lipoproteins (LDLs);
- very low-density lipoproteins (VLDLs).

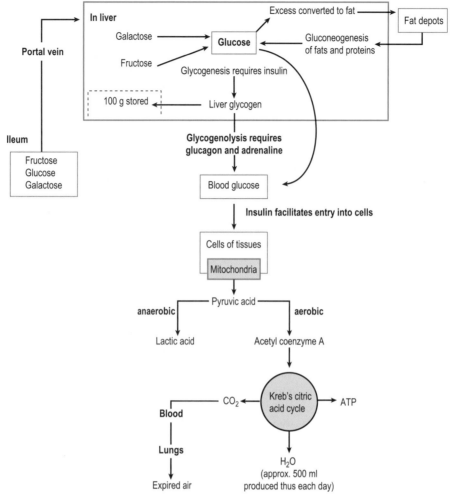

Figure 21.7 Metabolic pathways for glucose (from Hinchliff S M, Montague S E 1990, with permission).

Cholesterol (in the form of LDLs and VLDLs) is laid down in arterial walls as atheromatous plaques. A high ratio of HDLs to LDLs and VLDLs may offer protection against ischaemic heart disease. An increased ratio of HDLs to LDLs and VLDLs has been shown in vegetarians, in those whose fat intake is largely unsaturated and in those who take regular exercise. The ratio is reduced in those who smoke cigarettes.

Fat can be utilised by the body to form energy and any excess fat is stored as adipose tissue. When fat stores are needed for energy production they are mobilised under the influence of growth hormones or cortisol and taken to the liver where the triglycerides are broken down into free fatty acids and glycerol. The fatty acids are converted to acetyl CoA in the presence of oxygen and glucose and these enter the Kreb's citric acid cycle (Fig. 21.9). If glucose is not available, acetyl CoA metabolism is deranged and the ketone bodies acetoacetic acid and beta (β)-hydroxybutyric acid accumulate in the blood. These can be oxidised to release energy but metabolic acidosis will occur.

Sodium, potassium and water

About 2 L of fluid are ingested daily. A further 8–9 L of fluid are added to the gut during the production of digestive juices. Only 50–200 ml are lost in the faeces, the rest being absorbed from both the small and large intestine at a rate of 200–400 ml/min. The jejunum, ileum and colon actively reabsorb sodium ions, which are followed passively by chloride and water. Some potassium is actively secreted into the gut and reabsorbed from the ileum and colon along a concentration gradient.

Vitamins

The water-soluble vitamins, with the exception of vitamin B_{12} (absorbed as a complex with the intrinsic factor in the terminal ileum), are passively absorbed with water. The fat-soluble vitamins, A, D, E and K, enter the enterocytes in the micelles. Bile and lipase are necessary for their absorption.

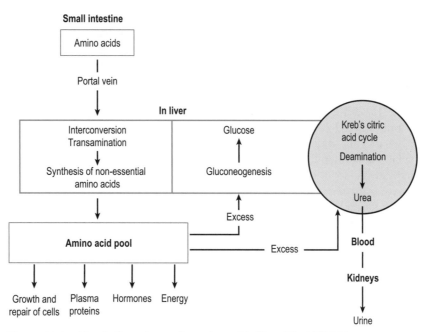

Figure 21.8   Metabolic pathways for amino acids (from Hinchliff S M, Montague S E 1990, with permission).

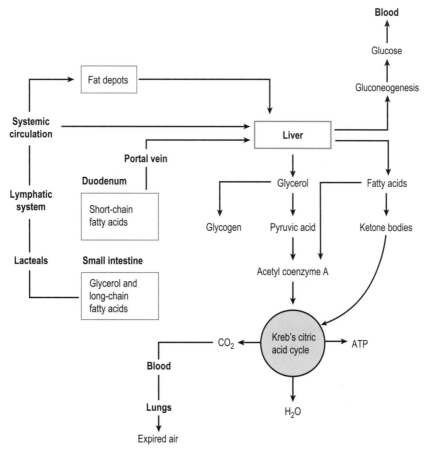

Figure 21.9   Metabolic pathways for fats (from Hinchliff S M, Montague S E 1990, with permission).

Most calcium is absorbed in the upper part of the small intestine under the influence of parathyroid hormone and calcitonin. The active process is facilitated by vitamin D.

Iron

In developed countries about 15–20 mg of iron is ingested daily, mostly as ferric salts, but only 5–10% is absorbed into the blood. There is a daily loss of 1 mg/day from desquamation of the skin and in the faeces. Women lose about 25 mg each month during menstruation. Iron is more readily absorbed in the ferrous form and the ferric form is reduced to the ferrous form by gastric juice and vitamin C.

Iron is actively absorbed in the upper part of the small intestine and is stored in the enterocytes when their cellular stores are low. The enterocytes discharge iron into the bloodstream when serum levels fall. Iron travels in the blood bound to **apoferritin**, which is known as **ferritin** when iron is bound to it. About 70% of iron in the body is in haemoglobin and 3% in myoglobin in muscle protein. The rest is stored in the liver as ferritin or as **haemosiderin**.

THE LARGE INTESTINE

The adult large intestine is about 1.5 m long, consisting of the caecum, appendix, colon and rectum (Fig. 21.10). It has a diameter of 5–6 cm and can store large quantities of food residues. The large intestine has no villi and a much smaller internal surface than the small intestine. The colon differs from the generalised structure of the gastrointestinal tract as the longitudinal muscle bands are incomplete and the wall is gathered into three longitudinal bands, the **taenia coli**. These bands are shorter than the remaining colon, so that the wall pouches outwards into **haustrations** (buckets) between the taeniae, when the circular muscles contract. The filling and emptying of the haustrations help to mix the colonic contents. Patches of lymphoid tissue are scattered throughout the length of the large intestine, providing a protection against pathogens.

About 1 L of porridge-like chyme enters the large intestine daily through the ileocaecal valve. This valve, normally closed because of back pressure from the colon's contents, opens in response to peristaltic waves. The caecum relaxes and the ileocaecal valve opens, a reflex called the **gastro-colic reflex**. The colonic peristalsis that follows fills the rectum with faeces, resulting in the urge to defecate.

The **caecum**, a blind pouch between the ileocaecal valve and the colon, is about 7 cm long. This has no known function in humans although it is involved in cellulose digestion in herbivores. The **vermiform appendix**, a worm-like blind-ending sac projecting from the end of the caecum about the size of an adult's little finger, contains lymphoid tissue and enlarges in the presence of infection or inflammation (appendicitis). An enlarged appendix may rupture so that faecal material and bacteria enter the abdominal cavity, leading to peritonitis.

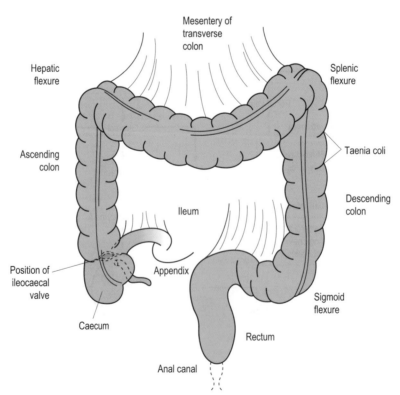

Figure 21.10 The large intestine (from Hinchliff S M, Montague S E 1990, with permission).

The colon

The large intestine is divided anatomically into three regions:

- The **ascending colon**, about 15 cm long, commences at the caecum and extends upwards on the right of the abdominal cavity as far as the lower border of the liver.
- The **transverse colon** begins at the hepatic flexure and traverses the abdominal cavity below the liver and stomach to the slightly higher splenic flexure.
- The **descending colon**, about 25 cm long, descends along the left side of the abdominal cavity. The sigmoid (S-shaped) colon, about 40 cm long, is a continuation of the descending colon and empties into the rectum.

The large intestine has five functions:

1. Storage of unabsorbed food residues prior to defecation. About 70% of food residues are excreted within 72 h of ingestion, but the remainder may stay in the colon for 1 week. Non-absorbable dietary fibre gives bulk to the faeces.

2. Absorption of water, electrolytes and some vitamins. Sodium is actively reabsorbed into the hepatic portal vein, followed passively by water and chloride. The amount of water reabsorbed depends on how long the residue remains in the colon. In constipation the residue may stay in the colon for several days, resulting in removal of most of the water.

3. Synthesis of vitamin K and some B vitamins – thiamine, folic acid and riboflavin – by commensal colonic bacteria. Bacterial fermentation of food residues results in the formation of flatus, which consists of nitrogen, carbon dioxide, hydrogen, methane and hydrogen sulphide. Between 500 and 700 ml of flatus is produced daily depending on the type of food eaten; legumes lead to an increase in flatus production.

4. Secretion of mucus, which acts as a lubricant for elimination of faeces. The mucus contains bicarbonate, which gives the contents of the colon a pH of 7.5–8.0.

5. Secretion of potassium ions.

Movements of the colon

Contraction of the circular muscle fibres occurs about once every 30 min. This causes **segmentation**, a non-propulsive movement in the colon, which mixes the colonic contents and facilitates absorption. Peristalsis moves the faeces towards the rectum. Following meals, there is an increase in colonic activity due to the gastrocolic reflex. Associated with the gastrocolic reflex is **mass movement**, which propels the faeces towards the rectum. The haustrations in the midcolon disappear and the tube becomes flattened and shortened by waves of rapid, powerful contractions, moving the colonic contents rapidly into the sigmoid colon.

The rectum

The rectum is a muscular tube about 15 cm long. It is capable of great distension but is usually empty until just before defecation. The sudden distension of the rectal walls brought about by filling of the rectum during mass movement brings about the urge to defecate. The rectum opens to the exterior by the anal canal, which has both internal and external sphincters.

The anal canal

The anal canal is about 3 cm long and begins where the rectum perforates the levator ani muscle of the pelvic floor. It has a sphincter at both ends. The **internal anal sphincter** is composed of smooth muscle fibres and is not under voluntary control. When nerve fibres from the sympathetic system are stimulated, the muscle fibres in the internal anal sphincter contract. Fibres from the parasympathetic system inhibit contractions and the sphincter relaxes. The **external anal sphincter** is made up of striated voluntary muscle and is supplied by fibres from the pudendal nerve. The sphincter is under conscious control from about 18 months of age. Damage to the sphincter or its nerve supply may occur in childbirth, resulting in incontinence of faeces.

The mucosa of the anal canal hangs in long ridges called **anal columns** and is made of stratified squamous epithelium. Mucus is secreted from the anal recesses between the columns, which aids in defecation. Two superficial venous plexi, the haemorrhoidal veins, are associated with the anal canal. These may become distended, resulting in varicosities or haemorrhoids.

Defecation

Afferent nerves impulses travel to the sacral spinal cord when faeces enter the rectum. Impulses then travel back from the spinal cord in a reflex arc to the terminal ileum and anal sphincter to allow defecation. The cerebral cortex receives nerve messages, which allow inhibition of the spinal reflex arc if it is not convenient to defecate. Defecation is usually assisted by voluntary effort, which raises intra-abdominal pressure. A deep breath is taken and is expired against a closed glottis. This is called **Valsalva's manoeuvre**. The levator ani muscles contract and the pressure in the rectum is raised to about 200 mmHg (26 kPa). The anal sphincters relax and the contents of the rectum are expelled. During straining there is a sharp rise in blood pressure followed by a sudden fall.

Faeces

About 100–150 g of faeces are eliminated each day, consisting of 30–50 g solids and 70–100 g water. The solid portion consists mainly of cellulose, shed epithelial cells, bacteria, some salts and stercobilin, which gives it the brown colour. The characteristic odour of faces is caused by bacterial break-down of amines.

MATERNAL ADAPTATIONS TO PREGNANCY

The gastrointestinal and hepatic systems during pregnancy have dramatic anatomical and physiological alterations that are essential in supporting the nutritional demands of the mother and fetus. The related alterations are often accompanied by upsets of the gastrointestinal function, which are probably the commonest cause of complaint by pregnant women (Enkin et al 2000). These minor disorders are discussed in Chapter 30.

The mouth

Pregnant women usually find that they have an increased appetite, cravings or aversions for certain food, and pica, which is a craving for non-food substances. Specific changes in food consumption and food habits are strongly influenced by cultural and economical factors and may also change to meet the needs of the fetus. Progesterone is a known appetite stimulant and evidence for this is supported by changes in appetite, which closely follow the hormonal changes during the menstrual cycle. During pregnancy, alterations in the balance of oestrogen, progesterone, glucagon and insulin contribute to the changes in food intake.

The gums and teeth

The gums may become swollen and spongy and bleed easily. This results from oedema due to the effects of oestrogen on blood flow and the consistency of connective tissue. There is an increase in gingivitis and periodontal disease, caused by the oedema rather than by an increased presence of irritant particles of food. This is often more extreme with increased maternal age and parity and where there are pre-existing dental problems. About 3–5% of pregnant women will develop an **epulis** (pregnancy tumour), which is a friable growth or hyperplasia of the gum usually found on the palatal side of the maxillary gingiva (Blackburn 2003). It may bleed or interfere with chewing and will usually regress after delivery, although occasionally excision of the growth may be necessary.

Although dentists and women believe that pregnancy damages teeth, there is no evidence to suggest that demineralisation of teeth occurs from pregnancy. The calcium needs for the fetus are drawn from maternal stores (skeleton) and not from maternal teeth (Blackburn 2003).

Saliva

Ptyalism or excess salivation may occur but there is no evidence to suggest that more saliva is actually produced. The problem is due to a reluctance of women to swallow because of the associated nausea. This is often a particular problem in Afro-Caribbean women. Ganglion-blocking drugs may be required if ptyalism becomes a major problem. There is uncertainty as to the changes in the pH of saliva. It is more likely that the pH drops and saliva becomes more acid in pregnancy.

The oesophagus

Heartburn affects about two-thirds of all women at some stage in pregnancy (Enkin et al 2000). It is probably due to reflux oesophagitis due to the effects of progesterone on the muscle tone of the cardiac sphincter between the oesophagus and stomach. The competence of the sphincter is impaired and regurgitation of gastric acid is more likely. This may not be the single cause as acid reflux has also been found to be present in 40% of people with no heartburn. There is an increased risk of **hiatus hernia** where there is displacement of the cardiac sphincter into the thorax. Displacement of the sphincter has probably a minor role to play in heartburn and the more likely factor to be considered is the strength of the sphincter (Hytten 1991).

The stomach

Acid secretion

Gastric acid secretions tend to decrease during pregnancy, beginning in the early weeks and becoming even less in late pregnancy. This may explain why a peptic ulcer is rarely detected in pregnancy and those women with an ulcer have a clear remission during pregnancy, with a return to the symptoms experienced by the 3rd month after delivery.

Emptying time

Gastric muscle tone and motility are reduced during pregnancy due to the effect of progesterone. However, low levels of circulating motilin have been found during pregnancy. This results in delay in emptying, which is probably due to the lower secretion rate of gastric juices. The digestion time for solid food is prolonged although watery food is digested and passed on to the small intestine with little delay. Drinks containing high levels of glucose such as those administered in glucose tolerance tests have a high osmotic effect and gastric emptying is delayed in hyperosmotic foods. The reduced activity of the gastric muscle may exaggerate the effect and result in nausea. During labour, reduced stomach motility leads to a delay in emptying and a risk of acid aspiration.

The small intestine

There is no increase in the absorption of food even though metabolism is anabolic during pregnancy. Any increased nutrition must come from increased intake and there is facilitated absorption of nutrients such as iron and calcium. The prepregnant levels of calcium absorption (20–25%) increase early in pregnancy, to a 50% absorption by 24 weeks, and then remain stable until delivery (Hosking 1998). Phosphate and magnesium absorption is assumed to follow calcium in terms of intestinal absorption. The transit time of food and waste products through the intestine is prolonged due to reduced mobility and a decrease in the tone of the intestine musculature. Hytten (1991) discusses a case reported by Montgomery & Pincus (1955) where a young woman, following an ileostomy, demonstrated increased absorption of food during pregnancy while the number of daily stools decreased. The delay in passage of food through the gut was probably responsible for both phenomena.

The large intestine

The colon shares in the general relaxation of smooth muscle found throughout the body. Constipation is a common complaint during pregnancy and is made worse by the prolonged transit time of waste materials and the resulting increased absorption of water in the colon. Increased flatulence may also occur.

MAIN POINTS

- The gastrointestinal tract is a continuous, coiled, fibromuscular tube extending from the mouth to the anus. It consists of the mouth, pharynx, oesophagus, stomach, small intestine and large intestine.

- The function of the gastrointestinal tract is controlled by the autonomic nervous system (ANS). Parasympathetic activity leads to an increase in both the motility and secretory functions of the tract and to relaxation of the gut sphincters. Sympathetic activity leads to a decrease in blood supply to the gut with a decrease in secretions and in gut motility.

- The gastrointestinal tract processes the food to be used by the body cells. Six processes can be described: ingestion, propulsion, mastication, digestion, absorption and elimination.

- Digestion of food begins in the stomach and is completed in the small intestine. Saliva contains the digestive enzyme salivary amylase, which acts upon starch to convert polysaccharides into disaccharides.

- Gastric acid inactivates salivary amylase, alters the molecular structure of proteins to tenderise them, curdles milk and converts pepsinogen to pepsin. Pepsin converts proteins to polypeptides. Once chyme leaves the stomach, there is a change to an alkaline medium and pepsin's activity ceases.

- Both neural and hormonal aspects are involved in the control of gastric juice secretion. The neural control has two phases: the cephalic phase, mediated by the vagus nerve, stimulates both parietal and chief cells; and the gastric phase, mediated by stretch and chemoreceptors responding to the presence of food within the stomach. Hormonal influences contribute most to the gastric phase of secretion.

- The three sections of the small intestine comprise the duodenum, the jejunum and the ileum. Digestion is completed and absorption of nutrients and most of the water takes place in the small intestine.

- Pancreatic digestive enzymes are secreted into the duodenum (pH 8). Pancreatic juice contains three proteolytic enzymes: trypsinogen, trypsin and carboxypeptidase. Bile emulsifies fats so that fat-soluble vitamins and iron can be absorbed. Cholecystokinin (CCK) is the major controller of bile release, causing contraction of the gall bladder and relaxation of the sphincter of Oddi.

- Juices secreted in the duodenum and jejunum complete digestion. Basic nutrients are then absorbed into the circulating blood through intestinal villi.

- About 2 L of fluid are ingested daily. A further 8–9 L of fluid are added to the gut during the production of digestive juices. Only 50–200 ml are lost in the faeces, the rest being absorbed from both the small and large intestine.

- Most calcium is absorbed in the upper part of the small intestine under the influence of parathyroid hormone and calcitonin. The active process is facilitated by vitamin D. About 15–20 mg of iron is ingested daily but only 5–10% is absorbed. There is a daily loss of 1 mg/day from desquamation of the skin and in the faeces and women lose about 25 mg during menstruation.

- The large intestine is about 1.5 m long in an adult and consists of the caecum, appendix, colon and rectum. It can store large quantities of food residues. The gastrocolic reflex and colonic peristalsis fill the rectum with faeces, resulting in the urge to defecate.

- The colon absorbs most of the remaining water and electrolytes, synthesises vitamin K and some B vitamins, secretes mucus and acts as a lubricant for elimination of faeces. Sudden distension of the rectum results in the urge to defecate. The rectum opens to the exterior by the anal canal. About 100–150 g of faeces are eliminated each day.

- Pregnant women usually find that they have an increased appetite and food consumption, craving of certain foods and avoidance of others. Pica is a craving for non-food substances. The gums may become swollen and spongy in pregnancy and bleed easily. There is an increase in gingivitis and periodontal disease, caused by oedema rather than by an increased presence of irritant particles of food.

- Gastric acid secretion tends to be reduced during pregnancy, beginning early in pregnancy and increasing in late pregnancy. Peptic ulceration is rare in pregnant women. Gastric muscle tone and motility are reduced during pregnancy due to the effect of progesterone. The delay in emptying may also be due to the lower secretion of gastric juices, resulting in prolonged digestion time for solid food. Watery food is digested and passed on to the small intestine with little delay.

- Absorption of food does not increase even though the metabolism of pregnant women is anabolic. Any increased nutrition must come from increased intake. Iron and calcium appear to be absorbed more readily. Constipation is a common complaint as the colon shares in the general relaxation of smooth muscle found throughout the body.

References

Blackburn S T 2003 Maternal, Fetal and Neonatal Physiology: A Clinical Perspective, 3rd edn. W B Saunders, Philadelphia.

Enkin M, Keirse M J N C, Neilson J 2000 A Guide to Effective Care in Pregnancy, 3rd edn. Oxford University Press, Oxford.

Hinchliff S M, Montague S E, Watson R (eds) 1996 Physiology for Nursing Practice, 3rd edn. Ballière Tindall, London.

Hosking D J 1998 Calcium Metabolism. In Chamberlain G, Broughton Pipkin F (eds) Clinical Physiology in Obstetrics, 3rd edn. Blackwell Science, Oxford.

Hytten F 1991 The alimentary system. In Hytten F, Chamberlain G (eds) Clinical Physiology in Obstetrics, 2nd edn. Blackwell Science, Oxford.

Marieb E N 2000 Human Anatomy and Physiology, 5th edn. Benjamin/Cummings, New York.

Montgomery T L, Pincus I J 1955 A nutritional problem in pregnancy resulting from extensive resection of the small bowel. American Journal of Obstetrics and Gynecology 69:865.

Tortora G J, Grabowski S R 2000 Principles of Anatomy and Physiology, 9th edn. John Wylie, Chichester.

Annotated recommended reading

Sherwood L 2001 Human Physiology: From Cells to Systems, 4th edn. Brookes Cole, New York.
This is one of a range of human physiology text books that provide an in-depth introduction to the function of human body systems for undergraduate students in health-related studies.

Chapter 22

The accessory digestive organs

INTRODUCTION

The alimentary system contains not only the gastrointestinal tract discussed in the previous chapter but also the associated and accessory organs for digestion. It is an artificial division to separate out these accessory organs, as their function is integrated into the system. However, the sheer complexity of the physiology may be better understood by this format. This chapter discusses the contribution of the salivary glands, the pancreas and the liver to the process of digestion. The role of the liver in detoxification of drugs and ingested substances and the limitations to the protective role of the placenta are also discussed. Readers are referred to the selection of referenced textbooks if more detailed information is required.

THE SALIVARY GLANDS

Three pairs of salivary glands produce the saliva that aids speech, chewing and swallowing. They are the parotid, submaxillary and sublingual glands. The **parotid glands** are the largest pair and are situated by the angle of the jaw. These glands produce a watery solution forming 25% of the daily saliva secretion. The **submaxillary glands** lie below the upper jaw and produce thicker saliva which forms 70% of the total daily output. The **sublingual glands** lie under the tongue on the floor of the mouth and produce only 5% of the daily output. Their solution is rich in glycoproteins, called mucins, which are primarily responsible for the lubricating action of saliva. Salivary glands produce 1–1.5 L of saliva each day. Saliva consists of 99.5% water and 0.5% solutes and has a pH value of 6.75–7.0.

The functions of saliva

- It cleanses the mouth. It contains lysozyme, which has an antiseptic action and the immunoglobulin IgA as a defence against microorganisms.
- It provides oral comfort, reducing friction and allowing speech.

- It ensures that food is in solution so that the taste buds can recognise the contained chemicals.
- It facilitates the formation of a bolus of partly broken up food ready to swallow. The mucins present in saliva help to mould and lubricate the bolus.
- It contains a digestive enzyme, salivary or α amylase (formerly know as ptyalin), which acts upon starch to convert the polysaccharides into disaccharides.

Control of saliva production

The secretion of saliva is controlled primarily by parasympathetic supply from the facial (VII cranial) nerve and glossopharyngeal (IX cranial) nerve. Normally, parasympathetic stimulation produces continuous moderate watery amounts of saliva while sympathetic activity produces a sparse viscid secretion and the dry mouth most of us experience during times of stress or following the administration of atropine or hyoscine, which block receptor sites for the neurotransmitter acetylcholine.

Saliva is produced as a conditioned reflex in response to the cerebral perception of the thought, sight or smell of food. The salivary nuclei are situated in the reticular formation in the floor of the fourth ventricle and, when stimulated by the thought, sight or smell of food, secretion of saliva occurs. The presence of food in the mouth will also lead to saliva production – an unconditioned reflex where the impulse created by the physical presence of the food in the mouth directly stimulates the salivary nuclei without the cerebral cortex being involved. The process of deglutition propels the food into the stomach and the next stage in the digestion of food can continue.

THE PANCREAS

The pancreas is a gland lying just below the stomach that has both endocrine and exocrine functions. It is a soft friable pink gland, is 'tadpole' shaped, with a head surrounded by the C-shaped loop of the duodenum and a tail which extends towards the right side of the abdomen. Most of the pancreas is retroperitoneal. Through the centre of the pancreas runs the **pancreatic duct**, which fuses with the common bile duct just before it enters the duodenum at the hepatopancreatic ampulla.

Exocrine functions of the pancreas

Within the pancreas are the acini, which are clusters of cells surrounding small ducts. These provide the exocrine function and play a major role in digestion. The cells form and store zygomen granules, consisting of a wide range of digestive enzymes that act on all nutrients. The enzymes are secreted into the pancreatic duct and then into the duodenum.

Pancreatic juice

The pancreatic enzymes were briefly mentioned in Chapter 21. About 1.5–2 L of pancreatic juice are secreted daily with a pH of 8–8.4. A mixture of two types of secretions are produced: a copious watery solution and a scanty solution rich in enzymes. The profuse watery solution contains the ions hydrogen carbonate (bicarbonate), sodium, potassium, calcium, magnesium, chloride, sulphate, phosphate and some albumin and globulin proteins. The enzyme-rich secretion contains the three proteolytic enzymes of trypsinogen, trypsin and carboxypeptidase. Enzyme activity is summarised in Figure 22.1. Other enzymes are pancreatic amylase, pancreatic lipase, ribonuclease and deoxyribonuclease.

Control of pancreatic juice secretion The hormones secretin and cholecystokinin (CCK) were mentioned in Chapter 21. Secretin is produced by the S cells in the duodenum and upper jejunum, when acid chyme enters the duodenum. This enters the venous systemic circulation and arrives back at the pancreas via the pancreatic artery. Its presence results in the secretion of the watery component, which is rich in bicarbonate but low in enzymes.

Cholecystokinin secreted by the columnar cells of the duodenum and jejunum in response to the presence of the products of protein and fat digestion, also circulates and return to the pancreas via the pancreatic artery. Its presence causes the release of the enzyme-rich secretion. CCK has many important functions:

- stimulation of the enzyme-rich pancreatic secretion;
- augmentation of the activity of secretion;
- the slowing of gastric emptying and inhibition of gastric secretion;
- stimulation of the secretion of enterokinase;
- stimulation of glucagon secretion;
- stimulation of motility of the small intestine and colon;
- contraction of the gall bladder with the release of bile.

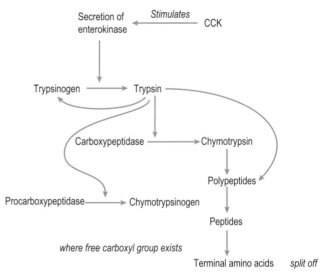

Figure 22.1 Summary of activity of the pancreatic proteolytic enzymes (from Hinchliff S M, Montague S E 1990, with permission).

Endocrine functions of the pancreas

Scattered among the acini are the **islets of Langerhans**, which can be called mini-endocrine glands (Marieb 2000). About 1% of the pancreas consists of the islet cells. There are two types of cells: the α cells synthesise glucagon and a more numerous population of cells; the β cells produce insulin. The normal human pancreas produces about 40 international units (IU) of insulin in 24 hours. The other cells produce somatostatin, which acts to suppress islet cell hormone production. A hormone called **amylin** appears to be an insulin antagonist.

Glucagon

Glucagon is a short polypeptide of 29 amino acids and a strong hyperglycaemic agent. Marieb (2000) writes that one molecule of glucagon causes the release of 100 million molecules of glucose into the blood. Glucagon acts mainly in the liver to promote:

● glycogenolysis (the breakdown of glycogen to glucose);
● lipolysis;
● gluconeogenesis (the formation of glucose from fatty acids and amino acids).

The liver releases the glucose into the bloodstream, raising the blood sugar level. There is a fall in serum amino acid levels as the liver then takes up amino acids to synthesise new glucose molecules.

Falling blood sugar levels stimulate secretion of glucagons from α cells. Increasing amino acid levels also stimulates glucagon release. Glucagon release is suppressed by increasing blood sugar levels and by somatostatin.

Insulin

Insulin is also a small polypeptide consisting of 51 amino acids. It begins as the middle part of a larger polypeptide chain called **proinsulin**. Enzymes cut amino acid bonds to release the functional hormone just before the insulin is secreted from the beta cell. Insulin affects the metabolism of fat and protein as well as glucose (Table 22.1).

Production of insulin   Insulin production is stimulated by glucose, amino acids and fatty acids in blood and hyperglycaemic agents such as glucagon, adrenaline (epinephrine), growth hormone, thyroxine or glucocorticoids. Insulin production is inhibited by somatostatin. Insulin binds firmly to a receptor site on the cell membrane. It appears to modify cellular activity without entering the cell. The presence of calcium is necessary for its functioning. A high carbohydrate diet leads to increased sensitivity of tissues to insulin and this may be due to a rise in the number of insulin receptors in the cell walls.

The role of insulin at cellular level   Insulin assists the entry of glucose into muscle cells, connective tissue cells and white blood cells. It does not facilitate entry of glucose into liver, kidney and brain cells. Those cells have easy access to glucose regardless of insulin (Marieb 2000). Insulin counters any metabolic activity that would increase plasma glucose levels such as glycogenolysis and gluconeogenesis. These last effects are probably due to insulin inhibition of glucagon. Once glucose has entered the cells, insulin triggers enzyme activity which:

● catalyses the oxidation of glucose to produce ATP;
● joins glucose molecules together to form glycogen;
● converts glucose to fat, particularly in adipose tissue.

These processes will be considered in more detail in Chapter 23.

THE LIVER AND GALL BLADDER

The liver, which is one of the accessory organs and is associated with the small intestine, is one of the body's most important organs. While it has many metabolic roles (see Ch. 23), its only digestive function is to secrete **bile**, which it stores in the gall bladder and discharges into the duodenum. Bile acts on fats to emulsify them; i.e. to break fat up into tiny particles so that it is more accessible to digestive enzymes.

Anatomy

The liver is a very large gland and weighs on average 1.4 kg. It is located in the abdominal cavity under the diaphragm, extending more to the right of the midline than

Table 22.1	The effects of insulin on foods		
On glucose	**On fat**	**On protein**	**On electrolytes**
Stimulates glucose utilisation Stimulates glycogen synthesis Inhibits glycogen breakdown Inhibits gluconeogenesis	Stimulates fatty acid and triglyceride synthesis Inhibits triglyceride breakdown	Stimulates incorporation of amino acids into protein molecules	Stimulates the entry of potassium into cells

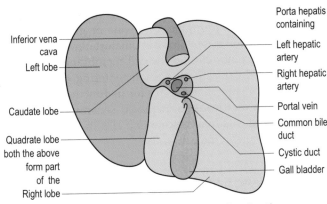

Figure 22.2   The inferior surface of the liver showing the position of the four lobes (from Hinchliff S M, Montague S E 1990, with permission).

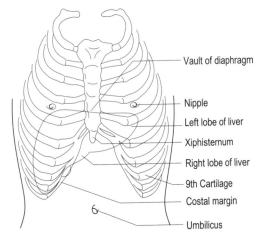

Figure 22.3   The position of the liver in relation to the rib cage (from Hinchliff S M, Montague S E 1990, with permission).

the left, obscuring the stomach (Fig. 22.2). It lies totally protected by the rib cage. The liver has four lobes (Fig. 22.3):

1. the right lobe, which is the largest;
2. the smaller left lobe;
3. the caudate lobe which is the posterior lobe;
4. the quadrate lobe, which lies inferior to the left lobe.

The right lobe is the largest and is separated from the left lobe by a deep fissure. The right and left lobes are also separated by the **falciform ligament**, a cord of mesentery which suspends the liver from the diaphragm and the anterior abdominal wall. A fibrous remnant of the left umbilical vein, called the **ligamentum teres**, runs along the free edge of the falciform ligament. The superior aspect of the liver, or bare area, is fused to the diaphragm while the remainder of the organ is enclosed in visceral peritoneum. The lesser omentum anchors the liver to the lesser curvature of the stomach.

Microscopic anatomy

The liver is composed of small units called liver lobules. Lobules are small hexagonal cylinders consisting of plates

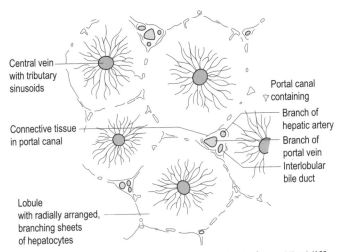

Figure 22.4   The main features of the portal vein (from Hinchliff S M, Montague S E 1990, with permission).

of **hepatocytes** (epithelial liver cells). The hepatocytes produce bile, process bloodborne nutrients, and play an important role in detoxification (see below). The hepatocytes radiate outwards from a central vein running along the longitudinal axis of the lobule. At each of the six corners of a lobule is a **portal triad**. The three structures present in the triad (Fig. 22.4) are:

1. a branch of the hepatic artery, supplying arterial blood to the liver;
2. a branch of the hepatic portal vein (Fig. 22.5), carrying nutrient-rich blood from the digestive tract;
3. a bile duct.

The hepatic artery and the hepatic portal vein enter the liver at the **porta hepatis**. Between the hepatocyte plates are enlarged capillaries called **sinusoids**. Blood percolates through the sinusoids from both the hepatic artery and the hepatic portal vein and is collected up into the central veins. Inside the sinusoids are the **Kupffer cells**, hepatic macrophages which remove debris such as worn-out blood cells and bacteria from the blood.

Digestive functions of the liver

The liver produces bile and also many enzymes that are able to detoxify the many noxious substances arriving at the organ via the bloodstream.

The production of bile

Bile produced by the hepatocytes flows into tiny channels called **bile canaliculi** and enters the bile duct branches in the portal triads. Collectively, the hepatocytes produce as much as 1000 ml of bile daily, with more being produced if a fatty meal is taken. Blood and bile flow in opposite directions in the liver lobules (Fig. 22.6). The bile flows into the hepatic duct and, if needed by the digestive system, flows into the duodenum. If no bile is needed, the sphincter of

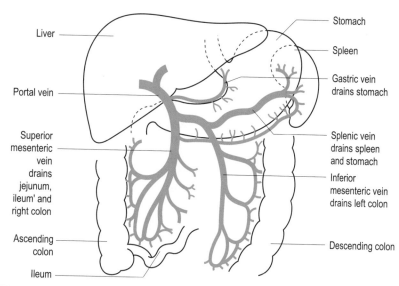

Figure 22.5   The general features of the liver lobules at low magnification, showing the portal triad (from Hinchliff S M, Montague S E 1990, with permission).

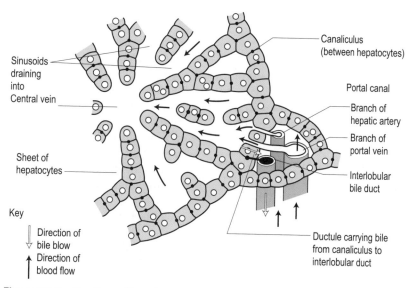

Figure 22.6   The flow of blood and bile within the liver lobule (from Hinchliff S M, Montague S E 1990, with permission).

Oddi is tightly closed and bile flows through the cystic duct to be stored in the gall bladder (Fig. 22.7).

The gall bladder is a thin-walled muscular bag about 10 cm long, situated in a fossa on the inferior surface of the right lobe of the liver. It stores secreted bile and concentrates it by absorbing water and ions. When empty, its walls are thrown into rugae to allow for distension. When the muscular wall contracts, bile is ejected into the cystic duct, leading to the common bile duct. It is covered with visceral peritoneum.

Bile contains no digestive enzymes and its chief role in digestion is to emulsify fats so that they and the fat-soluble vitamins and iron can be absorbed. Bile is a viscous fluid coloured greeny-yellow to brown. It contains 97% water, 0.7% bile salts, mucin and bicarbonate. Also present in bile are fatty acids, lecithin, inorganic salts, alkaline phosphatase and the excretory products of steroid-based hormones. Bile is alkaline with a pH of 7.8–8.0.

Bile salts   Bile salts are formed from the steroids cholic acid and deoxycholic acid, manufactured in the liver from cholesterol. In the liver, cholic acid is **conjugated** (joined together with the elimination of water) with the amino acids taurine and glycine to form taurocholic acid and glycocholic acid. The bile acids form salts with sodium and potassium, which are in solution in the bile.

The functions of the bile salts are to:

- deodorise faeces;
- activate lipase and proteolytic enzymes in the duodenum;
- reduce the surface tension of fat droplets which helps to emulsify them.

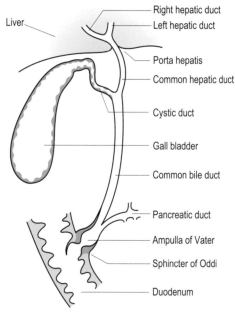

Figure 22.7   The drainage of bile from the liver to the intestine (the biliary tract) (from Hinchliff S M, Montague S E 1990, with permission).

Bile salts combine with lipids, lecithin and cholesterol to form micelles that are water-soluble and allow fat to be more easily absorbed. If bile salts are absent, about 25% of ingested fat will be lost in the stools. These stools will be bulky and have an offensive odour.

Bile pigments   Bile pigments make up 0.2% of the composition of bile. They are produced from the breakdown of red blood cells and are mainly bilirubin with a small amount of biliverdin. The pigments are taken to the liver bound to plasma albumin where they are conjugated with glucuronic acid in the presence of the enzyme glucuronic transferase. This forms the water-soluble bilirubin diglucuronide which enters bile to give it the golden colour. In the gut stercobilinogen is formed and, following conversion by bacterial action, is excreted as stercobilin. Some stercobilinogen is absorbed by the bloodstream and is then excreted as urobilinogen by the kidneys.

Control of bile secretion   As with other secretions into the gastrointestinal tract, the control of bile secretion involves neural and hormonal factors. CCK is the major controller, causing contraction of the gall bladder and relaxation of the sphincter of Oddi. Once the gall bladder has emptied its contents, further flow of bile into the duodenum occurs directly from the liver. Vagus nerve stimulation will bring about a similar action. About 97% of bile salts are reabsorbed into the portal circulation, following their passage through the intestine, and are returned to the liver: this is called the **enterohepatic circulation of bile salts**. The production of bile by the liver depends on the blood level of bile salts. High blood levels of bile salts stimulate the liver cells to secrete more bile.

Detoxification of ingested material

A second important function of the liver is the detoxification of ingested substances. Systems have evolved to protect humans from ingested poisons found especially in plants (see Ch. 8). This involves detoxification by enzyme systems and subsequent excretion of the by-products by the liver. Any alteration in liver or kidney function may reduce the ability of the body to handle harmful chemicals. Many drugs are simply purified naturally occurring chemicals and even those synthesised in the laboratory will have similar chemical structures to naturally occurring substances.

The role of the liver in metabolism

The liver processes nearly every type of nutrient absorbed from the digestive tract. It also plays a major part in controlling plasma cholesterol levels. The hepatocytes carry out at least 500 metabolic functions. It would take a textbook devoted to the topic to begin to explore all of the functions of the liver. That is why the liver is such an important organ. Major metabolic roles include:

- packaging fatty acids into forms that can be stored and transported;
- synthesising plasma proteins;
- synthesising non-essential amino acids;
- converting ammonia, from the deamination of amino acids, to urea for excretion;
- storing glucose as glycogen;
- regulating blood sugar level by glycogenolysis and gluconeogenesis;
- storing vitamins;
- conserving iron from the breakdown of red blood cells;
- detoxifying substances such as alcohol or drugs.

THE ABSORPTION, DISTRIBUTION AND FATE OF DRUGS

There are two main ways of describing drugs in the body:

- **pharmacokinetics**, which is concerned with the way the body handles drugs;
- **pharmacodynamics**, which is concerned with the effect drugs have on the body function (Rang et al 2001).

Drugs are often given to patients because of a need to support a failing system or organ. Examples are the administration of insulin when the pancreas is unable to make sufficient or no insulin of its own in diabetes mellitus, or the use of antibiotics to support the immune system in bacterial invasion. Drugs may also be used to control a function: for example, the administration of the contraceptive pill to control reproductive function. Drugs usually have the following attributes:

- they bind to protein targets;
- they exert chemical influences on one or more cellular components;

- they may affect one or more tissues;
- they may have agonist or antagonist effects.

The protein targets of drugs may be enzymes in metabolic reactions, carrier molecules on cell membranes, receptor molecules on cell membranes or ion channels in cell membranes.

Drug disposition

Drug disposition is the process of drug molecule behaviour in the body. There are four stages:

1. absorption from the site of administration;
2. distribution within the body;
3. metabolic alteration;
4. excretion from the body.

Absorption

Absorption is the passage of a drug from the site of administration into the plasma. Except for some topical applications and some inhaled substances, most drugs must enter the plasma to travel to target tissues. Drugs are absorbed at different rates from sites and some may be unsuitable for some routes.

Distribution within the body (translocation)

There are two main phases in drug distribution. The first is **bulk flow transfer**, which is the transport of drugs around the body by the circulatory system. Some drugs may be transported freely in solution but many are carried around the blood attached to a carrier molecule such as plasma albumin. At cellular level **diffusional transfer** describes the carriage of drugs into the cells in a specific tissue. Diffusional transfer may be by:

- diffusion through the lipid cell membrane;
- diffusion through aqueous pores which traverse the lipid membrane;
- combination with a carrier molecule to ferry the drug across the membrane;
- pinocytosis to engulf the substance.

There is controversy as to whether aqueous pores exist; if they do, they are probably too small to allow entry of most molecules. Pinocytosis, where a piece of cell membrane surrounds the substance and draws it into the cell, concerns large biological molecules only.

Diffusion through the lipid membrane

This is one of the most important pharmacokinetic characteristics of a drug. Fat-soluble drugs diffuse across capillary walls and through cell membranes easily. Other determinants of diffusion include the pH of body fluids (acids and alkalis neutralise each other to precipitate a salt and water) and ionisation (drugs that are strongly ionised are not lipid soluble and may not be able to enter cells unaided).

Carrier mediation

Many drugs have specialised transport mechanisms to regulate entry and exit from cells. This usually involves a carrier molecule incorporated into the cell membrane. In facilitated diffusion, energy is not needed, but in active transport, the cell must use energy. Some pharmaceutical effects are the result of interference with the function of carrier proteins.

Drug metabolism in the liver

Drugs pass through the liver several times while they are in the circulation. Metabolic alteration of drug molecules involves two kinds of biochemical reactions brought about by liver enzymes:

1. **Phase 1 reactions**, which may result in a more active or toxic metabolite of the drug, involve:
   - oxidation – adding oxygen or removing hydrogen;
   - reduction – adding hydrogen or removing oxygen;
   - hydrolysis – splitting of the molecule into separate parts by water.
2. **Phase 2 reactions** involve conjugation by liver enzymes, resulting in a water-soluble inactive product ready for excretion.

Excretion of drugs

Drugs are mainly excreted by the kidney but may also be excreted in expired air, perspiration, faeces and breast milk. In pregnancy, they may cross the placental barrier to the fetus. In the kidney there are three processes for excretion of drugs:

1. **glomerular filtration** – if drugs are free in the plasma, i.e. not bound to plasma proteins and if their molecular weight is below 20 000;
2. **active tubular secretion/reabsorption** – independent carrier systems are present in the cells of the proximal tubule for non-lipid-soluble drugs or ionised drugs (one for acids and one for bases);
3. **passive diffusion across the tubular epithelium** – diffusion of lipid-soluble drugs occurs across the tubular and capillary cell membranes in the distal tubule and collecting tubule.

Drugs that are hydrophilic and poorly lipid soluble such as antibiotics do not enter cells readily. They have a lower density volume and are readily excreted by the kidney. Lipid-soluble drugs are readily reabsorbed in the renal tubule and need breaking down to water-soluble by-products, usually in the liver, in order to be excreted.

MATERNAL ADAPTATIONS TO PREGNANCY

The pancreas

Although there is a slight decrease in serum amylase and lipase, this seems to have no significance. The alterations in glucose metabolism, due to increasing insulin resistance, are much more significant. This may be enough to precipitate diabetes mellitus in susceptible women. Glucose metabolism will be discussed in Chapter 23 and diabetes in pregnancy in Chapter 35.

The gall bladder

The decrease in muscle tone and motility of the gall bladder during pregnancy is probably due to the effects of progesterone on smooth musculature. As a result, the volume is increased and the emptying rate is decreased. An increased fasting volume is probably due to decreased water absorption by the mucosa of the gall bladder. This change is due to reduced activity of the cell wall sodium pump, which is a function of the increased circulating oestrogens. Alterations in gall bladder tone lead to a retention of bile salts, leading to pruritus (Blackburn 2003). Pregnancy may predispose to gall stones but there is little empirical evidence to support this belief.

The liver

Liver size and liver blood flow appear to be unchanged and no histological changes have been seen in pregnancy (Reynolds 1998). However, as pregnancy progresses, the liver is displaced superiorly, posteriorly and anteriorly by the growing uterus. Although there is no change in blood flow to the liver there may be a reduction in the proportion of cardiac output to the liver of about 30% (Blackburn 2003).

There is an alteration in the production of plasma proteins, bilirubin, serum enzymes and serum lipids by the liver. Some changes arise from the presence of oestrogen and some from haemodilution. The changes reduce liver function and make normal testing of liver function less useful.

There may be a reversible disturbance of liver function in pregnancy in women who are otherwise healthy (Hytten 1991). A small proportion of women taking the contraceptive pill show the same effect. There will be jaundice, histologically dilated bile canaliculi and increased bile viscosity. Increased phagocytosis by the Kupffer cells, under the stimulus of oestrogen, has been seen in primate studies and may occur in humans. Storage and mobilisation of liver glycogen may occur more rapidly because of the 50% increase in glomerular filtration rate.

PHARMACOKINETICS AND PREGNANCY

Health professionals who prescribe drugs must consider the likelihood of a woman being pregnant. Drugs taken in early pregnancy may be teratogenic, a prime example being the tragedy of thalidomide in the 1960s (Reynolds 1998). Drugs given in late pregnancy may cause behavioural anomalies in children. Many women are unaware of the danger of taking over-the-counter drugs. Taking drugs in pregnancy may be essential for some women, and their life and the life of the fetus may be endangered if the drugs are discontinued even though the drugs may be involved in causing abnormalities in the fetus. A good example would be the use of Epanutin (phenytoin) in epilepsy, which may cause oral deformities.

Modification of pharmacokinetics

Ingestion

Many knowledgeable women will not comply with taking medicines in pregnancy. Nausea and vomiting may cause rejection of the drug.

Absorption

Most drugs are taken orally and are absorbed by the stomach and small intestine. Gastric motility is reduced throughout pregnancy and especially in labour. This slows down absorption of some drugs but may increase absorption of others. Most common drugs show little change from normal. Taking antacid preparations will lead to the absorption of some drugs being reduced.

Distribution

Increased extracellular fluid and body fat may alter the compartmental distribution of drugs. The fetus is considered to be a compartment and, although probably resistant to bolus doses, may be at risk in long-term drug therapy of some chemicals.

Protein binding

Many drugs circulate around the body bound to plasma proteins, especially albumin, which is reduced in pregnancy. There is an increase in some specific proteins such as transferrin and thyroid-binding hormone. Some drugs which bind to α_1 acid glycoprotein are more likely to cross the placenta.

Elimination

Drugs that act within the central nervous system or within cells are lipid soluble. These cannot be effectively excreted without conjugation to water-soluble by-products in the liver. The kidney will excrete those drugs excreted by the renal tubules. The rule of the placenta as a barrier to drugs is discussed in Box 22.1.

Box 22.1 The placenta and fetus

Almost all drug reactions carried out by the liver have been identified in placental tissue. However, no studies have been carried out in vivo. This means we cannot trust the placenta to protect the fetus from the effect of drugs. The main trophoblastic layer in the placenta is a syncytium, covered by a continuous lipid membrane. This membrane acts in a similar way to the blood–brain barrier so that lipid substances of low molecular weight (below 1000) can readily diffuse across the membrane. Water-soluble molecules of up to 100 MW can also diffuse easily but charged ionic molecules cannot pass unless they are bound to a carrier protein. Therefore drugs that affect the central nervous system will readily cross the placental barrier.

Other drugs such as barbiturates, non-steroidal anti-inflammatory agents, warfarin and anticonvulsants are weak acids while narcotics, local anaesthetics, beta blockers or beta stimulants are weak bases. These act as non-ionic substances and will cross the placental barrier slowly. Polar drugs such as the penicillins and cephalosporins are transferred so slowly that the fetus has no problem eliminating the drugs faster than they are transferred. Heparin is a large molecule and cannot cross the placenta. The fetus and neonate have a much reduced ability to handle drugs because of immaturity of liver enzyme systems.

Maternal elimination of polar non-lipid drugs is much faster during pregnancy, as the kidney excretes them. This means that the dose requirements of some drugs, such as anticonvulsants, may rise during pregnancy. Some of these drugs cannot cross the placental barrier while others are excreted rapidly by the fetus and pose no problem. Some drugs such as anticonvulsants build up slowly in the fetus and may cause malformations. Maternal breakdown of lipid-soluble drugs is slower in pregnancy and these drugs readily cross the placenta and into fetal tissues and may be excreted very slowly (Reynolds 1998).

MAIN POINTS

- Salivary glands (three pairs) produce saliva, which aids speech, chewing and swallowing. Saliva contains lysozyme and immunoglobulin IgA as defence against microorganisms. A digestive enzyme, salivary or α amylase, acts upon starch to convert polysaccharides into disaccharides.

- The secretion of saliva is controlled primarily by parasympathetic supply, producing continuous moderate amounts of watery saliva. Saliva is produced as a conditioned reflex in response to the perception of the thought, sight or smell of food.

- The pancreas has both endocrine and exocrine functions. The pancreas produces 1.5–2 L of alkaline pancreatic juice daily. Pancreatic juice secretion is divided into a cephalic phase in response to food stimuli and a gastric phase stimulated by the release of gastrin.

- About 1% of the pancreas consists of the islet of Langerhans cells. The α cells synthesise glucagon and the β cells produce insulin. The δ cells produce somatostatin, which acts to suppress islet cell hormone production.

- Glucagon acts in the liver to promote glycogenolysis, lypolysis and gluconeogenesis. Insulin stimulates glucose utilisation, glycogen synthesis, inhibition of glycogen breakdown and inhibition of gluconeogenesis. Insulin assists the entry of glucose into muscle, connective tissue and white blood cells.

- The liver is composed of lobules, consisting of plates of hepatocytes radiating outwards from a central vein. The hepatocytes produce bile, process bloodborne nutrients and play an important role in detoxification.

- Bile produced by the hepatocytes flows into tiny channels called bile canaliculi and enters the bile duct branches in the portal triads. If no bile is needed, the sphincter of Oddi is tightly closed and bile flows through the cystic duct to be stored in the gall bladder.

- Bile salts manufactured in the liver, from cholesterol, deodorise faeces, activate lipase and proteolytic enzymes in the duodenum and reduce the surface tension of fat droplets, which helps to emulsify them. Bile pigments are produced from the breakdown of red blood cells.

- The control of bile secretion involves neural and hormonal factors. CCK is the major controller, causing contraction of the gall bladder and relaxation of the sphincter of Oddi. High blood levels of bile salts stimulate the liver cells to secrete more bile.

- The liver detoxifies ingested substances by enzyme systems and excretes the by-products. The liver processes nearly every type of nutrient absorbed from the digestive tract.

- Pharmacokinetics is concerned with the way the body handles drugs and pharmacodynamics is concerned with the effect drugs have on the body function. Drug disposition is the process of drug molecule behaviour in the body. There are four stages: absorption from the site of administration, distribution, metabolic alteration and excretion.

- Liver size and liver blood flow seem to be unchanged in pregnancy and no histological changes have been found. The growing uterus displaces the liver as pregnancy progresses.

- Increased extracellular fluid and body fat during pregnancy may alter the compartmental distribution of drugs. The fetus is considered to be a compartment and, although probably resistant to bolus doses, may be at risk in some long-term drug therapy. Many drugs circulate around the body bound to plasma proteins, especially albumin. Some drugs are likely to cross the placenta.

- Almost all drug reactions carried out by the liver have been identified in placental tissue. This means we cannot trust the placenta to protect the fetus from the effect of drugs. The fetus and neonate have a reduced ability to handle drugs because of immaturity of liver enzyme systems.

- Maternal elimination of polar non-lipid drugs is much faster during pregnancy, as the kidney excretes them. This means that the dose requirements of some drugs such as anticonvulsants may rise during pregnancy. Maternal breakdown of lipid-soluble drugs is slower in pregnancy and these drugs readily cross the placenta into fetal tissues and may be excreted very slowly.

References

Blackburn S T 2003 Maternal, Fetal and Neonatal Physiology: A Clinical Perspective, 3rd edn. W B Saunders, Philadelphia.

Hytten F 1991 The alimentary system. In Hytten F, Chamberlain G (eds) Clinical Physiology in Obstetrics, 2nd edn. Blackwell Science, Oxford.

Marieb E N 2000 Human Anatomy and Physiology, 5th edn. Benjamin/Cummings, New York.

Rang H P, Dale M M, Ritter J M et al (eds) 2001 Pharmacology, 4th edn. Churchill Livingstone, Edinburgh.

Reynolds F 1998 Pharmacokinetics. In Chamberlain G, Broughton Pipkin F (eds) Clinical Physiology in Obstetrics, 3rd edn. Blackwell Science, Oxford.

Annotated recommended reading

Marieb E N 2000 Human Anatomy & Physiology, 5th edn. Benjamin/Cummings, New York.
This textbook presents a detailed overview of human anatomy and physiology and is well illustrated with diagrams and pictures.

Coad J, Dunstall M 2001 Anatomy and Physiology for Midwives. Mosby, Edinburgh.
This is an excellent textbook that provides detailed information on the adaptations made during pregnancy and is applicable to midwifery practice.

Chapter **23**

Nutrition and metabolism during pregnancy

INTRODUCTION

There has been considerable progress in nutritional science as well as significant changes in the reproductive life cycle. Over recent decades the average age of menarche has been reduced to 12.5 years and the average menopause age is about 50 years, leading to a 40-year span for female reproduction. In addition, the number of women delaying their first pregnancies until their thirties has increased and there are huge lifestyle changes. In line with the above alterations in the pattern of reproduction and lifestyle, there is more emphasis on the importance of nutrition in maternity care (Edelmann & Mandle 1998). Nutrition, alongside other advancements in health care, can have a pivotal effect in optimising a successful pregnancy outcome. Its importance lies in prevention of birth defects, promoting appropriate gestational weight to long-term health outcome for the baby as well as the mother.

Nutritional advice for pregnant women has recently changed from eating for two to more careful consideration of dietary quality as well as quantity on a need basis. Adequate energy and nutrient intake during pregnancy has significant impact on the wellbeing of the mother and her growing fetus, both in the short and long term. However, some health professionals do not feel confident enough to give nutritional advice to their clients. In this chapter, the principles of general nutrition as well as pregnancy specific nutritional requirements and metabolic adaptation will be discussed.

NUTRITION

Nutrition is based on two fundamental areas of science: biochemistry and physiology. For practical purposes, this section will focus on a brief overview of basic nutrition physiology: general food groups, energy and nutrients and metabolism. Nutrients are utilised by the body for tissue growth, maintenance and repair. They can be divided into six categories – three major nutrients (macronutrients) are carbohydrates, lipids and proteins; vitamins and minerals are required in small amounts and water is usually considered

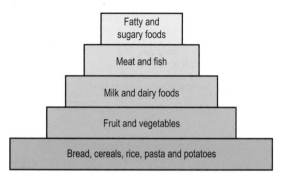

Figure 23.1   The 'good food guide', showing the five main groups of food (from Sweet B 1997, with permission).

as a food because of its role as a solvent. Most foods provide a combination of nutrients, and water makes up 60% of the volume of food intake.

There are hundreds of molecules involved in maintaining good health. Many cells, especially those in the liver, can convert one type of food molecule to another but there are about 50 essential nutrients which cannot be manufactured by the body cells. These must be provided in the diet if the body is to synthesise the remainder (Marieb 2000).

Food groups

There are four food groups which must be eaten in order to provide a balanced diet. The types and a general guide on the daily food choices are:

- Grains, bread, cereal, rice and pasta, 6–11 servings.
- Fruits, 2–4 servings, and vegetables, 2–3 servings.
- Meat, poultry and fish, 2–3 servings.
- Dairy products, milk, cheese and yoghurt, 2–3 servings.

Tiran (1997) adds a fifth group – fats and sugary foods. These can be arranged in a pyramid, showing the quantities in relation to the health benefits of consumption (Fig. 23.1).

Carbohydrates

Carbohydrate is the main source of energy in our food although the other macronutrients can also be metabolised to yield energy. According to their structure, there are three types of carbohydrates: monosaccharides (single sugars), disaccharides (double sugars) and polysaccharides (multiple sugars or complex carbohydrates). Most of the carbohydrate we eat comes from plants. The main food sources of carbohydrates according to their classes are given below.

1. Monosaccharides:
   - glucose, which is the ultimate example (corn syrup, processed foods);
   - fructose (fruits, honey);
   - galactose (milk).
2. Disaccharides:
   - sucrose, which is made from glucose and fructose (sugar);
   - lactose, which is made from glucose and galactose (milk);
   - maltose, which is made from two glucoses (commercial malt product of starch breakdown, intermediate sweetener in food products).
3. Polysaccharides:
   - starch (grains, legumes, root vegetables);
   - glycogen (liver and muscle meats);
   - Dietary fibre (whole grain, fruit and vegetables, seeds and nuts).

Carbohydrates play a fundamental role in the physiology of the body: glucose, for example, is the ultimate common refined body fuel that is oxidised in cells to give energy. It is important to maintain a certain range in the blood of between 3.9 and 7.8 mmol/L to allow normal functioning. Cellulose is a form of plant carbohydrate (dietary fibre) that the human digestive system cannot process. It provides roughage to increase the bulk of faeces, thus facilitating defecation. Dietary fibres are also believed to have a role in the management of serum lipid and glucose levels; therefore, they are helpful in prevention and management of chronic diseases such as diabetes and cardiovascular disease.

Carbohydrate metabolism

The Krebs (tricarboxylic acid or citric acid cycle)   When glucose in the circulating blood arrives at the tissues it is taken up by the cells by facilitated diffusion under the influence of insulin. Glucose is taken to the cells' mitochondria where it is oxidised to form energy in the Krebs cycle (Figs 23.2 and 23.3). A series of reactions are involved when glucose, a 6-carbon molecule, is broken down into two 3-carbon molecules of pyruvic acid, in a process called glycolysis.

Pyruvic acid is broken down further to a 2-carbon molecule called acetic acid and the released carbon atom forms carbon dioxide by combining with oxygen. The acetic acid now combines with coenzyme A (a derivative of a B complex vitamin, pantothenic acid) to form the enzyme acetyl coenzyme A (acetyl CoA). Acetyl CoA enters the Krebs cycle to undergo changes mediated by enzymes; ATP, water and carbon dioxide are formed in the process of oxidation.

The Krebs cycle consists of a series of eight separate biochemical reactions. This cycle of reactions is like one revolution of a wheel with acetyl CoA sitting at the top. Each glucose molecule produces two pyruvic acid molecules and allows two turns of the cycle. Carbon dioxide produced when the excess carbon atoms unite with oxygen and surplus hydrogen atoms need to be disposed of. Two hydrogen carrier molecules, nicotinamide adenine dinucleotide (NAD) and flavin adenine dinucleotide (FAD), perform this function. The transfer of the hydrogen atoms converts the compounds into NADH and $FADH_2$, respectively.

ATP synthesis   Energy is stored in carbon–hydrogen bonds in food but cells cannot use energy in this form. They must convert it into the high-energy phosphate bonds of

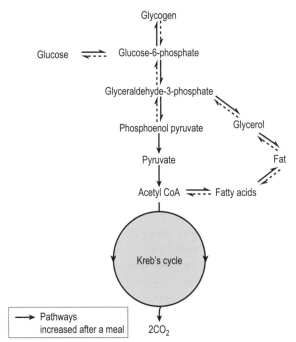

Figure 23.2   A summary of glucose metabolism after a meal (from Hinchliff S M, Montague S E 1990, with permission).

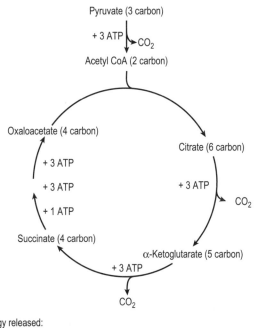

Energy released:
    from pyruvate 15 ATP
    from 2 x pyruvate formed from 1 glucose molecule   30 ATP
    from glycolysis of 1 glucose molecule to 2 x pyruvate   8 ATP

    Total from aerobic metabolism of 1 glucose molecule   38 ATP

Figure 23.3   A summary of the Krebs cycle (from Hinchliff S M, Montague S E 1990, with permission).

adenosine triphosphate (ATP) (Sherwood 1989). ATP consists of adenosine with three phosphate groups attached. When a bond between adenosine (a nucleotide) and one of the phosphate groups is split, large amounts of energy are released and adenosine diphosphate + an inorganic phosphate molecule (P_i) is formed. Some of the energy produced is in the form of heat and helps to maintain the temperature of the body. This can be written as:

$$\text{Splitting by hydrolysis}$$
$$ATP \rightarrow ADP + P_i + energy$$

Cellular respiration

Aerobic cellular respiration   The main role of the Krebs cycle is to prepare the hydrogen acceptors for entry into the electron transport chain (respiratory chain) in the inner mitochondrial membrane. Electron transfer molecules are mostly brightly coloured protein-bound iron-containing pigments called cytochromes. These are arranged in a specific order which allows high-energy electrons to pass through a chain of reactions, resulting in a lowering of the energy levels at each step. At the end of this chain, the electrons are passed to the final electron acceptor, which is inspired oxygen.

The stepwise release of energy during the progression through the electron transport chain is used to pump protons into the intermembrane space. This creates an electrochemical proton gradient across the mitochondrial inner membrane which temporarily stores the energy. Protons flow back across the membrane through the enzyme ATP synthetase, providing the energy to attach a phosphate group to ADP to create a further 32 ATP molecules for each glucose molecule processed. The total production of ATP for one turn of the cycle is therefore 38 molecules. NAD and FAD are released to capture more hydrogen and begin the energy transfer again. This process, which uses oxygen and phosphate, is called oxidative phosphorylation or aerobic respiration (Marieb 2000).

Anaerobic cellular respiration   If there is no oxygen available, a few molecules of ATP are synthesised during glycolysis but the process cannot proceed further. Only two molecules of ATP are available for each glucose molecule. This is called substrate-level phosphorylation (Marieb 2000). The energy remains trapped in the molecules of pyruvic acid, and lactic acid is formed (anaerobic respiration). An oxygen debt arises and metabolic acidosis is created (Sherwood 1989). When oxygen is available, the lactic acid is gradually converted to pyruvic acid and fed into the Krebs cycle.

Lipids

Lipid is the chemical name for fats and fat-related compounds. The most common source of lipids is in the form of triglycerides. Triglycerides are made up of fatty acids and glycerol. Fats provide the highest-density source of energy for the body. Carbohydrates can also be converted to fat and stored in the adipose tissue. Fat is essential for maintaining health; what is harmful is excess fat intake (more than 30% of the total calories). Fatty acids, the common structural units of lipids, are also a refined fuel form which is preferred by some cells (e.g. heart muscle) over glucose.

Fatty acids consist of carbon, hydrogen and oxygen atoms. If a given fatty acid is filled with as much hydrogen as it can take, the fatty acid is saturated with hydrogen and the lipids containing them are called saturated fats. Saturated fats are mainly in animal fats such as meat and dairy products. Monounsaturated fats are fats containing fatty acids with one less hydrogen atom, creating one double bond between carbon atoms. The main sources of such fats are olive oils and canola oil, which is derived from the rape seed. Finally, lipids mainly made from unsaturated fatty acids with two or more places unfilled with hydrogen, creating double bonds, are called polyunsaturated. These are also from plant sources (see Rodwell-Williams 1999).

Despite common perception, cholesterol is not a fat itself but is a fat-related compound vital in human metabolism. Cholesterol belongs to the steroid family and helps in production of vitamin D, formation of bile acids, digestion and absorption of fats. Cholesterol is found in all animal foods, mainly in egg yolk and organ meats such as kidneys and liver. Even with no dietary intake of cholesterol, it is synthesised in our liver.

There are some fatty acids that the liver cannot synthesise so that they are an essential dietary component. These include linolenic and alpha-linolenic, arachidonic, eicosapentanoic and decosahexanoic acids. They can all be synthesised from linoleic and alpha-linolenic acid, but if the supply of linoleic and alpha-linolenic acid is limited, they can become essential fatty acids. These fatty acids, are also found in vegetable oil.

Body fat stores and functions

Body fat is mainly stored under the skin and around the abdominal organs. It is continually being interchanged with the fats circulating in the bloodstream and being metabolised for use as fuel. The dietary reference values for total fat intake are that 35% of energy should be provided by fat. Fats are essential for many of the body's functions.

- They are a source of energy.
- They are involved in the absorption of the fat-soluble vitamins.
- Triglycerides provide the major fuel for energy for hepatocytes and skeletal muscle.
- Phospholipids are a component of myelin sheaths that surround larger nerves and all cell membranes.
- Fatty deposits act as protective cushions for the vital organs such as eyes and kidneys
- Fats provide an insulating layer under the skin.
- Prostaglandins are formed from linoleic acid. They play a role in smooth muscle contraction and inflammatory responses.
- Fats are part of the cell membrane structure.

- Fats are involved in cell metabolism. Combinations of lipids and protein, called lipoproteins, carry lipids in the blood to cells.
- They are involved in nerve impulse transmission.

Lipid metabolism

The energy obtained from fat breakdown or lypolysis is twice that obtained from the metabolism of glucose or protein (4 kcal/g each), providing 9 kcal/g. About 80 g of fat is absorbed daily, mainly in the duodenum. Any excess fat is stored as adipose tissue in subcutaneous tissues and retroperitoneal tissue. When fat stores are needed for energy production, as in glucose shortage, they are mobilised from the stores under the influence of growth hormones or cortisol. They are taken to the liver where the triglycerides are broken down into free fatty acids and glycerol which are released into the blood.

Glycerol is converted to one of the intermediate products of glycolysis called glyceraldehyde phosphate and is thus assimilated into the energy-releasing process. Further oxidation of the fatty acids releases the 2-carbon acetic acid which is fused to coenzyme A to form acetyl CoA, which enters the Krebs cycle. Fatty acids cannot be used for gluconeogenesis (glucose synthesis) because they enter the cycle beyond the pyruvic acid stage when the changes are irreversible.

In the presence of oxygen and glucose, fatty acids are converted to acetyl CoA, which enters the Krebs cycle. If no glucose is available (e.g. in starvation, diabetes mellitus, some slimming diets or hyperemesis gravidarum) metabolism of a large amount of fat may occur, acetyl CoA accumulates and the liver converts the molecules to ketone bodies, i.e. acetoacetic acid and β-hydroxybutyric acid, which accumulate in the blood. These can be oxidised to release energy but metabolic acidosis will occur.

Cholesterol   Bile salts, steroid hormones and cell membranes are formed from cholesterol. Cholesterol is found in the blood – mainly in combination with a protein carrier – as lipoproteins, of which there are three types:

1. high-density lipoproteins (HDLs);
2. low-density lipoproteins (LDLs);
3. very low-density lipoproteins (VLDLs).

It is also thought that cholesterol is laid down as atheromatous plaques in arterial walls in the form of LDLs and VLDLs. A high ratio of HDLs to LDLs and VLDLs may offer protection against ischaemic heart disease (Marieb 2000). The ratio of HDLs to LDLs and VLDLs has been shown to be increased in vegetarians, people whose fat intake is largely unsaturated and who take regular exercise and reduced in smokers.

Proteins

Animals (including humans) can synthesise protein from amino acids but are unable to synthesise amino acids de novo. Plants can synthesise amino acids from carbon dioxide, water and nitrogen. Therefore, human dietary sources of amino acids/proteins are plants or other animals. Amino acids can be converted to each other through a process in the liver called transamination. Those amino acids that the body either cannot make or cannot make in sufficient amount are called essential or semi-essential amino acids. The best source of essential amino acids is animal products.

Protein foods which have all the essential amino acids such as eggs, meat and human breast milk are said to have a high biological value. Protein foods from plant sources tend to have a lower biological value and should be eaten as a mixture, for their proteins complement each other, hence improving their biological values. Strict vegetarians can obtain all the essential amino acids by varying their diet carefully. For instance, cereals and legumes contain all the essential amino acids when taken together. Examples of such meals are West Indian rice and peas or the Middle Eastern meal of a meat dish with a mixture of peas and beans eaten with bread.

The functions of proteins

Proteins include important structural molecules such as muscle protein, collagen and elastin in connective tissue and keratin in skin. They produce new tissue and are therefore essential for growth, recovery from injury, pregnancy and lactation. Proteins also function as hormones, enzymes and transport molecules such as haemoglobin. Amino acids can be used to synthesise proteins or can be converted to glucose to provide energy. These uses depend on:

1. the presence within the cell at the same time of all the amino acids needed to manufacture a protein;
2. adequacy of calorie intake in the form of carbohydrates and fats for energy production;
3. nitrogen balance, which is the balance between protein synthesis and protein breakdown;
4. the influences of hormones – anabolic hormones such as growth hormone and the sex hormones stimulate tissue growth while the glucocorticoids produced in stress enhance protein breakdown and the conversion of amino acids to glucose.

The amount of protein needed in the diet is influenced by the age, size, metabolic rate and nitrogen balance. The recommended daily intake is 0.8 g per kg body weight in non-obese individuals. This is equivalent to 60 g of fish or meat and a glass of milk daily. Meat eaters in developed countries eat far in excess of the daily amount needed while some people in developing countries rarely eat meat.

Amino acids

At least 50 g a day is needed to maintain nitrogen balance and to provide for growth and repair of tissues. Amino acids cannot be stored by the body. However, the liver can interconvert amino acids by utilising the eight essential amino acids to synthesise the non-essential amino acids. Any excess amino acids are broken down by the liver by a process of deamination. The nitrogen portion is converted into urea, which enters the blood and is excreted by the kidney.

Proteins are needed by the body for the following functions:

- development and growth and the formation of new cells;
- the manufacture of enzymes, hormones and antibodies;
- the transport molecules such as haemoglobin;
- plasma proteins which act as buffers to maintain acid–base balance;
- the control of osmotic pressure between body fluid compartments;
- amino acids can be used in gluconeogenesis once glucose stores are depleted.

Vitamins

Vitamins were discovered in the first half of the 1900s and were called vitalamines at first. They are non-energy yielding organic micronutrients needed in small amounts for growth and health (Marieb 2000). Both vitamin deficiency and excess intake may be associated with adverse pregnancy outcome. They mainly function as coenzymes to assist in the catalysis of chemical processes and metabolism in the body. The human body is unable to synthesise most vitamins with the exception of vitamin K and some of the B vitamins. Vitamins are distinguished usually according to their solubility in either fat or water. Some vitamins are fat-soluble, such as vitamins A, D, E and K, and are absorbed bound to digested lipids. The water-soluble vitamins, such as most of the B complex and vitamin C, are absorbed with water from the gastrointestinal tract. A normal varied diet should provide them all. Excessive intake can create as many health problems as insufficient intake. Details of the vitamins are given in Box 23.1.

Minerals, trace elements and water

Minerals and trace elements known as micronutrients are inorganic elements that are widely distributed in nature. The mineral content of the human body is very similar to that of the Earth. There are seven minerals that the human body requires in greater amount, comprising calcium, phosphorus, potassium, sulphur, sodium, chloride and magnesium. The remaining 18 elements, called trace elements, include iron, iodine and zinc and are no less important, but they occur in very small amounts, contributing to 20–40% of the total inorganic elements in the body.

Minerals constitute about 4% of the body's weight. Most minerals are found in solution in body fluids or are bound to organic molecules such as iron in haemoglobin. Calcium and phosphorus are found in bone, adding strength to the structure, and they make up three-quarters of the amount (see Ch. 24). Iron is discussed in Chapter 16 and sodium

Box 23.1 The vitamins

Fat-soluble vitamins

Vitamin A

Vitamin A is available in two forms: β-carotene and the active form, retinol. Beta-carotene is found in plant food, whereas retinol is from animal food sources. Beta-carotene is converted to retinol in the intestines, liver and kidneys and provides two-thirds of required vitamin A in human nutrition. Several substances aid in absorption of vitamin A, including bile salts, pancreatic lipase and dietary fat. It is stored in liver, easily oxidised and destroyed rapidly by light. Retinol is found in fish liver oils, egg yolk, liver and fortified milk; butter and commercial products such as margarine are fortified with vitamin A. Good sources of beta-carotene are carrots and deep green leafy vegetables (broccoli, spinach).

Importance   Vitamin A is involved in vision, growth and bone development, tooth formation, maintenance of strong epithelial tissue and reproduction. It has a role in adaptation of eyes to light and dark through synthesis of photoreceptor pigments as well as prevention of infection because of its role in stability of cell membranes, skin and mucous membranes. Absorption is impeded by alcohol, coffee and vitamin D deficiency. Beta-carotene has also been shown to have an antioxidant capacity, helping to neutralise free radicals in the cell, and it may protect against the ageing process.

Deficiency   The early sign of vitamin A deficiency is a poor dark adaptation or night blindness. Severe deficiencies may lead to blindness, skin disorders, tooth decay and gastrointestinal disorders. Birth defects have occurred in women taking supplements or eating excessive amounts, such as found in liver. It is thought that retinol is a teratogenic agent (Ranjan 1991).

Vitamin D

Vitamin D (7-dehydrocholesterol) is a sterol hormone precursor ingested from animal products. The precursor obtained from plants is called ergosterol. Following ingestion these two substances are transported to the skin where 7-dehydrocholesterol is changed in the skin by the action of ultraviolet (UV) light to an intermediate product Vitamin D_3 (cholecalciferol) and ergosterol is converted to vitamin D_2 or ergocalciferol. The most important one is cholecalciferol, which is modified firstly by the liver and then by the kidneys to produce physiologically active Vitamin D_3 calcitriol (1,25-dihydroxycholecalciferol). It is absorbed in the small intestine with the aid of bile. Vitamin D is stored in liver and skin and is stable to heat and light. Dark-skinned people or those who avoid dairy products may be prone to deficiency. The major source of vitamin D is that formed in the body as a result of ultraviolet irradiation of skin. Dietary sources of vitamin D are fish liver oils, egg/egg yolk, liver and fortified milk. Laxatives and antacids may inhibit gut absorption.

Importance   The predominant role of vitamin D is in the metabolism of calcium and phosphorus. It activates absorption of calcium and promotes bone mineralisation. It is also needed for renal, cardiac and nervous system functions and is involved in blood clotting.

Deficiency   Deficiency causes poor mineralisation of bones and teeth such as rickets in children and osteomalacia in adults. There may be poor muscle tone, restlessness and irritability.

Vitamin E (tocopherol)

Vitamin E is chemically related to the sex hormones. It is stored in muscle and adipose tissue and is heat and light resistant. It is an antioxidant that is unstable in oxygen. Vitamin E is widely distributed in foods and wheat germ and wheat germ oil are particularly rich in it. Vitamin E is found in vegetable oils, margarine, whole grains and dark green leafy vegetables. It is destroyed by food processing and its absorption is reduced by the contraceptive pill.

Importance   Vitamin E deficiency in rats has been shown to be related to failure of reproduction but its role in humans is not fully understood. It may assist in reproduction and has antioxidant effects, so it is important in the prevention of cancers and cardiovascular disease and in maintaining the integrity of the cell membrane.

Deficiency   In vitamin E deficiency, cell membranes are more in danger of oxidation and breakdown; therefore, there is more risk of haemolytic anaemia. In particular, its deficiency can occur in premature infants, as vitamin E stores are normally built up the last month or two of fetal life. It may also cause neurological symptoms, as it is involved in myelin, the protective fat covering for the long axons of nerve cells (Ch. 25). Deficiency may result in spontaneous abortion, preterm labour and stillbirth.

Vitamin K – coagulation vitamin

There are different forms of vitamin K, including vitamin K_1 (phylloquinone), the dietary form found in green leaves, vegetables (and small amounts in fruit, meat, dairy products and cereal) and vitamin K_2 (menaquinone), which is mainly produced by intestinal bacteria. The approximate recommended dietary allowance (RDA) for men is 80 μg/day and 65 μg/day for women. No additional amount is advised for pregnancy or lactation. It is stored in the liver, is heat resistant but is destroyed by acids, alkalis, light and oxidising agents.

Importance   Vitamin K is essential for maintaining and activating blood clotting factors (e.g. prothrombin) and some other proteins in the liver.

Deficiency   Deficiency is rare in normal health but easy bruising and bleeding occur due to prolonged clotting time. Deficiency occurs as a result of anticoagulant or antibiotic therapy.

Water-soluble vitamins

Vitamin C – ascorbic acid

Vitamin C is a 6-carbon crystalline substance derived from glucose. Unlike other primates, humans cannot synthesise vitamin C and must obtain it from food. It is rapidly destroyed by heat, light and alkalis so that food containing vitamin C should be cooked with minimum water for brief periods and kept covered. It is easily absorbed from the small intestine and is not stored in a single tissue, but is distributed throughout body tissues. Sufficient vitamin C is present in mother's milk (with a balanced diet) but very little exists in cow's milk so it is added to formula milk.

Vitamin C is found in fruits and vegetables, particularly in citrus fruits, strawberries, tomatoes and fresh potatoes. Some drugs such as aspirin, anticoagulants, antibiotics, diuretics, cortisone, the contraceptive pill and antidepressants may interfere with absorption. Other factors that interfere with absorption are pollution, industrial toxins, overcooking or poor food storage (Tiran 1997).

Importance   Along with vitamin A and E, vitamin C is an antioxidant. It is essential to build and maintain body tissues, especially collagen. It is involved in the formation of haemoglobin and development of red blood cells by facilitating the absorption of iron and removal of iron from ferritin. It also assists in other vital processes such as the metabolism of amino acids and synthesis of peptide hormones.

Deficiency   Vitamin C deficiency can cause poor resistance to bacterial infections, anaemia, bruising and haemorrhage, oedema, poor digestion and gum disease. This combination of symptoms is called scurvy. Vitamin C is important in wound healing, fever and infection, growth period, stress and body defence. Recent research appears to suggest that a very low intake of vitamin C may more than double the risk of women developing pre-eclampsia (Zhang et al 2002). Supplementation with antioxidants (vitamins C and E) was associated with a reduced incidence of pre-eclampsia (Alexander 2002).

Vitamin B₁ – thiamine

This vitamin is a fairly stable antioxidant but is destroyed by alkalis and high temperature. A small amount only can be stored (a continuous supply is necessary); excess is eliminated in urine. Its requirement depends on carbohydrate and energy intake. The RDA for adults is 0.5 mg/1000 kcal daily. It is not necessary to increase intake during pregnancy and lactation. Vitamin B_1 is found in lean meat, liver, eggs, whole grains, nuts, leafy green vegetables and legumes. Its absorption in the small intestine is reduced by alcohol, coffee, food additives and overcooking and it is lost in cooking water.

Importance   Vitamin B_1 helps to maintain healthy nerves, cardiac muscle and digestive tract and forms part of an enzyme which is energy metabolism-related and specifically acts in the metabolism of carbohydrate, alcohol, fat and pyruvic acid (produced during the metabolism of glycogen in muscles).

Deficiency   As it is involved in energy and glucose metabolism, deficiency of thiamine can affect the gastrointestinal (deficiency of hydrochloric acid), nervous, cardiovascular and musculoskeletal systems. Its deficiency causes the disease beriberi (I can't, I can't) with pain, weakness, degeneration of muscles and inability to perform coordinated movements. The full disease is rarely seen in developed countries. The other disease due to thiamine deficiency is Wernicke–Korsakoff syndrome which could occur in people with long-term vomiting (e.g. hyperemesis gravidarum) or in alcoholics. Its symptoms include poor memory, confusion, apathy and ataxia.

Vitamin B₂ – riboflavin

This vitamin contains a sugar named ribose and is yellow (flavin means yellow in Latin). A small amount can be stored and excess is eliminated in urine. It is stable to heat but sensitive to light. Vitamin B_2 is found in lean meat, yeast, liver, eggs, whole grains, nuts, meats, legumes and mainly in milk. Its absorption will be reduced by the contraceptive pill and antibiotics.

Importance   Riboflavin forms part of enzymes which help in energy metabolism and tissue building.

Deficiency   Poor wound healing and cracks in lips, corner of mouth and tongue are typical signs of vitamin B_2 deficiency. Because of the sensitivity of riboflavin to light, attention should be given to premature infants who are getting phototherapy treatment for the symptoms of riboflavin deficiency.

Vitamin B₃ – niacin

Niacin exists in two forms: nicotinic acid, which is easily converted to its amide form, and nicotinamide, which is a simple, stable organic compound. A small amount can be stored and daily intake is desirable. Excess is eliminated in urine. It is found in any protein food: meat, peanuts, dry beans and peas. It can easily be synthesised in the body from the amino acid tryptophan. Its absorption will be reduced by alcohol, coffee, antibiotics and antitubercular drugs.

Importance   It has two coenzyme forms involved in catabolic and anabolic functions which help to metabolise fats, carbohydrates and proteins.

Deficiency   Deficiency of vitamin B_3 causes the disease pellagra with headache, weight loss, loss of appetite and later, soreness and redness of the lips and tongue, vomiting and diarrhoea and skin ulceration. Neurological symptoms may also occur. This disease is rarely seen in developed countries.

Vitamin B_6 – pyridoxine

This vitamin occurs in free and phosphorylated forms in the body. It is stable to heat and acids but destroyed by alkalis and light. Body stores are limited and excess is eliminated in the urine. The RDA standard is 2 mg/day for men and 1.6 mg/day for women, with additions for pregnancy and lactation. Vitamin B_6 is found in grains, seeds, meat, liver and kidney. Its absorption is reduced by antibiotics and antitubercular drugs.

Importance   Pyridoxine forms part of enzymes which help to metabolise proteins, fats and carbohydrates. It is important for the nervous system, amino acid formation, sulphur transfer, formation of niacin from tryptophan and formation of antibodies and haemoglobin. A dosage of vitamin B_6 of up to 100 mg/day is likely to be beneficial in treating premenstrual symptoms and premenstrual depression (Wyatt et al 1999).

Deficiency   Deficiency of vitamin B_6 causes anaemia, convulsions, irritability, vomiting and abdominal pain in infants and dermatitis and depression in adults. It could be toxic in large amounts (up to 5 g/day).

Vitamin B_{12} – cyanocobalamin

This vitamin is complex and contains cobalt. It is stable to heat but inactivated by acids and alkalis. Vitamin B_{12} is found mainly in meat, but milk, eggs, butter and cheese are also valuable sources. Some synthesis is done by human intestinal bacteria and it is found in some seaweeds. It is not found in any vegetable or fruit.

Importance   It is the intrinsic factor necessary for the transportation of iron across the intestinal membrane. It is stored in the liver, with stores sufficient to last 3–5 years in normal health. It is also involved in enzymes working in bone marrow in the formation of DNA. In its absence, erythrocytes do not divide. It is necessary for normal protein metabolism and production of myelin sheath around nerve cells.

Deficiency   Vitamin B_{12} deficiency causes pernicious anaemia and neurological symptoms. Vegans and vegetarians may have a diet deficient in vitamin B_{12}.

Folic acid

Folic acid is not a stable vitamin, so considerable losses occur in cooking. It is stored mainly in the liver. It is toxic in excessive amounts. Folic acid is widely distributed in food sources such as liver, yeast, eggs, whole grain, deep green vegetables and nuts. It is also synthesised in the gut by enteric bacteria. Absorption is hindered by alcohol and drugs that are folic acid antagonists such as anticonvulsants, aspirin and sulphonamides.

Importance   Folic acid is essential for the formation of red blood cells. It is necessary for the health of the nervous system and for the development of the fetus.

Deficiency   Folic acid is needed for the production of the red cell membranes and in deficiency megaloblastic anaemia occurs. An increased incidence of fetuses with neural tube defects occurs in women who are deficient in folic acid and perinatal supplementation has a strong protective effect (Lumley et al 2001 and see Ch. 15).

and potassium in Chapter 20. Generally, minerals and trace elements function as structural and catalyst substances. These include regulation of fluid balance and acid–base balance, transmission of action along nerves and contraction of muscle fibres. They are also important as components of enzymes and hormones essential for energy metabolism and functioning of the immune system.

REGULATION OF FOOD INTAKE AND ENERGY BALANCE

As discussed earlier, energy is produced from oxidation of macronutrients in the body and is essential to maintain life. When there is a balance between energy intake and energy output, the body weight remains stable. Obesity occurs when energy intake exceeds energy output. However, this is more complicated than a straightforward equation, as two people with the same energy intake may have totally different body type and size. Genetic as well as environmental factors are believed to have a role in causing obesity. There appear to be body mechanisms that control intake which enable most people to maintain a steady weight. Factors that influence food intake may include (Marieb 2000):

- nutrient signals related to body energy stores;
- hormones;
- body temperature;
- psychological factors.

NUTRITIONAL STATES

There are two nutritional states: the absorptive state when nutrients are being eaten and absorbed by the digestive tract and the postabsorptive state when the gastrointestinal (GI) tract is empty and energy requirements are met by breakdown of body stores. The absorptive state lasts for about 4 h after a reasonable meal has been eaten. If three meals are eaten in the day there is a balance between the two states, each occupying about half of a 24-hour period. Insulin directs the events of the absorptive state, mainly by its control of blood glucose levels.

The body can be maintained in the postabsorptive state for days or weeks in a famine or during illness as long as sufficient water is taken. Glucose is made available to cells via the bloodstream by glycogenolysis in the liver. Muscle glycogen cannot be broken down to glucose because it lacks the enzymes. It is partly oxidised to pyruvic acid or, in anaerobic conditions, to lactic acid. These substances enter the blood and are converted to glucose by the liver. The hormone glucagon is released when blood sugars become too low. Glucagon targets the liver and adipose tissue to enable glucose to be released into the blood.

Total energy expenditures (TEE)

The total energy requirements in the body are to support three main energy uses: the basal metabolic rate (BMR) or resting metabolic rate (RMR), which are used interchangeably (BMR and RMR are slightly different in measurement but practically the same); the thermic effect of food; and variable amounts of physical activities.

Metabolic rate

BMR is the amount of energy required for the body's internal organs to maintain resting activities; it is measured after an overnight fast in a normal environmental temperature. In general, the younger the person, the higher the BMR, and males have a higher BMR than females because of the ratio of metabolically active muscle to the metabolically sluggish fatty tissue. Four main factors that positively influence BMR are lean body mass, growth, fever and disease condition as well as cold climate. BMR makes the largest contribution to TEE (about 60–70%).

The effect of food intake and body heat production

The ingestion of food stimulates metabolism and requires energy to meet the needs of the processes involved: digestion, absorption and transport of nutrients. This is called the thermic effect of food (TEF) and comprises 10–15% of TEE.

Regulation of body temperature

Humans are homeothermic: i.e. they are warm blooded. The maintenance of body temperature depends on the balance between heat production and heat loss. The body temperature of humans is usually maintained within a range of 36.1°–37.8°C independently of external environment or internal heat production. Body temperature rarely varies during the day by more than 1°C and is usually lowest in the early morning and highest in the afternoon or early evening. This temperature is optimum for enzyme activity.

A raise in body temperature increases enzyme activity and most adults will have convulsions when their temperature reaches 41°C and die if their temperature exceeds 43°C. Temperature varies slightly depending on where in the body it is recorded. The body's core (organs within the body cavities) has the highest temperature and the shell (heat loss surface of the skin) has the lowest temperature. Rectal temperature is nearer the core than oral temperature. The hypothalamus (Ch. 26) is the major heat-regulating centre. It receives input from both peripheral thermoreceptors in the skin and central thermoreceptors from the core. Like a thermostat, the hypothalamus responds to any heat change by initiating heat-promotion or heat-loss mechanisms.

Body composition and body weight

In simple terms, body composition can be divided into two main compartments: lean mass and fat mass. Other more detailed models classify the body to three, four or five compartments (including lean, fat, water, mineral mass: bones and glycogen stores). In the concept of weight and health, the emphasis has been too much on the anthropometric side of measurements rather than body composition. However, what is important is the amount of excess fat and its distribution rather than just excess weight. Central obesity (accumulation of excess fat around the abdomen and upper body) is related to diseases such as diabetes and cardiovascular disease.

MATERNAL ADAPTATION TO PREGNANCY

Nutrition

Nutritional advice during pregnancy has had little supporting research-based evidence to date: for instance, restricted diets have been advised for pregnant women in an attempt to produce smaller babies and facilitate an easier delivery. However, more recent research into the effects of poor nutrition on the fetus (Tiran 1997) has suggested that nutrition is an essential foundation for a happy and healthy mother and baby. There is a relationship between poor intake of essential nutrients and a higher-than-normal perinatal morbidity and mortality. Fetal growth may be compromised with an increase in preterm delivery and a decrease in weight for gestational age. Luke (1994) suggests this may be due to low placental weight. The implications of low birth weight in the causation of adult diabetes mellitus and hypertension have been postulated by Barker (1992). The importance of diet in preconception care is discussed in Chapter 8.

Specific requirements of pregnancy

Maternal weight increases significantly, which includes the products of conception, increased water and excess uterine and breast tissue. There is a need for increased nutrients to meet both the increase in maternal tissue and fetal needs. Additional factors that influence nutritional requirement during pregnancy include age, gravidity and parity. Age has an important role in pregnancy nutrition, as teenage mothers have their growth requirements to meet as well as those of the fetus and older mothers have a higher risk of complications. Gravidity and parity, as well as the time interval between pregnancies, influence maternal nutritional reserves.

Energy

Factors influencing energy needs during pregnancy include metabolic cost, prepregnancy fat and weight, level of activity and the stage of pregnancy. The significant differences between the pattern of changes in BMR between women from developing and developed countries indicate that there may be some energy-sparing mechanism in process that causes variation in estimation of energy requirements during pregnancy.

The average total energy cost of pregnancy is estimated to be about 70 000 kcal for a woman with a prepregnancy weight of 60 kg and fat deposition of 2–2.4 kg during pregnancy. The UK dietary reference value (DRV) for extra energy requirement in pregnancy is 200 kcal/day, but only during the last trimester. This recommendation varies in different countries: e.g. 300 kcal/day during the second and third trimester in the USA. These are guidelines and the actual requirements depend on the individual basis: e.g. size, activity and original nutritional status of the woman.

Protein

The quality of protein intake depends on both the type and quantity of food eaten and the conditions under which it is eaten. For example, if the total energy supplied by the diet is so low that gluconeogenesis utilises amino acids to provide energy, the ability to construct new tissue will be reduced. The average pregnant woman in Britain will need an extra 6 g of dietary protein daily, a total of 51 g/day. However, Kramer (2000) concluded that there appeared to be no long-term benefits to the babies when mothers significantly increased their protein intake above normal. This is probably because most women in developed countries eat far more protein than is needed for health.

Carbohydrates and fats

There is little need to increase either glucose or fats for energy but the absorption of fat-soluble vitamins must be considered when advising women about diet in pregnancy. During pregnancy women should have adequate dietary intakes of essential fatty acids (EFAs) and their longer derivatives, omega-6 (mainly arachidonic acid) and omega-3s (mainly docosahexaenoic acid (DHA)). The omega-3 polyunsaturated fats found primarily in fish oils may have specific benefit for the pregnant woman and her baby. These EFAs are among the main material requirements for the growth of the fetal brain and central nervous system (Rice 1996).

Vitamins

In developed countries for healthy women with a balanced diet there is usually no need for vitamin supplementation. However, in women with restricted dietary intake or those with gastrointestinal surgery, especially ileostomy, supplementation may be necessary. In particular it is important to remember the role of folic acid in the cause or prevention of neural tube defects (Wald & Bower 1995). There has been an effort to add folic acid to basic foods to ensure compliance with intake, especially prior to conception. Reference values for some of the vitamins are summarised below.

Vitamin A The DRVs for retinol during pregnancy are an extra 100 μg (Barker 2002). However, because of the teratogenic effects of retinol, the Department of Health and Social Security (DHSS 1990) recommend that the RDA should not be exceeded and pregnant women should avoid liver and liver products.

Vitamin D Routine supplementation of vitamin D in pregnancy is not recommended. Asian women in the UK, in particular those who are vegetarian, may be prone to vitamin D deficiency and need consideration.

Thiamine riboflavin and folate The need for thiamine increases by increased requirements of energy. The increment for average riboflavin intake is 0.3 mg/day throughout pregnancy. The reference nutrient intake (RNI) for folic acid is 200 μg/day for adults and it should be increased during pregnancy (+100) and lactation (+60).

Vitamin C To ensure sufficient maternal stores, an increment of 10 mg/day during the last trimester of pregnancy is recommended.

Calcium The adult average requirement is 700 mg but no increment is established for pregnancy since calcium absorption increases and maternal stores meet the requirement. However, for teenage pregnant mothers, calcium-rich diets are particularly advisable since they have their own growth requirements to deal with as well.

Iron The iron requirements are met by utilisation of maternal stores, cessation of menstrual losses and increased absorption. Therefore, no extra iron is required in a healthy woman with a balanced diet. Iron supplementation during pregnancy is discussed in Chapter 16, p. 209.

Metabolism

Metabolic and physiological processes are altered significantly during pregnancy to accommodate maternal and fetal requirements. Increased endocrine activity and placental hormones have major influences on maternal metabolism to allow provision of nutrients for fetal growth. Human placental lactogen (hPL), oestrogen and progesterone affect metabolism mainly by antagonising insulin.

Plasma T_3 and T_4 (thyroxine) are increased, leading to a physiologic state of hyperthyroidism (Ch. 35). Maternal insulin plasma level is also increased to ensure availability of glucose for placental take up. An increased state of maternal insulin resistance assists glucose availability for fetal utilisation. The changes in glucose tolerance and insulin levels during pregnancy make it a diabetogenic condition. Women who have predisposing factors may develop gestational diabetes (Ch. 35, p. 458).

The BMR rises during pregnancy, reflecting increased oxygen demands of the fetus, placenta and mother. Metabolism of carbohydrate, protein and fat alters, with a major shift in the fuel sources: fat becomes the maternal fuel, whereas glucose becomes the major fetal fuel. Approximately 50–70% of energy required daily by the fetus in the third trimester is derived from glucose, about 20% of it from amino acids and the remainder comes from fat (Worthington-Roberts & Rodwell-Williams 1996).

Carbohydrates

Blood glucose levels are generally between 10 and 20% lower than in the non-pregnant state. This decrease leads to lower insulin levels in the postabsorptive state and a tendency towards ketosis. As pregnancy progresses, there is less peripheral use of glucose by the mother because of increasing insulin antagonism (blockage of cellular uptake). Glucose therefore becomes more readily available to the fetus. Insulin resistance is thought to be due to a decrease in sensitivity of cell receptors, resulting from the effects of hPL, progesterone and cortisol. In response, the pancreatic beta islet cells undergo hyperplasia and hypertrophy to produce increased insulin during meals. The results of changes in the above hormones are listed briefly below:

- Progesterone also helps to increase insulin secretion, decreases peripheral insulin usage and increases insulin levels after meals.
- Oestrogen increases the level of plasma cortisol, which is an insulin antagonist, stimulates beta-cell hyperplasia and enhances peripheral glucose usage.
- Cortisol depletes hepatic glycogen stores through glycogenolysis and increases hepatic glucose production.
- Human placental lactogen correlates with fetal and placental weight. It increases in the plasma as pregnancy progresses and is higher in multiple pregnancy. It antagonises insulin to increase glucose availability and increases the synthesis and availability of lipids which can be used as an alternative fuel to glucose.

Proteins

Pregnancy is an anabolic state with significant nitrogen retention, particularly in the first 20 weeks. Serum amino acid and protein levels are decreased in pregnancy because of placental uptake, increased insulin levels and hepatic use of amino acids for gluconeogenesis. The 50% expansion of plasma volume as well as changes in hormone levels account for the reduction of biochemical substances such as plasma albumin and haemoglobin.

Lipids

Every aspect of lipid metabolism changes in pregnancy. During the first two trimesters, triglyceride synthesis and fat storage (lipogenesis) increase, mediated by the increase in insulin production and enhanced by progesterone. About 60% of fat storage occurs in the first 16 weeks of gestation (Forsum et al 1988). There is an overall store of 3.5 kg in normal pregnancy.

During the third trimester lipolysis increases further, probably due to the increase in hPL. There is accelerated ketogenesis in the liver due to increased oxidation of free fatty acids for conversion into energy. Fats are therefore acting as an alternative source of energy so that the mother can conserve glucose for the fetus. At the same time in the last trimester, when glucose transfer to the fetus is maximal, there is decreased lipogenesis in adipose tissue and the balance is tipped in the direction of lypolysis (Blackburn 2003). Blood cholesterol increases steadily as pregnancy progresses and stays stationary for the last few weeks before delivery. This is unrelated to diet.

Changes in the absorptive and postabsorptive states

During the absorptive state ingested nutrients are digested and absorbed by the gastrointestinal tract. The absorptive state in pregnancy is characterised by relative hyperinsulinaemia and hyperglycaemia due to reduced liver uptake. There is also hypertriglyceridaemia and increased lipogenesis due to the conversion of glucose to fat for storage.

In the postabsorptive or fasting state, energy has to be supplied from the body stores. Most of this comes from the catabolism of fat. Fat and protein synthesis are decreased and catabolism exceeds anabolism. The central nervous system has no alternative but to carry on using available glucose but other organs move to production of energy from lipids. Triglycerides are broken down and fed into the Krebs cycle with the production of ketone bodies. If these accumulate, ketoacidosis will occur. After an overnight fast, maternal plasma glucose falls significantly below that of a non-pregnant woman because of extra demand by the fetus and impaired gluconeogenesis. Gluconeogenesis and circulating free fatty acids are decreased. The reduced gluconeogenesis capacity preserves maternal muscle mass.

Maternal weight gain and body composition

The amount of weight gain may vary to a great extent among individual pregnant women. However, the average weight gain for most mothers is about 11–15 kg for a full-term pregnancy. About 35% of weight gain is accounted for by the weight of the fetus and placenta unit in developed countries, compared with 50% in less-developed countries (Norgan 1992). Of the total weight gain, approximately 62% represents water, 30% fat and 8% protein. Fat distribution is not uniform and mostly accumulates in abdominal, subscapular and upper thigh areas (Forsum et al 1988).

A wide range, from weight loss to a weight gain of 30 kg, is reported during pregnancy. A greater incidence of poor outcome is associated with the extreme of this range. Higher risk of low birth weight is reported more in women with a low net weight gain during pregnancy. Maternal prepregnancy weight, socioeconomic status, genetic factors (to a small degree) and pregnancy weight gain have all been shown to influence infant birth. High net weight gain during pregnancy is also problematic as it leads to complicated pregnancy, prolonged labour, retained weight after birth and increased birth weight. Most excess weight is lost within the first 3 months after birth. Factors that influence postpartum weight loss are maternal age, prepregnancy weight, mothers' desired weight and length of lactation.

It is not advisable to encourage a strict diet for pregnant women in general (Enkin et al 2000). Nonetheless, a modest reduction in energy intake for some women seems most unlikely to have any adverse effect on the birth weight, yet it may prevent the problem of excessive fat gain by the woman. A study by Mathews et al (1999) showed that maternal nutrition (intake of macronutrients), at least in industrial countries, seems to have only a very small effect on the placental and infant birth weight.

MAIN POINTS

- Hundreds of molecules are involved in maintaining good health. Many cells, especially in the liver, can convert one type of food molecule to another but there are about 50 essential nutrients which cannot be manufactured by the body cells and must be provided in the diet.

- Four food groups provide a balanced diet – grains; fruits and vegetables; meat and fish; and milk products.

- Proteins have many important roles in the body. The best source of essential amino acids is animal products. The proteins found in legumes, nuts and cereals are nutritionally incomplete and are low in one or more of the essential amino acids. Strict vegetarians can obtain all the essential amino acids by varying their diet carefully.

- Vitamins may be fat soluble or water soluble. Their main role is to function as coenzymes to assist in the catalysis of chemical processes in the body. The human body is unable to synthesise most vitamins with the exception of vitamin K and some of the B vitamins.

- Body cells must convert ingested food into the high-energy phosphate bonds of ATP. When glucose arrives at the tissues it is taken up by the cells by facilitated diffusion under the influence of insulin. Glucose is taken to the mitochondria where it is oxidised to form energy in the Krebs cycle.

- Excess fat is stored as adipose tissue. When fat is needed for energy production it is mobilised from the stores under the influence of growth hormones or cortisol, taken to the liver and broken down into free fatty acids and glycerol which are released into the blood.

- Cholesterol, found in the blood in combination with a protein carrier such as lipoproteins, exists as three types: high-density lipoproteins (HDLs), low-density lipoproteins (LDLs) and very low-density lipoproteins (VLDLs).

- The ratio of HDLs to LDLs and VLDLs is increased in those whose fat intake is largely unsaturated and who take regular exercise and reduced in cigarette smokers.

- At least 50 g of protein/day is needed to maintain nitrogen balance and to provide for growth and repair of tissues.

- The basal metabolic rate (BMR) is the rate needed to maintain the body at rest with no energy expenditure to maintain body warmth. Even slight increases in muscle work can cause remarkable leaps in metabolic rate and heat production. Ingestion of food also increases the metabolic rate.

- In pregnancy, increased nutrients are needed to supply the increase in maternal and fetal needs although reducing energy expenditure without increased intake may be sufficient. More protein is required but there is little need to increase glucose or fats. In women with restricted dietary intake or those with ileostomy, vitamin supplementation may be necessary. Folic acid deficiency is implicated in the cause of neural tube defects.

- Metabolic processes in the pregnant woman are closely linked with the function of endocrine glands and there are changes in carbohydrate, lipid and protein metabolism. As pregnancy progresses, there is less peripheral use of glucose by the mother because of increasing insulin antagonism. Glucose becomes more readily available to the fetus.

- There are decreased serum amino acid and protein levels in pregnancy because of placental uptake, increased insulin and gluconeogenesis. In the first half of pregnancy, protein storage increases and, during the second half, protein breakdown occurs to provide amino acids for the fetus and energy for the mother.

- During the first two trimesters fat storage increases due to increased insulin production and progesterone.

During the third trimester lipolysis increases due to the increase in hPL. Fats act as an alternative source of energy to conserve glucose for the fetus.

- The central nervous system can only use available glucose but other organs move to production of energy from lipids. Triglycerides are broken down and fed into the Krebs cycle with the production of ketone bodies. If these accumulate, ketoacidosis will occur.

- A wide range, from weight loss to a weight gain of 30 kg, is reported during pregnancy. A greater incidence of poor outcome is associated with the extreme of this range.

References

Alexander S 2002 On the prevention of preeclampsia: nutritional factors back in the spotlight. Epidemiology 13(4):382–383.

Barker D J P (ed.) 1992 Fetal and Infant Origins of Adult Disease. BMJ Books, London.

Barker H M 2002 Nutrition and Dietetics for Health Care, 10th edn. Churchill Livingstone, Edinburgh.

Blackburn S T 2003 Maternal, Fetal and Neonatal Physiology, 2nd edn. W B Saunders, Philadelphia.

DHSS 1990 Vitamin A and pregnancy, PL/C (90) 10 and 11. DHSS, London.

Edelmann C L, Mandle C L 1998 Health Promotion Throughout the Lifespan, 4th edn. Times Mirror–Mosby, London.

Enkin M, Keirse M J N C, Renfrew M, Neilson J 2000 A Guide to Effective Care in Pregnancy and Childbirth, 3rd edn. Oxford University Press, Oxford.

Forsum E, Sadurskis A, Wager J 1988 Resting metabolic rate and body composition of healthy Swedish women during pregnancy and lactation. American Journal of Clinical Nutrition 47:942–947.

Kramer M S 2000 Balanced protein/energy supplementation in pregnancy. Cochrane Review: In The Cochrane Library, Issue 1. Update Software 2003, Oxford.

Luke B 1994 Nutrition during pregnancy. Current Opinion in Obstetrics and Gynaecology 6(5):402–407.

Lumley J, Watson L, Watson M, Bower C 2001 Periconceptual supplementation with folate and/or multivitamins for preventing neural tube defects. Cochrane Review: In The Cochrane Library, Issue 1. Update Software 2003, Oxford.

Marieb E N 2000 Human Anatomy and Physiology, 5th edn. Benjamin/Cummings, New York.

Mathews F, Yudkin P, Neil A 1999 Influence of maternal nutrition on outcome of pregnancy: prospective cohort study. British Medical Journal 319:339–343.

Norgan N G 1992 Maternal body composition: methods for measuring short term changes. Journal of Biosocial Science 24:367–377.

Ranjan V 1991 Vitamin A and birth defects. Professional Care of Mother and Child 1(1):3–4.

Rice R 1996 Fish and healthy pregnancy: more than just a red herring! Professional Care of Mother and Child 6(6):171–173.

Rodwell-Williams S 1999 Essentials of Nutrition and Diet Therapy, 7th edn. Mosby, St Louis.

Sherwood L 1989 Human Physiology – From Cells to Systems. West Publishing, Maine.

Tiran D 1997 Maternal nutrition. In Sweet B R, Tiran D (eds) Mayes Midwifery, 12th edn. Baillière Tindall, London.

Wald N J, Bower C 1995 Folic acid and the prevention of neural tube defects. British Medical Journal 310:1019–1020.

Worthington-Roberts B S, Rodwell-Williams S 1996 Nutrition Throughout the Life Cycle, 6th edn. Mosby, St Louis.

Wyatt K M, Dimmock P W, Jones P W, O'Brian P M S 1999 Efficacy of vitamin B_6 in the treatment of premenstrual syndrome: systematic review. British Medical Journal 318:1371–1381.

Zhang C, Williams M A, King I B et al 2002 Vitamin C and the risk of preeclampsia – results from dietary questionnaire and plasma assay. Epidemiology 13(4):409–416.

Annotated recommended reading

Edelmann C L, Mandle C L 1998 Health Promotion Throughout the Lifespan, 4th edn. Mosby, St Louis.
This book is informative about health promotion throughout the life span, including concepts of lifestyle choices in preconception, antenatal and postnatal periods.

Soltani H, Fraser R B 2002 Pregnancy as a cause of obesity – myth or reality? RCM Midwives Journal 5(5):193–195.
This paper is accessible and worth reading for both the content and conclusions and also to demonstrate the necessity for good research to be carried out by midwives.

Worthington-Roberts B S, Rodwell-Williams S 1996 Nutrition Throughout the Life Cycle, 6th edn. Mosby, St Louis.
This book provides an excellent source about nutritional needs before and during pregnancy and for lactation. It includes practical advice for those involved in supporting breastfeeding mothers.

Chapter **24**

The nature of bone – the female pelvis and fetal skull

CHAPTER CONTENTS

INTRODUCTION

The successful outcome of childbearing depends on the relationship between the size and shape of the maternal pelvis and the fetal skull. The evolution of bipedalism (walking on two legs) and the large size of the human brain have increased the risk to both mother and fetus. This chapter looks at the general structure and function of bone and calcium and phosphorus metabolism. A detailed description of the bones of the pelvis and of the fetal skull will be given.

THE NATURE OF BONE

Functions of bone

Bone is a highly vascular, constantly changing, hard mineralised connective tissue (Aiello & Dean 1990) which contains depositions of calcium and phosphorus. It performs important functions for the body, including support and protection of the soft organs of the body; movement, by acting as anchorage for muscles and levers; storage of fat, but mainly of minerals such as calcium and phosphorus and smaller amounts of potassium, sulphur, magnesium and copper; and blood cell formation.

Structure of bone

Bone is a living tissue that consists of three basic components: an organic matrix of **collagen**, known as **osteoid**; a mineral **matrix** of calcium and phosphorus; and **bone cells**. The cells include **osteoblasts**, **osteoclasts**, **osteocytes** and **fibroblasts**. Calcium (Ca^{2+}), the commonest mineral in the body, and phosphorus are present in bone as crystals of **hydroxyapatite** or $(Ca_3(PO_4)_2)_3 \cdot Ca(OH)_2$. These crystals are attached to collagen fibres, resulting in the hardness of bone. Bone is continuously remodelled by bone cells, with calcium and phosphorus slowly exchanged between bone and the extracellular fluid (ECF). Bone can be divided into **compact** or lamellar bone and **spongy** bone (trabecular, cancellous bone) (Marieb 2000).

Compact bone

Compact bone forms the outer rim or cortex of all bones and consists of units called **osteons** or **Haversian systems**. There is a central Haversian canal oriented to the long axis of the bone. A second type of canal called perforating or Volkmann's canals run at right angles to the long axis of the bone and carry nerves, blood vessels and lymphatic vessels. Around the central canal are concentric hollow tubes of bone known as **lamellae**. Each lamella has small concavities at its junctions with others called **lacunae**, which contain the spider-shaped osteocytes. Hair-like canals called **canaliculi** connect the lacunae to each other and to the central canal, linking all the osteocytes in an osteon together to facilitate exchange of nutrients and removal of waste products.

Spongy bone

Spongy bone contains far fewer Haversian systems and is made up of a lattice of **trabeculae** with red or fatty bone marrow filling the cavities (Figs 24.1 and 24.2). The trabeculae are only a few cell layers thick and contain irregularly arranged lamellae and osteocytes connected by canaliculi. There are no osteons present. Nutrients arrive at the osteocytes by diffusing through narrow spaces between the bony spicules. Although the tissue looks disorganised, the tiny struts of bone are arranged to combat the stress placed on the bone during activity.

Periosteum and endosteum

Most bones have a tough outer covering of fibrous connective tissue, the **periosteum**, which does not cover the articular surfaces of joints. Periosteum transmits blood vessels and acts as an attachment surface for ligaments and muscles. It is supplied abundantly with nerve fibres. Beneath this is a layer of **osteoblasts**. Lining the marrow cavity of a bone is a fine layer of tissue called the **endosteum**, which contains the bone cells (**osteoblasts**, **osteoclasts** and their precursor cells).

Bone cells

- **Osteoblasts** are present on all bone surfaces in single layers next to the unmineralised osteoid of newly forming bone. Osteoblasts may be differentiated from haemopoietic stem cells and are uniformly sized. They are linked to each other by fine cytoplasmic processes. They synthesise and secrete the constituents of the organic matrix and promote mineralisation.

- **Osteocytes** are derived from osteoblasts that have become trapped in lacunae. They maintain the bone matrix and if they die the surrounding matrix is resorbed.

- **Osteoclasts** resorb bone and are found on or near surfaces undergoing erosion. They may have developed separately to osteoblasts and derive from mononuclear phagocytic cells. They vary a great deal in size and in nuclear form and are very mobile. Osteoclasts contain many enzymes which remove both the organic and mineral matrix.

Calcium and phosphorus metabolism

There is a total of about 1000 g of calcium in an adult, of which the skeleton contains 99%. This leaves only 10 g of calcium available for other cellular processes (Brook & Marshall 2001). The small amount of calcium found in body fluids and cells plays a very important part in the metabolic processes of the body and needs to be maintained within narrow limits. Phosphorus is also crucial to body function and the skeleton contains 85% (Boore 1996). The normal plasma concentration of calcium is 2.10–2.70 mmol/L and of phosphate is 0.70–1.40 mmol/L.

Functions of calcium

Calcium is an important intracellular and extracellular ion with many functions. It is present in the ECF in two forms: half is bound to the proteins albumin and globulin and half is in ionised form. The ionised form Ca^{2+} is important in many cell activities (Brook & Marshall 2001):

- nerve and muscle function;
- hormonal actions;
- blood clotting;
- cell motility;
- acting as a secondary messenger between environmental stimulus and cell function by modulation of enzyme response function when bound to the protein **calmodulin**.

Functions of phosphorus

In the form of phosphates, phosphorus plays a large role in cell function:

- as a component of nucleic acids;
- by regulating energy storage as adenosine triphosphate (ATP).

Hormonal control of calcium and phosphorus metabolism

Regulation of calcium balance is closely associated with that of phosphate. There is continuous exchange of calcium between different sites (calcium pools) in the body. Three hormones are involved in the control of calcium and phosphorus metabolism, mainly by maintaining the concentration of calcium in ECF. These are **parathyroid hormone (PTH)**, **vitamin D** and **calcitonin**. Plasma inorganic phosphate is more loosely controlled than calcium (Brook & Marshall 2001).

If there is no change in the amount of calcium in the skeleton, ECF calcium level depends on the balance between calcium absorption in the gut and its excretion in urine and

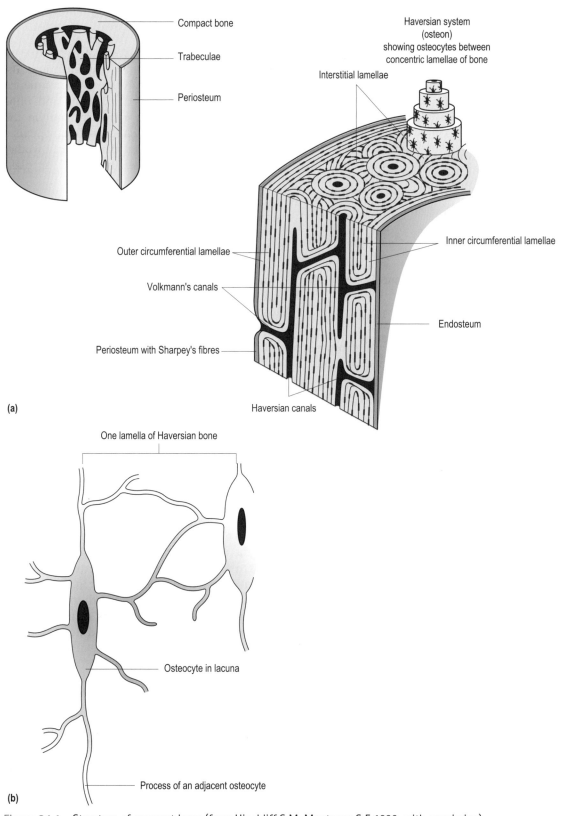

Figure 24.1   Structure of compact bone (from Hinchliff S M, Montague S E 1990, with permission).

faeces. About 50% of the calcium in the blood passing through bone capillaries is exchanged in a single passage and about 300 mmol of calcium is involved in the exchange of calcium between blood and bone every day.

Parathyroid hormone   Four parathyroid glands which are embedded in the thyroid gland secrete parathyroid hormone. It increases the concentration of Ca^{2+} in the blood and depresses plasma phosphate concentration by acting

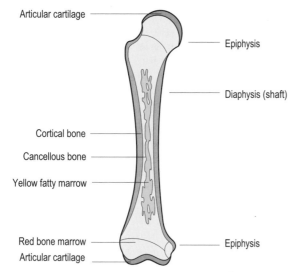

Figure 24.2 Anatomical features of a long bone (from Hinchliff S M, Montague S E 1990, with permission).

on bone and kidneys. PTH increases osteocyte reabsorption of bone with a rapid release of calcium and phosphorus into the blood. Calcium reabsorption in the kidney tubules is increased but the excretion of phosphate is increased. This results in a rise in plasma calcium level and a fall in phosphate level. PTH activity is directly related to serum calcium concentration. When the level of calcium rises, PTH production falls, resulting in calcium deposition in bone, and vice versa (Brook & Marshall 2001).

Vitamin D   The D vitamins are steroid substances formed from **ergosterol** in plants and **7-dehydrocholesterol** in animals. Ultraviolet radiation modifies these to **ergocalciferol** (**vitamin D$_2$**) and **cholecalciferol** (**vitamin D$_3$**). Humans can either ingest vitamin D from plant and animal sources or manufacture it by the action of sunlight on the skin to form cholecalciferol. Vitamin D has to be further metabolised by adding hydroxyl groups before it can be active. The first step occurs in the liver where it is converted to **25-hydroxycholecalciferol**. The active form, called **1,25-dihydroxycholecalciferol** (**calcitriol**), is produced by the kidney in response to PTH stimulation and is released into the circulation to be transported to its target organs of intestine, bone and kidneys (Brook & Marshall 2001).

The overall effect of calcitriol is to stimulate calcium absorption by having a direct effect on the intestinal mucosa. In the kidney calcium and phosphate reabsorption are increased but phosphate reabsorption is masked by the effect of PTH, which increases its excretion. As calcitriol is secreted by the kidney and acts on distant targets, it can be thought of as a hormone (Brook & Marshall 2001). The feedback mechanism is as follows; hypocalcaemia increases the secretion of PTH, which in turn increases the production of active vitamin D by the kidney. Once the level of plasma calcium has returned to normal, the secretion of

PTH decreases and the level of active vitamin D secretion falls.

Calcitonin   Calcitonin is secreted by the **parafollicular cells** (**clear or C cells**) of the thyroid gland. Its main effect is opposite to that of parathyroid hormone, causing a fall in plasma concentration of calcium and phosphate. This hormone may play an important part in the regulation of skeletal growth in children but appears to have no major role in adults other than pregnant women. The secretion of calcitonin is directly related to plasma calcium concentration.

THE PELVIC GIRDLE

The pelvic girdle is for attachment of the lower limbs and for support of the pelvic and to some extent abdominal organs (Aiello & Dean 1990). The continuous bony basin is important in an upright posture as it transmits the weight of the trunk to the legs. The sacroiliac joints must be strong and stable. The size, shape and rigidity of the pelvic girdle is related directly to bipedal locomotion and the human pelvis compared to other primates is short, squat and basin shaped (Trevathen et al 1999).

The mammalian spine is highly efficient for walking on four legs. In **quadrupeds** the abdominal organs are suspended from a single horizontal arch (the backbone). This single arch is still present in the human neonate but when babies learn to sit up their spines develop a forward curve near the top of the spine. When babies stand their spines develop a second forward curve near the base. The curved spine is essential for maintenance of an upright posture (Morgan 1990).

The evolving changes in pelvic shape placed constraints on the limits of the baby's head size, limiting gestation length and resulting in an immature baby (Morgan 1990), a feature referred to as **altricial**. In humans, the gynaecoid pelvis is adapted for giving birth to a comparatively large-headed baby but **mechanisms of labour** are necessary to facilitate the descent of the head through the pelvis. These include passive alterations to fetal position and **moulding** of the skull bones.

Bones of the pelvis

Although diagrams and text can illustrate the features of the pelvis, there is no substitute for handling a life-sized pelvic model. The reader is strongly encouraged to handle a pelvis repeatedly. Familiarity with the shape and size of the pelvis may enable life-saving decisions to be made. Whenever vaginal examinations are carried out, relevant pelvic features must be identified in vivo.

The bony ring of the pelvis is made up of four irregularly shaped bones: **two innominate bones** forming the lateral and anterior walls and the **sacrum** and **coccyx** forming the posterior wall. Each innominate bone consists of three fused

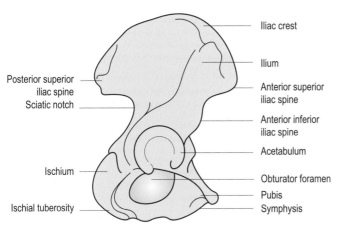

Figure 24.3   The outer or lateral surface of the right innominate bone (from Sweet B 1997, with permission).

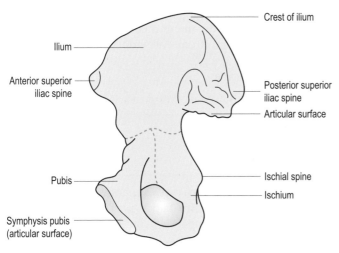

Figure 24.4   The inner or medial surface of the right innominate bone (from Sweet B 1997, with permission).

bones – the **ilium**, **ischium** and **pubis**. The three bones were formed as cartilage in the fetus and their ossification centres fuse at puberty. Ossification in the pelvis is not completed until about 25 years of age. The description of these three bones given below is mirrored to the left and right of the pelvis.

The ilium

The ilium has an upper flat plate of bone and forms part of the **acetabulum** below (Figs 24.3 and 24.4). The external part of the plate of bone is curved and has a roughened surface for attachment of the **gluteal muscles**, which form the buttocks. The inner surface forms the **iliac fossa**, which is smooth and concave. The **iliacus muscle**, which forms a platform on which the abdominal organs rest, originates from this surface. The upper ridge of the ilium is called the **iliac crest** and is shaped like the letter S. The muscles of the abdominal wall have attachments to this surface.

At the anterior end of the iliac crest is the **anterior superior iliac spine**, which can be identified under the skin, and at the posterior end is the **posterior superior iliac spine**, which is marked externally by a dimple at the level of the second sacral vertebra. Two **inferior iliac spines**, anterior and posterior, can be found below the superior spines. The lower margin of the ilium forms two-fifths of the acetabulum, where it fuses with the ischium and pubis. Behind the acetabulum, the ilium forms the **greater sciatic notch**, through which the nerves from the sacral plexus pass. Above the greater sciatic notch is the area of ilium which articulates with the sacrum at the **sacroiliac joint**.

The ischium

The ischium forms the lowest aspect of the innominate bone. The upper part forms two-fifths of the acetabulum, where it fuses with the ilium and ischium. Below the acetabulum, a thick buttress of bone called the **ischial tuberosity** takes the weight of the seated body. The **hamstring muscles** in the thigh arise from this bone. Passing upwards and inwards from the ischial tuberosity, a shaft of ischium meets the **inferior ramus of the pubis** to form the **pubic arch**.

The ischium also forms the lower boundary of the **obturator foramen**, a large opening in the lower part of each innominate bone below the acetabula. On its internal surface, protruding from its posterior edge and about 5 cm above the tuberosity, is a protuberance called the **ischial spine**, an important landmark to be found on vaginal examination. The ischial spine separates the **greater sciatic notch** from the **lesser sciatic notch**.

The pubis

This bone forms the anterior aspect of the innominate bone and is a square bone. The two pubic bones articulate medially to form the joint called the **symphysis pubis**. Laterally, the **superior ramus of the pubic bone** passes to the acetabulum and forms one-fifth of this structure. The superior ramus also forms the upper boundary of the obturator foramen. The inferior ramus passes downwards and outwards to join the ischium and form the pubic arch. The upper surface of the pubis forms the **pubic crest**, which ends laterally in the **pubic tubercle**.

The sacrum

The sacrum is a shield-shaped mass of bone formed from five fused sacral vertebrae (Fig. 24.5). It articulates with the two innominate bones at the sacroiliac joints. The anterior surface is smooth and concave both from above downwards and from side to side. This curvature is called the **hollow of the sacrum**. The first sacral vertebra overhangs the sacral hollow and the central point of this projection is called the **sacral promontory**. Through the centre of the

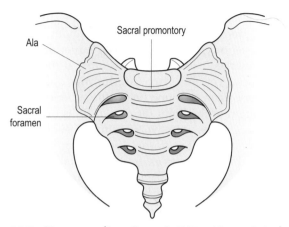

Figure 24.5   The sacrum (from Sweet B 1997, with permission).

bone the sacral and coccygeal nerves pass through the **sacral canal**.

Four pairs of **foramina** (openings) are present anteriorly between the five fused sacral vertebrae where the sacral nerves exit to form the **sacral plexus**. Posteriorly, eight small foramina are present through which posterior branches of the sacral nerves exit to supply the skin of the buttocks and the muscles of the lower part of the back. On its upper surface a smooth oval area forms an articular surface for the fifth lumbar vertebra to form the **lumbosacral point**. Lateral masses of bone on either side of the sacrum are called the **wings of the sacrum** or **sacral alae**.

The coccyx

This small bone is triangular in shape with its base uppermost. It is formed of four fused coccygeal vertebrae. The first coccygeal vertebra articulates with the lower end of the sacrum at the **sacrococcygeal joint**. The rudimentary vertebrae forming the rest of the coccyx are smooth on their inner surface and support the rectum. The external anal sphincter is attached to the lowest point.

Joints of the pelvis

There are four joints – one symphysis pubis, two sacroiliac joints and one sacrococcygeal joint.

- The **sacroiliac joints** are synovial joints with a joint cavity filled with synovial fluid, a capsule formed of synovial membrane and tough external supporting ligaments. Special features include very strong posterior ligaments which transmit the weight of the trunk, head and arms to the legs. Movement at these joints is normally slight but increases in range during pregnancy when the ligaments become softened under the influence of the hormone relaxin.

- The **symphysis pubis** consists of an oval disc of fibrocartilage about 4 cm long lying between the bodies of the two pubic bones. The joint is reinforced by ligaments crossing from one pubic bone to the other.

- The **sacrococcygeal joint** lies between the sacrum and coccyx. There is sometimes a small synovial joint cavity present. Slight movement can occur backwards and forwards and the backwards movement is greatly increased as the baby's head passes through the pelvis in the second stage of labour.

Ligaments of the pelvis

Besides the ligaments supporting each of the pelvic joints, there are three other pairs of ligaments:

- The **sacrotuberous ligament** crosses from the posterior superior iliac spine and the lateral borders of the sacrum and coccyx to the ischial tuberosity. It bridges the greater and lesser sciatic notches.

- The **sacrospinous ligament** passes in front of the sacrotuberous ligament from the side of the sacrum and coccyx, crosses the greater sciatic notch and is attached to the ischial spine.

- The **inguinal ligament** (Poupart's ligament) runs from the anterior superior iliac spine to the pubic tubercle and forms the groin.

Regions of the pelvis

There is a clear line of bone separating the upper flare of the iliac fossae from the basin-shaped part of the pelvis. This line of bone is called the **pelvic brim**. The area above this is called the **false pelvis** and is of no consequence in childbearing, while below the brim is the **true pelvis** with a **cavity** and **outlet** through which the fetus must pass in order to be born.

The pelvic brim

Landmarks are identifiable on the pelvic brim or inlet and it is important to be aware of these as important measurements are made between them. In the normal **gynaecoid (female) pelvis** the brim is oval in shape with the anteroposterior diameter reduced by the sacral promontory. Starting at the centre of the sacral promontory and tracing the brim round to the symphysis pubis, the landmarks (Fig. 24.6) are:

- the sacral promontory;
- the sacral ala;
- the upper border of the sacroiliac joint;
- the iliopectineal line;
- the iliopectineal eminence;
- the inner upper border of the superior pubic ramus;
- the inner upper border of the body of the pubis;
- the upper inner border of the symphysis pubis.

If a piece of paper was placed across the landmarks, a flat surface would be formed. This imaginary flat surface is

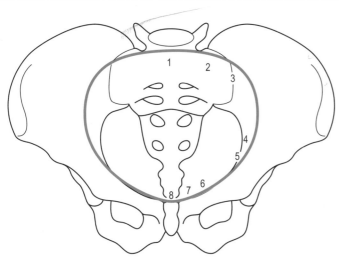

Figure 24.6   The pelvic brim. 1, sacral promontory; 2, sacral ala; 3, sacroiliac joint; 4, iliopectineal line; 5, iliopectineal eminence; 6, superior pubic ramus; 7, body of pubic bone; 8, symphysis pubis (from Sweet B 1997, with permission).

called a **plane** and the concept can also be applied to the cavity and outlet. The **diameters** of the pelvis are measured from the landmarks across the planes.

The cavity of the pelvis

The cavity is that part of the pelvis between the brim and the outlet. It is a **curved canal** with a short anterior surface measuring 4.5 cm, formed by the inner aspect of the pubic bones and symphysis pubis, and a longer posterior surface measuring 12 cm, formed by the hollow of the sacrum. The lateral walls are formed from the greater sciatic notch, the inner surface of part of the ilium, the body of the ischium and the obturator foramen. The plane of the pelvic cavity is taken from the midpoint of the symphysis pubis anteriorly to the junction of the second and third sacral vertebrae posteriorly.

The outlet of the pelvis

Two pelvic outlets, the anatomical and the obstetric outlets, may be described. The anatomical outlet is traced from the lower border of the symphysis pubis along the pubic arch to the inner border of the ischial tuberosity and along the sacrotuberous ligament to the tip of the coccyx. It is of no value in labour as it is not a flat surface but the lower border of the pelvis. It varies in size during labour because of the range of backwards tilting of the coccyx in different women. The obstetric outlet, which is the constricted lower portion of the true pelvis, is a more useful landmark. The structures making up the obstetric outlet are:

- the lower border of the symphysis pubis;
- a line passing along the pubis, obturator foramen and ischium to the ischial spine;
- the sacrospinous ligament;
- the lower border of the sacrum.

Table 24.1   Pelvic measurements in centimetres

	Anteroposterior	Oblique	Transverse
Brim	11 cm	12 cm	13 cm
Cavity	12 cm	12 cm	12 cm
Outlet	13 cm	12 cm	11 cm

The plane of the outlet is the imaginary flat surface between these structures. It is occupied by the muscles of the pelvic floor (Ch. 25, p. 339).

The dimensions of the pelvis (diameters)

Measurements are taken of the planes of the pelvic brim, cavity and outlet using the landmarks described above. These are taken in three directions – anteroposterior, oblique and transverse. The measurements given in Table 24.1 are average for a gynaecoid pelvis.

The brim

- The smallest diameter of the brim is the **anteroposterior diameter**, which is measured from the upper part of the symphysis pubis to the sacral promontory. This is the **anatomical conjugate**, which measures 12 cm. However, this is not available for accommodating the fetal head. If the measurement is taken from the inner border of the symphysis pubis to the sacral promontory, the measurement is 11 cm; this is the **obstetric conjugate**. Both of these two measurements can be referred to as the **true conjugate**. The **diagonal conjugate**, measured during a pelvic assessment, is taken from the lower border of the symphysis pubis to the sacral promontory and measures about 13 cm. It is normally difficult to measure because of its length but, if the sacral promontory is reached, the obstetric conjugate is calculated by subtracting 2 cm.

- The **two oblique diameters** are taken from one sacroiliac joint to the opposite iliopectineal eminence. They are named left and right after the corresponding sacroiliac joint. All the oblique diameters throughout the pelvis are 12 cm.

- The **transverse diameter** is taken between points on the two iliopectineal lines that are farthest apart and measures 13 cm. However, the descending colon passes near to the left sacroiliac joint and may limit the space available for passage of the fetus.

- The **sacrocotyloid diameter** is another diameter measured at the brim and is taken from the sacral promontory to the iliopectineal eminence. This measures about 9.5 cm and is important if the fetus is presenting with the occiput posteriorly. The parietal eminences may become caught in this diameter, causing the head to extend.

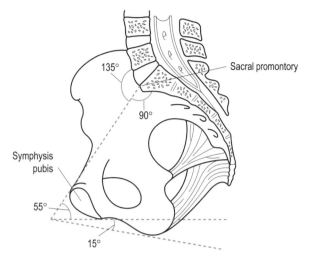

Figure 24.7 The pelvis, showing the degrees of inclination. Inclination of the pelvic brim to the horizontal, 55°; inclination of pelvic outlet to the horizontal, 15°; angle of pelvic inclination, 135°; inclination of the sacrum, 90° (from Sweet B 1997, with permission).

The cavity

- The cavity is considered to be circular in diameter and the measurements taken through the plane of the cavity are all 12 cm.

The obstetric outlet

- The outlet is diamond shaped with its longest diameter in the anteroposterior direction. This is measured from the lower border of the symphysis pubis to the sacro-coccygeal joint and is 13 cm.
- The oblique diameter has no fixed points but is between the obturator foramen and the opposite sacrospinous ligament. It is 12 cm.
- The transverse diameter is measured between the two ischial spines. It measures 11 cm.

The planes of the pelvis and pelvic inclination

When a person stands up the pelvic basin is tilted so that the plane of the brim forms an angle of 60° to the horizontal. This concept can be checked if the reader stands facing and pressed up against a vertical surface. The two points of the pelvis which would touch the vertical surface are the pubic bones and the anterior superior iliac spines. The plane of the cavity forms an angle of 30° and that of the outlet 15° (Fig. 24.7). Another angle which indicates the adequacy of the pelvic size is the subpubic angle of the pubic arch, which measures 90°. Two other angles which measure 90° in an adequate pelvis are:

1. the sacral angle, which lies between the plane of the brim and the anterior surface of the first sacral vertebra;
2. the greater sciatic notch, which is the large indentation on the sacral margin of the ileum.

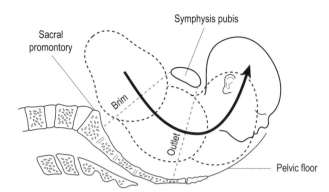

Figure 24.8 The axis of the birth canal (from Sweet B 1997, with permission).

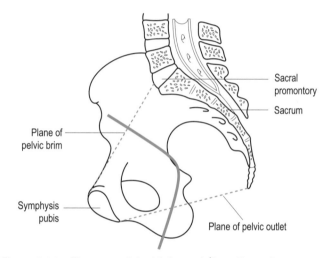

Figure 24.9 The curve of the birth canal (from Sweet B 1997, with permission).

Axes of the pelvic canal

If imaginary lines are drawn at right angles through the pelvic planes, axes will be created. If these lines are joined together a curve can be traced because each plane is at a different angle to the horizon. This curve is the space that the fetus must pass through and is called the curve of Carus. This is unique to the human and is the price paid for our upright posture as it makes delivery of the fetus more difficult. Instead of an easy journey through a relatively large, straight pelvic canal the fetus must be moved passively by mechanisms to overcome the changing curves and diameters (Figs 24.8 and 24.9).

Basic types of pelvis

There are four basic types of pelvis described according to the shape of the brim and other features (Fig. 24.10). These are gynaecoid, android, anthropoid and platypelloid. However, many pelves cannot be classified so easily and may contain features of different types. It is now considered that

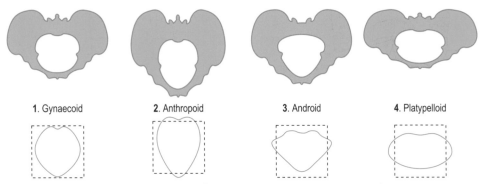

Figure 24.10   Shapes of the pelvic brim (from Sweet B 1997, with permission).

the size of the pelvis in relation to the fetus that must pass though it is more important than a slight abnormality of shape and there is a saying that the fetal head is the best pelvimeter.

The gynaecoid pelvis

This is the ideal female pelvis. Its main features are a rounded brim, large forepelvis (that portion in front of the widest transverse diameter), a transverse diameter that bisects the anteroposterior diameter, parallel side walls, a shallow cavity, blunt ischial spines, a wide sciatic notch and a pubic angle of 90°. It is associated with women of average height and shoe size of 4 or over.

The android pelvis

The name android suggests that the pelvis has male features. Its brim is more heart shaped with a narrow forepelvis and a widest transverse diameter set towards the back. The side walls converge and the sacrum is straight, making the cavity funnel shaped. The ischial spines are prominent and the subpubic angle and the angle of the greater sciatic notch are less than 90°. Women with this type of pelvis may be of short stature, heavily built and have a tendency to be hirsute. There may be an occipitoposterior position of the head at the commencement of labour and this type of pelvis is the least suitable for childbearing as it becomes narrower as the fetus descends (Fig. 24.11).

The anthropoid pelvis

This pelvis has a long oval brim with the anteroposterior diameter greater than the transverse as is found in other primates; hence the name anthropoid or ape-like. This results from a reduction in the transverse diameter but the pelvis is generally large all over. The side walls diverge and the sacrum is long and deeply concave. There may be a sixth sacral vertebra present, especially in tall African women. This is called a **high assimilation pelvis**. The ischial spines are not prominent and the angle of the greater sciatic notch

is wide while the subpubic angle may be normal or wide. The fetus may present with the occiput either anterior or posterior but the pelvis is so large that delivery may occur without rotation.

The platypelloid pelvis

This pelvis is flat with a reduced anteroposterior diameter. It is usually called kidney shaped. The side walls diverge, the sacrum is flat and the cavity shallow (Fig. 24.12). The ischial spines are blunt and the sciatic notch and subpubic angle are wide. The fetal head may have difficulty negotiating the brim, a feature that will be discussed later, but once through the brim there should be no further difficulty.

MATERNAL PHYSIOLOGICAL ADAPTATIONS IN PREGNANCY

Calcium and phosphorus metabolism

Maternal calcium metabolism is altered to meet fetal needs for calcium and phosphorus to enable skeletal growth and development but these changes are largely reversible following delivery and cessation of lactation (Prentice 2000). Although studies have shown that bone mineral density falls temporarily during lactation, even grand multiparity with prolonged breastfeeding does not lead to permanent osteoporotic changes (Henderson et al 2000).

The total extra calcium by term is about 25–30 g, most of which is used for fetal bone formation (Blackburn 2003). Fetal plasma calcium level exceeds that of the mother, suggesting that the mineral is actively transported across the placenta. The hormones PTH and calcitonin cannot pass across the placenta so that the fetus must manufacture his own. The placenta can transfer vitamin D to the fetus and can also synthesise vitamin D. During pregnancy maternal calcium, phosphate and magnesium levels fall due to the increased production of PTH, calcitonin and vitamin D. These changes occur under the influence of oestrogen and human placental lactogen (hPL). Calcium metabolism is

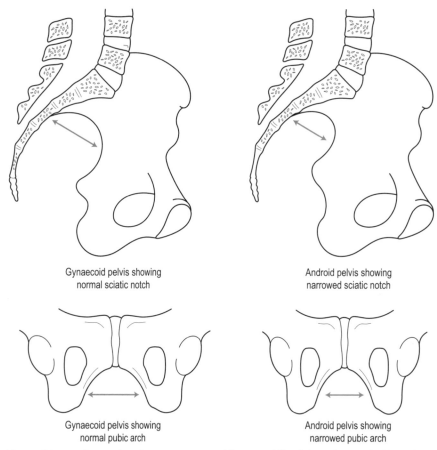

Gynaecoid pelvis showing
normal sciatic notch

Android pelvis showing
narrowed sciatic notch

Gynaecoid pelvis showing
normal pubic arch

Android pelvis showing
narrowed pubic arch

Figure 24.11   Comparison between a normal (gynaecoid) pelvis and an android pelvis. An android pelvis has a narrower outlet because of the narrow sciatic notch and pubic arch (from Sweet B 1997, with permission).

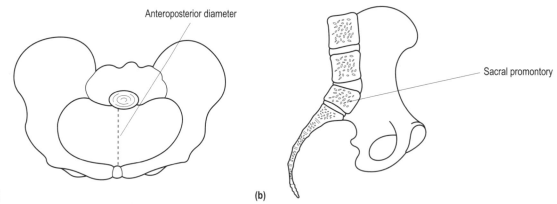

Anteroposterior diameter

Sacral promontory

(a)

(b)

Figure 24.12   A rachitic flat pelvis. (a) Reduced anteroposterior diameter; widened and irregular transverse diameter. (b) Sacral promontory pushed forwards and downwards; sacrum pushed backwards (from Sweet B 1997, with permission).

related to the changes in ECF volume, renal function and fetal needs.

Calcium

Calcium absorption and urinary calcium excretion are increased during pregnancy. These increases precede fetal demand for calcium. Maternal bone resorption and new bone formation are also elevated (Prentice 2000). Serum calcium levels begin to fall soon after fertilisation and reach their lowest levels at about 30 weeks of pregnancy (Blackburn 2003). These parameters are evidence of a greater mobilisation of calcium in order to supply the needs of the fetal skeleton.

Phosphorus and magnesium

Serum inorganic phosphate levels and magnesium levels fall slightly until 30 weeks of pregnancy and return to non-pregnant levels by term. These changes are related to haemodilution.

Control of calcium metabolism in pregnancy

Levels of active vitamin D (1,25-dihydroxycholecalciferol), also called calcitriol, show a small rise by 10 weeks of pregnancy although staying within recognised normal limits. They rise above the normal limit in the last few weeks of pregnancy. However, there is little elevation in either **intact parathyroid hormone** or **calcitonin** levels (Cross et al 1995). Intestinal absorption of vitamin D is enhanced throughout pregnancy. Elevated amounts of vitamin D ensure both maternal and fetal demands for calcium are met.

CLINICAL IMPLICATIONS

Maternal calcium and phosphorus intake

Although there may be an increase in calcium storage in preparation for lactation, an increase in dietary calcium does not appear to increase bone density. Any increase in bone calcium due to hPL is counterbalanced by the effect of oestrogen, causing a decrease in reabsorption. These changes are independent of maternal calcium intake and there is no need to provide supplements in countries where dietary intake is adequate. Supplementation may be needed by pregnant adolescents or by women in groups where dietary insufficiency is suspected.

Adequate vitamin D is essential to ensure absorption and 400 IU/day is advised. Supplementation is recommended if dietary intake is poor or there is poor exposure to sunlight. Milk is an excellent source of calcium, phosphorus and vitamin D and women who cannot drink milk can be encouraged to take cheese, yoghurt, sardines, whole grain foods or green leafy vegetables.

Some foods, such as those which contain excessive fats, phytates (found in many vegetables) and oxalates, interfere with the absorption of calcium by forming insoluble calcium salts within the intestine, which are excreted. High sodium intake may also interfere with calcium absorption. Although phosphorus is essential during pregnancy, high intake levels limit calcium absorption while high plasma phosphorus levels increase the urinary excretion of calcium. Processed meats, snack foods and cola drinks all have high phosphorus but low calcium levels (Blackburn 2003).

Leg cramps

Women may suffer from intense sudden cramping pain in the calf muscles, especially during the third trimester of pregnancy. These tend to occur in bed. Lowered serum ionised calcium and increased phosphates are thought to be responsible for the muscle contractions. Respiratory alkalosis may precipitate muscle spasm. Thrombophlebitis must be eliminated as a possible alternative cause of pain. Cramps may be prevented by reducing milk and processed food intake (reducing phosphate intake) and performing stretching exercises before retiring. Jimenez (1994) suggests that taking calcium salts that are free of phosphates or taking the antacid aluminium hydroxide may prevent phosphorus absorption and correct the balance.

Restless leg syndrome

This disorder is seen in about 10–15% of pregnant women and occurs usually about 15 min after going to bed (Blackburn 2003). There is a burning, twitching feeling in the lower leg and the more the wish to fidget is resisted the worse the sensation becomes. The cause of this syndrome, either in pregnancy or in non-pregnant women and men, is unknown. Iron and/or folic acid deficiency have been implicated and replacement therapy has helped. Circulatory problems may also be involved. Walking about and the application of a cold compress may relieve symptoms.

Backache in pregnancy

Davis (1996) reports that about 50% of pregnant women experience backache and that it was more likely to be reported in very young women, women who had back pain before pregnancy and multiparous women. Postural changes, overstretched abdominal muscles, strained back muscles and the effect of relaxin on the pelvic ligaments may contribute to backache. Before advising a pregnant woman on ways of preventing or managing the pain, other causes should be ruled out by a medical practitioner. A urinary tract infection may be present and occasionally the woman may be in labour. More rarely, demineralisation of bone may cause backache and hip pain.

The effects of relaxin

Relaxin is a small peptide with a similar structure to insulin. It probably acts as a growth-controlling hormone which affects collagen and appears to be a potent stimulator of uterine growth in pregnancy. It is involved in the softening and effacement of the cervix and in the onset of labour. During pregnancy it plays a major role in restraining uterine muscle contractability.

With progesterone, relaxin causes relaxation of the ligaments and muscles, reaching its maximum effect in the last few weeks of pregnancy. Relaxation of the symphysis pubis and sacroiliac joints of the pelvis leads to instability of the pelvic girdle, and relaxation of the sacrococcygeal joint allows extra backwards movement. These changes facilitate engagement of the presenting part in late pregnancy and delivery by increasing the pelvic diameters. Some women develop a rolling gait and, as the developing weight and position of the uterus changes the centre of gravity, the woman leans backwards to compensate, exaggerating the normal lumbar curve and leading to backache.

Assessment of backache will include:

- location and extent of pain;
- onset and duration of pain;
- nature and degree of pain;
- any other symptoms;
- relationship to activities;
- self-treatment strategies.

In the absence of serious pathology, localised heat application may help as may massage. The woman is advised to rest and take analgesics. A supporting elasticated sacroiliac belt may help and a maternity girdle will support the uterus and relieve strain. Early advice on posture with careful exercise to tone and strengthen the back muscles may be preventative. Shoes with heels no higher then a 0.5–1.0 inch should be worn.

Rickets and osteomalacia

Malabsorption of calcium is brought about by a deficiency in vitamin D caused by low intake but sometimes combined with decreased exposure to sunlight. The bones are poorly ossified and soft and become deformed. In childhood the condition is called rickets and in adults osteomalacia. Distortion of the pelvis may occur, leading to severe problems in childbirth. Both rickets and osteomalacia may be more common in the Asian population in Great Britain (Dunnigan et al 1982).

Spinal cord injury

Women who are paraplegic or quadriplegic can have a successful outcome to their pregnancy. Although there are dangers of urinary tract infections, constipation and pressure sores, most of these problems can be avoided. Uterine contractions in labour are mainly independent of neurological control and labour should progress normally. Pain may be perceived if the spinal lesion is below T10. Delivery of the baby may need to be aided if the control of muscles used in expulsion is lost.

THE FETAL SKULL

The shape and size of the human pelvis creates difficulties in the birthing process not found in other primates. This is further compounded by the large human brain. At birth the average human baby weighs 3300 g, of which its brain constitutes about 385 g and continues to grow at fetal rates for the next 20 months to reach 1000 g. Brain growth slows down, achieving its adult size of 1400 g by age 8. In contrast, a newborn gorilla weighs 2000 g and has a correspondingly

smaller brain of 225 g, already half the adult size of 450 g after a gestation only 6 days shorter than human pregnancy (Morgan 1994). Gorillas have very easy births! To overcome the tight fit between the human pelvis and the fetal skull the following evolutionary changes have developed:

- birth while the fetus is very immature;
- continuation of fetal rate of brain growth after delivery;
- flexion of the head on the neck so that the narrowest diameters pass through the pelvis;
- moulding of the skull to change the shape (but not the size) from globular to cylindrical.

Anatomy of the skull

The fetal skull is ovoid in shape and the bones can be divided into the vault, the face and the base. The vault extends from the orbital ridges to the base of the occiput and contains the brain, which sits in the bones forming the base of the skull. The fetal skull differs from the adult skull in its proportions as the vault is large in relation to the face (Sweet 1997). For the purposes of measurement and to describe the degree of flexion and extension in the different presentations, the fetal skull is divided into regions of face, brow, vertex and occiput (Fig. 24.13):

- the **face** extends from the chin to the orbital ridges;
- the **brow or sinciput** is the area of the two frontal bones, extending from the orbital ridges to the anterior fontanelle;
- the **vertex** is bounded by the anterior fontanelle, the posterior fontanelle and the two parietal eminences;
- the **occiput** is the area over the occipital bone, extending from the posterior fontanelle to the nape of the neck.

The face and base of the skull are laid down in cartilage and are almost completely ossified by birth. The vault of the fetal skull is composed of flat bones which develop from

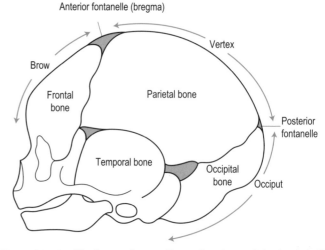

Figure 24.13   The bones, fontanelles and regions of the fetal skull (from Sweet B 1997, with permission).

membrane. Ossification centres within the membrane lay down bone around them. The ossification centre of each bone is visible on the ossified bone (Bennett & Brown 1996).

Bones – the vault

Five main bones make up the vault, with two others helping to form the lateral walls – the squamous (flattened) parts of the temporal bones. Each bone is named for the lobe of the brain lying beneath it:

- two frontal bones from ossification centres indicated by the frontal bosses;
- two parietal bones from ossification centres indicated by the parietal eminences;
- two squamous portions of the temporal bones;
- one occipital bone from an ossification centre indicated by the occipital protruberance.

The process of ossification is incomplete at birth so that membranous sutures remain between the bones and membranous fontanelles where two or more sutures meet. These areas of membrane facilitate moulding of the fetal skull during birth. They also provide landmarks on the skull for identification during vaginal examination (Fig. 24.14).

The sutures

- The **frontal** suture lies between the two frontal bones.
- The **sagittal** suture runs from the anterior to the posterior fontanelle, uniting the two parietal bones.
- The **lambdoidal** suture (after its resemblance to the Greek letter lambda – λ) lies between the posterior edges of the parietal bones and the occipital bone.

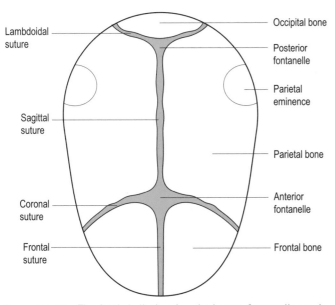

Figure 24.14   The fetal skull, showing the bones, fontanelles and sutures (from Sweet B 1997, with permission).

- The **coronal** suture separates the posterior edges of the two frontal bones from the anterior edges of the two parietal bones.

The fontanelles

There are two main fontanelles:

- The **anterior** fontanelle or **bregma** is roughly diamond shaped and is formed at the junction of four sutures – the frontal, parietal and two halves of the coronal sutures. It measures 2.5 cm across by 3 cm long and is not fully closed by ossification until 18 months of age.
- The **posterior** fontanelle or **lambda** is much smaller and triangular in shape and is formed at the junction of three sutures – the sagittal suture and the two halves of the lambdoidal suture. It closes by the 6th week after birth.

Besides these two main fontanelles, four minor fontanelles form on the side walls of the vault. These are the two temporal fontanelles at the ends of the coronal suture and two mastoid fontanelles at the ends of the lambdoidal suture. These are not of any significance in childbearing.

Bones – the base

The fused bones of the base of the skull are perforated by the foramen magnum, which allows passage of the spinal cord leading from the brain.

Diameters of the fetal skull

Measurements of the skull are used to assess its size in relation to the maternal pelvis. Longitudinal diameters are taken between key landmarks so that the diameters presenting at the pelvis in different degrees of flexion or extension of the head on the neck can be estimated (Figs 24.15 and 24.16):

1. **Suboccipitobregmatic** is measured from the nape of the neck to the centre of the anterior fontanelle. It is 9.5 cm and presents when the head is fully flexed.
2. **Suboccipitofrontal** is measured from the nape of the neck to the centre of the frontal suture. It is 10 cm and presents when the head is almost completely flexed.
3. **Occipitofrontal** is measured from the glabella (bridge of the nose) to the occipital protruberance. It is 11.5 cm and presents when the head is deflexed in an occipitoposterior position.
4. **Mentovertical** is measured from the point of the chin to the highest point of the vertex. It is 13.5 cm and presents when the head is midway between flexion and extension in a brow presentation.
5. **Submentovertical** is measured from the junction of the chin with the neck to the highest point on the vertex.

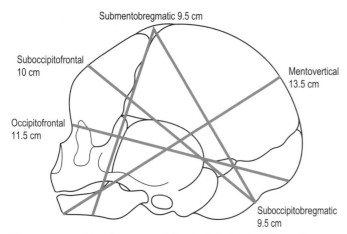

Figure 24.15   The diameters of the fetal skull (from Sweet B 1997, with permission).

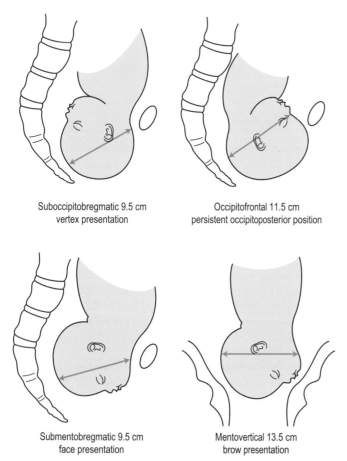

Suboccipitobregmatic 9.5 cm
vertex presentation

Occipitofrontal 11.5 cm
persistent occipitoposterior position

Submentobregmatic 9.5 cm
face presentation

Mentovertical 13.5 cm
brow presentation

Figure 24.16   The diameters of the fetal head in relation to the maternal pelvis (from Sweet B 1997, with permission).

It is 11.5 cm and presents when the head is not fully extended in a face presentation.

6. **Submentobregmatic** is measured from the junction of the chin with the neck. It is 9.5 cm and presents when the head is fully extended in a face presentation.

Transverse diameters are also taken:

1. The biparietal is measured between the parietal eminences. It is 9.5 cm and is the widest transverse diameter of the skull.
2. The bitemporal is measured between the widest aspects of the coronal suture. It is 8 cm.

Circumferences of the skull are:

- **Suboccipitobregmatic** – 33 cm presents when the head is well flexed. The head engages, fits well onto the cervix and labour should be easy.
- **Occipitofrontal** – 35 cm presents when the head is deflexed. Engagement is delayed, the membranes may rupture early and labour may be difficult.
- **Mentovertical** – 39 cm presents when the head is fully extended. The head cannot descend into the pelvis and labour is obstructed.

Moulding

Moulding of the fetal skull results in a change in shape but not size of the vault brought about by the pressures of the pelvis and pelvic floor during labour. The diameters which are compressed reduce in size by at least 0.5 cm while those at right angles to them are elongated (Table 24.2). *Note that vertex and brow presentations affect the same diameters but in opposite ways, as do face presentation and occipitoposterior position.* The skull changes shape from ovoid to cylindrical to facilitate passage through the cylindrical birth canal. The sutures and fontanelles allow overlap of the bones of the vault in a typical way:

- the frontal bones are pushed under the anterior edge of the parietal bones;
- the occipital bone is pushed under the posterior part of the parietal bones;
- the medial edge of the leading parietal bone is pushed under the other parietal bone.

Table 24.2   Involvement of diameters of the fetal skull in moulding

Presentation	Diameters decreased	Diameters increased
Vertex presentation	Suboccipitobregmatic Biparietal	Mentovertical
Brow presentation	Mentovertical Biparietal	Suboccipitobregmatic
Face presentation	Submentobregmatic Biparietal	Occipitofrontal
Occipitoposterior position	Occipitofrontal Biparietal	Submentobregmatic

Moulding is abnormal if it involves wrong diameters (Fig. 24.17), if it is too rapid or if it is too extreme so that the brain is compressed, all carrying a risk of intracranial damage.

Caput succedaneum

During labour and especially after rupture of the membranes, the fetal head is pressed against the ring of the dilating cervix. In cephalic presentations venous return in the circulation to the scalp is impeded and oedema forms in the loose tissues. This is called a caput succedaneum and varies in size with the length and difficulty of the delivery. Caput forms on the leading parietal bone, which is the left one when the occiput is to the right and vice versa. It forms on the anterior part if the position is occipitoanterior and on the posterior part of the parietal bone if the position is occipitoposterior.

External structures of the fetal skull

The scalp of the fetal skull consists of five layers. From the inside out these are:

1. The **pericranium**, which covers the outer surface of the bones and is firmly attached to the edges of the bones. Bleeding may occur between the bone and the pericranium to form a swelling called a **cephalhaematoma**. The size of the haematoma is limited to that of the bone over which it forms because of the attachment of the pericranium to the bony edges.
2. A loose layer of **areolar tissue** that permits limited movement of the scalp over the skull.
3. A layer of tendon known as the **galea** that is attached to the **frontalis muscle** anteriorly and the **occipitalis muscle** posteriorly.
4. A layer of subcutaneous tissue that contains blood vessels and hair follicles. This is the part of the scalp affected by the caput succedaneum (Fig. 24.18).
5. The skin.

Internal structures of the fetal skull

The meninges

The brain is surrounded by three membranes: from the inside these are the **pia mater**, which is closely applied to the surface of the brain; the **arachnoid mater**, which contains cerebrospinal fluid; and the outer, tough **dura mater**.

The dura mater covers the outer surface of the brain and dips down to form compartments (Fig. 24.19). There are two main folds of the dura mater. The **falx cerebri** is a double fold forming a partition between the two cerebral hemispheres. It is attached to the skull following the line of the frontal and sagittal sinuses from the root of the nose to the internal aspect of the occipital protruberance. Its lower edge is unattached and is sickle shaped.

The **tentorium cerebelli** lies horizontally, separating the cerebrum from the cerebellum. It is at right angles to the

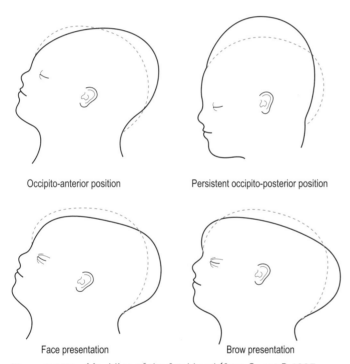

Occipito-anterior position   Persistent occipito-posterior position

Face presentation   Brow presentation

Figure 24.17   Moulding of the fetal head (from Sweet B 1997, with permission).

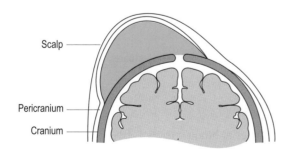

Scalp

Pericranium

Cranium

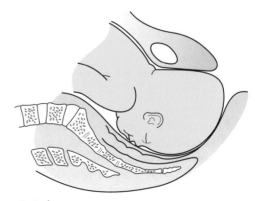

Figure 24.18   Caput succedaneum (from Sweet B 1997, with permission).

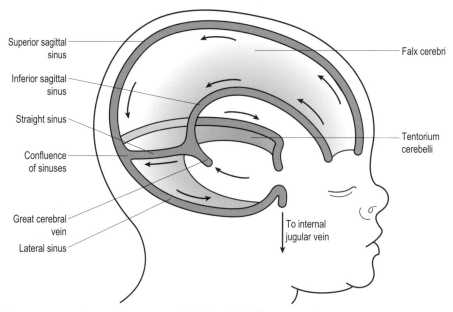

Figure 24.19   Internal structures of the fetal skull (Sweet 1997).

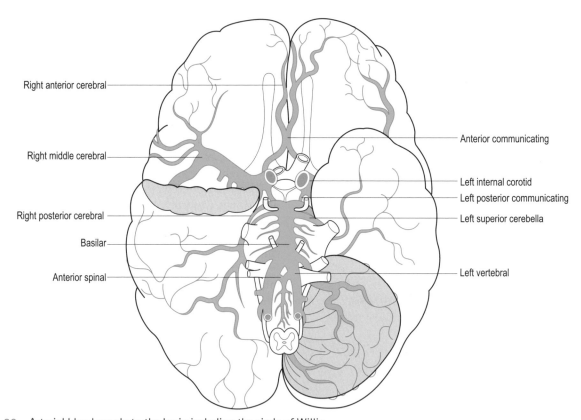

Figure 24.20   Arterial blood supply to the brain including the circle of Willis.

falx cerebri and is horseshoe shaped. Each side of the horseshoe is attached laterally to the sphenoid bone and along the inner surface of the petrous portion of the temporal bone. It meets the falx at the internal occipital protruberance. The brainstem passes in front of the junction of the two folds of dura mater (Fig. 24.20).

Blood supply of the brain

The arterial blood supply is by two **internal carotid** arteries and two **vertebral arteries**. The internal carotid arteries give off pairs of **anterior**, **middle** and **posterior cerebral arteries**. Each vertebral artery gives off a branch which supplies the cerebellum and medulla oblongata before uniting with its partner to form the **basilar artery**. The basilar artery gives off two pairs of arteries to the cerebellum and upper brainstem before dividing into two terminal branches that link up with the ends of the internal carotids. Twenty-five per cent of the population maintain three cerebral arteries on both sides of the brain, while in the majority of people the vertebral arteries take over the posterior cerebral arteries. These intercommunicating arteries at the base of the brain are known as the **circle of Willis** (Fig. 24.20).

The venous drainage is by channels in the dural folds called sinuses:

1. the superior longitudinal (or sagittal) sinus runs along the upper border of the falx cerebri;
2. the inferior longitudinal (or sagittal) sinus runs along the lower border of the falx cerebri;
3. the straight sinus is a continuation of the inferior longitudinal sinus which runs posteriorly to join the superior longitudinal sinus;
4. the great vein of Galen joins the straight sinus at the junction with the inferior venous sinus;
5. from the confluence of sinuses, the lateral sinuses pass along the line of attachment of the tentorium cerebelli and emerge from the skull to become the internal jugular veins of the neck.

When moulding is severe, rapid or in the wrong direction, these membranes and sinuses may be torn, especially at the junction of the two folds of dura. The tentorium is most likely to be damaged and bleeding involves the great vein of Galen, the straight sinus and the inferior longitudinal sinus.

MAIN POINTS

- Bone is a connective tissue which contains depositions of calcium and phosphorus and performs important functions for the body. It consists of an organic matrix of collagen known as osteoid, a mineral matrix of calcium and phosphorus and bone cells. Bone can be divided into compact or lamellar bone and spongy bone.

- Most bones have a tough outer covering called the periosteum. Lining the marrow cavity of a bone is the endosteum, which contains the osteoblasts, osteoclasts and their precursor cells. Osteoblasts synthesise and secrete the constituents of bone and promote mineralisation of the matrix. Osteocytes maintain the bone matrix. Osteoclasts contain enzymes which can remove both the organic and mineral matrix.

- The skeleton contains 99% of the calcium and 85% of the phosphorus present in the body. Three hormones are involved in the control of calcium and phosphorus metabolism: parathyroid hormone (PTH), vitamin D and calcitonin.

- The pelvic girdle provides attachment for the lower limbs and supports the pelvic abdominal organs. The size, shape and rigidity of the pelvic girdle and the curved spine are related to bipedal locomotion, essential for maintaining an upright posture.

- The bony ring of the pelvis is made up of two innominate bones: the sacrum and the coccyx. Each innominate bone consists of three fused bones – the ilium, ischium and pubis. The four joints are the symphysis pubis, two sacroiliac joints and the sacrococcygeal joint. Besides the ligaments supporting each of the pelvic joints, there are three other pairs: the sacrotuberous ligament, the sacrospinous ligament and the inguinal ligament.

- The pelvic brim separates the upper flare of the iliac fossae from the basin-shaped part of the pelvis. The area above this is called the false pelvis while below the brim is the true pelvis forming the birth canal. Measurements are taken of the planes of the pelvic brim, cavity and outlet in three directions – anteroposterior, oblique and transverse.

- In the upright posture the pelvic basin is tilted in relation to the horizontal. Imaginary lines drawn at right angles through the planes of the pelvis and joined together form a curve that the fetus must pass through during birth: the curve of Carus. There are four basic types of pelvis: gynaecoid, android, anthropoid and platypelloid.

- Maternal calcium metabolism alters to meet fetal needs for calcium and phosphorus to enable skeletal growth and development. Serum calcium begins to fall soon after fertilisation and reaches its lowest level at about 30 weeks of pregnancy. Serum inorganic phosphate levels and magnesium levels fall slightly until 30 weeks of pregnancy and return to non-pregnant levels by term.

- Adequate calcium, phosphorus and vitamin D are essential in pregnancy. Some foods which contain excessive fats, phytates and oxalates interfere with the absorption of calcium. Pregnancy problems related to calcium include intense cramping pain in the calf muscles, restless leg syndrome and backache. Serious problems are rickets, osteomalacia and spinal cord injury.

- The bones of the fetal skull are divided into vault, face and base. The face and base of the skull are laid down in cartilage and are almost completely ossified by birth. The vault of the fetal skull is composed of flat bones which develop from membrane. The fetal skull is divided into regions of face, brow, vertex and occiput.

- The process of ossification is incomplete at birth so that membranous sutures remain between the bones and membranous fontanelles where two or more sutures meet. Measurements of the skull are used to assess its size in relation to the maternal pelvis.

- Moulding of the fetal skull results in a change in shape but not size of the vault brought about by the pressures of the pelvis and pelvic floor during labour. Moulding is abnormal if it involves wrong diameters is extreme or too rapid.

- The brain is surrounded by three meninges: the pia mater, the arachnoid mater and the dura mater. The dura mater covers the outer surface of the brain and dips down to form compartments. There are two main folds of the dura mater: the falx cerebri and the tentorium cerebelli.

- The arterial blood supply to the brain is by two internal carotid arteries and two vertebral arteries. The internal carotid arteries give off pairs of anterior, middle and posterior cerebral arteries. The intercommunicating arteries at the base of the brain are known as the circle of Willis. The venous drainage is by channels in the dural folds called sinuses.

References

Aiello L, Dean C 1990 An Introduction to Human Evolutionary Anatomy. Academic Press, New York.

Bennett V R, Brown L K 1996 Myles Textbook for Midwives, 12th edn. Churchill Livingstone, Edinburgh, pp 57–64.

Blackburn S T 2003 Maternal, Fetal and Neonatal Physiology. W B Saunders, Philadelphia.

Boore J R P 1996 Endocrine function. In Hinchliff S M, Montague S E, Watson R (eds) Physiology for Nursing Practice, 2nd edn. Baillière Tindall, London, pp 202–244.

Brook G D, Marshall N J 2001 Essential Endocrinology, 4th edn. Blackwell Science, Oxford.

Cross N A, Hillman L S, Allen A H, Krause G F, Vieira N E 1995 Calcium homeostasis and bone metabolism during pregnancy, lactation and post-weaning: a longitudinal study. American Journal of Clinical Nutrition 61:514–523.

Davis D C 1996 The discomforts of pregnancy. JOGNN January:73–80.

Dunnigan M G, McIntosh W B, Ford J A, Roberson I 1982 Acquired disorders in vitamin D metabolism. In Heath D, Marx S J (eds) Calcium Disorders. Butterworths, London.

Henderson P H, Sowers M F, Kotuku K E, Jannausch M L 2000 Bone mineral density in grand multiparous women with extended lactation. American Journal of Obstetrics and Gynecology 182(6):1371–1377.

Jimenez S 1994 If you can't get comfortable. Childbirth 11(1):37–40.

Marieb E N 2000 Human Anatomy and Physiology, 5th edn. Benjamin/Cummings, New York.

Morgan E 1990 The scars of evolution. Penguin Books, Harmondsworth.

Morgan E 1994 The Descent of the Child. Souvenir Press, London.

Prentice A 2000 Maternal calcium metabolism and bone mineral status. American Journal of Clinical Nutrition 71(suppl):13112S–13126S.

Sweet B R 1997 The fetal skull. In Sweet B R, Tiran D (eds) Mayes Midwifery, 12th edn. Baillière Tindall, London.

Trevathen W R, Smith E O, McKenna J J 1999 Evolutionary Medicine. Oxford University Press, Oxford.

Annotated recommended reading

Brook G D, Marshall N J 2001 Essential Endocrinology, 4th edn. Blackwell Science, Oxford.
This endocrinology textbook is presented in a straightforward accessible manner. While the content is of adequate depth for degree students, the text ensures that those with no previous knowledge can understand the principles. Chapter 7 gives an excellent overview of calcium metabolism.

Morgan E 1994 The Descent of the Child. Souvenir Press, London.
This book is written by a specialist in human evolution. She discusses why our babies are so small and helpless at birth compared with other species. It has insights into the relationships between mother, infant and family.

Prentice A 2000 Maternal calcium metabolism and bone mineral status. American Journal of Clinical Nutrition 71 (suppl):13112S–13126S.
Prentice has collated what is currently known about calcium in pregnancy and lactation in a very succinct manner. Although detail is given it is in a well set out, readable form at the right level for midwifery students.

Trevathen W R, Smith E O, McKenna J J 1999 Evolutionary Medicine. Oxford University Press, Oxford.
This book integrates evolutionary theories with health and disease and Chapters 1–8 discuss aspects of childhood and childbearing. In particular, in Chapter 8, Travathen discusses childbirth and the effects of pelvic shape and fetal size on human childbearing.

Chapter **25**

Muscle – the pelvic floor and the uterus

INTRODUCTION

Muscle makes up almost half of the body's mass and is specialised tissue which generates forces and enables movement to occur. It has the ability to transform the chemical energy in adenosine triphosphate (ATP) into mechanical energy. This section will describe the nature of muscles and, for the purpose of this text, only the individual muscles of the pelvic floor and uterus will be described in detail.

Three basic muscle types can be identified on the basis of structure, contractile properties and control mechanisms: skeletal muscle, smooth muscle and cardiac muscle. Most skeletal muscle is attached to bone and is responsible for supporting and moving the skeleton. Smooth muscle is found in the walls of the hollow viscera of the gastrointestinal, genitourinary and respiratory tracts and the specialised cardiac muscle propels blood through the circulation. Although there are significant differences in these types of muscle, the force-generating mechanism is similar in all of them.

All muscle cells are elongated and therefore referred to as fibres and they all contain two kinds of protein filaments – **actin** and **myosin**. Muscles have **four functions**: they produce movement, maintain posture, stabilise joints and generate heat. They have **four properties**: excitability, which is the ability to receive and respond to a stimulus; contractility, or the ability to shorten when stimulated; extensibility, or the ability to be stretched or extended beyond its resting length; and elasticity, or the ability of muscle to recoil back to its resting length.

SKELETAL MUSCLE

Skeletal muscles, as the name implies, are attached to and cover the bony skeleton. The longest muscle fibres are found in skeletal muscle. One striking feature of the fibres are obvious bands or **striations**: hence the term **striated muscle**. Another term used for skeletal muscle is **voluntary** as this is the only muscle type under voluntary control. Skeletal muscle can contract rapidly but tires easily and must be rested after short bursts of activity. Each skeletal

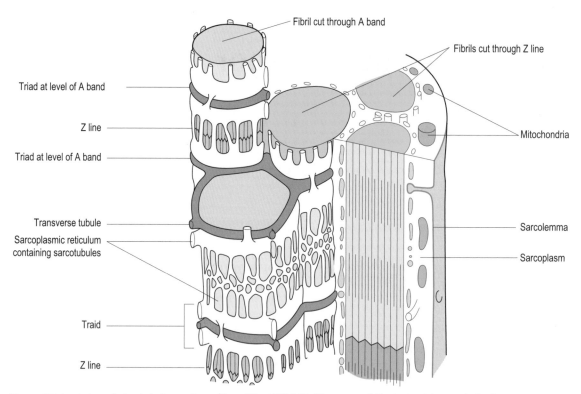

Figure 25.1 Intracellular tubular systems (from Hinchliff S M, Montague S E 1990, with permission).

muscle is a discrete organ made up of multiple muscle fibres. Other tissues found in the individual muscles include connective tissue, blood vessels and nerve fibres. Muscle fibres are gathered into functional units by a network of fibrous connective tissue (Fig. 25.1). This connective tissue condenses into the **tendons** which form the muscular origins and insertions onto bone.

The activity of skeletal muscle depends on its rich blood supply and nerve supply. While the other muscle types can contract without nerve stimulation, each skeletal muscle fibre is supplied with a nerve ending. The blood supply is essential to deliver the large amounts of oxygen and nutrients and to remove equally large amounts of metabolic waste. The smaller blood vessels are long and winding, which permits the changes in muscle length to occur.

Microscopic anatomy of a skeletal muscle fibre

Skeletal muscle fibres are long cylindrical cells which taper at both ends. The plasma membrane is called the **sarcolemma** and there are multiple oval nuclei arranged just below the surface. Skeletal muscle fibres are huge. The fibre length is variable, ranging from a few millimetres in short muscles to lengths of 300 mm in longer muscles (1 ft in length). Their diameter ranges from 10 to 100 μm which is up to 10 times that of other body cells. The presence of multiple nuclei indicate that each muscle fibre is a **syncytium** (fusion of many cells) formed during embryonic development. The cytoplasm in muscle cells is called **sarcoplasm**

and the endoplasmic reticulum is referred to as **sarcoplasmic reticulum**. The sarcoplasm contains large amounts of stored glycogen and a unique oxygen-binding protein called **myoglobin** similar to haemoglobin (Marieb 2000).

Myofibrils

Each muscle fibre contains a large number of rod-like **myofibrils** extending the full length of the cell and parallel to each other. Myofibrils are densely packed and form 80% of the cellular content. Mitochondria, the energy-producing organelles, and other organelles are packed in between the myofibrils. Myofibrils are the contractile elements of the cell and each myofibril consists of smaller contractile units called **sarcomeres**. Several sarcomeres are arranged along each myofibril.

Myofibrils appear to be made of alternate dark or **A bands** and light or **I bands**, giving the characteristic striped appearance under the light microscope. The bands are named according to how they refract (bend) polarised light (light waves with a definite direction): **A** bands (**anisotropic**) refers to their ability to refract light, depending on its angle; **I** bands (**isotropic**) refers to their ability to refract light, whatever its angle (Marieb 2000).

The A band is interrupted in mid-section by the highly refractive **H zone** (H stands for helle, which means bright). Each H zone is bisected by a dark line called the **M line**. The I bands also have a midline interruption called the **Z line** (Figs 25.1 and 25.2). A sarcomere is the region of a

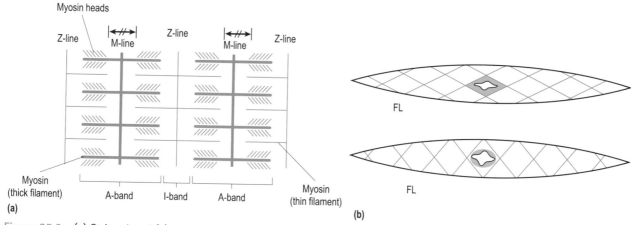

Figure 25.2   (a) Striated and (b) smooth fibres. A, actin; M, myosin; FL, filaments. (Reproduced with permission from Huszar & Roberts 1982.)

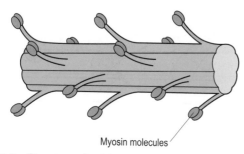

Figure 25.3   Structure of a thick filament (from Hinchliff S M, Montague S E 1990, with permission).

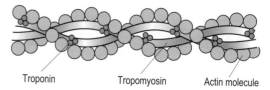

Figure 25.4   Structure of a thin filament (from Hinchliff S M, Montague S E 1990, with permission).

myofibril that extends from one Z line to the next. Brief explanations of these other features are as follows:

- the Z line is a network of interconnecting proteins that form a point of attachment for thin filaments;
- the H zone is only visible in relaxed muscle when the thick filaments are not overlapped by the thin filaments;
- the M line in the centre of the H zone appears darker because it is slightly thicker due to the presence of fine strands that connect adjacent thick filaments together.

The higher magnifying power of the electron microscope shows that the A bands are formed of thick **myosin** filaments (Fig. 25.3). The thin filaments are formed of three different proteins: **actin**, **troponin** and **tropomyosin**. These run the length of the I band, overlapping the thick filaments (Fig. 25.4). In an intact muscle fibre the bands are aligned horizontally across the width of the cell. Each myosin molecule has a rod-like tail (axis) and two globular heads (cross-bridges) that interact with special sites on the thin filaments. Each thick filament within a sarcomere contains about 200 myosin molecules.

The thin filaments are mainly composed of actin. Subunits called **globular** or **G actin** bear the active sites to which the **myosin cross-bridges** attach themselves during muscle contraction. The backbone of each actin molecule is formed by two strands of **fibrous** or **F actin** arranged in a helical structure. Regulatory proteins include tropomyosin, which spirals around the F actin to stiffen it. In resting muscle the orientation of the tropomyosin blocks the myosin-binding sites on the actin molecules. This prevents the formation of cross-bridges. Troponin actually consists of three polypeptides: one binds to actin and another to tropomyosin helping to position it on the actin, while the third binds calcium.

Intracellular tubular systems

The muscle cell is penetrated by two tubular systems (see Fig. 25.1), both ending near the A–I band junctions. One tubular system is called the **transverse** or **T system**, extending from the cell exterior into the sarcoplasm where they branch and terminate. The other is the **internal system** formed by fine tubules called **sarcotubules** of the **sarcoplasmic reticulum**. These sarcotubules end in terminal sacs called the **terminal cysternae**. Both systems play a key role in muscle contraction. T tubules conduct electrical stimuli deep within the muscle cell to the sarcomeres. The sarcoplasmic reticulum regulates the calcium (Ca^{2+}) ions.

Muscle contraction

There are several theories of how muscle fibres contract but most evidence supports the **sliding filament theory**. The theory explains that during contraction the thin filaments slide past the thick ones, increasing the amount of overlap. This allows the thin filaments to penetrate more deeply into the central region of the A band. Overlapping is brought

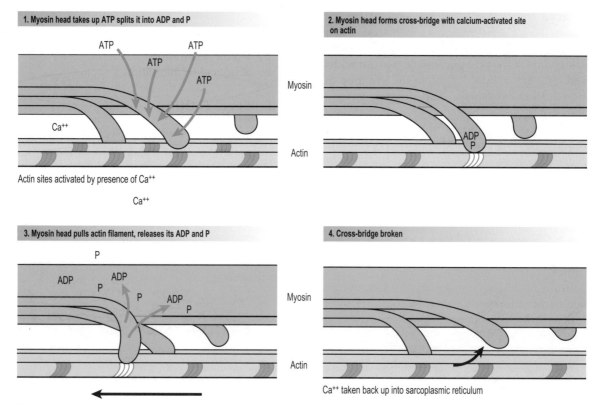

Figure 25.5 Diagrammatic representation of the sliding-filament theory showing how the thick filaments of skeletal muscle move relative to one another as cross-bridges are formed and broken (from Hinchliff S M, Montague S E, Watson R 1996, with permission).

about by the cross-bridges of the sarcomeres acting simultaneously as a ratchet to pull the thin filaments towards the centre of the sarcomeres. This results in shortening of the muscle cell. The myosin heads are said to 'walk up' the actin filaments step by step from one binding site to the next (Fig. 25.5). This requires the presence of calcium, which binds to the troponin to form a complex. The configuration of tropomyosin is changed to move it away from the myosin-binding sites. As calcium is removed by the sarcoplasmic reticulum, the contraction comes to an end and the muscle cell relaxes.

Regulation of contraction Skeletal muscles contract in response to nerve stimulation, which results in an **action potential** being sent along the sarcolemma. This electrical event results in a rise in intracellular calcium (Ca^{2+}) ion levels that triggers off the contraction. The axon of a **lower motor neuron** (Ch. 27, p. 368) branches profusely as it enters the muscle and each mound-shaped unmyelinated axonal terminal forms a junction with a single muscle fibre, approximately in the middle of the cell. This is called a neuromuscular junction or **motor end plate** (Fig. 25.6). The plasma membrane of the axonal ending does not actually touch the muscle fibre; between them is a small fluid-filled extracellular space called the **synaptic cleft**. The action potential must be transmitted across the space and this happens by the release of the neurotransmitter substance **acetylcholine (ACh)** from small membranous sacs in the axon terminal called **synaptic vesicles**.

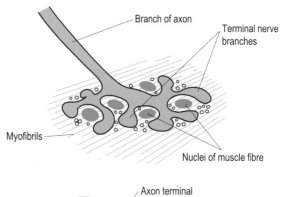

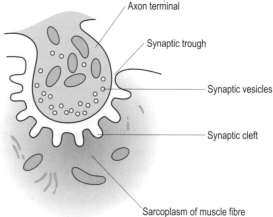

Figure 25.6 The neuromuscular junction (from Hinchliff S M, Montague S E, Watson R 1996, with permission).

When a nerve impulse reaches the end of an axon, **voltage-regulated calcium channels** open and calcium flows in from the extracellular fluid (ECF). The entry of the calcium causes some of the synaptic vesicles to fuse with the plasma membrane and release ACh into the synaptic cleft. This process is called **exocytosis**. ACh diffuses across the synaptic cleft and attaches itself to ACh receptors on the sarcolemma. All plasma membranes are polarised with a **voltage gradient** (membrane potential) across the membrane. The inside of the cell is negative. This attachment of ACh molecules opens chemically regulated ion gates. The positively charged ion sodium (Na^+) passes from its higher concentration in the ECF fluid down a gradient into the cell, leading to a slight decrease in the negative potential. This event, called **depolarisation**, allows a muscle cell action potential to be generated and to pass in all directions across the sarcolemma.

Repolarisation of the sarcolemma occurs following the wave of the muscle action potential when sodium channels close and potassium channels open. Potassium (K^+) ions rapidly diffuse out of the cell into the ECF down a gradient to restore the negativity inside the cell. The normal ionic balance of sodium and potassium is restored during the refractory period when the muscle cannot respond to stimuli. After the release of ACh and its binding to the ACh receptors, it is quickly destroyed by the enzyme **acetylcholinesterase**. This prevents the muscle contraction lasting longer than the stimulus requires.

Excitation–contraction coupling This is the process whereby the generation of an action potential is followed by activation of the contractile machinery in the myofibrils. It involves the exposure of the binding sites on the actin to allow the formation of cross-bridges. Energy released from ATP is used to fuel the muscle contraction. As action potentials continue to arrive, the process is repeated many times, allowing sustained muscle contraction. Calcium ions are continuously released and taken up by troponin. This also requires energy from ATP. However, muscles store very little ATP and the supply is soon exhausted. If contraction is to continue, ATP must be regenerated. This can occur in three ways:

1. by the interaction of ADP with creatine phosphate;
2. by aerobic respiration;
3. by lactic acid fermentation.

THE PELVIC FLOOR

The bony pelvis provides protection to the pelvic organs while the **pelvic floor** holds them in position. The pelvic floor is primarily composed of soft tissues which fill the outlet of the pelvis. The most important of these is the strong funnel-shaped diaphragm of muscle attached to the pelvic walls. The posterior part of the diaphragm of muscles lies higher than the anterior. Through it passes the urethra, vagina and anal canal (Fig. 25.7).

The pelvic floor consists of six layers of tissue. From the inside outwards:

1. pelvic peritoneum;
2. visceral layer of pelvic fascia thickened to form pelvic ligaments which support the uterus;
3. **deep muscles** encased in fascia;
4. **superficial muscles** encased in fascia;
5. subcutaneous fat;
6. skin.

Superficial muscles

These muscles lie external to the deep muscles and provide additional strength – a little like the webbing beneath the cushion on some chairs. They consist of:

- the transverse perinei;
- the bulbocavernosus;
- the ischiocavernosus;
- the external anal sphincter;
- the external urethral meatus, sometimes called the membranous sphincter of the urethra (Fig. 25.8).

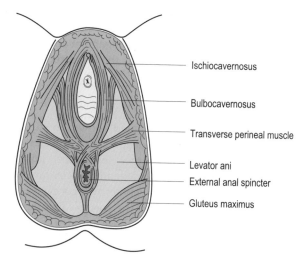

Figure 25.8   The perineal muscles (from Sweet B 1997, with permission).

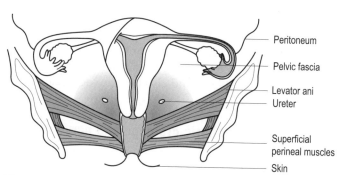

Figure 25.7   The layers of the pelvic floor (from Sweet B 1997, with permission).

The transverse perinei

One muscle arises from the inner surface of each **ischial tuberosity** of the pelvis and passes transversely to meet its fellow, inserting into the **perineal body**. Some fibres pass posteriorly to blend with the anal sphincter.

The bulbocavernosus

This arises in the centre of the perineum and fibres pass on either side of the vagina and urethra, encircling them both, to insert into the corpora cavernosa (body) of the clitoris just under the pubic arch. This muscle is responsible for erection of the clitoris and contraction of the vaginal walls.

The ischiocavernosus

A muscle runs from each ischial tuberosity along the pubic arch to the corpora cavernosa of the clitoris and fibres interweave with the membranous sphincter of the urethra.

External anal sphincter

This is a circle of muscle surrounding the anus formed by merging of muscle fibres from deep and superficial layers. The sphincter is attached behind the anus to the coccyx.

External urinary meatus

The membranous sphincter of the urethra is a weak and not too important muscle. It is composed of muscle fibres passing above and below the urethra and attached to the pubic bones. It is not a true sphincter since it is not circular, but it acts to close the urethra.

The superficial muscles do not form a continuous sheet and there are gaps filled with other tissues. Anteriorly is the **triangular ligament** bounded by the ischiocavernosus and the transverse perinei. It consists of two layers of fascia. Where the triangular ligaments stretch across the **pubic arch**, they help to support the bladder neck. Posteriorly, the gap is filled with fat and is bounded by the gluteus maximus muscle, the sacrotuberous ligament and the transverse perinei. This area is known as the **ischiorectal fossa**.

Deep pelvic floor muscles

The deep floor muscles are situated above the superficial muscles and are about 5 cm deep. Deep muscles called **levator ani** are by far the largest and most important muscles of the pelvic floor. The levator ani muscles raise or elevate the anus. They are collectively termed coccygeus muscles because they insert around the coccyx. Together with the fascia covering their surfaces, these muscles are referred to as the pelvic diaphragm. The arrangement of muscle gives the appearance of a funnel or sling suspended from its attachments on the pelvic wall (Fig. 25.9). These muscles are *vital* to the control of bladder and bowel function.

It is conventional to describe the levator ani in three pairs of deep muscles:

1. pubococcygeus;
2. iliococcygeus;
3. ischiococcygeus.

The pubococcygeus

These are the most medial muscles. Fibres arise from the inner border of the body of the pubis and from the white line of fascia (arcus tendineus fasciae). They sweeps posteriorly in three bands:

1. a central band of fibres surrounding the urethra;
2. some fibres form a U-shaped loop around the vagina and insert into the lateral and posterior vaginal walls in the perineum;
3. other fibres loop around the anus and insert into the lateral and posterior walls of the anal canal and the coccyx.

These muscles support and maintain position of the pelvic viscera; resist increased intra-abdominal pressure during forced expiration, vomiting, coughing, urination and defecation; constrict the anus, urethra and vagina; and support the fetal head during childbirth. During childbirth the muscles may be injured as a result of a difficult childbirth or trauma during an episiotomy.

The iliococcygeus

These muscles arise from the inner border of the white line of fascia on the iliac bone and also from the ischial spines and run to the coccyx, some crossing over in the perineal body. They support and maintain position of the pelvic viscera; resist increased intra-abdominal pressure during forced expiration, vomiting, coughing, urination and defecation; and pull the coccyx anteriorly following defecation or childbirth. During childbirth the muscles may be injured as a result of a difficult childbirth or trauma during an episiotomy.

The ischiococcygeus

Fibres arise from each ischial spine and insert into the upper edge of the coccyx and lower border of the sacrum. These muscles help to stabilise the sacroiliac and sacrococcygeal joints of the pelvis and also flex the coccygeal joints.

Blood supply, lymphatic drainage and nerve supply

Blood supply

Arterial supply is by branches of the two internal iliac arteries and drainage is by corresponding veins.

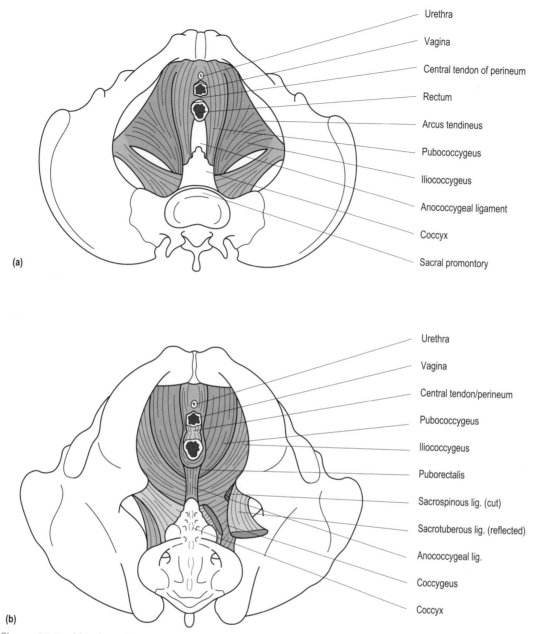

Figure 25.9 Muscles of the pelvic diaphragm. (a) Superior view. (b) Inferior view. (Reproduced with permission from Gabbe et al 1991.)

Lymphatic drainage

Lymph drainage is widespread, both laterally and medially.

Nerve supply

The pelvic floor muscles are under voluntary control. The nerve supply is by branches of the pudendal nerve via the sacral plexus.

The **perineal body** is a wedge-shaped mass of muscular and fibrous tissue situated between the vaginal and anal canals. Both the superficial and deep pelvic floor muscles are involved in its structure. The wedge of tissue is pyramidal or triangular in shape; the apex is uppermost and is the central point of the pelvic floor. The perineal body measures 4 cm in each direction (Bennett & Brown 1999).

Functions

Effective functioning is dependent on the integrity of the muscle fibres and maintenance of muscle tone. The pelvic floor has the following functions:

- supports the weight of the abdominal and pelvic organs;
- maintains intra-abdominal pressure;
- voluntary control of defecation and micturition;
- facilitates the movements of the fetus through the birth canal;
- enables flexion of the sacrum and coccyx.

Clinical implications

Loss of integrity and trauma to the pelvic floor can often be associated with childbearing (Stanton 1999). In the event of damage to the pelvic floor, the following reproductive anomalies may occur.

Uterovaginal prolapse

Prolapse of the pelvic organs with the possibility of urinary and faecal incontinence may cause women much anxiety, embarrassment and discomfort. Symptoms may occur with ageing due to loss of muscle tone and withdrawal of oestrogen, prolonged immobility due to muscle atrophy and congenital weakness of the muscles. However, the problems are most often related to childbearing and damage to the pelvic floor during childbirth may lead to long-term problems. This includes uterine prolapse, which is downward displacement of the uterus to varying degrees. It is now rare to see **procidentia**, which is total prolapse of the uterus outside the body.

Vaginal prolapse – anterior wall

A **cystocele** is a herniation of the bladder which may present with bladder irritation or a feeling of a lump in the vagina. This is often symptomless but, if large, may lead to collection of residual urine, infection and pyelonephritis. A **urethrocele** is a displacement of the urethra with loss of the acute angle between it and the bladder. This angle helps to maintain continence so the result may be urinary stress incontinence, which is the involuntary loss of small amounts of urine during coughing, sneezing or any other activity that increases intra-abdominal pressure.

Vaginal prolapse – posterior wall

A **rectocele** is a prolapse of the posterior middle vaginal wall, allowing herniation of the rectum. As in the cystocele, this may be symptomless unless very large, when faeces become lodged in the herniated sac. Defecation will be difficult unless digital pressure is applied on the vaginal side of the sac. An **enterocele** is a herniation higher in the vagina and on examination will not be palpable per vaginam.

Dyspareunia (painful sexual intercourse)

This may occur depending on the degree of prolapse.

Treatment

Treatment of reproductive anomalies is usually by surgical repair. In a few women, such as those who refuse surgery or are too ill or frail, insertion of a ring pessary may be the treatment of choice.

Prevention of prolapse

A midwife can minimise the risk by careful practice:

- attempt to avoid pushing until full dilatation of the cervix;
- prevent delivery of the baby before full dilatation of the cervix;
- ensure that the second stage is not prolonged without obvious progress;
- avoid fundal pressure to deliver the placenta;
- ensure careful repair of any perineal trauma;
- ensure early ambulation of the woman;
- encourage pelvic floor exercises in the puerperium.

SMOOTH MUSCLE

Smooth muscle has two common characteristics: it lacks the cross-striated banding pattern found in skeletal and cardiac fibres, and nerve supply is derived from the autonomic division of the nervous system rather than the somatic division. Hence, the muscle is described as smooth, **non-striated**, **involuntary** and is often referred to as **visceral muscle** (Vander et al 2000). Smooth muscle, like skeletal muscle, uses cross-bridge movements between actin and myosin filaments to generate force and calcium ions to control cross-bridge activity. However, there are differences between the two types of muscles in the organisation of the contractile filaments and in the excitation–contraction coupling process. There is also diversity within the range of smooth muscle types in respect of the mechanism of excitation–contraction coupling.

The contractions of smooth muscle are slow and sustained. The fibres of smooth muscle are small, spindle-shaped cells with a central nucleus. They have no striations and have a large surface area, allowing calcium ions to enter the cells easily. There are notably fewer myosin fibres than actin fibres in smooth muscle. The myosin heads are arranged along the length of the myosin fibre so that each myosin fibre is attached to many actin fibres.

The fibres are arranged in a spiral around the muscle cell and can change their lengths much more than skeletal muscle fibres. The fibres are arranged in two (or more) sheets, usually at right angles to each other. For instance, there are three layers in the body of the uterus – an outer, mainly longitudinal layer; an oblique middle layer; and an inner, mainly circular layer (Romanini 1994). Muscle fibres in the cervix are mainly circular with only a few longitudinal fibres.

There are no clear neuromuscular junctions in smooth muscle. The innervating fibres have bulbous varicosities and release their neurotransmitter substance directly onto many fibres. This allows a slow, **synchronised contraction** of the whole muscle sheet. Action potentials are transmitted from cell to cell until the whole muscle sheet is contracting. Some fibres act as **pacemaker cells** to set the contractile pace for the whole muscle sheet. It is thought that such fibres in the uterus are beneath the cornua so that the fundus dominates. Both the rate and intensity of smooth muscle contraction can be modified by neural and chemical stimuli.

Calcium triggers the onset of contractions and ATP provides the energy. Contraction in smooth muscle is slow, sustained and resistant to fatigue. Smooth muscle fibres take 30 times longer to contract and relax than skeletal muscle fibres. The same muscle tension can be maintained for long periods at less than 1% of the energy cost in skeletal muscle. In many parts of the body smooth muscle tone is maintained continuously with low energy expenditure and often by anaerobic ATP production.

Special features of smooth muscle include:

- less vigorous contractile response to being stretched so that distension of a hollow organ can occur without provoking expulsive contractions;
- ability to change more in length and create more tension than skeletal muscle;
- ability to divide – hyperplasia;
- secretion of the connective tissue proteins collagen and elastin.

UTERINE MUSCLE DURING PREGNANCY

Like most other smooth muscle the uterus is spontaneously contractile. When required, it has the ability to perform considerable muscular feats to expel its contents such as during menstruation and delivery. At other times it is prevented from contracting and must remain quiescent to allow development and growth of the fetus and placenta during pregnancy (Steer & Johnson 1998). The uterus is unique among smooth muscular organs in that it undergoes profound, largely reversible, changes during pregnancy. In early pregnancy, muscle fibres become more compliant and growth of fibres is mainly due to hyperplasia. This occurs under the influence of oestrogen and independently of fetal growth. If the fetus embeds outside of the uterus (ectopic gestation), this early growth of the uterus would still occur.

The size of the non-pregnant uterus is 7.5 cm in length, 5 cm in width and 2.5 cm in depth but by term the uterus has grown to 30 cm long, 22.5 cm wide and 20 cm deep. There is 20-fold increase in weight of the uterus from 50 g to 1100 g (Steer & Johnson 1998). The main part of uterine growth during the second half of pregnancy is almost entirely due to hypertrophy (increase in size) in response to various stimuli. The growth of the fetus stretches the uterus and this acts as a powerful stimulator of growth-promoting synthesis of the contractile proteins of the myometrium (Steer & Johnson 1998). By 3–4 months the uterine wall has thickened from 10 to 25 mm but by term the wall has thinned to between 5 and 10 mm (Blackburn 2003). The lower part of the uterus, consisting of the isthmus, softens and elongates from its original 7 mm until about 10 weeks of pregnancy when it measures 25 mm. This is the beginning of differentiation of the lower uterine segment (Dunlop 1999).

Uterine shape and position: uterine growth

The uterus is expected to follow a predicted rate of growth during pregnancy. However, this is only a reliable indicator of gestational age in the first 20 weeks of pregnancy. Routine measurement of fundal height of the uterus is used to assess the growth of the fetus and the umbilicus and xiphisternum are useful landmarks for this purpose.

By 12 weeks the uterus has risen out of the pelvis and has become an abdominal organ. It is no longer anteverted and anteflexed. As it becomes upright, the uterus often inclines to and rotates to the right. This may be because the colon occupies the space in the left side of the pelvic cavity. This is known as **right obliquity of the uterus** and increases as pregnancy progresses. At this time the conceptus fills the uterine cavity and the isthmus opens out. The fundus of the uterus can be palpated abdominally just above the symphysis pubis.

As pregnancy progresses, the shape and position of the uterus changes to accommodate the growing fetus. Following implantation, the embedded blastocyst does not require much space but the upper part of the uterus begins to enlarge due to the influence of oestrogen. The uterus becomes globular in shape until about 20 weeks and then pear shaped or cylindrical until term. The fundus may be palpated at the level or just below the level of the umbilicus at 20 weeks and midway between the umbilicus and xiphisternum at 30 weeks. At this time the lower uterine segment (LUS) is identified but is not complete. By 36 weeks, the fundus reaches its maximum height at the xiphisternum. A reduction in fundal height may now occur as the presenting part of the fetus enters the pelvis. This is due to softening of the pelvic floor tissues together with good uterine tone and further formation of the LUS (Dunlop 1999). Lay people generally know this as 'lightening'.

Hormonal influences on the uterus in pregnancy

Oestrogen and progesterone, initially from the corpus luteum and then the placenta, are mainly the hormones responsible for influencing the uterus. Oestrogen promotes growth of muscle fibres and progesterone maintains the quiescence of the myometrium by possibly blocking the excitation and conduction mechanisms of the muscle cells. In particular, the interaction of these hormones has a growth-promoting effect and increases uterine muscle compliance. By term, each muscle fibre increases three-fold in diameter and 10-fold in length.

Actions of oestrogen and progesterone on target cells

The hormone probably enters the target cell by passive diffusion across the cell membrane and then binds to specific receptor proteins present in the cellular cytoplasm. The complex formed between the steroid and the receptor is transferred to the nucleus where gene function is regulated.

The hormone estradiol stimulates RNA synthesis. The RNA is transferred to the cytoplasm where it is responsible for the synthesis of new protein. The role of progesterone is less understood mainly due to the lack of thorough research. It may be responsible for increasing membrane resting potential in pregnancy so that muscle fibre contractions are less likely to occur.

The uterus at term

The uterus at term is generally described as having two main structural compartments: the upper uterine segment (UUS), formed of the body and fundus, and the lower uterine segment (LUS), formed of the isthmus and cervix. The uterus cannot simply be divided in this way as there is a gradual fall in the smooth muscle content from the fundus to the cervix. The muscle content of the cervix is estimated to be 10% and the functional significance of this cervical muscle is not understood. The physiological mechanisms regulating these functions are becoming clearer but there remains uncertainty about the pathophysiology, for example in incompetent cervix (Calder 1994).

The decidua

During pregnancy the endometrium becomes thicker, richer and more vascular in the upper part of the body of the uterus and the fundus, the normal site for implantation. It is now termed the decidua, because it is similar to the deciduous tree in that it sheds at the end of pregnancy. The decidua is thinner and less vascular in the lower pole of the uterus. The decidua provides a glycogen-rich environment for the blastocyst until the placenta is able to fulfil its functions. As the zygote embeds, the following changes occur in the endometrium due to increased progesterone production by the corpus luteum:

- Endometrium hypertrophies to become 6–8 mm in thickness.
- Stroma become more vascular and oedematous and the functional layer becomes organised into two distinct areas.
- Stroma cells enlarge and become more closely packed together to form the compact layer. They are now known as **decidual cells** and become polygonal in shape because of the pressure they exert on each other.
- Tubular glands become dilated and more tortuous in their deeper parts and the lumen becomes packed with secretion. This dilatation below the compact layer gives the stroma a cavernous spongy appearance and is known as the spongy or cavernous layer.
- The basal layer remains unchanged.

The myometrium

The myometrium forms the greater part of the uterine wall and the detailed arrangement of muscular tissue is highly

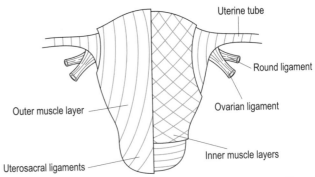

Figure 25.10 The outer and inner layers of uterine muscle (from Sweet B 1997, with permission).

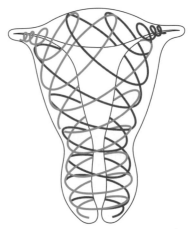

Figure 25.11 The spiral arrangement of the uterine muscle fibres (from Sweet B 1997, with permission).

effective, especially for evacuation of uterine contents. During pregnancy, the muscle fibres of the myometrium become more differentiated and organised in order to fulfil their roles in labour (Figs 25.10 and 25.11). The myometrium is composed of at least three inter-digitating muscle layers: an outer, middle and inner layer (Romanini 1994). Each layer performs a different function.

The middle layer forms the bulk of the organ and is composed of obliquely inter-digitating strands of muscle fibres forming a network around blood vessels. It is involved with expulsion of the fetus and the control of bleeding after delivery of the placenta. The outer and inner layers contain both circular and longitudinal fibres and functional and structural studies indicate that these layers may be continuous (Garfield & Yallampalli 1994). The outer layer, with mainly longitudinal fibres, contracts and retracts during labour. The inner layer, with mainly circular fibres, is more evident around the cornua and lower uterine segment and cervix. It is involved in distension of the lower uterine segment and dilatation of the cervix during labour.

The muscle cells of the myometrium are grouped into bundles with thin sheets of connective tissue including collagen, elastic fibres, fibroblasts and mast cells between the bundles. The collagenous connective tissue probably serves two functions: a support for the muscle fibres and a transmission network for the tension developed by smooth muscle contraction (Steer & Johnson 1998). Around the bundles of smooth muscle cells are fibroblasts, blood and lymphatic vessels and nerve cells.

The perimetrium

This outer layer of peritoneum does not totally cover the uterus. It drapes over the bladder anteriorly to form a fold called the uterovesical pouch and posteriorly it drapes over the rectum to form the pouch of Douglas (Ramsay 1994). It forms the broad ligament, thus maintaining the anatomical position of the uterus. This loosely applied layer allows for unrestricted growth of the uterus during pregnancy.

Cervical changes

In line with the gradual build-up of uterine activity in pregnancy, changes take place in the cervix. Its function changes from a firm structure to an elastic tissue which can stretch to a diameter of 10 cm or more during labour and then almost return to its original state. During pregnancy the cervix increases in mass, water content and vascularity (Blackburn 2003). It remains 2.5 cm long throughout pregnancy until effacement begins. Early in pregnancy cervical softening occurs and some opening of the external os is detectable from 24 weeks and of the internal os in about one-third of primigravidae by 32 weeks (Steer & Johnson 1998). **Effacement** or shortening of the cervix and its gradual inclusion in the LUS occurs in the last few weeks of pregnancy. Tension exerted by the outer longitudinal muscle fibres of the fundus may contribute to the process of effacement (O'Lah 1996). These changes are seen only in the human cervix; the cervices of most other animals studied remain closed until the onset of parturition (Steer & Johnson 1998).

Dramatic changes need to occur in the cervix at time of delivery to allow uterine contractions to influence dilatation of the cervix. The changes involve degradation of the collagen content by enzymes such as collagenase and elastase. Changes also occur in the proteoglycans ground substance matrix which attracts water, and smooth muscle fibres which become more stretchable (Blackburn 2003). Oestrogen causes increased vascularity and the cervix appears purple when viewed through a speculum.

Myometrial contractions have little effect on the ripening of the cervix which usually occurs prior to the onset of labour. Hormonal control of cervical ripening may involve multiple changes in oestrogen, progesterone, relaxin and prostaglandins and seems to correlate well with a gradual rise in circulating oestrogens. PGE_2 and $PGF_{2\alpha}$ have a localised action on cervical softening that is independent of uterine activity and PGE_2 is used to improve the cervical state prior to induction of labour (Blackburn 2003). However, there is much variation in individual women in the changes in the cervix outlined above. Labour may begin in some women when the cervix is long, firm, uneffaced and undilated. In others, the cervix may be soft, effaced and partly dilated for some weeks prior to the onset of labour.

The cervix also acts as an efficient barrier to infection. Under the influence of progesterone the mucus secreted by the endocervical cells becomes thicker and more viscous. It forms a cervical plug called the **operculum** which prevents ascending infection.

Uterine blood flow

Increased vessel diameter and lowered resistance cause an increase in uterine blood flow during pregnancy. Prostacyclin (PGI_2) is produced by the pregnant and non-pregnant myometrium as well as by the placental blood vessels. This acts as a potent vasodilator to inhibit platelet aggregation and also to protect the vascular epithelium. It is therefore important in maintaining blood flow to the placenta and the uterus during labour. Unlike other prostaglandins, PGI_2 has little effect on uterine contractability.

Innervation of the human uterus

The uterus is innervated by sympathetic and parasympathetic fibres of the autonomic nervous system. In comparison to other smooth muscle cells, the uterus is poorly innervated with a low density of nerves to smooth muscle. The physiological result of the innervation of the uterus is unknown as labour will occur even if complete spinal transection is present. It is probable that central nervous system connections are not essential to the onset and progress of labour.

Sympathetic fibres

Preganglionic fibres leave the spinal cord and enter a chain of ganglia running alongside the spinal column from T1 to L5 vertebrae. In the ganglia they synapse with postganglionic fibres that synapse with the target organ. The uterus is unusual, as the preganglionic fibres leaving T10–T12 run directly to the uterus to synapse with the postganglionic fibres. Preganglionic fibres release acetylcholine into the synapse from their endings and postganglionic fibres release noradrenaline (norepinephrine) onto the target organ from their terminals.

There are two types of adrenergic receptors in target organs, alpha (α) receptors, which are normally excitatory, and beta (β) fibres, which are normally inhibitory. There are two types of beta receptors – beta-1 (β_1) and beta-2 (β_2). Beta-1 (β_1) receptors are cardiospecific and are excitatory, while beta-2 (β_2) receptors are present in the uterus and are inhibitory. Drugs such as salbutamol and ritodrine inhibit uterine contractions in preterm labour but will excite cardiac muscle, causing a rise in pulse rate, leading to increased cardiac output and blood pressure. The beta-blocking agent propranolol will enhance uterine activity.

Parasympathetic fibres

The parasympathetic innervation to the pelvis is through the sacral outflow from S2, 3 and 4. The preganglionic fibres end in or near the target organs and synapse with short postganglionic fibres. Acetylcholine is the neurotransmitter substance in both pre- and postganglionic fibres. The fibres innervating the uterus synapse in two nerve plexi on either side of the pouch of Douglas. These are the **paracervical plexi** (Lee–Frankenhäuser's plexi).

Changes in the vagina in pregnancy

Oestrogen produces changes in both the muscle layer and the epithelium. There is hypertrophy of the muscle layer and changes in the surrounding connective tissue allow the vagina to become more elastic, allowing it to distend during the second stage of labour. There is a marked desquamation of the superficial cells of the epithelium giving rise to an increased amount of normal vaginal discharge called **leucorrhoea** because of its white colour (Beischer et al 1997).

The epithelial cells also have an increased glycogen content and interaction with Döderlein's bacillus produces a more acid environment which adds to the protection against many microorganisms. Unfortunately, this means an increased susceptibility to the organism *Candida albicans*, which causes moniliasis or thrush. There is increased vascularity and the vagina appears reddish purple in colour, a change in pregnancy referred to as **Jacquemenier's sign**. The increased vascularity of the pelvic organs gives rise to another sign of pregnancy called **Osiander's sign**, which is increased pulsation in the lateral vaginal fornices.

Uterine activity in pregnancy

As in skeletal muscle, myosin-containing thick filaments interact with the actin-containing thin filaments and the energy source is from ATP. There are no clear neuromuscular junctions in smooth muscle and innervating neurons release their neurotransmitter substance directly onto many fibres, resulting in a change in intracellular calcium concentration and allowing a slow, synchronised contraction of the whole muscle sheet. As pregnancy progresses, the timing and speed of the myometrial action potentials change and the muscle cells increase their content of contractile proteins, gap junctions, sarcoplasmic reticulum and mitochondria.

Calcium is a key ion in the contraction process and mainly comes from the ECF where its concentration is 10 000 times that of the myometrial cell. At rest the cell membrane does not allow calcium to enter the cell but after a contraction calcium enters the cell through ion channels. Action potentials are transmitted from cell to cell until the whole sheet is contracting. The uterus at term appears to have enhanced communication between cells and the action potential can spread across the entire uterus in only 2–3 s.

The role of pacemakers in uterine activity

Some fibres may act as pacemaker cells to set the contractile pace for the whole sheet. Specific pacemaker cells have not yet been identified. It was previously thought that fibres beneath the cornua of the uterus acted as pacemakers so that the fundus dominates. Investigations no longer support this theory and although it is likely that cells near the cornua may initiate contractions it is now thought that any myometrial cell would have this property (Garfield & Yallampalli 1994). Both the rate and intensity of smooth muscle contraction can be modified by neural and chemical stimuli. Contraction in smooth muscle is slow, sustained and resistant to fatigue. The action potential is conducted from the cell membrane down the sarcoplasmic reticulum so that there is a rapid release of calcium deep in the cell.

In pregnancy, uterine activity gradually evolves, with activity being seen as early as 7 weeks with high frequency (about two contractions per minute) but very low intensity (about 1–1.5 kPa) (Steer & Johnson 1998). This pattern continues until about 20 weeks when uterine contractions increase in both frequency and amplitude until term. These tend to occur more rapidly in the last 6–8 weeks of pregnancy. This is thought to be facilitated by the development of gap junctions within the myometrium where the plasma membranes of adjacent cells are closely applied, which act as areas of low resistance so that conduction of electrical impulses can spread rapidly from one cell to another. They are important in the spread of action potentials and the development of the coordinated uterine activity that is seen in efficient labour.

Gap junctions The appearance of gap junctions seems to depend on changes in the levels of oestrogen, progesterone and prostaglandins occurring in late pregnancy. The absence of gap junctions may be important for the maintenance of pregnancy and their appearance may be necessary to allow the development of effective uterine contractions in labour. Low-frequency but high-pressure Braxton–Hicks contractions are perceived by the mother. They may be as strong as labour contractions but are not painful and the cervix does not dilate.

Sensitivity to oxytocin and prostaglandins

Sensitivity to oxytocin is dependent on both gestational age and the level of spontaneous uterine activity. Up to about 30 weeks the uterus is very insensitive to oxytocin and it is necessary to give very high infusion rates of oxytocin in order to stimulate uterine activity (up to 128 mU/min). After 30 weeks the uterus will respond to much smaller concentrations of oxytocin of 8 mU/min and by 40 weeks as little as 4 mU/min will cause uterine activity similar to that seen in spontaneous labour. In contrast to this variable response, prostaglandins E_2 and $F_{2\alpha}$ will induce uterine contractions at any gestational age. Therefore, prostaglandins are probably the final mediator of uterine contractions.

MAIN POINTS

- Muscle is specialised tissue with the ability to transform chemical energy to mechanical energy to produce force and enable movement to occur. All muscle cells are elongated and contain two kinds of protein filaments – actin and myosin.

- The three basic muscle types are skeletal muscle, smooth muscle and specialised cardiac muscle. The four functions of muscle comprise the production of movement, maintenance of posture, stabilisation of joints and the generation of heat. The four properties of muscle are excitability, contractility, extensibility and elasticity.

- Skeletal muscles are attached to and cover bones. Fibres have obvious bands or striations. Skeletal muscle contracts rapidly, tires easily and must be rested after short bursts of activity. Activity depends upon a rich blood supply to deliver oxygen and nutrients and remove metabolic waste.

- The sliding filament theory of muscle action is commonly supported. Skeletal muscles contract in response to nerve stimulation, resulting in an action potential being sent along the sarcolemma. This electrical event results in a rise in intracellular calcium ion levels that triggers off the contraction.

- The pelvic floor is formed by the soft tissues (six layers) which fill the outlet of the pelvis. The most important tissue is the strong funnel-shaped diaphragm of skeletal muscle attached to the pelvic walls. Through it passes the urethra, vagina and anal canals.

- The superficial muscles lie external to the deep muscles and provide additional strength. The deep muscles called the levator ani are the major muscles of the pelvic floor. The deep muscles, because of their insertion, are also collectively known as the coccygeus muscles and are vital for bladder and bowel function.

- The perineal body is a wedge-shaped mass of muscular and fibrous tissue situated between the vaginal and anal canals. Superficial and deep pelvic floor muscles are both involved in its structure.

- Effective functioning of the pelvic floor depends on the integrity of the muscle fibres and maintenance of muscle tone. The pelvic floor supports the abdominal and pelvic organs, maintains intra-abdominal pressure, enables defecation and micturition, facilitates the fetus through the birth canal and enables flexion of the sacrum and coccyx. The pelvic floor muscles may become traumatised in childbirth.

- Prolapse of the pelvic organs with the possibility of urinary and faecal incontinence may cause physical and emotional discomfort for women. Treatment is usually by surgical repair. The risk of prolapse can be minimised by careful management of labour, careful repair of any perineal trauma, ensuring early ambulation and encouraging pelvic floor exercises in the puerperium.

- Smooth muscle is non-striated and involuntary and is referred to as visceral muscle. Contractions are slow and sustained. There are no clear neuromuscular junctions in smooth muscle. Innervating fibres release their neurotransmitter substance directly onto many fibres, allowing slow, synchronised contraction of the whole muscle sheet.

- Smooth muscle has special features which include a less vigorous contractile response to being stretched so that distension of a hollow organ can occur without provoking expulsive contractions; ability to divide and change more in length and width than skeletal muscle; and ability to secrete collagen and elastin (connective tissue proteins).

- Smooth muscle fibres in the uterus undergo hyperplasia in early pregnancy but the main part of uterine growth is due to hypertrophy. Uterine growth is a reliable indicator of fetal gestation in the first 20 weeks. It is less reliable as a predictor of gestational age as pregnancy progresses.

- The uterus at term has two main structural compartments: the upper uterine segment formed of the body and fundus; and the lower uterine segment formed of the isthmus and cervix.

- During pregnancy the endometrium becomes thicker, richer and more vascular in the upper part of the body of the uterus and the fundus, the normal site for implantation. It is now called the decidua, which is thinner and less vascular in the lower pole of the uterus.

- The smooth muscle fibres of the myometrium are arranged in two (or more) sheets, usually at right angles to each other. The body of the uterus has three muscle layers: an outer layer with mainly longitudinal fibres, a middle oblique layer and an inner layer with mainly circular fibres.

- Changes in the cervix include an increase in mass, water content and vascularity. Under the influence of progesterone, endocervical cell mucus thickens, becomes more viscous and forms the operculum which prevents ascending infection.

- Under the influence of oestrogen the muscle layer in the vagina hypertrophies and the surrounding connective tissue becomes more elastic, allowing distension during the second stage of labour. Increased desquamation of superficial epithelial cells leads to leucorrhoea.

- Contraction of uterine smooth muscle involves a slow, synchronised contraction of the whole muscle sheet. Some fibres may act as pacemaker cells. Sensitivity to oxytocin and prostaglandins depends on gestational age and the level of spontaneous uterine activity. Prostaglandins are probably the final mediator of uterine contractions.

References

Beischer N, Mackay E, Colditz P 1997 Obstetrics and the Newborn. W B Saunders, London.

Bennett V R, Brown L K 1999 The reproductive organs. In Bennett V R, Brown L K (eds) Myles Textbook for Midwives, 13th edn. Churchill Livingstone, Edinburgh.

Blackburn S T 2003 Maternal, Fetal and Neonatal Physiology: A Clinical Perspective, 3rd edn. W B Saunders, Philadelphia.

Calder A A 1994 The cervix during pregnancy. In Chard T, Grudzinskas J G (eds) The Uterus: Cambridge Reviews in Human Reproduction, 2nd edn. Cambridge University Press, Cambridge.

Dunlop W 1999 Normal pregnancy: physiology and endocrinology. In Edmonds D K, Dewhurst J (eds) Textbook of Obstetrics and Gynaecology for Postgraduates, 6th edn. Blackwell Science, Oxford.

Garfield R E, Yallampalli C 1994 Structure and function of uterine muscle. In Chard T, Grudzinskas J G (eds) The Uterus: Cambridge Reviews in Human Reproduction, 2nd edn. Cambridge University Press, Cambridge.

Marieb E N 2000 Human Anatomy and Physiology, 5th edn. Benjamin/Cummings, New York.

O'Lah K 1996 The cervix in pregnancy and labour. In Studd J (ed.) Progress in Obstetrics and Gynaecology. Churchill Livingstone, Edinburgh.

Ramsay E M 1994 Concepts of the uterus: a historical perspective. In Chard T, Grudzinskas J G (eds) The Uterus: Cambridge Reviews in Human Reproduction, 2nd edn. Cambridge University Press, Cambridge.

Romanini C 1994 Measurement of uterine contractions. In Chard T, Grudzinskas J G (eds) The Uterus: Cambridge Reviews in Human Reproduction, 2nd edn. Cambridge University Press, Cambridge.

Stanton J 1999 Vaginal prolapse. In Edmonds D K, Dewhurst J (eds) Textbook of Obstetrics and Gynaecology for Postgraduates, 6th edn. Blackwell Science, Oxford.

Steer P J, Johnson M R 1998 The genital system. In Chamberlain G, Broughton Pipkin F (eds) Clinical Physiology in Obstetrics, 3rd edn. Blackwell Science, Oxford.

Vander A, Sherman J, Luciano D 2000 Human Physiology: The Mechanisms of Body Function, 8th edn. McGraw-Hill, New York.

Annotated recommended reading

Chard T, Grudzinskas J G (eds) 1994 The Uterus: Cambridge Reviews in Human Reproduction, 2nd edn. Cambridge University Press, Cambridge (reprinted 2003.)
This text is at postgraduate level and provides a wide-ranging and authoritative account of the uterus and its physiological role in fertility, normal pregnancy and delivery.

Coad J, Dunstall M 2001 Anatomy and Physiology for Midwives. Mosby, Edinburgh.
This is an excellent text for related midwifery practice issues.

Chapter 26

The central nervous system

INTRODUCTION

The ability to respond appropriately to environmental change depends on the rapid communication achieved by two systems in the body: the **nervous system** and the **endocrine system**. The nervous system communicates by the rapid transmission of electrical signals. The endocrine glands secrete hormones into the bloodstream which modify the working of target organs (Ch. 28). Normal functioning of these systems is critical for the maintenance of **homeostasis** in both the non-pregnant and pregnant population.

The nervous system controls every system of the body – every thought, action and emotion. It is only possible to give a brief outline of this complex system and to elaborate on some of the important aspects such as pain perception. This chapter concentrates on tissues and the central nervous system and Chapter 27 considers the peripheral and autonomic nervous systems and neural integration.

ORGANISATION OF THE NERVOUS SYSTEM

The **central nervous system** (CNS) consists of the **brain** and **spinal cord**. It has an integrating function and receives messages from and sends messages to all parts of the body via the **peripheral nervous system** (PNS). That part of the PNS that innervates the smooth muscle and glands of the viscera and cardiac muscle is called the **autonomic nervous system** (ANS) and can be subdivided into the **sympathetic nervous system** and **parasympathetic nervous system**. Sensory organs such as the eyes and ears feed information about the environment back to the brain (Allan et al 1996).

NEUROANATOMY

Nervous tissue is made of two cell types: the *neurons* (Fig. 26.1) and a group of cell types collectively known as *neuroglia*, the connective tissue of the nervous system (Fitzgerald & Folan-Curran 2002). The tissue is supplied by blood vessels and supported by connective tissue.

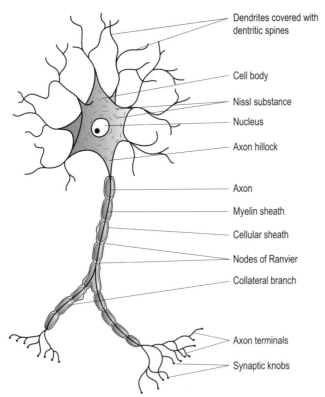

Figure 26.1   Structure of a whole nerve fibre (from Hinchliff S M, Montague S E, Watson R 1996, with permission).

Neurons

The structural units of the nervous system are the **neurons**. These specialised cells have the following characteristics (Marieb 2000):

- they have processes called **axons** and **dendrites** which communicate with other cells;
- they conduct messages by nerve impulses from one part of the body to another;
- they are extremely long lived but cannot undergo mitosis and divide;
- they have a very high metabolic rate and need continuous glucose and oxygen;
- they cannot survive for more than a few minutes without oxygen.

Structure of neurons

The cell body   Each neuron has a cell body (**soma**) which has a large spherical nucleus surrounded by granular cytoplasm. **Neurotransmitters** (NTs) are synthesised in the soma, which contains all the usual organelles except for centrioles. Most neuron cell bodies are located in the CNS, where they are clustered together in groups called **nuclei**. There are far fewer neuron cell bodies in the PNS and its clusters are called ganglia.

Dendrites   Dendrites are short, diffusely branching extensions which receive messages from other cells at synapses.

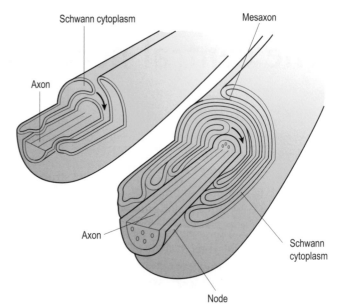

Figure 26.2   Myelination in peripheral nervous system. Arrows indicate movement of flange of Schwann cytoplasm (from Fitzgerald M J T 1996, with permission).

Dendrites are the input part of the neuron and there may be hundreds clustering close to the cell body. They provide an enormous surface area for the reception of signals from other neurons. Dendrites conduct electrical signals called graded potentials towards the cell body (Marieb 2000).

Axons   Each cell has only one axon arising from the **axon hillock** on the cell body. Each axon is the same diameter along its length and some are over a metre long such as those travelling from the spine to the foot. Axons may give off branches called axon collaterals and usually have terminal branches ending in **synaptic knobs** or **boutons** (Marieb 2000). Axons contain **microtubules** and **microfilaments** for the transport of substances to the cell body (**anterograde**) and from the cell body (**retrograde**). Axons conduct messages to other cells by electrical nerve impulses and by neurotransmitters which excite or inhibit other neurons by attaching to receptors in their plasma membrane.

Myelin sheaths   Larger nerve fibres are covered in a white fatty segmented sheath called the **myelin sheath** which protects and insulates fibres and increases the rate of impulse transmission; messages can be transmitted up to a 100 times more rapidly than unmyelinated fibres (Fig. 26.2). Myelin sheaths in the PNS are formed by the **Schwann cells** which wrap themselves around the axon. As the Schwann cell protoplasm is squeezed out of the cell, the axon remains wrapped in a multilayered membrane. The external portion is called the **neurolemma** or Schwann sheath. Adjacent Schwann cells along the axon do not touch and the gaps between them, which occur at regular intervals, are called the **nodes of Ranvier**. **Axon collaterals** can only emerge at these nodes.

The myelin sheaths in the central nervous system are produced by cells called **oligodendrocytes**. Myelinated fibres form the white matter in the brain and spinal cord and the cell bodies form the grey matter. Cell bodies are outside the white matter in the brain and inside the white matter in the spinal cord.

Classification of neurons

Neurons may be classified structurally or functionally (Marieb 2000).

Structural classification Neurons are grouped structurally according to the number of processes extending from their cell body. There are three major groups:

- Multipolar neurons are the most common type found in the human nervous system and have at least three processes, usually multiple dendrites and one axon. However, some do not have an axon.
- Bipolar neurons have two processes: an axon and a dendrite. They are rare but are found in some special sense organs such as in the retina or in the olfactory mucosa.
- Unipolar neurons have a single, very short process emerging from the cell body. They are found in the ganglia of the PNS where they function as sensory neurons.

Functional classification

- Motor neurons with cell bodies mainly in the CNS carry impulses to control effector organs such as muscles or glands.
- Sensory neurons whose cell bodies are located in the sensory ganglia outside the CNS often have very long dendritic branches which gather impulses from the periphery of the body such as the ends of the toes and fingers.
- Association neurons, often called **interneurons**, carry signals between motor and sensory neurons in complex networks.

Neuroglia

Neuroglial cells support and protect neurons and outnumber them in a ratio of 5 to 1. As there are billions of neurons in the brain, the number of neuroglial cells is enormous. These cells are subdivided into four basic types (Fitzgerald & Folan-Curran 2002):

- **Astrocytes** are star-shaped cells with long, fine processes arising from their cell body. They have one process against a neuron and other processes close to capillary walls.
- **Oligodendrocytes** in the CNS and Schwann cells in the PNS are smaller than astrocytes and have fewer processes. They form the myelin sheaths around nerve fibres.
- **Ependyma** form a continuous layer of cells lining the ventricles of the brain and central canal of the spinal cord. They help to produce the cerebrospinal fluid.
- **Microglia** are small cells which are part of the immune system, acting as macrophages.

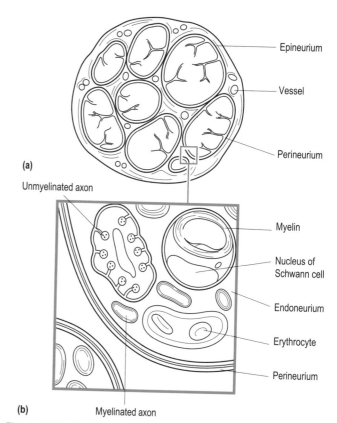

(a)

Unmyelinated axon

Epineurium

Vessel

Perineurium

Myelin

Nucleus of Schwann cell

Endoneurium

Erythrocyte

Perineurium

(b) Myelinated axon

Figure 26.3 Transverse section of a nerve trunk. (a) Light microscopy; (b) electron microscopy (from Fitzgerald M J T 1996, with permission).

The structure of a nerve

The axons from single neurons are bound together to form **nerves** (Fig. 26.3). Nerves may contain afferent fibres (to the CNS), efferent fibres (from the CNS) or both. Those with both types of fibres are referred to as mixed nerves. Each separate nerve fibre is embedded in a fibrous connective tissue sheath called the **endoneurium**. These are bound in groups by the **perineurium**, a connective tissue sheath, and the complete nerve is surrounded by the **epineurium**. Each nerve has an arterial blood supply and venous drainage.

NEUROPHYSIOLOGY

The nerve impulse

Both nerve fibres and muscle fibres are excitable tissues which conduct electrochemical signals. When a neuron is stimulated, an electrical impulse is sent along the length of its axon (Fig. 26.4). The human body is electrically neutral (positive and negative charges are equal). Potential electrical energy is called **voltage**, which is measured in volts (V) or millivolts (mV). The flow of electricity from one point to another is called a **current**. Substances that hinder the flow are said to provide **resistance**. Ions, which are electrically charged particles, provide the currents, and usually flow

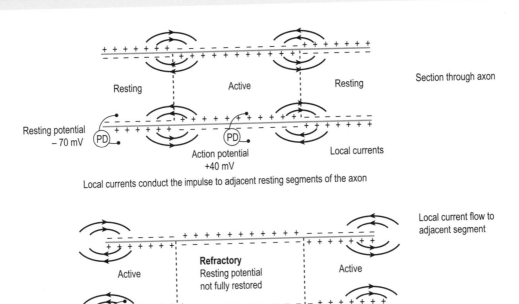

Figure 26.4 Propagation of an action potential along a nerve fibre (from Hinchliff S M, Montague S E 1990, with permission).

through an aqueous solution across a plasma membrane. Plasma membranes are studded with proteinaceous ion channels.

Polarisation

When a membrane is resting its potential is polarised, i.e. the inside of the cell has a different electrical potential than the interstitial fluid. The resting potential of neurons averages −70 mV. This is maintained by the distribution and relative concentration of negative and positive ions. Inside the cell, the positive ion is potassium and the negative ion is protein. In the interstitial fluid, the positive ion is sodium and the negative ion is chloride.

The role of sodium ions

When the cell is stimulated, sodium channels open in the membrane and sodium ions rush into the cell. This changes the membrane potential to +40 mV, a process called depolarisation. This action potential is the sum of all negative and positive charges stimulating the cell and proceeds down the axon in a wave. Behind the wave the cell pumps three sodium ions out in exchange for two potassium ions. The membrane potential falls to −90 mV (hyperpolarisation) and then recovers.

Depolarisation increases the chance of a nerve impulse being generated but hyperpolarisation decreases it. The period of hyperpolarisation is known as the refractory period, during which the cell cannot generate an action potential. Firing of a neuron is an all or nothing phenomenon, occurring only if the potential reaches a threshold. Strong stimuli will result in more impulses rather than stronger impulses being generated.

Saltatory conduction of the impulse

Nerve fibres can be classified according to their speeds of conduction of the action potential. The larger the nerve, the more rapidly it can conduct its impulses. Myelinated nerves conduct nerve impulses more rapidly than unmyelinated nerves. The myelin sheath increases the electrical resistance of a nerve but it is more leaky at the nodes of Ranvier. The electrical current flows smoothly along each section of the sheath between nodes of Ranvier and it is only necessary to generate an action potential at the nodes. The impulse seems to jump from node to node. This is called **saltatory conduction** (Fig. 26.5). In a non-myelinated nerve, new action potentials have to be generated across each adjacent section of the nerve membrane.

Classification of nerves by speed of impulse conduction

Nerves are classified as follows:

- Group A fibres are myelinated and can conduct impulses at up to 120 metres per second (m/s). They are further subdivided into α, β, γ and δ fibres.
- Group B fibres are also myelinated. They are all preganglionic fibres of the autonomic nervous system.
- Group C fibres are non-myelinated and conduct impulses as slowly as 1 m/s.

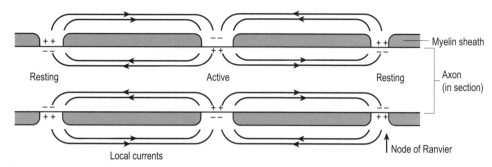

Figure 26.5   Saltatory conduction in a myelinated nerve fibre. Local currents conduct the impulse from node to node. The action potential is regenerated at each node of Ranvier (from Hinchliff S M, Montague S E 1990, with permission).

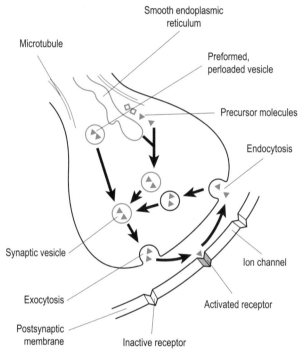

Figure 26.6   Diagram to show origin and fate of synaptic vesicle and transmitter–receptor binding (from Fitzgerald M J T 1996, with permission).

The synapse

Synapses are junctions between the terminal bouton of the axon and its target tissue, which may be a neuron cell body, a gland or a muscle (Fig. 26.6). Synapses enable transfer of information between one cell and another. They may be electrical or chemical (Fitzgerald & Folan-Curran 2002). The presynaptic neuron conducts impulses towards the synapse and the postsynaptic neuron transmits information away from the synapse.

Electrical synapses

These synapses are bridged junctions that correspond to the gap junctions found in other cell types. Protein channels connect the cytoplasm of adjacent neurons, providing electrical pathways through which ions can flow from one neuron to another. Such neurons are electrically coupled and communication between the cells is extremely rapid. They provide a means of synchronising all the interconnected neurons and are rare in the adult body. They are responsible for stereotyped movements such as the jerky movements of the eyes. They are much commoner in the embryo but are gradually replaced by chemical synapses. They remain abundant in some non-nervous tissues such as cardiac and smooth muscle (Marieb 2000).

Chemical synapses

Between the neuron and its target cell the synaptic cleft is a fluid-filled space into which NTs are released from the presynaptic membrane. These open and shut ion channels in the postsynaptic membrane. The electrical message of the action potential is conducted chemically across the gap. This is a reversible change and the NT is removed:

- enzymes which degrade the NT are released into the synaptic cleft;
- the NT is retaken up by the presynaptic membrane;
- the NT diffuses away from the synapse.

Neurotransmitters

Neurotransmitters are molecules which help neurons to communicate messages and regulate body activities and states (Marieb 2000). Over 100 different chemicals act as NTs in the body. They are classified according to chemical structure and are synthesised by the body with the help of enzymes.

Acetylcholine

Acetylcholine (ACh) was the first neurotransmitter to be identified. It has been easy to study because it is the NT released at neuromuscular junctions and is accessible. ACh is synthesised and stored within synaptic vesicles in the presence of the enzyme **choline acetyltransferase**. Acetic acid is bound to coenzyme A to form **acetylCoA**; this compound then combines with choline and the coenzyme is released:

$$\text{Choline acetyl transferase}$$
$$\text{Acetyl CoA + choline} \rightarrow \text{ACh + CoA}$$

The released ACh binds to the postsynaptic membrane and is degraded to acetic acid and choline by the enzyme **acetylcholinesterase** (AChE). The released choline is captured by the presynaptic membrane and used to synthesise more ACh, which is released by some neurons of the ANS and is found in the CNS.

The biogenic amines

Biogenic amines include **catecholamines** such as **dopamine**, **noradrenaline** (norepinephrine) and **adrenaline** (epinephrine) and the **indolamines**, *serotonin* (5-hydroxytryptamine, 5-HT) and **histamine**. Catecholamines are synthesised from the amino acid **tyrosine** in a common pathway. Neurons produce only the enzymes which control the steps necessary to produce the NT they need. The common pathway for the synthesis of the catecholamines is:

$$\text{Tyrosine} \rightarrow \text{L-Dopa} \rightarrow \text{dopamine} \rightarrow$$
$$\text{noradrenaline (norepinephrine)} \rightarrow \text{adrenaline (epinephrine)}$$

NTs are widely distributed in the brain and are involved in emotional behaviour and in regulation of the body clock. Catecholamines, especially noradrenaline (norepinephrine), are also released by some motor neurons of the ANS. Serotonin is synthesised from tyrosine by a different pathway. Histamine is synthesised from the amino acid histidine.

Amino acids

The most important amino acids involved in neurotransmission are γ-aminobutyric acid (GABA) and glutamate.

Peptides

The neuropeptides include many molecules with diverse effects. These include the endorphins and encephalins involved in pain perception (Ch. 38).

THE BRAIN

During the course of evolution there has been an increasing tendency to elaboration of the brain, reaching its greatest complexity in humans (Aiello & Dean 1990). The average adult brain weighs 1500 g and is slightly heavier in men than women. However, it is the complexity of the wiring that determines the power of the brain, not its size. Although the brain is described as a single organ (Figs 26.7 and 26.8), an analogy can be made with the gastrointestinal system, with individual parts performing discrete functions.

The brain can be subdivided into four main parts (Marieb 2000):

1. the cerebral hemispheres;
2. the diencephalon, comprising the thalamus and hypothalamus;
3. the brainstem, comprising the midbrain, pons and medulla;
4. the cerebellum.

The cerebral hemispheres

The two **cerebral hemispheres** form 85% of the total weight of the brain and sit like an umbrella over the **diencephalon** and **brainstem**. The neurons are organised with their cell bodies outermost, forming the **grey matter** or cortex (outer rind), and their fibres innermost, forming the **white matter**.

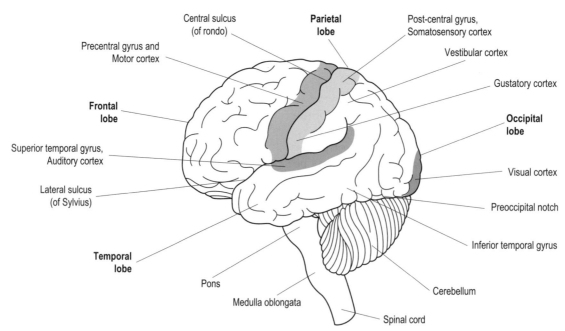

Figure 26.7 Lateral aspect of the human brain (from Hinchliff S M, Montague S E 1990, with permission).

The cortex is thrown into elevated ridges called **gyri** which are separated by shallow grooves called **sulci**. This vastly increases the surface area of the cortex. The deepest of these grooves are called **fissures** and form important landmarks. There is a midline longitudinal fissure called the midsagittal fissure that separates the two cerebral hemispheres and the transverse fissure separates the cerebral hemispheres from the cerebellum.

Each hemisphere is divided into six main **lobes**. Four of these have the same names as the bones under which they lie and are the frontal, parietal, occipital and temporal lobes. The other two lobes are buried in the hemispheres. These are the **insula**, revealed if the frontal and temporal lobes are eased apart, and the **limbic lobe**, which can be seen if the brain is divided along the midsagittal fissure.

The cerebral cortex

The **cerebral cortex** enables conscious behaviour such as perception, communication, memory, understanding, appreciation and initiation of voluntary movements. It can be divided into three functional areas:

1. the **primary sensory area**, which receives stimuli from the periphery of the body;
2. the **primary motor area**, which sends out impulses that control the periphery;
3. the **association areas**.

Sensory areas are posterior to the central sulcus as they are posterior in the spinal columns. The motor areas are anterior to the central sulcus and in the spinal column.

The association areas integrate diverse information to allow appropriate actions to be taken. These include the **prefrontal cortex**, which is concerned with intellect; the **diffuse gnostic area**, which contributes memory of sensation and emotional response; and the **language areas**, which are usually in the left hemisphere. There is insufficient space to discuss brain lateralisation and the reader is referred to an excellent book by Springer & Deutsch (1998).

Prefrontal cortex

The prefrontal cortex is concerned with higher mental functions such as abstract thinking, decision making, social behaviour and anticipating the effects of actions. It has two-way connections with the cortex on the same side of the brain (**ipsilateral**), except the primary motor and sensory areas, the cortex of the opposite side of the brain (**contralateral**), the **thalamus** and the **hypothalamus** (Fitzgerald & Folan-Curran 2002).

Sensory cortex

Thalamic nerve fibres project to the sensory areas of the cerebral cortex. It is essential that nerves coming into the spinal cord from the periphery of the body maintain their **somatotopic organisation** so that a representation of the body is faithfully organised in the sensory cortex. The size of an area of the sensory cortex given over to receiving input from the body depends on its degree of innervation. This results in a peculiarly shaped **homunculus** represented upside down in the sensory cortex. Those parts of us that are most sensitive such as the tongue, lips, fingers and toes are well represented.

The control of movement

Motor cortex

Movement of the body by the skeletal muscles is controlled by input from the nervous system. Motor control can be

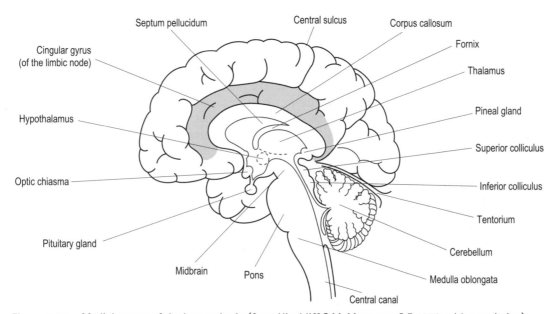

Figure 26.8   Medial aspect of the human brain (from Hinchliff S M, Montague S E 1990, with permission).

divided into three neural systems (Allan et al 1996):

- the **pyramidal system**, a fast and usually direct descending pathway from the cortex;
- the **extrapyramidal system** with multiple synapses involving many brain structures, the **basal ganglia** being the most important;
- the **cerebellum**.

Traditionally, the order in which the above are named has represented the relative importance of the system to motor control. Recently, research has shown that the extrapyramidal system is very important and the intention to act is developed by the integration of widespread neuronal impulses. The motor cortex is involved at the end of the integration and development of intent. Efferent fibres from the motor cortex project to the basal ganglia, the thalamus, the red nucleus, the lateral reticular formation and the spinal cord in a topographically organised manner.

The extrapyramidal system

The basal ganglia The basal ganglia consist of large nuclei lying laterally to the thalamus. These are the globus pallidus, the subthalamic nucleus, the pars compacta (including the substantia nigra) and the striatum (including the caudate nucleus and the putamen), which is the largest subcortical mass of cells in the brain. Motor activity is strongly influenced by the basal ganglia, which constitute the main extrapyramidal control. Four basic circuits have been demonstrated Fitzgerald & Folan-Curran 2002):

1. a motor loop concerned with learned movements;
2. a cognitive loop concerned with motor intentions;
3. a limbic loop concerned with emotional aspects of movement;
4. an oculomotor loop concerned with voluntary saccades.

The red nucleus The **red nucleus** is found between the substantia nigra and the aqueduct of Sylvius. It is an oval-shaped structure involved in the control of limb flexion.

The cerebellum

This large brain structure lies beneath the occipital lobes and is separated from them by a fold of dura mater called the **tentorium cerebelli**. The cerebellum is bilaterally symmetrical, divided by a midline structure called the **vermis**. There are no interhemispheric nerve fibres so that messages are not relayed between the two halves. The cerebellum monitors the strength and execution of movements and therefore motor coordination. It is able to do this because of incoming sensory stimuli. Its function is entirely inhibitory in nature and is controlled by the inhibitory NT **GABA**.

The limbic system

The limbic system consists of nuclei and fibres located on the medial aspect of each cerebral hemisphere. Its structures encircle the upper part of the brainstem (**limbus** means ring) and include the **cingulate gyrus**, the **parahippocampal gyrus**, the **hippocampus**, the **amygdala**, the hypothalamus, part of the thalamus, the **insula** and the **septum**. It is closely related to the reticular formation. Its function is concerned with emotional (affective) feelings. The limbic system interacts with higher brain centres and facilitates a close relationship between cognition and emotion. All the 'Trekkies' out there should wonder about the limbic system of Mr Spock and the limitations of logic without emotional reactions!

The cingulate gyrus

The cingulate gyrus involves part of the cortex and part of the limbic system. A bundle of fibres form a neural network interconnecting parts of the limbic lobe. The cingulate gyrus receives fibres from the parahippocampal gyrus, the temporal lobe, the thalamus and visual and tactile areas of the cortex. Its function is the emotional interpretation of pain and vision.

The hippocampus

The hippocampus, situated in the temporal lobe, has a complex three-dimensional trumpet shape and is called '**Ammon's horn**'. It communicates with the neocortex, the thalamus and other subcortical regions. Its functions include memory, learning, spatial awareness and cognitive mapping.

The amygdala

The amygdala consists of a pair of nuclei in the temporal lobes. It is a focal point between incoming sensory systems and outgoing effector systems responsible for emotion. Lesion studies suggest a different role for each nucleus. The right seems to be involved in the strength of emotion and in negative emotions, the left in unemotional response and positive emotions.

The hypothalamus

This structure is involved in homeostasis and survival. It contains centres involved in the regulation of food intake, water intake, sleep–wake cycles, sexual behaviour and defence against attack. The hypothalamus controls the output of anterior pituitary hormones by producing releasing and inhibiting factors. It secretes the posterior pituitary hormones directly.

The thalamus

The thalami are a pair of organs joined in the midline at the centre of the brain. It could be said to be a traffic conductor. The thalami contain multiple nuclei, each with a specific function. These include hearing, vision, memory, cognition, judgement and mood. There are multiple projections to the cortex and it is continuous with the reticular formation.

The insula

The insula lies deep in the brain. The anterior insula is a cortical centre for pain. The posterior insula is continuous with the entorrhinal cortex and the amygdala and may be involved in emotional responses to pain. The central region is continuous with the frontoparietal and temporal cortex and may have a language rather than a limbic function (Fitzgerald & Folan-Curran 2002).

The septum

The connections of the septum lie central to the brain. Fibres are received from the amygdala, olfactory tract, hippocampus and brainstem. Fibres from the septum connect with the hypothalamus, brainstem and hippocampus. The septum controls sensations of pleasure and wellbeing and appetites that stimulate those feelings. It is also involved in memory.

The medulla oblongata and pons

The medulla is the conical-shaped lowest part of the brainstem that blends into the spinal cord at the level of the foramen magnum in the base of the skull. The central canal of the spinal cord broadens out in the medulla to form the fourth ventricle. It functions as an autonomic reflex centre, maintaining homeostasis. Its nuclei include the **cardiac**, **vasomotor** and **respiratory centres** and nuclei that control vomiting, swallowing, coughing and sneezing.

The **pons** forms a bulbous structure between the medulla and the midbrain and forms part of the anterior wall of the third ventricle. It is a bridge formed of nerve fibres running between the spinal cord and the higher brain centres.

The reticular formation

The reticular formation (RF) is an old part of the brain, sometimes called the reptilian brain. In the human brain the RF is important in automatic and reflex activities (Fitzgerald & Folan-Curran 2002). It extends through the medulla, pons and midbrain and is closely related to the olfactory and limbic systems. Its neurons have long, branching dendrites and its fibres run in three columns: the main column or **midline raphe**, the **medial nuclear group** and the **lateral nuclear group**.

The part of the RF that makes multiple synapses throughout the brainstem is called the reticular activating system (RAS) and is involved in the level of consciousness and alertness and the sleep–wake cycle (Box 26.1). RF neurons maintain homeostasis by controlling the cardiac centre, the vasomotor centre, the respiratory centre and vomiting, swallowing, coughing and sneezing.

The following summary of the functions of the reticular formation demonstrates the extent of its links to other brain

centres (Fitzgerald & Folan-Curran 2002):

- pattern generation and patterned cranial nerve activities;
- posture and locomotion;
- salivation and lacrimation;
- bladder control;
- involvement in vital centres such as circulation and respiration and blood pressure control;
- conveys both somatic and visceral sensory information to the cerebellum;
- sleeping and waking, attention and mood and arousal.

Protection of the brain

Nervous tissue is very delicate and neurons can be injured by even a slight pressure. The brain is protected by the bony skull (Ch. 24), by three membranes called the **meninges**

Box 26.1 The sleep–wake cycle

Conscious awareness allows the nervous system to interact deliberately with the environment. The neural processes that underlie altered states of consciousness, even the normal sleep–wake cycles are not well understood. Dark and light cycles are known to play a role in the sleep–wake cycle. Waterhouse (1991), an expert on **circadian rhythms**, wrote that left to its own devices the body clock will complete its cycle in a period of about, but not exactly 24 h. However, in our everyday life, the cycle is driven by environmental cues called **zeitgebers** which synchronise the clock with the 24 h solar cycle. Zeitgebers include light, social activity and diet.

Sleep is a complex phenomenon and involves many physiological processes (Allan et al 1996). The pattern of sleep has been studied by measuring the electrical activity of the brain by means of an **electroencephalogram** (EEG). Characteristic patterns in the electrical activity of the cerebral cortical neurons accompany varying states of consciousness (Fitzgerald & Folan-Curran 2002). Normal sleep consists of two types: **synchronised** (S) sleep and **desynchronised** (D) sleep, also known as **rapid eye movement** (REM) sleep. In the normal waking state there are rapid, low-amplitude waves while the onset of sleep is accompanied by slow, high-amplitude waves due to the synchronisation of many neurons (S sleep). This lasts for about 90 min before being replaced by D sleep where REMs and dreams occur. Several S and D phases occur during a normal night's sleep.

Sleep may have two purposes: it may be restorative, a necessary part of replenishing energy and restoring tissues; or it may be protective to ensure safety for a daytime species by limiting activity during the hours of darkness. D sleep may allow the integration of the day's events into long-term memory, promoting learning, species-typical reprogramming or brain development.

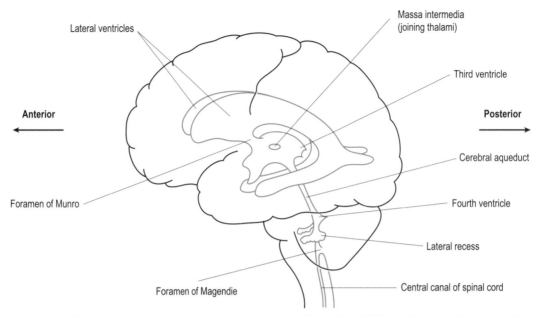

Figure 26.9   The ventricular system of the brain, lateral view (from Hinchliff S M, Montague S E 1990, with permission).

which surround the brain and by a watery cushion of cerebrospinal fluid (CSF). It is also protected from harmful substances by the **blood–brain barrier** (Marieb 2000).

The meninges

The meninges are made of connective tissue that cover and protect the brain and spinal cord, protect blood vessels, enclose venous sinuses and contain CSF. They are the pia, arachnoid and dura maters.

1. The **pia mater** is very delicate and has many tiny blood vessels. It clings tightly to the surface of the brain, following every convolution.

2. The **arachnoid mater** forms a loose brain covering and is attached to the pia mater by thread-like arachnoid extensions which cross the subarachnoid space which is filled with CSF. The knob-like extensions of the arachnoid are called arachnoid villi and protrude into the dura mater into the dural sinuses which carry venous blood.

3. The **dura mater** is the double-layered membrane that lines the skull with its periosteal layer and is reflected onto the surface of the brain as the meningeal layer. In places the dura extends inwards to form septa that anchor the brain to the skull and limit movement. These include:
   - the **falx cerebri**, which runs vertically in the sagittal plane of the skull;
   - the **falx cerebelli**, another small vertical septum in the sagittal plane that runs along the vermis of the cerebellum;
   - the **tentorium cerebelli**, which is a horizontal fold of dura extending into the transverse fissure between the cerebral hemispheres and the cerebellum.

The ventricles

Four fluid-filled ventricles help to cushion and protect the brain (Fig. 26.9): the two **lateral ventricles** and the **third** and **fourth ventricles**. The ventricles are continuous with each other and with the central canal of the spinal cord via the **aqueduct of Sylvius**. The hollow chambers are filled with CSF and lined by ependymal cells. Three apertures in the wall of the fourth ventricle connect the ventricles to the fluid filled subarachnoid space surrounding the brain (Marieb 2000).

Tufts of capillaries called **choroid plexi** hang from the roof of each ventricle and manufacture CSF, which moves freely through the ventricles and into the central canal of the spinal cord (Fig. 26.10). Most of the CSF enters the subarachnoid space, bathing the outer surfaces of the brain and cord and returning to the blood via arachnoid villi to the dural sinuses. An obstruction to the flow will result in CSF accumulating in the ventricles and putting pressure on the brain. In a neonate, the skull bones are not fused and a collection of fluid in the ventricles causes enlargement of the skull (**hydrocephalus**).

The blood–brain barrier

The blood–brain barrier ensures that the brain's internal environment remains stable by providing a chemically optimum environment for neuronal function (Fitzgerald & Folan-Curran 2002). It selectively allows substances needed by the brain such as glucose, amino acids and some electrolytes to cross by facilitated diffusion while keeping toxic chemicals within the capillary network. In other body regions, extracellular concentrations of hormones, amino acids, ions and other substances are in constant flux. If the brain was exposed to these variations, neurons could fire

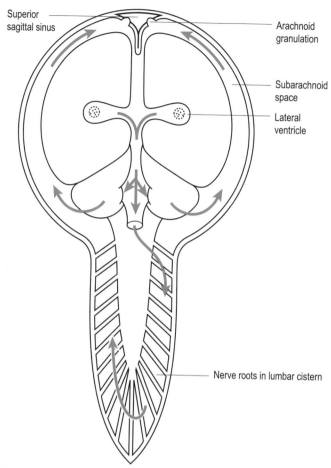

Figure 26.10   Circulation of cerebrospinal fluid (from Fitzgerald M J T 1996, with permission).

uncontrollably, as many of the substances act as neurotransmitters, especially potassium. Bloodborne substances within the brain's capillaries are separated from the extracellular space and the neurons by:

- a continuous endothelial capillary wall with tight junctions;
- a thick basal lamina surrounding the external face of the capillary;
- the bulbous feet of astrocytes clinging to the capillaries and signalling them to maintain tight junctions.

The cranial nerves

Twelve pairs of cranial nerves are associated with the brain and pass through foramina in the skull. The first two pairs originate from the forebrain and the rest are in the brainstem. All but the vagus nerve target structures in the head and neck. The cranial nerves are:

   I olfactory, which is concerned with the sense of smell;
  II optic, which is the nerve concerned with vision;

  III oculomotor, which moves four of the extrinsic muscles of the eye;
  IV trochlear, which also innervates an extrinsic muscle of the eye;
  V trigeminal, which supplies facial sensory fibres and motor fibres for chewing muscles;
  VI abducens, which controls the extrinsic muscle that turns the eyeball laterally;
  VII facial, which innervate the muscles of facial expression;
  VIII vestibulocochlear, which is the sensory nerve for hearing and balance;
  IX glossopharyngeal, which innervates the tongue and pharynx;
  X vagus nerve, which innervates thoracic and abdominal viscera;
  XI accessory, which helps the vagus nerve;
  XII hypoglossal, which innervates the tongue moving muscle.

THE SPINAL CORD

Knowledge of the anatomy of the spinal cord is important to those caring for childbearing women because of the use of epidural analgesia (Ch. 38). The spinal cord is enclosed within the vertebral column and extends from the **foramen magnum** of the skull to the level of the first **lumbar vertebra**. It is about 42 cm long and 1.8 cm thick and carries ascending and descending nerve pathways (Fig. 26.11). There are enlargements of the spinal cord in **the cervical** and **lumbo-sacral regions** where the nerves supplying the limbs arise (Fitzgerald & Folan-Curran 2002).

Like the brain, it is protected by bone, cerebrospinal fluid and meninges. The dura mater here is a single layer only and is not attached to the bony walls of the vertebral column. Between the bones and the dural sheath is the epidural space filled with fat and blood vessels. The subarachnoid space between the pia and arachnoid maters is filled with CSF. The dura and arachnoid meningeal membranes extend beyond the end of the spinal cord to the second sacral vertebra.

The spinal nerves

Thirty-one pairs of spinal nerves arise from the cord and leave the vertebral column by the **intervertebral foramina** to target specific areas of the body (Fitzgerald & Folan-Curran 2002). The spinal cord is segmented and each segment is defined by a pair of spinal nerves, each of which conducts sensory information from a specific body area called a dermatome (Fig. 26.12).

Inferiorly, the spinal cord ends in a cone-shaped structure, the **conus medullaris**, and nerve roots fan outwards and downwards to exit through relevant vertebrae. This collection of nerve roots is called the **cauda equinae** (horse's tail). There is a fibrous extension of the pia called

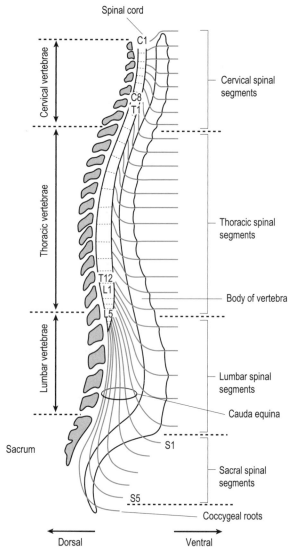

Figure 26.11   The relationship between the spinal cord and the vertebral column (from Hinchliff S M, Montague S E 1990, with permission).

the **filum terminale**, extending downwards to attach to the posterior surface of the coccyx.

A cross-section of the anatomy of the spinal cord

The grey matter and the spinal roots

The grey matter of the cord consists of neuronal cell bodies, their unmyelinated process and neuroglia (Marieb 2000). It is central to the white matter and looks like a letter H. There are two posterior or dorsal horns which contain interneurons and two anterior or ventral horns which house the nerve cell bodies of the somatic motor neurons (Fig. 26.13).

The ventral roots of the spinal cord contain the axons of the somatic motor neurons on their way to the skeletal muscles. Small lateral horns are columns of grey matter

found in the thoracic and upper lumbar segments of the cord. These carry the neurons of the autonomic motor system. Their axons leave via the ventral roots. Afferent fibres of the peripheral sensory nerves form the dorsal roots of the spinal cord. The cell bodies of these nerves are found in the dorsal root ganglion, an enlargement of the dorsal root. The dorsal and ventral roots are short and fuse laterally to form the spinal nerves.

The white matter

The white matter of the spinal cord is composed of myelinated and unmyelinated nerve fibres running in three directions:

1. ascending tracts of sensory inputs going to the higher centres;
2. descending tracts of motor outputs coming from the brain;
3. across from one side of the spinal cord to the other (commissural fibres).

The white matter on each side of the cord is divided into three white columns or funiculi – the posterior, lateral and anterior funiculi. These spinal tracts connect the periphery of the body to the brain. Some generalisations can be made (Marieb 2000).

1. Most pathways cross from one side to the other of the spinal column. This is decussation.
2. Most consist of a chain of two or three neurons, contributing to successive tracts of the pathway.
3. Most show somatotopy, reflecting an orderly mapping of the body.
4. All pathways and tracts are paired right and left.

Ascending sensory pathways

Ascending pathways take sensory impulses upwards to the brain through small chains of neurons. These are called first-, second- and third-order neurons. Incoming information is transmitted to the brain for conscious interpretation by six main pathways:

- The fasciculus cuneatus and fasciculus gracilis in the posterior funiculus, also known as the dorsal white column, transmit information from fine touch receptors and joint proprioceptors. These tracts decussate in the medulla. The pathway is called the dorsal column–medial lemniscal pathway.
- The lateral and anterior spinothalamic tracts convey information about pain (Ch. 38), temperature, deep pressure and course touch. These tracts decussate in the cord.
- The anterior and posterior spinocerebellar tracts convey information from the proprioceptors to the cerebellum and do not contribute to conscious sensation.

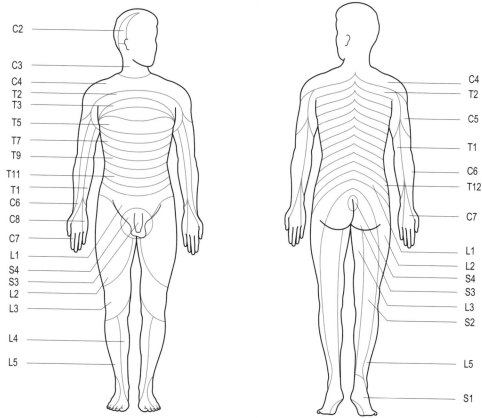

Figure 26.12   Adult dermatome pattern (from Fitzgerald M J T 1996, with permission).

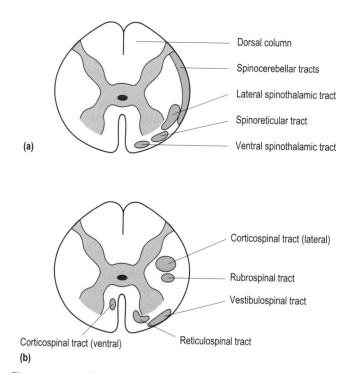

Figure 26.13   Major nerve tracts of the spinal cord. (a) Ascending nerve tracts. (b) Descending nerve tracts (from Hinchliff S M, Montague S E 1990, with permission).

ADAPTATION TO PREGNANCY

The function of the central nervous system and brain is complex and covers all activities from basic reflex actions to detailed cognitive and emotional changes. Blackburn (2003) includes the following list of changes, many due to the altered output from the endocrine system:

- musculoskeletal discomforts;
- sleep disturbances;
- alterations in sensation;
- the experience of pain.

The central nervous system

Pregnancy hormones affect the CNS, but these effects are not well understood. The ways that hormones alter the sensory systems are better documented. An anaesthetist called Anita Holdcroft described findings from magnetic resonance imaging (MRI) in a small group of 10 healthy women (Moore 1997). Women often report that their cognitive ability diminishes in pregnancy, with difficulty in concentration and poor memory top of the list. Holdcroft believes that women's brains shrink during pregnancy and return to normal following delivery, brought about by changes in individual cell volume and not by a reduction of cell numbers.

This shrinkage of the brain and the reduction in cognitive abilities could be linked but more research is needed.

Sleep

Sleep patterns change during pregnancy and in the post-partum period. From about 25 weeks the pregnant woman experiences more D sleep. This decreases to non-pregnant levels by term. There is a corresponding decrease in S sleep when the body undertakes tissue repair and recovers from fatigue (Blackburn 2003). This returns to normal immediately after delivery. During the first trimester sleep time and napping both increase but later night wakening occurs because of the minor disorders of nocturia, dyspnoea, heartburn, nasal congestion, muscle aches and anxiety.

Alterations in sensation

Nasal symptoms

Changes in the ear, nose and larynx occur because of the changes in fluid dynamics and vascular permeability. This is related to the increase in circulating oestrogen. Congestion and hyperaemia of the nasal mucosa cause nasal stuffiness and rhinorrhoea, which may lead to nose bleeds or to loss of sleep. Blocked ears and ear stuffiness may also occur. Similar laryngeal changes may result in voice changes or persistent cough.

The perceptions of smell and taste are closely related and a reduction in the sense of smell may lead to altered taste sensations and a change in food preference. Alterations in taste perception may be a factor in nausea and food aversions, especially for foods that taste bitter in pregnancy. Profet (1992) believes these aversions are protective, as bitter foods in nature are often poisonous or teratogenic.

MAIN POINTS

- The central nervous system receives messages from and sends messages via the peripheral nervous system to all parts of the body. It communicates by the rapid transmission of electrical signals. The autonomic nervous system innervates the smooth muscle and glands of the viscera and cardiac muscle and is subdivided into the sympathetic and parasympathetic nervous systems.

- Nervous tissue consists of neurons and the supporting neuroglia which provide support and protection for the neurons. Neurons have axons and dendrites which communicate with other cells by nerve impulses and neurotransmitters.

- Large nerve fibres are covered in a myelin sheath which protects and insulates fibres and increases the rate of impulse transmission up to a 100 times more rapidly than unmyelinated fibres. Axons from single neurons are bound together to form nerves.

- Nerve electrical activity is maintained by the distribution and relative concentration of negative and positive ions. Synapses are junctions between the terminal bouton of the axon and its target tissue. The synaptic cleft is a fluid-filled space into which neurotransmitters are released from the presynaptic membrane.

- The average brain weighs about 1500 g and is slightly heavier in men than women. The brain can be subdivided into the cerebral hemispheres; the diencephalon, comprising the thalamus and hypothalamus; the brainstem, comprising the midbrain, pons and medulla; and the cerebellum.

- Each hemisphere is divided into the frontal, parietal, occipital and temporal, the insula and the limbic lobes. The cerebral cortex is divided into the primary sensory area, the primary motor area and the association areas.

- Nerve fibres from the thalamus project to the sensory areas of the cerebral cortex. Nerves coming into the spinal cord from the periphery of the body maintain their somatotopic organisation so that a representation of the body is faithfully organised in the sensory cortex. The system is concerned with emotional feelings and it links with higher brain centres forming a close relationship between cognition and emotion.

- The hypothalamus is involved in homeostasis and survival. It controls the output of anterior pituitary hormones by releasing and inhibiting factors but secretes posterior pituitary hormones directly.

- The functions of the thalamic nuclei include hearing, vision, memory, cognition, judgement and mood. The insula is involved in olfaction, taste and autonomic reflexes. The functions of the septum are sensations of pleasure and wellbeing and memory.

- The medulla maintains homeostasis. Its nuclei include the cardiac centre, the vasomotor centre, the respiratory centre and nuclei that control vomiting, swallowing, coughing and sneezing. The pons is a bridge formed of nerve fibres running between spinal cord and higher brain centres.

- The reticular formation is involved in the level of consciousness and alertness. Some reticular formation neurons maintain rhythmic movements. Conscious awareness allows the nervous system to interact with the environment. Sleep may be restorative or it may ensure safety for a daytime species by limiting activity during darkness.

- The pia, arachnoid and dura maters protect the brain and spinal cord, protect blood vessels, enclose venous sinuses and contain cerebrospinal fluid (CSF). The dura extends inwards to form septa that anchor the brain to the skull. These include the falx cerebri, the falx cerebelli and the tentorium cerebelli.

- The four ventricles are filled with CSF and are continuous with each other and with the central canal of the spinal cord via the aqueduct of Sylvius. Choroid plexi form the CSF.

- The blood–brain barrier ensures that the brain's internal environment remains stable. It is selective so that substances needed by the brain cross by facilitated diffusion while toxic chemicals are kept within the capillary network.

- Twelve pairs of cranial nerves pass through foramina in the skull. The first two pairs originate from the forebrain and the rest in the brainstem. All but the vagus nerve target structures in the head and neck.

- The spinal cord carries ascending and descending nerve pathways. Thirty-one pairs of spinal nerves arise from the spinal cord and leave the vertebral column to target specific areas of the body. Each segment conducts sensory information from a specific body area called a dermatome. The cord is protected by bone, CSF and meninges.

- Inferiorly, the spinal cord ends in the conus medullaris and a collection of nerve roots called the cauda equinae fan outwards and downwards to exit through relevant vertebrae. The filum terminale extends downwards to attach to the posterior surface of the coccyx.

- The grey matter of the spinal cord is central to the white matter and looks like a letter H. There are two posterior or dorsal horns and two anterior or ventral horns. The white matter is composed of nerve fibres running in three directions: ascending tracts, descending tracts and across from one side of the spinal cord to the other.

- Musculoskeletal discomforts, sleep disturbances, alterations in sensation and in the experience of pain occur in pregnancy. Women report that their cognitive ability is worse, with difficulty in concentration and poor memory.

- Congestion and hyperaemia of the nasal mucosa cause nasal stuffiness and rhinorrhoea, which may lead to nose bleeds or to loss of sleep. Blocked ears and ear stuffiness may also occur, as may voice changes or persistent cough. Alterations in taste perception may lead to nausea and food aversions, especially for bitter tastes. This may protect against the ingestion of teratogens.

References

Aiello L, Dean C 1990 An Introduction to Human Evolutionary Anatomy. Academic Press, New York.

Allan D, Nie V, Hunter M 1996 Control and co-ordination. In Hinchliff S M, Montague S E, Watson R (eds) Physiology for Nursing Practice, 2nd edn. Baillière Tindall, London.

Blackburn S T 2003 Maternal, Fetal and Neonatal Physiology. W B Saunders, Philadelphia.

Fitzgerald M J T, Folan-Curran J 2002 Clinical Neuroanatomy and Related Neuroscience, 4th edn. W B Saunders, Philadelphia.

Marieb E N 2000 Human Anatomy and Physiology, 5th edn. Benjamin/Cummings, New York.

Moore P 1997 Pregnant women get that shrinking feeling. New Scientist 11 January:5.

Profet M 1992 Pregnancy sickness as adaptation: a deterrent to maternal ingestion of teratogens. In Barkow J, Cosmides L, Tooby J (eds) The Adapted Mind: Evolutionary Psychology and the Generation of Culture. Oxford University Press, New York, pp 327–365.

Springer S P, Deutsch G 1998 Left Brain, Right Brain, 5th edn. W H Freeman, New York.

Waterhouse J 1991 Light dawns on the body clock. New Scientist 26 October:30–34.

Annotated recommended reading

Greenfield S (ed.) 1996. The Human Mind Explained. Cassell, London.
This book, by the well-known researcher into the human mind, presents an easily read with an up-to-date overview of the human brain. It is written in clear concise language and has many illustrations, making it an excellent guide for students wishing to understand how the brain controls functions as far apart as movement, thought and male/female brain differences.

Marieb E N 2000 Human Anatomy and Physiology, 5th edn. Benjamin/Cummings, New York.
This textbook was a major source for this chapter and provides a multi-chaptered deeper and very lucid account of the anatomy and physiology of the nervous system. It is an excellent source book for students of anatomy and physiology.

Springer S P, Deutsch G 1998 Left Brain, Right Brain, 5th edn. W H Freeman, New York.
This textbook examines all theories about left- and right-handedness in humans. For interested students, sections include preferred neonatal head turning (to the right) and parental infant holding patterns.

Chapter 27

The peripheral and autonomic nervous systems

THE PERIPHERAL NERVOUS SYSTEM

Introduction

The **peripheral nervous system** (PNS) detects changes in the external or internal environment of the body, codes them into nerve impulses by sensory receptors and passes the information back to the central nervous system (CNS) so that appropriate action can be instituted (Allan et al 1996). Some messages are not passed back to the brain; they influence reflex actions at the level of the spinal cord or brainstem. The PNS includes all the neural structures outside the brain and spinal cord, i.e. sensory receptors, peripheral nerves and associated ganglia and efferent motor endings (Marieb 2000).

Ascending sensory tracts

Categories of sensation

There are two kinds of sensation (Fig. 27.1): **conscious** and **non-conscious** (Fitzgerald & Folan-Curran 2002). Conscious sensation can be divided into **exteroception** and **proprioception**. Exteroception involves messages from the outside world which are perceived in the cerebral cortex.

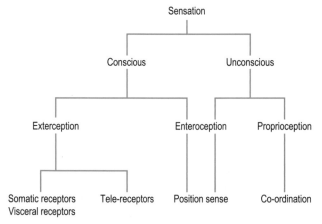

Figure 27.1 Categories of sensation.

Sensations may originate in body surface somatic receptors or in telereceptors of the special senses such as vision and hearing. **Proprioceptors** in the locomotor system and the labyrinth of the inner ear inform the brain of position when stationary (**position sense**) and during movement (**kinaesthetic sense**).

Non-conscious sensation can also be divided into two kinds: Non-conscious proprioception, which has its effect in the cerebellum and involves messages essential for smooth motor coordination received through spinocerebellar pathways and the brainstem; enteroception, which refers to non-conscious signals from visceral reflexes.

Somatic sensory perception

Two major pathways are involved in somatic perception sensations: the **posterior column–medial lemniscal pathway** and the **spinothalamic pathway** (Fig. 27.2). Both have common features (Fitzgerald & Folan-Curran 2002):

- they contain first-order, second-order and third-order sensory neurons;
- the cell bodies of the first-order neurons are in the posterior root ganglia;

- the cell bodies of the second-order neurons are on the same side of the CNS grey matter as the first-order neurons;
- second-order axons cross the midline to ascend and terminate in the thalamus;
- the third-order neurons project to the somatosensory cortex;
- both pathways are somatotopic, meaning that they represent the body parts in an orderly fashion up to the sensory cortex;
- the pathways can be modulated, either by inhibition or enhancement, by other neurons.

The posterior column–medial lemniscal pathway

The first-order nerve fibres enter the dorsal columns without synapsing. They are usually large **A fibres** with conduction velocities about 70 m/s. As nerve fibres from higher levels in the cord are added, they take up lateral positions so that the higher the level of origin is, the more lateral the position of the fibre in the column. The fibres of the cell bodies of second-order neurons at the level of the brainstem cross the midline to project to the thalamus. Crossing over is the reason why one side of the brain controls the opposite or **contralateral side** of the body. Cells in the sensory relay

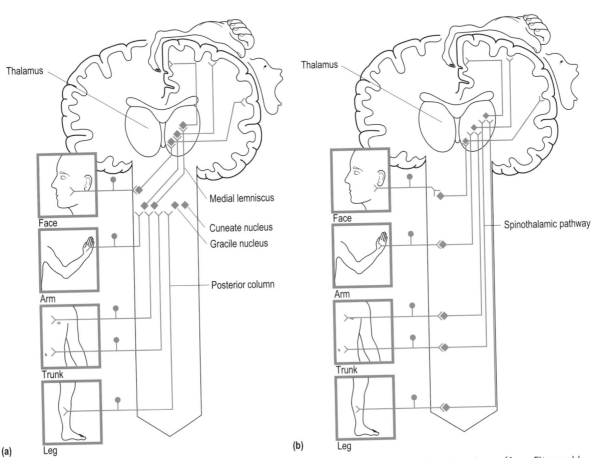

Figure 27.2 Basic plans of: (a) posterior column–medial lemniscal pathway; (b) spinothalamic pathway (from Fitzgerald M J T 1996, with permission).

nucleus of the thalamus are third-order neurons and project their fibres to the **somatosensory cortex**.

Functions The chief functions of this pathway are conscious proprioception and discriminatory touch. These provide the parietal lobe with an instantaneous body image so that we are aware of our position both at rest and while moving. Disturbances of this pathway cause multiple sclerosis and other demyelinising diseases.

The spinothalamic tract

The **dorsal root fibres** of this pathway tend to be the smaller A-δ or unmyelinated **C fibres** with slow conduction velocity. The dorsal root fibres enter the spinal cord and may ascend or descend a few segments of the cord before synapsing with cells of the dorsal horn in the **substantia gelatinosa**. The dorsal horn cell second-order fibres ascend or descend a few segments before crossing over the midline to ascend in the spinothalamic tract. These fibres terminate on third-order neurons in the thalamus. The fibres of these third-order neurons synapse on the cells of the sensory cortex.

Functions The role of this pathway is the perception of heat, cold and touch on the other side of the body. The role of the substantia gelatinosa in the gate control theory of perception of pain is discussed in Chapter 38, p. 498.

Somatosensory receptors

Sensory receptors are mostly adapted nerve fibre endings that respond to environmental changes. Sensory afferent nerves arising from the body are grouped together as the somatosensory system and include sensation from the skin, muscles, joints or viscera. The special senses are associated with organs in the head and include vision, hearing, balance, taste and smell; they are not discussed in this book. Anatomical and physiological aspects of vision and hearing can be found in Marieb (2000).

Types of somatosensory receptors

- **Mechanoreceptors** – respond to touch, pressure, vibrations and stretch.
- **Thermoreceptors** – respond to temperature change.
- **Photoreceptors** – respond to light.
- **Chemoreceptors** – respond to smell, taste and changes in blood chemistry.
- **Nociceptors** – respond to damage by causing pain (see Ch. 38).

For an explanation of general sensory receptors, the reader is referred to Marieb (2000). Nearly all receptors will function as nociceptors if overstimulated.

Descending motor pathways

The descending tracts carry efferent messages from the brain down the spinal cord and are divided into four main pathways (Fitzgerald & Folan-Curran 2002):

- **corticospinal** (pyramidal);
- **reticulospinal** (extrapyramidal);
- **vestibulospinal**;
- **tectospinal**.

The corticospinal tract

The corticospinal tract (Fig. 27.3) is the major motor pathway involved with voluntary movement. It contains about 1 million nerve fibres, about 60–80% of which originate in the primary motor cortex. The tract descends through the internal capsule to the brainstem. It continues through the pons to the medulla oblongata where about 80% of the pyramidal tract fibres **decussate**. The fibres, which are arranged

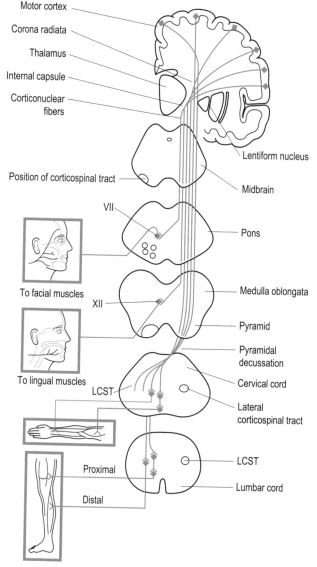

Figure 27.3 Corticospinal tract viewed from the front. At spinal cord level, only the lateral corticospinal tract is shown. LCST, lateral corticospinal tract; VII, nucleus of facial nerve; XII, hypoglossal nucleus (from Fitzgerald M J T 1996, with permission).

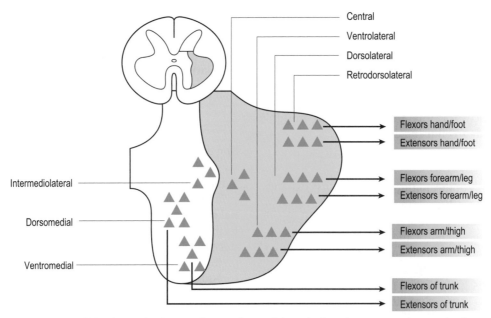

Figure 27.4 Cell columns in the anterior grey horn of the spinal cord: somatotopic organisation (from Fitzgerald M J T 1996, with permission).

somatotopically (Fig. 27.4), synapse with interneurons or directly with anterior horn neurons.

The reticulospinal tract

The reticulospinal tract is partially crossed and originates in the reticular formation of the pons and medulla. This system is involved in two different kinds of motor behaviour: locomotion, where it controls bilateral rhythmicity (try moving the arm and leg of the same side together when walking); and postural control.

The vestibulospinal tract

The vestibulospinal tract is an uncrossed paired pathway originating in the vestibular nucleus of the medulla oblongata. It maintains balance when the head is tilted to one side.

The tectospinal tracts

The tectospinal tract is a crossed pathway descending from the tectum of the midbrain to the medial part of the anterior grey horn at cervical and upper thoracic levels. In reptiles it is important in orienting the head and trunk towards sources of visual or auditory stimulation and may have a similar function in humans.

Upper and lower motor neurons

The neurons of the motor cortex are called the pyramidal cells because of the shape of their cell bodies. They are referred to as the upper motor neurons. The anterior horn neurons whose axons leave the cord to innervate the skeletal muscles are called the lower motor neurons. Damage to one or the other of these neuronal pathways will cause different symptoms.

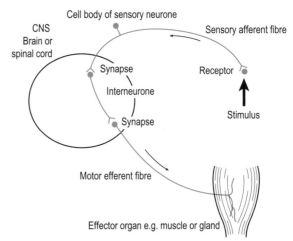

Figure 27.5 The component structures of a reflex arc (from Hinchliff S M, Montague S E 1990, with permission).

REFLEX ACTIVITY

A reflex is a rapid, predictable unlearned, involuntary response to a stimulus. Some reflex activity is protective, such as the rapid removal of a part of the body from a noxious stimulus like heat. Other reflexes occur without any awareness of change. These control visceral activities. There can be learned reflexes that come from practice or repetition (Marieb 2000), such as driving a car. In fact, many reflex actions are modifiable by learning and conscious effort.

The reflex arc

Reflexes occur over specific neural paths called **reflex arcs** (Fig. 27.5) which have five main components:

1. The receptor at the site where the stimulus occurs.
2. The sensory neuron, which takes the message to the CNS.

3. The integration centre within the CNS, which may be a single synapse or may involve a chain of interneurons.
4. The motor neuron, which conducts efferent impulses from the integration centre to an effector organ.
5. The effector, which may be a gland or a muscle fibre and acts to complete the reflex action. Reflexes may be somatic or autonomic. Somatic reflexes can be tested to confirm normal neural function.

Spinal reflexes

Many spinal reflexes occur with little or no brain input:

- Stretch and deep tendon reflexes, where the message from the proprioceptors in the muscles and joints are transmitted to the cerebellum and cerebral cortex. These allow normal muscle tone and activity to be maintained.
- The flexor reflex, which causes automatic withdrawal of the body from a painful stimulus.
- The crossed extensor reflex consists of an ipsilateral withdrawal reflex and a contralateral extensor reflex. These are important in maintaining balance.
- Superficial reflexes can be elicited by gentle stroking of the body. The best known are the plantar reflex, with incurling of the toes occurring in response to stroking the sole of the foot. Babinski's reflex, with extension of the toes, occurs in

infants less than 1 year old. The abdominal reflex occurs when the skin on one side of the trunk is stroked.

THE AUTONOMIC NERVOUS SYSTEM

The **autonomic** (self-regulating) nervous system or ANS is responsible for maintaining the stability of the body's internal environment (Clarke et al 1996). Motor neurons of the ANS innervate smooth muscle, cardiac muscle and glands, making adjustments to alter function in response to messages from the viscera sent to the CNS. Systemic changes brought about by the ANS include making adjustments to:

- shunting of blood to the needy areas;
- the heart rate;
- the blood pressure;
- the respiratory rate;
- body temperature;
- stomach secretions.

The role of the two divisions

There are differences between the somatic and autonomic nervous systems in their pathways and neurotransmitters (NTs). The ANS is divided into two arms: the sympathetic system (Fig. 27.6), which prepares the body for emergency

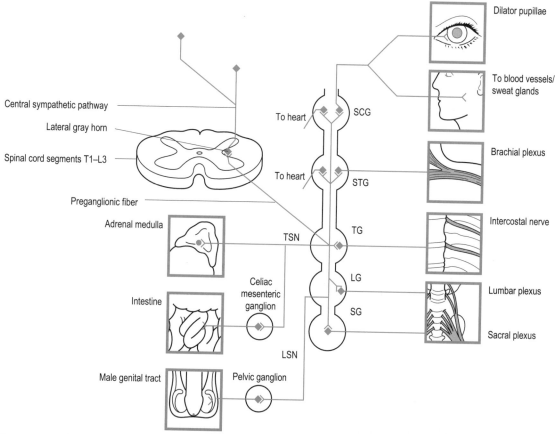

Figure 27.6   General plan of the sympathetic system. Ganglionic neurons and postganglionic fibres are shown in red. LG, lumbar ganglia; LSN, lumbar splanchnic nerve; SCG, superior cervical ganglion; SG, sacral ganglia; STG, stellate ganglion; TG, thoracic ganglia; TSN, thoracic splanchnic nerve (from Fitzgerald M J T 1996, with permission).

action, and the parasympathetic system (Fig. 27.7), which counterbalances the sympathetic system and has a calming effect, allowing general body maintenance and the conservation of energy to occur. There is usually a dynamic interaction between the two systems aimed at maximising homeostasis.

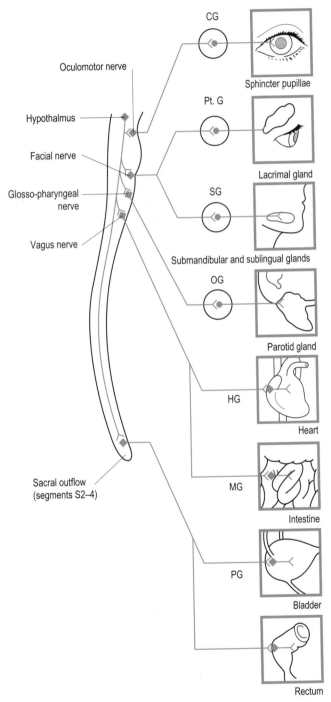

Figure 27.7　General plan of the parasympathetic system. Ganglionic neurons and postganglionic fibres are shown in red. CG, ciliary ganglion; HG, heart ganglia; MG, myenteric ganglia; OG, otic ganglion; PG, pterygopalatine ganglion; SG, submandibular ganglion (from Fitzgerald M J T 1996, with permission).

The sympathetic nervous system

The sympathetic system is so-called because it acts in sympathy with the emotions (Fitzgerald & Folan-Curran 2002). It is sometimes referred to as the **'fight or flight'** system and is activated if we are excited or in a threatening situation. The heart rate increases, there is rapid breathing, a cold sweaty skin and dilated eye pupils. Visceral blood vessels are constricted and digestion ceases. Blood is shunted to the heart and skeletal muscles and the liver releases glucose into the blood so that the cells are provided with energy.

The parasympathetic nervous system

The parasympathetic division is active when the systems are unstressed. It has been called the **'resting and digesting system'** and is active during digestion of food and elimination of waste. Blood pressure, heart rate and respiratory rate are low. The skin is warm as the skeletal muscles do not require extra blood supply. The eye pupils are constricted and the eye lenses are adjusted for close vision.

Anatomy of the ANS – pathways

The motor unit of the ANS is a two-neuron chain:

- The first neuron is called the preganglionic neuron. Its cell body is found in the brain or spinal column. It synapses with:
- The second motor neuron or postganglionic neuron, which has its cell body in the autonomic ganglion outside the CNS. The postganglionic neuron extends to the target tissue.

Preganglionic neurons are thin and lightly myelinated while postganglionic fibres are even thinner and unmyelinated. Both types of fibre may run with somatic nerves in spinal or cranial nerves.

Differences between the two divisions

1. Parasympathetic fibres emerge from the brain and sacral spinal cord (craniosacral division) while the sympathetic fibres originate from the thoracolumbar region of the spinal cord.
2. The parasympathetic division has long preganglionic and short postganglionic fibres. The sympathetic division has short preganglionic and long postganglionic fibres.
3. Parasympathetic ganglia are located in terminal ganglia within or close to the visceral target organs. Sympathetic ganglia lie close to the spinal cord.

Sympathetic division

The sympathetic division is more complex because it innervates more organs. Sympathetic activity tends to inhibit the activity of visceral organs, some body wall structures such as sweat glands and smooth muscles such as the hair-raising muscles (erector pili). Also, all arteries and veins, superficial and deep, are innervated by sympathetic fibres.

Preganglionic fibres Preganglionic fibres arise from cell bodies of neurons located in thoracic and lumbar spinal cord segments from T1–L2 (**thoracolumbar division**). The presence of these preganglionic sympathetic neurons produces the lateral horns (visceral motor horns) of the spinal cord, found in these sections. The fibres leave the spinal cord via the ventral root and pass through a myelinated **white ramus communicans** to enter the appropriate paravertebral (chain) ganglion which forms part of the sympathetic chain. Two sympathetic chains flank the vertebral column, one on each side. The fibres arising from the thoracolumbar region innervate 23 pairs of **ganglia** running from neck to pelvis:

- 3 cervical;
- 11 thoracic;
- 4 lumbar;
- 4 sacral;
- 1 coccygeal.

A preganglionic fibre reaching a paravertebral ganglion may:

- synapse with a postganglionic neuron in the same ganglion;
- ascend or descend within the sympathetic chain to synapse in another ganglion:

Fibres from T5–L2 pass through the ganglion and emerge as preganglionic **splanchnic nerves** (Fitzgerald & Folan-Curran 2002).

The splanchnic nerves – thoracic, lumbar and sacral – contribute to **plexi** such as the abdominal aortic plexus, the coeliac plexus, the superior and inferior mesenteric plexi and the hypogastric plexi from which postganglionic fibres fan out to their target organs (Table 27.1). The lumbar and sacral nerves send most of their fibres to the inferior mesenteric and hypogastric ganglia from where postganglionic fibres supply the distal half of the large intestine, the urinary bladder, the ureters and reproductive organs such as the uterus.

Postganglionic fibres From the synapse, postganglionic axons join the spinal nerves by non-myelinated branches called grey rami communicantes. They are then distributed to the sweat glands and smooth muscle of the hair roots and blood vessels.

Some postganglionic fibres travelling in the thoracic splanchnic nerves synapse with the adrenal medullary cells and are stimulated to produce adrenaline (epinephrine) and noradrenaline (norepinephrine) into the blood.

Parasympathetic division

The cranial outflow The cranial parasympathetic preganglionic fibres run in several cranial nerves:

- Oculomotor nerve parasympathetic fibres innervate smooth muscle within the eyes causing the pupils to constrict and the lenses to shorten and thicken to focus at near objects.

- Facial nerve parasympathetic fibres stimulate the large glands in the head such as the nasal and lacrimal glands and the submandibular and sublingual salivary glands.

- Glossopharyngeal parasympathetic nerves activate the parotid salivary glands.

- Vagus nerve parasympathetic activity accounts for 90% of preganglionic parasympathetic nerve activity. Preganglionic axons synapse on intramural (within walls) ganglia of target organs. Thoracic organs are the heart, lungs and oesophagus. Abdominal organs receiving innervation are the liver, stomach, small intestine, kidneys, pancreas and the proximal half of the large intestine.

The sacral outflow The sacral outflow arises from neurons in the lateral grey matter of sacral spinal cord segments S2–S4. The axons of these neurons run in the ventral roots of the spinal cord and branch off to form the splanchnic nerves. Most fibres synapse in intramural ganglia in the distal half of the large intestine, the urinary bladder, the ureters and reproductive organs such as the uterus.

Visceral sensory neurons

Although the ANS is considered to be a motor system, there are **visceral pain afferents** in autonomic nerves which travel along the same pathways as somatic pain fibres. Visceral pain is caused by mechanisms such as inflammation, smooth muscle spasm, ischaemia and distension. It is usually vague and deep seated and is often accompanied by sweating and nausea. As it increases in severity, the pain perception is referred to the somatic structures innervated from the same embryological segmental level. Labour pains are referred to the sacral area of the back and the pain of a heart attack is felt in the chest wall and along the medial aspect of the left arm (Fitzgerald & Folan-Curran 2002).

Table 27.1 Segmental sympathetic supply to the organs

Organ	Spinal cord segment
Head and neck + heart	T1–T5
Bronchi and lungs	T2–T4
Upper limb	T2–T5
Oesophagus	T5–T6
Stomach, spleen and pancreas	T6–T10
Liver	T7–T9
Small intestine	T9–T10
Kidney and reproductive organs	T10–L1
Lower limb	T10–L2
Large intestine, bladder and ureter	T11–L2

Physiology of the ANS

As described, an autonomic nerve pathway consists of a two-neuron chain, with the terminal neurotransmitter differing between the sympathetic and parasympathetic nerves. Neurotransmitters (NTs) are molecules which help neurons to communicate messages and regulate body activities and states (Marieb 2000). The major NTs of the ANS are acetylcholine (ACh) and noradrenaline (norepinephrine).

ACh is released by all preganglionic axons and by the postganglionic axons of the parasympathetic system. ACh-releasing fibres are called **cholinergic fibres**. Most sympathetic postganglionic fibres release noradrenaline (norepinephrine) and are called **adrenergic fibres**. The exceptions to the above rule are sympathetic postganglionic fibres innervating sweat glands, some skeletal muscle blood vessels and the external genitalia which release ACh. ACh and noradrenaline (norepinephrine) do not consistently produce excitation or inhibition on their target tissues. The response of visceral effectors depends on the type of receptor to which the NTs attach: there are at least two receptors for both NTs.

Cholinergic receptors

The two types of ACh-binding receptors have been given names for the drugs which bind to them and mimic ACh's effects: they are **nicotinic receptors**, to which nicotine binds, and **muscarinic receptors** (muscarine is a mushroom poison).

Site of nicotinic receptors

- Motor end plates of skeletal muscle cells (somatic targets).
- All postganglionic neurons, both sympathetic and parasympathetic.
- The hormone-producing cells of the adrenal medulla.

The effect of ACh binding to nicotinic receptors is always excitatory.

Site of muscarinic receptors

- All cells stimulated by postganglionic cholinergic fibres targeted by the parasympathetic system and a few sympathetic targets such as the sweat glands and some blood vessels of skeletal muscles.

The effect of ACh binding to muscarinic receptors may be excitatory or inhibitory, depending on the target organ.

Adrenergic receptors

There are two major classes of adrenergic receptors: alpha (α) and beta (β). In general, noradrenaline (norepinephrine) binding to α receptors is excitatory while binding to β receptors is inhibitory. There are notable and medically important exceptions. Binding of noradrenaline (norepinephrine) to β receptors of cardiac muscle induces vigorous activity in the heart. This is due to both α and β receptors having subclasses, i.e. α_1 and α_2, β_1 and β_2 (Marieb 2000).

Interactions of the autonomic divisions

Most visceral organs receive innervation from both sympathetic and parasympathetic fibres. They are said to receive dual innervation. If, as normal, both divisions are partially active, a dynamic antagonism is present that allows precise control of visceral activity. Antagonistic effects are more easily seen on the activity of the heart, respiration and gastrointestinal organs as discussed above: i.e. the fight or flight versus the rest and digest modes.

Sympathetic and parasympathetic tone

The sympathetic division controls blood pressure, even at rest. The vascular system is innervated by sympathetic fibres. The partial constriction of blood vessels maintaining sympathetic or vasomotor tone is under sympathetic control. If blood flow needs increasing, sympathetic impulses increase, vessels constrict and blood pressure rises. If blood pressure needs decreasing, impulses decrease, smooth muscle relaxes and the vessels dilate. However, the heart, along with the gastrointestinal tract and urinary tract, is dominated by parasympathetic effects. The smooth muscles of these organs exhibit parasympathetic tone. The sympathetic division overrides this parasympathetic tone in times of stress.

Cooperative efforts

This is best demonstrated during sexual intercourse. The parasympathetic division causes dilatation of the blood vessels of the external genitalia and results in erection of the penis and clitoris. Sympathetic stimulation then results in the rhythmic contractions that result in ejaculation in men and reflex rhythmic contractions of the pelvic floor in women.

Effects unique to the sympathetic division

Some physiological functions are not under parasympathetic influences and are controlled totally by the sympathetic division. These include:

- control of the adrenal medulla;
- the sweat glands;
- the erector pili muscles;
- the production of renin by the kidney;
- thermoregulatory response to heat;
- mobilisation of glucose and fats to be used as fuel.

Control of autonomic functioning

Several levels in the CNS contribute to the regulation of the ANS. These include controls in the brainstem, hypothalamus and cerebral cortex.

Brainstem controls

The most direct influence appears to be via the reticular formation. Most sensory impulses that cause the autonomic reflexes arrive in the brainstem via afferents from the vagus nerve. Centres in the medulla that are influenced include the cardiac, vasomotor, respiratory centres and those controlling gastrointestinal activities. Control of micturition and defecation are reflexes that can be overcome by conscious control.

Hypothalamic controls

The hypothalamus coordinates heart activity, blood pressure, body temperature, water balance, endocrine activity, emotional states such as rage or pleasure and biological drives such as hunger and thirst. It can influence and be influenced by the higher cortical centres. The hypothalamus is the main integration centre for the ANS. Medial and anterior hypothalamic regions direct parasympathetic activities while the posterior and lateral areas direct sympathetic

functions. The route of influence is:

$$\text{Hypothalamus} \rightarrow \text{Reticular formation} \\ \rightarrow \text{Preganglionic ANS motor neurons}$$

Cortical controls

There is growing knowledge and interest in the effect of the higher brain centres on regulation of the autonomic system. This is an expanding research area and includes such behaviours as meditation, biofeedback, neuropsychoimmunity and psychosomatic illness (Watkins 1997).

ADAPTATION TO PREGNANCY

Changes in the functioning of the peripheral and autonomic nervous systems are related to changes in the endocrine system during pregnancy and the relevant neurohormonal reflexes such as that involved in lactation will be discussed in relevant chapters. The role of the sympathetic nervous system in the stress response is important for understanding uterine muscle activity and cervical dilatation in labour.

MAIN POINTS

- The peripheral nervous system (PNS) detects changes in the external or internal environment and passes the information back to the central nervous system (CNS) so that appropriate action can be instituted. Sensory afferent nerves include sensation from the skin, muscles, joints or viscera. Large bundles of first-order nerve fibres arranged somatotopically enter the dorsal columns without synapsing. They cross the midline to synapse with second-order neurons at the level of the medulla. These project second-order fibres to the thalamus. Thalamic third-order neurons project fibres to the sensory cerebral cortex.

- The dorsal root fibres of the spinothalamic tract ascend or descend a few segments before crossing over the midline to ascend in the spinothalamic tract and terminate on third-order neurons in the thalamus. The fibres of these third-order neurons synapse on the cells of the sensory cortex.

- The descending tracts carry efferent messages from the brain down the spinal cord. The pyramidal cells of the motor cortex are the upper motor neurons. The anterior horn neuron axons which leave the cord to innervate the skeletal muscles are the lower motor neurons.

- Reflexes occur over reflex arcs and may be somatic or autonomic. Many spinal reflexes occur with little or no brain input.

- The autonomic nervous system (ANS) maintains stability of the body's internal environment. Its motor neurons innervate smooth muscle, cardiac muscle and glands,

making functional adjustments in response to visceral messages sent to the CNS.

- The ANS is divided into the sympathetic system, which prepares the body for emergency action, and the parasympathetic system, which has a calming effect. There is a dynamic interaction between the two divisions of the ANS, aimed at maximising homeostasis. Sympathetic activity tends to inhibit the activity of visceral organs. Sympathetic fibres innervate sweat glands, smooth muscles such as erector pili and all arteries and veins.

- Visceral pain afferents in autonomic nerves respond to ischaemia, distension, smooth muscle spasm and inflammation and travel along the same pathways as somatic pain fibres.

- The neurotransmitters of the ANS are acetylcholine (ACh) and noradrenaline (norepinephrine). ACh is released by all preganglionic axons and by parasympathetic postganglionic axons. Most sympathetic postganglionic fibres are adrenergic. Most visceral organs are innervated by both sympathetic and parasympathetic fibres.

- The sympathetic division is the main controller of blood pressure. The partial constriction of blood vessels to maintain sympathetic or vasomotor tone is under the control of the sympathetic division. The heart, the gastrointestinal tract and urinary tract are dominated by parasympathetic effects.

- Several levels in the CNS contribute to the regulation of the ANS. These include controls in the brainstem, hypothalamus and cerebral cortex.

References

Allan D, Nie V, Hunter M 1996 Control and co-ordination. In Hinchliff S M, Montague S E, Watson R (eds) Physiology for Nursing Practice, 2nd edn. Baillière Tindall, London.

Clarke M 1996 The autonomic nervous system. In Hinchliff S M, Montague S E, Watson R (eds) Physiology for Nursing Practice, 2nd edn. Baillière Tindall, London.

Fitzgerald M J T, Folan-Curran 2002 Clinical Neuroanatomy, and Related Neuroscience, 4th edn. W B Saunders, Philadelphia.

Marieb E N 2000 Human Anatomy and Physiology, 5th edn. Benjamin/Cummings, New York.

Watkins A 1997 Mind–Body Medicine, A Clinician's Guide to Psychoneuroimmunology. Churchill Livingstone, Edinburgh.

Annotated recommended reading

Marieb E N 2000 Human Anatomy and Physiology, 5th edn. Benjamin/Cummings, New York.
This textbook was a major source for this chapter and provides a multi-chaptered deeper and very lucid account of the anatomy and physiology of the nervous system. It is an excellent source book for students of anatomy and physiology.

Watkins A 1997 Mind–Body Medicine, A Clinician's Guide to Psychoneuroimmunology. Churchill Livingstone, Edinburgh.
Although not specifically related to childbearing, this book is an excellent primer for students who are interested in the way the body and mind work together to influence health.

Chapter 28

The endocrine system

INTRODUCTION

The nervous system (Chs 26 and 27) is the rapid controller of the body while the endocrine system provides a much slower control. By coordinating the body's internal physiology and modifying cell function, the endocrine system helps it to adapt to external environmental changes (Brook & Marshall 2001). The two systems are closely related and the hypothalamus provides a major link between them. Adaptations to pregnancy will be discussed after the anatomy and physiology of each gland.

THE ENDOCRINE SYSTEM – THE HYPOTHALAMUS

The **hypothalamus** controls the function of the **endocrine glands** and has wider links with parts of the nervous system. The hypothalamus can therefore be called a **neuroendocrine** organ – producing, releasing and inhibiting hormones to influence the production of hormones by the anterior pituitary gland. Endocrine glands include the thyroid, parathyroid, adrenal and pineal glands. These are discussed below. Other organs produce hormones, including the pancreas (Ch. 22), ovaries (Ch. 4), testes (Ch. 5) and placenta (Ch. 12). Functions of the endocrine glands include reproduction, growth and development, mobilisation of body defences against stress, maintenance of fluid and electrolyte balance, nutrient content in the blood, regulation of cell metabolism and energy balance. Tissue responses to hormones may take only a few seconds or may take days.

HORMONES

Hormones are regulatory molecules synthesised in specialist cells which may be collected into distinct endocrine glands or found as single cells within an organ: for example, in the gastrointestinal tract. Hormone-secreting cells in a gland are arranged in cords and branching networks to maximise the contact between cells and the capillaries that receive the secretions (Marieb 2000). In contrast, exocrine glands pass their products through ducts into a body cavity or onto the surface of the skin.

Hormones affect tissues by binding to specific receptors on the surface of target cells. They are released into the adjacent extracellular space and enter a local blood vessel to be taken to their target tissue. Some hormones act locally in the gland without entering the bloodstream, either on adjacent cells (**paracrine hormones**) or on the cell of origin (**autocrine hormones**) (Brook & Marshall 2001).

Types of hormones

Hormones can be classified into three groups of molecules: those derived from the amino acid tyrosine; peptide and protein molecules; and steroid hormones (Brook & Marshall 2001).

Hormones derived from tyrosine

These hormones include **adrenaline** (epinephrine) and **noradrenaline** (norepinephrine) produced in the adrenal medulla. **Dopamine** acts as a hormone when it suppresses **prolactin** secretion. The thyroid hormones, **thyroxine** and **triiodothyronine**, are derived from tyrosine.

Protein and peptide hormones

These hormones vary in size; the smallest include the hypothalamic-releasing hormones. Gastrointestinal hormones such as **secretin** from the duodenum and **gastrin** from the stomach are much larger (Ch. 21, p. 282). Others include **parathyroid hormone**, **oxytocin**, **vasopressin**, **insulin** and the glycoprotein hormones from the anterior pituitary gland such as the gonadotrophins, follicle-stimulating hormone and luteinising hormone.

Steroid hormones

Steroids, which are a class of lipids derived from **cholesterol**, include cortisol and aldosterone from the adrenal cortex and the sex hormones testosterone, progesterone and oestrogens.

Eicosanoids

Eicosanoids, which are formed from the essential fatty acid **arachidonic acid**, also influence cell activity locally. These are biologically active lipids found in nearly all cell membranes and include **prostaglandins**. They are not hormones and do not appear to circulate in the blood to influence distant tissues (Boore 1996). Their role in the onset of labour is discussed in Chapter 36, p. 473.

Target cells

Hormones circulate to nearly all tissues but a particular hormone can only influence cells with specific receptors in their plasma membranes. Some hormones only influence a few tissues – for example, **adrenocorticotrophic hormone** only affects certain cells of the adrenal cortex – while others such as thyroxine are essential for the metabolism of all cells.

The half-life of a hormone is the time taken for half of it to be removed from the plasma (Boore 1996). The catecholamines and insulin are transported in plasma in the free state and have very short half-lives. Hormones such as thyroxine and the corticosteroids are bound to specific carrier proteins and have a much longer half-life. The extent of cellular activity depends on blood levels of the hormone, the numbers of receptors on the target cells and the affinity of the receptor for the hormone.

Cell surface receptors and intracellular signalling

Hormone–receptor binding is a first step to target cell interaction. There are two major groups of cell surface receptors: tyrosine kinase receptors and G-protein coupled receptors.

Tyrosine kinase receptors There are two subgroups of tyrosine kinase receptors – those which use tyrosine kinase locally at the hormone-binding site (integrated) and those which recruit tyrosine kinase activity following binding (recruited):

- Insulin is a hormone member of the integrated receptors. These receptors typically bind ligands which stimulate cell growth and proliferation and are therefore known as growth factor receptors.
- The second subgroup includes growth hormone and prolactin. These hormones share a similar structure with cytokines and erythropoietin and are commonly referred to as cytokine/erythropoietin receptors (Brook & Marshall 2001).

G-protein coupled receptors These receptors (GPCRs) couple with G (guanine) proteins associated with the inner surface of the cell membrane. This mechanism utilises intracellular second messengers such as cyclic adenosine monophosphate (cAMP). The most striking difference from tyrosine kinase receptors is the complexity of the receptor structure which 'crosses the lipid bilayer of the plasma membrane seven times' (Brook & Marshall 2001).

Second messengers Most amino acid-based hormones cannot penetrate cell membranes and have to utilise intracellular second messengers such as cyclic AMP. When a hormone (first messenger) binds to a receptor which is coupled with the membrane-bound enzyme adenylate cyclase, it uses a G-protein signal to activate the adenylate cyclase which catalyses the conversion of ATP to cyclic AMP. This initiates a cascade of enzyme-controlled chemical reactions, resulting in the correct cellular response. Cyclic AMP is rapidly degraded by the enzyme phosphodiesterase so that its action persists only briefly and cellular activity can be ended as necessary.

Other amino acid-based hormones involve a third messenger, calcium, in their pathway. Calcium either acts directly by altering the activity of specific enzymes or indirectly by binding to an intracellular protein called calmodulin.

Intracellular receptors

Steroid and thyroid hormones bind to protein members of a super-family of intracellular receptors. These hormones are hydrophobic and lipid soluble and diffuse across the plasma membrane of their target cells to gain access to intracellular receptors in the cytosol or nucleus. Compared with the hormones which act via cell surface receptor/second messenger systems, responses to steroid and thyroid hormones are sluggish (Brook & Marshall 2001).

When steroid and thyroid hormones bind to a receptor in the cell nucleus, the activated hormone–receptor complex binds to a DNA-associated receptor protein. This switches on DNA transcription of RNA and the specific receptor protein molecule is produced, triggering the metabolic activity that the hormone induces (Marieb 2000).

The mechanisms of hormone action

Hormones increase or decrease cell activity by producing one or more of the following (Marieb 2000):

1. changes in cell membrane permeability and/or electrical potential;
2. enzyme synthesis, activation or deactivation;
3. induction of secretory activity;
4. stimulation of mitotic cell division.

Regulation of receptors

Target cells may make more receptors in response to high levels of hormone: this is up-regulation. Other cells may respond to high levels of hormones by loss of receptors or down-regulation. Hormones may also influence receptors responsive to other hormones. For example, the presence of progesterone causes a loss of oestrogen receptors but oestrogen causes an increase in progesterone receptors, causing the cells to have an enhanced ability to respond to progesterone.

Control of hormone release

The synthesis and release of hormones depends on inhibition by a system of negative feedback. Hormone secretion is triggered by an internal or external stimulus and blood levels rise until they reach the required level when further hormone release is inhibited. This maintains blood levels within a narrow range. The stimuli that induce hormone release may be hormonal, humoral or neural.

Hormonal stimuli The hypothalamic releasing and inhibiting hormones regulate anterior pituitary gland production of hormones, some of which in turn induce other glands to secrete their hormones. The rise in blood levels of the hormones produced by the final target glands inhibits the release of anterior pituitary hormones.

Humoral stimuli Changing blood levels of ions and nutrients may affect hormone release: for example, the production of parathyroid hormone (PTH) is prompted by decreasing blood calcium levels.

Neural stimuli In a few cases hormones are released in response to neural stimuli. An example is the release of catecholamines by the sympathetic nervous system in response to stress.

THE PITUITARY GLAND

The pituitary gland (**hypophysis**) is a small ovoid gland weighing 500 mg that is situated in the **sella turcica** of the sphenoid bone. It has a stalk called the **infundibulum** which connects the pituitary gland to the hypothalamus. The pituitary gland has two lobes:

- The posterior lobe (**neurohypophysis**) consists of nerve fibres and neuroglia and is derived from a downward growth of the hypothalamus. It does not manufacture hormones but acts as a storage unit for hypothalamic hormones, releasing them as necessary.

- The anterior lobe (**adenohypophysis**) is composed of glandular tissue and manufactures and releases its own hormones.

The gland has a very rich blood supply derived from the internal carotid artery via superior and inferior hypophyseal branches. Venous drainage is by short vessels into the dural venous sinuses. The rich blood supply makes the gland vulnerable to blood loss in haemorrhage, particularly in pregnancy.

The pituitary–hypothalamic axis

A nerve bundle called the hypothalamic–hypophyseal tract runs through the infundibulum (Fig. 28.1). The tract neurons are situated in two groups of nuclei in the hypothalamus:

- The paired supraventricular and supraoptic nuclei are responsible for posterior pituitary function. Oxytocin is secreted from the paraventricular nuclei and antidiuretic hormone from the supraoptic nuclei. These hormones are transported along axons to their terminals in the neurohypophysis.

- The hypothalamic–hypophyseal nuclei are responsible for anterior pituitary function. There is no direct neural connection between the adenohypophysis and the hypothalamus. A vascular connection, the hypophyseal portal system, carries the hypothalamic releasing and inhibiting hormones to the adenohypophysis.

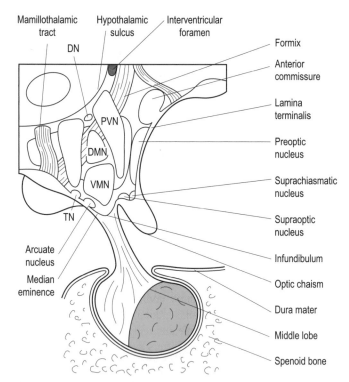

Figure 28.1 Hypothalamic nuclei and hypophysis, viewed from the right side. DN, dorsal nucleus; DMN, dorsomedial nucleus; MB, mamillary body; PN, posterior nucleus; PVN, periventricular nucleus; TN, tuberomamillary nucleus; VMN, ventromedial nucleus (from Fitzgerald M J T 1996, with permission).

Table 28.1 Actions of hypothalamic neurohormones

Name	Major functions
Thyrotrophin-releasing hormone (TRH)	Stimulates release of TSH and PRL Minor stimulation of FSH release
Gonadotrophin-releasing hormone (GnRH)	Stimulates release of LH and FSH
Growth hormone-releasing hormone	Stimulates release of GH
Growth hormone release inhibiting hormone (somatostatin – SMS)	Inhibits release of GH, gastrin, VIP, glucagons, insulin, TSH, and PRL
Corticotropin-releasing hormone (CRH)	Stimulates release of ACTH
Dopamine (DA)	Inhibits release of PRL

ACTH, adenocorticotropic hormone; FSH, follicle-stimulating hormone; GH, growth hormone; LH, luteinising hormone; PRL, prolactin; TSH, thyroid-stimulating hormone (thyrotrophin); VIP, vasoactive intestinal peptide.

Regulation of function

A number of hypothalamic neurohormones regulate anterior pituitary function. They have short half-lives in the circulation and act rapidly on their specific anterior pituitary target cells. Their actions are summarised in Table 28.1.

Anterior pituitary hormones

The anterior lobe of the pituitary gland has been called the 'master endocrine gland' because of its control of other glands. There are six anterior pituitary hormones – four of them regulate the hormonal functioning of other glands:

- thyroid-stimulating hormone (TSH);
- adrenocorticotropic hormone (ACTH);
- follicle-stimulating hormone (FSH);
- luteinising hormone (LH).

The other two hormones influence non-endocrine targets:

- growth hormone (GH);
- prolactin (PRL).

These hormones all utilise the second messenger system. Growth hormone, prolactin and the posterior pituitary hormones will be discussed next. The tropic hormones are considered with their target glands.

Growth hormone

Growth hormone (GH) stimulates cells to grow and divide. It promotes growth of bone, soft tissue and viscera with a direct action on fibroblast differentiation. An indirect action promotes clonal expansion of newly differentiated cells mediated by **insulin-like growth factors** (IGF-1 and IGF-2). The total amount secreted daily declines with age. GH has a diurnal cycle, with the highest levels occurring during sleep. It is anabolic and stimulates protein synthesis, facilitates the use of fats for fuel and conserves glucose.

Regulation of GH secretion Two hypothalamic hormones with antagonistic effects regulate the production of GH: these are GH-releasing hormone and GH-inhibiting hormone (**somatostatin**). Hypersecretion of GH in childhood results in **gigantism** and the person may reach a height of 2.4 m (8 ft). After cessation of longitudinal bone growth, enlargement of bony areas of the hands, feet and face occurs, a condition known as acromegaly. Hyposecretion of GH in children leads to **pituitary dwarfism**. Such people have normal body proportions but a maximum height of 1.2 m (4 ft).

Prolactin

Prolactin (PRL) is similar to GH. The only known effect in humans is the stimulation of milk production by the breasts (Ch. 54). PRL is regulated by the negative control of dopamine (DA) in men and non-lactating women.

Regulation of PRL Prolactin levels are influenced by the effect of oestrogen on the breast. The release of PRL just before a menstrual period accounts for premenstrual breast swelling and tenderness but the stimulation is so brief that no milk is produced. Hypersecretion of prolactin will cause inappropriate lactation (galactorrhoea) and is seen in both sexes, mostly due to an anterior pituitary gland tumour. Women will have amenorrhoea and men may become impotent.

Posterior pituitary hormones

Oxytocin

Oxytocin is a strong stimulator of uterine action. Its synthesis and release are important in childbirth and in nursing women.

Regulation of oxytocin Oxytocin is released by the pituitary gland during the final stages of labour due to the stretching of the lower genital tract, a phenomenon called Ferguson's reflex (Ch. 37). It is also secreted during the puerperium as a response to suckling (Ch. 54).

Antidiuretic hormone

Antidiuretic hormone (ADH) inhibits or prevents urine formation by targeting the renal tubules, which respond by reabsorbing more water. Less urine is produced and blood volume rises.

Regulation of ADH Osmoreceptors in the hypothalamus monitor the solute concentration in blood and if too much is detected, as in inadequate fluid intake, they send excitatory messages to the ADH-secreting neurons in the hypothalamus. ADH release is also stimulated by pain, low blood pressure and drugs such as nicotine, morphine and barbiturates. In large blood loss situations, enormous amounts of ADH are released, causing vasoconstriction and a rise in systemic blood pressure. That is why ADH is sometimes referred to as vasopressin.

Inhibition of ADH Inhibition of ADH is caused by ingestion of alcohol so that a diuresis occurs, accounting for the thirst and dry mouth the following morning! Drinking large amounts of water will also suppress ADH release. A rare disorder resulting in inadequate release of ADH is diabetes insipidus. There is excessive urination and thirst and it can be life threatening if the individual cannot take in enough fluid.

ADH changes during pregnancy Antidiuretic hormone production is similar in pregnant and non-pregnant women. However, the osmoreceptors are reset to accommodate the extra blood volume of pregnancy (Blackburn 2003).

Anterior pituitary changes during pregnancy

A functioning pituitary gland is not essential for the maintenance of pregnancy once conception has occurred. Women who have had removal of the pituitary gland after 12 weeks of pregnancy have delivered healthy babies (Jacobs 1991). However, there are changes in both structure and function of the gland during a normal pregnancy.

Box 28.1 Sheehan's syndrome

The increase in size of the anterior pituitary gland in pregnancy necessitates an increased oxygen supply carried to it by an increased circulation. The unique blood supply to the pituitary gland makes it vulnerable to a reduction in arterial blood supply if there is vasospasm of the superior hypophyseal artery leading to swelling and necrosis of the gland (Sheehan & Stanfield 1961). This may be why the pituitary gland is more readily damaged in pregnancy.

Sheehan's syndrome or anterior pituitary necrosis is a rare condition associated with severe and prolonged obstetric shock. The usual cause is severe haemorrhage during labour, resulting in postpartum **hypopituitarism**. The symptoms are caused by loss of the anterior pituitary hormones. The earliest sign is failure to lactate due to prolactin deficiency, followed by amenorrhoea due to deficiency of the gonadotrophic hormones. The activity of the thyroid and adrenal glands gradually diminishes and the woman becomes lethargic and feels cold. Her hair and skin become coarser and she suffers loss of libido. Her genitalia and breasts atrophy. Adequate and prompt treatment of obstetric shock will prevent the syndrome developing (Sleep 1996). If the diagnosis is not made, the woman may die. Treatment is by total hormone replacement.

The pituitary gland in non-pregnant women is about 20% heavier than in men. During pregnancy its weight increases by 30% in first pregnancies and 50% in subsequent pregnancies, almost entirely due to an increase in the number of prolactin-secreting cells known as **lactotrophs**. The increase in size leads to an enhanced blood supply. The pituitary gland is then vulnerable to a reduced blood supply if there is arterial vasospasm. This may lead to Sheehan's syndrome (see Box 28.1) with swelling and necrosis of the pituitary gland (Sheehan & Stanfield 1961). The number of GH-producing cells falls, probably due to the presence of **human placental lactogen**. Growth hormone secretion returns to normal within a few weeks of pregnancy. The number of cells is paralleled by blood levels of the two hormones.

During pregnancy the fetoplacental hormones greatly influence the pituitary gland and the secretion of FSH and LH are inhibited, possibly due to human chorionic gonadotrophin. However, hyperprolactinaemia of pregnancy also contributes to the fall in gonadotrophic secretion. The pattern of hormone production by the anterior pituitary changes in the puerperium to accommodate lactation.

THE THYROID GLAND

The thyroid gland lies in the neck in front of the trachea and below the larynx. It has two lateral lobes joined by a medial isthmus. It is the largest endocrine gland, weighing 10–20 g in an adult, and is well supplied with blood via the superior and inferior thyroid arteries. It concentrates **iodide** from the bloodstream to synthesise its hormones (Brook & Marshall 2001).

The internal structure of the thyroid gland consists of hollow spherical structures called **follicles**, lined by cuboidal epithelial cells. These follicle cells produce thyroglobulin, a glycoprotein. The follicles store an amber-coloured sticky material consisting of thyroglobulin molecules attached to iodine. This material gives rise to two thyroid hormones – thyroxine or T_4 and triiodothyronine or T_3. Another group of cells, **the parafollicular cells**, produce the hormone **calcitonin** (Ch. 24).

Thyroid hormones

Thyroxine is the major hormone and more of it is secreted than triiodothyronine. The structure of the two hormones is similar, each consisting of two tyrosine molecules linked together. Thyroxine binds four iodine atoms (hence T_4) and triiodothyronine binds three iodine atoms (hence T_3). Although both T_3 and T_4 bind to tissues, T_3 is 10 times more active. Most of the T_3 is formed in the target tissues by enzymatic removal of an iodine group from T_4, which may be a prohormone.

Iodine molecules are attached to a tyrosine molecule to make **iodotyrosines**. If two iodine atoms are attached to a tyrosine molecule, **diiodotyrosine** (DIT) is produced. The attachment of one iodine atom to a tyrosine produces **monoiodotyrosine** (MIT). A coupling of DIT + DIT within the thyroglobulin molecule forms T_4, while a coupling of a DIT + MIT forms T_3. Enzymes split the thyroid hormones off from the thyroglobulin molecule.

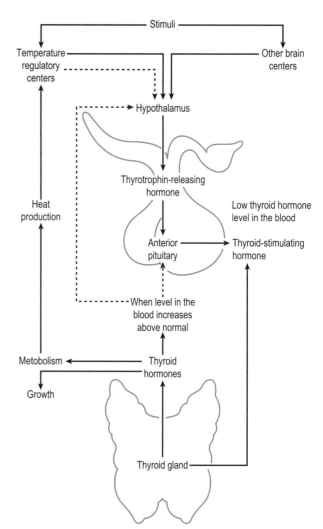

Figure 28.2   The regulation of thyroid hormone secretion by negative feedback loop.

Secretion of thyroid hormones

In the adult about 1.2 mmol of dietary iodine is required for the manufacture of the thyroid hormones. The iodine removed from the bloodstream is concentrated in the gland, combined with thyroglobulin. Transfer of iodide into follicular cells occurs against a steep iodide concentration gradient by a mechanism similar to the sodium pump (Brook & Marshall 2001). The hormones circulate around the body bound to a plasma protein, **thyroid-binding globulin** (TBG). Less than 1% of the hormones remain free in the blood and it is this that stimulates tissues. Thyroid hormones are broken down in the tissues and some iodine is returned to the thyroid gland to be reused while some is excreted.

Regulation of thyroid hormone secretion is by a negative feedback loop from T_3 so that blood levels are maintained within a narrow limit. TRH from the hypothalamus influences the secretion of TSH from the anterior pituitary gland (Fig. 28.2).

Functions of thyroid hormones

Thyroid hormones affect most cells except the tissues of the brain, spleen, testes, uterus and the thyroid gland itself and seem to be essential for the maintenance of normal metabolic functions. Their only definitive action is to increase basal metabolic rate, possibly by increasing intracellular concentrations of enzymes involved in catabolic processes (Brook & Marshall 2001). Cellular thyroid hormone receptors are nucleic acid proteins which can bind to specific DNA sequences. After binding, the hormone–receptor complex directly induces transcription of the genes responsive to thyroid hormones.

Changes in the thyroid gland during pregnancy

Secretion of TSH is reduced in the first trimester, returning to normal for the remainder of pregnancy. Thyroid function remains normal during pregnancy, although some women exhibit some of the signs associated with an overactive thyroid gland, including thyroid hyperplasia or goitre. During pregnancy, a balance is achieved by alterations in the metabolism of iodine. Renal iodide clearance doubles, plasma inorganic iodide falls and thyroid clearance of iodine trebles. The absolute uptake of iodine remains within normal limits (ACOG 2001).

From 12 weeks there is an increase in plasma concentration of TBG, probably influenced by reduced hepatic clearance and oestrogenic stimulation of production, and free thyroxine due to the influence of human chorionic gonadotrophin or hCG (ACOG 2001). The ability of TBG to bind thyroxine doubles (Blackburn 2003). Basal metabolic rate increases by 25% from 4 months.

The above alterations have been linked with nausea and vomiting in early pregnancy, especially in hyperemesis gravidarum (Vitoratos et al 2000). Maternal immunological reactiveness also appears to be involved (Leylek et al 1999). The changes revert to normal in the puerperium but it may take up to 12 weeks for them to be completely reversed. Thyroid gland disorders are considered in Chapter 35.

THE ADRENAL GLANDS

The two pyramid-shaped adrenal glands each weigh about 4 g and are situated on the superior poles of each kidney. The inner medulla is derived from the neural crest and is functionally part of the sympathetic nervous system. It is composed of chromaffin cells, which give it a reddish-brown colour. The outer cortex forms 80–90% of each gland and is derived from embryonic mesoderm similar to the ovary and testis. It is yellow due to its high lipid content.

Adrenal blood supply

The adrenal gland blood supply is derived from a circle of arteries arising from the superior, middle and inferior adrenal arteries. These give off three types of artery: capsular vessels, cortical vessels and medullary vessels. The medulla has a double blood supply: a systemic one derived from medullary arterioles and one derived from cortical capillaries. The latter is similar to a portal system and ensures that blood arriving in the medulla is rich in the corticoid hormones necessary for the production of adrenaline (epinephrine) (Brook & Marshall 2001). Medullary venules empty blood into the central vein. The central vein of the right adrenal gland empties into the inferior vena cava while the left venous drains into the left renal vein.

The adrenal cortex

The cortex consists of large, lipid-filled cells arranged in three concentric regions which synthesise the corticosteroids from cholesterol (Brook & Marshall 2001):

- The outer **zona glomerulosa** produces mineralocorticoids;
- The middle **zona fasciculata** makes up 5–10% of the cortex and secretes glucocorticoids;

- The inner **zona reticularis** forms about 75% of the cortex and produces glucocorticoids and small amounts of the sex hormones or gonadocorticoids.

The mineralocorticoids

Mineralocorticoids regulate the amount of electrolytes and water in extracellular fluid. In particular, they affect sodium and potassium concentrations. **Aldosterone** makes up more than 95% of the total output and is the most potent of the mineralocorticoids. It regulates sodium balance by targeting the distal tubules of the kidneys and stimulates reabsorption of sodium ions from the urine and returns them to the bloodstream. Aldosterone is also involved in sodium reabsorption from perspiration, saliva and gastric juice. Potassium, hydrogen, bicarbonate and chloride ions are coupled to sodium regulation and water follows sodium passively.

Four mechanisms help to regulate its secretion (Fig. 28.3):

1. The renin–angiotensin mechanism.
2. Rising levels of potassium ions and low levels of sodium in the blood.
3. Release of atrial natriuretic factor by the heart when blood pressure rises.
4. Decreasing blood volume and blood pressure stimulate aldosterone secretion. In severe stress the hypothalamus releases corticotropin-releasing hormone which steps up ACTH production, leading to increased aldosterone production.

The glucocorticoids

Glucocorticoids include **cortisol** (hydrocortisone), **cortisone** and **corticosterone**. Only cortisol is secreted in significant amounts in humans (Marieb 2000). The control of glucocorticoid secretion is by feedback mechanism (Fig. 28.4). CRH from the hypothalamus causes ACTH release by the anterior pituitary gland, which in turn causes the release of cortisol.

The functions of cortisol Cortisol affects the metabolism of most body cells. It converts the intermittent intake of food into a steady level of glucose in the plasma by the stimulation of gluconeogenesis, the mobilisation of fatty acids and the breakdown of proteins for repair of tissues or enzyme manufacture.

Other functions of cortisol include:

- reducing inflammation following injury;
- enhancing the vasoconstrictive effects of noradrenaline (norepinephrine);
- increasing blood pressure and circulatory efficiency;
- helping to maintain fluid balance by preventing the shift of water into tissue cells.

In severe stress due to haemorrhage, infection, physical trauma or emotional distress, the output of glucocorticoids

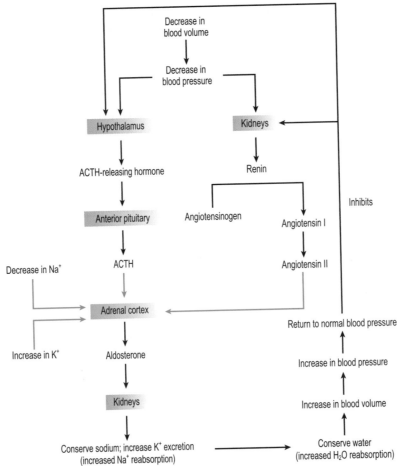

Figure 28.3   Regulation of aldosterone secretion (from Hinchliff S M, Montague S E, Watson R 1996, with permission).

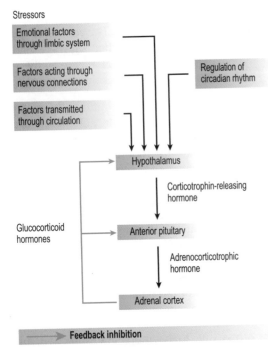

Figure 28.4   Regulation of glucocorticoid secretion.

rises dramatically to help the body through the crisis. Continuing high levels of glucocorticoids will:

1. depress cartilage and bone formation;
2. inhibit the inflammatory response;
3. depress the activity of the immune system;
4. cause changes in cardiovascular, neural and gastrointestinal function (Watkins 1997).

Gonadocorticoids

The main gonadocorticoids secreted are androgens. Small amounts of oestrogen and progesterone are also secreted. In adult women, adrenal androgens are thought to be responsible for libido. Adrenal oestrogens may replace ovarian oestrogens at the menopause.

The role of the fetal cortex

In the term fetus the adrenal gland is 20 times larger in relation to other organs than that of an adult. It regresses after birth and reaches normal proportions by 1 year. The fetal cortex appears to produce mainly **dehydroepiandrosterone sulphate** (DHEAS) which is the substrate for placental oestrogen synthesis. It cannot synthesise the glucocorticoids essential for important fetal processes. They may be obtained from the mother or synthesised by the placenta for:

1. surfactant production;
2. development of the hypothalamo–pituitary axis;
3. changes in placental structure and amniotic fluid composition during development;
4. initiation of endocrine changes in the fetus and mother that are responsible for the onset of labour;
5. the development of liver enzymes;
6. induction of thymic gland involution.

The adrenal medulla

The **chromaffin cells** produce the adrenal medullary hormones. The two main hormones, adrenaline (epinephrine) and noradrenaline (norepinephrine), are known as the **catecholamines**. About 80% of hormone production is adrenaline (epinephrine). Sympathetic nerve endings stimulate the adrenal medulla to produce the fight or flight response. Adrenaline (epinephrine) stimulates the heart and metabolic activity while noradrenaline (norepinephrine) affects peripheral vasoconstriction and blood pressure. Unlike cortical hormones, catecholamines produce short-term responses. During short-term stress the main effects of the sympathetic nervous system are a rise in blood sugar levels and constriction of blood vessels. The heart beats faster, blood pressure rises and blood is diverted to the brain and muscles.

Changes in the adrenal gland during pregnancy

Cortical function in pregnancy

ACTH plasma concentrations rise progressively during pregnancy, associated with a doubling of plasma cortisol, but still remain in the range for non-pregnant women.

Normally, a rise in plasma cortisol would suppress ACTH production, but the feedback mechanism appears to change during pregnancy. The placenta may contribute to the increase in plasma ACTH. The myometrium and decidua convert cortisone to cortisol, resulting in a local cortisol concentration of nine times normal. This may contribute to the immunological protection of the fetus.

Cortisol   There is a steady rise in plasma cortisol due to a doubling of CBG. Free plasma cortisol is increased with loss of diurnal variation so that there is a greater exposure of maternal tissues, especially in late pregnancy. It has been suggested that the cushingoid appearance in pregnancy with striae gravidarum, impaired carbohydrate tolerance and hypertension is due to excess cortisol. There is increased cortisol production in labour, probably due to stress.

Aldosterone   There is an increase in renin substrate due to the higher level of oestrogens. Excretion of sodium and chloride is increased in response to the presence of progesterone. Alterations in the renin–angiotensin mechanisms lead to increased aldosterone production, which enhances the reabsorption of sodium to maintain balance (Thomson 1996).

THE PINEAL GLAND

The minute **pineal gland** hangs from the floor of the third ventricle. Its secretory cells are called **pinealocytes**. Neural connections between the retina and pineal gland allow a light-regulated secretion of the hormone **melatonin** which waxes and wanes in a diurnal cycle; it is highest during the night and lowest about noon. In animals, melatonin controls reproduction and changes in the periods of light and dark affect gonadal size and mating behaviour. In humans, melatonin causes the hypothalamus to inhibit release of gonadotrophin-releasing hormone. It also causes daily variations in temperature, sleep and appetite.

MAIN POINTS

- Endocrine glands comprise the pituitary, thyroid, parathyroid, adrenal and pineal glands. The hypothalamus controls endocrine function. It has links with other parts of the nervous system. Hypothalamic releasing and inhibiting hormones influence the production of hormones by the anterior pituitary gland.

- Most amino acid-based hormones cannot penetrate cell membranes and utilise intracellular second messengers. Other amino acid-based hormones involve a third messenger, calcium, in their pathway. Steroid and thyroid hormones bind to intracellular receptors found in the cytosol or nucleus.

- Cellular activity depends on blood levels of the hormone, the relative numbers of target cell receptors and the affinity of the receptor for the hormone. Target cells may up-regulate or down-regulate receptors in response to levels of hormone. The synthesis and release of hormones depends on a system of negative feedback.

- The posterior pituitary gland does not manufacture hormones but acts as a storage unit, releasing the hypothalamic hormones. There are six anterior pituitary hormones: four regulate the hormonal functioning of other glands – TSH, ACTH, FSH and LH. The other two, GH and PRL, influence non-endocrine targets.

- Fetoplacental hormones influence the pituitary gland; the secretion of gonadotrophins, FSH and LH are inhibited. The pattern of hormone production by the anterior pituitary changes in the puerperium to accommodate lactation.

- ACTH plasma concentrations rise during pregnancy, associated with a doubling of plasma cortisol. The placenta may contribute to the increase in plasma ACTH. There is a local uterine cortisol concentration nine times normal, which may contribute to fetal immunological protection.

- The increase in size of the anterior pituitary gland during pregnancy makes the gland vulnerable to a reduction in blood supply due to vasospasm of the superior hypophyseal artery. The gland is more readily damaged in pregnancy, resulting in Sheehan's syndrome.

- Antidiuretic hormone production is similar in pregnant and non-pregnant women but osmoreceptors are reset to accommodate the extra blood volume of pregnancy.

- The thyroid gland produces the hormones thyroxine and triiodothyronine, which maintain normal metabolic functions. Thyroid function remains normal during pregnancy although some women develop thyroid hyperplasia. During pregnancy a balance is achieved by alterations in the metabolism of iodine. The uptake of iodine remains within normal limits.

- There are significant increases in plasma concentrations of the thyroid hormones and of TBG during pregnancy, probably influenced by oestrogen and human chorionic gonadotrophin. The changes have been linked with nausea and vomiting in pregnancy.

- In the adrenal cortex the outer zona glomerulosa produces mineralocorticoids, the middle zona fasciculata secretes glucocorticoids and the inner zona reticularis produces glucocorticoids and small amounts of gonadocorticoids.

- Aldosterone regulates sodium balance by stimulating reabsorption of sodium ions from the urine in the renal tubules and returning them to the bloodstream.

- Cortisol affects cellular metabolism by converting the intermittent intake of food into a steady level of glucose in the plasma. It reduces inflammation, enhances the vasoconstrictive effects of noradrenaline (norepinephrine), increases blood pressure and circulatory efficiency and maintains fluid balance by preventing the shift of water into cells.

- In severe stress the output of glucocorticoids rises to combat the crisis. However, continuing high levels of glucocorticoids will depress bone formation, inflammatory response and immune system function and cause changes in cardiovascular, neural and gastrointestinal function.

- The fetal adrenal glands appear to produce mainly DHEAS, the substrate for placental oestrogen synthesis. The fetal cortex cannot synthesise glucocorticoids, which may be obtained from the mother or synthesised by the placenta.

- Adrenaline (epinephrine) and noradrenaline (norepinephrine) are produced by the adrenal medulla. Adrenaline (epinephrine) stimulates the heart and metabolic activity while noradrenaline (norepinephrine) affects peripheral vasoconstriction and blood pressure. Their main effects are a rise in blood sugar and constriction of blood vessels.

- ACTH concentrations rise progressively during pregnancy, associated with a doubling of plasma cortisol, although they still remain in the range for non-pregnant women. The placenta may contribute to ACTH increase.

- There is a greater exposure of maternal tissues to cortisol in late pregnancy, which may cause striae gravidarum, impaired carbohydrate tolerance and hypertension. Cortisol production is increased in labour, probably due to stress.

- There is an increase in renin substrate due to the rise in circulating oestrogens. Excretion of sodium and chloride is increased in response to progesterone. Alterations in the renin–angiotensin mechanisms lead to increased aldosterone production, which enhances the reabsorption of sodium.

- Melatonin secretion is highest during the night and lowest at noon. In humans, melatonin inhibits the release of gonadotrophin-releasing hormone. Melatonin affects variations in temperature, sleep and appetite.

References

ACOG 2001 Thyroid disease in pregnancy. Practice Bulletin No 32. American College of Obstetrics and Gynecology 98(5):879–888.

Blackburn S T 2003 Maternal, Fetal and Neonatal Physiology: A Clinical Prespective, 3rd edn. W B Saunders, Philadelphia.

Boore J R P 1996 Endocrine function. In Hinchliff S M, Montague S E, Watson R (eds) Physiology for Nursing Practice, 2nd edn. Baillière Tindall, London.

Brook G D, Marshall N J 2001 Essential Endocrinology, 4th edn. Blackwell Science, Oxford.

Jacobs H S 1991 The hypothalamus and pituitary gland. In Hytten F, Chamberlain G (eds) Clinical Physiology in Obstetrics, 2nd edn. Blackwell Scientific, Oxford.

Leylek A, Toyaksi M, Arselcan T, Dokmetas S 1999 Immunologic and biochemical factors in hyperemesis gravidarum with or without hyperthyroxaemia. Gynecological and Obstetric Investigations 47:299–334.

Marieb E N 2000 Human Anatomy and Physiology, 5th edn. Benjamin/Cummings, New York.

Sheehan H L, Stanfield J P 1961 The pathogenesis of postpartum necrosis of the anterior lobe of the pituitary gland. Acta Endocrinologica 37:479.

Sleep J 1996 Complications of the third stage of labour. In Bennett V R, Brown L K (eds) Myles Textbook for Midwives, 12th edn. Churchill Livingstone, Edinburgh.

Thomson V 1996 Psychological and physiological changes of pregnancy. In Bennett V R, Brown L K (eds) Myles Textbook for Midwives, 12th edn. Churchill Livingstone, Edinburgh.

Vitoratos N, Salamalekis E, Kassanos D et al 2000 Hyperemesis gravidarum: its relationship to maternal immune response

and thyroid function. Prenatal Neonatal Medicine 5:363–367.

Watkins A 1997 Mind/Body Medicine. A Clinician's Guide to Psychoneuroimmunity. Churchill Livingstone, Edinburgh.

Annotated recommended reading

ACOG 2001 Thyroid disease in pregnancy. Practice Bulletin No 32. American College of Obstetrics and Gynecology 98(5):879–888.
Thyroid disease is the second most common endocrine problem seen in pregnancy after diabetes mellitus. This paper provides an excellent overview of thyroid disease in pregnancy and its management.

Brook G D, Marshall N J 2001 Essential Endocrinology, 4th edn. Blackwell Science, Oxford.
Although there are no references cited within the text of this book, it is an excellent source for students needing concise information about endocrinology. The chapters are well organised and content is easy to find.

Vitoratos N, Salamalekis E, Kassanos D et al 2000 Hyperemesis gravidarum: its relationship to maternal immune response and thyroid function. Prenatal Neonatal Medicine 5:363–367.
This paper presents a small research project considering a possible link between vomiting in pregnancy and hCG levels. The mechanisms by which thyroid function and changes in the immune system may influence the onset of nausea and vomiting in hyperemesis gravidarum were studied.

Chapter 29

The immune system

CHAPTER CONTENTS

INTRODUCTION

The immune system protects the individual from environmental factors such as microorganisms, irritants and abnormal cells. Pathogens such as viruses, bacteria and fungi constantly mount invasions of the body, both on its surface and internally (Roitt et al 2001). Larger organisms such as worms are parasitic, living by tapping into bodily metabolic processes (Kendall 1998). Many microorganisms do not cause disease in the healthy person but may threaten life if the immune system is defective.

In developed countries, infection accounts for fewer than 2% of deaths. However, there are new problems such as the development of resistant strains of bacteria such as methicillin-resistant *Staphylococcus aureus* (MRSA). Almost 50% of travellers to tropical countries suffer with diarrhoea (Kendall 1998). Global travel makes the transfer of deadly diseases much more rapid. The outbreak of severe acute respiratory syndrome (SARS) in April 2003 is an example.

DIVISIONS OF THE IMMUNE SYSTEM

The immune system recognises pathogens and mounts an immune response to eliminate them. Because there are many different pathogens, a wide variety of immune responses are needed (Roitt et al 2001). There are three lines of defence in the immune system: the first two, **surface barriers** and the **inflammatory response**, are **non-specific** and the third is a **specific** response to a particular foreign protein. Non-specific immunity (**innate**) immediately protects the body from a range of substances while specific immunity (**acquired**, **adaptive**) acts against a particular invader but must be primed by its presence and takes time to develop. A high level of interdependence exists between the two categories of immune response and they work together to either destroy the invading organism or reduce its harmful effects (Fig. 29.1).

CELLS OF THE IMMUNE SYSTEM

Immune responses are mediated by a variety of cells and the soluble molecules which they secrete. **Leucocytes** (white

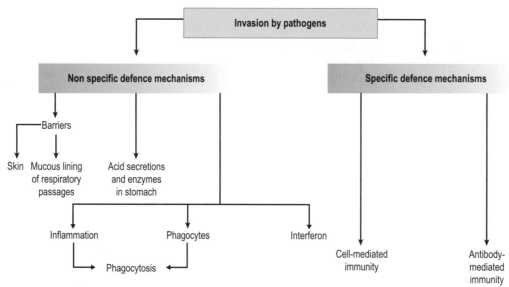

Figure 29.1   Summary of specific and non-specific defence mechanisms. Non-specific mechanisms prevent entry of many pathogens and act rapidly to destroy those that manage to cross the barriers. Specific defence mechanisms take longer to mobilise but they are highly effective in destroying invaders (from Hinchliff S M, Montague S E, Watson R 1996, with permission).

blood cells, WBCs) are protective against bacteria, viruses, parasites, toxins and tumour cells. There are normally about 4000–11 000 per cubic mm ($4–11 \times 10^9$/L). Most leucocytes are in the tissues and there is a wide variation in the blood count as cells enter and leave the circulation from hour to hour. All leucocytes are produced in the bone marrow from **haemopoietic stem cells** (Roitt et al 2001).

Types of leucocyte

Several types of leucocyte are distinguished by their shape, appearance and function. **Granulocytes** (polymorphonuclear leucocytes) have granules in their cytoplasm which contain substances that fight infection. They are 10–14 μm in diameter and have a lobed nucleus. They are divided into three groups, **neutrophils**, **eosinophils** and **basophils**, by the size of their granules. All are **phagocytic**, engulfing and destroying foreign proteins. **Natural killer cells** (NK cells) are a specialised type of large granular lymphocyte. **Agranulocytes**, which include **lymphocytes** and **monocytes**, do not contain granules.

Granulocytes

- Neutrophils contain granules that stain violet because they take up both acidic red dyes and basic blue dyes. They account for more than 50% of granulocytes and have the most lobular nucleus. Neutrophils migrate to sites of inflammation. They are short-lived cells that engulf foreign material such as bacteria, destroy it and die.

- Eosinophils have large granules which stain red with acidic dyes. They make up about 1–4% of the leucocyte population. They attack parasitic worms by surrounding

them and releasing granular enzymes onto the parasite's surface to digest it from the outside. Eosinophils also deal with allergy by destroying antigen–antibody complexes.

- Basophils have large granules that take up a basic dye and stain blue-black. They account for only 0.5% of white cells. Their large granules contain histamine, an inflammatory substance that acts as a vasodilator and draws other white blood cells to the site of inflammation. Mast cells are similar to basophils and are present in connective tissue. Both types of cell release histamine when they bind to immunoglobulin E.

The production of granulocytes   The process of **granulopoiesis** takes about 14 days but is considerably reduced if cells are urgently needed. There is progressive condensation and lobulation of the nucleus, loss of organelles and development of granules in the cytoplasm. Within 7 h of reaching the circulation, half of the granulocytes will have migrated into tissue and will not return. They survive about 5 days and are eliminated from the body in faeces and respiratory secretions and form pus at infection sites. For every granulocyte in the circulation, there may be 50 in bone marrow.

Natural killer cells are present in blood and lymph and destroy cancer cells and virus-infected body cells. They account for 15% of blood lymphocytes. Unlike other lymphocytes which only react to specific virus-infected or tumour cells, NK cells react against cells which do not express **major histocompatibility complex (MHC) class 1 molecules** (see below), an important factor in the immunology of pregnancy.

Agranulocytes

Lymphocytes are round cells with large round nuclei and are the second most common type of leucocyte. Immature cells migrate to the **thymus** and other **lymphoid tissue** to divide and mature. Large numbers exist in the body but most are found in lymphoid tissue. They recirculate between blood and lymph and are subdivided into small and large lymphocytes. There are two types of lymphocytes: **T** and **B lymphocytes**. Some lymphocytes leave the bone marrow and migrate to the thymus gland where they become T cells. They are selected so that they will not attack **self-antigens** present on the surface of the individual's own cells. B cells were first identified in the **bursa of Fabricius**, a pocket of lymphatic tissue associated with the digestive tract in birds. T cells are involved in cell-mediated immune responses and account for 80% of the lymphocytes present in blood. B cells are involved in humoral immunity and produce antibodies.

Monocytes are large cells produced in the bone marrow from **myeloid progenitors**. Mature cells spend about 30 h in the blood and then migrate to the tissues, where they develop into phagocytic **macrophages** (giant eaters). Macrophages regulate the immune response by presenting antigens to activate B and T cells.

Non-specific defences

These can be divided into surface barriers, such as the skin and mucous membranes, and cellular and chemical defences.

Surface barriers include:

- a thickly keratinised unbroken skin;
- intact mucous membranes lining the organs;
- acidic secretions, such as in the vagina, gastric juices and urine;
- sticky mucus to trap organisms;
- ciliated cells that sweep particles towards the outside;
- lysozyme, an enzyme that destroys bacteria, in saliva and tears.

Phagocytes

If the intact surfaces are breached, cellular and chemical non-specific defence mechanisms are triggered. In most cases, phagocytic cells (Fig. 29.2) will be involved. These are amoeba-like and travel though tissue spaces in search of invading organisms or other debris to engulf and destroy.

Macrophages are the main phagocytic cells but neutrophils become phagocytic if an infection is present. Macrophages are long-lived cells but neutrophils are destroyed during phagocytosis. Both cells destroy microbes by producing **free radicals**. Neutrophils also produce antibiotic-like chemicals called **defensins**. **Complement proteins** and antibodies coat foreign particles and provide binding sites for attachment of phagocytes, a process called **opsonisation**.

Inflammation

Inflammation is a local response which occurs when there is tissue injury due to trauma or invasion by microorganisms.

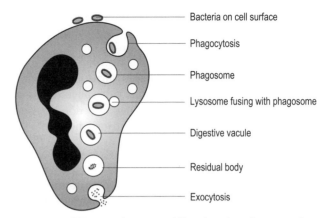

Figure 29.2 Diagram of a neutrophil undergoing phagocytosis (from Hinchliff S M, Montague S E 1990, with permission).

The inflammatory response prevents the spread of damaging substances to nearby tissues, disposes of cell debris and pathogens and allows repair to begin. There are four **cardinal signs** of inflammation: heat, redness, swelling and pain. Depending on the site and type of tissue damage, chemicals are released into the extracellular fluid by injured cells, phagocytes, lymphocytes, mast cells and blood proteins. Four major plasma enzyme systems are involved in the control of inflammation (Roitt et al 2001):

- the clotting system;
- the fibrinolytic system;
- the kinin system;
- the complement system.

The most important molecules are **histamine**, **kinins**, **prostaglandins**, **complement** and **lymphokines**. They induce vasodilation of localised small blood vessels, causing heat and redness. Capillary wall permeability increases, allowing a fluid exudate containing clotting factors and antibodies to seep into the tissue spaces and cause oedema and swelling. Clotting proteins form a **fibrin mesh** which limits the spread of harmful agents and acts as scaffolding for tissue repair. Pain results from pressure on local nerve endings, release of bacterial toxins, lack of cellular nutrition and the effects of prostaglandins and kinins. Loss of function may occur, forcing the person to rest the injured part to aid healing.

The damaged area is first invaded by phagocytes. Rapid release of neutrophils by the bone marrow is caused by **leucocyte-inducing factors** so that four times as many neutrophils may be in the bloodstream after a few hours. These cells are attracted to the injury site by chemicals called **chemotactic agents**. At the site, they cling to the capillary walls (**margination** or **pavementing**) and squeeze through capillary walls (**diapedesis**) to the site where they devour bacteria, toxins and dead tissue. Monocytes now enter the tissue, swell and mature into macrophages.

If the infection is severe, pus – which is a mixture of dead neutrophils, living and dead pathogens and damaged tissue cells – is produced. If this becomes walled off by collagen fibres, an abscess forms. Some bacteria like the tuberculosis bacillus are resistant to digestion by macrophages because of their waxy outer coat and remain alive inside the macrophage. Infectious **granulomas** develop which have a central core of infected macrophages surrounded by uninfected macrophages and an outer fibrous capsule. The person only becomes ill if his resistance to infection is reduced when the bacteria may break out and cause disease.

Fever

Fever is an elevation of the body temperature in response to chemicals called **pyrogens** such as the **interleukins**. High fevers are dangerous because they inactivate enzymes and disrupt cellular metabolic processes but mild to moderate fevers are helpful to the body in stimulating the immune system (Kendall 1998). Fever speeds up both metabolic rate of tissue and defensive actions to aid repair. Other antibacterial responses include the sequestering of iron and zinc in the liver and spleen to prevent the bacteria using these essential nutrients to proliferate.

Complement

Complement is a system of about 30 antimicrobial plasma proteins constituting 10% of total plasma proteins. They normally circulate in the blood in an inactive state. In evolutionary terms they are very old and developed long before the adaptive immune system (Roitt et al 2001). Their functions are:

- control of inflammatory reactions;
- chemotaxis;
- clearance of immune complexes;
- cellular inactivation;
- antimicrobial defence;
- development of antibody responses.

The proteins are named **C1–C9**. Activation of the complement system releases chemical mediators that support and increase most parts of the inflammatory process and enhance the specific immune system. Complement can be activated by three pathways, all of which activate C3, causing it to split into two fragments, C3a and C3b:

- the evolutionary younger **classical pathway** (Fig. 29.3) is activated by the formation of antigen–antibody complexes;
- the **lectin pathway** is similar to the classical pathway and is activated by bacterial carbohydrates;
- the older alternative pathway provides non-specific immunity and is triggered by the presence of microbial pathogens.

An orderly **cascade** of complement protein activation occurs and C3b binds to the target cell's surface. This results in the insertion of a group of complement proteins called the **membrane attack complex** (MAC) into the bacterial cell wall, forming a hole and allowing solutes to leak from the cell and destroying it (Roitt et al 2001).

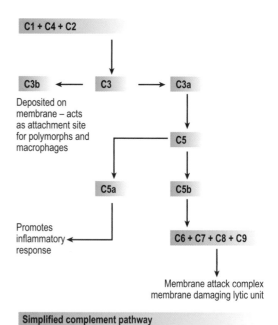

Simplified complement pathway

Figure 29.3 Simplified complement pathway (from Hinchliff S M, Montague S E, Watson R 1996, with permission).

Specific defence – the immune system

Tissues of the lymphatic system

The lymphatic system consists of two parts: a network of lymphatic vessels and lymphoid organs and tissues throughout the body. The organs and tissues are divided into **primary lymphoid organs** such as the bone marrow and thymus gland where B cells and T cells mature and the **peripheral lymphoid system** where they spend most of their active lives (Fig. 29.4). The peripheral lymphoid system includes encapsulated organs such as the spleen, tonsils and lymph nodes. Unencapsulated lymphoid tissue is found in association with mucosal surfaces in the gut, lungs and urogenital tract (Roitt et al 2001).

Lymph nodes The immune response takes place in the lymphatic system. **Lymph nodes** (Fig. 29.5) are encapsulated kidney-shaped glands (about 2–10 mm in diameter) which filter lymph. They consist of a radial network of fibres in which lymphocytes are embedded. The inner medulla contains macrophages, T cells, B cells and plasma cells. B cells are concentrated in primary and secondary follicles in the outer cortex. Cells at the centre of a follicle actively divide while those at the periphery produce antibodies. T cells are found in the paracortical area.

Macrophages tend to be fixed in the lymphoid organs, whereas lymphocytes also circulate throughout the body. Lymph capillaries pick up pathogens and other foreign proteins. The presence of immune cells in lymph nodes is protective: for instance, lymphocytes and macrophages in the tonsils combat organisms that invade the nasal and oral cavities.

The spleen The **spleen** is the largest lymphoid organ and is located on the left side of the body just below the diaphragm.

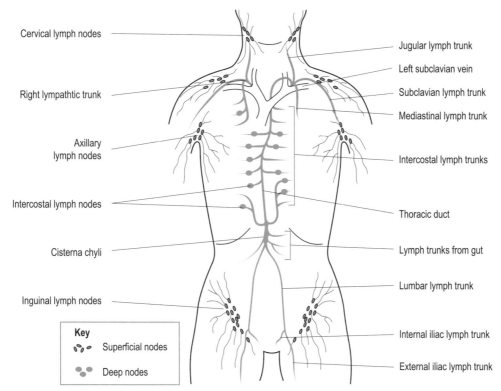

Figure 29.4   General arrangement of the lymphatic system (from Hinchliff S M, Montague S E 1990, with permission).

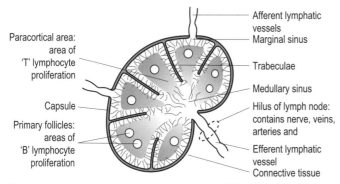

Figure 29.5   Section through a lymph gland (from Hinchliff S M, Montague S E 1990, with permission).

It is about 18 cm × 8 cm in size and weighs 200 g. It is composed of venous sinuses and reticular connective tissue forming the **red pulp** where removal of ageing and defective red cells, cellular debris and microorganisms from the blood takes place. There are areas of reticular fibres with attached lymphocytes called the **white pulp**, which provide sites for the proliferation of lymphocytes. The spleen stores the products from broken-down red cells and blood platelets. During fetal life, it is a site of red cell production.

The thymus gland   This bilobed gland, found in the mediastinum of the thorax, is more active in the early years of life. It is organised into lobules separated by connective tissue. Within each lobule, the lymphoid cells (**thymoytes**) are arranged in an outer cortex and inner medulla. The cortex contains immature cells and the medulla contains densely packed, more mature cells. During adolescence it decreases in size and starts to atrophy. The thymus is involved in the differentiation of the T lymphocytes. In the embryo, stem cells migrate from the bone marrow to the thymus, where they mature and differentiate.

Lymphatic vessels   An extensive network of lymphatic vessels connects the body's tissues to lymphoid organs. Lymphatic capillaries are like blood capillaries but the endothelial cells of their walls do not lie on a basement membrane. They join up to make larger lymphatic vessels which contain smooth muscles in their walls and have one-way valves. The flow of lymph is ensured by skeletal muscle contraction and negative intrathoracic pressure. Unlike veins, lymphatic vessels contract rhythmically to help the lymph flow.

Lymph

Lymph originates as plasma which leaks from the blood capillaries. It transports water and small molecules and contains proteins which enter the capillary lumen between the endothelial cells. Fluids and solutes enter lymphatic capillaries along their length and dietary fat is absorbed as triglycerides from the small intestinal villi. Up to 4 L of lymph accumulates over 24 h and is returned to the blood.

Lymph enters lymph nodes by afferent vessels and leaves via an efferent vessel. Lymph is returned to the blood into the large veins in the neck via the thoracic duct, which arises anterior to the second lumbar vertebra as an enlarged sac called the cisterna chyli. It drains the lower limbs, digestive system, the left arm and left side of the thorax, neck and head. The smaller right lymphatic duct accepts lymph from the right arm and right side of thorax, neck and head.

THE IMMUNE RESPONSE

There are three important aspects of the immune response:

1. it is antigen-specific – directed against particular pathogens or foreign substances;
2. it is systemic – not restricted to the initial site of infection;
3. it has memory – once it has recognised a foreign antigen, it responds by producing antibodies to subsequent invasion by the same molecule.

Immunity can be divided into two types. **Humoral immunity** or antibody-mediated immunity is provided by the presence of antibodies in body fluids (humors). When lymphocytes attack the invader directly, the process is called **cellular immunity** or **cell-mediated immunity** (Fig. 29.6). Three cell types are involved in the immune response:

- B lymphocytes produce antibodies and are responsible for humoral-mediated immunity;
- T lymphocytes do not produce antibodies and are involved in cell-mediated immunity;
- macrophages support the two sets of lymphocytes.

The humoral immune response

Antigens

Recognition of a foreign antigen is the basis for specific, adaptive immunity (Roitt et al 2001). Two different types of molecule are involved: immunoglobulins and T-cell antigen receptors. The first encounter between an invading antigen and an immunocompetent lymphocyte involves the activation of a B cell and the collaboration of T cells. Foreign antigens such as proteins, nucleic acids, lipids and large polysaccharides are non-self, i.e. not usually present in the

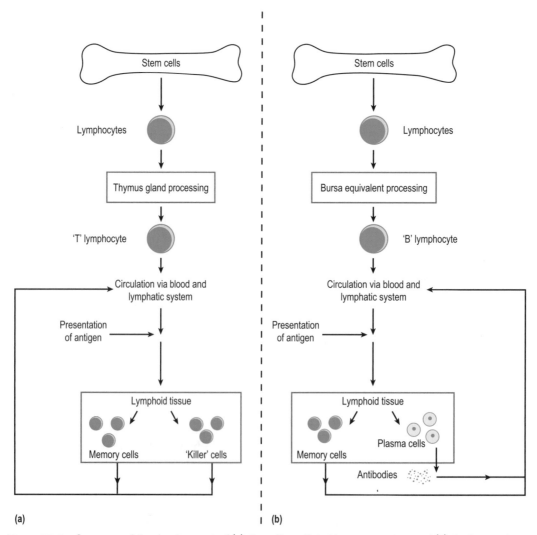

Figure 29.6 Summary of the development of (a) the cell-mediated immune system and (b) the humoral immune system (from Hinchliff S M, Montague S E 1990, with permission).

body. A small area on an antigen called the **epitope** is recognised by a small area on a B-lymphocyte cell membrane receptor called the **antigen-binding site**.

Pollen grains and microorganisms are the strongest antigens. Small molecules such as peptides, nucleotides and hormones are not immunogenic but may form a complex with the body's proteins to cause allergies. Such molecules are called **haptens** and include drugs, detergents, plant products and industrial pollutants. The immune system responds by antibody production.

Clonal selection

The binding of the antigen and the lymphocyte stimulates the B cell to divide rapidly, forming a **clone** of identical cells that are able to recognise that antigen. As the response is so specific, a huge variety of lymphocytes are available to recognise the enormous number of antigens met throughout life. This response to a particular antigen by a specific lymphocyte is called clonal selection.

Most clone cells differentiate into **antibody-forming cells** (AFCs or plasma cells), which secrete antibody molecules at about 2000 per second for 5 days before the cell dies. Antibodies circulate in blood and lymph, where they bind to antigens and present them to phagocytes for destruction. This primary immune response occurs the first time the body meets the antigen. There is a lag of about 3–6 days as

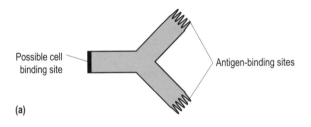

Possible cell binding site — Antigen-binding sites

(a)

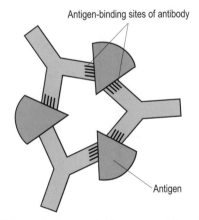

Antigen-binding sites of antibody

Antigen

(b)

Figure 29.7   Schematic diagram (a) to represent the structure of a simple (IgG type) antibody and (b) to illustrate the way in which this bivalent structure enables antigens to be clumped together (from Hinchliff S M, Montague S E 1990, with permission).

the B cells proliferate and form AFCs. Plasma antibody levels then rise, reaching a peak at 10 days.

Immunological memory

Those clone cells that do not differentiate into plasma cells become long-lived **memory cells**, able to mount a rapid humoral response if the antigen is encountered again. Then, a secondary immune response occurs that is faster, prolonged and more effective because the memory cells produce a new clone of plasma cells within hours. Peak levels are reached within 2 days.

Antibodies

Antibodies, also called immunoglobulins (Igs), are a group of glycoproteins present in the blood and tissue fluid (Fig. 29.7). Some are present on the surface of B cells, where they act as receptors for specific antigens. Others, secreted by the activated B cell and the cloned AFCs following an encounter with a specific antigen, are free in blood and lymph. Individuals come into contact with a great number of antigens and there is a need for tremendous antibody diversity to combat them (see Box 29.1).

Antibody classes

The five classes of **immunoglobulin** (Ig) are given Greek alphabet names, depending on their heavy chain structure. They are:

1. Gamma (γ) – IgG is produced in large quantities in the secondary response, diffuses easily through blood vessel walls and is the major class of antibody found in tissue fluids. IgG is quite successful at activating the classical complement pathway. It crosses the human placenta to confer passive immunity to the fetus and is found in colostrum and breast milk.

2. Alpha (α) – IgA protects the exposed surfaces of the body against bacteria and fungi. It is found in the secretions of mucous membranes lining the organs and in watery secretions such as tears, saliva and perspiration.

3. Mu (μ) – IgM is a large immunoglobulin found mainly in serum and is the first and most abundant antibody to be secreted during the primary response. It can bind to multiple antigens and causes them to agglutinate so that they are more easily recognised by phagocytes. IgM is a potent trigger of the classical complement pathway.

4. Delta (δ) – IgD is mainly found attached to B cells and may be involved in their differentiation.

5. Epsilon (ε) – IgE precipitates inflammatory reactions around parasites. It is mainly bound by its constant region to the surface of basophils and mast cells in skin, lungs and mucous membranes and responds to inhaled antigens. IgE is implicated in allergy and hypersensitivity reactions.

Box 29.1 Generation of antibody diversity

The following facts help to explain antibody diversity:

1. a small number of immunoglobulin genes are recombined in individual B cells so that each mature B cell contains a unique antibody molecule;
2. the genes are found on different chromosomes so that the antibody chains are made separately and recombined inside the cell.

Antibodies are grouped into five classes, each with a specific function. There is a basic antibody structure made of four polypeptide chains linked together by disulphide bonds. There are two identical **heavy chains** and two identical **light chains** about half as long. The heavy chains are structurally distinct for each antibody class and are hinged about half way along their length. There are two distinct types of light chains: λ (lambda) and κ (kappa). The chains form a Y-shaped molecule.

Each of the four chains is made up of different regions joined together. Each has a **variable** or V region, which differs between antibodies and forms the binding site at one end, and a much larger **constant** or C region. Between the V and C sections of light chains is the **joining** or J region. In heavy chains there is an additional region between the J and V sections called the **diversity** or D region. These multiple regions greatly increase the number of antibodies available to counteract antigens (Fig. 29.8).

Recombination of the immunoglobulin genes can be understood by thinking about Lego bricks. If a box held five bricks of each of five colours – red, black, blue, yellow and white – and these could be combined in any order from all one colour through to five different colours, think how many combinations of five bricks could be achieved! As the light and heavy chains, with all their variable sites, are combined separately from each other, millions of antibody configurations are possible.

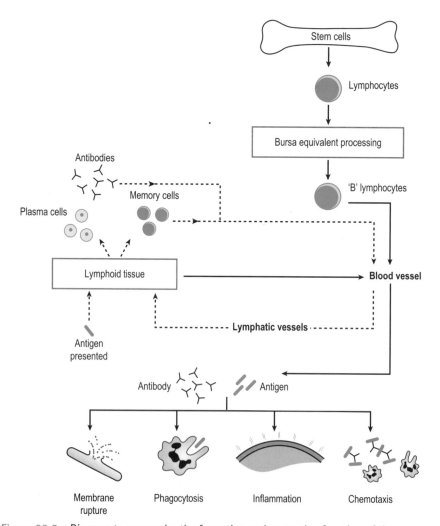

Figure 29.8   Diagram to summarise the formation and protective function of the humoral immune system (from Hinchliff S M, Montague S E 1990, with permission).

Antibody functioning

Antibodies do not destroy antigens directly but inactivate them and tag them for other parts of the immune system to destroy by forming **antigen–antibody (immune) complexes**. The destruction of antigen-bearing molecules is accomplished by mechanisms including complement fixation, neutralisation, agglutination and precipitation. The first two of these are most important:

- **Complement fixation** is the main protection against cellular antigens such as bacteria. When antibodies bind to the target cell, their shape changes and this exposes complement-binding sites on their constant regions, which triggers the complement cascade.

- **Neutralisation** is a mechanism whereby antibodies block specific sites on viruses or chemicals secreted by bacteria (**exotoxins**), thus preventing them from binding to cells. Phagocytes destroy the resulting immune complexes.

- **Agglutination** of cell-bound antigens occurs because antibodies have more than one binding site and molecules have more than one antigenic site. Large lattices are formed by the cross-linkage of immune complexes.

- **Precipitation** is a similar mechanism whereby soluble molecules are cross-linked into large complexes that settle out of solution. The large complexes caused by agglutination or precipitation become a target for engulfing by phagocytes.

Antigen–antibody interaction

Formation of non-covalent bonds Antibodies form multiple non-covalent bonds (Ch. 1, p. 4) with antigens. The hypervariable regions at the end of the two arms of the Y shape form bonds with the antigen. Although the hydrogen and electrostatic bonds and van der Waals and hydrophobic forces acting at the site are weak, the large number of interactions adds up to a large total binding energy. The strength of non-covalent bonds depends on proximity. The antigen epitope and antibody paratope must have close complementary configurations to accomplish successful neutralising of the antigen. Ideally, they would be perfect mirror images of each other, as in a well-cut jigsaw puzzle.

Cell-mediated immune response

T lymphocytes

T lymphocytes form the basis for cellular immunity. They are much more complex than B cells in their classification and function. There are two major groups of T cells: **cytotoxic T cells**, T_C or killer cells, and **helper T cells** or T_H cells (Fig. 29.9). All T cells have glycoproteins on their cell surfaces, which are the **CD4** and **CD8 surface receptor molecules** (CD means cluster of differentiation). Generally, T_H cells have CD4 proteins and are also known as T4 cells, especially in the HIV and AIDS literature, and T_C cells have CD8 molecules on their surfaces and are known as T8 cells. Although there is evidence that suppressor T cells (T_S) exist, they probably do not form a functionally separate subset. Both CD4 and CD8 cells can suppress immune responses (Roitt et al 2001).

The T-cell antigen receptor T cells are also distinguished by the type of **T-cell antigen receptor** (TCR) on their cell surface. Antigen recognition by T cells is central to the generation and regulation of an effective immune response (Roitt et al 2001). The TCR recognises antigen fragments which are bound and presented by specialised antigen-presenting molecules. They do not recognise free antigen: that is the role of antibodies. The most important of these molecules are the **class I** and **class II molecules** of the **major histocompatibility complex** (MHC). TCRs and antibodies are structurally related and both reproduce by cloning.

T-cell differentiation – the major histocompatibility complex For T cells to be selected and cloning to occur there must be a double recognition of **antiself** (the antigen) and **self**. Every cell has surface proteins that identify it as self. These are coded for by the MHC, which is a very large gene complex. This provides the basis of human uniqueness, as the genes can be combined in millions of ways. Tissue transplants from one person to another are difficult because they are unlikely to have identical MHC proteins unless they are identical twins.

There are two main classes of MHC protein important in T cell activation: MHC class I and MHC class II (Engelhard 1994). MHC I proteins are present on most body cells to enable self recognition but MHC II proteins are found only on the surfaces of mature B cells, macrophages and some T cells. MHC proteins are the self part of the self–antiself complex which activates T cells. MHC cells are shaped like a hammock, so that the antigenic fragment to be displayed sits inside them. T_H and T_C cells prefer different classes of MHC protein, a phenomenon called MHC restriction:

- T_H cells bind only to complexes which include MHC II proteins on the surfaces of macrophages;
- T_C cells are activated by complexes which include MHC I proteins on any cell.

Immunologic surveillance T cells crawl over other cells searching for antigens, a process called **immunologic surveillance**. When the T cell is activated by binding to the self–antiself complex, it enlarges and forms a clone. After the primary response, as with B cells, some are left as memory cells. T_C cells act mainly against virus-infected cells but can kill cells invaded by some bacteria such as the tubercle bacillus. T_H cells stimulate the proliferation of other T cells and B cells by releasing a **lymphokine** called **interleukin II**. Some T cells release lymphokines that inhibit the activated B cells and T cells, ensuring that the immune response is brought to an end after the successful destruction of an antigen.

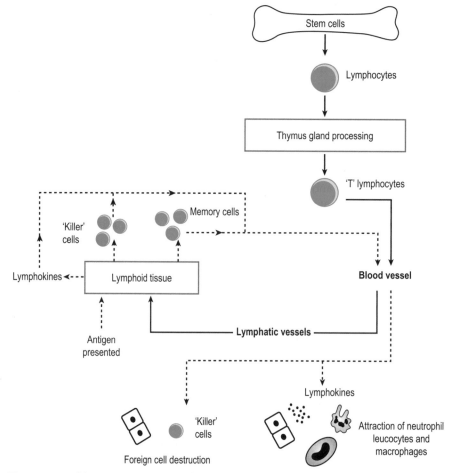

Figure 29.9   Diagram to summarise the formation and protective function of the cell-mediated immune system (from Hinchliff S M, Montague S E 1990, with permission).

Most T-cell activity is by T_C cells attacking cells infected by microorganisms, cancerous cells or transplanted tissue.

Cytokines

The cells of the immune system release chemicals called **cytokines** (from cells) to stimulate each other. These soluble glycoproteins fall into different categories: e.g. they are called lymphokines when released by lymphocytes. Lymphokines enhance the activity of immune system cells including the T cells themselves, B cells and macrophages.

The principal sets of cytokines (Roitt et al 2001)

- **Interferons** (IFNs) limit the spread of intracellular viral infections. They are produced by certain T cells early in a viral infection and may be the first line of resistance. They diffuse to nearby cells and stimulate them to produce proteins that inhibit viral replication. There are α (alpha) interferons produced by most white cells and γ (gamma) interferons produced by lymphocytes. NK cells produce gamma interferons which can activate macrophages.

- **Interleukins** (ILs) are a large group; 22 have been found. They are named IL-1, IL-2, etc., and are produced mainly by T cells. They mainly direct other immune system cells to divide and differentiate.

- **Colony-stimulating factors** (CSFs) are primarily involved in directing the division and differentiation of bone marrow stem cells.

- **Chemokines** are chemotactic cytokines which direct cell movement around the body: for example, movement of immune cells out of the blood into the tissues to combat infection.

- **Tumour necrosis factors** (TNFs) are important in mediating inflammation and cytotoxic reactions.

The brain's immune system

White cells secrete substances capable of killing neurons but these are prevented from entering the brain by the blood–brain barrier unless blood vessels are damaged. Microglia can become phagocytic and are the cells that HIV attacks in the brain; their activation is implicated in AIDS dementia.

PHYSIOLOGICAL CHANGES IN PREGNANCY

The immune system in the pregnant woman undergoes minor alterations to both primary and secondary defence mechanisms but they can still respond immunologically to the fetus. The fetus is antigenically unique as are all humans and an unsolved mystery is why the fetus is not rejected as foreign tissue. While helping to protect the fetus, the changes may increase the severity of some maternal infections and influence the progress of autoimmune diseases (Blackburn 2003).

White cell count

The total white cell count rises early in pregnancy mainly due to an increase in neutrophils and probably caused by circulating oestrogen. A peak is reached at 30 weeks and a plateau maintained until delivery. There is a further rise in labour and the count returns to normal by the 6th postnatal day. There is a slight rise in circulating eosinophils in ratio to the increased white cell count but a sharp fall occurs during labour. They are absent at delivery, returning to normal by the 3rd postnatal day. The basophil and monocyte counts appear to remain unchanged.

Cell-mediated immunity

Although the lymphocyte count remains unchanged in pregnancy, there is a change in cell-mediated immunity. T_H cells decline in relation to T_C cells able to suppress the immune response, possibly due to circulating pregnancy hormones. However, these changes are insufficient to prevent fetal rejection and other mechanisms must be present (Johnson & Everitt 2000). It is likely that both maternal and fetoplacental mechanisms help prevent fetal rejection during pregnancy.

IMMUNOLOGY OF THE FETOPLACENTAL UNIT

Any theory of maternal immunological tolerance of the fetus must explain why the normal mechanisms of graft rejection do not occur. The alterations in the woman's immune system during pregnancy are insufficient to prevent the rejection of the fetus, so there must be other explanations. The fetoplacental unit is an **allograft** (foreign tissue from the same species) with different MHC cell surface receptors as paternal antigens are expressed on fetal cells as early as the eight-cell stage (Roitt et al 2001).

Local inhibition of immune response

There may be local immune regulation in the uterus. T cells are low in number in the decidua and may not recognise the antigens on the invading trophoblast cells. High local levels of progesterone, corticosteroids, and/or human chorionic gonadotrophin (hCG) may moderate local immune response. A high local metabolism of the amino acid **tryptophan** might reduce maternal immune response but there is no evidence as to how these mechanisms might work (Roitt et al 2001).

Protective immunological barrier

The fetus and its circulating blood are separated from the mother by the fetal membranes. The trophoblast at the feto-maternal interface may be important in protecting the fetus from the maternal immune system. If the chorionic trophoblast could prevent maternal immune cells and antibodies from entering the fetal circulation, fetal protection could be achieved (Johnson & Everitt 2000).

Studies have shown that neither the villous cytotrophoblast nor the syncytiotrophoblast express class I MHC antigens. However, the trophoblast cells which invade the uterus, especially in the spiral arteries, express other MHC molecules – namely human leucocyte antigens HLA-C and HLA-G – not expressed by either fetal or maternal cells. Most MHC receptors are downgraded in trophoblastic cells, except for HLA-C and HLA-G. This appears to confer resistance to destruction by NK cells by inhibiting cytokine production.

The fetal immune response

Although the barrier is effective against most cells and antibodies in humans, IgG crosses to the fetus to protect it against any infectious diseases the mother has suffered. Other antibodies may cross the placental barrier (e.g. rhesus incompatibility). The fetal immune system may be able to destroy such proteins. The rhesus antigen only exists as a cell surface antigen and is never found as a free molecule. As red blood cells are too large to cross the placental barrier, there is no possibility of raising fetal antibodies unless there is an escape of maternal red cells into fetal blood, usually at delivery. Unlike the rhesus antigen, other fetal cell surface antigens such as the ABO system and major MHC molecules are naturally present as soluble molecules in fetal blood or tissue fluids. If any maternal immune cells or antibodies cross the placental barrier, they are likely to be mopped up by free fetal antigens before they can damage fetal cells.

Johnson & Everitt (2000) summarise the above theories of non-rejection:

1. there is an antigenically inert trophoblast together with local, hormonally mediated depression of immune reactivity;
2. special populations of NK cells can recognise trophoblast-specific HLAs;
3. a highly selective barrier blocks transmission of immune cells or antibodies from mother to fetus;
4. any maternal immune cells or antibodies that do get across the placental barrier are mopped up before they can cause extensive fetal damage.

The immunology of breast milk

Colostrum and breast milk during the 1st week following delivery contain enormous quantities of immunoglobulin capable of reacting against many microorganisms. Bacteria that may cause gastroenteritis in the neonate are especially protected against. After the 1st week, it is mainly IgA which is present. A wider discussion on the anti-infective benefits of breastfeeding is found in Chapter 54.

CLINICAL IMPLICATIONS

Active and passive humoral immunity

Active immunity

Immunity to infectious diseases is naturally acquired when a person's B cells produce antibodies against a bacterium or virus during an infection. However, the symptoms of the disease may cause serious illness or even death. Edward Jenner noticed that people who caught cowpox were unaffected by smallpox. In 1796 he inoculated James Phipps with liquid from a pustule on the hand of a milkmaid who had cowpox. He then inoculated him with pus from a smallpox sufferer and James did not develop the disease. This technique is now used on a massive scale: protection of a person against infectious diseases by raising antibodies. The word **vaccine** derives from this experiment (the Latin for cow is *vacca*). Most vaccines contain dead or attenuated (weakened) pathogens which actively challenge the immune system without producing symptoms.

Passive immunity

Just as active immunity can be naturally or artificially acquired, so can passive immunity. The antibodies are not actively produced by a person's immune system but are obtained from another source. Protection against disease is limited to the survival time of the acquired antibodies, at most 2–3 weeks. Naturally occurring passive immunity is acquired by the fetus from the mother with the transfer of IgG across the placenta and by the breastfed baby because of the antibodies in breast milk. Injection of immune serum such as gamma-globulin can offer passive immunity to a person needing short-term protection from a pathogen with which they have been in contact, such as hepatitis virus.

Autoimmune disorders

There may be improvement, deterioration or no change in the status of **autoimmune disorders** during pregnancy. The pathology of autoimmune disorders may involve failure to deselect thymic T cells which are potentially **autoreactive**. There may also be populations of autoreactive B cells. Both T cells and autoantigens (self cells) are needed to allow production of autoantibodies. The resulting immune complexes activate the complement system, mediating phagocytosis and an inflammatory response (Roitt et al 2001).

The changes in the immune system in pregnancy are exactly opposite to the above events, so that women with autoimmune disorders should experience relief from their symptoms. Most women with **rheumatoid arthritis** improve during pregnancy. However, women with **systemic lupus erythematosus** (SLE), particularly those with renal involvement, may have an exacerbation of their condition, affecting the fetus and neonate adversely (Classen et al 1998). SLE is also associated with an increase in stillbirth and abortion (Johnson & Everitt 2000).

Maternal antibodies and the fetus

The fetus of a woman with autoimmune disease may develop transient autoimmune symptoms. In **Graves' disease** a thyroid-stimulating immunoglobulin passes across the placenta and may cause neonatal hyperthyroidism. **Myasthenia gravis** is associated with an antibody against acetylcholine receptors, resulting in profound muscle weakness. These antibodies can cross the placenta to produce transient myasthenia gravis in about 15% of neonates.

A drug effect on immunity

Between 1940 and 1970 the drug **diethylstilbestrol** was given to one and a half million women in the USA to prevent miscarriages. Many of their daughters developed **clear cell carcinoma** of the vagina as teenagers, and had increased incidences of infertility, fetal anomalies, ectopic pregnancies, miscarriages, stillbirths and premature deliveries. Now they have been found to have a higher risk of autoimmune disorders. Researchers believe these have a common factor: alterations in their T-cell mediated immunity (Burke et al 2001).

MAIN POINTS

- The immune system protects individuals from environmental factors such as microorganisms, irritants and abnormal cells. Its cells and molecules work together to either destroy an invading organism or reduce its harmful effects.

- The immune system is divided into non-specific immunity and specific immunity. Non-specific defences include surface barriers such as skin and mucous membranes and some cellular and chemical defences, usually with involvement of the phagocytic cells.

- The lymphatic system consists of primary lymphoid organs, where B cells and T cells differentiate and mature, and the peripheral lymphoid system, which includes encapsulated organs and unencapsulated lymphoid tissue.

- Specific immunity is divided into humoral and cellular immunity or cell-mediated immunity. The three main cell types involved in the immune response are B lymphocytes, T lymphocytes and macrophages. Macrophages present antigens to T cells for recognition and secrete substances that activate them. T cells secrete chemicals that activate macrophages.

- The immune response targets antigens that are recognised as non-self. Small molecules such as penicillin and pollutants which are not immunogenic can link up with the body's own proteins to form haptens, which may cause allergies.

- The binding of an antigen and lymphocyte stimulates the formation of a clone of identical cells which recognise that antigen. Most clone cells differentiate into plasma cells, secreting large numbers of antibodies for 5 days then dying; a few become memory cells able to mount a secondary response if the antigen is encountered later.

- Antibodies are grouped into five classes, each with a specific function – IgG, IgA, IgM, IgD and IgE. Mechanisms that complete the destruction of the antigen-bearing molecules include complement fixation, neutralisation, agglutination and precipitation.

- There are two major groups of T cells: cytotoxic T cells and helper T cells. Generally, helper T cells have CD4 proteins and cytotoxic T cells have CD8 molecules on their surfaces. Both types of cell suppress immune responses.

- Class I and class II molecules of the MHC on cell surfaces define self. MHC I proteins are present on most body cells to enable self recognition but MHC II proteins are found only on the surfaces of mature B cells, macrophages and some T cells.

- Helper T cells bind only to complexes which include MHC II proteins on macrophage surfaces. Cytotoxic T cells are activated by complexes which include MHC I proteins on any cell.

- The immune system cells release cytokines to stimulate each other. Cytotoxic T cells act mainly against virus-infected cells but also attack abnormal or cancerous cells or transplanted tissue. Helper T cells stimulate the proliferation of other T cells and B cells by releasing interleukin II.

- Microglia in the brain behave like macrophages. HIV attacks microglia and their activation is implicated in AIDS dementia.

- The immune system in the pregnant woman undergoes alterations to both primary and secondary defence mechanisms but the mother can still respond immunologically to the fetus: though protecting the fetus, the changes may increase the severity of some maternal infections and influence the progress of autoimmune diseases.

- The total white cell count rises early in pregnancy, mainly due to an increase in neutrophils. There is a slight rise in circulating eosinophils while basophil and monocyte counts remain unchanged.

- Cell-mediated immunity changes in pregnancy possibly due to pregnancy hormones. T_H cells decline in relation to T_C cells which may suppress the immune response. As these changes are insufficient to prevent fetal rejection, other mechanisms must be present. Both maternal and fetoplacental mechanisms may help prevent fetal rejection.

- There may be local immune regulation in the uterus. Decidual T cells are low in number and may not recognise the antigens on invading trophoblastic cells. High local levels of hormones may moderate local immune response as may high local metabolism of tryptophan.

- The trophoblast may prevent most maternal immune cells and antibodies except IgG from entering the fetal circulation. Neither the cytotrophoblast nor the syncytiotrophoblast express class I MHC antigens. Most MHC receptors are downgraded in trophoblastic cells, which may confer resistance to destruction by maternal NK cells.

- Most fetal cell surface antigens (except the rhesus factor) such as the ABO system and major MHC molecules are naturally present as soluble molecules in fetal blood or tissue fluids. Any maternal immune cells or antibodies that cross the placental barrier may be mopped up by fetal antigens.

- Colostrum and breast milk contain large quantities of immunoglobulins capable of reacting against many microorganisms. After the 1st week IgA predominates.

- Active immunity to infectious diseases can be acquired during an infection. Vaccines contain dead or attenuated pathogens which challenge the immune system without producing symptoms.

- Passive immunity is acquired by the fetus from the mother by placental transfer of IgG and by the breastfed baby via antibodies in breast milk.

- There may be improvement, deterioration or no change in the status of autoimmune disorders during pregnancy. Both T cells and autoantigens are needed to allow production of autoantibodies.

References

Blackburn S T 2003 Maternal, Fetal and Neonatal Physiology: A Clinical Perspective, 3rd edn. W B Saunders, Philadelphia.

Burke L, Segall-Blank M, Lorenzo C et al 2001 Altered immune response in adult women exposed to diethylstilboestrol in utero. American Journal of Obstetrics and Gynecology 185:78–81.

Classen S R, Paulson P R, Zacharias S R 1998 Systemic lupus erythamatosus: perinatal and neonatal complications. Journal of Obstetric and Neonatal Nursing 27(5):493–500.

Engelhard V H 1994 How cells process antigens. Scientific American August 1994:44–51.

Johnson M H, Everitt B J 2000 Essential Reproduction, 5th edn. Blackwell Science, Oxford.

Kendall M D 1998 Dying to Live. How our Bodies Fight Disease. Cambridge University Press, Cambridge.

Roitt I, Brostoff J, Male D 2001 Immunology, 6th edn. Mosby, St Louis.

Annotated recommended reading

Engelhard V H 1994 How cells process antigens. Scientific American August 1994:44–51.
This well-written and beautifully illustrated article is makes it easy to visualise how invisible cellular actions take place.

Johnson M H, Everitt B J 2000 Essential Reproduction, 5th edn. Blackwell Science, Oxford.
This textbook places human reproduction in the wider context and represents an integrated approach to the subject. Wherever appropriate, descriptions and discussions centre on the human reproductive system. Chapter 12 includes a clear discussion about the non-rejection of the human fetus.

Roitt I, Brostoff J, Male D 2001 Immunology, 6th edn. Mosby, St Louis.
The first half of this book covers basic immunology while the second half is geared to clinical application of concepts. The plentiful use of paragraph headings and 'thinking boxes' coupled with a glossary of terms ensures that concepts are well explained. Colour illustrations are excellent.

Section 2C

PREGNANCY – THE PROBLEMS

Although pregnancy is a normal physiological function, some women may develop illnesses independently of their pregnancy. Some minor health problems are caused by the pregnancy but are not life threatening. These are discussed in Chapter 30. Long-term health problems such as diabetes mellitus are influenced greatly by the pregnancy and, perhaps the most widespread danger to pregnant women, pregnancy itself may precipitate a hypertensive condition in up to 10% of women. Chapters 31–35 discuss pathological states relevant to the pregnant woman. Chapter 31 examines the possible causes and management of bleeding in pregnancy. Chapters 32–35 utilise a systems approach and each disorder is discussed in depth with its management in terms of diagnosis and treatment.

Chapter **30**

Minor disorders of pregnancy

INTRODUCTION

During pregnancy women suffer inconvenient but not life-threatening symptoms referred to collectively as the minor disorders of pregnancy. It should also be considered that a minor disorder may suddenly become a much more serious illness. For these two reasons, it is essential for the midwife or doctor caring for women to pay attention to these symptoms and to offer safe and sensible advice on their alleviation.

MAINTENANCE OF PREGNANCY

Maternal physiological recognition of pregnancy begins with the presence of the blastocyst in the uterine cavity. The development of the embryo and placentation are described in Chapters 9–12. The corpus luteum normally regresses after about 14 days if a fertilised ovum does not reach the uterus. The maintenance of the **corpus luteum of pregnancy** has been ascribed to the production of **human chorionic gonadotrophin** (hCG) by the cells of the **syncytiotrophoblast** as they invade the endometrium. This is secreted into maternal blood and taken to the ovary where it augments the action of **luteinising hormone** from the anterior pituitary gland to continue production of **progesterone** from the corpus luteum. The role of the corpus luteum is to maintain the pregnancy by secreting steroid hormones, mainly progesterone, until the placenta can take over the major role about 4–5 weeks after the last menstrual period (Johnson & Everitt 2000). The corpus luteum continues to secrete progesterone but this only plays a minimal role in later pregnancy.

The hormone hCG can be identified in the blood 6–7 days post fertilisation and before the first missed period; its excretion in the urine forms the basis of the widely available and highly efficient **immunological pregnancy tests**. There is no ovulation, and endocrine production is changed to maintain the pregnancy.

Another mechanism important in maintaining early pregnancy is the suppression of **prostaglandin** concentrations in decidual tissue. In the menstrual cycle these play a role in **luteolysis**, the breakdown of the corpus luteum.

Prostaglandin concentrations in early pregnancy are lower than those measured in the endometrium during the menstrual cycle. It is possible that prostaglandin production is reduced by a substance which inhibits the biosynthesis of arachidonic acid, their precursor substance. The hormone **relaxin**, a small polypeptide, seems to be produced by the corpus luteum in early and late pregnancy. It inhibits myometrial activity and may play a role in the maintenance of early pregnancy (Fig. 30.1) (Johnson & Everitt 2000). Other important factors **include inhibin, interferon, cytokines** and **growth factors** which assist in the early development of the conceptus (Coad & Dunstall 2001).

MINOR DISORDERS OF PREGNANCY

The minor disorders occur because of physiological adaptation of the woman's body to pregnancy, in particular the

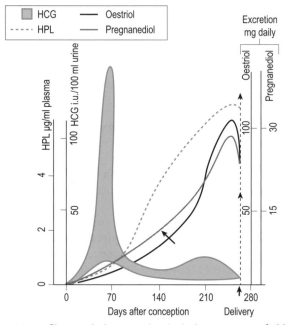

Figure 30.1 Changes in hormone levels during pregnancy (hCG, human chorionic gonadotrophin; hPL, human placental lactogen) (from Hinchliff S M, Montague S E 1990, with permission).

effect of progesterone and other hormones on the smooth muscle and connective tissue. Davis (1996) divides the disorders into which trimester of pregnancy they are most likely to occur (Table 30.1). The list is impressive but some of the disorders may be present throughout pregnancy, especially those associated with psychological wellbeing.

The digestive system

Nausea and vomiting

This troublesome complaint begins early in pregnancy at the 4th week and persists until about the 12th week in most sufferers; a few continue to have symptoms until the 16th week. Although commonly referred to as morning sickness, many women feel nauseous but may not vomit. Others will vomit at any time of day. In a prospective study of 160 women, 80% found nausea lasted all day, and sickness occurred in 1.8% (Lacroix et al 2000). The duration of these symptoms in 90% of women lasted 22 weeks. Nausea and vomiting for approximately two-thirds of women is an expected and normal feature of pregnancy (Flaxman & Sherman 2000, Furneaux & Langley-Evans 2001). A few women will develop severe vomiting known as **hyperemesis gravidarum**, which is life threatening to the woman and is discussed in Chapter 34, p. 450.

The aetiology of nausea and vomiting is not fully understood. It may be that a combination of physical and emotional factors is involved (Furneaux & Langley-Evans 2001). However, this period of time is close to the peak presence of hCG, which may be a trigger. Oestrogen and progesterone may also be involved. Early studies supported a psychological component but this may be a simplistic concept of the manner in which the mind and body work in unison. Flaxman & Sherman (2000) reviewed the literature and mentioned other facts:

- peak sickness occurred at 6–18 weeks, the period of embryonic organogenesis – increasing hormone levels;
- women who experience sickness are less likely to miscarry;
- aversions to some foods may be protective.

Huxley (2000) suggested that the nausea and vomiting stimulated placental growth by dividing nutrient factors

Table 30.1 Minor disorders of pregnancy by trimester

Trimester	Weeks	Minor disorder
First	0–14	Breast tenderness, morning sickness, increased urinary frequency, fatigue
Second	15–28	Fainting/dizziness, mild skin irritation
Third	29 onwards	Slight nausea, increased urinary frequency
Second and third	15 onwards	Constipation, heartburn, dyspnoea, varicose veins, oedema of the ankles, excessive weight gain, leg cramps, restless leg syndrome, carpal tunnel syndrome, increased vaginal discharge
Throughout pregnancy	Physical changes	Skin changes, backache, ligament pain, headache, stuffy nose, bleeding gums
Throughout pregnancy	Emotional changes	Mood swings, changing body image, depression, fearfulness, increased sensitivity, indecisiveness, alterations in libido

from the mother to the benefit of the growing embryo. Alterations in thyroid function have been suggested (Mori et al 1988). The severity of morning sickness has been correlated with the increased amount of free thyroxine (T_4), and decreased thyroid-stimulating hormone (TSH). There is a link between altered thyroid gland function and nausea and excessive vomiting in pregnancy (Asakura et al 2000).

Profet (1992) believes morning sickness is **adaptive** in an evolutionary sense and nausea and food aversions minimise fetal exposure to toxins during the period of **organogenesis**. Women are inclined to eat bland food without strong odours and flavours. This avoids the ingestion of spicy plant toxins and foods produced by bacterial and fungal decomposition. She supports this theory with a statistical observation that women who have no pregnancy nausea are more likely to miscarry. If this is correct, pregnancy nausea is unlikely to be unique to humans (Nesse & Williams 1995).

There have been anxieties about the safety of **antiemetic drugs**. Non-pharmacological measures are best used and are usually sufficient to combat pregnancy nausea. Light snacks instead of large meals and carbohydrate snacks at bedtime and before rising can prevent the hypoglycaemia that appears to be the cause. The avoidance of iron supplements is advisable. Ginger capsules and ginger root tea has been found to combat nausea and vomiting in some diseases but Davis (1996) warns that the safety of this substance taken in quantity has not been established (Vutyavanich et al 2001). If vomiting persists or becomes severe, a medical practitioner should be consulted. The use of pressure bands has been found to be beneficial to some women (Steele et al 2001).

Heartburn

Heartburn (**reflux oesophagitis**) is a burning sensation felt behind the sternum caused by reflux of acid gastric contents into the oesophagus. It is most problematic after 30 weeks of pregnancy, increasing in intensity until term and disappearing after delivery. Some 30–70% of women at some time in their pregnancy complain of heartburn, with 25% of those complaining of symptoms daily in the latter half of pregnancy (Blackburn 2003).

The main cause is the relaxing effect of progesterone on the smooth muscle of the cardiac sphincter between stomach and oesophagus. In the non-pregnant woman, sphincter tone increases in response to raised intragastric pressure to prevent reflux. This ability is greatly diminished in pregnancy as peristaltic activity is slowed and gastric emptying time is lengthened. Pressure from the growing uterus increases the intragastric pressure and flattening of the diaphragm distorts the shape of the stomach and decreases the angle at the gastrojejunal junction (Girling 2000).

The anatomical changes may cause the sphincter to become incompetent, causing a **temporary hiatus hernia** (Coad & Dunstall 2001). Reflux can be prevented by avoiding bending over when doing housework such as cleaning the bath, particularly with a full stomach. Sleeping in a more upright position by using additional pillows helps at night. A balanced diet, not spicy, with small regular meals, is recommended. Antacids may be taken after meals and at bedtime under medical supervision (Lloyd 2000).

Ptyalism

This disorder, which is more common in women with an Afro-Caribbean background, is excess salivation and is the equivalent of morning sickness. In some cases the woman must continuously wipe saliva from her mouth with a tissue. It is referred to as 'spitting' and is a sign of pregnancy, particularly in the West Indies. If severe, it may lead to loss of fluids and electrolytes and dehydration. Similar advice as for morning sickness may help. It may also accompany heartburn (Girling 2000).

Pica

This is the medical term for the craving for foods or substances such as coal that some women experience during pregnancy. There is a belief that the craving occurs because of a need of the fetus for certain minerals but this has not been substantiated by research (Girling 2000). Hormones and metabolic changes have also been implicated. Some substances if eaten in excess may be dangerous for the fetus so the person caring for the pregnant woman needs to know and to give advice if necessary (Cooksey 1995).

Constipation

Constipation is a common and troublesome disorder of pregnancy and may lead to the development of haemorrhoids, which in turn may increase constipation because of a fear of pain. The increased production of progesterone in pregnancy causes relaxation and reduced peristalsis in the smooth muscle of the digestive tract. This increases the transit time of food through the gut and a greater time for water to be absorbed in the large intestine. A dryer bulkier stool is then more difficult to defecate. The gut is also displaced upwards and outwards by the growing uterus. Faulty diet and disregarding the need to defecate add to the problem.

Oral iron therapy is also implicated by some women. Advice should be given to pregnant women as soon as they have had their pregnancies confirmed to avoid the situation if possible. It is necessary to ensure that they have an adequate fluid intake, maintain regular bowel habits and take in enough roughage in the form of fruits, vegetables and grains. Live yoghurt also is a natural laxative because of its **bifidus** content. Exercise is also useful. A stool softener or mild laxative can be useful as an adjunct to the above advice (Girling 2000).

Skin

Anterior pituitary production of **melanocyte hormone** is increased by the progesterone and oestrogen levels of pregnancy. This increases skin pigmentation in pregnancy, which may lead to a condition called **chloasma** or 'pregnancy mask', typically found on the face. **Palmar erythema** may be seen, due to increased circulation and the palms may feel hot. The skin changes very common to all are the **striae gravidarum** of pregnancy due to the rupturing of small amounts of tissue under the skin caused through stretching of the skin layers. Although pink in pregnancy, as the skin returns to normal and after time the striae become mauve and less noticeable. Pruritus or itching of the skin is not a problem in itself but of great nuisance to the woman. It only becomes a problem when the liver enzymes are raised and **cholestasis of pregnancy** is suspected (Coggins 2002).

The cardiovascular system

Fainting

The effect of progesterone on smooth muscle increases the incidence of fainting in pregnancy. Although the increase in circulating blood volume partly compensates, there is decreased vascular resistance. This alters the blood pressure and the venous return, permitting the pooling of blood in the lower extremities. Standing erect for long periods and the increased vasodilatation by being too warm may precipitate a faint. Later in pregnancy **supine hypotension** can be a problem; it is caused by the gravid uterus pressing on the inferior vena cava, preventing venous return to the heart and thus reducing cardiac output. It is easily prevented or reversed by avoiding the total supine position or turning the woman quickly onto her side if she begins to feel faint.

Varicosities

Varicosities occur as an outcome of the relaxing effect of progesterone on the smooth muscle of the walls of the veins. Circulation in the lower limbs becomes sluggish and the veins dilate, reducing valvular efficiency. The situation is exacerbated by pressure from the growing uterus, causing pelvic congestion and poor venous return. Other factors that contribute are increased weight of the pregnant uterus and also weight gain in the woman. **Varicose veins** may occur in the legs, in the anus as haemorrhoids and in the vulva (Turner 2001). Varicose veins of the leg can be made more bearable with the use of support tights applied in the morning and gentle walking to maintain circulation. Where possible, women should sit with their legs elevated and uncrossed.

Haemorrhoids occur as an outcome of the relaxing effect of progesterone on the veins of the anus, the reduction of venous return by the growing uterus and the incidence of constipation. They can be helped by the prevention and treatment of constipation. If needed, topical applications can be suggested and medical advice sought. As the haemorrhoids often disappear after delivery and because of the alteration in venous tone, surgery would not be performed in pregnancy.

Vulval varicosities, while rare, are very painful. A sanitary pad or sometimes a panty girdle may give support. Lying down will help to prevent congestion in the area. Care must be taken during delivery as there is a risk of haemorrhage from the distended veins, especially if cut through during an episiotomy (Turner 2001).

The musculoskeletal system

Backache

At least 50% of women may experience backache in pregnancy. It is essential to differentiate the cause of back pain so that appropriate treatment can be obtained. Some contributing factors are postural changes resulting in lumbar lordosis with overstretched abdominal muscles and strained back muscles (Ostgaard et al 1991). Also, the relaxing effect of progesterone and relaxin on the pelvic ligaments allows movement of the symphysis pubis and lumbosacral joints. Relaxin may make the intervertebral joints unstable as they try to support the increased weight of pregnancy. Once the more worrying causes of backache are excluded, the woman is advised on back care to minimise pain. The following advice may be helpful.

Sitting   She should choose a comfortable chair which supports both back and thighs when sitting. She should sit well back and it may be necessary to place a small cushion behind the lumbar spine.

Standing   It is advised that standing tall with tummy and buttocks tucked in and weight evenly distributed on both legs with a flat shoe would be of benefit to prevent backache.

Lying   Lying in the lateral position is preferable to supine with a good supportive mattress. Care should be taken when changing from lying down to sitting up to avoid strain on back and abdominal muscles. When getting off the examination couch, rolling on to the side and allowing the legs to fall over the side of the couch will place less strain on the back. The arms should be used to push up into a sitting position.

Work   Lifting or dragging heavy objects should be avoided and women should discuss the best position for managing their work both in business and at home.

The nervous system

Carpal tunnel syndrome

Women who develop **carpal tunnel syndrome** complain of numbness and tingling, often called pins and needles, in their fingers and hands. This is most likely to be present in the morning but can occur at any time of day. The cause is fluid retention of pregnancy and swelling of connective tissue which compresses the median nerve as it runs through the carpal tunnel in the wrist. It may be necessary for the woman to wear a splint at night and elevate the hand, to prevent fluid collecting in the night. Occasionally, the doctor may prescribe diuretics.

Fatigue

Reeve (1991) reported on an exploratory study on fatigue in early pregnancy. It was found that the symptom of fatigue necessitated changes in the daily routine of 70% of the sample of 30 women. The women had reduced the amount of housework they did and reported an increased need for sleep. The women reported that they had begun to experience fatigue within 4 weeks of the first missed menstrual period and that the symptom continued into the second trimester of pregnancy.

Fatigue was associated with the younger women in the above study and correlated positively with nausea (Reeve 1991). Associated factors in the aetiology of fatigue include poor nutrition, anaemia, slowed circulation and sleep disturbances caused by urinary frequency, leg cramps, breathing problems and vomiting (Lee & DeJoseph 1992). Advice regarding these problems can alleviate them but adequate sleep at night and a rest during the day is often the remedy.

Emotional changes

Emotional changes in pregnancy include mood swings, changing body image, depression, fearfulness, increased sensitivity, indecisiveness and alterations in libido with either an increased or decreased increase in sexual activity. These changes are complex and involve the personality type of the woman, her knowledge base, her response to physical symptoms and fears and anxieties about the outcome of pregnancy as well as psychological and social factors (Davis 1996).

The genitourinary system

Frequency of micturition

Urinary frequency affects women most in the first and third trimesters of pregnancy, mainly because of pressure on the bladder of the growing uterus. During the second trimester the uterus is displaced upwards over the pelvic brim and the incidence of frequency is lower.

The increased reabsorption of sodium and water increases the need to pass urine through the night (**nocturia**). During the day excess water is trapped in the lower extremities because of venous stasis. When the woman lies down at night, pressure on the large veins is reduced and there is increased cardiac return, cardiac output and renal blood flow with a subsequent increase in urinary output, particularly in the left lateral position. There is an increased risk of urinary tract infection because of progesterone's effect on ureteric smooth muscle. This may cause **urinary reflux** or **stasis** (Turner 2000).

Small lifestyle changes can reduce nocturia:

- restrict fluids in the evening by increasing the fluid intake earlier in the day;
- limit the intake of natural diuretics such as caffeine;
- lie down in the left lateral recumbent position during the evening to encourage a diuresis.

Leucorrhoea

There is an increase in white, non-irritant vaginal discharge in pregnancy. Once the possibility of vaginal moniliasis or trichomonal infection has been excluded, simple personal hygiene will ensure comfort for the woman. Wearing cotton pants and avoiding tights will also increase comfort.

Conclusion

Midwives play an important role in the management of minor disorders of pregnancy. Women often discuss their discomforts with the midwife, who can reassure women that their problem is not health threatening and offer simple advice to minimise the particular problem. Occasionally, a more serious condition may be present and midwives should be vigilant about seeking medical advice in such cases.

MAIN POINTS

- Maternal physiological recognition of pregnancy begins with the presence of the blastocyst in the uterine cavity. There is no ovulation and the endocrine production is changed to maintain the pregnancy. The corpus luteum continues to secrete progesterone until term.

- A minor disorder of pregnancy may suddenly become a much more serious illness. Minor disorders include breast tenderness, morning sickness, increased urinary frequency, leg cramps, carpal tunnel syndrome, increased fatigue, fainting/dizziness, constipation, heartburn, dyspnoea, varicose veins, haemorrhoids, ankle oedema, vaginal discharge, skin changes, backache, ligament pain, headache,

stuffy nose, bleeding gums, mood swings, changing body image, depression, increased sensitivity, indecisiveness and alterations in libido.

- Midwives play an important role in the management of minor disorders of pregnancy. Women often discuss their discomforts with the midwife, who can reassure women that their problem is not health threatening and offer simple advice to minimise the particular problem.

- Occasionally a more serious condition may be present and midwives should be vigilant about seeking medical advice in such cases.

References

Asakura H, Watanabe S, Sekiguchi A, Power GG, Araki T 2000 Severity of hyperemesis gravidarum correlates with serum levels of T3. Archives Gynaecology Obstetrics 264(2):57–62.

Blackburn S T 2003 Maternal, Fetal and Neonatal Physiology, 3rd edn. W B Saunders, Philadelphia.

Coad J, Dunstall M 2001 Anatomy and Physiology for Midwives. Mosby, St Louis.

Coggins J 2002 Early pregnancy care. The Practising Midwife 5(9):14–17.

Cooksey N R 1995 Pica and olfactory craving of pregnancy: how deep are the secrets? Birth 22(3):129–137.

Davis D C 1996 The discomforts of pregnancy. Journal of Gynecological and Neonatal Nursing January:73–81.

Flaxman S M, Sherman P W 2000 Morning sickness: a mechanism for protecting mother and embryo. Quarterly Review Biology 75(2):113–148.

Furneaux E C, Langley-Evans A J 2001 Nausea and vomiting of pregnancy. Obstetrical and Gynaecological Survey 56:775–782.

Girling J C 2000 Physical adaptation to pregnancy. In Page L (ed.) The New Midwifery. Churchill Livingstone, Edinburgh.

Huxley R R 2000 Nausea and vomiting in early pregnancy: its role in placental development. Obstetric Gynaecology 95(5):779–782.

Johnson M H, Everitt B J 2000 Essential Reproduction, 5th edn. Blackwell Science, Oxford.

Lacroix R, Eason E, Melzack R 2000 Nausea and vomiting during pregnancy: a prospective study of its frequency, intensity and pattern changes. American Journal of Obstetric Gynecology 182(4):931–937.

Lee K A, DeJoseph J F 1992 Sleep disturbances, vitality and fatigue among a select group of employed childbearing women. Birth 19:208–213.

Lloyd N 2000 How to cope with heartburn during pregnancy. British Journal of Midwifery 8(4):254.

Mori M, Amino N, Tamaki H et al 1988 Morning sickness and thyroid function in normal pregnancy. Obstetrics and Gynaecology 72(3) part 1:355–359.

Nesse R M, Williams G C 1995 Evolution and Healing. Weidenfeld and Nicolson, London.

Ostgaard H C, Andersson G B, Karlson K 1991 Prevalence of back pain in pregnancy. Spine 16:549–552.

Profet M 1992 Morning sickness – an adaptive response in pregnancy. In Barkow J H et al (eds) The Adapted Mind. Oxford University Press, New York, pp 327–365.

Reeve J 1991 Calcium metabolism. In Hytten F, Chamberlain G (eds) Clinical Physiology in Obstetrics, 2nd edn. Blackwell Scientific, Oxford, pp 213–223.

Steele NM, French J, Gatherer-Boyles J 2001 Effect of acupressure by sea-bands on nausea and vomiting of pregnancy. Journal of Gynaecologic and Neonatal Nursing 30(1):61–70.

Turner A 2000 How to manage urinary tract infection in pregnancy. British Journal of Midwifery 8(12):777.

Turner A 2001 Varicose veins during pregnancy. British Journal of Midwifery 9(7):464.

Vutyavanich T, Kraisarin T, Ruangsri R A 2001 Ginger for nausea and vomiting in pregnancy: randomised, double masked, placebo-controlled trial. Obstetrics and Gynaecology 97(4):577–582.

Annotated recommended reading

Coggins J 2002 Early pregnancy care. The Practicing Midwife 5(9):14–17.
This is part 2 of two articles covering all aspects of antenatal care with application to the physiological and psychological changes women experience.

Girling J C 2000 Physiological adaptation to pregnancy. In Page L (ed.) The New Midwifery. Churchill Livingstone, Edinburgh.
This chapter covers adaptation to pregnancy, including the minor ailments women complain of. It is well set out and easy to read.

Smith C, Crowther C, Beilby J 2002 Acupuncture to treat nausea and vomiting in early pregnancy: a randomised controlled trial. Birth 29(1):1.
This is a report of a trial in Australia to help women with vomiting in pregnancy.

Chapter 31

Bleeding in pregnancy

BLEEDING IN EARLY PREGNANCY

Bleeding from the genital tract during pregnancy is abnormal and a doctor should see all women who report bleeding, irrespective of the amount. Bleeding prior to the 24th week of pregnancy may be caused by implantation bleeding, abortion, ectopic pregnancy, trophoblastic disease and lesions of the cervix or vagina. Axelsen et al (1995) examined the characteristics of bleeding during pregnancy. They found that the overall incidence was 19%, with the median being 8 weeks. Duration of bleeding was about 2 days and there was usually only one episode. Two-thirds of the women had no abdominal pain accompanying the bleeding and only one in five women were admitted to hospital.

Implantation bleeding

Normal implantation is thought to occur in three stages:

- apposition – the blastocyst sits adjacent to the endometrium, an unstable situation;
- stable adhesion – increased activation of the syncytiotrophoblast with the endometrium;
- invasion.

As the syncytiotrophoblast cells erode the maternal endometrium during embedding, a small amount of bleeding may occur at about 6–7 days (Norwitz et al 2001). By 10 days the blastocyst is completely covered by the decidua; this is just before the next menstrual period is due. Women may think this is a normal but short menstruation, which then often mars the true last menstrual cycle date and the calculation of the expected date of delivery will be inaccurate. Implantation is a complex interaction between the blastocyst and the endometrium which has been previously prepared by the hormones. At this early stage women often do not know they are pregnant. If the blastocyst does not implant, then menstruation begins, although a little late, and the conceptus is lost with menstrual debris.

Abortion

Spontaneous abortion is the complete loss of the products of conception prior to the 24th week of pregnancy. Human reproduction is not very efficient and it has been estimated that 45% of conceptions may be lost before the 20th week (Arias 1993). However, most of them are lost before implantation and only a quarter of them are clinically recognised as abortions. The risk of a recognisable spontaneous abortion is about 15% in women with no previous pregnancy loss and 19% for a repeated abortion in women with no living children. If two consecutive pregnancies are lost in spontaneous abortion, the risk rises to 35% and 47% after three consecutive abortions (Zinaman et al 1996). The aetiology of abortion is shown in Table 31.1.

About 80% will occur before 12 weeks gestation; the early abortions and the rest will occur between 13 and 24 weeks and are referred to as late abortions. The majority of early abortions are due to anembryonic pregnancies or blighted ova suggestive of genetic faults, while those with a formed fetus suggest the possibility of many causes and occur after 13 weeks. Fifty per cent of conceptions are lost before the next menstruation, 30% soon after the missed cycle and 65–90% of these losses are recognised as chromosomally abnormal (Lockwood 2000). This may be linked to older women and pregnancy loss.

Classification of spontaneous abortion (Fig. 31.1)

Threatened abortion In threatened abortion, painful or painless bleeding occurs, the cervical os is closed and ultrasound will define a live fetus when conservative treatment such as bed rest is advised. The outcome may be resolution and continuance of the pregnancy or proceed to an inevitable abortion.

Inevitable abortion A diagnosis of inevitable abortion is made on the fact that the cervical canal is open; ultrasound will define if the fetus is alive. Blood loss may be heavy and cause maternal collapse with increasing abdominal pain. The uterus may spontaneously evacuate its contents or surgical or medical removal with **mifepristone** (RU46) may be necessary to remove retained products. The use of ultrasound has tended to alter treatment and expectant management

Table 31.1 Aetiology of abortion

Cause	Percentage of total
Genetic abnormalities – mainly chromosomal abnormalities arising during meiosis of ovum or sperm	50–60
Endocrine abnormalities – progesterone deficiency, thyroid deficiency, diabetes, increased androgens, elevated leutinising hormone as in polycystic ovary	10–15
Chorioamniotic separations – there may be bleeding beneath the chorion or between the amnion and chorion	5–10
Incompetent cervix – usually the result of cervical trauma	8–15
Infections – usually ascending, but occasionally due to systemic microbial infections such as rubella, Listeria, Toxoplasmosis, Chlamydia.	3–5
Abnormal placentation – failure of the trophoblastic invasion of the spiral arteries, linked to raised blood pressure	5–15
Immunological abnormalities – may be the cause of repeated spontaneous abortions and have recognisable serum antibodies	3–5
Uterine anatomic abnormalities caused mainly by failure of the Mullerian ducts to unite in the embryonic stage resulting in septate uterus. A fibroid uterus may also cause abortion	1–3
Unknown reasons	Less than 5

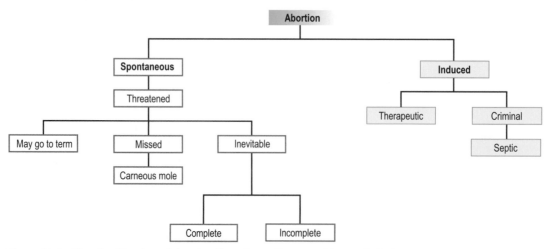

Figure 31.1   The classification of abortion (from Sweet B 1997, with permission).

is sometimes an alternative to operative measures for removing retained products of conception. Ultrasound measures endometrial thickness and the presence of a gestational sac. If left to nature, most women will lose the retained products naturally. This management requires regular follow-up as an outpatient and access to the clinic by phone (Luise et al 2002, Cahill 2001).

Missed abortion   In a missed abortion, now termed **early fetal demise** (Cahill 2001), a blood stained or brown loss may be evident, the woman may or may not still feel pregnant and the signs of pregnancy may disappear. Low levels of human chorionic gonadotrophin (hCG) may be found, in which case the conceptus has died or ultrasound confirms fetal death. A suction curette or oral mifepristone may be used. If the uterus is larger than 13 weeks, a combination of vaginal prostaglandins and intravenous Syntocinon (oxytocin) may be prescribed. Although the uterus would eventually expel the mole, there is a risk of disseminated intravascular coagulation because of the toxins produced by a dead fetus.

Recurrent abortion   Recurrent abortion is the term used for three or more consecutive abortions. Only 0.4% of women suffer in this way but they have a 55% increased risk of having a fourth miscarriage (Eblen et al 2000). In some women the cause is unknown but there is a specific group of women who are suffering from **antiphospholipid antibodies (Hughes syndrome)**: some 10–16% who will continually abort. In other words, the mother produces antibodies against the fetus. These antibodies also affect clotting factors and the process of abortion is thought to involve the activation of clotting mechanisms on the endothelial decidual cell surface (Singh 2001).

Induced abortion (therapeutic)   Therapeutic abortions have been available in the UK since 1967 but there are other countries where the procedure is illegal. The lack of an abortion law leads to the risk of women seeking illegal abortions, often carried out in unfavourable conditions by unskilled practitioners, including the woman herself. In the past this often resulted in a septic abortion, which occurred because of infection, and the woman suffered from **septicaemia**, **endotoxic shock** and **disseminated intravascular coagulation**. Liver and renal damage and pelvic infection may have led to the formation of adhesions, salpingitis and infertility. Fatalities were common. As for long-term health problems, there seems to be no connection between induced abortion and later early pregnancy loss or the incidence of ectopic pregnancy, but the risk of preterm birth and placenta praevia in subsequent pregnancies is increased (Thorp et al 2003).

It should be considered that if a woman is pregnant and the pregnancy is unwanted, then she may choose the route to abort the baby. Other women abort because of fetal abnormality and this in itself is difficult for the woman and her partner. Some women are treated as outpatients using mifepristone or prostaglandins followed by a suction evacuation under a general anaesthetic.

Gestational trophoblastic tumours (GTT)

Chorionic tumours deriving from the placenta include **hydatidiform mole** (partial or complete), **placental site tumours** and **choriocarcinoma** with varying degrees of the diseased tissue spreading and causing malignancy, which is highly treatable (Berkowitz & Goldstein 1996). Persistent disease occurs in 0.5% of partial moles, whereas complete moles have an incidence of 8% and GTT can also occur after a normal pregnancy in approximately 1:40 000 pregnancies.

Hydatidiform mole

Hydatidiform mole is a benign neoplastic disease, an abnormal growth of the trophoblast where the chorionic villi proliferate, become avascular and are filled with fluid. The mole looks like a bunch of grapes, often filling the uterus, which clinically palpates large for dates (Fig. 31.2). Complete and partial moles have abnormal sets of chromosomes (Fig. 31.3), a complete mole will have a 46XX where all chromosomes are of paternal origin, partial moles where a fetus may be present is usually triploid, either 69XXX or 69XXY (Berkowitz & Goldstein 1996, Blackburn 2003). During early pregnancy a partial moles fetus will die because of the proliferation of the molar tissue from the abnormal placenta.

Aetiology   There are wide variations in incidence: 2:1000 in Japan; 1:1000 in Europe and North America; and 1:1945 in Ireland. It is suggested that diet and socioeconomic factors may play a role in this, particularly the lack of carotene and animal fats (Berkowitz & Goldstein 1996). Women over 35, and who have had a previous mole, have an increased risk of a complete mole. Acaia et al (1988) found that women

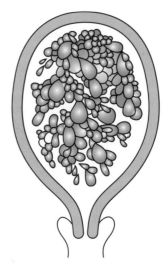

Figure 31.2   A hydatidiform mole (from Sweet B 1997, with permission).

Paternal chromosomal origin of a complete hydatiform mole (46XX)

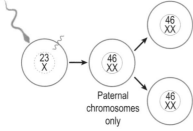

Triploid chromosomal origin of a partial mole (69XX-dispermy)

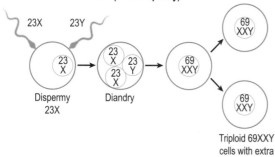

Figure 31.3 Genetic origins of complete and partial hydatidiform moles.

with two consecutive abortions were at an increased risk of a complete mole to the factor of 32.

Signs and symptoms

- Intermittent vaginal bleeding with increasing bleeding as the mole is aborted.
- Early onset of pre-eclampsia.
- The uterus is large for dates and no fetal parts will be palpated in a complete mole.
- There may be mild signs of thyrotoxicosis and hyperemesis gravidarum due to the action of hCG, which is similar to thyroid-stimulating hormone (TSH) (Misra et al 2002).
- Diagnosis is confirmed by ultrasound scan, which will show a snowstorm effect of multiple vesicles.
- Urinary or serum hCG is very high, exceeding that of a multiple pregnancy.

Management Complete emptying of the uterus by suction and then curettage to eliminate all diseased tissue is essential. The molar tissue always expresses the RhD factor, therefore Rh-negative women require rhesus immunoglobulin following evacuation (Berkowitz & Goldstein 1996). Follow-up at one of the three centres in the UK for the measurement of hCG until hCG levels are normal (urine hCG, 0–24 IU/L; serum hCG, 0–4 IU/L) will be routine. A 2-year follow-up will continue if hCG levels do not return to normal in 8 weeks. Hormonal contraception should be avoided, as it increases the chance of developing malignant disease.

Choriocarcinoma and placental site tumours

The diagnosis of a choriocarcinoma is the presence of a persistently raised level of hCG more than 2000 IU/L; the tumour consisting of placental tissue and haemorrhage debris and the spread to lung and brains is typical. Other symptoms such as haemorrhage and rising levels of hCG are also diagnostic. The tumour is very invasive and treatment must be commenced immediately following diagnosis. Placental site tumours can be difficult to diagnose, with hCG levels elevated but not markedly as in choriocarcinoma; irregular bleeding may be a first sign.

Treatment Choriocarcinoma in all its presentations responds very well to **chemotherapy**. To assist in the treatment process a scoring system is used: women scoring 0–8 are low risk and are administered methotrexate and folinic acid; those scoring above 8 receive etoposide, methotrexate, cyclophosphamide and vincristine (McNeish et al 2002). The problem of toxicity is as for every use of cytotoxic drugs with malaise, stomatitis, pharyngitis, diarrhoea, leucopoenia and alopecia occurring. Follow-up treatment will continue for life with some women opting for hysterectomy.

Ectopic pregnancy

An ectopic pregnancy occurs when the fertilised ovum implants outside the uterine cavity. In 95% of cases the site of implantation is the uterine tube. More rarely, the implantation site may be the ovary, the cervical canal or the abdominal cavity. Ectopic pregnancy is a serious condition and is the major cause of maternal death. The incidence is 11.1 per 1000 pregnancies, with 0.4 per 1000 deaths in that figure. Reasons for death have been stated as, in the main, missed diagnosis in primary care and accident and emergency. The Royal College of Obstetricians and Gynaecologists (RCOG) recommend the use of the urinary hCG dipstick test to ascertain pregnancy to prevent missed diagnosis (RCOG 2002).

Tubal pregnancy

There is a rise in the incidence of tubal pregnancies due to the increase in sexually transmitted diseases, in particular by *Chlamydia trachomatis* (Tay et al 2000), to the use of the oral contraceptive pill and the intrauterine device and to the delay in starting a family until later in reproductive life. Any condition that delays the transport of the zygote along the uterine tube may lead to a tubal pregnancy (Fig. 31.4). This may be due to malformation of the tubes but is more likely due to tubal scarring and the loss of cilia due to pelvic infection.

Risk factors Risk factors for tubal pregnancy include (Tay et al 2000):

- an older woman;
- women of low gravidity or parity;

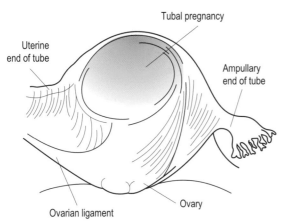

Figure 31.4   Tubal pregnancy (from Sweet B 1997, with permission).

- previous tubal pregnancy;
- tubal surgery;
- salpingitis;
- intrauterine contraceptive device;
- hormonal stimulation of ovulation;
- in-vitro fertilisation and embryo transplant;
- tubal endometriosis;
- pelvic inflammatory disease (PID);
- pelvic or abdominal surgery;
- progestogen-only pill (interferes with the action of the cilia).

Pathophysiology   Implantation may occur in various sites along the genital tract (Table 31.2).

The outcome varies depending on where in the tube implantation occurs, its ability to distend and the size of blood vessels eroded. If the pregnancy occurs in the fimbriated end or the ampulla, the conceptus may continue to grow until 10 weeks. The gestation sac may be expelled into the abdominal cavity as a tubal abortion (Fig. 31.5). Blood clot may be organised around the separated sac to form a tubal mole, which may remain in the uterine tube or be expelled from the fimbriated end as a tubal abortion. Tubal rupture (Fig. 31.6) may lead to devastating haemorrhage. The most severe haemorrhage occurs if the zygote implants at the level of the isthmus where the mucosa is thinner and the blood vessels larger. Tubal rupture is likely to occur between the 5th and 7th weeks of pregnancy.

Diagnosis   The condition may be subacute or acute with signs of shock and collapse. The condition is serious and should always be suspected in women of childbearing age, especially if there is a history of amenorrhoea or previous salpingitis. The likely signs and presenting history of ectopic pregnancy are given in Table 31.3 (Tay et al 2000).

Delay in diagnosis may be fatal as the clinical picture is similar to PID or threatened abortion:

- the woman will give a history of early pregnancy signs;
- the uterus will have enlarged but feel soft;

Table 31.2   Sites of ectopic implantation

Position	Percentage occurrence
The fimbriated part of the tube	17
The ampulla	55
The isthmus	25
The ovary	0.5
The abdominal cavity	0.1

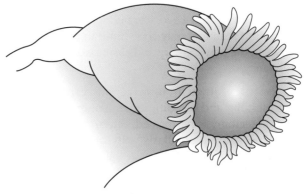

Figure 31.5   Tubal abortion (from Sweet B 1997, with permission).

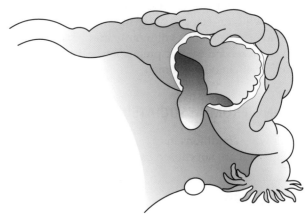

Figure 31.6   Rupture of the uterine tube (from Sweet B 1997, with permission).

Table 31.3   Signs and presenting history of ectopic pregnancy

Sign	Percentage occurrence
Abdominal pain	97
Abdominal tenderness	91
Vaginal bleeding	79
Adnexal tenderness	54
History of infertility	15
Use of intrauterine device	14
Previous ectopic pregnancy	11

- abdominal pain may occur as the tube distends and uterine bleeding may be present as the endometrium begins to degenerate;
- the abdomen is tender and may be distended;
- shoulder tip pain may be due to referred pain;
- the woman may appear pale, complain of nausea and collapse;
- severe pain may be felt during pelvic examination, especially if the cervix is moved;
- a mass may be felt in the adnexa on one or other side of the uterus;
- hormonal assay will find progesterone levels to be low and hCG levels may be low or falling;
- ultrasound scanning may show fluid in the pelvic cavity, a mass in the pelvic cavity and absence of an intrauterine pregnancy.

Management   Although an acute emergency when rupture of the tube and bleeding occurs, surgery is indicated and salpingectomy is performed, ectopic pregnancy can be treated expectantly, particularly with early ultrasound diagnosis. Observation of hCG titres less than 1000 IU/L in 88% of patients, the ectopic resolves naturally (Tay et al 2000). The use of systemic methotrexate in women who have not ruptured and are haemodynamically stable has been beneficial; however, it is not without side-effects.

Prognosis   About 40% of women may never become pregnant following an ectopic pregnancy. About 75% of these women avoid pregnancy voluntarily and 25% are infertile. The risk of a second ectopic pregnancy is 10% as compared with only 0.4% in other women.

BLEEDING FROM ASSOCIATED CONDITIONS

The following conditions may cause bleeding at any time in pregnancy but are not caused by the pregnancy.

Cervical polyps

Cervical polyps are benign growths which are bright red, fleshy and attached by a pedicle. They usually originate in the cervical canal and can be seen on speculum examination. Polyps may have been present before the onset of pregnancy but bleed during pregnancy because of the increased blood supply.

Cervical erosion

Cervical erosion (eversion, ectropion) forms when the columnar epithelium lining the cervical canal proliferates because of the influence of the pregnancy hormones. Columnar epithelium secretes mucin and the woman may complain of profuse vaginal discharge. This may be blood stained because of rupture of capillaries, especially following sexual intercourse. The epithelium should recede after

delivery but, if it persists, treatment by diathermy or cryosurgery can be given (Hefner 2001).

Carcinoma of the cervix

Carcinoma of the cervix if diagnosed early is a very treatable condition; the incidence is 1:2000–5000 women (Shires 1999). Diagnosis is made with a Papanicolaou smear and treatment may depend on the stage of pregnancy and the severity of the findings. Prospective parents have a difficult choice to make and must be guided to make an informed decision. Cellular dysplasia (abnormal growth of cells) and nuclear dyskaryosis (abnormal chromosomes) are associated with human papillomavirus (HPV) infection types 6, 16 and 18 and between 10 and 30% of women have been affected by age 30. HPV is transmissible and is a cause of genital warts. About 60% of the partners of women with HPV infection of the cervix have penile infection. HPV virus acts with a coagent to cause carcinoma of the cervix. Clinical findings may show cervical intraepithelial neoplasia (CIN invasive carcinoma of the cervix).

Cervical intraepithelial neoplasia

Cervical cytology may show normal cells, mild, moderate or severe dysplasia or carcinoma in situ. When carried out in the antenatal period, 1 in 200 mothers have abnormal cell changes. If these are consistent with CIN, a repeat Papanicolaou smear is taken and the cervix is assessed by colposcopy. A small cervical biopsy may be carried out. If the tissue is precancerous, treatment can be deferred until after delivery (Hefner 2001).

Invasive carcinoma of the cervix

Invasive carcinoma of the cervix occurs in about 1 in 5000 women of childbearing age. It is an aggressive cancer and may progress rapidly. The cervix feels hard and nodular and bleeds when touched. Decisions about treatment should be discussed with each woman and will depend on the degree of invasion and the duration of pregnancy.

Vaginitis

Occasionally the use of vaginal deodorants may lead to inflammation and bleeding from the vaginal epithelium. Infections by organisms such as Candida albicans or Trichomonas vaginalis are more likely causes of vaginitis, which may be accompanied by slight bleeding. Following culture of the organism, the correct antibiotic should be given.

ANTEPARTUM HAEMORRHAGE

Antepartum haemorrhage is bleeding after the 24th week of pregnancy and before the birth of the baby. Bleeding during labour can be called **intrapartum haemorrhage**. Bleeding is from the placental site and may be severe enough to cause the death of the woman or the fetus. The two main types of antepartum haemorrhage are **placenta praevia**, where the bleeding occurs from a placenta implanted wholly or partly in the lower uterine segment, and **placental abruption**, where there is premature separation of a normally situated placenta.

Placenta praevia

Normally, the chorionic villi surround the whole embryo but later degenerate under the decidua capsularis to form the chorion laeve. The fetus grows to fill the uterine cavity and the decidua capsularis fuses with the decidua vera by about 4 months. If the chorionic villi near the lower pole of the uterus fail to degenerate as the decidua capsularis fuses with the decidua vera, the area will become part of the placenta, encroaching on the lower uterine segment (Blackburn 2003).

The incidence of placenta praevia ranges between 0.5% and 1% at term, rising to 2% in grandmultiparity (Enkin et al 2000). Although a low-lying placenta may be detected on routine ultrasound scanning in early pregnancy, it may be detected in as many as 25% of pregnancies in the second trimester. Growth of the lower segment in later pregnancy appears to remove the placental site away from the internal os. In the later weeks of pregnancy sheering stresses may detach the placenta from the uterine wall, resulting in haemorrhage. When the placenta is found to be covering the internal os in early pregnancy, the woman is most at risk of

haemorrhage and the earlier the first episode of bleeding the worse the prognosis (Arias 1993).

Classification of placenta praevia

The standard classification of placenta praevia is shown below although in practice such precision between types I–III is not always possible (Fig. 31.7):

- type I – the placenta lies mainly in the upper uterine segment but encroaches on the lower segment;
- type II – the placenta reaches to the edge of the internal os;
- type III – the placenta covers the internal os when it is closed but not completely when it is dilated;
- type IV – the placenta completely covers the internal os.

The use of ultrasound has improved the diagnosis and allows prognosis of outcome (Arias 1993).

> *Vaginal examination is an extremely dangerous procedure in placenta praevia and must never be carried out unless in theatre with the ability to perform an immediate caesarean section.*

Aetiology of placenta praevia

In most cases of placenta praevia no specific cause can be assigned. However, Table 31.4 lists the conditions which are associated with its presence.

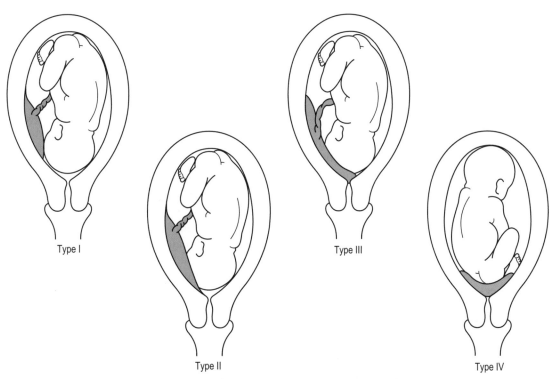

Figure 31.7   Placenta praevia, types I to IV (from Sweet B 1997, with permission).

Table 31.4 Conditions associated with the presence of placenta praevia

Condition	Cause
Conditions which may damage the endometrium and myometrium	Previous caesarean section (Obed & Adewole 1996, Hendricks et al 1999) Previous placenta praevia Previous uterine curettage (Rose & Chapman 1986) Spontaneous abortion (Hendricks et al 1999) Endometriosis Multiparity Closely spaced pregnancies
Maternal health	Age (Zhang & Savitz 1993) Anaemia Smoking – possibly due to enlargement of the placenta as a response to hypoxia (Chelmow et al 1996, Andres 1996)
Fetoplacental causes	Multiple pregnancy, as the larger placental site is more likely to encroach on the lower segment Congenital malformations Presence of a male fetus (James 2000) Placental abnormality: bipartite placenta, placenta membranacea

Signs and symptoms

In units where early ultrasound scanning is routine, at-risk women will be identified. Women with low-lying placentae should be rescanned at about 30 weeks gestation. If the placenta is still considered to be low-lying placenta praevia should be diagnosed and subsequent care modified. Other indications result because the placenta occupies space in the lower uterine segment and include:

- malpresentations of the fetus;
- non-engagement of the presenting part;
- the presence of a loud maternal pulse that originates in the placental bed below the umbilicus.

Blood loss

In 98% of cases painless fresh recurrent vaginal bleeding occurs after 24 weeks due to stretching of the lower uterine segment and detachment of the placenta, although it may occur earlier. Blood loss usually stops after a few hours and is rarely dangerous. Subsequent episodes of bleeding due to increased development of the lower uterine segment and further detachment of the placenta tend to become worse and may need a blood transfusion. Torrential maternal haemorrhage may occur at any time especially if labour commences and the cervix begins to dilate. The fetus may

be compromised if maternal bleeding is severe enough to reduce the uterine blood supply. The placenta may be torn and fetal bleeding occurs. Severe bleeding may occur after 34 weeks when most women with placenta praevia will be delivered (Sundle 2002).

Management

Management may be conservative or active. Any woman bleeding in her own home should be transferred to hospital by ambulance. Vital signs should be assessed and intravenous fluids used to stabilize condition. The amount of blood lost should be estimated.

General examination

- There may be a history of spotting or small blood losses.
- Observations of maternal pulse and blood pressure should correspond with the amount of blood loss and the degree of shock.
- Temperature should be normal.

Abdominal examination

- The uterus should feel soft and should not be tender.
- The size will correspond to the period of gestation.
- There may be a malpresentation, an unstable lie and a high presenting part.
- Usually the fetus is in good condition with a fetal heart of normal rate and rhythm.

Blood is taken for cross-matching and at least two units placed on standby. Full blood count and Kleihauer estimation is needed if the woman is rhesus negative. An intravenous infusion of Hartmann's solution is commenced if bleeding is persistent. Blood loss is estimated. The woman remains on bed rest until the bleeding ceases. On no account is a vaginal examination performed.

Conservative management If bleeding is slight to moderate and occurs before the 38th week of pregnancy and both maternal and fetal conditions are satisfactory, conservative treatment is commenced. The aim is to maintain the pregnancy until 38 weeks to avoid preterm delivery of an immature fetus. When bleeding ceases the obstetrician may carry out a speculum examination of the cervix to exclude incidental bleeding.

Ultrasound examination is used to identify the placental site and, if this is found to be normal, the woman is allowed home. If placenta praevia is diagnosed the woman will be advised to remain in hospital to reduce any risk of severe bleeding in the absence of immediate medical help. Fetal growth will be monitored and any women who are rhesus negative will receive anti-D γ-globulin after each episode of bleeding (Chamberlain & Steer 1999).

However, Love & Wallace (1996) reviewed the outcome of 58 pregnancies complicated by placenta praevia in Edinburgh. Of these women, 42 (72%) had one or more episodes of bleeding. Repeated episodes of bleeding did not affect the outcomes of pregnancy. Both diagnosis and delivery occurred earlier in the women who bled and delivery by caesarean section was more common in the women who were bleeding. Only three women required emergency delivery because of bleeding. They concluded that as the clinical outcome of placenta praevia is so variable in both women who have no bleeding and those who bleed, outpatient management is safe and appropriate.

Delivery   If no serious haemorrhage occurs, the fetus is delivered at 38 weeks. If placental localisation is not clear, an examination under general anaesthetic in theatre should be made. The surgical team should be ready to carry out an immediate caesarean section. The obstetrician performs a gentle vaginal examination through the fornices. If the placenta is felt, a caesarean section is carried out. If the placenta is not palpable, the cervical os is examined; if no placenta is felt, the membranes will be swept and ruptured. An oxytocin infusion will be commenced. Vaginal delivery should be possible in type I placenta praevia although many clinicians believe caesarean section should be carried out in all cases of placenta praevia.

Enkin et al (2000) list the hazards of vaginal delivery as:

- profuse maternal haemorrhage;
- malpresentation;
- cord accidents;
- placental separation;
- fetal haemorrhage;
- dystocia if the placenta is situated posteriorly.

Active management   This is more likely to be needed in the last 2 weeks of pregnancy. If bleeding is severe or continuous or there is deterioration in maternal or fetal condition or if labour has commenced, the woman's condition is stabilised and an emergency caesarean section is carried out. Blood must be cross-matched but it may be necessary to give the woman a transfusion of O-negative blood in a dire emergency. Surgery can be complicated if the placenta underlies the site of normal surgical incision. Even if the fetus has died, caesarean section will be needed in types III and IV to prevent torrential maternal haemorrhage and death.

Third stage   The lack of oblique fibres in the lower uterine segment may fail to control bleeding and postpartum haemorrhage may occur. Placenta accreta is often associated with placenta praevia as the thin decidua over the lower uterine segment increases the likelihood of myometrial invasion. Hysterectomy may be required to control haemorrhage and to save life.

Placental abruption (abruptio placentae)

Placental abruption (accidental haemorrhage) is bleeding due to the separation of normally situated placenta (Fig. 31.8). It may occur at any stage in pregnancy or labour in about 1% of all deliveries and bleeding occurs into the decidua basalis beneath the placenta. A haematoma is formed which separates the placenta from the maternal vascular system

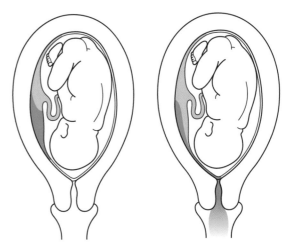

Figure 31.8   Abruptio placentae (from Sweet B 1997, with permission).

and the fetus is deprived of oxygen and nutrients. Most maternal complications arise from hypovolaemia and collapse of the systems (Yerby 2002). The haemorrhage may be secondary to degenerative changes in the arteries supplying the intervillous spaces (Blackburn 2003). Enkin et al (2000) suggest that the perinatal mortality may be as high as 30%. Some fatalities occur because bleeding is profuse, the mother is at home and neonatal death occurs because of prematurity.

Causes

In the majority of cases bleeding is slight and no cause may be found. The following risk factors are associated with this serious complication of pregnancy:

- **hypertensive states** – essential hypertension or preeclampsia are present in 50% of severe cases (Hladky et al 2002);
- sudden decompression of the uterus, as when membranes rupture in **polyhydramnios** (Hladky et al 2002);
- preterm, prelabour rupture of the membranes (Ananth et al 1996, Major et al 1995);
- previous history of placental abruption, increasing parity (Ananth et al 1996, Hladky et al 2002);
- trauma, as in a fall or road traffic accident;
- smoking (Andres 1996, Hladky et al 2002);
- illegal drug abuse, such as cocaine (Hladky et al 2002).

Previously accepted causes such as short cord, uterine anomalies, inferior vena caval occlusion and dietary folate deficiency are probably not significant (Arias 1993).

Blood loss

Blood loss comes from the maternal venous sinuses and may be revealed, partly revealed or concealed (Fig. 31.9). The blood is darker than that seen in placenta praevia, because

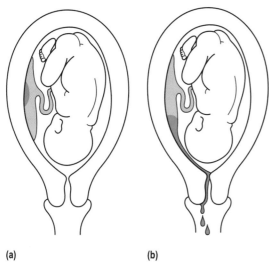

(a)   (b)

Figure 31.9   (a) Concealed abruptio placentae. (b) Revealed abruptio placentae (from Sweet B 1997, with permission).

Table 31.5   The main features of bleeding in abruptio placentae

	Mild	Moderate	Severe
Blood loss	Slight	More than 1000 ml	More than 2000 ml
Uterus on abdominal examination	Soft, not tender	Firm and tender	Hard (woody) and tender; backache if the placenta is posterior
Pain	None or mild	Quite severe	Severe
Shock	No sign	Tachycardia, hypotension	Extreme shock
Fetus	Fetal heart normal	Signs of fetal distress	Fetal heart absent

of the time taken to trickle out of the vagina. Vaginal bleeding is present in 78% of cases (Arias 1993). Some experts believe that the magnitude of placental separation is determined at the outset and that no further separation occurs. Others believe that abruption causes progressive placental separation.

- Revealed bleeding occurs when the site of placental detachment is at the margin. The blood escapes between the membranes and decidua and is seen at the vulva. The condition of the woman is directly related to the observed blood loss.

- Partially revealed bleeding occurs when some of the blood remains in the uterus. The bleeding may exceed that which is visibly lost and the degree of shock may be greater than expected.

- Concealed bleeding occurs when the site of detachment is near to the centre of the site of placental attachment. Blood cannot escape and a large retroplacental clot forms. Extravasated blood may also infiltrate the full-thickness myometrium, a condition known as **Couvelaire uterus**. Under direct observation, the uterus would appear bruised and oedematous. There may be no vaginal blood loss and pain and shock is usually severe (Crafter 1999, Sundle 2002).

As shown in Table 31.5, depending on the amount of placental separation and blood lost, either revealed or concealed, placental abruption may be mild, moderate or severe (Crafter 1999):

- Mild includes situations where the mother and fetus are not compromised in any way. Ultrasound will define where the placenta lies. Observation of the blood loss

and fetal wellbeing will continue in hospital until bleeding stops. Discharge home will occur if before 37 weeks.

- Moderate blood loss may be greater than 1000 ml and the fetus may be alive. Immediate caesarean section may be necessary if the fetus is distressed. The mother may show signs of hypovolaemia and require stabilisation with intravenous fluids. The uterus may be tender and the mother in pain. Clotting screens should be undertaken. If the fetus is dead, a vaginal delivery could be possible if the mother is stable.

- Severe separation of the placenta is life threatening for the mother, the fetus is nearly always dead, and blood loss may be in the region of 2000 ml or more. The uterus will be hard and woody and blood loss may not be totally revealed, giving a false impression of less blood loss. The maternal condition is poor with severe shock and pain. Complications which may arise from this are coagulation defects, kidney failure and Sheehan's syndrome. Most maternal deaths occur in this latter group of women and it is important to monitor cardiovascular and renal status closely to ensure a good maternal outcome. If the fetus is alive, the maternal condition should be stabilised and caesarean section performed.

The amount of bleeding per vaginam is no guide to the degree of placental separation.

Management of placental abruption

When bleeding is slight and there is no effect on maternal or fetal condition, it may be difficult to differentiate the cause of bleeding, especially if there is no sign of hypertension. Because of the risk of placenta praevia, the woman is treated as if that condition is present until it is excluded by ultrasound scan. If the placenta is localised in the upper uterine segment, the bleeding stops and the condition of mother and fetus are satisfactory, the woman may go home.

Moderate or severe placental abruption is usually easy to diagnose and is an obstetric emergency. The woman is resuscitated if necessary and an intravenous infusion commenced. Morphine 15–20 mg may be ordered to relieve pain and shock and the woman is then transferred to hospital. The aim is to restore blood loss and deliver the baby as quickly as possible to avoid complications such as renal failure and blood clotting defects.

Blood is taken for grouping and crossmatching and it is wise to have at least 6 units standing by. Full blood count with urea and electrolytes, clotting studies and fibrin degradation products should be routine. Central venous pressure is monitored to avoid under- or overtransfusion and the woman's blood pressure, pulse and respiratory rate are monitored frequently. A Foley urinary catheter is inserted to observe urinary output and allow urine to be tested.

The only way to stop the bleeding is to empty the uterus. Vaginal delivery may be achieved if the fetus has died or is in a good enough condition to allow the time for induction. The membranes are ruptured and an oxytocic infusion is commenced. Caesarean section will be carried out if the fetus is alive but in poor condition. Postpartum haemorrhage is likely due to the poor ability of the uterine muscle to contract when it is infiltrated by blood; intravenous Syntocinon (oxytocin) infusion may be continued for some hours following delivery.

Blood coagulation disorders

Damage to tissue causes the release of **thromboplastins** from the cells. In normal circumstances thromboplastin activates the clotting mechanism and **fibrinogen** is converted to **fibrin**, forming a clot to seal any broken blood vessels. This clot is later dispersed by **plasmin**, releasing **fibrin degradation products** (FDPs). The tissue damage in placental abruption is so severe that there is a massive release of thromboplastin into the circulation. Widespread clotting occurs within the vascular tree, a condition called disseminated intravascular coagulation (DIC). At the same time, the anticlotting mechanisms are affected and shut down, preventing dissolution of the clots. The **microthrombi** produced occlude small blood vessels, which results in ischaemic damage in organs (Crafter 1999). The damaged tissue then releases more thromboplastins and a vicious circle commences. DIC will affect about 13% of women (Arias 1993).

- Damage to the kidney results in reduced urinary output and may result in **anuria**.
- The liver may be damaged, leading to **jaundice**.
- Damage to the lungs may result in **dyspnoea** and **cyanosis**.
- Brain involvement may result in **convulsions** or **coma**.

- The retina may be affected and cause **blindness**.
- If the pituitary gland is damaged, **Sheehan's syndrome** may occur.

Platelets and clotting factors are depleted and no further coagulation can occur. Spontaneous bleeding begins from puncture wound sites, mucous membranes, petechiae develop in the skin and there will be uncontrollable uterine bleeding. Transfusions of fresh frozen plasma, packed cells and platelets will be needed. Specific tests for coagulation failure are:

- partial thromboplastin time (normal = 60–90 s);
- prothrombin time (normal = 11–16 s);
- thrombin time (normal = 10–15 s);
- fibrinogen levels (normal = 150–400 mg/dl);
- fibrin degradation products;
- whole blood film and platelet count.

Other complications

The complications of acute renal failure, Sheehan's syndrome, postpartum haemorrhage, infection, anaemia and mental disturbances are discussed in relevant chapters. Women who have had a placental abruption have a higher risk of complications such as spontaneous abortion or repeated abruption in later pregnancies.

Vasa praevia

Vasa praevia is an unusual cause of bleeding in pregnancy where the blood lost is fetal. It is associated with **velamentous insertion** of the umbilical cord where one of the fetal vessels crosses the membranes between the presenting part of the fetus and the internal os of the uterus. The vessel may be torn when the membranes rupture and fetal bleeding may be severe. There is a high incidence of perinatal mortality with this condition and the incidence is said to be 1:2500 (Oyelese et al 1999). Diagnosis has been possible since transvaginal ultrasound and Doppler ultrasound has been used. It is possible to diagnose the condition by feeling a pulsating vessel on examination.

If the condition is suspected during a vaginal examination, the membranes are left intact and the fetus delivered by emergency caesarean section. If the woman is in the second stage of labour, rapid delivery is made by forceps. Any sudden vaginal bleeding accompanied by fetal distress following rupture of the membranes should alert the practitioner and the blood should be tested for fetal cells. Although this sounds sensible, in reality there may be no time and the fetus should be immediately delivered as above. A blood transfusion may be needed to restore the baby's blood volume. A much higher incidence of velamentous cord insertion following IVF pregnancies has been noted (Schachter et al 2002).

MAIN POINTS

- Any bleeding from the genital tract during pregnancy is abnormal and all women who bleed should be seen by a doctor. The causes of bleeding prior to the 24th week of pregnancy are implantation bleeding, abortion, ectopic pregnancy, cervical lesions, vaginitis and bleeding from trophoblastic disease. Spontaneous abortion is a common serious cause of bleeding in early pregnancy.

- Inevitable abortion is accompanied by cervical dilatation. The bleeding is severe with increasing abdominal pain and may result on maternal collapse. The uterus may spontaneously evacuate its contents or it may be necessary to surgically evacuate the uterus. In women who have recurrent abortions, investigations to ascertain the cause are made in order to plan treatment.

- Abortions may be induced in unwanted pregnancies. Sepsis may follow any type of abortion, when the term septic abortion is used. This is a serious condition and is potentially fatal. Antibiotics are commenced before surgical intervention.

- Hydatidiform mole is an abnormal growth of the trophoblast. The uterus must be emptied by suction curettage. Following the emergency treatment, follow-up must be continued for 1 year to ensure that there is no progression to choriocarcinoma.

- Between 5 and 10% of women may go on to develop choriocarcinoma, which responds well to chemotherapy. Follow-up treatment will continue for life, with some women opting for hysterectomy.

- In 95% of cases of ectopic pregnancy the implantation site is the uterine tube. Ectopic pregnancy may be subacute with most of the signs but without the shock and collapse that is present with the classical acute picture with sudden collapse. Tubal rupture is an obstetric emergency; bleeding is heavy and can only be stopped surgically.

- Cervical polyps, vaginitis, cervical erosion and carcinoma of the cervix may cause associated bleeding and require treatment in pregnancy.

- The two main types of antepartum haemorrhage are placenta praevia and placental abruption. Placenta praevia causes bleeding from an abnormally sited placenta. In units where early ultrasound scanning is routine, at-risk women will be identified. If the placenta is still low-lying at 30 weeks, placenta praevia should be diagnosed and subsequent care modified. In 98% of cases, painless fresh recurrent vaginal bleeding occurs.

- Risk factors for placental abruption include hypertensive states, sudden decompression of the uterus, preterm prelabour rupture of the membranes, previous history of placental abruption, trauma, smoking and abuse of cocaine. The bleeding is from maternal venous sinuses and may be revealed, partly revealed or concealed.

- Moderate or severe placental abruption is an obstetric emergency. The aim is to restore blood loss and deliver the baby as quickly as possible to avoid renal failure and blood clotting defects. The only way to stop the bleeding is to empty the uterus.

- Vasa praevia is associated with a velamentous insertion of the umbilical cord where one of the fetal vessels crosses the membranes between the presenting part of the fetus and the internal os of the uterus. The vessel may be torn when the membranes rupture and fetal bleeding may be severe. There is a high incidence of perinatal mortality with this condition.

References

Acaia B, Parazzini F, LaVechia C, Fedele L, Battista Candiani G 1988 Increased frequency of complete hydatidiform mole in women with repeated abortion. Gynaecology Oncology 31:310–314.

Ananth C V, Savitz D A, Williams M A 1996 Placental abruption and its association with hypertension and prolonged rupture of the membranes: a methodologic review and meta-analysis. Obstetrics and Gynecology 88(2):309–318.

Andres R L 1996 The association of cigarette smoking with placenta praevia and abruptio placentae. Seminars in Perinatology 20(2):154–159.

Arias F 1993 Practical Guide to High Risk Pregnancy and Delivery, 2nd edn. Mosby Year Book, Chicago.

Axelsen S M, Hendriksen T B, Hedegaard M et al 1995 Characteristics of vaginal bleeding in early pregnancy. European Journal of Obstetrics and Gynecology and Reproductive Biology 63(2):131–134.

Berkowitz R, Goldstein D 1996 Chorionic tumours. New England Journal of Medicine 335(23):1740–1748.

Blackburn S T 2003 Maternal, Fetal and Neonatal Physiology: A Clinical Perspective, 3rd edn. W B Saunders, Philadelphia.

Cahill D J 2001 Managing spontaneous first trimester miscarriage: we don't yet know the optimal treatment. British Medical Journal 322(7298):1315–1316.

Chamberlain G, Steer P 1999 ABC of labour care: obstetric emergencies. British Medical Journal 318(7194):1342–1345.

Chelmow D, Andrew E, Baker E R 1996 Maternal cigarette smoking and placenta praevia. Obstetrics and Gynecology 87(5):703–706.

Crafter H 1999 Problems of pregnancy. In Bennett V R, Brown L K (eds) Myles Textbook for Midwives, 3rd edn. Churchill Livingstone, Edinburgh, pp 253–278.

Eblen A, Gercel-Taylor C, Shields L et al 2000 Alterations in humoral responses associated with recurrent pregnancy loss. Fertility and Sterility 73(2):305–313.

Enkin M, Keirse M J, Neilson J et al 2000 A guide to effective care in pregnancy and childbirth. Oxford University Press, Oxford.

Hefner L 2001 Human Reproduction at a Glance. Blackwell Science, Oxford.

Hendricks M, Chow Y, Bhagavath B, Singh K 1999 Previous caesarean section and abortion as risk factors for developing placenta praevia. Journal of Obstetrics and Gynaecology Research 25(2):137–142.

Hladky K, Yankowitz J, Hanson W 2002 Placental abruption. Obstetrical and Gynaecological Survey 57(5):299–305.

James W H 2000 Placenta praevia: preponderance of male sex at birth. American Journal of Epidemiology 152(2):195–196.

Lockwood C 2000 Prediction of pregnancy loss. Lancet 355(9212):1292–1293.

Love C D B, Wallace E M 1996 Pregnancies complicated by placenta praevia: what is appropriate management? British Journal of Obstetrics and Gynaecology 103(9):864–867.

Luise C, Jermy K, Collins W 2002 Expectant management of incomplete spontaneous first trimester miscarriage: outcome according to initial ultrasound criteria and value of follow-up visits. Ultrasound in Obstetrics and Gynaecology 19(6):580–582.

McNeish I, Strickland S, Holden L et al 2002 Low risk persistent gestational trophoblastic disease: outcome after initial treatment with low dose methotrexate and folinic acid from 1992–2000. Journal of Clinical Oncology 20(7):1838–1844.

Major C A, de Vaciana M, Lewis D F et al 1995 Preterm premature rupture of the membranes and abruptio placentae: is there an association between these pregnancy complications? American Journal of Obstetrics and Gynaecology 172(2) part 1:672–676.

Misra M, Levitsky L, Lee M 2002 Transient hyperthyroidism in an adolescent with hydatidiform mole. Journal of Paediatrics 140(3):362–366.

Norwitz E R, Schust D, Fisher S J 2001 Mechanisms of disease: implantation and survival of early pregnancy. New England Journal of Medicine 345(19):1400–1408.

Obed J Y, Adewole I F 1996 Placenta praevia: a late sequela of previous lower segment caesarean scars, as manifest in subsequent pregnancies. Journal of Obstetrics and Gynaecology of Eastern and Central Africa 12(1):15–17.

Oyelese K, Turner M, Lees C, Campbell S 1999 Vasa praevia: an avoidable obstetric tragedy. Obstetrical Gynaecological Survey 54(2):138–145.

Rose G L, Chapman M G 1986 Aetiological factors in placenta praevia – a case-controlled study. British Journal of Obstetrics and Gynaecology 93(6):586–588.

RCOG 2002 Why Mothers Die. 1997–1999. Royal College of Obstetricians and Gynaecologists, London.

Schachter M, Tovbin Y, Arieli S et al 2002 In vitro fertilization is a risk factor for vasa previa. Fertility and Sterility 78(3):642–643.

Shiers C V 1999 Abnormalities of early pregnancy. In Bennett V R, Brown L K (eds) Myles Textbook for Midwives, 13th edn. Churchill Livingstone, Edinburgh, pp 235–251.

Singh A 2001 Immunopathogenesis of the antiphospholipid antibody syndrome, an update. Current Opinion in Nephrology and Hypertension 10(3):355–358.

Sundle H 2002 Antepartum haemorrhage. In Boyle M (ed.) Emergencies Around Childbirth. Radcliffe Medical Press, Abingdon, Oxfordshire.

Tay J, Moore J, Walker J 2000 Ectopic pregnancy. British Medical Journal 320:916–919.

Thorp J, Hartmann K, Shadigian E 2003 Long-term physical and psychological health consequences of induced abortion: review of the evidence. Obstetrical and Gynaecological Survey 58(1):67–79.

Yerby M 2002 In Boyle M (ed.) Emergencies around Childbirth. Chapter 2. Radcliffe Medical Press.

Zhang J, Savitz D A 1993 Maternal age and placenta previa: a population-based case-control study. American Journal of Obstetrics and Gynecology 168(2):641–645.

Zinaman M, Clegg E, Brown C, O'Connor J, Selevan S 1996 Estimates of human fertility and pregnancy loss. Fertility and Sterility 65(3):503–509.

Annotated recommended reading

Long L 2000 Antepartum haemorrhage. The Practising Midwife 3(5):32–35.
This article provides a sound base for students learning about antepartum haemorrhage.

Norwitz E R, Schust D J, Fisher S J 2001 Mechanisms of disease: implantation and survival of early pregnancy. New England Journal of Medicine 345(19):1400–1408.
This is a review paper that covers normal implantation, maintenance of early pregnancy and implications for infertility and loss of pregnancy.

Sundle H 2002 Antepartum haemorrhage. In Boyle M (ed.) Emergencies around Childbirth. Radcliffe Medical Press, Abingdon, Oxfordshire.
This excellent chapter covers all aspects of antepartum haemorrhage, is worth reading and has some good references.

Website: http://www.hmole-chorio.org.uk
This website is clearly set out and is full of very readable information on trophoblastic disease and hydatidiform mole.

Chapter **32**

Cardiac and hypertensive disorders

INTRODUCTION

Heart disease in pregnancy is a serious medical condition and may lead to maternal death (Lewis 2001). Each year it has been estimated that there are approximately 6000 new patients reaching their 16th birthday who have had heart lesions and require medical supervision (Chambers & Hunter 2000). This has implications within the maternity service for those women of childbearing years. The most dangerous cardiac lesions are those that involve pulmonary hypertension such as **primary pulmonary hypertension** and **Eisenmenger's syndrome** where there is a 30–50% and 30% risk, respectively, of dying in pregnancy. Other dangerous cardiac conditions include **Marfans' syndrome**, an autosomal dominant disorder of connective tissue where aortic dilatation is present. Rupture of the aorta may occur in late pregnancy or in labour.

Rheumatic heart disease is still fairly common despite the reduction in rheumatic fever in the British population. The most common lesion is **rheumatic mitral stenosis** with the most common complication being **pulmonary oedema** occurring in late pregnancy or immediately after delivery. It is important to consider that although the indigenous population may have a changing pattern of heart disease, we see many immigrants who may have not been diagnosed with a condition.

CARDIAC DISORDERS IN PREGNANCY

The incidence of heart disease in the pregnant population ranges between 0.5% and 2% (Gilbert & Harmon 1998). It is important to understand the physiological adaptation of the heart and circulation in pregnancy in order to understand the detrimental effects in pregnancy on the health of a woman with diagnosed heart disease. The changes in the cardiovascular system begin early, reach their maximum at about 30 weeks and are maintained until term. They include:

- an increase in cardiac output by 40%;
- an increase in blood volume up to 50%;

- a heart rate increase of 10–20 beats/min (bpm);
- a decrease in total peripheral resistance;
- a lowering of blood pressure in the first and second trimesters.

The changes in cardiac output in normal pregnancy may produce signs and symptoms of cardiac disease: for example, dyspnoea, orthopnoea, breathlessness on exertion, oedema and occasional palpitations (Gilbert & Harmon 1998). Heart sounds may change and confuse diagnosis (Prasad & Ventura 2001).

Risk factors

In some women the adaptive changes may exceed the ability of the heart to function and **congestive cardiac failure** with pulmonary oedema may occur. More rarely, sudden death may be the outcome. Arias (1993) discussed periods during pregnancy when the danger of **cardiac decompensation** is higher:

- The first period is between 12 and 32 weeks when the **haemodynamic changes** are increasing towards their maximum, with the most critical time between 28 and 32 weeks.
- The second dangerous period is during labour and delivery. During labour every uterine contraction injects blood from the uteroplacental circulation into the maternal bloodstream, which temporarily increases the cardiac output by 15–20%. The continuous demand on the heart may precipitate heart failure. Pushing during the second stage of labour increases the risk further by reducing venous return. Intravenous fluids should be accurately calculated, as overperfusion will be increased by the sudden injection of 300–500 ml of blood into the maternal circulation at delivery of the placenta. Congestive heart failure is frequent at this time (Gilbert & Harmon 1998).
- Finally, 4–5 days following delivery is a danger period, with thrombus formation and pulmonary embolism being a problem as blood constituents rapidly return to normal levels.

Main types of cardiac disorder

Rheumatic heart disease

The main effect of this disease is to cause valvular lesions. Mitral and aortic incompetence may be improved during pregnancy because of the lower pressure within the arterial tree. However, there is a risk of **endocarditis**. Mitral stenosis requires an increase in left atrial pressure to push blood into the left ventricle and will require an even greater effort in pregnancy. Women with mitral stenosis may develop increasing breathlessness. The heart rate increases, which decreases diastolic filling time, and there is a rise in left atrial pressure which causes pulmonary oedema – hence, the breathlessness (Williams 1999).

To prevent pulmonary oedema, **diuretics** should be given with **β blockers** to aid diastolic filling (Prasad & Ventura 2001). **Anticoagulation** is important and warfarin is used only after the first trimester to prevent embryopathy. Williams (1999) discusses the use of prophylactic antibiotics to prevent bacterial endocarditis in women with heart lesions, suggesting it should be routine for operative or normal delivery. He presents research stating that, in a series of 2000 women given antibiotic cover, there were no cases of bacterial endocarditis.

A study in India of 486 women with rheumatic heart disease showed the commonest lesion was mitral stenosis. There were 10 maternal deaths and 48 **valvotomies** performed in pregnancy. Preterm birth and small for gestational age infants were 12% and 18% respectively. It was concluded that the condition was associated with high risks for both mother and fetus (Sawhney et al 2003).

Congenital heart disease

If there is a family history of congenital heart defect, there will be a higher incidence of a heart defect in the baby (Gilbert & Harmon 1998). These defects are present in 1% of births and are the commonest abnormality. The cause is often not found but if the mother has rubella in the first trimester, this could be responsible (American Heart Association website 2002).

Categorisation of congenital heart disease
- **Septal defects:** atrial septal defect (ASD), ventricular septal defect (VSD), patent ductus arteriosus, Eisenmenger's complex (Ammash & Warns 2001). Obstruction defects: pulmonary stenosis, aortic stenosis, coarctation of the aorta (Brickner et al 2000a).
- **Cyanotic defects:** tetralogy of Fallot, transposition of great vessels (American Heart Association 2002, Brickner et al 2000b).

Some of the defects mentioned in the above list will not be problematic in pregnancy if the woman has been treated in childhood. There is a need to prevent bacterial endocarditis; thus, antibiotics in labour are necessary, as even though defects are repaired, some impairment may be present following the surgery. The greatest area for concern is for women with pulmonary vascular disease; they may have a poor outcome (Chambers & Hunter 2000).

Women with prosthetic valve replacement are at risk of **thromboembolism** and should be anticoagulated (Williams 1999). Oral anticoagulants carry a risk of 3–4% of first trimester embryopathy. This is related to warfarin: the higher the dose, the higher the risk (Williams 1999, Meschengieser et al 2000). Also, anticoagulants may cause fetal haemorrhage. Meschengieser et al (2000) suggest that the use of low-molecular-weight heparin is far safer. Most regimes use heparin for the first trimester, changing to warfarin until 2 weeks before the due date, when heparin is recommended. This prevents the warfarin affecting fetal blood clotting time.

Eisenmenger's syndrome

Eisenmenger's syndrome with pulmonary hypertension has a high risk of maternal mortality and termination of pregnancy may be suggested. The syndrome consists of several defects: VSD, a right-to-left shunt causing the pulmonary hypertension and there may be an overriding aorta receiving blood from both ventricles (American Heart Association 2002). Cyanosis may be marked. During the third trimester, at birth and for 2 weeks postnatally the woman is at greatest risk of death and should stay in hospital for at least 2 weeks post delivery.

Pregnancy adaptation causes the right-to-left shunt to increase cyanosis and creates backpressure on the pulmonary circulation. Intrauterine growth restriction is seen in 30% of cases, with a high incidence of abortion and preterm birth (Siu & Colman 2001). During labour, haemodynamic monitoring should take place, but internal heart pressure measurements are not recommended in Eisenmenger's syndrome as there are more complications with catheter insertion. Vaginal delivery is preferable to caesarean section, with the second stage shortened with an instrumental delivery.

Marfan syndrome

Marfan syndrome is an inherited condition involving connective tissue which causes skeletal, eye and heart abnormalities. High oestrogen levels present in pregnancy affects the structure of the aorta, where spontaneous rupture may take place, particularly in labour, where pressures within the vascular system may be variable (American Heart Association 2002, Blackburn 2003). Again, termination of the pregnancy may be advised, but, if there has been no pre-existing heart disease, pregnancy should not pose a problem.

Assessment of mothers with heart disease

Heart disease can present itself in pregnancy for the first time, or be known about. Assessment is made jointly by the cardiologist and obstetrician so that counselling and decision making can be considered. If a termination of pregnancy is suggested, this should take place in the first trimester as, after 16 weeks continuing with the pregnancy, it may be the safer option. To assess client condition in heart diseases the following system has been widely used.

New York Heart Association classification

It is traditional to use the New York Heart Association classification (Hurst et al 1999) to describe the severity of heart disease but in practice this has little predictive value of the effect of pregnancy on the disease process.

Class 1 No symptoms during ordinary physical activity
Class 2 Symptoms during ordinary physical activity
Class 3 Symptoms during mild physical activity
Class 4 Symptoms at rest

A client in class 4 would need more care in pregnancy than one in class 1 (Siu & Colman 2001).

Management of women with heart disease

The major maternal complications and the treatments aimed at avoiding them are:

- bacterial endocarditis – routine antibiotics;
- thromboemboli – anticoagulation;
- cyanosis – rest, hospital admission;
- arrhythmias – β blockers, digoxin;
- heart failure – hospital admission, diet restriction of salt, diuretics;
- urinary tract infection, and respiratory infection – antibiotics;
- hypertension;
- anaemia.

Care should be directed towards prevention of complications rather than treating them. An assessment of risk can be made during pregnancy, by using electrocardiography (ECG), echocardiography and maternal function in everyday circumstances. Counselling is important, especially if the woman is high risk. Assessment of the heart lesion is important, by examining ventricular function, pulmonary pressure, persistence of shunts and valvular obstruction (Siu & Colman 2001).

SPECIFIC ASPECTS OF CARE

Intrapartum care

Labour should take place in a unit with full resuscitation facilities and an intensive care unit. The cardiologist, obstetrician and anaesthetist should collaborate. If possible, labour should be spontaneous in onset with a vaginal delivery. The use of intravenous fluids could increase circulating blood volume, which may result in pulmonary oedema, so accurate fluid balance is essential. If it is necessary to induce labour, prostaglandin pessaries are advocated. Blood should be crossmatched and oxygen and adult resuscitation equipment available. The heart may be monitored by ECG or internal catheterisation to measure pressures within the heart. During active labour, the left lateral position is advantageous to assist venous return and prevent aortocaval compression.

Pain relief

Epidural is the best form of pain relief to assist women in labour, as it assists in relaxation (Chamberlain & Steer 1999, Siu & Colman 2001).

Second stage

This stage should be kept short and without exertion. A forceps or vacuum extraction should be used.

Third stage

To prevent blood loss a continuous Syntocinon (oxytocin) infusion should be used instead of intramuscular Syntocinon for the third stage. When the uterus empties, approximately 500 ml of blood is returned to the central circulation.

Postnatal care

The risk of cardiac failure with pulmonary oedema is greatest in the early puerperium. Signs include tachycardia, cyanosis, oedema and distension of the liver. If pulmonary oedema occurs, acute dyspnoea with frothy sputum and haemoptysis may occur. In most units the woman will be admitted to a high dependency unit to stabilise her condition.

HYPERTENSION IN PREGNANCY

Terminology

- **Chronic hypertension** involves 1–5% of pregnancies; the blood pressure is greater than 140/90 mmHg. It is present before pregnancy and occurs before 20 weeks (Magee et al 1999). Some 15–20% of these women will develop pre-eclampsia (Pridjian & Puschett 2002a).

- In **gestational hypertension** blood pressure is raised, which may show a predisposition for raised blood pressure in later life but could lead on to pre-eclampsia (Magee et al 1999). It is generally resolved by 6 weeks postnatal (Chari et al 1995).

- **Pregnancy-induced hypertension** (PIH) is a condition specific to pregnancy that occurs mainly after the 20th week in some 5–10% of pregnancies (Magee et al 1999).

- **Pre-eclampsia** is more severe, with raised blood pressure, and is also associated with proteinuria of more than 500 mg/L/24 h (Broughton Pipkin 1995). There may be multiorgan involvement.

- **Eclampsia** is when convulsions occur, often with disseminated intravascular coagulation (DIC) and multisystems involvement (Broughton Pipkin 1995). It may occur postnatally for the first time (Zhang et al 1997) and the incidence is approximately 1:2000 pregnancies.

- **HELLP syndrome** (Nutt 1997) is an acronym for Haemolytic anaemia, Elevated Liver enzymes and Low Platelet count. This condition complicates 1:1000 pregnancies and both eclampsia and HELLP carry 1:50 morbidity. This may present on its own or as part of pre-eclampsia.

The above terminologies may seem clear but may be blurred at diagnosis and are used as guidelines only. Zhang et al (1997) discuss the various centres that have endeavoured to define this multisystem disorder, which adds greater confusion to the subject. In order to aid diagnosis, an attempt has been made to classify the disorders in a progressive manner.

Classification

It is generally accepted that hypertension in pregnancy may be defined as a diastolic pressure of greater than 90 mmHg. Davey & MacGillivray (1986) gave a clear definition:

> *the occurrence of a blood pressure of 140/90 mmHg on at least two occasions four hours apart after the 20th week of pregnancy – the woman is normotensive before this time.*

If proteinuria of 500 mg/L or more is present, the condition is described as pre-eclampsia. Pre-eclampsia may be mild or severe, depending on the rise in blood pressure and the clinical or laboratory results (Chari et al 1995):

- mild – blood pressure greater than 140 mmHg systolic or 90 mmHg diastolic, mild proteinuria less than 5.0 g in 24 h, no other abnormalities.
- severe – blood pressure greater than 160 mmHg systolic and 110 mmHg diastolic, proteinuria greater than 5.0 g in 24 h, platelet count less than 100 000/ml, elevated liver enzymes, haemolytic anaemia, headache, epigastric pain.

Incidence

The incidence of PIH in primigravidae is four to five times higher than multigravidae, some of whom may be misdiagnosed. Arias (1993) reported that while 75% of primigravidae who had kidney biopsy showed the typical endothelial changes, only 1 in 10 of the multigravidae did and there is reason to suspect chronic renal disease as the cause of their hypertension. The above statement is supported by Broughton Pipkin (1995), who says that as parity increases a diagnosis of PIH or pre-eclampsia is increasingly likely to be erroneous and underlying renal disease is more likely to be present.

This supports the theory that pre-eclampsia is mainly a disease of primigravidae. However, PIH may occur in a multiparous woman in a first pregnancy by another partner. There is also evidence that women in a prolonged sexual relationship develop an immune response to sperm and are therefore immunologically protected in later pregnancies (Robillard et al 1994). There is a genetic predisposition to this disease, women being more likely to develop the disorder if their mothers or sisters did (Zhang et al 1997). Multiple pregnancies predispose to pre-eclampsia. Women who experience a hydatidiform mole may develop symptoms of PIH before 20 weeks due to hyperplacentation. Women who were hypertensive before pregnancy may develop pre-eclampsia superimposed on the existing condition.

A major problem is that PIH can really only be diagnosed in retrospect by a post-delivery return to normal blood pressure (Hearnshaw 1996). There is also difficulty in predicting which woman is likely to progress to a more serious condition. Severe pre-eclampsia can rapidly fulminate to eclampsia before blood pressure or proteinuria reach levels of concern (Zhang et al 1997). Blood pressure returns to normal within weeks. It is believed that there is no long-term link between hypertension in pregnancy and later onset of chronic hypertension, although this may occur. Proteinuria may persist for longer than the hypertension and may indicate underlying renal disease.

Pathogenesis

The cause of PIH is still not completely understood and it has been described as a disease of theories. It is difficult to use animal models as there is no comparable process to make analogies. Pridjian & Puschett (2002a) hypothesise that pre-eclampsia is an immunologic phenomenon of primiparity.

In normal pregnancy the spiral arterial walls are invaded by trophoblasts and are transformed into large tortuous channels that carry large amounts of blood to the intervillous space. This occurs by 22 weeks, leading to a fall in peripheral resistance. In PIH this does not occur and the spiral arteries may only dilate to 40% of a normal pregnancy (Ghidini et al 1998).

In women with pre-eclampsia there is inadequate invasion of the spiral arterioles by trophoblastic cells so that a decreased uteroplacental perfusion occurs. The symptoms of PIH are a maternal response to poor placentation and an attempt to prevent poor oxygenation of the fetus. Maternal compensatory mechanisms may break down, causing the woman symptoms such as DIC. This disruption of normal placentation may lead to altered endothelial cell function throughout the body, causing generalised vasoconstriction.

In normal pregnancy, the renin–angiotensin–aldosterone system increases in activity, maintaining salt and water balance. In PIH this system is depleted (Pridjian & Puschett 2002b). Vasomotor tone depends on the relative influences of prostacyclin (a vasodilator) and thromboxane (a vasoconstrictor), which are substances from the prostaglandin family found in all tissues. In normal pregnancy there is an increase in substances that cause vasodilatation, including nitric oxide, which is a potent relaxing factor within the endothelium (Zhang et al 1997, Pridjian & Puschett 2002b).

The reduced volume of trophoblasts in the spiral arterioles leads to an underproduction of prostacyclin and a relative overproduction of thromboxane, which encourages vasospasm of the spiral arteries. The damaged endothelium of the spiral arteries undergoes acute atherosclerosis (thickening of the vessel walls), thus narrowing the lumen. This causes a rise in blood pressure to overcome the increased resistance.

Proteinuria is a serious sign in pre-eclampsia, resulting from a swelling of the kidney glomeruli partly due to the raised blood pressure causing leakage of protein through enlarged capillaries. Uric acid clearance is reduced and plasma urates rise, indicating kidney involvement and a need to deliver the woman (Redman et al 1976). The cardiac index (the ratio of cardiac output to body surface area) is reduced by 22% in established pre-eclampsia while systemic vascular resistance is raised (Broughton Pipkin 1995).

This raised systemic resistance is not due to the action of the sympathetic nervous system. It is associated with vasoconstriction, a reduced plasma volume and haemoconcentration, and oedema usually develops. The reduced plasma volume is associated with intrauterine growth restriction (Ghidini et al 1998).

Oxidative stress

Another theory is that **atherosclerosis** caused by **oxidative stress** is the link, as this affects endothelial cells, causing clotting defects and microthrombi. There is a link between oxidative stress and early-onset cardiac disease (Stephens et al 1996). Oxidative stress produces circulating free oxygen radicals as a metabolic by-product. This influences **lipid peroxidation** and damages proteins, nucleic acids and the endothelium. Prostaglandin production is affected, disturbing the balance between thromboxanes and prostacyclins and thus diminishing the vasodilatory effect that pregnancy requires (Broughton Pipkin 1995). Excess **free radicals** affect the endothelium, causing vasoconstriction and platelet aggregation and initiating clotting mechanisms (Chappell et al 1999).

The blood system has naturally occurring antioxidant substances which act against the mechanism of the free radicals. Research by Mikhail et al (1994) suggested that in pregnant women with pre-eclampsia there were lower than usual levels of these antioxidants, namely vitamins E and C, which work in tandem. Supplementing women at risk of pre-eclampsia with vitamins E and C was beneficial in preventing the development of pre-eclampsia (Briley et al 2001).

Outcomes

This multisystems disorder eventually affects the kidneys, the liver and the placental bed. The kidney changes are only distinguishable from acute **glomerulonephritis** by electron microscopy. Narrowing of the capillary lumen by vasospasm is worsened by the deposition of **fibrinous material** between the endothelial cells and the basement membrane as the disease progresses. In glomerulonephritis the narrowing is caused by swelling of the basement membrane. The same fibrinous deposits have been found in the liver of patients with pre-eclampsia. **Intracapsular haemorrhages** and necrosis occur and oedema of the liver cells may produce **epigastric pain** and impairment in liver function, showing diagnostically as raised liver enzymes.

The vessels supplying the placental bed may become constricted and the reduction in uterine blood flow along with placental vascular lesions may result in placental abruption. The reduced maternal capillary blood flow in the placental villi may result in the placental tissue becoming ischaemic. These changes have grave implications for fetal growth and survival. The release of thromboplastin into the maternal circulation results in DIC. The brain becomes oedematous with the development of headache and visual disturbances. As blood pressure continues to rise, fitting may occur. Thrombosis and necrosis of the cerebral blood vessel walls may result in a **cerebrovascular accident**. Seven deaths were reported in the maternal mortality report 1997–9 (Lewis 2001).

Eclampsia

If pre-eclampsia is of sudden onset or if the woman has not attended for antenatal care, about 1 in 2000 women develop the generalised tonic–clonic convulsions and coma of eclampsia. It is an obstetric emergency and immediate care is necessary to prevent death. About 70% of convulsions occurred within 1 week of seeing a doctor or midwife. In the UK many women had a convulsion before a notable rise in blood pressure or the presence of proteinuria developed and 40% of convulsions occurred in the postnatal period (Douglas & Redman 1994). Pre-term eclampsia is associated with more complications for both mothers and fetuses (Leitch et al 1997).

Prediction

As the disease process may be quite extensive by the time the signs and symptoms become obvious, there have been many studies aimed at predicting in early pregnancy which women will develop the disorder. To be of use a test must be non-invasive to mother or fetus, be easy to perform and have a high predictive value. None have been found to be successful and research is ongoing in this area, particularly in the genetic field (Pridjian & Puschett 2002b). Those involved in antenatal care must be vigilant in detecting early signs and symptoms to prevent severe pre-eclampsia and eclampsia developing.

HELLP syndrome

There is uncertainty about whether the HELLP syndrome is a serious complication of pre-eclampsia or a process in itself. Women may present with malaise, nausea, vomiting and epigastric pain, typically before term. They may have normal blood pressures and no proteinuria. If these symptoms, which imitate gastric flu, are present, women may be sent home to recover but the practitioner should think again and take blood specimens for platelets, liver enzymes and await results before sending them home (Nutt 1997).

The resultant pathophysiology may be present alone or together with pre-eclampsia. The severe decrease in platelets alters clotting mechanisms and the haemolysis damages the internal strata of the blood vessels. The multisystems involvement causes kidney failure, hepatic failure and neurological problems in the form of multiple emboli which block capillaries. The placenta is involved and abruptio placentae may occur with the death of the fetus. The HELLP syndrome is a serious condition and delivery is essential to prevent the above complications. Criteria for diagnosis are perhaps a

selection of abnormalities and not always all of them (Martin et al 1999).

Management of hypertensive conditions

Rest and observation

Women with mild PIH can rest at home but, if the disease is moderate to severe or worsening with proteinuria, hospitalisation is recommended. The mother is admitted to hospital where bed rest may be encouraged but this has never been found to be positively beneficial to the management of PIH (Enkin et al 2000). However, admission to hospital allows greater surveillance of maternal and fetal conditions.

A prime method of observing women antenatally is the assessment of blood pressure and urinalysis with estimation of maternal and fetal wellbeing. When proteinuria is present, hospital admission is generally advised once urinary tract infection is eliminated. Plasma urate concentrations are the only useful biochemical indicator of deterioration and severe disease is present if platelet counts begin to fall. Assessment of urinary output may be useful. As the blood pressure rises, visual disturbances, headache and epigastric pain may be experienced by the woman; these signs need investigating and acting on.

The measurement of blood pressure must be accurate and consistent. Doctors and midwives should be guided by the research into the taking and recording of blood pressure and the machines used for its measurement (Shennan & Shennan 1996). Errors are created by observer technique or bias, the sphygmomanometer and the stethoscope and the client's anxiety and fear (white coat hypertension).

Good practice pointers

- Sit client up; machine level with heart (if using mercury manometers).
- Always record on the same arm and use a correctly sized cuff.
- Automated blood pressure machines can underrecord the pressure.
- Let cuff down slowly; read to the nearest 2 mmHg; do not round up or down.
- Korotkoff sound V should be recorded; the disappearance of the sound; if this is 0, then Korotkoff 1V may be used; both should be noted on records.
- If raised measurement, allow a rest before retaking; record findings of both observations.

Fetal observations

Fetal observations will include twice-daily cardiotocograph (CTG) recordings, serial ultrasonic assessments of growth and Doppler measurements of blood velocity in placental bed and umbilical arteries. Any signs of impending eclampsia may necessitate rapid delivery. It is essential to prevent the onset of convulsions, which are life threatening to both mother and fetus.

Delivery

The only treatment for pre-eclampsia is delivery of the baby. A decision on when to deliver the baby will depend partly on how effective the treatment is considered to be, which depends on interpretation of the observations. The timing can be a fine line drawn between maternal condition and fetal maturity. The mode of delivery similarly depends on the risks to mother and baby. Whether delivery is by induction of labour or caesarean section depends on the urgency and suitability, including cervical ripeness, of the individual situations.

Control of blood pressure

There may be alternative therapies in an attempt to prevent complications and in some situations to control high blood pressure. **Methyldopa**, which affects noradrenaline (nor-epinephrine) synthesis (Rang et al 1999), reduces systemic peripheral resistance without changing heart rate or cardiac output (Chari et al 1995). It has been used safely for many years, particularly for women with chronic hypertension, who may have been prescribed **angiotensin-converting enzyme** (ACE) inhibitors prepregnancy; these are contraindicated in pregnancy. The aim is to maintain blood pressure below 100 diastolic, if blood pressure was raised early in pregnancy, to improve fetal outcome (Chari et al 1995).

Labetalol, a **β-adrenoreceptor antagonist** which lowers cardiac output by reducing heart rate and stroke volume, may give better control of blood pressure. However, it may impair maternal and fetal circulation, especially as stroke volume has already been impaired by reduced blood volume. It is probably best used in essential hypertension without pre-eclampsia. Use in the third trimester may prevent fetal growth restriction (Rang et al 1999).

Calcium channel blockers such as **nifedipine** have been used to try to achieve vasodilation (Lopez-Jaramillo et al 1990). There is a significant rise in intracellular free calcium in pre-eclampsia with urinary calcium excretion falling in direct proportion to the severity of the condition (Broughton Pipkin 1995). Many trials have compared therapies to lower blood pressure; the calcium channel blockers may be more effective than other hypotensive drugs but this is not conclusive (Magee et al 1999). A combination of agents may be used – for example, oral nefedipine, parenteral labetalol and parenteral **hydralazine** – in order to control severe pre-eclampsia, particularly where the pregnancy is preterm and time is needed for the fetus to mature (Chari et al 1995).

Hydralazine directly relaxes arterial smooth muscle, resulting in increased heart rate and contractility with decreased placental blood flow and consequent fetal distress (Chari et al 1995), but may cause maternal hypotension. In trials discussed by Magee et al (1999), parenteral labetalol had fewer side-effects and was as effective at lowering the blood pressure.

Anticonvulsive therapy

Magnesium sulphate is widely used in the USA to control the convulsive state. In the UK **diazepam** and **phenytoin** were used to prevent or treat fits in pre-eclampsia. Duley (1995) in the Eclampsia Study compared diazepam and phenytoin with magnesium sulphate, finding that magnesium sulphate reduced the risk by 52% and 67%, respectively, than when the above two drugs were used. There is overwhelming evidence in favour of magnesium sulphate (Duley et al 2003). Magnesium sulphate is toxic and monitoring blood levels and reflexes to test nervous system involvement is crucial. Calcium gluconate should be available in case toxicity is evident (Garovic 2000).

Diuretics are contraindicated in pre-eclampsia as they can aggravate plasma volume and balance of fluids. There is a place for them in women with chronic hypertension prepregnancy and hypertension in renal and heart failure, although they may adversely affect electrolyte imbalance (Garovic 2000).

Prevention

Aspirin prevents platelet aggregation by inhibiting thromboxane production. The multicentre Collaborative Low-Dose Aspirin Study trial (CLASP 1994) set out to show that, used prophylactically, it would prevent pre-eclampsia. The use of low-dose aspirin (60–150 mg) was not proven to be beneficial. There have been many follow-up studies and Duley et al (2001) systematically reviewed 39 trials of over 30 000 women. They found a 15% reduction in pre-eclampsia and a 14% reduction in stillbirth and neonatal death and an 8% reduction in preterm births. There is some benefit from starting early before 12–16 weeks and it was concluded that there was a small-to-moderate benefit in its use.

MAIN POINTS

- There is a changing pattern of heart disease, with increasing numbers of women surviving congenital heart disease and an increase in coronary artery disease. About 6000 new patients will reach their 16th birthday having had heart lesions and requiring medical supervision. The woman may already be aware of her heart disease and may have sought preconception advice. There will be a higher incidence of a heart defect in the baby if there is a family history of congenital heart defect.

- The main effects of rheumatic heart disease are to cause valvular lesions. Mitral stenosis requires an increase in left atrial pressure to push blood into the left ventricle and will require a greater effort in pregnancy.

- It is traditional to use the New York Heart Association classification to describe the severity of heart disease but in practice this has little predictive value of the effect of pregnancy on the disease process.

- Labour should take place in a unit with full resuscitation facilities and an intensive care unit. It should be spontaneous in onset, with a vaginal delivery where possible. The use of intravenous fluids increases circulating blood volume, which may result in pulmonary oedema, and an epidural reduces the risk. To prevent bacterial endocarditis antibiotic prophylaxis is necessary in labour. Anticoagulants could avoid the risk of developing thromboemboli.

- The second stage should be kept short and without exertion. Elective forceps delivery and avoiding the supine position should be advocated.

- Hypertension which develops for the first time in the second half of pregnancy and is caused by the pregnancy is common. Pre-eclampsia is associated with proteinuria and may lead to eclampsia. It is a multisystem disorder, which may result in maternal and fetal morbidity and mortality.

- Pre-eclampsia is mainly a disease of primigravidae but may occur in a multiparous woman in a first pregnancy by a new partner.

- In pre-eclampsia there is inadequate invasion of the spiral arterioles by trophoblastic cells and decreased uteroplacental perfusion occurs. Associated with vasoconstriction is a reduced plasma volume and haemoconcentration and oedema usually develop. There are two common features of pre-eclampsia – vasoconstriction and DIC – leading to changes in the kidney, liver and placental bed.

- The aim of care is to prolong the pregnancy until the fetus is mature enough to survive. Antihypertensive drugs are useful at protecting the woman's circulation against the risk of cerebrovascular accident but have no effect on the disease or on fetal growth.

- Maternal observations include urinalysis for protein, fluid balance, presence of oedema, blood pressure and abdominal examination for pain and tenderness. Plasma urate concentrations are the only useful biochemical indicator of deterioration and severe disease is present if platelet counts fall.

- Deciding when to deliver the baby depends partly on how effective the treatment is considered to be, which will depend on the interpretation of the observations. The timing can be a fine line drawn between maternal condition and fetal maturity. The mode of delivery similarly depends on the risks to mother and baby.

- In a few women severe pre-eclampsia may affect the liver and be complicated by the HELLP syndrome. Immediate delivery will resolve the abnormal blood picture but there may be a need to give platelets or packed red cells to lessen the risk of haemorrhage. The long-term prognosis is that the blood pressure returns to normal within weeks. It is believed that there is no long-term link between hypertension in pregnancy and later onset of chronic hypertension.

References

American Heart Association 2002 Congenital cardiovascular disease: http://www.americanheart.org.

Ammash N, Warnes C 2001 Ventricular septal defect in adults. Annals of Internal Medicine 35(9):812–824.

Arias F 1993 Practical Guide to High Risk Pregnancy and Delivery, 2nd edn. Mosby Year Book, Chicago.

Blackburn S T 2003 Maternal, Fetal and Neonatal Physiolog: A Clinical Perspective, 3rd edn. W B Saunders, Philadelphia.

Brickner E, Hillis D, Lange A 2000a Medical progress: congenital heart disease in adults (Part 1). New England Journal of Medicine 342(4):256–263.

Brickner E, Hillis D, Lange A 2000b Medical progress: congenital heart disease in adults (Part 2). New England Journal of Medicine 342(5):334–342.

Briley A, Chappell L, Kelly F, Shennan A, Poston L 2001 The vitamins in pre-eclampsia study. RCM Midwives Journal 4(9):288–291.

Broughton Pipkin F 1995 The hypertensive disorders of pregnancy. British Medical Journal 311:609–613.

Chamberlain G, Steer P 1999 ABC of labour care: labour in special circumstances. British Medical Journal 318(7191):1124–1127.

Chambers T, Hunter S 2000 Congenital heart disease and adolescents. Journal of the Royal College of Physicians of London 34(2):150–152.

Chappell L, Seed P, Briley A et al 1999 Effects of anti-oxidants on the occurrence of pre-eclampsia in women at increased risk: a randomised trial. Lancet 354(9181):810–815.

Chari R, Friedman S, Sibai B 1995 Antihypertensive therapy during pregnancy. Maternal Medicine Review No. 7:71–75.

CLASP 1994 Collaborative Low-dose Aspirin Study in Pregnancy, Collaborative Group. Lancet 343(8898):619–629.

Davey D, MacGillivray I 1986 The classification of the hypertensive disorders of pregnancy. Clinical and Experimental Hypertension B5:97–133.

Douglas K A, Redman C W G 1994 Eclampsia in the United Kingdom. British Medical Journal 309(6966):1395–1400.

Duley L 1995 The Eclampsia Trial Collaborative Group. Which anticonvulsant for women with eclampsia? Evidence from the collaborative eclampsia trial. Lancet 345:1455–1463.

Duley L, Henderson-Smart D, Knight M, King J 2001 Antiplatelet drugs for the prevention of pre-eclampsia and its consequences: systematic review. British Medical Journal 322(7782):329–333.

Duley L, Gulmezoglu A M, Henderson-Smart D J 2003 Anticonvulsants for women with pre-eclampsia. Cochrane Review: In The Cochrane Library, Issue 2. Update Software 2003, Oxford.

Enkin M, Keirse M, Neilson J et al 2000 A Guide to Effective Care in Pregnancy and Childbirth, 3rd edn. Oxford University Press, Oxford.

Garovic V 2000 Hypertension in pregnancy: diagnosis and treatment. Mayo Clinic Proceedings 75(10):1017–1076.

Ghidini A, Salfia C M, Pijnenborg R 1998 Lesions of the placental bed and placenta in relation to pre-eclampsia. Contemporary Reviews in Obstetrics and Gynaecology June:85–90.

Gilbert E, Harmon J 1998 High Risk Pregnancy and Delivery. Mosby, St Louis.

Hearnshaw A 1996 The trouble with terminology. APEC Newsletter No. 11 (Spring):17.

Hurst J, Morris D, Wayne A 1999 The use of the New York Heart Association's Classification of Cardiovascular Disease as part of the patient's complete problem list. Clinical Cardiology 22(June):385–390.

Leitch C, Cameron A, Walker J 1997 The changing pattern of eclampsia over a 60 year period. British Journal of Obstetrics and Gynaecology 104:917–922.

Lewis G (ed.) 2001 Why mothers die. Fifth Report of Confidential Enquiries into Maternal Deaths in the United Kingdom 1997–99. Royal College Obstetricians and Gynaecologists Press, London.

Lopez-Jaramillo P, Navarez M, Felix C, Lopez A 1990 Dietary calcium supplementation and prevention of pregnancy induced hypertension. Lancet 335:293.

Magee L, Ornstein M P, von Dadelszen P 1999 Management of hypertension in pregnancy. British Medical Journal 318:1332–1336.

Martin J, Rinehart B, Warren L et al 1999 The spectrum of pre-eclampsia: comparative analysis of HELLP syndrome classification. American Journal of Obstetrics and Gynaecology 180(6):1373–1384.

Meschengieser S, Fondevila C, Santarelli M, Lazzari M 2000 Anticoagulation in pregnant women with heart valve prosthesis. Obstetrical and Gynaecological Survey 55(2):72.

Mikhail M, Anyaegbunam A, Garfunkel D et al 1994 Pre-eclampsia and antioxidant nutrients, decreased plasma levels of reduced ascorbic acid, alpha-tocopheral and beta-carotene in women with pre-eclampsia. American Journal of Obstetrics and Gynecology 171:150–157.

Nutt J 1997 HELLP syndrome. British Journal of Midwifery l5(1):8–11.

Prasad A, Ventura H 2001 Valvular heart disease and pregnancy. Postgraduate medicine: online 110 (2) August: http://www.postgraduatemed.com/issues/2001/08/prasad.htm.

Pridjian G, Puschett J 2002a Pre-eclampsia part 1, clinical and pathophysiological considerations. Obstetrical and Gynaecological Survey 57(9):598–618.

Pridjian G, Puschett J 2002b Pre-eclampsia part 2, experimental and genetic considerations. Obstetrical and Gynaecological Survey 57(9):619–640.

Rang H P, Dale M M, Ritter J M 1999 Pharmacology, 4th edn. Churchill Livingstone, Edinburgh.

Redman C, Beilin L, Bonnar J 1976 Renal function in pre-eclampsia. Journal of Clinical Pathology (10, Supp. Royal College of Pathologists):91–94.

Robillard P Y, Hulsey T C, Perianin J 1994 Association of pregnancy induced hypertension with duration of sexual cohabitation before conception. Lancet 344(8928):973–975.

Sawhney H, Aggarwal N, Suri V et al 2003 Maternal and perinatal outcomes in rheumatic heart disease. International Journal of Gynaecology and Obstetrics 80(1):9–14.

Shennan C, Shennan A 1996 Blood pressure in pregnancy: the need for accurate measurement. British Journal of Midwifery 4(2):102–108.

Siu S, Colman J 2001 Heart disease in pregnancy. BMJ Heart 85(6):710–715.

Stephens N, Parsons A, Schofield P et al 1996 Randomised controlled trial of vitamin E in patients with coronary artery disease: Cambridge Heart Antioxidant Study (CHAOS). Lancet 347:781–786.

Williams D 1999 Pregnancy and the heart. Hospital Medicine 60(2):100–104.

Zhang J, Zeisler J, Hatch M, Berkowitz G 1997 Epidemiology of pregnancy-induced hypertension. Epidemiologic Review 19(2):218–232.

Annotated recommended reading

American Heart Association 2002 Congenital cardiovascular disease: http://www.americanheart.org.
Within this site is a clearly written account of congenital heart defects and also there are many links to other pertinent sites about heart disease.

Broughton Pipkin F 1995 The hypertensive disorders of pregnancy. British Medical Journal 311:609–613.
This paper is a must read as it is an overview of hypertension in pregnancy with clear physiological explanations of this puzzling disorder.

Magann E, Martin J 1999 Twelve steps to optimal management of HELLP syndrome. Clinical Obstetrics and Gynaecology 42(3):532–550.
This paper gives the reader a depth of understanding of HELPP syndrome. It includes classification, pathophysiology, assessment of maternal health and treatment.

Oakley C (ed.) 1997 Heart Disease in Pregnancy. BMJ Books, London.
This edited textbook gives a detailed account of all aspects of heart disease in pregnancy.

Zhang J, Zeisler J, Hatch M, Berkowitz G 1997 Epidemiology of pregnancy-induced hypertension. Epidemiologic Review 19(2):218–232.
This paper defines pregnancy-induced hypertension. It contains a depth of physiology which clarifies many aspects of the cause of hypertension in pregnancy.

Chapter 33

Anaemia and clotting disorders

ANAEMIA

Worldwide, the effects of anaemia and clotting disorders on maternal and fetal morbidity and mortality are enormous. This chapter examines these two clinical problems in detail. Anaemia is reduction in the oxygen-carrying capacity of the blood, which may be due to a reduced number of red blood cells, a low concentration of haemoglobin (Hb) or a combination of both (Lloyd & Lewis 1999). The effects of anaemia involve both mother and fetus. The mother may develop symptoms such as dyspnoea, fainting fatigue, tachycardia and palpitations. She may have reduced resistance to infection and her life may be threatened by antepartum or postpartum haemorrhage.

The fetus may suffer intrauterine hypoxia and growth restriction although it is difficult to separate the effects of anaemia from other factors such as social class, smoking and maternal age. Godfrey et al (1991) found that large placental weight with a reduction in fetal weight was associated with iron deficiency anaemia. This correlated the change in placental/fetal weight ratio with a risk of hypertension in later life (Godfrey & Barker 1995).

Recognition of anaemia

The World Health Organisation (WHO 1979) set criteria for diagnosis of anaemia in pregnancy as an Hb of less than (<) 11 g/dl but because of increased understanding of the physiological changes in pregnancy many doctors only investigate women with an Hb of <10.0 or 10.5 g/dl (Letsky 1995). Most cases of anaemia in pregnancy are due to iron deficiency but the following anaemias are associated with pregnancy (Schwartz & Thurnau 1995):

- iron deficiency anaemia (IDA);
- folic acid deficiency;
- hereditary haemoglobinopathies, sickle cell anaemias and the thalassaemias;
- anaemia due to blood loss.

Iron deficiency anaemia

Incidence

Iron is essential for the bioavailability of oxygen to cells. Iron deficiency is a common pathology of pregnancy, but may be asymptomatic and difficult to diagnose. The physiological changes of pregnancy make it difficult to use normal criteria such as haemoglobin level, except as an indicator of a potential problem. The WHO state that the prevalence of anaemia in pregnancy in developing countries is between 35% and 75% (Allen 1997). In developed countries this is lower, at 18%. IDA is the most common nutrient deficiency in the world (Schwartz & Thurnau 1995). The high rate in developing countries may be due to nutritional deficiencies or to infections such as malaria, dysentery and parasite infestation (Allen 1997).

Causes

In pregnancy there is a greater demand for iron for haemoglobin synthesis. If haemoglobin is low, there is a poor red cell uptake of oxygen and poor oxygen delivery to the placental bed and fetus. The fetus obtains its iron from transferrin in the maternal blood across the placental–maternal interface, usually after 30 weeks of pregnancy. In the earlier weeks maternal iron consumption increases and should meet the later demands, but if iron stores as ferritin are low the demand may not be met (Allen 1997). To ascertain those women at risk of IDA, the midwives' booking interview should highlight the following factors (Coggins 2001):

- reduced food intake or malabsorption of iron or protein;
- blood loss from previous heavy menses;
- iron deprivation from previous pregnancies or short pregnancy gap;
- multiple pregnancy;
- chronic urinary tract infection (low iron status affects immunity);
- previous antepartum or postpartum haemorrhage;
- women from low social groups.

In a multicultural society such as Britain the likelihood of the **inherited haemoglobinopathies** should be considered as well as the effects of nutrition and infection on iron status.

Investigations

Identification of IDA involves screening, blood counts, history taking and investigations. Screening all pregnant women for Hb concentration regularly indicates the presence of anaemia but will not identify the cause. However, normal non-pregnant reference values may not consider the haemodilution of pregnancy and there may be a danger of overdiagnosing asymptomatic women with low haemoglobin. Women who are identified as having a low Hb should be questioned about nutritional habits, gastrointestinal upset, and excessive menstrual bleeding prior to pregnancy.

IDA is a **microcytic anaemia** with a fall in mean cell volume (MCV), and a fall in **serum ferritin** (iron stores) before a fall in Hb. A fall in Hb is a late sign when iron stores have already been depleted. A urine sample should be obtained to exclude urinary tract infection. Coggins (2001) outlines the parameters considered when making a diagnosis of IDA (Table 33.1).

Management

An oral iron preparation is usually given once IDA has been diagnosed. Absorption is maximised if taken with orange juice (Coggins 2001). The daily iron needed to treat IDA is 60–120 mg in divided doses. Oral ferrous salts are more absorbable than ferric salts but all iron preparations tend to have side-effects such as nausea, vomiting and constipation (Frewin et al 1997). Letsky (1997) argues that all women are deficient in iron stores at some point in pregnancy and prophylactic dispensing of iron preparations to all women would prevent this. In most units in the UK, women are only given iron preparations if IDA has been diagnosed. Iron can be given by intramuscular injection or intravenous infusion if necessary (Lloyd & Lewis 1999):

- Intramuscular iron is given in the form of **iron sorbitol** 50 mg/ml. The dose is 1.5 mg/kg body weight and it can

Table 33.1 Blood tests used to diagnose iron deficiency anaemia (IDA)

Blood test	Normal reference range	Validity in diagnosis
Haemoglobin	11–15 g/dl (pregnant)	Lacks specificity, affected by haemodilution and smoking
Mean cell volume (MCV)	75–99 fl (femtolitres)	Raised in pregnancy, decreased in IDA
Reticulocyte count	25–75 × 10^9/L	Increased by pregnancy, decreased by IDA
Serum ferritin	15–300 μg/L	Signifies iron stores, early indication of iron deficiency
Total iron-binding capacity (TIBC)	45–72 μmol/L	Non-specific in pregnancy, TIBC raised by pregnancy, false-positive if infection present
Serum iron	13–27 μmol/L	Decreased by pregnancy, diurnal rhythm, non-specific in pregnancy

be given daily or weekly. A deep intramuscular injection should be given to avoid staining the skin and fat necrosis.

- Intravenous iron is given as a total dose iron infusion in the form of **iron dextran** 50 mg/ml. It is given slowly in normal saline and the dose depends on body weight and the degree of iron deficiency. Rang et al (1999) suggest that anaphylactic shock is a major side-effect and intravenous iron should only be given if absolutely necessary.

- Blood transfusion may be given late in pregnancy if Hb levels are extremely low but care must be taken to avoid circulatory overload. Further investigations should take place if treatment is not effective.

The treatment for IDA has been reviewed by Cuervo & Mahomed (2003) who looked at 53 trials. Evidence about the effects of iron therapy in pregnancy was inconclusive as there was a shortage of quality trials. Intravenous iron was associated with an increased risk of venous thrombosis.

Folic acid deficiency anaemia

Incidence

Folic acid is necessary for red cell proliferation and deficiency may occur in pregnancy unless folic acid intake is increased. It is difficult to measure folate levels as dietary folate intake varies and levels could be normal one day and low the next. Severe folate deficiency may lead to megaloblastic anaemia.

Megaloblastic anaemia is caused by vitamin B_{12} deficiency and iron deficiency may conceal a mild megaloblastic anaemia. Deficiency is most likely to occur in late pregnancy or in the puerperium. Folic acid deficiency may cause pallor, lassitude and gastrointestinal symptoms such as anorexia, nausea and vomiting, glossitis and gingivitis and diarrhoea. Mental depression may also occur (Letsky 1997).

Investigations

The red cells are macrocytic but less in number so that the Hb level is low. Plasma folate and red cell folate can be estimated. There may be a low platelet and white cell count. Serum folic acid is lower than 4 μg/ml. Diagnosis of true megaloblastic anaemia is by bone marrow aspiration (Letsky 1997).

Management

The anaemia usually responds to folic acid supplementation of 5–15 mg folic acid daily. Prevention by administration of prophylactic folic acid 300–500 μg daily can be given to:

- those with malabsorption syndrome;
- those with haemoglobinopathies (see below);
- those who are on anticonvulsant therapy;
- those with a multiple pregnancy.

Folate deficiency is involved in the causation of neural tube defects (Box 33.1).

Box 33.1 Neural tube defects in the fetus and folate deficiency

Neural tube defects (NTDs) include conditions such as anencephaly and **spina bifida** with or without a **meningocele**, most of which occur from failure of closure of the caudal neuropore between 22 and 30 days of pregnancy. This leaves the spinal cord unprotected by the spinal column. α–Fetoprotein (AFP) is a fetal protein found in small amounts in maternal serum in normal pregnancies. Any open fetal defect leads to the leaking of AFP into the amniotic fluid, with higher levels than usual entering maternal serum. Higher levels of AFP occur if the gestational age is overassessed or if more than one fetus is present.

About 1000 cases of NTD are detected through screening each year (Whyte 1996). The routine use of ultrasound at booking, then a further anomaly scan, identifies most of these defects so the parents can make a choice between continuing the pregnancy or termination (Devane & Devane 2000). The cause may involve both genetic and environmental triggers. A dietary factor has been suspected for a long time and **folic acid** was implicated as early as 1964 (Wald 1991). Two studies in the 1980s suggested that folic acid supplementation might reduce the risk of recurrence of NTDs.

The Medical Research Council's (MRC) Vitamin Study Group (1991) undertook a multicentred, double-blind, randomised trial

across 33 centres in seven countries to see if supplementation with folic acid or a mixture of seven other vitamins around the time of conception could prevent NTDs. The findings were that folic acid supplements prevented three-quarters of the cases of NTD recurrence. They concluded that it was unlikely that the effect would be restricted to recurrences and that folic acid would probably prevent first-time occurrences of NTD.

Folic acid is used in the metabolic chain to provide the chemical bases of three of the essential **DNA components**: guanine, adenine and thymine. Vitamin B_{12} is necessary to form an enzyme in the metabolic pathway of folate. Women who are epileptic tend to have more congenital abnormalities, in part due to the antiepileptic medication altering the absorption of folate (Steegers-Theunissen 1995).

Following the findings of the above study the expert advisory group to the Department of Health (1992) recommended the use of 4 mg of folic acid three months prior to conception continued until the early months of pregnancy. The fortification of food with folic acid was also discussed but there are concerns about intake of too much folic acid if folic acid was added to many foods such as flour, rice and pasta (Mason & McNabb 2000). The incidence of NTD has definitely declined in the last ten years; perhaps due to folic acid supplements.

HAEMOGLOBINOPATHIES

The World Health Organisation estimated that 7% of the world's population may be carriers of single gene defects of the red cell by the year 2000. Two of the commonest diseases are the recessively inherited **sickle cell disease** and **thalassaemias** which affect haemoglobin synthesis. In utero, the fetus is not affected as it carries fetal haemoglobin (HbF), but soon after birth the switch between fetal and adult haemoglobin (HbA) begins. As the ratio of HbF to HbA changes, the symptoms of inherited disease become evident (Stephen & Cunningham 1998).

The globin chains

The gene for the α-globin chain family is located on chromosome 16 and for the β-globin chain family on chromosome 11. The α-globin chain is 141 amino acids long and the β-globin chain is 146 amino acids long. All haemoglobin variants have a tetramic structure with four protein chains in association with four haem molecules. The four protein chains in normal haemoglobin take up a particular shape which allows maximum uptake, delivery and release of oxygen into the tissues (Stephen & Cunningham 1998).

Inherited genes produce abnormal proteins that cannot carry out their function efficiently and the result is ill health with anaemia, hypoxia, tissue damage and haemolysis (Fig. 33.1). There are three forms of inherited haemoglobinopathies:

● structural Hb variants, where there is a fault in either the α-globin chain or β-globin chain;
● the thalassaemias, where there is reduced production of either α-globin chain or β-globin chain;
● failure to switch from the production of HbF to HbA, which is clinically insignificant, although in some instances helps the sufferer because oxygen is absorbed more easily by HbF.

Sickle cell disease

Sickle cell disease is the commonest of the structural haemoglobin variants (Weatherall 1997b) (Table 33.2). A single amino acid substitution of **valine** for **glutamic acid** results in a haemoglobin molecule that is less soluble. When oxygen is low, the molecules form long, linear stacks that distort the red cells into a sickle shape. The inheritance of one gene from each parent (homozygous genotype for HbSS) makes the individual sickle cell positive. Those who inherit one gene (heterozygote) have the **sickle cell trait** (HbAS) and usually do not display signs of the disease. They do, however, have some protection against the organism *Plasmodium falciparum*, the cause of a severe form of malaria. The malarial parasite enters the red blood cell and makes it sickle. This cell and its parasite are destroyed by the spleen, protecting the individual from malaria (Bloom 1995).

Heterozygote parents have a 1 in 4 chance of producing a baby who is HbSS, sickle cell positive. These couples must be offered prenatal diagnosis. The diagnosis of sickle cell disease prenatally was undertaken by cordocentesis at 20 weeks of pregnancy, necessitating a late abortion. However, DNA technology permits diagnosis earlier. The advent of pre-implantation genetic diagnosis makes it possible for families with a history of inheritable haemoglobinopathies to have in-vitro fertilisation (IVF) treatment and only implant healthy conceptions (Layton 2003, Modell et al 1998).

Incidence

The incidence of sickle cell disease varies from country to country and is about 1 in 4 in parts of Africa and 1 in 10 of the black population of the USA and UK. It is estimated that 50 000 Americans have sickle cell disease. Amongst African-Americans 1:375 have HbSS, 1:832 have HbSC, 1:1667 have Hb β-thalassaemia (Website gscc.genetics). Heterozygote incidence ranges from 0.9% in Europe to 13.3% in Africa. The incidence of sickle cell births in the UK is 0.23 per 1000 (Layton 2003).

Pathophysiology

Deoxygenation is the most common cause of **sickling**; HbSS reacts by creating non-pliable intracellular fibres which pull the cells into a banana shape or holly leaf shape. These block capillaries, creating the pain of a sickle cell crisis (Bunn 1997). Decreased plasma volume, hypothermia, infection and acidosis also precipitate sickling. This will occur with minor degrees of oxygen shortage in people with sickle cell disease, but lack of oxygen has to be severe to cause sickling in people with sickle cell trait.

Vascular occlusion occurs anywhere but especially in the kidney and brain. In pregnancy the placental bed may be affected. Pain is severe and death of tissues may occur within affected organs. Sickled cells are haemolysed in the spleen, resulting in anaemia. Sickling is not permanent and most of the red cells regain their normal shape after reoxygenation and rehydration. The extent and clinical manifestations of sickling will depend on the percentage of haemoglobin that is HbS. This is why it is rare for a heterozygous person to suffer much sickling (McCance & Huether 2002).

Pregnancy outcomes

In general, women with sickle cell trait have uncomplicated pregnancies, whereas sickle cell-positive women may have complications. A US study compared HbSS and HbSC women with a group of women with normal haemoglobin. The HbSS and HbSC women were at increased risk of fetal growth restriction, antenatal admissions, preterm labour and postpartum infections, although women with HbSS had more complications (Sun et al 2001). An English study of 81 pregnancies in several centres observed there were

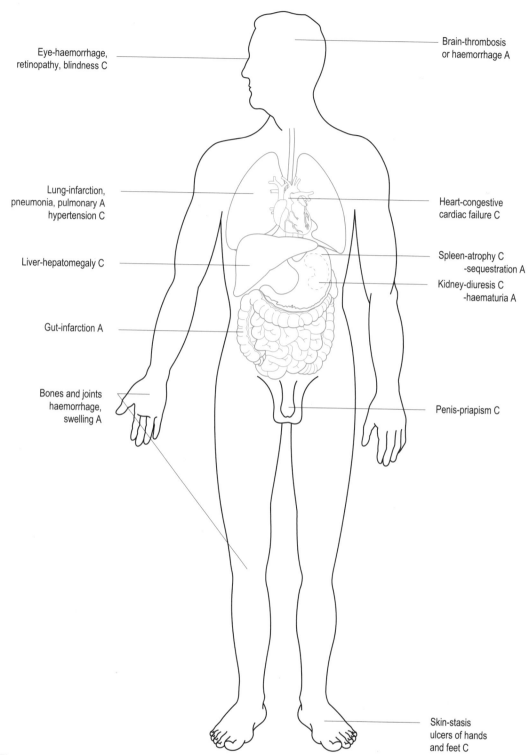

Eye-haemorrhage,
retinopathy, blindness C

Brain-thrombosis
or haemorrhage A

Lung-infarction,
pneumonia, pulmonary A
hypertension C

Heart-congestive
cardiac failure C

Liver-hepatomegaly C

Spleen-atrophy C
-sequestration A

Kidney-diuresis C
-haematuria A

Gut-infarction A

Bones and joints
haemorrhage,
swelling A

Penis-priapism C

Skin-stasis
ulcers of hands
and feet C

Figure 33.1   Major clinical manifestations of sickle cell anaemia. Acute (A) and chronic (C).

46.2% sickling crises in the antenatal period and 7.7% post-natal sickling episodes. These women were more likely to have anaemia, proteinuric hypertension and low birth weight babies. Prophylactic blood transfusion was used to prevent problems but there was no significance in preventing complications when compared with the untransfused women (Howard et al 1995).

Principles of treatment in pregnancy
(Lloyd & Lewis 1999)

- anaemia may be prevented by prophylactic use of folic acid and iron.
- blood transfusion may be necessary if Hb is extremely low.
- avoidance of infection.

Table 33.2 Common combinations of haemoglobin in sickle cell disease

Haemoglobin	Disease
HbSS	Homozygous sickle cell disease (sickle cell anaemia)
HbSC	Heterozygous sickle cell disease (sickle cell C disease), mild anaemia, and fewer crises, risk of retinal damage and thromboembolic problems in pregnancy
HbCC	Homozygous CC disease (not a sickling disorder)
HbS β-thalassaemia	Sickle–β-thalassaemia, generally produces sickle Hb
HbAS	Sickle cell trait, generally no problems

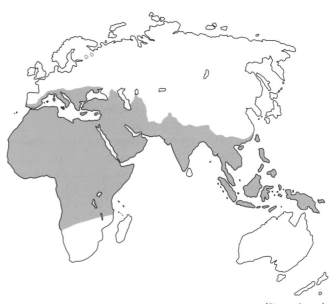

Figure 33.2 The world distribution of thalassaemia. (Reproduced with permission from Weatherall 1991.)

- avoidance of cold and stress.
- in labour keep hydrated and prevent acidosis by intravenous therapy; use prophylactic antibiotics; oxygen may be necessary; this will prevent crisis.
- if crisis occurs, give pain relief; this may be the first sign of sickling.

Anyone with sickle cell disease needs specialised care by both the haematologist and the obstetrician with back up from laboratory and a sickle cell centre (Lloyd & Lewis 1999). Treatment may include a blood transfusion every 6 weeks to maintain a high proportion of normal haemoglobin or it may be necessary to carry out an exchange transfusion (Boyle 2002).

Thalassaemia

Incidence

This disease is caused by the reduced rate of synthesis of either α-globin chains or β-globin chains. The heterozygote (**thalassaemia minor**) with one normal haemoglobin gene is generally asymptomatic but with reduced haemoglobin levels. The homozygous condition (**thalassaemia major**) is life threatening and if untreated leads to death in childhood. Homozygotes have severe anaemia that requires regular blood transfusions. There are more than 150 variants of the thalassaemia gene. These may be due to deletions along the gene as well as to mistakes in the sequencing of bases. This makes detection and counselling difficult (Savona-Ventura & Bonello 1994, Weatherall 1997a).

Thailand has a total population of about 50 million and about 500 000 children suffer severe ill health due to the interactions of different thalassaemias. Another haemoglobin variant, **HbE**, is carried by up to 50% of the population in parts of the country and people who inherit HbE and **β-thalassaemia**, a common genotype in Thailand, can be quite ill (Weatherall 1997a).

α-thalassaemia causes severe health problems in parts of China, Cambodia and Vietnam and β-thalassaemia in the Mediterranean countries of Italy, Greece, Cyprus and Sardinia (Fig. 33.2). About 7% of the population of the Greek mainland carry the gene for β-thalassaemia and about 250 homozygous babies are born annually. In Cyprus and Sardinia the carrier state reaches 15–20% and about 1 in 100 homozygous babies are born. Each new wave of immigration may lead to increased incidence of inherited disorders in the UK. As children mature, there will be greater mixing of hereditary diseases and screening programmes will need to be widened. Women and their partners who carry the gene for β-thalassaemia come from many countries and the provision of a prenatal diagnosis programme may be expensive.

Pathophysiology

The thalassaemias can be categorised as:

1. α+ thalassaemia with low production of α-globin chains due to one defective gene.

2. α° thalassaemia, where neither gene is producing α-globin chains. Tetramers of β chains and γ chains are produced. β_4 (HbH) and γ_4 (Hb Bart's) are formed but the absence of α-globin chains means that oxygen cannot be released and the condition is incompatible with life.

3. β+ thalassaemia with low production of β-globin chains, due to one defective gene.

4. β° thalassaemia, where neither gene is producing β-globin chains. There is production of HbF and α-globin chains. These cells are destroyed by the immune system, leading to ineffective erythropoiesis (Savona-Ventura & Bonello 1994).

Clinical signs and symptoms

β-thalassaemia is much more common than α-thalassaemia and in the carrier state leads to mild **microcytic hypochromic** anaemia and hyperplasia of bone marrow, due to increased haemopoiesis. Haemolysis of immature erythrocytes may cause a slight rise in serum iron. The spleen may be enlarged because of the increased haemolysis.

Homozygotes have severe anaemia and HbF levels are always raised. Bone growth may be stunted in young children due to the hyperplasia. Regular blood transfusions shut off the bone marrow overgrowth. The accumulation of iron may result in death from damage to heart muscle, liver and pancreas. Blood transfusions can increase the life span by up to 20 years (Weatherall 1997b). People who inherit the α-thalassaemia trait are usually symptom-free with a milder anaemia than seen in β-thalassaemia trait. However, homozygous α-thalassaemia leads to intrauterine congestive cardiac failure and **hydrops fetalis** with intrauterine death (Letsky 1995).

Treatment

Heterozygotes seldom need treatment and the treatment for homozygous β-thalassaemia is only partially successful. It involves:

- blood transfusions to top up the haemoglobin and haematocrit levels;
- iron chelation therapy with an agent such as desferrioxamine to allow the excess iron to be excreted from the body;
- splenectomy to reduce the amount of haemolysis;
- monitoring of hepatic iron and ferritin levels is essential.

Care in pregnancy

Anyone with thalassaemia trait is likely to develop anaemia that is similar to iron deficiency with microcytic cells. However, iron deficiency is not usually a problem as the reduced number of red cells and mild haemolysis ensure that iron is available. Iron therapy is inappropriate unless deficiency is proven. Folic acid supplements are given.

Girls with homozygous β-thalassaemia die in childhood but treatment increases the likelihood of them living long enough to become pregnant. They need care, shared between the haematologist and obstetrician, preferably in a specialised centre (Lloyd & Lewis 1999).

Kumar et al (1997) reported a study of transfusion-dependent women in India. There were 20 spontaneous conceptions and 12 induced ovulations, 24 delivered normally with 8 caesarean sections. There were multiorgan effects of iron deposition due to multiple blood transfusions. Induced ovulation was sometimes necessary because of **hypogonadism** and low estriol levels. Heart function may be altered in these women due to low Hb. Kumar et al (1997) comment that these pregnancies would not have occurred

except for good care that provided the thalassaemic women with better chances. Fetal testing was necessary as the severity of the effect on the child's health will depend on the abnormal genes inherited from each parent.

Glucose 6-phosphate dehydrogenase (G6PD) deficiency

G6PD deficiency is a rare X-linked enzyme deficiency found in people of African, Asian and Mediterranean origin. The enzyme protects the haemoglobin molecules from oxidation and certain drugs precipitate haemolytic crises, such as antimalarial preparations, sulphonamides, some antibiotics such as nitrofurantoin, nalidixic acid and chloramphenicol and also drugs acquired by a breastfeeding infant (Johnston 1998). A gene frequency of 11% has been found in the American black male population (McCance & Huether 2002). The gene is also present in the Sephardic Jewish population. Neonates who inherit the gene may have prolonged jaundice.

THROMBOEMBOLISM AND PREGNANCY

Thrombosis in childbearing women is serious because of its association with deep vein thrombosis and pulmonary embolism, which remains the most common cause of maternal death. There were 16.5 deaths per million maternities in the 1997–99 triennium (Lewis 2001). Thromboembolic diseases are much more likely to occur in the puerperium as the diuresis which occurs in the first 24 h following delivery changes the blood viscosity. This becomes significant now that the rate of operative deliveries is rising. Thrombosis can be divided clinically into superficial **thrombophlebitis** and **deep vein thrombosis** (DVT).

Superficial thrombophlebitis

The superficial veins of the legs are affected. The vein is tender and may be reddened and hard. It is usually a varicose vein that is affected and there is no risk of pulmonary embolism unless there is a concomitant deep vein thrombosis. Women who are at risk tend to be older, overweight and of high parity. Applying supportive bandages or the use of supportive tights assists in the treatment of this condition. The woman should elevate her legs when resting but there is no need to restrict movement and anticoagulant therapy is not necessary.

Deep vein thrombosis

The deep veins of the calf, thigh or pelvis are usually affected, particularly on the left side. If there is no accompanying inflammation (**phlebitis**) and the blood clot (thrombus) does not obstruct the blood vessel, there may be no clinical signs. If the clot is friable and pieces become detached from the vessel wall, they will travel around the circulation (**embolus**), through the heart and into the pulmonary circulation, leading to a **pulmonary embolism**. This may be fatal, but recovery could be complete (Bewley & Bradshaw 2001).

Factors associated with pregnancy predisposing women to thromboembolism

- Caesarean section.
- Age over 30 years; high parity.
- Weight over 80 kg.
- Family history or personal history of DVT.
- Thrombophilias; deficiency of antithrombin, protein C and protein S; antiphospholipid syndrome; Factor V Leiden mutations.
- Smoking.
- Immobility, from paralysis or medical problems; admission to intensive care.
- Reduced plasma volume as in dehydration or pre-eclampsia (Greer 1999).

Pathogenesis

During physiological adaptation to pregnancy some clotting factors are altered to prevent detrimental blood loss at delivery: factors von Willibrand, VIII and V and fibrinogen are increased. There is impaired fibrinolysis and the placenta produces plasminogen 1 and 2 activator inhibitors which prevent clotting at the placental bed (Greer 1999). Women with an inherited thrombophilia are at increased risk of developing DVT in pregnancy, over and above the normal risk (Gherman & Goodwin 2000). The triad of factors described by Virchow of hypercoagulability, vascular damage and venous stasis which predispose to thrombosis exist in pregnancy (Auter 1996).

Prevention of thrombosis

Exercise encourages the return of blood to the heart and helps to prevent stasis. Any treatment which immobilises women increases their risk of DVT, whether antenatally, intrapartum or postnatally. High-risk women with previous thrombosis may be given prophylactic treatment antenatally and postnatally with low-dose heparin. Oral warfarin may be prescribed to continue for 6 weeks following birth and is safe to use in breastfeeding, as is heparin (RCOG 1995). Some women could be treated with low-dose aspirin as a preventative measure (De Swiet 1999). The side-effects of heparin and warfarin include osteoporosis and embryopathy, respectively. De Swiet suggests low-dose aspirin until due, then heparin during and after birth until 6 weeks postnatal, when heparin or warfarin can be used (Greer 1999).

Diagnosis

DVT is most common in the first few days after delivery. The woman may complain of pain or discomfort in the leg, which is increased when the foot is dorsiflexed (**Homan's sign**). The affected leg may be swollen and measures 2–3 cm more than the unaffected leg. There may be a slight rise in systemic temperature. Diagnosis on clinical signs alone is difficult and there may be up to 50% error in diagnosing DVT of the lower extremity. Therefore, ultrasound examination by listening for the **Doppler effect** and **venography** by injecting a radiopaque dye prior to X-ray may be used to confirm the clinical picture. Although venography is the most accurate method, it can be painful and lead to local chemical phlebitis, so is not preferred. In 80% of pregnant women the thrombosis starts in the iliac and femoral veins and can be diagnosed by non-invasive methods such as ultrasound (Bothamley 2002). Blood estimation of **D-dimers** (fibrin degradation products) may be made but are inaccurate antenatally and of no value postnatally.

Treatment

Intravenous heparin will be commenced and may be followed by oral warfarin, especially if the woman has delivered her baby. The danger of haemorrhage and haematoma formation should be kept in mind and the effects of warfarin can be monitored by serial estimation of blood prothrombin time.

Pulmonary embolism

Diagnosis

Chest pain, dyspnoea, cyanosis, and hypotension are suggestive of pulmonary embolism and require action immediately. Oxygen may be given with intravenous (IV) heparin. The woman's physiological response depends on the size of the clot or clots. If she collapses and has a cardiac arrest the situation has a poor outcome. Resuscitation should continue as this may disperse the clot and IV heparin of 20 000 units given (de Swiet 1995). Subsequent treatment should centre on positive diagnosis and immediate dissolution of the clot with streptokinase, urokinase or plasminogen activator. Anticoagulation over several months is necessary. Rarely, surgery may be needed to remove the embolus (de Swiet 1995).

CONSUMPTIVE COAGULOPATHIES DURING PREGNANCY

Disseminated intravascular coagulation

Disseminated intravascular coagulation (DIC) is always secondary to some other occurrence: for example, abruptio placentae, postpartum haemorrhage, pre-eclampsia, a dead fetus or sepsis. Local activation of the clotting system releases thromboplastin into the circulation, leading to intravascular formation of fibrin. **Microthrombi** are released into the circulation, occlude blood vessels and may lead to **multiple organ failure** (Levi et al 2000). Consumption and reduction of clotting factors and platelets lead to severe bleeding.

Fibrinolysis stimulated by DIC results in the formation of **fibrin degradation products** (FDPs). These interfere with the formation of firm fibrin clots and a vicious circle is established increasing the blood loss. FDPs are also thought to interfere with myometrial contraction and cardiac function (Letsky 1995).

Diagnosis

Clinical condition and laboratory tests will accurately diagnose DIC such as the observation of the loss of blood from an IV site or the nose or the presence of **haematuria** (Crafter 2002). In laboratory tests (Levi et al 2000), the following tests will all deviate from normal:

- platelet count;
- clotting times (in series);
- levels of antithrombin III;
- fibrin degradation products.

Treatment

The replacement of blood cells and clotting factors is a priority, but treating the underlying disorder may in itself resolve DIC. A transfusion of fresh frozen plasma or plasma substitutes such as dextran and platelet concentrates will assist in preventing bleeding. Whole blood is not usually given but stored blood components are given separately (Letsky 1995).

Idiopathic thrombocytopenia

Idiopathic thrombocytopenia (ITP) is a rare disorder that is characterised by an autoimmune destruction of maternal and fetal platelets. Women sufferers are usually asymptomatic but may report that they bruise easily and bleed excessively. There may be bleeding from the gastrointestinal and urinary tracts. Intracranial haemorrhage may be a complication. There may be an increased rate of miscarriage.

Maternal platelets are low, at less than $5000/mm^3$, and the condition is diagnosed following a full blood count. Bone marrow aspiration used to be measured to aid diagnosis but now antiplatelet antibodies may be identified in the blood for a definitive diagnosis. In pregnancy, the aim is to maintain a platelet level greater than $100\,000/mm^3$ by administering corticosteroids. Intravenous γ-globulin may be used to suppress **antiplatelet antibodies**. There is a possibility of postpartum haemorrhage with platelets less than $100\,000/mm^3$. Fetal **thrombocytopenia** is due to transplacental passage of antiplatelet antibodies, which may cause neonatal haemorrhage (Duerbeck et al 1999).

MAIN POINTS

- Iron deficiency anaemia (IDA), folic acid deficiency, hereditary haemoglobinopathies and anaemia due to blood loss are associated with pregnancy. Most cases of anaemia in pregnancy will be due to IDA. Iron can be given by oral preparation, or intramuscular or intravenous infusion. In late pregnancy or if the iron deficiency is severe, blood transfusion may be given.

- Folic acid deficiency or vitamin B_{12} deficiency in pregnancy can lead to megaloblastic anaemia. Folic acid deficiency responds to folic acid supplementation.

- Two studies in the 1980s suggested that folic acid supplementation might reduce the risk of recurrence of neural tube defects (NTDs). The Department of Health (1992) recommended the use of 4 mg of folic acid 3 months prior to conception, continued until the early months of pregnancy to prevent NTDs.

- The World Health Organisation estimated that, by the year 2000, 7% of the world's population may be carriers of single gene defects of the red cell. Two of the commonest diseases seen are the recessively inherited sickle cell disease and thalassaemias.

- In sickle cell disease, when oxygen availability is low, the red cells are distorted into a sickle shape and cannot pass through the capillaries. Vascular occlusion occurs, especially in the kidney and brain. Normally, the sickle cell trait is asymptomatic and there is no anaemia, even with the added stress of pregnancy.

- Fetal blood can be tested for abnormal haemoglobin genes by cordocentesis. Chorionic villus sampling may also be used for DNA analysis. Cord blood may be taken at birth for screening purposes.

- β-thalassaemia is much more common than α-thalassaemia and in the carrier state leads to mild microcytic hypochromic anaemia and hyperplasia of bone marrow. Homozygous people have severe anaemia and death from cardiac failure, which is common in untreated people. Blood transfusions can increase the life span by up to 20 years.

- Pregnant women with homozygous β-thalassaemia need specialised care shared between the haematologist and obstetrician. Treatment may include repeated blood transfusions and folic acid supplementation. Prenatal diagnosis and genetic counselling should be available to couples susceptible to having an affected child.

- Glucose 6-phosphate dehydrogenase (G6PD) deficiency is a rare X-linked enzyme deficiency. It affects women of African, Asian and Mediterranean origin. Certain drugs precipitate haemolytic crises. Neonates may have prolonged jaundice if they carry this gene.

- Thrombosis in childbearing women is serious because of its association with deep vein thrombosis (DVT) and pulmonary embolism (PE), which remains the commonest cause of maternal death.

- In DVT the deep veins of the calf, thigh or pelvis are affected. If there is no accompanying inflammation and the thrombus does not obstruct the blood vessel, there may be no clinical signs. If the clot is friable, pieces detach from the vessel wall and travel round the circulation, leading to a pulmonary embolism. Women with an inherited thrombophilia are at increased risk of developing a DVT in pregnancy.

- Exercise encourages the return of blood to the heart and helps to prevent stasis. Any treatment which immobilises women will increase their risk of DVT, whether antenatal, intrapartum or postnatally. Those women with previous thrombosis (high risk) may be given prophylactic treatment antenatally and postnatally, with low-dose heparin.

- Massive release of thromboplastin into the circulation leads to intravascular formation of microthrombi with consumption of clotting factors and platelets and severe bleeding leading to organ failure. Fibrinolysis is stimulated by DIC. Replacement of blood cells and clotting factors is a priority.

- Idiopathic thrombocytopenia (ITP) is an autoimmune disease with destruction of platelets. It is usually asymptomatic but there may be easy bruising and excessive bleeding from the gastrointestinal and urinary tracts. Intracranial haemorrhage may be a complication.

References

Allen L 1997 Pregnancy and iron deficiency: unresolved problems. Nutrition Review 55(4):91–101.

Auter R 1996 Deep Vein Thrombosis; The Silent Killer. Quay Books, Dinton.

Bewley C, Bradshaw C 2001 Thromboembolic disorders during pregnancy, birth and the puerperium. MIDIRS Midwifery Digest 11(1):56–59.

Bloom M 1995 Sickle Cell Disease. University Press of Mississippi, Mississippi.

Bothamley J 2002 Thromboembolism in pregnancy. In Boyle M (ed.) Emergencies Around Childbirth. Radcliffe Medical Press, Oxford.

Boyle M 2002 Other causes of potential maternal collapse. In Boyle M (ed.) Emergencies Around Childbirth. Radcliffe Medical Press, Oxford.

Bunn F 1997 Mechanisms of disease: pathogenesis and treatment of sickle cell disease. New England Journal of Medicine 337(11):762–769.

Coggins J 2001 Iron deficiency anaemia: a complication of pregnancy or a foregone conclusion? MIDIRS Midwifery Digest 11(4):469–474.

Crafter H 2002 Intrapartum and primary postpartum haemorrhage. In Boyle M (ed.) Emergencies Around Childbirth. Radcliffe Medical Press, Oxford.

Cuervo L, Mahomed K 2003 Treatments for iron deficiency anaemia in pregnancy. Cochrane Review: In The Cochrane Library, Issue 1. Update Software 2003, Oxford.

Department of Health 1992 Report from an expert maternity group: folic acid and the prevention of neural tube defects. Health Publications Unit, Lancashire.

De Swiet M 1995 Thromboembolism. In de Swiet M (ed.) Medical Disorders in Obstetric Practice, 3rd edn. Blackwell Science, Oxford.

De Swiet M 1999 Thromboembolic disease. In James D, Steer P, Weiner C, Gonik B (eds) High Risk Pregnancy. W B Saunders, London.

Devane D, Devane M 2000 Termination for fetal defects? The debate must go on. British Journal of Midwifery 8(8):475–479.

Duerbeck N, Chaffin D, Coney P 1999 Platelet and haemorrhagic disorders associated with pregnancy, a review. Part 1. Obstetrical and Gynaecological Survey 54(11):96–105.

Frewin R, Henson A, Proven D 1997 ABC of clinical haematology, iron deficiency anaemia. British Medical Journal 314(7077):360–363.

Gherman R, Goodwin M 2000 Obstetric implications of activated protein C resistance and factor V Leiden Mutation. Obstetrical and Gynaecological Survey 55(2):117–125.

Godfrey K, Barker J 1995 Maternal nutrition in relation to fetal and placental growth. European Journal of Obstetrics and Gynaecology and Reproductive Biology 61:15–22.

Godfrey K M, Redman C W G, Barker D J P, Osmond C 1991 The effect of maternal anaemia and iron deficiency on the ratio of fetal weight to placental weight. British Journal of Obstetrics and Gynaecology 98:886–891.

Greer I 1999 Thrombosis in pregnancy: maternal and fetal issues. Lancet 353(9160):1258–1265.

Howard R, Tuck S, Pearson T 1995 Pregnancy in sickle cell disease in the UK: results of a multicentre survey of the effect of prophylactic blood transfusion on maternal and fetal outcome. British Journal of Obstetrics and Gynaecology 102(12):947–951.

Johnston P 1998 The Newborn Child. Churchill Livingstone, Edinburgh.

Kumar R, Riszk D, Khuranna A 1997 Maternal and fetal outcome of transfusion dependent beta thalassaemia major. Journal of Reproductive Medicine 42(5):294–298.

Layton M 2003 Website: Prenatal diagnosis and therapy of haemoglobinopathies. The Web Journal of Laboratory Haematology, Kings College, London: http://www.haem.net/clinical/clinical 014.asp.

Letsky E 1995 Blood volume, haematinics and anaemia. In de Swiet (ed.) Medical Disorders in Obstetric Practice, 3rd edn. Blackwell Science, Oxford.

Letsky E 1997 Haematological changes in pregnancy. In Oakley C (ed.) Heart Disease in Pregnancy. BMJ Books, London.

Levi M, de Yonge E, van der Poll, ten Cate H 2000 Novel approaches to the management of disseminated intravascular coagulation. Critical Care Medicine 28(9):S20–S24.

Lewis G (ed.) 2001 Fifth Report of the confidential enquiries into maternal deaths in the UK: Why Mothers Die. RCOG, London.

Lloyd C, Lewis V 1999 Common medical diseases associated with pregnancy. In Bennett V R, Brown L K (eds) Myles Textbook for Midwives, 13th edn. Churchill Livingstone, Edinburgh.

McCance K L, Huether S E 2002 Pathophysiology, The Biologic Basis for Disease in Adults and Children, 4th edn. Mosby Year Book, Chicago.

Mason J, McNabb M 2000 Folic acid supplementation: is it a safe option? British Journal of Midwifery 8(9):581–585.

Modell M, Wonke B, Anionwu E et al 1998 A multidisciplinary approach for improving services in primary care: randomised controlled trial of screening for haemoglobin disorders. British Medical Journal 31(7161):788–791.

MRC Vitamin Study Group 1991 Prevention of neural tube defects. Lancet 238:131–137.

Rang H P, Dale M M, Ritter J M 1999 Pharmacology, 4th edn. Churchill Livingstone, Edinburgh.

RCOG 2001 Thromboembolic disease in pregnancy and the puerperium: acute management. Guideline 28, Royal College of Obstetricians and Gynaecologists Press, London.

RCOG 1995 March, Report of the RCOG working party on prophylaxis against thromboembolism in gynaecology and obstetrics. Royal College of Obstetricians and Gynaecologists Press, London.

Savona-Ventura C, Bonello F 1994 Beta-thalassaemia syndromes and pregnancy. Obstetric and Gynaecological Survey 49(2):129–137.

Schwartz W J (III), Thurneau G R 1995 Iron deficiency anaemia in pregnancy. Clinical Obstetrics and Gynaecology 38(3):443–454.

Steegers-Theunissen R 1995 Folate metabolism and neural tube defects: a review. European Journal of Obstetrics and Gynaecology and Reproductive Biology 61:39–48.

Stephen J, Cunningham J 1998 Understanding fetal haemoglobin gene expression: a step towards effective HbF reactivation in haemoglobinopathies. British Journal of Haematology 102:415–422.

Sun P, Wilburn W, Raynor B, Jamieson D 2001 Sickle cell disease in pregnancy: twenty years of experience at Grady Memorial Hospital, Atlanta, Georgia. American Journal of Obstetrics and Gynaecology 184(6):1127–1130.

Wald N 1991 Prevention of neural tube defects: results of the Medical Research Council Vitamin Study. Report of the MRC Vitamin Study Research Group. Lancet 338(8760):131–137.

Weatherall D 1997a Fortnightly review: the thalassaemias. British Medical Journal 314(7095):1675–1678.

Weatherall D 1997b ABC of clinical haematology: the hereditary anaemias. British Medical Journal 314(7079):492–496.

Website: http://gsl.genetics.utah.edu/units/newborn/infosheets/sicklecelldisorder.cfm.

WHO 1979 The Prevalence of Nutritional Anaemia in Developing Countries. World Health Organisation, Geneva.

Whyte A 1996 Fortifying the pregnancy message. MIDIRS Midwifery Digest 6(1):38–40.

Annotated recommended reading

Devane D, Devane M 2000 Termination for fetal defects? The debate must go on. British Journal of Midwifery 8(8):475–479.
This article discusses the debate around termination for fetal abnormality, such as the ethical, moral and psychological issues.

Godfrey K, Barker J 1995 Maternal nutrition in relation to fetal and placental growth. European Journal of Obstetrics and Gynaecology and Reproductive Biology 61:15–22.
This paper provides a basis for the understanding of the Barker hypothesis.

Hall J 2002 Screening for sickle cell disorders Part 1. British Journal of Midwifery 10(4):233–237.

Hall J 2002 Screening for sickle cell disorders Part 2. British Journal of Midwifery 10(5):307–312.
These articles cover the issues concerning antenatal and neonatal testing for sickle cell disease. Race and ethnicity are discussed and whether or not midwives understand the issues surrounding this. The provision of care and the inequality of services outside city centres are addressed.

Jilma B, Kamath S, Lip G 2003 Antithrombic therapy in pregnancy and cancer. British Medical Journal 326(7379):37–40.
This paper is a clinical review of antithrombic therapy, giving the risks and benefits of various drugs in pregnancy, a small section of application to cancer patients.

Levi M, de Yonge E, van der Poll, ten Cate H 2000 Novel approaches to the management of disseminated intravascular coagulation. Critical Care Medicine 28(9):S20–S24.
This paper is well worth reading. It provides an in depth account of DIC and its management.

Schwartz W J (III), Thurneau G R 1995 Iron deficiency anaemia in pregnancy. Clinical Obstetrics and Gynaecology 38(3):443–454.
This chapter is an excellent basis for the subjects of anaemia and clotting disorders.

Chapter **34**

Respiratory, renal, gastrointestinal and neurological problems

RESPIRATORY TRACT PROBLEMS

Asthma

Asthma is the most common respiratory problem found in pregnancy, with an incidence of between 0.4% and 1.3% (Liu et al 2001), although de Swiet (1995) quotes 5%. Asthma is an inflammatory disease with **hyperresponsiveness** of the airways characterised by constriction of the smooth muscle in the bronchioles, hypersecretion of mucus and mucosal oedema (McCance & Huether 2002). The work of breathing is increased and excessive negative intrapleural pressures can increase the demands on the right ventricle. There is a rise in pulmonary arterial pressure and a decrease in arterial systolic pressure and pulse pressure.

Aetiology

Asthma is a complex disorder, involving biochemical, autonomic nervous system, immunological, endocrine and psychological factors which differ from person to person. Airway inflammation is present even when the person is symptom-free. There is a familial incidence and environmental factors such as dust, pollens, moulds, animal dandruff and foods interact with inherited factors to cause **bronchospasm**. About half of sufferers develop asthma in childhood and another third before age 40. Complete remission is quite common in children but less so in adults, in whom symptomatic episodes tend to occur more frequently (Liu et al 2001).

Pathophysiology

Bronchoconstriction occurs within minutes of exposure to the allergen and usually resolves in a short time although there may be a secondary episode called the **late reaction**, 6 hours later. Kumar & Busse (1995) highlight the pivotal role played by **mast cells**. Exposure to the allergen causes immunoglobulin E (IgE) antigen to bind to mast cell surface receptors. These release inflammatory substances such as **histamine**, **bradykinin**, **prostaglandins** and **thromboxane A_2** and **chemotactic factors** which attract eosinophils, neutrophils, T lymphocytes and platelets. In **extrinsic asthma**, eosinophils produce a protein that stops epithelial cell cilia from beating, disrupts mucosal integrity and causes damage and sloughing of epithelial cells.

Asthma in pregnancy

During pregnancy some asthmatic women improve, some deteriorate and some experience no change in lung function. It is difficult to predict events, so close monitoring and ensuring compliance with treatment is essential. Pregnancy is a state of slight immunosuppression so the asthmatic may be slightly more prone to chest infections, depending on the season; it is less likely in the summer months (Ie et al 2002). Women with asthma may have more complications in pregnancy such as preterm birth, small for gestational age and hypertension and more caesarean births and longer hospital stays (Liu et al 2001).

Treatment considerations

Asthma requires long-term administration of **bronchodilators** and **anti-inflammatory agents** and the effect of these on early fetal development must be considered. Women sometimes decrease their medication for fear of harming their babies to the detriment of treating their asthma. They must be encouraged to recognise the early symptoms of an attack to avoid hypoxia. Up to 15% of pregnant asthmatic women require hospitalisation for **status asthmaticus** or recurrent asthmatic episodes (Blackburn 2003). Women must understand the necessity for compliance with prescribed treatment and of avoiding over-the-counter (OTC) drugs. Anxiety exacerbates asthma attacks but sedative drugs are contraindicated, as these may cause respiratory depression.

Normal inhalation medications may continue, with regular examination of peak flow levels. **Aminophylline** is safe in pregnancy and may be used in acute-to-severe asthma attacks to aid breathing and **oral steroids** may be used to treat repeated asthma attacks. Medications in labour that cause vasoconstriction such as prostaglandin $F_{2\alpha}$ and ergometrine should not be used. Syntocinon (oxytocin) should be used for the third stage of labour (de Swiet 1995).

Tuberculosis

The prevalence of **pulmonary tuberculosis** (TB) in some areas of London exceeds 50 per 100 000. It is a global health problem (Watson & Moss 2001) and 50% of UK cases were born overseas. In a survey of asylum seekers screened at Heathrow Airport in 1995–9 the incidence was 241 per 100 000, with high rates from the Indian subcontinent and sub-Saharan Africa (Callister et al 2002).

Improvements in urban conditions during the 19th century decreased the incidence of TB. However, with the increase of travel and immigration, the incidence rose from 1986 to 1993, particularly in the more deprived areas of London. Elsewhere in the UK, it has fallen (Catchpole 1995). The TB survey in 1998 showed a further increase of 11% of cases since the 1993 survey, but with less children infected. The white population cases declined, with an increase in the ethnic groups particularly black African and Chinese. Coinfection with the **human immunodeficiency virus** (HIV) occurred in 3.3% of the TB-infected population (Rose et al 2001).

Some statistics

Around the world between 1985 and 1991 (Karlen 1995):

- there was a 12% increase in cases in the USA, a 30% increase in cases in Europe and a 300% increase in cases in parts of Africa where HIV is prevalent;
- 1.7 billion people, about a third of all humans are thought to be infected;
- 10 million people have active tuberculosis;
- 3 million people die every year from TB – 9000 people a day.

Aetiology

The disease is caused by the bacillus *Mycobacterium tuberculosis*, a soil-living organism pathogenic to some animals such as cattle. It infects far more people than it causes to be ill and infected people have a 10% lifetime risk of developing TB. It may manifest as **pulmonary** or **extrapulmonary** TB. Pulmonary TB with infected sputum is more contagious. It is a slow-growing bacterium with a waxy outer coat that protects it from immune system attack. The body responds by forming **fibrinous tubercles** to contain the microbe. The bacillus can lie dormant for years inside macrophages, but lowered resistance causes it to become active and the host becomes sick.

TB exploits the vulnerable, with poverty, overcrowding, institutionalisation, the presence of other disease and immune suppression leading to an increase in active disease. A study attempted to link poverty with ethnic groups, finding that it was positively correlated to the white population with TB but not the Asian groups (Hawker et al 1999). It is highly contagious: all contacts with tuberculosis should be followed up and vaccinated (Joint Tuberculosis Committee 2000).

Signs and symptoms

Although pregnancy increases the demands on the respiratory system, debilitation rather than dyspnoea may be the principal problem. There is a rare possibility of transplacental fetal infection (Ormerod 2001). The woman's poor health may affect fetal growth adversely. In 27 pregnant women who were culture-positive, signs and symptoms were (Good et al 1981):

- 74% cough;
- 41% weight loss;

- 30% fever, malaise or fatigue;
- 19% haemoptysis;
- 20% asymptomatic, but had abnormal X-rays.

Management of tuberculosis

A chest physician should be involved in the woman's care. If there are clinical signs of TB or the woman has been in contact with active TB, a chest X-ray is performed. Sputum specimens and pleural effusions may be cultured to confirm the presence of the bacillus. If the sputum contains the organism, the woman may need to be admitted to hospital but drug therapy is usually carried out at home. After 2 weeks of therapy there is no risk of infection to others.

Tuberculin skin tests are performed in the USA on those who have been at risk of TB and the family are investigated. The sole manufacturer of tuberculin in the UK has recently put in its data sheet that tuberculin testing should not be carried out in pregnancy but does not supply any data to support this recommendation. This has not been backed up by the Vaccination and Immunisation Committee (Ormerod 2001). However, BCG vaccination should not be performed in pregnancy as it is a live vaccine.

Treatment

- **Isoniazid** is given during the first trimester although fetal abnormalities have been seen in animals. The drug interferes with the absorption of pyridoxine so that supplementation is necessary. It is found in significant amounts in breast milk.

- **Ethambutol hydrochloride** freely crosses the placenta. Although fetal malformations were 2.2% in 638 infants, it is felt safe to use in the first trimester of pregnancy.

- **Rifampicin** is added after the first trimester when organogenesis is complete with **pyrazinamide**, which rapidly clears the sputum of bacteria. No trials have confirmed any fetal side-effects of these two drugs. Nine months treatment will be necessary, except when using pyrazinamide, when it may be shortened to 6 months.

- Intramuscular **streptomycin** is contraindicated in pregnancy because of the incidence of hearing loss in those neonates exposed to it in utero.

It is not necessary to discontinue drugs during pregnancy, neither is termination appropriate.

The baby

If the mother is on effective treatment and has negative sputum, there is no reason for the baby to be isolated from her. Staff will be protected by vaccination, which is prerequisite before employment. If treatment commenced late in pregnancy and sputum is still positive, the baby will need prophylactic isoniazid and a **tuberculin test** should be performed at 6 weeks. If the mother has a multiple drug-resistant strain (MDR) of TB, the infant will need to be separated from her. The mother would also need to be isolated and staff use dust mist fume masks. TB drugs cross into breast milk but there is no contraindication to breastfeeding, except where the neonate is separated from its mother (Ormerod 2001).

Vaccination – BCG

The bacillus Calmette-Guérin (BCG), a live attenuated strain developed from cattle TB, is given by injection into the skin to stimulate an immune response. In babies, care must be taken to inject intradermally to prevent abscess formation. The vaccine is effective in the prevention of tuberculosis in children but of variable value when given to adults. It can reduce the incidence of pulmonary tuberculosis by up to 80% and minimises the risk of complications.

The effectiveness of BCG programmes remains controversial. In the USA, vaccination is thought to create difficulties in interpreting the results of any future use of the tuberculin test performed to establish whether a person is infected with TB. In the UK, BCG vaccination is carried out in children aged 10–14 years if they demonstrate a negative tuberculin test (Joint Tuberculosis Committee 2000). Some areas with an incidence of less than 1% have discontinued routine vaccination.

Children and adults who have contact with someone suffering from active pulmonary tuberculosis should be tuberculin tested and given BCG if the test is negative. Babies in contact with active TB should be vaccinated without having a tuberculin test as their immune systems may be too immature to show a response. In the UK it is recommended that all immigrants from countries with a high incidence of TB are tested and BCG vaccination given to those with a negative result and that all babies born to recent immigrants are vaccinated (BNF 2003). All neonates born in an area of high TB incidence and neonates of health care workers are offered BCG soon after birth (Joint Tuberculosis Committee 2000).

Contraindications   Harmful effects of BCG are rare. However, ulcers and abscess formation may occur at the site of the vaccination, sometimes with swollen lymph glands and inflammation of the underlying bone. Healing of such an ulcer may be slow and result in a **kelloid scar**. The vaccine should not be given to people who have leukaemia, cancer, acute illness (including TB) or to patients taking corticosteroids or immune suppressant drugs. It is also contraindicated in those who are HIV positive (Joint Tuberculosis Committee 2000).

RENAL DISORDERS

Acute pyelonephritis

Pregnant women are more susceptible to renal tract infections than other women and there is an incidence of unsuspected asymptomatic bacteriuria in between 4 and 10% of them: if not diagnosed and treated, about 25% develop pyelonephritis. Ascending infection caused by perineal bacteria is the commonest route and the most common causative organisms are Gram-negative bacilli such as *Escherichia coli*, *Klebsiella pneumoniae* and *Proteus mirabilis* with *E. coli* present in at least 80% of cases. Some strains of *E. coli* have fimbriae that bind to specific receptors on the surface of epithelial cells, increasing their selection of the urinary tract and their virulence (Lindsay 2000).

Screening for asymptomatic bacteriuria

Women who have had previous episodes of asymptomatic bacteriuria or urinary tract infection should have a mid-stream specimen of urine cultured. If the presence of a specific bacterium exceeds 10^5 organisms/ml of urine (100 000 organisms/ml) asymptomatic bacteriuria is diagnosed. Appropriate antibiotics should be successful in treating the condition (Lindsay 2000).

Clinical implications of acute pyelonephritis

Fetal risks
- Intrauterine growth restriction, even with asymptomatic bacteriuria alone.
- Preterm labour is more common.
- There may be an associated risk of congenital abnormality.

Maternal risks
- Endotoxic shock.
- Chronic renal infection.
- Renal failure.

Signs and symptoms

Acute pyelonephritis occurs in 1–2% of pregnancies, usually in the second and third trimesters. It begins with the onset of malaise, fatigue, chills and back pain located in the upper lumbar region, accompanied by muscle guarding. The pain follows the path of the ureters and may radiate round to the suprapubic area. Some women complain of nausea, vomiting and uterine contractions. Affected women may have a temperature as high as 40°C with a corresponding increase in pulse rate. There may be dehydration and frequency of micturition with scalding on voiding. The urine appears cloudy and even bloodstained and on urinalysis red blood cells, leucocytes and casts may be present as well as bacteria (Gardner 2000).

Management

It is essential to treat acute pyelonephritis immediately to avoid serious side-effects. The woman is admitted to hospital and the following treatment is instigated:

- A midstream specimen of urine should be sent to the laboratory for culturing and sensitivity tests.
- A blood specimen (for full blood count and electrolytes) is taken if the woman is obviously very ill.

- Intravenous fluids may be required to correct any dehydration.
- Antibiotic therapy should be commenced, intravenously if women are nauseated. Oral medication may be commenced after 48 h. *E. coli* is becoming increasingly resistant to **ampicillin** and a combination of antibiotics may be prescribed until the sensitivity reports are returned.
- Pain relief may be necessary and an antiemetic to counter-act nausea.
- Renal function should be assessed both during the acute illness and as a follow-up.
- Maternal observations of temperature, pulse and blood pressure should be recorded at least 4 hourly. Tachycardia and hypotension may indicate the development of endotoxic shock.
- Fetal observations are as important as maternal and the early onset of labour should be recognised.

Most women will respond to the combination of rehydration and antibiotics. In cases of persistent problems, there may be an abnormality of the renal tract and such women should be referred appropriately (Gardner 2000).

Acute renal failure

Diagnosis

The onset of acute renal failure (ARF) has occurred if the urine output falls below 400 ml in 24 h or to less than 20 ml/h. There is a reduced glomerular filtration rate (GFR) and a rise in blood urea and creatinine. The incidence is 1 in 10 000 pregnancies, a decline since abortion has been legalized (Poole & Thorsen 1999). Acute renal failure usually results from a severe deficit in cortical renal blood flow that results in ischaemia to the kidneys. Pregnancy conditions associated with ARF are shown in Table 34.1 (Poole & Thorsen 1999).

If cortical hypoperfusion is allowed to persist, **acute tubular necrosis** (ATN) or **cortical necrosis** may follow. Renal cortical necrosis is a severe form of ARF that usually results from large, sudden blood loss or vascular collapse such as

Table 34.1   Pregnancy conditions associated with acute renal failure

Prerenal hypoperfusion	Hypotension and coagulopathy	Urinary tract obstruction
Haemorrhage	Abruptio placentae	Polyhydramnios
Spontaneous abortion	Pre-eclampsia	Damage to ureters
Hyperemesis gravidarum	Incompatible blood transfusion	Pelvic haematoma
Adrenocortical failure	Drug reaction	Calculus or clot in ureter
	Acute fatty liver of pregnancy	
	Sepsis	

in severe pre-eclampsia or haemorrhage. There is sudden onset of oliguria (less than 400 ml in 24 h) or anuria and a rise in serum creatinine (Poole & Thorsen 1999). Immediate treatment of ARF prevents necrosis occurring.

In a study of 72 pre-eclamptic women with renal failure, median gestation was 32 weeks and perinatal mortality was 38%. Twelve women had previous renal disease and only seven women required short-term dialysis. In the long term there was no need for dialysis or transplantation (Drakeley et al 2002). Those women with renal impairment had HELLP syndrome or abruptio placenta.

Management

The aims are to re-establish urinary output and treat the underlying condition. Blood is taken for estimation of urea, electrolytes and plasma proteins. Haematocrit and blood osmolality findings indicate the degree of dehydration. Blood culture and liver function tests help to identify a cause. Urine is tested for culture and sensitivity of organisms, protein estimation, specific gravity and osmolality. Maternal and fetal safety is paramount and immediate delivery is unavoidable. The incidence of fetal growth restriction is high. If the fetus is not viable, termination of the pregnancy may be necessary (Gilbert & Harmon 1998).

Re-establishing kidney function: principles of treatment
Treatment is guided by laboratory tests of kidney function and blood biochemistry results and includes:

- Control of bleeding, stabilising of raised blood pressure or sepsis.
- Intravascular volume expansion with packed red cells, fresh frozen plasma, and crystalloid solutions, guided by intake and output measurement. **Mannitol**, a plasma expander and diuretic, may be used.
- Restrict fluid intake to the volume of fluid lost in the previous 24 h plus 500 ml to replace insensible fluid loss. If the woman is pyrexial, an extra 200 ml may be added.
- Dialysis if there is cardiovascular overload, **hyperkalaemia**, electrolyte imbalances, metabolic acidosis or **uraemia**.
- Diet should be low in potassium and chloride, 1500 calorie, protein-free, fat/carbohydrate diet.

Chronic renal disease

The chances of a woman becoming pregnant are reduced as renal function declines, and pregnancy is rare when the kidneys function with less than 50% efficiency (Davison & Baylis 1995). Pregnancy is risky for these women and in 1:3 whose prepregnancy creatinine levels are greater than 170 μmol/L and GFR 30 ml/min/L, kidney function will decline during pregnancy (Williams 1999).

Pregnant women with chronic renal impairment may present with proteinuria, raised blood pressure and oedema, symptoms which need distinguishing from pre-eclampsia.

These women are more prone to pre-eclampsia, preterm labour and delivering a small for dates baby (Fink et al 1998). Oedema is present because of loss of protein in the urine and electrolytes become imbalanced because kidney excretion of urine is low. Blood acid–base balance is compromised. Erythropoietin and red cell production are decreased and anaemia occurs. A history of prior kidney problems or associated medical conditions is common, causing kidney function to deteriorate (Davison & Baylis 1995). These include:

- glomerulonephritis;
- chronic pyelonephritis;
- renal calculi;
- polycystic kidney disease;
- nephrotic syndrome greater than 3 g/day, a serum albumin of less than 3 g/dl plus oedema;
- diabetic nephropathy;
- systemic lupus erythematosus.

Antenatal care and prognosis

The mother   Hypertension is the most reliable indicator of outcome. If the blood pressure is high, hypotensive medication should commence. The next important factor is the degree of renal impairment as measured by creatinine clearance; the better the clearance, the better the prognosis. The presence or absence of proteinuria is important when predicting the risks of poor outcome to mother or baby. A woman who has 3 g or more in 24 h at the beginning of pregnancy will tend to develop increasing proteinuria. The pathology of kidney function is important. Women with glomerulonephritis have serious maternal and fetal complications. Early recognition of urinary tract infection is essential.

The fetus   Regular assessments of fetal growth are made and delivery should be preterm if necessary. Fetal distress occurs both antenatally and in labour in pregnancies complicated by intrauterine growth restriction, and fetal mortality may occur because of poor placental blood flow, abruptio placentae or hypoxia. If kidney function diminishes, renal dialysis and peritoneal dialysis are possible. There is a 50% survival rate for the fetus (Hou 1999).

Pregnancy following renal transplant

Alston et al (2001) suggest that 1:20 women with a transplant of any organ will become pregnant and 90% will have a live birth. Following transplantation, fertility returns. If kidney function is adequate and there is no hypertension, women with renal transplants tolerate pregnancy well but it is important to continue **immunosuppressive medication**. Most women are prescribed azathioprine as an immunosuppressor and prednisolone to prevent rejection of the transplanted kidney (Armenti et al 2002). There have been no reports of congenital malformations due to these drugs. Ciclosporin, a more potent immunosuppressant agent, has been linked to fetal growth restriction (Alston et al 2001). These women are more prone to infections because of these drugs, which may increase problems for the fetus (Hou 1999). The more common complications are preterm labour and small for dates infant and pre-eclampsia. Outcomes are good if the transplanted kidney functions well.

Davison & Baylis (1995) suggest assessing the following factors before embarking on a pregnancy:

- good health for 2 years following transplant;
- stature compatible with good obstetric outcome;
- no proteinuria;
- no significant hypertension;
- no evidence of graft rejection;
- no evidence of distension of the renal pelvis or calyces;
- plasma creatinine of 180 μmol/L or less;
- limited drug therapy.

Pregnancies in women with chronic renal disease, on dialysis or following a renal transplant should be planned. Contraceptive and preconception advice is essential. Life survival following a transplant is variable. Some have quoted 5 years, others 10, without a pregnancy, which will put a strain on the allograft. Close liaison should take place between specialist and obstetrician and the woman should be aware of all the facts (Armenti et al 1998).

GASTROINTESTINAL PROBLEMS

Vomiting in pregnancy

Slight nausea and vomiting may affect up to 80% of women in the first trimester (Ch. 30). Causes and management of moderate to severe vomiting are discussed below.

Causes of vomiting

Pregnant woman may suffer from diseases causing vomiting not associated with pregnancy. These disorders, such as gastric ulceration or infection, must be ruled out before accepting that moderate to severe vomiting is due to the pregnancy alone. Vomiting is a reflex which occurs because of stimulation of two centres in the brain (Rang et al 1999). These are the **vomiting centre** (VC) in the medulla and the **chemoreceptor trigger zone** (CTZ).

The VC controls smooth muscle movements in the stomach wall and the related skeletal muscle of the respiratory and abdominal muscles. The CTZ lies outside the blood–brain barrier and responds to circulating chemical stimuli from ingested drugs and endogenous toxins produced in uraemia and radiation sickness. This centre also produces motion sickness. Stimuli arising in the CTZ are passed to the VC, which then activates the relevant respiratory and gastrointestinal muscles, resulting in vomiting. There is a lack of clarity in the aetiology of vomiting in pregnancy (Hod et al 1994, Low 1996). Vomiting can be triggered by the factors outlined in Table 34.2.

Hyperemesis gravidarum

Hyperemesis gravidarum (HG) is a severe condition that results in excessive vomiting in pregnancy. It may lead to maternal death if not treated actively. HG usually begins in the first trimester and is continuous, severe and often associated with excessive salivation. The incidence is about 0.3–2% (Moran & Taylor 2002). It is associated with multiple pregnancies and hydatidiform mole and these conditions should be suspected if the uterus appears large for dates.

Numerous studies have tried to clarify the aetiology of HG, ranging from high levels of hCG and increasing levels

Table 34.2 Causes of vomiting in pregnant women

Non–pregnancy causes	Causes due to pregnancy
Stimulation of the sensory nerve endings in the stomach and duodenum and of the vagal sensory endings in the pharynx	High levels of pregnancy hormones, such as hCG or oestrogen, with multiple pregnancy and hydatidiform mole (trophoblastic disease)
Some stimuli to the heart and viscera, such as distension, damage or infection of the uterus, renal pelvis or bladder	Physiological changes in the gastrointestinal tract in pregnancy, resulting in decreased motility and in increased gastric reflux
Drugs or endogenous toxins produced as a result of radiation damage, infection or disease	Transient hyperthyroidism, causing high levels of hCG, stimulating thyroid secretion
Disturbance of the vestibular apparatus, as in motion sickness	Metabolic changes, including carbohydrate deficiency and alteration in lipid pathways
Raised intracranial pressure, migraine, cerebral tumour	Pre-eclampsia, HELLP syndrome
Nauseating smells, sights or thoughts	Renal tract infections
Endocrine factors such as increased oestrogen	Torsion of an ovarian cyst
A fall in blood pressure and reduced circulation to the brain (vasovagal events)	Genetic incompatibility between mother and fetus
Viral gastroenteritis	Psychological factors
Hepatitis, acute liver failure	
Gall bladder disease	

of oestrogen and progesterone to the slowing of gastro-intestinal peristalsis, which increases gastric reflux (Low 1996). Hyperthyroidism may be a cause of HG. Valentine et al (1980) found the use of antithyroid therapy abolished vomiting where hyperthyroidism and HG were present together. Studies do not agree on the hyperthyroid theory but it is noted that sometimes the two conditions coincide and require treatment (Hod et al 1994). When the two conditions occur together, women may present with vomiting, weight loss and increased thyroid activity which requires treatment to prevent adverse outcomes in pregnancy (Fantz et al 1999). The psychological aspect of the process must not be forgotten (Deuchar 1995).

Signs and symptoms

The woman complains of continuous nausea and vomiting throughout the day. Signs of dehydration are present. There is marked **oliguria** with dark urine of high specific gravity which may contain **ketones**, bile, protein and glucose. Electrolyte disturbances include **hyponatraemia** and **hypochloraemia** as sodium and chloride ions are lost in the vomit. The woman's breath smells offensive, she loses weight and her condition will deteriorate rapidly without treatment. The pulse will be rapid and the blood pressure reduced. Anaemia may occur because of the disruption in vitamin B_{12}, folic acid and vitamin C absorption (Hod et al 1994).

Complications

- Liver and renal damage, resulting in jaundice.
- Vitamin B deficiency, resulting in neuropathy such as **polyneuritis**.
- Rarely, **Wernicke's encephalopathy** may occur, signalled by confusion leading to coma because of hypothalamic lesions caused by haemorrhage in severe HG.
- **Hyperthermia** may occur due to disturbance of temperature control. The condition responds well to treatment with thiamine.
- Fetal growth may be impaired but there is no link to any other fetal condition (Fagan 1995).

Management

The woman is usually admitted to hospital for investigations and treatment. The cause of vomiting is identified, **antiemetics** given and fluids and electrolytes replaced by intravenous infusion of a solution such as Hartmann's. Vitamins B_{12}, and C, folic acid and iron will be needed to correct anaemia if present.

Observations of pulse, blood pressure and temperature enable the woman's condition to be monitored. Strict fluid balance should be maintained until rehydrated. There is usually a rapid response to treatment and oral fluids may be recommended when vomiting has ceased for 24 h. Solid food should be then introduced gradually. Moran & Taylor (2002) found that weight loss of more than 5% of prepregnancy weight in women with HG was effectively treated with 10 mg of prednisolone three times a day. This shortened the stay in hospital and stopped vomiting. This treatment was gradually decreased and discontinued at 20 weeks of gestation.

Appendicitis in pregnancy

The appendix is gradually displaced upwards by the growing uterus so that typical signs of appendicitis may not be present. In early pregnancy appendicitis may be difficult to differentiate from threatened abortion; however, there will be no bleeding. Later in pregnancy the pain may be mistaken for urinary tract infection, abruptio placentae or the onset of labour. A scan will confirm the diagnosis. The appendix must be removed to save life and prevent peritonitis.

The abdominal incision is made on **McBurney's point** although the appendix is slightly higher. In 94% of a small sample of 23 gravid women, the appendix was located through the normal incision point (Popkin et al 2002). **Laparoscopic surgery** is gaining favour and has been used in pregnancy to remove ovaries and the appendix. Evidence suggests that this is safe in pregnancy but more research is needed (Fatum & Rojansky 2001). There is a small risk of spontaneous abortion or preterm onset of labour but this has to be balanced against the need for surgery.

Peptic ulceration

Peptic ulceration is uncommon in childbearing years as oestrogen may protect the gastric lining against ulcer formation (Blackburn 2003). If peptic ulceration is present, up to 80% of women experience an improvement, possibly due to the reduction of gastric acidity (Fagan 1995). Almost all have a recurrence of their symptoms by 2 years following the pregnancy.

Pregnancy in women with a stoma

An ileostomy or colostomy for urinary or alimentary diversion should not affect the course of pregnancy. About 75% of women with stomas will have a normal vaginal delivery. The use of urinary diversion with an ileocaecal reservoir is now common treatment for congenital disorders, neurogenic disease or trauma and some women may require caesarean delivery in these circumstances (Schumacher et al 1997). Problems that may need careful management include:

- changes in shape and position of the stoma as the uterus enlarges;
- leaking from the stoma as the opening changes shape;
- hormonal changes that alter skin secretions, leading to reduced adhesiveness of the appliance;
- reduced absorption of nutrients – for example, vitamin B_{12} and folic acid – which may lead to anaemia;

- increased risk of gastrointestinal obstruction – the consequent abdominal pain is difficult to distinguish from appendicitis (Stables 1995).

Cholestasis

Cholestasis is a last trimester problem with the development of pruritus, abnormal liver enzymes and jaundice. The incidence in the UK is 0.5–1% (Burroughs 1998), whereas in other countries this is variable being high in Chile. Cholestasis may disappear postnatally but may reoccur when contraception or hormone replacement therapy (HRT) is commenced or when pregnant again. It is thought to be caused in the susceptible by raised oestrogen levels and may be an autoimmune response to pregnancy (Coombes 2000). There is a high incidence of stillbirth if left untreated. The recommended treatment is ursodeoxycholic acid (UDCA), which may assist in reducing the bile acid pool and serum bile acids (Davies et al 1995).

NEUROLOGICAL DISORDERS

Epilepsy

Epilepsy is a general term for a group of conditions that cause **seizures**. It occurs in approximately 1% of the population (Tortora & Grabowski 2000). There is a brief alteration in brain function with a high-frequency discharge that can involve motor, sensory, autonomic or psychic clinical features accompanied by an alteration in the level of consciousness. The area in the brain that the focus commences in determines the type of seizure.

Primary causes

Pathological processes lead to seizures although many seizures are **idiopathic** (no known cause). Some people may have a lower seizure threshold than others. Epilepsy may result from (Tortora & Grabowski 2000):

- birth injury;
- metabolic disorders;
- congenital malformation;
- genetic predisposition;
- postnatal trauma;
- motor syndromes;
- infection;
- brain tumour/head injury.

Seizures may be provoked by hypoglycaemia, lack of sleep, raised temperature, emotional or physical stress, drinking large amounts of water, constipation, drugs, hyperventilation, strobe lights, loud noises, some music and being startled.

Classification of seizures

- **Generalised seizures** involve neurons bilaterally, often without a focal onset and usually originating from a

subcortical or deeper brain focus. Consciousness is always impaired or lost. The term corresponds to grand mal and petit mal epilepsy.

- **Partial seizures (focal)** such as temporal lobe epilepsy and **Jacksonian epilepsy** often have a local onset and usually originate from cortical brain tissue. Consciousness is maintained if the seizure is limited to one cerebral hemisphere, but voluntary loss of muscular control occurs in the affected part of the body. **Temporal lobe epilepsy** is often characterised by continuous inappropriate rubbing of hands, or combing the hair (Rang et al 1999).

- In **status epilepticus** more seizures follow the first before consciousness is fully regained and the person is in the **postictal state** (a state following a seizure) when the next seizure begins. Cerebral hypoxia means that this state is a medical emergency and failure to treat adequately may result in dementia, mental retardation and death. The individual is also at risk of aspiration.

Pathophysiology of seizures

The abnormal discharge of electricity may rapidly spread throughout the brain to involve the cortex, basal ganglia, thalamus and brainstem, leading to a tonic phase with generalised muscle contraction and increased muscle tone. Respiration may stop, and involuntary urination or defecation may occur. This is followed by a clonic phase as inhibitory neurons begin to interrupt the seizure discharge, leading to an intermittent contract/relax pattern of muscle action. The clonic bursts gradually become more infrequent and the seizure ends. Immediately prior to the onset of a seizure there may be an aura which may involve a visual disturbance or sensing a peculiar smell (Rang et al 1999).

Treatment of epilepsy

Investigation to the background of seizures should be established in order to offer treatment. If no cause is found which is common, antiepileptic medication will be commenced. Drugs used in treatment:

- sodium valproate (Epilim);
- phenytoin sodium (Epanutin);
- phenobarbital benzodiazepines;
- carbamazapine and others.

Epilepsy in pregnancy

Epilepsy affects 1 in 200 of all pregnant women (Shorvon 2002). Many pregnancies are unplanned in women with epilepsy; antiepileptic drugs may increase the breakdown of oestrogens, rendering contraceptives less efficient. Pregnancy can affect the incidence of seizures. There may be an increase or decrease in seizures but there is no change for most women. The more severe the disorder, the greater the effect on pregnancy; however, 90% of pregnancies have a successful outcome.

Preconception advice is important but women who are epileptic perceive a lack of information and support in outpatient departments, particularly advice for pregnancy (Shorvon 2002). Preconception folic acid 4 mg daily is recommended to prevent neural tube defects when trying to conceive. The changing metabolism of pregnancy alters the effect of medication and there will be a need to increase the dose or change medication if it causes teratogenicity (Donaldson 1995). In trials it has been shown that epileptic women have more birth defects – not because they are epileptic but because of their medication. There is a two- to three-fold increased risk of deformity in these newborns. Specific abnormalities have been linked to specific drugs (Shorvon 2002):

- sodium valproate – neural tube and skeletal defects;
- carbamazapine – neural tube and cardiac anomalies;
- phenytoin – orofacial clefts, cardiac anomalies and digital defects.

Other problems associated with anticonvulsant drugs are anaemia, because of folate antagonism, and vitamin D deficiency. Seizures occurring during pregnancy may cause fetal hypoxia and there is a fetal bradycardia during most seizures which takes 20 min to recover. If status epilepticus occurs, there is a 50% chance of mortality for both mother and her baby (Donaldson 1995).

Fetus to neonate

Anticonvulsant drugs cross the placenta and decrease the production of vitamin K, which may lead to **haemorrhagic disease of the newborn**. Vitamin K should be administered to mothers from 36 weeks gestation (Shorvon 2002) and to all infants post delivery. During pregnancy it may be advisable to divide the dose of medication evenly through the day to prevent high fetal dosage. Blood medication levels should be assessed monthly. If the baby is formula fed it may have withdrawal symptoms from maternal medication at approximately 1 week, in the form of irritability, excessive crying and continuous hunger. Some babies may remain sleepy and difficult to feed. All the drugs are excreted in breast milk but as long as the dosage isn't high there is no contraindication to breastfeeding (Donaldson 1995).

MAIN POINTS

- Asthma is the commonest respiratory problem found in pregnancy. In pregnancy some asthmatic women improve, some deteriorate and some experience no change in lung function. Close monitoring and ensuring compliance with treatment ensures mother and fetus remain well.

- Asthma requires long-term administration of drugs such as bronchodilators and anti-inflammatory agents and it is necessary to consider the effect of these drugs on early fetal development. Women may decrease their medication for fear of harming their babies to the detriment of treatment.

- TB in some parts of London exceeds 50 per 100 000 and 50% of TB cases in the UK were born overseas. The bacillus lies dormant for years but lowered resistance activates it and the host becomes sick. TB exploits the socially vulnerable and presence of other disease and immune suppression leads to active disease.

- The signs of pulmonary tuberculosis include general malaise, anorexia, weight loss, low-grade fever and night sweats. Pulmonary specific symptoms include productive cough with purulent sputum and haemoptysis. Rest and drug therapy form the basis for treatment.

- There is a worldwide epidemic of multiple drug-resistant TB and many strains may resist up to seven different antibiotics. Vaccination is effective in the prevention of tuberculosis in children but of variable value in adults. In the UK, BCG vaccination is carried out in children who are aged 10–14 years if they demonstrate a negative tuberculin test.

- Pregnant women are more susceptible to renal tract infections than other women. There is an incidence of unsuspected asymptomatic bacteriuria in between 4 and 10% of pregnant women which if not diagnosed and treated results in about 25% of them developing pyelonephritis. If the culture of a specific bacterium exceeds 10^5 organisms per ml of urine, asymptomatic bacteriuria is diagnosed. An antibiotic regime should be successful in treating the condition. Acute pyelonephritis occurs in 1–2% of pregnancies, usually in the second and third trimesters.

- The onset of acute renal failure is diagnosed if the urine output falls below 400 ml in 24 h or less than 20 ml/h. The incidence is about 1 in 10 000 pregnancies.

- Pregnancy is rare when the kidneys are functioning with less than 50% efficiency. Women with chronic renal impairment may appear to have pre-eclampsia, from which it needs distinguishing. Hypertension is the most common and serious complication.

- Maternal mortality may occur because of cerebral haemorrhage, abruptio placentae or acute renal failure. Fetal mortality may occur because of poor placental blood flow, abruptio placentae or fetal hypoxia. If kidney function diminishes, renal and peritoneal dialysis are possible and there is a 50% fetal survival rate.

- Following kidney transplantation, fertility returns and pregnancy is likely. If kidney function is adequate and there is no hypertension, women with renal transplants tolerate pregnancy well. Common complications are preterm labour and delivery and pre-eclampsia.

- Pregnant women are as likely to suffer from vomiting not associated with pregnancy as the non-pregnant population. Hyperemesis gravidarum may lead to maternal death if not treated actively. Hyperemesis is treated by admission to hospital for investigations and treatment. The cause of vomiting should be identified, antiemetics should be given and fluids and electrolytes replaced by intravenous infusion. Vitamins B_{12}, and C, folic acid and iron will be needed to correct anaemia.

- In early pregnancy appendicitis may be difficult to differentiate from threatened abortion. Later in pregnancy the pain may be mistaken for urinary tract infection, abruptio placentae or the onset of labour. Careful consideration of the patient's symptoms should allow a correct diagnosis.

- An ileostomy or colostomy for urinary or alimentary diversion should not affect the course of pregnancy. About 75% of women with stomas will have a normal vaginal delivery.

- Cholestasis is a last trimester problem with the development of pruritus, abnormal liver enzymes and jaundice.

- Epilepsy occurs in approximately 1% of the population and affects 1 in 200 of pregnant women. Many pregnancies are unplanned in women with epilepsy, possibly because antiepileptic drugs increase the breakdown of oestrogens, rendering contraceptives less efficient. Preconception folic acid 4 mg daily will prevent neural tube defects. When pregnancy is confirmed, advice about type and dosage of antiepileptic medication is important. Epileptic women have more birth defects because of their medication.

- Anticonvulsants cross the placenta and decrease the production of vitamin K, which may lead to haemorrhagic disease of the newborn. Vitamin K should be administered to mothers from 36 weeks gestation and to all infants post delivery. Following birth, babies who are formula fed may have withdrawal symptoms at approximately 1 week. Some babies may remain sleepy and difficult to feed. As long as the maternal drug dosage isn't high there is no contraindication to breastfeeding.

References

Alston P K, Kuller J A, MacMahon M J 2001 Pregnancy in transplant recipients. Obstetrical and Gynaecological Survey 56(5):289–295.

Armenti V T, Moritz M J, Davison J M 1998 Medical management of the pregnant transplant patient. Advances in Renal Transplant Therapy 5(1):14–23.

Armenti V T, Moritz M J, Cardonick E H, Davison J M 2002 Immunosuppression in pregnancy: choices for infant and maternal health. Drugs 62(16):2361–2375.

Blackburn S T 2003 Maternal, Fetal and Neonatal Physiology: A Clinical Perspective, 2nd edn. W B Saunders, Philadelphia.

BNF 2003 BCG vaccines. British National Formulary March (46):582.

Burroughs A K 1998 Pregnancy and liver disease. Forum (Genova) 8(1):42–58.

Callister M E J, Barringer J, Thanbalasingam G, Gair R, Davidson R 2002 Pulmonary tuberculosis among asylum seekers screened at Heathrow Airport, London 1995–9. Thorax 57:152–156.

Catchpole M 1995 Tuberculosis in England and Wales (Letter). British Medical Journal 311:187.

Coombes J 2000 Cholestasis in pregnancy: a challenging disorder. British Journal of Midwifery 8(9):565–570.

Davies M H, da Silva E E, Weaver J B 1995 Fetal mortality associated with cholestasis of pregnancy and the potential benefit of therapy with ursodeoxycholic acid. Gut 37(4):580–584.

Davison J, Baylis C 1995 Renal disease. In de Swiet M (ed.) Medical Disorders in Obstetric Practice, 3rd edn. Blackwell Science, Oxford.

De Swiet M 1995 Diseases of the respiratory system. In de Swiet M (ed.) Medical Disorders in Obstetric Practice, 3rd edn. Blackwell Science, Oxford.

Deuchar N 1995 Nausea and vomiting in pregnancy: a review of the problem with particular reference to psychological and social aspects. British Journal of Obstetrics and Gynaecology 102:6–8.

Donaldson J O 1995 Epilepsy in pregnancy. In de Swiet M (ed.) Medical Disorders in Obstetric Practice, 3rd edn. Blackwell Science, Oxford.

Drakeley A J, Le Roux P A, Anthony J et al 2002 Acute renal failure complicating severe pre-eclampsia requiring admission to an obstetric unit. American Journal of Obstetrics and Gynaecology 186(2):253–256.

Fagan E A 1995 Disorders of the gastrointestinal tract. In de Swiet M (ed.) Medical Disorders in Obstetric Practice, 3rd edn. Blackwell Science, Oxford.

Fantz C R, Samuel DJ, Ladenson J H, Gronowski A M 1999 Thyroid function during pregnancy. Clinical Chemistry 45(12):2250–2258.

Fatum M, Rojansky N 2001 Laparoscopic surgery during pregnancy. Obstetrical and Gynaecological Survey 56(1):50–59.

Fink J C, Schwartz S M, Benedetti T J, Stehman-Breen C O 1998 Increased risk of adverse outcomes among women with renal disease. Paediatric and Perinatal Epidemiology 12(3):277–287.

Gardner J 2000 Acute pyelonephritis during pregnancy. American Journal of Nursing 100(3):24.

Gilbert E S, Harmon J S 1998 Renal disease. In High Risk Pregnancy and Delivery, 2nd edn. Mosby, St Louis.

Good J, Iseman M, Davidson P et al 1981 Tuberculosis in association with pregnancy. American Journal of Obstetrics and Gynaecology 140:492–498.

Hawker J I, Bakhshi S S, Shaukat A, Farrington C P 1999 Ecological analysis of ethnic differences in relation between tuberculosis and poverty. British Medical Journal 319:1031–1034.

Hod M, Orvieto R, Kaplan B, Friedman S, Ovadia J 1994 Hyperemesis gravidarum; a review. Journal of Reproductive Medicine 39:605–612.

Hou S 1999 Pregnancy in chronic renal insufficiency and end stage renal disease. American Journal of Kidney Diseases 33(2):235–252.

Ie S, Rubio E R, Alper B, Szerlip H M 2002 Respiratory complications of pregnancy. Obstetrical and Gynaecological Survey 57(1):39–46.

Joint Tuberculosis Committee of the British Thoracic Society 2000 Control and prevention of tuberculosis in the UK, Code of Practice 2000. Thorax 55(11):887–901.

Karlen A 1995 Plagues progress, a social history of man and disease. Victor Gollanz, London.

Kumar A, Busse W W 1995 Airway inflammation in asthma. Scientific American 'Science and Medicine' March/April:38–47.

Lindsay N E 2000 Asymptomatic bacteriuria – important or not? New England Journal of Medicine 343(34):1037–1039.

Liu S M B, Wen Shi Wu, Demissie K et al 2001 Maternal asthma and pregnancy outcome: a retrospective cohort study. American Journal of Obstetrics and Gynaecology 184(2):90–96.

Low K G 1996 Nausea and vomiting in pregnancy: a review of the research. Journal of Gender Culture and Health 1(3):151–172.

McCance K L, Huether S E 2002 Pathophysiology, The Biologic Basis for Disease in Adults and Children, 4th edn. Mosby, St Louis.

Moran P, Taylor R 2002 Management of hyperemesis gravidarum: the importance of weight loss as a criterion for steroid therapy. Queensland Journal of Medicine 95(3):153–158.

Ormerod P 2001 Tuberculosis in pregnancy and the puerperium. Thorax 56:494–499.

Poole J H, Thorsen M S 1999 Acute renal failure in pregnancy. The American Journal of Maternal/Child Nursing 24(2):66–73.

Popkin C A, Lopez P P, Cohn S M et al 2002 The incision of choice for pregnant women with appendicitis is through McBurney's Point. American Journal of Surgery 183(1):20–22.

Rang H P, Dale M M, Ritter J M 1999 Pharmacology, 4th edn. Churchill Livingstone, Edinburgh.

Rose A M C, Watson J M, Graham C et al 2001 Tuberculosis at the end of the 20th century in England and Wales: results of a national survey. Thorax l56:173–170.

Schumacher S, Fichtner J, Stein R et al 1997 Pregnancy after Mainz pouch urinary diversion. The Journal of Urology 158(4):1362–1364.

Shorvon S 2002 Antiepileptic drug therapy during pregnancy: the neurologist's perspective. Journal of Medical Genetics 39(4):248–250.

Stables D 1995 Mother and child nursing: stomas and pregnancy. In Heath H B M (ed.) Potter and Perry's Foundations in Nursing Theory and Practice. Mosby, St Louis.

Tortora G J, Grabowski S R 2000 Principles of Anatomy and Physiology. John Wiley and Sons, Chichester.

Valentine B V, Jones C, Tyack A J 1980 Hyperemesis gravidarum due to thyrotoxicosis. Postgraduate Medical Journal 56:746–747.

Watson J M, Moss F 2001 TB in Leicester: out of control, or just one of those things? (Editorial). British Medical Journal 322:1133–1134.

Williams D J 1999 The implications of pre-existing renal disease in pregnancy. Current Obstetrics and Gynaecology 9(2):75–81.

Annotated recommended reading

Joint Tuberculosis Committee of the British Thoracic Society 2000 Control and prevention of tuberculosis in the UK, Code of Practice 2000. Thorax 55(11):887–901.
This comprehensive guide to the control of tuberculosis in the UK includes management guidelines for health care workers in relation to open TB infection.

Low K G 1996 Nausea and vomiting in pregnancy: a review of the research. Journal of Gender Culture and Health 1(3):151–172.
This paper presents a comprehensive overview of nausea and vomiting in pregnancy.

Ormerod P 2001 Tuberculosis in pregnancy and the puerperium. Thorax l56:494–499.
This is an excellent overview of tuberculosis in pregnancy, including the use of medication.

Poole J, Thorsen M 1999 Acute renal failure in pregnancy. The American Journal of Maternal/Child Nursing 24(2):66–73.
Succinct and to the point, this paper gives salient facts of anatomical change in the kidneys to the recognition causes and treatment of renal failure in pregnancy.

Shorvon S 2002 Antiepileptic drug therapy during pregnancy: the neurologist's perspective. Journal of Medical Genetics 39(4):248–250.
The article is easy to understand and gives the main points about epilepsy and pregnancy.

Williams DJ 1999 The implications of pre-existing renal disease in pregnancy. Current Obstetrics and Gynaecology 9(2):75–81.
This article develops ideas in management and outcomes in chronic renal disease.

Chapter 35

Diabetes mellitus and other metabolic disorders in pregnancy

Dot Stables

INTRODUCTION

Pregnancy in some endocrine disorders is rare and management is sometimes based on limited observation and clinical judgement rather than on evidence-based criteria (Hague 2001). However, **diabetes mellitus** is by far the most common of these diseases and much progress has been made in its management. Normal metabolism is discussed in Chapter 23 and readers may wish to remind themselves of normal carbohydrate utilisation.

DIABETES MELLITUS

Diabetes mellitus is a group of disorders characterised by **impaired carbohydrate utilisation** caused by an absolute or relative deficiency of **insulin production** by the endocrine pancreas. The changes in uncontrolled diabetes are a rise in blood glucose (normal range 3–5 mmol/L), and increases in glycogen breakdown, gluconeogenesis, fatty acid oxidation, ketone production and urea formation. There is also a reduced production of glycogen, lipid and protein in tissue cells that are normally dependent on insulin such as muscle and adipose tissue (Brook & Marshall 2001).

Pathophysiology

The inability of the tissues to receive enough glucose results in inhibition of **glycolytic enzymes** and activation of the enzymes involved in **gluconeogenesis** (Bewley 1997). This results in more blood glucose than can be utilised. Excessive glucose passes into the renal filtrate and **glycosuria** occurs. Glucose is osmotically active and pulls water after it, resulting in **polyuria** and **dehydration**. **Thirst** increases to try and maintain adequate body fluids (Brook & Marshall 2001).

The body tries to mobilise energy from fats and proteins. Urea, produced as a by-product of amino acid metabolism, is excreted in the urine. Fatty acid release always results in **ketogenesis** but in the diabetic person excess ketones are produced and excreted in the urine. The ketones in the blood cause **metabolic acidosis** and lowering of pH

(Brook & Marshall 2001). The **buffer systems** attempt to correct this and become exhausted. Other metabolic processes are disturbed and all body systems are affected. If untreated, acidosis leads to shock, coma and death.

Diabetes mellitus in pregnancy

Diabetes mellitus in pregnancy includes type 1 or **insulin-dependent diabetes** (IDDM). Recently, more pregnant women are found to have type 2 or **non-insulin-dependent diabetes** (NIDDM) (Feig & Palda 2002). **Gestational diabetes** (GDM) is where diabetes develops for the first time in pregnancy.

Aetiology

Type 1 diabetes mellitus   Type 1 diabetes mellitus (IDDM) is rare before 9 months and peaks at 12 years of age and there is an almost total lack of insulin production. Hyperglycaemia, polyuria and ketosis are present at onset and insulin treatment is necessary. There are differences between populations both within and between countries. IDDM accounts for about 10% of diabetes in the developed countries. It is thought to be more prevalent amongst white people than non-white people and the incidence is highest in Finland and lowest in Japan. There is a seasonal variation in the onset of IDDM, with more new cases in the northern hemisphere being reported in autumn and winter.

The coxsackie virus B4 (CB4) may be implicated in the onset of type 1 diabetes (Saunders 2002). This common childhood infection causes a high fever, sore throat and headache which lasts for about 3 days. The CB4 virus may destroy pancreatic islet cells and trigger an autoimmune response in genetically susceptible children. There is a long period of subclinical diabetes as β cells are progressively destroyed and islet cell antibodies have been found years before the onset of clinical signs. There is evidence that α-cell function is impaired, leading to excess **glucagon**, which exacerbates hyperglycaemia. Autoantibodies have been found in most people with juvenile onset diabetes.

Type 1 diabetes mellitus is subdivided into 2 distinct types. **IDDM type 1A** develops in childhood and is thought to be due to a genetic–environmental interaction which results in destruction of pancreatic β cells. There is a link with a human leucocyte antigen – HLA-DR4. The predisposing gene is carried on chromosome 6. About 12% of newly diagnosed diabetics of this type have a first-degree relative with the disease. **IDDM type 1B** tends to occur later in life, between the ages of 30 and 50 years old, and is probably an autoimmune disorder linked to HLA-DR3.

Type 2 or non–insulin dependent diabetes mellitus   Type 2 diabetes mellitus (NIDDM) is four times as common as IDDM and the onset is usually in later life in obese people. Incidence is increasing globally and NIDDM occurs in pregnancy more frequently as women delay conception

(Hague 2001). It varies with ethnicity, suggesting a genetic–environment interaction (Feig & Palda 2002). A form of NIDDM called **maturity-onset diabetes of the young** (MODY) is caused by an autosomal dominant gene. Sufferers are usually of normal weight and under 25 years old.

Amyloid deposits associated with islet cell destruction are seen in about 25%, usually correlating with the person's age and severity of disease. The ratio of α to β cells is normal and there is no reduction of insulin in the blood but in obese people insulin has a decreased ability to influence cellular uptake of glucose. There is increased **insulin resistance** because of decreased **cellular insulin receptors**.

The incidence of NIDDM in pregnancy is difficult to assess as some women taking insulin may have type 2 diabetes, especially in susceptible populations such as East Asian women. Many women may be undiagnosed prior to pregnancy. Pregnant women with type 2 diabetes are likely to be obese and to suffer hypertension and hyperlipidaemia. Screening women before pregnancy or early in the first trimester of pregnancy might help to differentiate between women with NIDDM and those with gestational diabetes (Feig & Palda 2002) but the dangers are the same.

Gestational diabetes mellitus (GDM)

Some people have impaired glucose tolerance (IGT) and may develop diabetes in stressful situations. In pregnancy this is called gestational diabetes, although Jarrett (1993) concludes that gestational diabetes is no more than a special case of IGT temporarily associated with pregnancy. About 15% of such women will develop NIDDM in later life but if obesity is present the incidence rises to 70%. GDM occurs in 2% of all pregnancies, mostly in the third trimester. Following delivery, glucose metabolism may return to normal, stay impaired or diabetes mellitus may develop. Gestational diabetes may recur in subsequent pregnancies (Philipson & Super 1989).

Population differences in the incidence of GDM   Studies have been conducted into the incidence of gestational diabetes between different ethnic groups. Berkowitz et al (1992) in the USA found a higher risk of developing gestational diabetes in women from India and the Middle East, Oriental women and first-generation Hispanic women. There was an increased risk in women of lower socioeconomic class, older women, obese women and those with infertility. In Great Britain, Dornhurst et al (1992) found a high prevalence of gestational diabetes in women from ethnic minority groups, in older women, in increasing parity and in obesity.

Shelley-Jones et al (1993) in Australia compared the physiology of 15 women with normal glucose tolerance, 16 Caucasian women with GDM and 19 Asian-born women with GDM. They found:

- Caucasian women, unlike the Asian women, were obese compared to the control group of women.
- Both groups of women with GDM had a similar abnormal insulin response to a glucose load.

- Fasting serum triglycerides were increased in all women with GDM. Asian women had significantly lower serum cholesterol levels than the Caucasian women, with or without GDM.

They concluded that it is difficult to know whether the differences in obesity and serum cholesterol 'reflect a dietary difference or a major difference in lipid metabolism.'

Glucose tolerance test

A **glucose tolerance test** (GTT) will confirm the presence of diabetes. A drink containing 75 g of glucose is given in the morning after the patient has fasted. Venous blood samples are taken at intervals. Normally, blood glucose rises but returns to normal (3–5 mmol/L) within 2 hours. The following abnormalities occur in the diabetic:

- a fasting plasma glucose of over 7 mmol/L;
- a blood glucose level over 10 mmol/L after 2 h;
- if the 2 h blood glucose level is between 7 and 10 mmol/L, glucose tolerance is impaired.

Pathological effects of diabetes mellitus

The metabolic changes and physiological effects of diabetes mellitus are profound (Fig. 35.1). Seventy years ago young diabetics usually died within 2 years of onset. The identification of insulin by Banting and Best led to survival, but the acute and long-term effects of diabetes mellitus became apparent. Deaths from **cardiovascular disease** and **renal disease** are much commoner than in the general population. Acute complications include **hypoglycaemia** and **diabetic ketoacidosis**. Pregnant women who have had IDDM more than 10 years are significantly more at risk of associated cardiovascular, ophthalmic, renal and neuropathic problems if their diabetes is brittle or diabetic control has been less than ideal (Hague 2001).

Hypoglycaemia

Hypoglycaemia occurs in 90% of IDDM sufferers and is also known as **insulin shock** or **insulin reaction**. Diabetic patients aim to prevent hypoglycaemia by diet and insulin administration. In a review of the effects of glycaemic control, maternal hypoglycaemia was more common in women whose control was very tight compared with those in whom it was tight. There was no difference in perinatal outcome. This suggests that there is no need for very tight **glycaemic control** in pregnant women (Walkinshaw 1996).

Symptoms   Symptoms vary between individuals but tend to be consistent for an individual. If neurons cannot obtain enough carbohydrate to maintain normal function, tachycardia, palpitations, tremors, pallor and anxiety occur. Other symptoms include headaches, dizziness, irritability, confusion, visual disturbances, hunger, convulsions and coma.

Management   Emergency treatment is to provide glucose. If the person is conscious, ingestion of a fast-acting carbohydrate can be encouraged. If the individual has lapsed into coma, intravenous glucose is necessary.

Diabetic ketoacidosis

Ketoacidosis is a serious condition occurring when there is insufficient insulin and an increase in hormones antagonising the effect of insulin such as catecholamines, glucagon, cortisol and growth hormone. Liver glucose production increases and peripheral glucose usage decreases. Fat mobilisation increases and ketogenesis occurs and death may occur. The most likely precipitating causes are infection and trauma. Interruption of insulin administration can also lead to ketoacidosis.

Symptoms   Polyuria, polydipsia and dehydration will occur because of **osmotic diuresis**. Coma is rare. Sodium, magnesium and phosphorus deficits may occur but the most severe electrolyte disturbance is potassium deficiency. Hyperventilation (**Kussmaul respirations**) may occur to compensate for the acidosis. Postural dizziness, anorexia, nausea and abdominal pain may occur. Both glucose and ketones will be present in urine. There may be a smell of acetone on the breath.

Management   Treatment of diabetic ketoacidosis is to decrease blood glucose levels by continual administration of low-dose insulin. Fluids and electrolytes are replaced as needed, depending on laboratory findings.

Long-term complications

- Diabetic neuropathy with sensory deficits.
- Microvascular disease with thickening of capillary basement membrane appears to be directly linked to the duration of the disease and blood glucose levels. Retinopathy causes blood vessel changes, leading to loss of sight. Nephropathy may result in end-stage renal disease.
- Atherosclerosis appears at a younger age and progresses more rapidly in diabetic people, leading to hypertension, coronary artery disease and stroke. This is unrelated to the severity of diabetes and may occur in people who only have impaired glucose tolerance. Peripheral vascular disease, leading to gangrene and amputation may occur.
- Infection is more common as pathogens utilise the increased tissue glucose to multiply and the function of phagocytic white cells is impaired.
- Pre-eclampsia will develop in about 13% of pregnant women.

Effects of diabetes on pregnancy

Most women with abnormalities of carbohydrate metabolism cannot compensate for the **diabetogenic effect** of

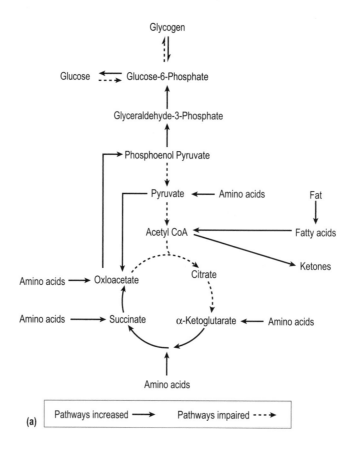

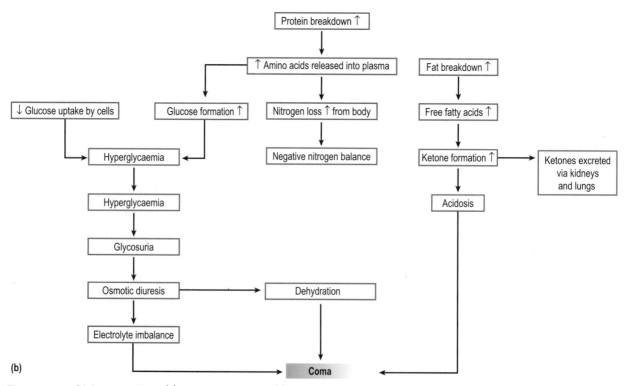

Figure 35.1   Diabetes mellitus: (a) metabolic changes, (b) physiological effects (from Hinchliff S M, Montague S E 1990, with permission).

pregnancy. Diabetes becomes more difficult to control in pregnancy although immediately after delivery women return to their prepregnancy needs. Although women with carbohydrate intolerance show no signs or symptoms, there is a significant increase in fetal and maternal morbidity.

Fetal problems

These include:

- First trimester abortions due to **congenital abnormalities** which are more common in poorly controlled diabetes due the metabolically abnormal environment. During the first 6 weeks following conception, congenital anomalies of the nervous, cardiovascular, renal and skeletal systems may occur.
- **Macrosomia** due to poor diabetic control in the second and third trimesters occurs with birth weights over the 90th centile (Buchanan & Kitzmiller 1994). This is not a simple relationship between blood glucose levels and fetal size, as both protein (Metzger 1991) and triglyceride (Knopp et al 1985) metabolism have been implicated in excessive fetal growth.
- Polyhydramnios.
- Traumatic delivery due to macrosomia.
- Stillbirth.
- Neonatal asphyxia and respiratory distress syndrome.
- Hyperviscosity syndrome.

Effect of pregnancy on the diabetes

Pregnancy with additional fetal requirements places large demands on maternal metabolism. This changes to allow more efficient storage of nutrients while minimising catabolism of protein stores (Buchanan & Kitzmiller 1994). There is progressive insulin resistance, which disappears immediately after delivery of the baby. Normally, the β cells increase the amount of insulin they release in the presence of insulin resistance but glucose metabolism in diabetic pregnant women becomes unstable and more insulin will be needed to achieve metabolic control.

Diabetic nephropathy   Diabetic nephropathy is present in 5% of pregnant women with IDDM and significant proteinuria in the first trimester is associated with poor outcome. Oedema, anaemia and hypertension further complicate the pregnancy. There is difficulty in choosing an appropriate antihypertensive drug. Although in non-pregnant patients a protein-restricted diet would be commenced, this is generally avoided in pregnancy because of fetal nutritional needs. In more than half of such pregnancies delivery is by caesarean section before 37 weeks (Garner 1995). The outcome may be satisfactory in that the woman has a live, healthy child but renal failure may affect her health.

Diabetic retinopathy   Progression of retinopathy has been associated with poor control of blood glucose and blood pressure, albuminuria and poor perinatal outcome (Lauszus et al 2000). Ophthalmologic examination and evaluation should be carried out at regular intervals and the Valsalva manoeuvre avoided in labour to prevent possible retinal haemorrhage. Pregnant women who have proliferative retinopathy with neovascularisation (new blood vessel growth) risk loss of vision. Neovascularisation can be prevented or treated by laser photocoagulation.

Care in pregnancy

IDDM complicates less than 0.5% of pregnancies and, prior to the availability of insulin, fetal and neonatal mortality was 60%. Vast improvements in care and outcomes have been made and the fetal/neonatal loss can be as low as 2%.

Preconception advice

Pregnancy should be discussed with the diabetic woman prior to conception (Hague 2001). Adequate blood glucose control prior to conception helps to reduce fetal loss due to early abortions, congenital abnormalities, fetal macrosomia, polyhydramnios and stillbirth. Research has shown that diabetic women whose blood sugar is well controlled around conception and during pregnancy have outcomes approaching the incidence of the non-diabetic population.

Management during pregnancy

Health professionals should collaborate with the diabetic woman in her care during pregnancy. The involvement of the **diabetic team**, the obstetrician and the midwife are essential. The woman should be booked for care and delivery in a consultant unit with attached neonatal care unit and is usually seen at least every 2 weeks (Hague 2001).

Diabetic control   The management of diabetes before and during pregnancy requires control of blood sugar and prevention of ketosis. If control is too extreme, hypoglycaemia may endanger the mother and cause fetal intrauterine growth retardation (Buchanan & Kitzmiller 1994, Hague 2001). Dietary intake and insulin dosage should be monitored with blood glucose levels. Because of the altered renal threshold for glucose, urinary glucose levels are unhelpful. Adjustment of insulin dosage during the antenatal period is managed better at home with normal food and energy usage rather than in the unusual hospital surroundings.

Glycaemic control   Ideally, plasma glucose levels should be below 5.0 mmol/L in the fasting state and less than 7.8 mmol/L after a meal (Garner 1995). Women must be told about the risk of nausea and vomiting likely to occur in the first trimester and how glucose metabolism is changed by the presence of the fetus. Instant reporting of problems to her doctor will help rapid adjustments to therapy to be made. The effect of the pregnancy on lifestyle, including the implications of maintaining a demanding job and the possible need for medical leave, should be discussed.

The role of haemoglobin A₁ (HbA₁) concentration

Glycosylated haemoglobin (HbA₁) is a type of adult haemoglobin where glucose is attached to part of the β chain. As this takes time to occur, HbA₁ levels indicate the blood glucose levels that were present about 2 months before the reading. They are increased in diabetes, especially if blood glucose control is inadequate. Pregnancy should be deferred until HbA₁ is less than 8% of the total (0.08 SI units). Following conception, HbA₁ readings once or twice a trimester will help to maintain adequate diabetic control (Hague 2001).

Insulin

Insulin is necessary for all women with type 1 diabetes and sometimes those with type 2 diabetes or gestational diabetes. Better control can be obtained by tailoring the insulin regime to the individual woman to avoid hypoglycaemia (Hague 2001). The regimen may be altered to twice-daily soluble and intermediate insulin. Women with gestational diabetes who require insulin may only need nocturnal medium-acting insulin. Ketoacidosis is mainly associated with hyperemesis gravidarum and infections (Garner 1995) but if it occurs there may be a fetal loss of 20%.

Oral hypoglycaemic agents

Data from South Africa suggest that the use of specific oral hypoglycaemic agents in pregnant women who are non-insulin dependent is safe to use where insulin therapy might create problems such as in non-compliant women. Unlike **chlorpropamide**, **Glyburide** (glabenclamide) does not cross the placenta. A recent study indicated that the use of **metformin** may be associated with increased risk of pre-eclampsia and perinatal mortality but the results may have been biased by the number of obese women in the study (Hague 2001). Further trials of the use of metformin during pregnancy are underway.

Diet

Dietary advice during pregnancy aims to achieve good diabetes control with optimum nutrition for both mother and baby. A calorie intake of 35 kcal per kg body weight is recommended (Garner 1995). An ideal dietary composition would be 55% carbohydrate, 20% protein and 25% fats, with polysaturated fats no more than 10%. This could be divided between three meals and three snacks. Ethnic differences in dietary habits should be discussed with the woman. Obese women may be asked to take a lower calorie intake as long as they do not lose weight or develop ketonuria.

Monitoring the fetus

Ongoing fetal wellbeing should be monitored closely using the methods discussed in Chapter 13. Although fetal macrosomia is the main problem, the babies of women with renal disease or superimposed preeclampsia may suffer from intrauterine growth retardation.

Delivery

Women with uncomplicated diabetes and no obstetric problems may be delivered vaginally at 38 weeks. Women with unstable diabetes, complications or obstetric problems may be delivered earlier by caesarean section to avoid the possibility of intrauterine death. Following induced or spontaneous onset of labour, blood glucose control needs to be maintained. In women with IDDM this is done by using a continuous dextrose 5% infusion and variable insulin infusion according to hourly blood glucose. Immediately following delivery, insulin requirements usually revert back to prepregnancy needs (Hague 2001).

Care in the puerperium

Control of diabetes

Insulin requirements fall and restabilisation is necessary. In women who choose to breastfeed, requirements may be less than prepregnancy. Women with type 2 diabetes or gestational diabetes can usually cease taking insulin and commence oral therapy if needed. In women who breastfeed, care must be taken with oral hypoglycaemic agents as they may cross into the milk and stimulate β-cell activity in the neonate, leading to hypoglycaemia, but no data are available according to Hague (2001).

Infection prevention

It is important to avoid infection in all postpartum women, but diabetic women are especially at risk. Data suggest that breast infection is higher in diabetic women, so care must be taken to control blood glucose level and to inspect the breasts for early signs (Whittaker 2001).

Breastfeeding

Breastfeeding is possible but it is necessary to remember that lactating women have a higher energy turnover and this means diet and insulin dosage need to be monitored carefully. Diabetic women gain the same benefits as all mothers who breastfeed, including protection against premenopausal breast and ovarian cancer (Chilvers 1993) and osteoporotic hip fractures in later life (Cumming & Klineberg 1993). Today women with diabetes of all types choose to breastfeed their babies as frequently as non-diabetic women (Whittaker 2001).

Contraceptive advice

Family planning methods must be discussed. The oral contraceptive pill can be taken but may mimic pregnancy, increasing the need for insulin. Intrauterine contraceptive devices may lead to infection and are not recommended for most diabetic women. A barrier method may be used by women wishing to add to their family.

Type 2 diabetes (NIDDM) and gestational diabetes

Gestational diabetes is 'the onset or recognition of glucose intolerance during pregnancy' (Berkowitz et al 1992). However, if women have not been screened before pregnancy or during the early part of the first trimester, it is difficult to differentiate this from prepregnancy-onset NIDDM. Gestational diabetes is associated with an increased risk of perinatal morbidity and mortality. There are usually no symptoms and diagnosis depends on abnormal blood glucose results, usually following a GTT.

Antenatal Screening for GDM   The Third International Workshop/Conference on GDM recommended screening of all pregnant women at 24–28 weeks gestation. Shamsuddin et al (2001) identified screening factors as positive family history of diabetes mellitus, history of spontaneous abortion, vaginal discharge and pruritus in the current pregnancy and maternal age greater than 35 years. However, they found that using screening factors only missed 25% of affected women. They concluded that the cost of an oral glucose tolerance test was marginal compared to its high sensitivity in detecting antenatal glucose intolerance and preventing associated problems.

Indicative clinical findings   Obstetricians may use clinical findings from history taking or from the present pregnancy to order tests for diagnosing the presence of GDM. These may include:

- a history of diabetes in close relatives;
- chronic hypertension;
- recurrent urogenital infections;
- age over 30 years;
- poor reproductive history (three or more spontaneous abortions);
- a previous baby weighing more than 4000 g;
- a previous unexplained perinatal death;
- a previous baby with unexplained congenital malformations;
- history of GDM in a previous pregnancy;
- obesity;
- glycosuria on two occasions at antenatal visit;
- the presence of polyhydramnios.

Complications of GDM   Macrosomia is twice as frequent, leading to a greater incidence of forceps delivery and caesarean section. Shoulder dystocia may result in injury to the mother or baby. Postnatally, women should be counselled about ways to minimise the risk of developing NIDDM later in life. They should be reminded to maintain normal body weight, to exercise regularly, to have annual blood glucose tests and to receive early care if they become pregnant again (Avery & Rossi 1994).

Management of GDM   Once GDM is diagnosed, treatment should aim to control blood glucose, carry out additional fetal surveillance and decrease the incidence of macrosomia. Dietary control is usually sufficient in GDM but occasionally insulin injections will be necessary. The need for insulin should disappear after delivery. Thompson et al (1990) carried out a randomised controlled research programme into the use of insulin prophylactically in the management of gestational diabetes. They found that insulin therapy had no apparent detrimental effect on pregnancy and there was no incidence of hypoglycaemia. The best results were seen in obese patients where larger reductions in birth weights were seen. However, routine use of insulin should not supersede its use in carefully selected women.

The baby of a diabetic mother   If there has been poor control of the diabetes mellitus the baby may be large, weighing over the 90th centile, and plethoric (Fig. 35.2). With the good control usually achieved in current practice, babies are more likely to be of a weight appropriate for gestational age (Bewley 1997). However, the baby may be physiologically immature and have problems similar to those of a preterm baby, including respiratory distress syndrome (Ch. 51, p. 657). Congenital defects are also related to the control of the diabetes around the time of conception. Birth injuries may occur if the baby is large (Ch. 53, p. 678).

Neonatal hypoglycaemia may occur because the islets of Langerhans hypertrophy during prenatal life and produce more insulin in response to high maternal blood glucose levels. Once delivered the baby no longer has access to this high glucose source. Careful monitoring of neonatal blood glucose and early feeding should help to prevent severe side-effects. Other problems encountered in this group of babies are skin infections, **polycythaemia with hyperbilirubinaemia**, weight loss and bleeding from the thick umbilical cord. The baby tends to be lethargic at first but development then proceeds normally.

ABNORMALITIES OF THYROID FUNCTION

Overactivity and underactivity of the thyroid gland can produce serious illness.

Hyperthyroidism (thyrotoxicosis) in pregnancy

Thyrotoxicosis occurs in about 0.2% of pregnancies and **Graves' disease** (Fig. 35.3) accounts for 95% of cases (Kilpatrick 2001). **Thyroid-stimulating immunoglobulins** (TSIgs) (antibodies) activate **follicular cell TSH receptors**, leading to increased production of **thyroid hormones**. Signs include raised basal metabolic rate (BMR), excessive perspiration, weight loss despite good calorific intake, a rapid irregular heart beat, palpitations, hypertension and nervousness. **Exophthalmos** (protrusion of the eyeballs) may

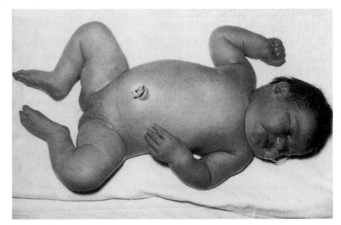

Figure 35.2   A large-for-gestational-age baby from a diabetic mother (from Kelnar C, Harvey D, Simpson C 1995, with permission).

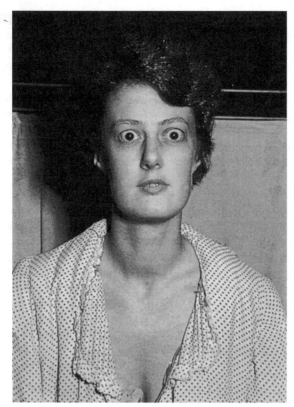

Figure 35.3   A person with Graves' disease (from Hinchliff S M, Montague S E 1990, with permission).

occur. Prepregnancy treatment may have been by surgical removal of the thyroid gland or ingestion of radioisotope-tagged iodine to destroy the most active thyroid cells.

Rarer conditions causing hyperthyroidism include **autonomous thyroid nodules**. **Biochemical thryotoxicosis** may occur in women who develop hyperemesis gravidarum because of the similarity between thyrotrophin (TSH) and human chorionic gonadotrophin (hCG) (Kilpatrick 2001, Vitoratos et al 2000). It may be difficult to diagnose thyrotoxicosis in pregnancy because of the normal thyroid changes. However, failure to gain weight despite a good appetite, a rapid sleeping pulse and lid lag are suspicious. Thyroxine (T_4) assays will be higher than in normal pregnancy.

Severe hyperthyroidism is associated with infertility but conception may occur if treatment has been successful or if the disease is mild (Bewley 1997). In mild hyperthyroidism, improvements may occur in pregnancy due to increase in thyroxine-binding globulin (TBG), which can offset the excess of thyroid hormones. Women with Graves' disease may also experience improvement due to altered immune system functioning, and drug dosages can often be reduced (Hague 2001). Relapse is common within several weeks of delivery.

Management

Inadequately managed thyrotoxicosis is associated with severe pre-eclampsia and maternal heart failure (Kilpatrick 2001). Pregnant women with hyperthyroidism need more calories to compensate for the higher metabolic rate. Fluid loss may occur if there is diarrhoea. If antithyroid drugs are used, their effects must be monitored carefully to avoid too high levels of drug. The drugs commonly used are **propylthiouracil** (PTU) or **carbimazole** (CBZ). PTU is the drug of choice in pregnancy and the puerperium. Failure to control the disease may necessitate a **partial thyroidectomy** if the disease is difficult to control or the woman has a large goitre (Hague 2001).

Thyroid storm

A **thyroid storm** is characterised by an extreme **hypermetabolic state**. It is a rare complication, occurring in 1% of hyperthyroid pregnancies, usually due to a stressful delivery or infection (Kilpatrick 2001). The woman develops hyperthermia, tachycardia, cardiac decompensation and mental disorientation. This carries a high rate of maternal morbidity and mortality. Therefore, treatment should be carried out in an intensive care unit whenever possible (Hague 2001).

Effect of maternal treatments on the fetus

Fetal loss   If hyperthyroidism is poorly controlled, intrauterine growth retardation, preterm labour and perinatal death may occur. No teratogenic effects have been reported for PTU or CMZ and perinatal mortality can be reduced by medical management of the mother (Hague 2001). Preterm labour should not be treated with β agonists such as salbutamol because of the risk of tachycardia. Calcium channel blockers such as nifedipine can be used instead.

Fetal hypothryoidism   Thionamide treatment of Graves' disease can suppress fetal and neonatal thyroid function (Kilpatrick 2001). There is a risk of 1 in 100 of fetal hypothyroidism as the drugs may cross the placenta and block the synthesis of thyroid hormones by the fetus so the lowest possible doses should be given.

Fetal hyperthyroidism   Women with Graves' disease who have been treated by surgical or **radioiodine ablation** of the thyroid, with or without thyroxine treatment, may have raised titres of TSIg. Their fetuses may develop uncontrolled hyperthyroidism with a heart rate above 160 beats/min. These women should be given thyroxine, which does not cross the placenta, to maintain their normal thyroid function and thionamides to treat the fetus, using its heart rate as a guide (Hague 2001). In pregnancies where there is placental transfer of **long-acting thyroid stimulator** (LATS) from mother to fetus, fetal hyperthyroidism may result. The baby's thyroid function will return to normal within 3 weeks.

Hypothyroidism in pregnancy

Hypothyroidism is more common than hyperthyroidism in pregnant women. It may be due to **autoimmune thyroiditis**

(Hashimoto's disease), viral thyroiditis or congenital absence of the thyroid gland (Hague 2001, Kilpatrick 2001). There may be a defect in the thyroid gland or in the control pathway of thyrotrophin-releasing hormone (TRH) or thyroid-stimulating hormone (TSH) release. In dietary iodine deficiency, the thyroid gland hypertrophies and a goitre occurs. The enlarged gland is stimulated by increasing amounts of TSH but produces unusable colloid. This used to be common in inland areas such as Derbyshire (hence **Derbyshire neck**).

Other causes of hypothyroidism in pregnancy are those secondary to immune disorders or following destruction of thyroid tissue either surgically or with radioactive iodine. Also, women with type 1 diabetes mellitus have a 5–8% incidence of hypothyroid disease and a 25% risk of developing postpartum thyroid dysfunction (Kilpatrick 2001).

Symptoms include a low BMR, feeling cold, constipation, thick, dry skin, puffy eyes, oedema, lethargy and mental sluggishness. Untreated hypothyroidism is often associated with infertility because TRH stimulation induces **hyperprolactinaemia**, which prevents ovulation (Hague 2001). Confirmation is by measurement of tri-iodothyronine (T_3) and T_4 levels. Treatment is by thyroxine medication, and assessment of thyroid function once in each trimester is usually sufficient (Hague 2001). As long as the fetus is not exposed to iodine deficiency or teratogenic drugs, development should be normal. Complications of increased fetal loss and prolonged pregnancy may occur.

ADRENAL DISORDERS IN PREGNANCY

Adrenal disorders in pregnancy are uncommon and most women will have had their disorder diagnosed and treated before pregnancy (Hague 2001).

Addison's disease

Addison's disease is caused by inadequate secretion of the adrenal cortical hormones with deficiency of both glucocorticoids and mineralocorticoids. Symptoms include falling plasma sodium and glucose levels, a rise in serum potassium levels, **skin hyperpigmentation** and weight loss. Severe dehydration and hypotension are common. The main cause is **autoimmune destruction** of the adrenal cortex and

it often occurs combined with other autoimmune endocrine disorders such as Graves' disease. In pregnancy, the condition is treated by replacement therapy of 20–30 mg/day of oral hydrocortisone (Hague 2001). In an acute episode, **intravenous hydrocortisone** is necessary.

Cushing's syndrome

Cushing's syndrome is rare in pregnancy because it is usually associated with amenorrhoea and anovulation (Hague 2001). It is caused by excessive levels of corticosteroids. The cause is often pituitary or adrenal carcinoma. Some normal pregnancy features mimic Cushing's syndrome but unless other signs such as a moon face, hirsutism, acne and proximal myopathy are present, it is unlikely that true Cushing's syndrome is present. In the rare cases seen, fetal loss has been 25% and preterm delivery occurred in up to 50%.

Congenital adrenal hyperplasia

Congenital adrenal hyperplasia (CAH) is a group of conditions with a block in the biosynthesis of **cortisol** (Brook & Marshall 2001). Women who remain undiagnosed tend to be infertile and few pregnancies occur (Hague 2001). Girls treated with hormones in childhood and adolescence may have clitoral and vaginal scarring, making vaginal delivery traumatic. Because of the masculinisation of the pelvis, **cephalopelvic disproportion** is a serious problem. Women with late-onset CAH usually have **polycystic ovary syndrome** and require adrenal suppression with glucocorticoids to allow ovulation to occur (Hague 2001). Any women who have been given prolonged steroid therapy should be given hydrocortisone during labour or at the time of caesarean section to avoid a hypoadrenal crisis.

Phaeochromocytoma

A phaeochromocytoma is a tumour of the adrenal medulla. It may be misdiagnosed as pre-eclampsia or essential hypertension. Symptoms include intermittent or sustained hypertension, postural hypotension, sweating, palpitations and tachycardia, anxiety, nausea and vomiting. The tumour and symptoms are treated medically until the fetus is viable when surgical removal of the tumour is carried out.

MAIN POINTS

- Diabetes mellitus is characterised by impaired carbohydrate utilisation caused by an absolute or relative deficiency of insulin production. In pregnancy abnormal carbohydrate metabolism occurs in women with IDDM, NIDDM or GDM. After delivery, glucose metabolism may return to normal, stay impaired or diabetes mellitus

may develop. Gestational diabetes is likely to recur in subsequent pregnancies.

- The Coxsackie virus B4 may destroy pancreatic islet cells and trigger an autoimmune response in genetically susceptible children. Type 1 diabetes mellitus is subdivided into two types: type 1A begins in childhood and may be due to destruction of the β cells in the pancreas. Type 1B occurs between the ages of 30 and 50 and may be an autoimmune disorder.

- Type 2 diabetes occurs mainly in obese people after the age of 40. MODY affects younger individuals, usually of normal weight. The incidence of NIDDM in pregnancy is difficult to assess, as some women taking insulin may have it. Many women may be undiagnosed prior to pregnancy.

- Long-term effects of diabetes mellitus include deaths from cardiovascular and renal disease. Chronic conditions include diabetic neuropathy; microvascular disease, leading to retinopathy and nephropathy; and atherosclerosis, leading to coronary artery disease and stroke. Peripheral vascular disease, leading to gangrene and amputation, may occur. Infection is more common.

- Acute complications include hypoglycaemia and diabetic ketoacidosis. The aim is to prevent hypoglycaemia. Emergency treatment is to provide glucose. Treatment of diabetic ketoacidosis is to decrease blood glucose levels by continual administration of low-dose insulin.

- Diabetes is difficult to control in pregnancy although immediately after delivery women return to their prepregnancy needs. Most women with carbohydrate intolerance show no signs or symptoms but there is a significant increase in fetal and maternal morbidity. Pre-eclampsia will develop in about 13% of pregnant women.

- Fetal problems include first trimester abortions, congenital abnormalities, macrosomia, polyhydramnios, traumatic delivery, stillbirth, neonatal asphyxia, respiratory distress syndrome and hyperviscosity syndrome.

- The management of diabetes requires control of blood sugar and prevention of ketosis. Adequate blood glucose control prior to conception helps to reduce fetal loss but, if control is too extreme, hypoglycaemia may endanger the mother and cause fetal intrauterine growth retardation. The diet and insulin dosage should be monitored by blood glucose levels.

- The need for insulin increases during pregnancy. Specific oral hypoglycaemic agents in pregnancies of women who are non-insulin dependent are safe to use where insulin therapy might create problems.

- Fetal complications include macrosomia with an increased incidence of shoulder dystocia, forceps delivery and caesarean section. It is usual to deliver the woman with uncomplicated diabetes and no obstetric problems vaginally at 38 weeks. Women with unstable diabetes, complications or obstetric problems may be delivered earlier by caesarean section to avoid intrauterine death.

- Women from India, and the Middle East and Oriental women have a higher risk of developing gestational diabetes. There is an increased risk in women of lower socioeconomic class, older women, obese women and those with infertility.

- In the puerperium, insulin requirements fall and restabilisation is necessary. In women who breastfeed, care must be taken with oral hypoglycaemic agents as they may cross into the milk and stimulate β-cell activity in the neonate, leading to hypoglycaemia. Breast infection is higher in diabetic women.

- The oral contraceptive pill may mimic pregnancy, increasing the need for insulin. Intrauterine contraceptive devices may lead to infection and are not recommended for most diabetic women.

- If there has been poor diabetic control, the baby may be large and plethoric and birth injuries may occur. The baby may be physiologically immature and have problems similar to those of a preterm baby. Congenital defects are related to the diabetic control around the time of conception.

- Hypoglycaemia may occur because the fetus produces more insulin in response to high maternal blood glucose levels and after delivery the baby has no access to this high glucose source. Other neonatal problems are skin infections, polycythaemia with hyperbilirubinaemia, weight loss and bleeding from the thick umbilical cord.

- Graves' disease accounts for 95% of cases of hyperthyroidism seen in about 0.2% of pregnancies. Thyrotoxicosis may be difficult to diagnose if it arises for the first time in pregnancy. Failure to gain weight despite a good appetite, a rapid sleeping pulse and lid lag should raise the possibility. T_4 assays higher than in the normal elevation of pregnancy will be present.

- Improvements may occur in pregnancy. If antithyroid drugs are used, their effects must be monitored carefully to avoid too high levels of drug treatment. A partial thyroidectomy may be necessary if there is failure to control the disease or the woman has a large goitre.

- Inadequately managed thyrotoxicosis is associated with severe pre-eclampsia and maternal heart failure. A thyroid storm with high maternal morbidity and mortality rate may occur if there is stress. Thionamide treatment of Graves' disease can suppress fetal and neonatal thyroid function, causing hypothyroidism.

- Neonatal hyperthyroidism may occur in women who have been treated by surgical or radioiodine ablation of the thyroid. These women should be treated with thyroxine to maintain their normal thyroid function and thionamides drugs to treat the fetus, using its heart rate as a guide. Placental transfer of LATS from mother to fetus may result in neonatal hyperthyroidism. The baby's thyroid function will return to normal within 3 weeks.

- Maternal hypothyroidism may be due to Hashimoto's disease, viral thyroiditis or congenital absence of the thyroid gland. It may result from a defect in the thyroid gland or in the control pathway of TRH or TSH release. Dietary iodine deficiency may be a cause. Hypothyroidism in pregnancy may be secondary to immune disorders or follow destruction of thyroid tissue. Treatment is by thyroxine medication.

- Addison's disease is mainly caused by autoimmune destruction of the adrenal glands. In pregnancy it is treated by oral hydrocortisone 20–30 mg/day. In an acute episode, intravenous hydrocortisone is necessary. Cushing's disease is rarely associated with pregnancy because amenorrhoea and anovulation are usually present. Fetal and neonatal loss is high. The cause is often pituitary or adrenal carcinoma.

- Women with congenital adrenal hyperplasia who remain undiagnosed tend to be hirsute and infertile. Girls treated with hormones in childhood and adolescence have a fertility rate of 64%. Because of the masculinisation of the pelvis, cephalopelvic disproportion is a serious problem.

- The symptoms of phaeochromocytoma, which include hypertension, postural hypotension, sweating, palpitations and tachycardia, anxiety, nausea and vomiting, are treated medically until the fetus is viable, when surgical removal of the tumour is carried out.

References

Avery M D, Rossi M A 1994 Gestational diabetes. Journal of Nurse-Midwifery 39(2):S9–S13.

Berkowitz G S, Lapinski R H, Wein R, Lee D 1992 Race/ethnicity and other risk factors for gestational diabetes. American Journal of Epidemiology 135(9):965–973.

Bewley C 1997 Medical conditions complicating pregnancy. In Sweet B R, Tiran D (eds) Mayes Midwifery, 12th edn. Baillière Tindall, London, pp 548–569.

Brook C G D, Marshall N J 2001 Essential Endocrinology, 4th edn. Blackwell Science, Oxford.

Buchanan T A, Kitzmiller J L 1994 Metabolic interactions of diabetes and pregnancy. Annual Review of Medicine 45:245–260.

Chilvers C 1993 Breast-feeding and risk of breast cancer in young women, United Kingdom case control study group. British Medical Journal 507:17–20.

Cumming R, Klineberg R 1993 Breast-feeding and other reproductive factors and the risk of hip fractures in elderly women. International Journal of Epidemiology 22(4):684–691.

Dornhurst A, Paterson C E, Nicholls J S D et al 1992 High prevalence of gestational diabetes in women from ethnic minority groups. Diabetic Medicine 9:820–825.

Feig D S, Palda A 2002 Type 2 diabetes in pregnancy: a growing concern. Lancet 359:1690–1692.

Garner P 1995 Type I diabetes mellitus and pregnancy. Lancet 346:157–161.

Hague W M 2001 Endocrine disease (including diabetes). Best Practice & Research Clinical Obstetrics and Gynaecology 15(6):877–889.

Jarrett R J 1993 Gestational diabetes: a non-entity? British Journal of Medicine 306:37–38.

Kilpatrick S 2001 Thyroid disease in pregnancy. ACOG Practice Bulletin Clinical Guidelines for Obstetrician–Gynecologists No 32 98(5):879–888.

Knopp R H, Bergelin R O, Wahl P W, Walden C E 1985 Relationship of infant birth size to maternal lipoproteins, apoproteins, fuels, hormones, clinical chemistries and body weight at 36 weeks gestation. Diabetes 34(suppl 2):71–77.

Lauszus F, Klebe J G, Bek T 2000 Diabetic retinopathy in pregnancy during tight metabolic control. Acta Obstetrica et Gynecologia Scandinavica 79:367–370.

Metzger B E 1991 Biphasic effects of maternal metabolism on fetal growth: quintessential expression of fuel-mediated metabolism. Diabetes 40(suppl 2):99–105.

Philipson E H, Super D M 1989 Gestational diabetes mellitus: does it recur in subsequent pregnancy? American Journal of Obstetrics and Gynaecology 160(6):1324–1331.

Saunders R 2002 Casualties of war. Balance (Diabetes UK) 189:42–44.

Shamsuddin K, Mahdy Z A, Siti Rafiaah I, Jamil M A, Rahimah M D 2001 Risk factor screening for abnormal glucose tolerance in pregnancy. International Journal of Gynecology and Obstetrics 75:27–32.

Shelley-Jones D C, Wein P, Nolan C, Beischer N A 1993 Why do Asian-born women have a higher incidence of gestational diabetes? An analysis of racial differences in body habitus, lipid metabolism and the serum insulin response to an oral glucose load. Australian and New Zealand Journal of Obstetrics and Gynaecology 33(2):114–118.

Thompson D J, Porter K B, Gunnells D J, Wagner P C, Spinnato J A 1990 Prophylactic insulin in the management of gestational diabetes. Obstetrics and Gynaecology 75(2):960–964.

Vitoratos N, Salamalekis D, Kassanos D et al 2000 Hyperemesis gravidarum: its relationship to maternal immune response and thyroid function. Prenatal and Neonatal Medicine 5:363–367.

Walkinshaw S 1996 Very tight versus tight control for diabetes in pregnancy. Cochrane Review: In The Cochrane Library, Issue 1. Update Software 2003, Oxford.

Whittaker K M 2001 Breast-feeding and the diabetic mother. British Journal of Midwifery 9(8):484–488.

Annotated recommended reading

Hague W M 2001 Endocrine disease (including diabetes). Best Practice & Research Clinical Obstetrics and Gynaecology 15(6):877–889.
This paper gives an excellent overview of all the endocrine disorders, including diabetes mellitus, their effects on pregnancy and their current management.

Kilpatrick S 2001 ACOG Practice Bulletin, Clinical Guidelines for Obstetrician–Gynecologists No 32 98(5):879–888.
This practice bulletin presents a highly readable account of thyroid disease in pregnancy. It discusses the aetiology of thyroid problems, the normal physiology of the thyroid in pregnancy and the diagnosis and management of the conditions.

Vitoratos N, Salamalekis D, Kassanos D et al 2000 Hyperemesis gravidarum: its relationship to maternal immune response and thyroid function. Prenatal and Neonatal Medicine 5:363–367.
This is an interesting paper to read because it underlines the similarities between some placental hormones and hormones found in the adult body and how metabolism may be affected.

Walkinshaw S 1996 Very tight versus tight control for diabetes in pregnancy. Cochrane Review: In The Cochrane Library, Issue 1. Update Software 2003, Oxford.
Like all Cochrane reviews, this paper on diabetes presents a summary of research and discusses the findings in relation to good practice.

Section 3A

LABOUR – NORMAL

Perhaps the most exciting aspect of childbearing is the birth. Midwives in the United Kingdom are privileged to be the major carer during this short but intensively meaningful time in the life of a woman and her family. There is no denial of the importance and social and psychological aspects of this major life event but these chapters concentrate on the management of labour that arises from a deep knowledge of physiology. Chapter 36 examines what is currently known about the causes of the onset of labour. Currently there is a strong tendency to a rise in the numbers of babies delivered by caesarean section. If a return to more normal deliveries is to be achieved it is imperative that midwives understand the progress and management of normal labour. Therefore, there is a chapter dedicated to each of the so-called three stages of labour. Chapter 37 discusses the physiology and management of the first stage of labour and Chapter 38 is dedicated to the important topic of pain relief in labour. Chapters 39 and 40 discuss the second and third stages of labour, respectively.

Chapter 36

The onset of labour

INTRODUCTION

The two main issues about providing care for women in labour are how to meet the social, psychological and spiritual needs and how to provide physiological safety for the woman and her baby. A major problem for anyone courageous enough to research the field of human behaviour, especially in physiological terms, is to place such behaviour in the context of cultural influences.

A great number of textbooks devoted to the social meaning of pregnancy and labour are worth reading for anyone considering how the management of childbearing is influenced by major changes and beliefs of society. The purpose of this chapter is to examine the physiological concepts associated with normal uncomplicated labour so that the reader can make caring decisions on the management of labour based on current concepts and theories.

TIMING OF THE ONSET OF LABOUR

In humans the timing of the onset of labour is less precise than in many other species. The mean day of onset of labour in humans is probably about 39.6 weeks with a range of 3 weeks on either side of the mean. The timing may be related to fetal brain activity via **adrenocorticotrophic hormone** (ACTH) and the pituitary–adrenal axis. Progesterone is then metabolised to oestrogen, which gradually increases the sensitivity of the uterus to prostaglandins and oxytocin produced by both the fetoplacental unit and maternal tissues. Large numbers of research projects into the onset of labour in cattle, sheep and humans have found that when there is an abnormality of the fetal hypothalamus and pituitary area of the brain, extreme prolongation of pregnancy may occur (Johnson & Everitt 2000, Steer & Johnson 1998).

The aetiology of labour is complex and at present is not understood and therefore there are numerous hypotheses and theories. Consequently, an outline only of key areas of discussion is given. If the sequence of events leading to the onset of labour were fully understood it might be easier to prevent the onset of preterm labour and the devastating fetal loss and morbidity resulting from extreme immaturity. There is good evidence for a central role for **prostaglandins** in the initiation of labour but the composition and biosynthesis of prostaglandins by the various tissues remains unclear (see below).

The role of the fetal endocrine system

There is evidence to support the concept that the fetus is largely responsible for triggering the onset of labour. However, there is still uncertainty about the role of the fetal hypothalamo–pituitary–adrenal axis in the initiation of labour in humans. It has become apparent that the extrapolation of experimental findings from one species to another is not reliable, as events may differ between species. In sheep, parturition is initiated by a surge of cortisol secreted by the fetal adrenal cortex. This acts on placental enzymes to convert progesterone to oestrogen. The rapid change in steroid balance stimulates the release of prostaglandins from both the placenta and the myometrium. There is increased sensitivity of the myometrium to oxytocin and uterine contractions are produced which are powerful enough to expel the fetus.

The adrenal cortex

Johnson & Everitt (2000) have summarised the research findings and suggest it is unlikely that increased production of cortisol plays a major part, as labour begins in the congenital absence of the fetal adrenals. Cortisol levels measured in the umbilical cord blood after delivery are difficult to assess, as they may increase because of the stress of labour rather than be responsible for initiating labour. Scalp blood cortisol measurements made in early labour showed no difference in spontaneous or induced labour, although there was a rise in fetal plasma cortisol as labour progressed. There is no dramatic rise in total cortisol level in fetal circulation prior to the onset of labour.

The administration of corticosteroids such as **betamethasone** to women in late pregnancy results in a fall in maternal circulating oestrogen levels but there is little effect on the placental progesterone synthesis or the duration of pregnancy. In the human placenta, although **glucocorticoids** do not induce the fall in progesterone and rise in oestrogen leading to labour, they are involved in the maturation of the fetus, in particular the fetal lung, allowing survival of a fetus born 6 weeks early. In sheep, cortisol produces both organ maturity and the onset of labour and a lamb born even 1 week or 2 weeks early may be too immature to survive.

One hormone that may be implicated in fetal control of the onset of labour is **dehydroepiandrosterone sulphate** (DHAS), which is the major precursor of placental estradiol and estrone synthesis. The human fetal adrenal gland is relatively large at birth with a fetal zone occupying 80% of the cortex and being responsible for the size. The function of the adrenal cortex is different in the fetus from the adult and the fetal zone atrophies after birth. It has been found that human chorionic gonadotrophin (hCG) is a major stimulator of the fetal zone during pregnancy and ACTH can also stimulate the production of DHAS.

The fetal posterior pituitary gland

Higher concentrations of the posterior pituitary hormones vasopressin and oxytocin have been found in the umbilical circulation than in the maternal circulation. Although the source of this fetal oxytocin is not clear, the levels are higher in fetal arterial blood than venous blood, which suggests fetal origin. It is possible that as much as 1–3 mU/min of oxytocin is transferred from fetus to mother, which is enough to promote uterine activity at term. An argument against the fetal role is that labour almost always follows fetal death in utero, depending on the gestational age of the fetus. Possibly the release of prostaglandins is more important and the mechanism of release differs when the fetus is dead, being provoked by the massive fall in progesterone level that accompanies fetal death.

The role of the placenta

Progesterone

It is now over 30 years since Csapo put forward a hypothesis that labour is initiated by the withdrawal of the progesterone block on myometrial activity. It has been difficult to prove or disprove this hypothesis (Steer & Johnson 1998). All attempts to use progesterone to prolong labour, postpone preterm labour or to prevent early abortion have been unsuccessful. Measurement of progesterone levels in the peripheral blood of women has not shown any withdrawal of progesterone at the end of pregnancy. However, this may not be significant if the progesterone acts locally and it may be an alteration in the binding of progesterone that is important rather than the level.

Oestrogens

Placental production of **oestrogens** rises as pregnancy progresses and DHAS of both maternal and fetal origin contributes to the placental production of oestrogens, most importantly of estradiol. However, women do go into labour without the rise in the concentration of estradiol and there is no dramatic rise in the levels of estradiol just prior to the onset of labour. It is probable that estradiol facilitates rather than causes the onset of labour. As yet, there is no clear evidence that changing concentrations of oestrogens and progesterone alters at the onset of labour. However, these changes in balance between the two steroid hormones facilitate increasing myometrial activity.

Fetal membranes

Steroid hormones

The fetal membranes are known to have a relatively high concentration of progesterone. Both the chorion laeve and the amnion have been shown to contain enzymes that can reduce the level of progesterone and also both chorion and amnion contain a protein which increases towards the end of pregnancy and that can bind progesterone. These two mechanisms would produce a local progesterone withdrawal effect. However, the membranes are avascular and any substance produced by them must travel by diffusion.

Prostaglandins

The amnion and chorion are both involved in the production of **prostaglandins (PGs)**. Karim (1966) first suggested that prostaglandins played a role in the initiation of labour. It is still unclear whether prostaglandins initiate labour or maintain it. Findings from earlier studies have been unusable because of prostaglandin production by tissue trauma during sample collection. Making measurements of prostaglandins is extremely difficult as storage or temperature can affect the findings. Drugs such as aspirin act as **prostaglandin inhibitors**, preventing the first step in the metabolism of **arachidonic acid**. The fetal membranes contain significant amounts of arachidonic acid and research indicates that the membranes are significantly involved in the synthesis of prostaglandins, but once again there seems to be no significant change at the onset of labour.

Maternal influences

The decidua

The decidua is also implicated in the production of prostaglandins. Evidence suggests that the decidua is a major source of prostaglandins during labour. In the 1970s Gustavii studied the role of the decidua in controlling the onset of labour (Steer & Johnson 1998). Gustavii (1977) proposed that the decidual cells have lysosomes which contain **phospholipase A_2**, an enzyme necessary for the synthesis of prostaglandins. These lysosomes are fragile and degenerate under the influence of oestrogen in late pregnancy when progesterone levels fall and oestrogen levels rise. Steer & Johnson (1998) find this hypothesis useful in the explanation of the onset of labour at term.

Work carried out by Keirse and his colleagues in the 1970s showed that the primary prostaglandins present were PGE_2 and $PGF_{2\alpha}$. The precursor of the two prostaglandins is an essential fatty acid called arachidonic acid derived from glycerophospholipids and involves several stages of conversion by enzymes. Both prostaglandins are known to stimulate myometrial contractions (McNabb 1997). Production rates of the two prostaglandins in decidual cells may be 30 times greater in labour than at elective caesarean section.

The endocrine system

The ovaries are not necessary for the initiation of labour and it seems that maternal oxytocin from the pituitary gland plays little part in the initiation of labour. The maternal adrenal glands do not seem to play any part in labour.

Neurohormonal control

The **Ferguson reflex** is a neurohormonal reflex (Fig. 36.1) arising from the genital tract that may be involved in the release of both oxytocin and prostaglandin in labour. The release of oxytocin could lead to increasing prostaglandin production as it does in some animal species. If this were so, then administration of epidural analgesia should block the spinal part of the reflex and oxytocin release, resulting in prolongation of the first stage of labour. Since there is no evidence to suggest this happens, prostaglandin release in human labour probably does not involve oxytocin release.

Control of cervical changes in labour

It is absolutely necessary that uterine contractions are coordinated with cervical dilatation. The increasing pressure placed on the cervix by the presenting part during active labour is said to aid dilatation of the cervix by the mechanism of Ferguson's reflex described above. Uterine contractions alone cannot bring about cervical softening and cervical dilatation. Changes in the collagen content of the cervix must occur and evidence is that it is the hormone estradiol that brings about the change. Prostaglandins also play a part in the ripening of the cervix and are often used prior to the induction of labour if the cervix is unfavourable.

DEFINITIONS OF LABOUR

The previous section considered the role of the myometrium, decidua, fetus, placenta and membranes in the initiation of labour and the maintenance of contractions resulting in progress. This progress must be achieved without compromising maternal or fetal safety. Cassidy (1999) defines concepts associated with labour:

- Labour is the process by which the fetus, placenta and membranes are expelled through the birth canal.
- Normal labour is spontaneous in onset at term, with the fetus presenting by the vertex, and is completed within 18 h with no complications arising.
- There are three stages:
  Stage 1 – is the stage of dilatation of the cervix and begins with the onset of regular rhythmic contractions and is complete when the cervix is fully dilated.

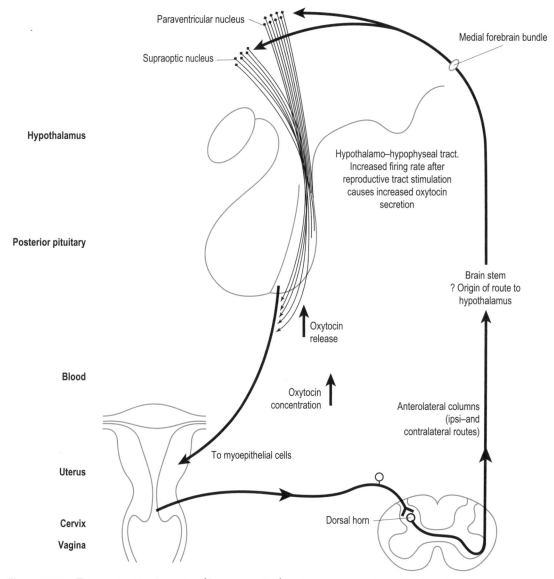

Figure 36.1 The neuroendocrine reflex (Ferguson reflex) underlying oxytocin synthesis and secretion. (Reproduced with permission from Johnson & Everitt 1995.)

Stage 2 – is the stage of expulsion of the fetus and begins when the cervix is fully dilated. It ends with complete expulsion of the fetus.

Stage 3 – is the stage of expulsion of the placenta and membranes and the control of bleeding. It begins following expulsion of the fetus and ends when the placenta and membranes are expelled.

The causes of onset of labour have been discussed above and the timing is important as it allows decisions to be made about the progress and ongoing management of labour, yet it is difficult to establish with accuracy. The concept of prelabour relates to the changes that occur in the last few weeks of pregnancy (Gibb 1988). It is often difficult to decide when the transition from the painless uterine contractions of prelabour develops into true labour. The length of labour

is variable and may be affected by parity, birth interval, psychological state, presentation and position, pelvic shape and size and the type of uterine contractions.

MATERNAL PHYSIOLOGICAL ADAPTATION IN LABOUR

The physiological changes in labour are examined separately to the process of labour so that sufficient depth can be achieved.

Cardiovascular system

There are profound changes in the cardiovascular system due to the effect of uterine contractions. The woman's emotional response to labour may affect the cardiovascular system, especially in primigravidae. The first stage of labour is associated with a progressive rise in cardiac output as each contraction adds 300–500 ml blood to the circulating blood volume. These changes are limited by epidural analgesia or supine position and by alleviation of pain and anxiety. Epidural analgesia appears to prevent the progressive increases in cardiac output while supine positioning lowers the cardiac output, decreases stroke volume but causes a compensatory increase in heart rate.

Pain, anxiety and apprehension may add to this effect, causing an increase in systolic and diastolic blood pressure and heart rate by increasing sympathetic tone. Blood pressure begins to rise 5 s before the contraction begins and returns to its baseline after the contraction has ended. During the first stage of labour there may be a rise in blood pressure of 35 mmHg systolic and it may rise even higher in the second stage. The diastolic pressure can rise 25 mmHg in the first stage of labour and up to 55 mmHg in the second stage. There is only a small change in peripheral vascular resistance in labour so the increase is probably due to the transient rise in cardiac output during the contraction.

Following the delivery of the fetus, placenta and membranes, there may be cardiovascular instability because of dramatic haematological changes. The changes occur because of blood loss at delivery and compensatory mechanisms. Within 10 min of the delivery, cardiac parameters fall to prelabour levels and may then take up to 4 weeks to return to prepregnancy levels.

Haematological system

There are changes in the haematological system and haemostasis to ensure that blood loss is kept to a minimum and tolerated. Haemoglobin levels tend to increase slightly in labour because of haemoconcentration. This is related to an increase in erythropoiesis due to stress, muscular activity and dehydration. White blood cell (WBC) count increases during labour and immediately postpartum and may reach levels of 25–$30 \times 10^9/L$. This is mainly due to an increase in neutrophils and is a probable response to stress.

The hypercoagulable state that is present in pregnancy is further magnified in labour. There is a transitory increase in the activity of the coagulation system during and immediately after placental separation so that clot formation in the torn blood vessels is maximised and blood loss from haemorrhage minimised. The placenta and decidua are rich in thromboplastin and release of this factor during separation activates coagulation via the extrinsic system.

There is also a decrease in fibrinolytic activity, enhancing clot formation at the placental site. The placental site is rapidly covered by a fibrin mesh which utilises about 5–10% of the circulating fibrinogen. Levels of fibrin/fibrinogen degradation products (FDPs) rise after delivery, increasing the risk of coagulation disorders in the immediate postpartum period.

Respiratory system

Maternal acidosis

There is an increase in the work of the uterine and other muscles during labour and therefore a greater need for oxygen. Alterations in ventilation and acid–base status occur. If the contractions are occurring too frequently, there will be a decrease in the oxygenation of the myometrium and metabolic acidosis. In the presence of strong, frequent uterine contractions, ischaemia and the resulting tissue hypoxia will occur with an increase in PCO_2 because of the change to anaerobic metabolism leading to a fall in pH (maternal acidosis). The ischaemia will increase the pain experienced during contractions.

In the second stage of labour, maternal PCO_2 may rise during pushing and also due to the use of voluntary muscles during bearing down. Fetal PCO_2 will rise if the mother is acidotic because the build-up of maternal PCO_2 will prevent placental transfer to the mother of fetal PCO_2. This will lead to significant fetal acidosis and distress.

Maternal alkalosis

In some women there is a tendency to hyperventilation, leading to respiratory alkalosis. This appears to be mainly caused by pain. Anxiety, drugs, breath holding, panic and excessive use of breathing exercises learned in the antenatal period will also add to the likelihood of hyperventilation. The end result will be a fall in PCO_2 and a level of 25 mmHg can commonly occur. Blackburn (2003) reports that levels as low as 17 mmHg have been seen in women during painful contractions. The woman may complain of tingling of the fingers and toes and dizziness due to overbreathing. She should be encouraged to change her respiratory rate, to lower it if necessary, to breathe when breath holding is inappropriate and to deep breathe if oxygen is needed, such as between contractions.

Renal system

The renin–angiotensin systems of mother and fetus are altered during labour and delivery. There is an increase in maternal and fetal renin and angiotensin which may be important in reducing uteroplacental blood flow following delivery. The changes in pregnancy outlined in Section 2 of the book affect fluid and electrolyte status so that administration of intravenous fluids and their electrolytic content must be carefully monitored to avoid water intoxication. Also, it is important to remember that oxytocin has an antidiuretic effect so that oxytocin infusion during labour reduces water excretion.

Gastrointestinal system

Gastric emptying

Gastric motility is decreased and gastric emptying is mildly delayed during labour, with or without epidural analgesia. Factors dramatically increasing this delayed gastric emptying include:

- fear and pain;
- the administration of opioid drugs;
- food intake during labour that contains high levels of fibre and fat.

There is also an increase in gastric acidity, thus increasing the risk of aspiration pneumonitis, commonly known as **Mendelson's syndrome**, should a woman require general anaesthesia. Nutrition and hydration in labour and the prevention of acid aspiration are discussed in the section on clinical implications below.

Metabolism

Generally, prior to labour, women have a degree of respiratory alkalosis and metabolic acidosis and a reduced ability to utilise glucose so that the main source of glucose for the fetus is met. Provision of glucose (gluconeogenesis) from the metabolism of body fat (lipolysis) occurs, causing an increase in plasma ketones throughout pregnancy. Labour has an effect on maternal metabolism and plasma electrolytes and these changes may affect the fetus.

The vigorous contractions of the uterus throughout labour require energy, and glucose is the main substrate for this. Most women have little reserve for aerobic metabolism and glucose stores are quickly used up, especially with the modern tendency to restrict oral intake in labour. The energy cost of active labour is estimated to be between 700 and 1100 calories/h. Compensatory lipolysis occurs to meet the body's energy requirements, resulting in the production of ketones which, in excess, may depress fetal pH and interfere with myometrial activity (Liu 2003). Anaerobic metabolism causes the accumulation of lactate (see Krebs cycle) and this produces a small drop in maternal plasma pH to about 7.34, a reduction in base excess to $-5\,\text{mEq/L}$ and a fall in PCO_2.

CLINICAL IMPLICATIONS

Recognition of the onset of labour

Women themselves usually recognise that labour has begun, especially if they have received antenatal education about what to expect. The woman may notice a **show**, although this may occur following a vaginal examination in the antenatal clinic. **Contractions** which are regular, rhythmic and increase in **length**, **strength** and **frequency** occur but the woman may only be aware of backache with hardening of her uterus. When the presenting part of the fetus is not well applied to the cervix, the membranes may rupture and the woman has a sudden gush of fluid. This must be reported to the midwife immediately as there is a small risk of cord prolapse. Sometimes a steady trickle of amniotic fluid may be difficult to distinguish from urine and it is possible to pass a speculum into the vagina and test the fluid with a nitrazine yellow swab (**amnistest swab**) or similar method. The swab changes from orange to dark blue if amniotic fluid is present.

Initial examination of the woman

Although this is a book on physiology, it is important to realise that the social and psychological background and approach to care may interfere with the process of labour. This interaction between the mind and body will be discussed in Chapter 57. For now, it is necessary to remember that the approach taken at this initial meeting of the woman and her midwife may influence not only her perception of labour but also her physical progress towards delivery. While it is desirable to provide a meaningful experience for the woman, it is of paramount importance that the physical safety of mother and fetus are ensured. This is the aspect of care that follows below.

The history

When a woman telephones her midwife, information may be obtained allowing the decision to be made either to visit at home, especially if there is to be a home confinement, or admit to hospital. If there are no complications and the woman is in early labour, it will be beneficial for her to remain in her own surroundings for the time being. The history of the woman's health, any previous pregnancies and this pregnancy up to the onset of labour should be carefully scrutinised for any indications that complications may occur. **True labour** can be recognised by the midwife from what is termed **spurious** or **false** labour by the nature of the contractions and the state of the cervix. In true labour, contractions will show a pattern of increase in length, strength and frequency and the state of the cervix will dilate progressively.

General examination

The general condition of the woman is important and her appearance may indicate aspects of her wellbeing to the midwife. Her general stance and gait may indicate pain or even imminent delivery. The midwife should look for any abnormality in skin colour such as flushing, pallor or cyanosis which may indicate underlying problems. Her behaviour may indicate how well she is coping with contractions and whether she is anxious or afraid. Observations of temperature, pulse rate and blood pressure, signs of oedema and urinalysis should be taken and recorded.

Abnormal findings may indicate a problem with the general health of the woman or be associated with an abnormality of labour. If the temperature and pulse rate are elevated, it is necessary to find the cause. Infection may be present and care must be taken to avoid passing this on to other women and their babies. A rise in blood pressure should be reported to the obstetrician. The presence of slight oedema of the feet and ankles may be normal, depending on the time of day but pretibial oedema or puffiness of the fingers or face, especially if there is a raised blood pressure, may indicate the presence of pregnancy-induced hypertension (PIH). Urine is tested for protein, which may indicate that the woman has had a show or that her membranes have ruptured, both easily confirmed, but may also indicate PIH or urinary tract infection. Glucose and ketones are also tested for and are considered in the light of the woman's past medical history, when she last ate and how her labour is progressing.

Assessing progress in labour

When as much detail as possible about the progress of labour prior to admission has been ascertained, the woman is examined to confirm details given verbally and to establish a baseline on which to judge further progress. An abdominal examination is made and this may be followed by a vaginal examination. Progress can be considered as a function of descent of the presenting part through the pelvis and dilatation of the cervix. The presence of one in the absence of the other suggests lack of progress and is a cause for concern if this persists. These factors will be discussed in the next chapter.

MAIN POINTS

- In humans the timing of the onset of labour is less precise than in many other species and may be related to fetal brain activity via ACTH and the pituitary–adrenal axis. Progesterone is metabolised to oestrogen, which gradually increases the sensitivity of the uterus to prostaglandins and oxytocin produced by both the fetoplacental unit and maternal tissues.

- Prostaglandins may play a central role in the initiation of labour but their composition and biosynthesis by various tissues remains unclear.

- Dehydroepiandrosterone sulphate (DHAS), the major precursor of placental estradiol and estrone synthesis, may be implicated in fetal control of the onset of labour. Higher concentrations of the posterior pituitary hormones vasopressin and oxytocin have been found in the umbilical circulation than in the maternal circulation. The source of this fetal oxytocin is not clear but the levels are higher in fetal arterial blood than venous blood, which suggests a fetal origin.

- One argument against the fetal role is that labour almost always follows fetal death in utero, depending on the gestational age of the fetus. Possibly the release of prostaglandins is more important, being provoked by the massive fall in progesterone level that accompanies fetal death.

- Placental production of oestrogens rises as pregnancy progresses but women go into labour without a rise in the concentration of estradiol and there is no dramatic rise just prior to the onset of labour. There is no clear evidence to suggest that concentrations of oestrogens and progesterone alter at the onset of labour but changes in balance between them facilitate increasing myometrial activity.

- The fetal membranes have a relatively high concentration of progesterone. Both the chorion and amnion contain enzymes that can reduce the level of progesterone and both chorion and amnion contain a protein which increases towards the end of pregnancy and that can bind progesterone. The debate continues as to whether prostaglandins initiate labour or maintain it.

- Uterine contractions are coordinated with cervical dilatation. The increasing pressure placed on the cervix by the presenting part during active labour is said to aid dilatation of the cervix by the mechanism of the Ferguson reflex, which may be involved in the release of both oxytocin and prostaglandin in labour. Prostaglandin release in labour seems not to involve oxytocin release.

- Uterine contractions alone cannot bring about cervical softening and cervical dilatation. Changes in the collagen content of the cervix must occur and evidence is that it is the hormone estradiol that brings about the change. Prostaglandins also play a part in the ripening of the cervix.

- Normal labour is spontaneous in onset at term with the fetus presenting by the vertex and is completed within 18 h with no complications arising. Factors affecting the length of labour include parity, birth interval, psychological state, presentation and position, pelvic shape and size and the type of uterine contractions.

- There are profound changes in the cardiovascular system due to the effect of uterine contractions. The woman's emotional response to labour may affect the cardiovascular system, especially in primigravidae. Pain, anxiety, apprehension and uterine contractions may cause an increase in systolic and diastolic blood pressures and heart rate. Within 10 min of delivery, cardiac parameters fall to prelabour levels and may take up to 4 weeks to return to prepregnancy levels.

- Observations of temperature, pulse rate, blood pressure, signs of oedema and urinalysis should be taken and recorded for baseline levels. Abnormal findings may indicate a problem with the general health of the woman or be associated with an abnormality of labour.

References

Blackburn S T 2003 Maternal, Fetal and Neonatal Physiology: A Clinical Perspective, 2nd edn. W B Saunders, Philadelphia.

Cassidy P 1999 The first stage of labour: physiology and early care. In Bennett V R, Brown L K (eds) Myles Textbook for Midwives, 13th edn. Churchill Livingstone, Edinburgh.

Gibb D 1988 A Practical Guide to Labour Management. Blackwell Science, Oxford.

Gustavii B 1977 Human decidual and uterine contractility. In Chamberlain G, Broughton Pipkin F (eds) Clinical Physiology in Obstetrics, 3rd edn. Blackwell Science, Oxford.

Johnson M H, Everitt B J 2000 Essential Reproduction, 2nd edn. Blackwell Science, Oxford.

Karim S M M 1966 Identification of prostaglandins in human amniotic fluid. Journal of Obstetrics and Gynaecology of the British Commonwealth 73:903.

Liu D T Y 2003 Labour Ward Manual, 3rd edn. Churchill Livingstone, Edinburgh.

McNabb M 1997 Hormone interactions in labour. In Sweet B R, Tiran D (eds) Mayes Midwifery: A Textbook for Midwives, 12th edn. Baillière Tindall, London. Reprinted 2002.

Steer P J, Johnson M R 1998 The genital system. In Chamberlain G, Broughton Pipkin F (eds) Clinical Physiology in Obstetrics, 3rd edn. Blackwell Science, Oxford.

Annotated recommended reading

Blackburn S T 2003 Maternal, Fetal and Neonatal Physiology: A Clinical Perspective, 2nd edn. W B Saunders, Philadelphia.
This book covers physiological changes that occur throughout the perinatal period, with the emphasis on the mother, fetus and the neonate and the relationship between them. It provides an in-depth study of the major body systems.

Cassidy P 1999 The first stage of labour: physiology and early care. In Bennett V R, Brown L K (eds) Myles Textbook for Midwives, 13th edn. Churchill Livingstone, Edinburgh.
This chapter provides a detailed description of the first stage of labour, an essential reference for any student of midwifery or obstetrics.

Chapter 37

The first stage of labour

CHAPTER CONTENTS

INTRODUCTION

It is essential to understand the physiology of any system or process so that observations and care are based on understanding. One problem of caring for women in labour is to define the acceptable parameters for progress and maternal and fetal responses so that women view the experience as being satisfactory while safety is assured. In the past these parameters were arbitrarily decided by empirical methods but, more recently, research is being increasingly utilised. Practitioners have a duty to women to ensure that they read widely, develop a discerning mind and base their practice on the best of this research.

PHYSIOLOGY OF THE FIRST STAGE OF LABOUR

Uterine activity in labour

In early labour, contractions may be 15–20 min apart and are fairly weak, lasting for about 30 s. These may not be recognised as labour pains by the mother for a while. In established labour, the uterus contracts 3–4 times every 10 min, and in advanced labour each contraction may last 50–60 s and is powerful. Contractions can be measured in mmHg (millimetres of mercury) by the pressure they exert on the amniotic fluid. This is called the **intrauterine hydrostatic pressure**. The resting pressure exerted by the muscular myometrium is about 5 mmHg. In pregnancy, the intensity of uterine contractions may reach 30 mmHg and up to 60–80 mmHg in labour.

Several concepts are described in relation to uterine activity in labour. The spread of each contraction across the uterine muscle is thought to begin in the fundus near the cornua, spreading outwards and downwards, remaining most intense in the fundus and being weakest in the lower uterine segment (LUS), a phenomenon known as **fundal dominance**. The spread of myometrial electrical activity to its maximum takes about 1 min and the same time is taken for the wave of contraction to pass off. This allows progressive dilatation of the cervix and, as the upper segment thickens and shortens, the fetus is propelled down the birth canal. During contractions, the upper and lower poles of the uterus act in harmony, with contraction and retraction of the upper **pole**, and dilatation of the lower pole to allow expulsion of the fetus. This is known as **polarity**.

Uterine muscle in labour has the unique property of **contraction** and **retraction** (Fig. 37.1). Following each contraction, the muscle fibres do not completely relax but retain some of the shortening of contraction. This is called **retraction** and leads to the progressive shortening and thickening of the upper uterine segment (UUS) and the diminishing of the uterine cavity. A ridge forms between the UUS and LUS, known as a **retraction ring**. The name **Bandl's ring** is usually applied only to the exaggerated pathological retraction

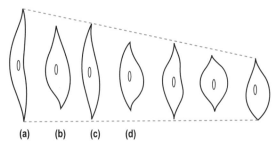

Figure 37.1 Retraction of the uterine muscle fibres. (a) Relaxed. (b) Contracted. (c) Relaxed but retracted. (d) Contracted but shorter and thicker than those in (b) (from Sweet B 1997, with permission).

ring that develops in obstructed labour and becomes visible above the symphysis pubis.

Effacement or 'taking up' of the cervix is the term used to describe the gradual mergence of the cervix into the LUS. In primigravidae, this process is sometimes complete before the onset of labour and before dilatation of the external cervical os occurs (Fig. 37.2a). In multigravidae, a perceptible cervical canal remains until labour is well established, a finding midwives refer to as a 'multip's os'. During labour there is **dilatation** of the external os (Fig. 37.2) until it is large enough for the widest diameter of the presenting part to pass through. In a fetus at term presenting by the vertex, the diameter of the cervix would normally have to reach 10 cm but this would be less in a preterm infant with a smaller head. As the cervix begins to dilate, the operculum or mucus plug formed in pregnancy is lost around the time of the commencement of labour and the woman will notice a mucoid discharge, which may be bloodstained. This is termed the **show**. The blood originates from ruptured capillaries when the lining of the cervix is stretched or where the chorion has become detached from the dilating cervix.

Mechanical factors

Besides uterine action, there are mechanical forces that aid dilatation of the cervix. As the lower uterine segment is stretched, the chorion is detached from it. In normal labour

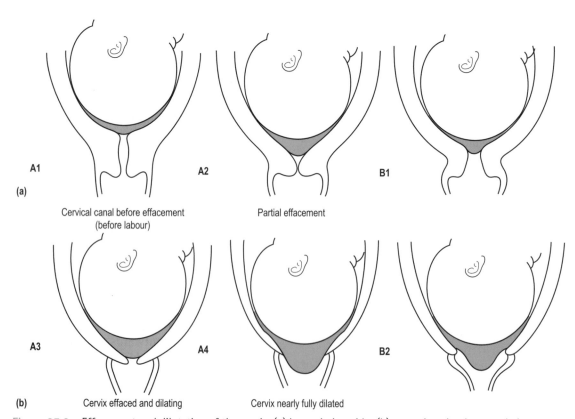

(a)   Cervical canal before effacement (before labour)   Partial effacement

(b)   Cervix effaced and dilating   Cervix nearly fully dilated

Figure 37.2 Effacement and dilatation of the cervix. (a) In a primigravida; (b) occurring simultaneously in a multigravida (from Sweet B 1997, with permission).

the increased intrauterine pressure during contractions forces a well-flexed head snugly against the cervix, trapping a small amount of amniotic fluid in front of the head separate from the rest of the fluid surrounding the body of the fetus. This small sac of fluid is known as the **forewaters** and the rest of the fluid as the **hindwaters**. The forewaters bulge through the cervix, becoming more tense during contractions (Fig. 37.2). This separation of the forewaters from the larger volume of the hindwaters keeps the membranes intact during the first stage of labour, providing a barrier against ascending infection.

When the membranes remain intact the pressure of each contraction is exerted on the fluid and, as fluid is not compressible, pressure is equalised throughout the uterus. This is known as **general fluid pressure**. If the membranes are ruptured and amniotic fluid is reduced, contraction pressure is applied directly to the fetus. The placenta is compressed between the uterine wall and the fetus, which further reduces the oxygen supply to the fetus. Therefore, there are two good reasons for maintaining intact membranes: to reduce the risk of infection and to maintain a good oxygen supply to the fetus. The physiological moment for the membranes to rupture is when the cervix is fully dilated and no longer able to support the forewaters and the force of the uterine contractions reaches maximum. The evidence remains clear that *routine amniotomy during the first stage of labour can never be justified* (Enkin et al 2000, World Health Organisation 2002).

During each contraction, the force of the fundal contraction is transmitted to the upper pole of the fetus, down the long axis of the fetal spine, causing increasing flexion of the head. This ensures that the smallest possible circumference, which is the circular vertex, is applied to the circular cervical os. This is known as **fetal axis pressure**. It becomes much more significant after the membranes have ruptured and during the second stage of labour.

Phases of the first stage of labour

The present understanding of labour is based on the work of Emanuel A Friedman. He developed the graphic representation of labour by plotting cervical dilatation and descent of the presenting part against time (Arias 1993). In normal labour, the rate of dilatation of the cervix follows a sigmoid-shaped curve. There are three distinct parts:

1. an initial part where there is little progress in cervical dilatation, which Friedman called the **latent phase**;
2. a part of the curve where there is rapid progress in dilatation, called the **active phase**;
3. a part of the curve where dilatation slows, called the **deceleration phase**.

The latent phase, which lasts until cervical dilatation is about 3–4 cm, can take 6–8 h in a primigravida. The active phase occurs with rapid dilatation of the cervix at about 1 cm/h in a primigravida and 1.5 cm/h in a multigravida. Plotting the rate of cervical dilatation has been commonly carried out in labour (a **cervicograph**) and an average duration is indicated in Figure 37.3.

Individualised care

Childbearing experience for women encompasses both a biological and a social event. The midwife should carefully consider these aspects when planning care with the labouring woman. This should include the following:

- assess the woman's needs and expectations;
- plan care accordingly to meet the specific needs and expectations;
- carry out the plan;
- evaluate the effect of the care and modify it if necessary.

The physiological aspects of care in labour include assessing progress, positioning of the woman, nutrition and hydration and monitoring the condition of mother and fetus.

ASSESSING PROGRESS IN THE FIRST STAGE OF LABOUR

When as much detail as possible has been ascertained about the progress of labour prior to admission, the woman is examined to confirm details given verbally and to establish a baseline on which to judge further progress. An abdominal examination is made and this may be followed by a vaginal examination. Progress can be considered as a function of descent of the presenting part through the pelvis and dilatation of the cervix. The presence of one in the absence of the other may suggest lack of progress and is a cause for concern.

Abdominal examination in labour

Most of the aims of abdominal examination, considered by Das (1999) in the context of antenatal care, apply equally

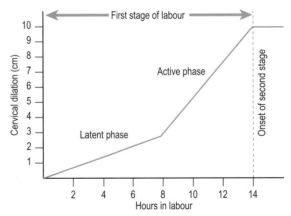

Figure 37.3   A cervicograph (from Sweet B 1997, with permission).

well to labour. These are to assess fetal size and wellbeing, to diagnose the location of fetal parts – in particular, lie, presentation, position and engagement – and to detect any deviation from normal. Abdominal examination should always be carried out prior to performing a vaginal examination and repeated abdominal examinations can be used to assess descent of the presenting part.

Inspection

The size and shape of the uterus can be of value in ensuring that there is a normal longitudinal lie. In the rare instance of a transverse lie, the uterus may appear to be low and broad. If there is a saucer-shaped depression below the umbilicus, the fetus may be lying in an occipitoposterior position. Fetal movements may be seen and can help in the diagnosis of position.

Palpation

The following terms are used to describe fetal palpation:

- **Lie** – the relationship of the long axis of the fetus and the long axis of the uterus. It may be longitudinal, oblique or transverse.

- **Presentation** – that part of the fetus which lies at the pelvic brim or in the lower pole of the uterus. This is usually cephalic but other possible presentations include breech, face, brow and shoulder.

- **Attitude** – the relationship of the fetal head and limbs to its body; it may be fully flexed, deflexed or partially or completely extended.

- **Denominator** – identifies the name of the part of the presentation used when referring to fetal position. Each presentation has a different denominator: occiput for cephalic presentation; sacrum for breech presentation; and mentum for face presentation.

- **Position** – the relationship of the denominator to six points on the maternal pelvic brim. These points are right and left anterior, right and left lateral and right and left posterior.

- **Engagement of the fetal head** – this occurs when the widest presenting transverse diameter has passed through the brim of the pelvis, i.e. biparietal diameter of 9.5 cm in cephalic presentation.

Practitioners often get the terms 'presentation' and 'presenting part' confused. The presenting part refers to that part of the fetus which lies over the cervical os during labour and on which the caput succudaneum may form.

Fundal palpation (Fig. 37.4), (taking into account the overall size of the uterus), allows a judgement of the gestational age to be made (Fig. 37.5). It is also a necessary part of

determining the lie of the fetus (Fig. 37.6). **Lateral palpation** is used to locate the fetal back to determine position. The length and frequency of contractions should be noted by palpation rather than by the reaction of the woman. The hardness of the abdomen may give a good indication of the strength of the contractions.

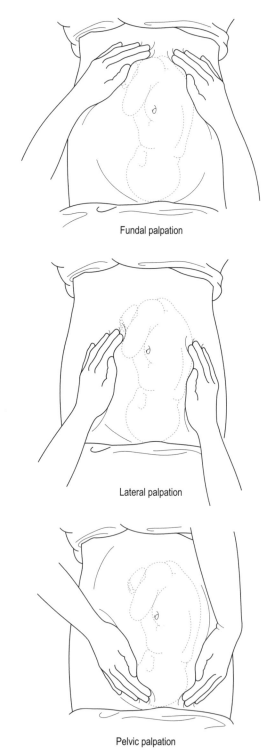

Fundal palpation

Lateral palpation

Pelvic palpation

Figure 37.4 Types of palpation per abdomen (from Sweet B 1997, with permission).

Pelvic palpation using both hands can identify the presenting part (Fig. 37.7) and the amount of flexion (Fig. 37.8) and engagement of the head can be assessed by estimating the amount of head still present above the pelvic brim.

If the head is engaged, it will be possible to feel less than half the fetal head above the pelvic brim and the head will not be mobile. It may not be possible to palpate the occiput if the head is deeply engaged (Fig. 37.9). Engagement is a good sign and indicates that the bony pelvis is adequate for the passage of the fetus and a vaginal delivery should follow. Stuart (2003) summarises descent of the head by abdominal assessment, which can be described in fifths of the head felt above the pelvic brim. Determination of the level of the fetal head by abdominal palpation excludes the variability due to caput and moulding and that produced by a different depth of pelvis.

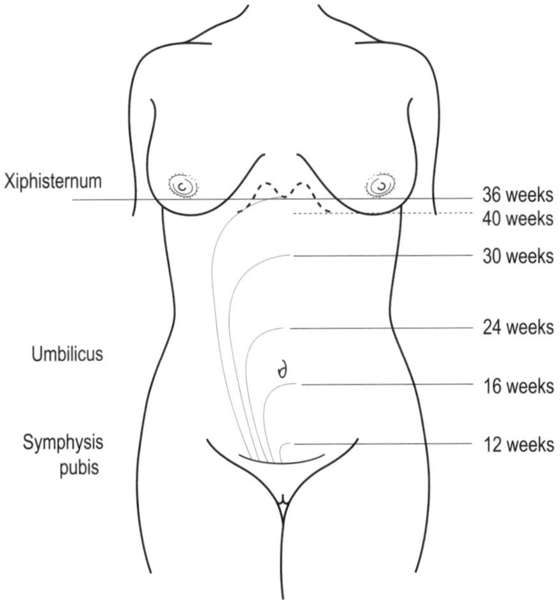

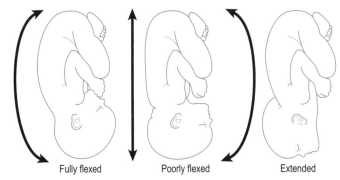

Figure 37.8   The attitude of the fetus (from Sweet B 1997, with permission).

Fully flexed   Poorly flexed   Extended

Xiphisternum

36 weeks
40 weeks

30 weeks

24 weeks

Umbilicus

16 weeks

Symphysis pubis

12 weeks

Figure 37.5   The height of the fundus at different stages of pregnancy (from Sweet B 1997, with permission).

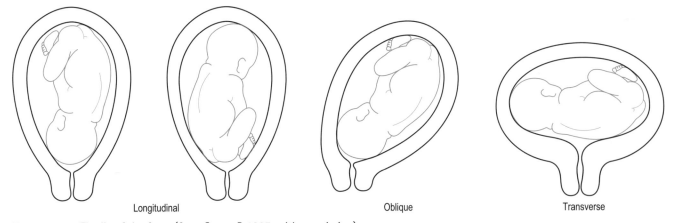

Longitudinal   Oblique   Transverse

Figure 37.6   The lie of the fetus (from Sweet B 1997, with permission).

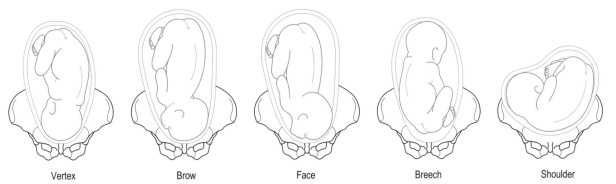

Vertex   Brow   Face   Breech   Shoulder

Figure 37.7   The presentation of the fetus (from Sweet B 1997, with permission).

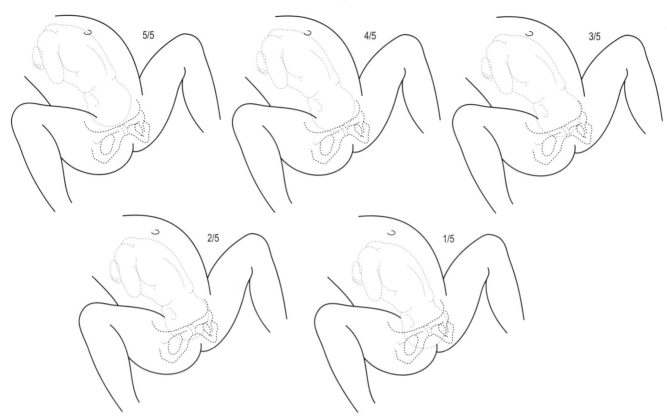

Figure 37.9 Examination per abdomen to determine the descent of the fetal head in fifths (from Sweet B 1997, with permission).

Auscultation

Listening to the fetal heart is an important part of any abdominal examination as it enables the practitioner to make an assessment of fetal wellbeing. The point of maximum intensity is located by considering the position of the fetus (Fig. 37.10). As labour progresses and descent takes place, the point of maximum intensity will change. The Pinard's stethoscope usually needs to be moved around the abdomen to ensure the best possible clarity of the fetal heartbeat and its regularity, strength and frequency can be assessed. Continuous monitoring of the fetal heart may be necessary where there is doubt about fetal wellbeing.

Vaginal examination in labour (VE)

Cassidy (1999) gives the following indications for vaginal examination in labour:

- to make a positive diagnosis of labour;
- to make a positive identification of presentation;
- to determine whether the head is engaged if there is doubt;
- to ascertain whether the forewaters have ruptured or to rupture them artificially;
- to exclude cord prolapse if the forewaters rupture and the presenting part is high;
- to assess progress or delay in labour;
- to apply a fetal scalp electrode;
- to confirm full dilatation of the cervix;

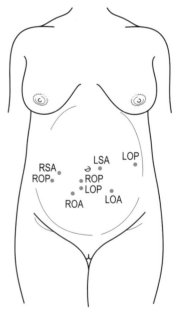

Figure 37.10 The approximate points of the fetal heart sounds in vertex and breech presentations. ROA, right occipitoanterior; ROP, right occipitoposterior; LOA, left occipitoanterior; LOP, left occipitoposterior; RSA, right sacroanterior; RSP, right sacroposterior; LSA, left sacroanterior; LSP, left sacroposterior.

- in multiple pregnancy, after the birth of the first baby, to confirm the lie and presentation of the second fetus and to rupture the second amniotic sac.

There is a way in which such a list, while comprehensive, does not do justice to the value of a well-performed and carefully timed vaginal examination. Firstly, it is the combination of abdominal and vaginal findings that enables a clear picture of the progress in labour to be made and, secondly, continuous careful observation of the mother will enable the avoidance of unnecessary vaginal examinations.

In any clinical examination, it is sensible to use the same order of findings each time. This ensures that there is less chance of missing an important feature. It is also important to continue with the examination until satisfied in all aspects, as it is essential to keep the number of vaginal examinations to a minimum to minimise the risk of infection and distress to the woman. Full aseptic technique should be used at all times to safeguard the lives of women in labour. The book *The Cry and the Covenant* (Thompson 1949) should be essential reading for anyone caring for women in labour.

The concept of a 'quick VE' is dangerous for more than one reason. Adequate care to prevent infection is unlikely to be present and important features of the examination are likely to be missed.

Findings

The following order is suggested for the performance and recording of a vaginal examination.

External genitalia Prior to inserting fingers into the vagina, the external genitalia should be inspected as some findings may influence the course and management of labour. The labia should be examined for any varicosities or warts and the presence of oedema noted. The perineum should be inspected for scarring which could indicate a previous tear or episiotomy and, in some cultures, female circumcision. Signs of vaginal discharge or bleeding and, if the membranes have ruptured, the colour and quantity of any amniotic fluid should be recorded. Any offensive odour should be reported as this is likely to indicate the presence of infection.

Condition of the vagina The normal vagina in labour should feel warm and moist. It is very rare but not impossible that the implications of a prolonged labour with obstruction would be seen. Women who have been cared for in pregnancy and have sought care early in their labour should never present with a hot and dry vagina but occasionally someone may have tried to conceal their pregnancy and labour and only ask for help when unable to deliver themselves. A cystocele and/or rectocele may be present in a multiparous woman. A loaded rectum can be easily felt through the posterior vaginal wall.

State of the cervix The cervix is palpated for length, consistency and dilatation to diagnose the length of the cervical canal and the degree of effacement. The position of the cervix relative to the fetal presenting part is noted – is it in the normal central position or, as is occasionally found in early labour, very posterior? A long closed cervix may indicate

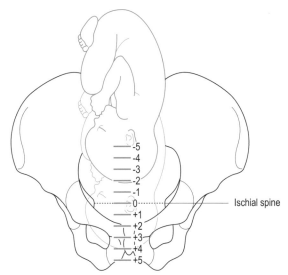

Figure 37.11   The stations of the head. Descent in relation to the maternal ischial spines is expressed in centimetres (from Sweet B 1997, with permission).

early stages of labour or that labour has not begun. The cervix in labour should feel soft and elastic and will usually be applied closely to the presenting part.

Assessing the dilatation of the cervical os The two examining fingers are gently inserted into the vagina and the cervical os is located. The fingers are then inserted into the os and parted gently to assess the diameter of cervical os dilatation in centimetres. This should be done gently to minimise discomfort to the mother. The cervix should be palpated in every direction, by a circular movement of the examining fingers to ensure a complete circle or that no lip of cervix remains; in particular, when assessing full cervical dilatation. Intact membranes can be felt through the dilating os. They feel a little like clingfilm and become tense during a contraction. If the membranes are absent, the slightly rougher fetal scalp can be felt.

Level or station of the presenting part The level of the presenting part is judged in relation to the ischial spines so that descent of the fetus through the pelvis can be monitored. The distance above or below the ischial spines is estimated in centimetres above or below the ischial spines (Fig. 37.11). If there is a caput succedaneum, care must be taken to establish the level of the bony skull above the swelling.

The presentation In 96% of cases this will be vertex and easily confirmed. Only rarely will it be difficult to confirm presentation on VE and this usually indicates a very abnormal labour or even more rarely a fetal abnormality such as an encephalocele which may have slipped through the vaginal os and feel too soft to be a head.

Position Landmarks such as sutures and fontanelles on the fetal skull can be felt to diagnose or confirm the position of the presenting part (Fig. 37.12). The most commonly identified landmark is the sagittal suture as it is found in a

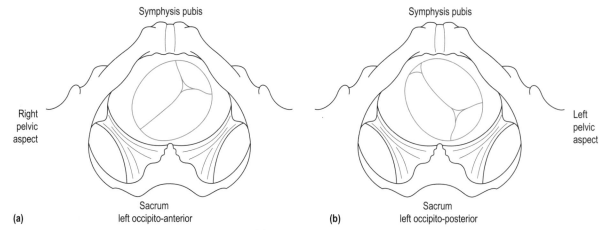

(a) Sacrum
left occipito-anterior

(b) Sacrum
left occipito-posterior

Figure 37.12   Identifying the position of the fetus. (a) Left occipitoanterior: the sagittal suture is in the right oblique diameter of the pelvis. (b) Left occipitoposterior: the sagittal suture is in the left oblique diameter of the pelvis (from Sweet B 1997, with permission).

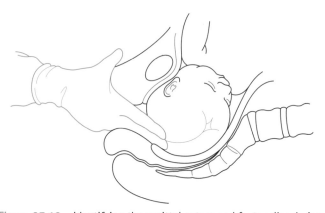

Figure 37.13   Identifying the sagittal suture and fontanelles during examination per vaginam (from Sweet B 1997, with permission).

vertex presentation (Fig. 37.13). It is identifiable by moulding that occurs with the leading anterior parietal bone over-riding the posterior parietal bone and is usually in one or other of the oblique diameters. The posterior fontanelle can be identified because of its small size and the three sutures that leave it. The anterior fontanelle is larger, diamond shaped and has four sutures leaving it.

Moulding of the fetal skull   Moulding is described in Chapter 24, p. 330. The most important aspect is to make a judgement on whether the amount of moulding is normal or excessive, suggesting disproportion between the fetal skull and the bony pelvis.

Pelvic capacity   An estimation of pelvic size has probably been made antenatally but the practitioner responsible for the safe conduct of the delivery should make her own estimation of the pelvic outlet by assessing the ischial spines and the angle of the subpubic arch. Prominent ischial spines often accompany a pubic arch that is less than 90° and the features suggest an android pelvis.

Fetal heart rate   An assessment of the fetal heart should always be made after the vaginal examination is completed,

especially if the membranes are ruptured, to ensure that the examination has had no adverse effect on the fetus. This aspect was brought home to the author while assisting the obstetric registrar in doing a 'controlled rupture of membranes' in a woman with a 'high head'. A large amount of liquor drained; this was immediately followed by severe fetal bradycardia, the fetal heart rate being recorded by continuous external monitoring. Bradycardia was resolved by encouraging the woman to turn to a left lateral position. The sudden reduction in intrauterine volume may have caused sudden compression of the umbilical cord, which in turn resulted in bradycardia. In some cases the fetal heart may become erratic or tachycardic before settling down to the original baseline and pattern. This is the fetus's response to having its head palpated.

MATERNAL POSITION IN THE FIRST STAGE OF LABOUR

Mobility and positions for labour and delivery have been an area of interest for a number of years. Where appropriate, most labouring women are encouraged to move about in labour and adopt the position they find to be most comfortable while still maintaining safety (Hughes 2003). Women remaining mobile in labour (Fig. 37.14) have shown this to be a core attribute of physiological labour (Gould 2000). As well as adding to the discussion on placental perfusion, it is proposed that there is better alignment between the descending presenting part and the pelvic brim so that engagement of the presenting part is facilitated and, in occipitoposterior presentation, rotation of the occiput to the anterior may be helped.

Labour normally begins with the fetal head in **asynclitism**. This means that the head is tilted so that one of the parietal bones enters the pelvis first. This tilting facilitates passage of the fetal head through the pelvic inlet. Once through the inlet, the head shifts to **synclitism** so that the vertex presents as the head descends further through the

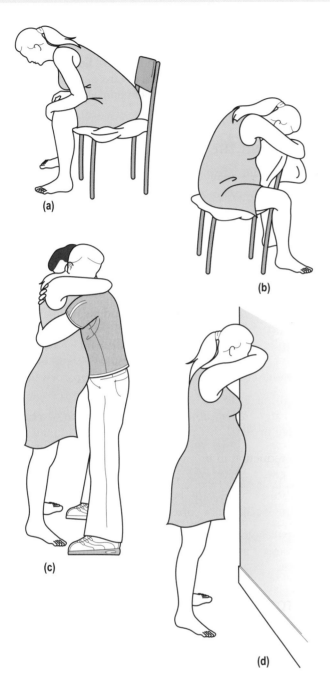

Women who remain ambulant and adopt an upright posture during labour report a greater level of maternal satisfaction, perceive less pain and backache and often request delivery in an upright position for a subsequent labour (Enkin et al 2000, Walsh 2000).

IMMERSION IN WATER

Immersion of the body in warm water has been in use for decades and is acceptable to many women. Although its main use is for relaxation and pain relief it may also shorten the labour and decrease the need for augmentation. The warmth of the water relaxes the muscles and enhances a state of mental relaxation, with women reporting a greater sense of satisfaction (Nikodem 2002) and a greater sense of control over their labour (Hall & Holloway 1998). There may be a decrease in the release of the stress hormones such as catecholamines, resulting in better uterine perfusion and more efficient contractions (Schorn et al 1993). The woman feels weightless, can support her body in whatever position she prefers and is helped to cope with the discomfort of contractions. However, there may be problems such as unrealistic expectations, restricted choice of analgesia, restriction of mobility, increase in perineal trauma, postpartum haemorrhage, infection to both the mother and the baby and severe blood loss of the neonate due to rupture of the umbilical cord (de Graaf et al 1999). Emergency interventions may be delayed if there is difficulty in emptying the water bath quickly or getting the mother out of the water. Overall, the reports on the safety aspects for mother and baby have been reassuring (Gilbert & Tookey 1999, Otigbah et al 2000).

NUTRITION AND HYDRATION IN LABOUR

Nutrition

The nutritional needs of labouring women are poorly understood. The process of labour uses energy and the body stores fat in pregnancy to use as fuel in longer labours (Odent 1998). If insufficient carbohydrate is available, then body fat will be utilised with the release of ketones and the development of ketoacidosis. Prior to admission, women can be advised to take carbohydrate foods such as toast, cereal and plain biscuits. The main problem with food intake in normal labour is the possible need for the administration of a general anaesthetic. Coupled with the delayed emptying of the stomach and the relative inefficiency of the cardiac sphincter brought about by the influence of progesterone is a risk of inhalation of acid gastric reflux, resulting in **inhalational pneumonitis** (Mendelson's syndrome).

Practices for eating and drinking in labour vary considerably across the world and within the UK (McCormick & Champion 2002). Fasting in labour has been a feature of management since the relationship between anaesthesia and Mendelson's syndrome was established more than 40 years

Figure 37.14 Resting positions in labour. (a) In chair. (b) Astride chair. (c) Supported by partner. (d) Leaning. (Illustrations courtesy of Jim Morrin 1993.)

pelvis. Encouraging women with firm abdominal muscles to adopt forward leaning positions can promote the fetal head to adopt more favourable positions (Simpkin & Ancheta 1999). The forces of gravity may also lead to better application of the presenting part to the cervix, promoting the Ferguson reflex. The strength and length of uterine contractions are increased, leading to a more rapid dilatation of the cervix, and the supine position should be avoided as it can compromise uterine blood flow (Enkin et al 2000).

ago. In a review of the literature, Sleutal & Golden (1999) noted that anaesthetic research has focused primarily on gastric emptying and that withholding of food does not necessarily ensure an empty stomach or reduce the acidity of stomach contents. They concluded that while death due to aspiration pneumonitis is rare, there was little difference on labour and birth outcomes between women who fasted or did not fast in labour and there was no evidence that fasting improved the outcome for mother and baby. Enkin et al (2000) suggest that there is no need to prevent women from eating and drinking sensible amounts in labour unless there is a reason why an epidural analgesia cannot be administered.

Policies for eating and drinking in labour may vary between maternity units. Some units continue to have restrictions on eating and drinking in labour, whereas women in other units may be allowed a low-residue, low-fat diet. On the subject of oral nutrition in labour, women who are considered high risk should have clear fluids only. Women considered low risk in the first stage of normal labour can eat and drink from a restricted range of food with characteristics such as low fat, high carbohydrate/high energy, low fibre and near isomolar (Micklewright & Champion 2002). Suggested food and drink includes toast with low-fat spread, jam or honey; cereals with skimmed milk; clear soup; tea with skimmed milk; squash drinks (dilute); and water.

A sensible protocol would be:

- where there is no risk of general anaesthetic or instrumental delivery, women should be allowed to eat a light diet and drink as required;
- when narcotic analgesia has been given, oral food should be withheld and sips of water given.

Hydration

In the early 1990s, work was undertaken to examine four of the situations which may lead to the administration of intravenous fluids in labour (Millns 1991). It was advocated that any administration of fluid in labour should be given intravenously. The following four situations remain relevant for current practice:

1. during the administration of epidural analgesia;
2. for the administration of oxytocic drugs;
3. to correct ketonuria which has occurred because of metabolism of fat stores;
4. to correct dehydration.

Nordstrom et al (1995) examined the effects of maternal glucose administration in labour by comparing continuous infusion of 5% dextrose with 0.9% saline solution. They found a significant rise in maternal and neonatal plasma glucose levels and maternal insulin levels during the administration of 5% dextrose but did not find evidence of fetal hyperinsulinism in healthy term fetuses. No differences were found in either maternal or fetal lactate levels and both regimes seemed to present no risk of increased fetal lactate levels or fetal hypoglycaemia. However, Stratton et al (1995) carried out similar research in women who required the administration of oxytocin. They found significantly lowered serum sodium levels in both mothers and babies where the oxytocin had been infused in 5% dextrose, suggesting that non-electrolyte solutions administered in labour may lead to hyponatraemia.

MONITORING THE MATERNAL CONDITION

Local protocols may vary but observations for maternal monitoring should include the following:

- Maternal temperature should be recorded 4 hourly and the pulse hourly unless there is an indication for more frequent recording.
- In the early part of labour, blood pressure can be taken every 2 h and then hourly as labour progresses.
- Fluid intake should be encouraged and the woman should be encouraged to pass urine regularly to ensure the bladder is empty. Where a woman is compromised – for example, in the case of pre-eclampsia/eclampsia – input and output should be accurately measured and recorded hourly.
- The urine is tested for protein, glucose and ketones. Small amounts of protein in the absence of known hypertensive or renal disease may indicate contamination by show or amniotic fluid. A small amount of ketosis is expected in normal labour and can be considered part of the physiological adaptation. Large amounts of ketones indicate exhaustion of the energy stores and may lead to uterine inertia if not corrected.
- The psychological response to labour and to pain should be assessed as any stress may interfere with the course of labour.

MONITORING THE FETAL CONDITION

The fetus in the first stage of labour

Blood vessels in the myometrium, which supply the fetus with oxygen and nutrients, are compressed during each uterine contraction. Delivery of nutrients and oxygen are impeded when the strength of a contraction exceeds 40 mmHg. Therefore, increased myometrial tone or rapidly occurring contractions may cause fetal hypoxia and distress. When the membranes remain intact, the pressure of each contraction is exerted on the fluid and, as fluid is not compressible, pressure is equalised throughout the uterus; this is known as **general fluid pressure**.

If the membranes are ruptured and the amniotic fluid is reduced, the pressure of contractions is applied directly to the fetus and the placenta is compressed between the uterine wall and the fetus, further reducing the oxygen supply to the fetus. Although there is a theoretical improvement in oxygenation by the avoidance of aortocaval compression, no research supports a clinical advantage to the fetus from any position taken in labour. The fetus is subjected to compression and hypoxic stress during uterine contractions and, if healthy, tolerates these conditions without a change in heart rate.

Distress in the fetus is indicated by alterations in heart rate, development of acidosis, passage of meconium, presence of excessive moulding and excessive movements. Information about fetal wellbeing is mainly obtained by recording fetal heart rate and rhythm, either intermittently or continuously. Amniotic fluid is inspected for the presence of meconium and, where the fetal heart rate is abnormal, a fetal blood sample is taken to check the pH of the fetal blood. A pH below 7.2 indicates fetal distress.

Heart rate

Intermittent monitoring

Intermittent monitoring of the fetal heart can be undertaken using Pinard's fetal stethoscope or a Doppler ultrasound apparatus such as Sonicaid. The **rate** is best counted over a full minute to allow for variations and should be between 110 and 150 beats per min (bpm). If a Doppler apparatus is used, the heart rate can be monitored throughout a contraction and the rate should usually be within normal limits. If there is bradycardia, hypoxia may be a problem. The **rhythm** of the fetal heart, as for any heart, is coupled and should remain steady. Any irregularity needs prompt action to establish the cause.

Continuous fetal heart recording

Continuous recording of the fetal heart (**cardiography**) is usually combined with continuous monitoring of maternal uterine activity (**tocography**) by using a **cardiotocograph apparatus (CTG)**. This allows a graphic response of the fetal heart to uterine activity to be recorded (Fig. 37.15). A baseline CTG is done for about 20 min, followed by intermittent auscultation. If the fetus is thought to be compromised, continuous monitoring is performed. It is important that an explanation is given to the mother if there is a need for continuous fetal heart monitoring. The woman should discuss antenatally what her feelings are concerning an urgent need to monitor the fetus arising in the course of her labour. Guidelines such as those from the National Institute for Clinical Excellence (NICE 2001) should be used as a basis for fetal heart monitoring.

External cardiotocography involves strapping on an ultrasound transducer to the abdominal wall over the point of maximum intensity of the fetal heart and the contraction transducer to the fundus of the uterus. The reading can be affected by maternal or fetal movement, the thickness of the abdominal wall and uterine contractions but is non-invasive. Internal cardiography (electrocardiogram) can be used by the application of a fetal scalp electrode to the fetal scalp. Membranes must be ruptured and the cervix should be at least 2–3 cm dilated. Wiring attaches the electrode to the CTG.

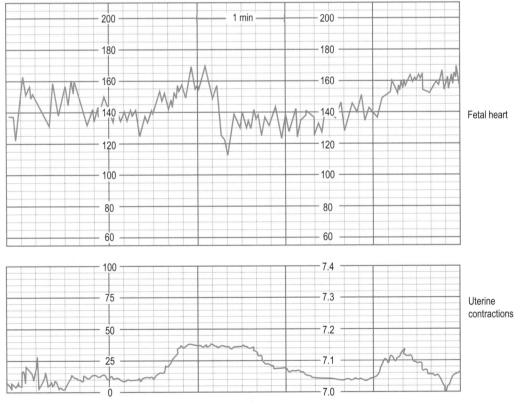

Figure 37.15   Normal cardiotocograph: the fetal heart rate is normal and reactive. (Courtesy of J. A. Jordan, Birmingham Maternity Hospital.)

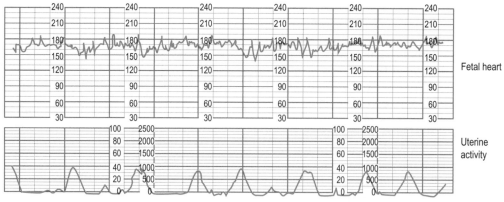

Figure 37.16   Uncomplicated baseline tachycardia. (Courtesy of Sonicaid, Abingdon, Oxon.)

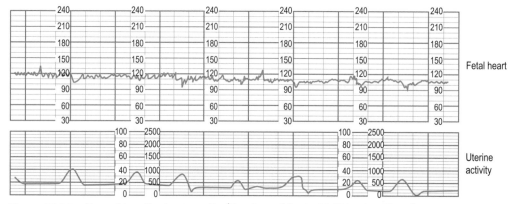

Figure 37.17   Normal baseline bradycardia. (Courtesy of Sonicaid, Abingdon, Oxon.)

Telemetry

If available, internal cardiography can be recorded by a portable battery-operated transmitter used to pick up the signal from the fetal heart and the mother can be ambulant (telemetry). However, no recording of uterine activity can be made and the woman is requested to press a button at the onset of each contraction, which will mark the strip chart accordingly.

Findings

The cardiotocograph provides information about:

- baseline fetal heart rate (FHR);
- baseline variability;
- fetal heart response to uterine contractions, i.e. accelerations or decelerations.

Each of the above measurements is now discussed and graphs are used to demonstrate the points and to begin to develop the skills of reading and interpreting recordings.

Baseline fetal heart rate

The definition of the normal range of FHR is 120–160 bpm but in practice this is often accepted as being 110–160 bpm

(RCOG 2001). The baseline FHR is the mean level of the FHR between contractions. If the heart rate is more than 160 bpm, it is termed **baseline tachycardia** (Fig. 37.16), while a baseline of less than 110 bpm is called **baseline bradycardia** (Fig. 37.17). These two features, with no other alteration, may indicate hypoxia, but tachycardia may be a response to maternal ketosis, infection or pyrexia. Some fetuses have a normal baseline of between 110 and 120 bpm. Continuous compression of the cord will cause a prolonged severe bradycardia.

Baseline variability

It is a normal function of hearts to have minute variations in the length of each beat. This is caused by electrical activity varying as a response to the environment and will produce a jagged rather than a smooth line on the graph called **baseline variability** (Fig. 37.18). The baseline rate should vary by at least 5 beats over a period of 1 min. Loss of this (Fig. 37.19) may indicate fetal hypoxia but has also been noted for a short period following the administration of pethidine to the woman, which depresses the cardiac centre in the fetal brain. Gibb (1988) found that periods of 'fetal sleep' will cause a loss of baseline variability lasting for about 20–30 min; sometimes this period can be longer than 30 min. Where there is very poor baseline variability in the absence of

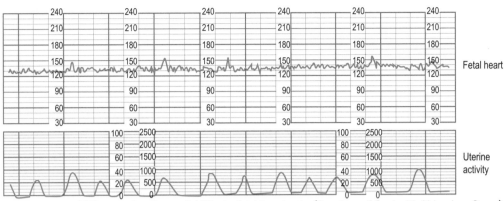

Figure 37.18   ECG trace showing variability in fetal heart rate. (Courtesy of Sonicaid, Abingdon, Oxon.)

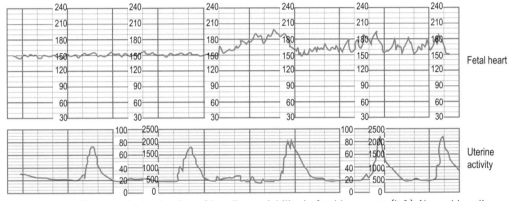

Figure 37.19   Physiological reduction of baseline variability in fetal heart rate (left). Normal baseline variability (right). (Courtesy of Sonicaid, Abingdon, Oxon.)

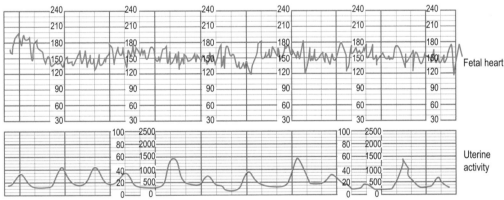

Figure 37.20   Fetal heart rate accelerations. (Courtesy of Sonicaid, Abingdon, Oxon.)

accelerations, the obstetrician will perform a fetal blood sampling procedure to ascertain the fetal blood pH.

Response of the fetal heart to uterine contractions

It is normal for the fetal heart rate to remain steady or to accelerate during contractions (Fig. 37.20). The relationship of decelerations to the occurrence of uterine contractions must be considered closely to assess their significance. **Early decelerations** (Fig. 37.21) begin at or after the onset of a

contraction, reach their lowest point at the peak of the contraction and return to the baseline rate by the time the contraction has finished. They are commonly associated with compression of the fetal head but may be an early sign of hypoxia.

A **late deceleration** (Fig. 37.22) begins during or after a contraction, reaches its lowest point after the peak of the contraction and has not recovered by the time the contraction ends. In severe deceleration the heart rate may not have returned to normal by the onset of the next contraction. The **time lag** between the peak of the contraction and

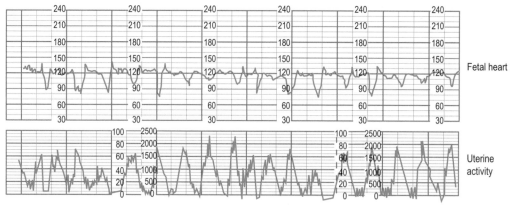

Figure 37.21   Early fetal heart rate decelerations. (Courtesy of Sonicaid, Abingdon, Oxon.)

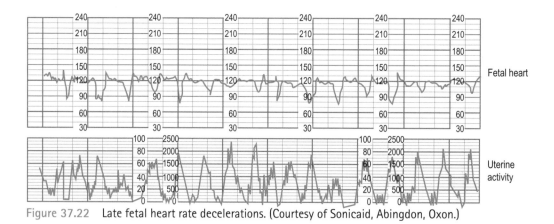

Figure 37.22   Late fetal heart rate decelerations. (Courtesy of Sonicaid, Abingdon, Oxon.)

the low point of the deceleration is more significant than the actual fall in rate. This always indicates fetal hypoxia and should be treated as an emergency. It is sensible to perform a vaginal examination to assess dilatation of the cervix and exclude cord prolapse prior to informing the obstetrician. The obstetrician will always do a fetal blood sampling procedure in all cases where there are late decelerations.

Fetal blood sampling

Hypoxia will lead to respiratory acidosis and a lowering of blood pH. The normal pH of fetal blood should be 7.35 or above. In the first stage of labour a pH of 7.25 calls for urgent action and in the second stage of labour a level of 7.2 can be accepted if delivery is imminent. Blood is taken by passing an amnioscope through the cervix and using a small blade to puncture the scalp skin (Fig. 37.23). A heparinised capillary tube is used to collect a blood sample for immediate analysis. The blood must not be allowed to clot or come into contact with atmospheric oxygen.

Amniotic fluid

If the membranes have ruptured there is a continuous escape of amniotic fluids available for inspection. The fluid

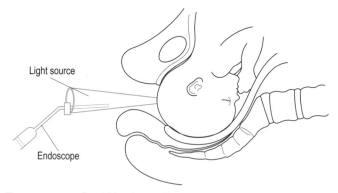

Figure 37.23   Fetal blood sampling.

should normally remain clear but the fetus may pass meconium; this is common at term but may also be due to fetal hypoxia. Fresh meconium stains the amniotic fluid green and it is likely that the fetus is hypoxic at that time, but a muddy yellow colour indicates old meconium. A full discussion on fetal distress and neonatal asphyxia is presented in Chapter 46.

MAIN POINTS

- In early labour, contractions may be 15–20 min apart and are fairly weak, lasting about 30 s. In established labour, the uterus contracts every 2.5–3 min, and in advanced labour each contraction may last 50–60 s, with contractions being powerful. Contractions can be measured in mmHg by the pressure they exert on the amniotic fluid.

- Fundal dominance allows progressive dilatation of the cervix and, as the upper segment thickens and shortens, the fetus is propelled down the birth canal. Polarity during contractions allows the upper and lower poles of the uterus to act in harmony with contraction and retraction of the upper pole and dilation of the lower pole. Contraction and retraction of the uterine muscle leads to the progressive shortening and thickening of the UUS and diminishing of the uterine cavity. A retraction ring forms between the UUS and LUS. The external os dilates until it is large enough for the widest diameter of the presenting part to pass through.

- When the membranes remain intact there is general fluid pressure. If the membranes are ruptured the placenta is compressed between the uterine wall and the fetus, reducing fetal oxygen supply.

- During each contraction, fetal axis pressure causes increasing flexion of the head. This is more significant during the second stage of labour. Upright postures facilitate engagement of the presenting part. Gravity may lead to better application of the presenting part to the cervix, promoting the Ferguson reflex and a rapid cervical dilatation.

- The process of labour uses energy. If insufficient carbohydrate is available, body fat will be utilised, with the release of ketones and the development of ketoacidosis. The main problem with food intake in labour is the possible need for a general anaesthetic and the subsequent risk of inhalation of acid gastric reflux, resulting in Mendelson's syndrome. The practice for eating and drinking in labour varies between maternity units.

- Blood vessels in the myometrium are compressed during each uterine contraction with impeded delivery of nutrients and oxygen when the strength of a contraction exceeds 40 mmHg. Fetal hypoxia and distress may occur, especially if the membranes are ruptured.

- Cardiotocography allows recording of the response of the fetal heart rhythm and rate to uterine activity. No research findings support the value of CTG in normal labour. In the first stage of labour, fetal blood with a pH of 7.25 calls for urgent action and in the second stage of labour pH of 7.2 may be accepted if delivery is imminent.

- If the membranes have ruptured, there is a continuous escape of amniotic fluid, which should normally remain clear. During episodes of fetal distress in labour, hypoxia results and the fetus passes meconium, which stains the fluid green. Presence of meconium requires closer vigilance on the condition of the fetus and the paediatrician should always be present at hospital delivery.

References

Arias F 1993 Practical Guide to High Risk Pregnancy and Delivery, 2nd edn. Mosby Year Book, Chicago.

Cassidy P 1999 The first stage of labour: physiology and early care. In Bennett V R, Brown L K (eds) Myles Textbook for Midwives, 13th edn. Churchill Livingstone, Edinburgh.

Das S 1999 Antenatal care. In Bennett V R, Brown L K (eds) Myles Textbook for Midwives, 13th edn. Churchill Livingstone, Edinburgh.

de Graaf J H, Haringa M P, Zweens M J 1999 Rupture of umbilical cord in water. British Medical Journal 319:483–487.

Enkin M, Keirse M J N C, Neilson J et al 2000 A Guide to Effective Care in Pregnancy and Childbirth, 3rd edn. Oxford University Press, Oxford.

Gibb D 1988 A Practical Guide to Labour Management. Blackwell Science, Oxford.

Gilbert R, Tookey P 1999 Perinatal mortality and morbidity among babies delivered in water. British Medical Journal 319:483–487.

Gould D 2000 Normal labour: a concept analysis. Journal of Advanced Nursing 31(2):418–427.

Hall S, Holloway M 1998 Staying in control: women's experiences of labour in water. Midwifery 14(1):30–36.

Hughes D 2003 Midwives and women – coping with pain together. In Wickham S (ed.) Midwifery: Best Practice. Elsevier, London.

McCormick C, Champion P 2002 Cultural and historic perspectives on eating and drinking in labour. In Champion P, McCormick C (eds) Eating and Drinking in Labour. Books for Midwives Press, Cheshire.

Micklewright A, Champion P 2002 Labouring over food: the dietician's view. In Champion P, McCormick C (eds) Eating and Drinking in Labour. Books for Midwives Press, Cheshire.

Millns J P 1991 Fluid balance in labour. Current Obstetrics and Gynaecology 1(1):35–40.

NICE (National Institute for Clinical Excellence) 2001 Electronic fetal heart monitoring: http://www.nice.org.uk.

Nikodem V 2002 Immersion in water during pregnancy, labour and birth. Cochrane Review: In The Cochrane Library, Issue 1. Update Software 2003, Oxford.

Nordstrom L, Arulkumaran S, Chua S et al 1995 Continuous maternal glucose infusion during labour: effects on maternal and fetal glucose and lactate levels. American Journal of Perinatology 12(5):357–362.

Odent M 1998 Labouring women are not marathon runners. The Practising Midwife 1(9):16–18.

Otigbah C, Dhanjal M, Harmsworth G 2000 A retrospective comparison of water births and conventional vaginal deliveries. European Journal of Obstetrics, Gynaecology and Reproductive Biology 9(1):15–20.

RCOG (Royal College of Obstetricians and Gynaecologists) 2001 Electronic fetal monitoring – the use and interpretation of CTG: evidence based clinical guideline No 8. RCOG, London.

Schorn M N, McCallister J L, Blanco J D 1993 Water immersion and the effect on labour. Journal of Nurse-Midwifery 38(6):338–342.

Simkin P, Anchetta R 1999 The Labour Progress Handbook. Blackwell Science, London.

Sleutal M, Golden S 1998 Fasting in labour: relic or requirement. Journal of Obstetric, Gynaecology and Neonatal Nursing 28(5):507–512.

Stratton J F, Stronge J, Boylan P C 1995 Hyponatraemia and non-electrolyte solutions in labouring primigravidae. European Journal of Obstetrics and Gynaecology and Reproductive Biology 59(2):149–151.

Stuart C C 2003 Invasive actions in labour – Where have all the 'old tricks' gone? In Wickham S (ed.) Midwifery: Best Practice. Elsevier, London.

Thompson M 1949 The Cry and the Covenant. Garden City Books, New York.

Walsh D 2000 Evidence based care series 5: Why should we reject the bed myth? British Journal of Midwifery 8(9):554–559.

World Health Organisation (WHO) 2002 Women's healthcare in normal childbirth: a report of a Technical Working Group. WHO/FRH/HSM96.24.

Annotated recommended reading

Liu D T Y 2003 Labour Ward Manual, 3rd edn. Churchill Livingstone, Edinburgh.
This book is a useful reference book for all those working on, or managing, the labour ward.

National Institute of Clinical Excellence (NICE) 2001 Clinical guidelines: the use and interpretation of cardiotography in intrapartum fetal surveillance: *http://www.nice.org.uk.*
The guidelines agree with the midwifery concept of fetal heart rate monitoring and emphasise the selective use of continuous electronic fetal heart monitoring. The responsibility of fetal surveillance still remains with health care professionals responsible for the care of labouring woman.

Thompson M 1949 The Cry and the Covenant. Garden City Books, New York.
This book highlights the importance of 'gowning and gloving up' as an infection control measure. It is essential reading for students in nursing, midwifery and medicine. Infection control issues highlighted in 1949 are just as valid today in the era of the super bug methicillin-resistant Staphylococcus aureus *(MRSA).*

Das S 1999 Antenatal care. In Bennett V R, Brown L K (eds) Myles Textbook for Midwives, 13th edn. Churchill Livingstone, Edinburgh.
This chapter provides a good reference for those providing antenatal care.

Chapter **38**

Pain relief in labour

INTRODUCTION

The experience of pain can be discussed on three levels: pain transmission and perception; pain reception; and pain modulation. Pain is a complex process and is experienced differently depending on the physiological process, the context and the previous experience of an individual. Pain can be modulated at different points in the physiological pathway and by education aimed at achieving an understanding of the accompanying events and the meanings attached to them by individuals and by their culture.

PAIN PERCEPTION

The nature of pain depends not just on physiological parameters such as the part of the body affected and the extent of the injury but also on the psychological reaction to the pain (Allan et al 1996). McCaffery (1983) reminded us of the cognitive and emotional inputs into pain perception, stating that pain is what the patient says it is and exists when he says it does. Telfer (1997) wrote that pain 'is a complex, personal, subjective, multifactorial phenomenon which is influenced by psychological, biological, sociocultural and economic factors.' In similar fashion, Carlson (1991) reminds us that pain is not purely physical. Pain can be modified by placebo drugs, emotions and other stimuli such as acupuncture. The translation of pain messages into unpleasant feelings ensures that an individual avoids repeating the experience if possible. These are important factors in the management of pain.

Whereas the physiological threshold for pain sensation appears to be similar in all people, the cognitive and emotive factors alter the individual's reaction to pain and the meaning attached to the experience. The anticipation of pain increases anxiety levels and the perceived intensity of pain. Hayward (1975) demonstrated that knowledge of events reduces anxiety and pain and this applies to pain in labour. Interesting work has been done by Walding (1991) on the 'locus of control' theory which suggests that pain is perceived as less threatening and with less intensity if women believe they are in control of events. Placing the woman at the centre of her care should therefore make labour less painful and less traumatic, even if problems such as occipitoposterior position occur.

Pain may also increase the level of catecholamines released into the blood. This in turn has the usual result of increased heart and respiration rate with decreased blood flow to the internal organs such as the uterus. The uterus in labour needs a good delivery of oxygen and nutrients to enable efficient contractions, and thus anxiety and fear increase pain, reduce uterine blood supply and may prolong labour.

PAIN RECEPTION

The principle of pain reception is that several million bare sensory nerve endings weave their way through all the tissues and organs of the body (except the brain) and respond to noxious stimuli.   (Marieb 2000).

A chemical released from damaged tissue seems to act as a universal pain stimulus. This is **bradykinin**, which in turn releases inflammatory chemicals such as **histamine** and **prostaglandin**. Bradykinin is thought to bind to receptor endings, resulting in an action potential. However, pain perception is much more than the simple sensation relayed by neurons.

Classification of pain

Pain can be classified as somatic or visceral. Somatic pain arising from skin, muscles or joints can be deep or superficial. **Superficial pain** tends to be brief, highly localisable and sharp or pricking in character. This pain is transmitted along large myelinated fibres – the A-δ fibres. **Deep somatic pain** is more likely to be described as burning or aching; it is more diffuse and longer lasting and always indicates tissue destruction. Impulses travel along small unmyelinated fibres called C fibres. A third type of fibre, the myelinated A-β fibre, relays light touch.

Pain pathways

Visceral pain results from the organs of the body cavities; it is described as burning, gnawing or aching. **Visceral sensory neurons** (afferents) accompany autonomic sympathetic and parasympathetic fibres and send information about chemical changes, distension or irritation of the viscera. Both somatic and visceral pain stimuli pass along the **dendrites** of the **first-order neurons** to their cell bodies in the **dorsal root ganglia**. Their **axons** leave the dorsal root ganglia to enter the spinal cord and synapse with **second-order neurons** in the dorsal horns of the spinal cord. The pain impulse causes the release of the pain neurotransmitter (NT), **substance P**, from the presynaptic membrane into the synaptic cleft.

The anatomy of the dorsal horn

The cells in the spinal cord are arranged in **laminae** (layers) in a dorsal–ventral direction and running the full length

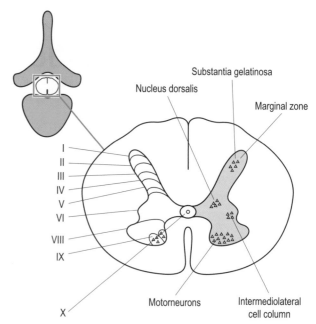

Figure 38.1   Laminae (I–X) and named cell groups at mid-thoracic level (from Hinchliff S M, Montague S E, Watson R 1996, with permission).

of the spinal cord (Fig. 38.1). The **dorsal horn** contains six laminae numbered from the tip of the horn inwards. The **ventral horn** contains three other laminae and another column of cells, lamina 10, is clustered around the central canal. Laminae 1 and 2 are visible to the naked eye as a clear zone and are together called the **substantia gelatinosa**.

Ascending pathways

Sensory fibres returning to the dorsal horns do so in an orderly fashion (Fig. 38.2). The rule is that the thicker the fibre, the deeper it penetrates. The unmyelinated C fibres do not penetrate past lamina 2; the small myelinated A-δ fibres mainly terminate in laminae 1 and 2 although a few make it to lamina 5. The large myelinated fibres from the skin end mainly in laminae 4, 5 and 6. The specialised large muscle stretch afferents reach level 6 (Melzack & Wall 1988).

The axons of most of the second-order neurons cross the cord and enter the **anterolateral spinothalamic tracts** to ascend to the thalamus (Fitzgerald 1992). There they synapse with **third-order neurons** to pass the pain message to the **sensory cortex** for interpretation. The second-order fibres may make abundant synapses in the brainstem, hypothalamus and limbic system before reaching the thalamus. This will add a state of arousal and emotion to the perception of pain.

PAIN MODULATION

Control systems descending from the brain

Nerve fibres descending in the white matter penetrate into the grey matter and innervate the nearest cells. The dorsolateral

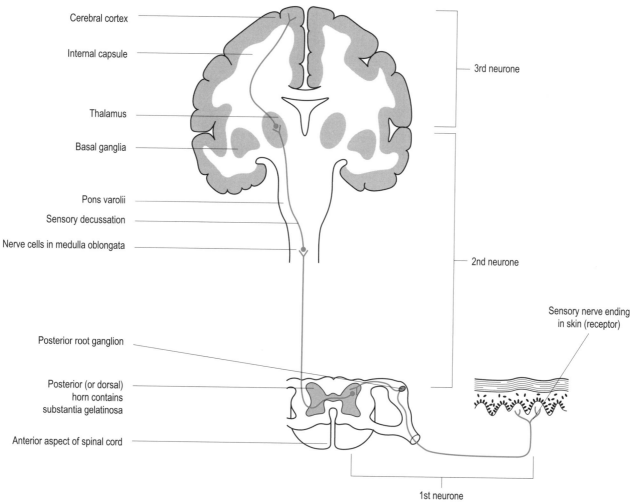

Figure 38.2   The sensory pathway showing the structures involved in the appreciation of pain. (Reproduced with permission from Bevis 1984.)

column is therefore able to send axons to the most dorsal laminae. In particular, fibres from the **raphe**, the **locus caeruleus** in the reticular formation and from the **hypothalamus** as well as the **pyramidal tract** from the cortex innervate the dorsal laminae 3–6. Descending fibres synapse in the dorsal horns and further modify the final ascending message by releasing endogenous opiates such as endorphins and encephalins, discovered by Hughes et al (1975), into the synaptic cleft. Endogenous opiates have been shown to inhibit prostaglandin production. Prostaglandin is thought to be a key chemical necessary for pain perception.

The gate control theory of pain

In order to understand the theory of Melzack & Wall (1988), it is necessary to keep the following in mind:

- the ascending and descending tracts in the spinal cord;
- the relative conduction speeds of sensory nerve fibres returning to the spinal cord;
- the anatomy of the dorsal horns of the spinal cord.

Any theory of pain must explain several facts about pain perception (Melzack & Wall 1988):

- the high variability between injury and pain;
- the production of pain by innocuous stimuli;
- the perception of pain in areas seemingly removed from the area of damage;
- the persistence of pain in the absence of injury or after healing;
- the change in the location and nature of pain over time;
- the multidimensional nature of pain;
- the lack of treatment for some types of pain such as arthritic pain and migraines.

Melzack & Wall (1988) described their updated **gate control theory of pain** which they first proposed in 1965 (Fig. 38.3). Although they would emphasise that there is still work to be done to complete their understanding, most people would agree that the gate control theory offers satisfactory explanations for some of the above unusual phenomena.

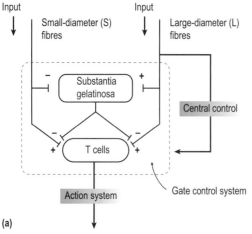
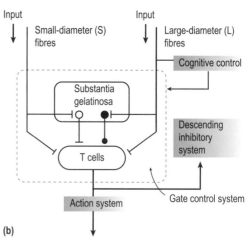

Figure 38.3   The gate control theory of pain. (a) Original formulation of the theory. Large diameter (L) and small diameter (S) peripheral nerve fibres input to the substantia gelatinosa (SG) and to the first central transmission (T) cells of the spinal cord. The inhibitory effect exerted by the SG on the T cells is increased by activity of the S fibres (pain fibres). The central control mechanisms are represented as running from the L fibre system and feeding back to the gate control, (b) Updated model. On the basis of subsequent evidence, Melzack and Wall formulated the gate control theory to include excitatory (white circle) links from the SG to the T cells, as well as descending inhibitory control from the brain-stem. All synaptic connections are excitatory except the inhibitory link from SG to T. The round knob at this inhibitory synapse implies that its action may be presynaptic, postsynaptic, or both. (Reproduced with permission from Melzack & Wall 1988.)

The essence of the gate control theory

Gating of the spinothalamic tract response to C fibre activity can be achieved by stimulating large myelinated mechanoreceptor afferents by rub or tickle. These impulses inhibit the ascending pain impulse. Inputs from the large myelinated fibres conveying touch and smaller A-δ and C fibres conveying pain interact at the level of the spinal cord. The large-diameter sensory nerve impulses come into the spinal cord more rapidly. This normally inhibits the slower smaller fibre pain impulses presynaptically. This inhibition constitutes the gate that is normally closed against small-diameter fibre impulses unless the stimulation is so great that it overcomes the gate (Fig. 38.3).

Other modifications of the ascending pain impulse take place in the substantia gelatinosa:

- Interneurons in the substantia gelatinosa can regulate and amplify the impulse conducted to the brain via the ascending pathways.
- Descending fibres synapse in the same area of the spinal cord and further modify the final ascending message by releasing endogenous opiates such as endorphins and encephalins into the synaptic cleft (see above).
- Virtually all of the brain plays a part in pain perception; the thalamus, reticular system, limbic system and cortex add their effects to the physical, emotional and cognitive experience of pain.

Knowledge of the multidimensional nature of pain perception allows the management of pain to be approached in an equally multidimensional manner. Techniques to inhibit the gate include stimulation of the large nerve fibres so that the pain impulses from the smaller fibres are blocked. Methods include heat, massage and pressure. Transcutaneous electrical nerve stimulation (TENS) works by applying a stimulating electrode to the skin at the level of the noxious C fibre activity and delivering an electrical current sufficient to cause a buzzing sensation (Fitzgerald 1992). **Descending fibre impulses** can also inhibit transmission of pain by release of natural opiates and concentration techniques may work in this way (Blackburn 2003).

Visceral sensory neurons

Although the autonomic nervous system (ANS) is considered to be a motor system, there are sensory neurons, mainly visceral pain afferents, in autonomic nerves. These visceral pain afferents travel along the same pathways as somatic pain fibres. Pain perception is referred to the somatic area of the specific dermatome of the surface of the body: for example, the pain of a heart attack is felt in the chest and along the medial aspect of the left arm.

PAIN PATHWAYS IN LABOUR

Both visceral and somatic pain are perceived in labour. Visceral pain is caused by the uterine contractions, the dilatation of the cervix and, later, by the stretching of the vagina and pelvic floor. The body of the uterus is served by autonomic nerves originating in thoracic 11 and 12 and lumbar 1 vertebrae (Fig. 38.4). Sensation from the body of the uterus is perceived as pain in response to stretch, infection and contraction and possibly ischaemia.

The cervix is innervated by the sacral plexus from sacral 2, 3 and 4 vertebrae nerves (Fig. 38.4), which then pass through the transcervical nerve plexi. Pain sensation from

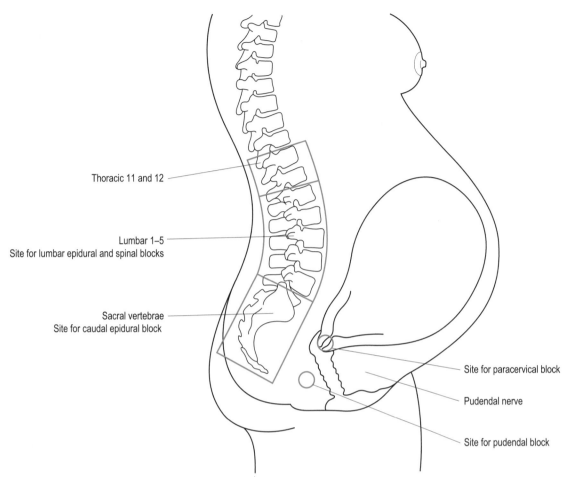

Thoracic 11 and 12

Lumbar 1–5
Site for lumbar epidural and spinal blocks

Sacral vertebrae
Site for caudal epidural block

Site for paracervical block

Pudendal nerve

Site for pudendal block

Figure 38.4   Pain pathways in labour, showing the sites at which pain may be intercepted by local anaesthetic technique. (Reproduced with permission from Bevis 1984.)

the cervix is in response to rapid dilatation. Somatic pain is caused by the pressure of the fetus as it distends the birth canal, vulva and perineum. Sensations from the pelvic floor are relayed from the pudendal nerve to the sacral plexus. Pain during the first stage of labour may be referred as nerve impulses from the uterus and cervix stimulate spinal cord neurons that innervate the abdominal wall. Pain may be felt between the umbilicus and the symphysis pubis, and around the iliac crests to the buttocks. It may radiate down the thighs and into the lumbar and sacral regions of the back.

THE EFFECT OF PAIN

Besides the physical, emotional and cognitive factors affecting pain quality and perception, abnormalities of labour may cause an increase in the pain perceived. Pain may be increased in labours complicated by prolongation, occipitoposterior position and borderline cephalopelvic disproportion.

Pain is a form of stress and may cause increased levels of catecholamine secretion and these substances will cause the following signs:

- increased cardiac output;
- increased heart rate;
- a rise in blood pressure;
- hyperventilation;
- maternal alkalosis;
- decreased cerebral and uterine blood flow due to vasoconstriction;
- decreased uterine contractions;
- delayed stomach emptying, leading to nausea and vomiting;
- delayed bladder emptying.

MANAGEMENT OF PAIN

Understanding of pain pathways and perception leads to the offering of a reasonable range of interventions. Care may include pharmacological and non-pharmacological methods of pain relief. Carers can offer:

- non-pharmacological support;
- transcutaneous electrical nerve stimulation (TENS);
- systemic analgesia;
- tranquillisers;
- inhalational analgesia;
- regional and local analgesia;
- alternative methods.

Non-pharmacological support

Antenatal preparation

Pain management ideally begins during the antenatal period. Women should be given the opportunity to discuss their anxieties and fears and be given information about pain relief at a level they are able to understand. Every person's needs are different but all women should participate in the planning of care in labour, including the choice of pain relief. There should be no feeling of finality in the choice made: women need to understand and feel reassured that they can change their minds during the course of labour, depending on their actual experience of pain. Some women may wish to attend preparation classes.

During labour

Environment   The environment is important. When women and their partners enter the labour environment it is essential that they find the atmosphere and attitude of staff to be relaxed, friendly and welcoming to them. This is often more powerful at putting them at ease than the physical surroundings themselves, which also have a role to play. The room should be furnished comfortably but in such a way that any emergency treatment needed can be carried out swiftly and efficiently (Bevis 1999). Wallpaper, curtains and screens can be useful in creating a restful atmosphere. There is a move towards informal furnishings such as beanbags, reclining chairs and rocking chairs in many units. Music and television can provide pleasure and distraction for some women in early labour.

Companionship   A companion of the woman's choice should be able to stay with her throughout labour. This may not be her partner as some men find the situation uncomfortable. Women may choose to give birth supported by a female relative or friend. If possible, a midwife known to the woman prior to labour should be available and should form a supportive relationship with the woman and her chosen companion.

Freedom of movement   Freedom to move about as and when she wants can give the woman control of her situation and shorten the process of birth. The perception of active participation in the birth is very important. The woman should be helped to find the position in which she is most comfortable, making full use of the range of furniture and equipment provided. Thus, she may walk about, lie down, sit astride a chair or kneel as she wishes.

Relaxation techniques   Relaxation techniques should be encouraged if the woman has learned them antenatally. It is also possible to teach women simple breathing techniques during the course of labour.

Communication of information   Communication of information about progress and encouragement to keep going will also reduce anxiety and add to the feeling of being in control.

The woman and her companion should participate in any decision making, such as the need for pain relief. Communication also includes physical contact but care should be taken to ascertain what the woman is comfortable with. Some women may appreciate hand holding, back rubbing, massage and cuddling while others prefer to be left alone.

Bathing   Bathing may be soothing for some women both as a direct reliever of pain and indirectly through making her feel fresher. If necessary, clean clothing should be available. Access to mouth cleansing such as brushing teeth or sucking ice can be most refreshing.

Transcutaneous electrical nerve stimulation

This non-pharmacological method of pain relief is based upon two hypotheses of pain physiology. First, is the gate control theory, according to which, cells in the posterior horn of the spinal grey matter have a gate function. Electrical stimulation by TENS is thought to increase A-β fibre input to the central pain pathways, thus producing inhibitory NTs which cause presynaptic inhibition, the closing of the 'gate' (Melzack & Wall 1965). Secondly, TENS is also thought to cause the production of endogenous opiates, which act as neuromoderators. A TENS unit is an electronic stimulus generator which transmits pulses of various configurations to electrodes which are attached to the skin. Electrodes are placed over the areas of the skin on the woman's back which overlie the thoracic (T10) and lumbar (L1) nerve endings and over the sacral nerves (S2–S4) (Fig. 38.5).

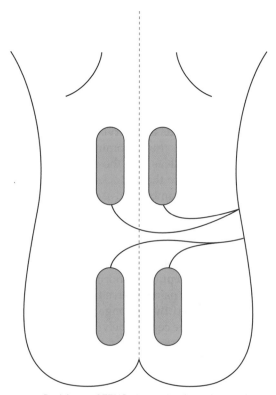

Figure 38.5   Positions of TENS electrodes for pain relief in labour (from Sweet B 1997, with permission).

Accurate placing of electrodes is important for maximising the pain relief (R Ndala unpublished work 2001). The woman operates the equipment herself and she should have been able to practice with it in the antenatal period. Pressing a button causes a small electrical current to pass through the electrodes. The current may be pulsed, that is intermittent and low frequency, or it may be continuous and high frequency. Low-frequency TENS is thought to stimulate the release of endogenous opiates while high-frequency TENS closes the pain gate (Bevis 1999). TENS is most effective when commenced early in labour but may not provide adequate analgesia for some women if used on its own. It is probably most useful in the shorter multigravid labours although many primigravidae find it useful. The TENS equipment may interfere with some electronic fetal monitors and may need to be switched off to obtain an accurate reading.

The use of TENS is within the midwives scope of practice (UKCC 1998) and practitioners should be responsible for keeping themselves updated in the use of TENS, the contraindications for its use, and that equipment conforms to current safety standards.

Systemic analgesia

An analgesic is a substance that reduces sensibility to pain without loss of consciousness and sense of touch. In labour the substance should not compromise the safety of mother or fetus and it is advisable that there should be a specific antagonist (Telfer 1997). A strong analgesic drug is called a narcotic and these include opioid drugs. The most commonly used of these is **pethidine**. Pethidine is a synthetic drug which has powerful analgesic, sedative and antispasmodic effects. The effect of intramuscular injection of pethidine is rapid and lasts up to 4 h. The dose is from 50 to 200 mg, depending on the route of administration, the mother's weight, the progress of labour and the degree of pain. Pethidine may be given by intramuscular injection, by intravenous injection or by self-administered infusion. In the case of self-administered infusions, there is a built-in time limitation so that the woman does not take an overdose.

Side-effects of pethidine include nausea, loss of self-control, a fall in blood pressure and perspiration. Pethidine crosses the placental membrane to affect the fetus and changes in fetal heart rate pattern, with a loss of baseline variability, may be seen within 40 min of administration. As it also depresses the fetal respiratory centre, it is preferably not given if delivery is expected within 2–3 h. Given within 1 h of delivery, or more than 6 h before delivery, its effect on the neonate's respiration is minimal.

However, Barrett (1983) found that changes in sleep and arousal patterns, attention, motor competence and sucking and feeding patterns followed the administration of analgesics, especially of pethidine. Babies were less alert, more likely to cry when disturbed and more difficult to settle. They were more difficult to attach to the nipple and sucked less efficiently. The antidote for pethidine is naloxone hydrochloride (Narcan) and the neonatal dose is 200 μg.

Meptazinol is an analgesic which has little effect on cardiovascular and respiratory function. The dose is 100–150 mg and it is administered intramuscularly. There is little difference in the analgesic properties of pethidine and meptazinol and both may cause vomiting in the woman.

Tranquillisers, which also have antiemetic properties, may be given with the narcotic. The most commonly used are promazine (Sparine) 25–50 mg and promethazine (Phenergan) 25–50 mg.

Inhalational analgesia

- The inhalation of a low dose of an anaesthetic agent will provide analgesia. **Entonox gas** contains a mixture of equal parts of oxygen and nitrous oxide (laughing gas) and is approved for use by midwives. Entonox may be available by cylinder or by piped supply (Fig. 38.6).

Entonox is colourless and odourless and the nitrous oxide is a heavier gas than oxygen. If stored at a temperature below −7°C, the gases may separate. Therefore, cylinders should always be stored above 10°C and on their side until needed, when the cylinder should be inverted several times to mix the contents. Entonox does not flow from the cylinder and must be obtained via the mouthpiece or facemask by inspiratory efforts. The analgesic begins to take effect after about 20 s, with maximum effect after 50 s. The mother is instructed to begin to breathe the gas as soon as the uterus begins to contract and before the sensation of pain is felt. Entonox can be used in conjunction with narcotic drugs. It is excreted rapidly via the lungs as the mother exhales and therefore toxic levels do not build up to affect the fetus. Entonox does cross the placental barrier in both directions following a concentration gradient.

Anaesthetics are used to make a patient unaware of and unresponsive to painful stimulation (Rang et al 2001). They

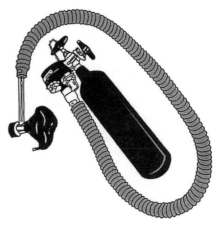

Figure 38.6   The Entonox inhaler (from Sweet B 1997, with permission).

are given systemically and have their effect on the central nervous system. In order to be a useful anaesthetic a drug must induce anaesthesia rapidly, be easily adjustable and be reversible. The use of the inhaled gaseous agent nitrous oxide (laughing gas) was suggested by Humphrey Davy in 1800. Like ether, it was first used in dental extractions.

James Simpson used the agent chloroform to relieve the pain of childbirth, which was opposed at first by the clergy. The administration of chloroform to Queen Victoria during the birth of her seventh child silenced the opposition. Inhalation anaesthetics include a wide variety of substances with no common chemical structure such as halothane, nitrous oxide and xenon and the mechanism for their action is not clear despite much research.

Stages of anaesthesia

When inhalational anaesthetics are given on their own, four well-defined stages are passed through as the blood concentration increases:

- **Stage 1 – analgesia.** The person is conscious but drowsy and response to painful stimuli is reduced.
- **Stage II – excitement.** The subject loses consciousness and does not respond to non-painful stimuli but will respond in a reflex manner to painful stimuli. Cough and gag reflexes are also present. Irregular breathing may occur and this is a dangerous state that modern procedures are designed to eliminate.
- **Stage III – surgical anaesthesia.** Spontaneous movement ceases and respiration becomes regular. If the anaesthesia is light, some reflexes are still present and muscle tone is still good. As the anaesthesia deepens, muscles become flaccid and reflexes disappear. Respirations become progressively shallower.
- **Stage IV – medullary paralysis.** Respiration and vasomotor control disappear and death would occur in a few minutes.

Obstetric use of inhalational anaesthetics

An important characteristic of an inhalational anaesthetic is the rapidity at which the arterial blood concentration changes as the amount of drug inhaled changes. These drugs are generally used as anaesthetics in obstetrics in two ways: either as pain relief or as part of a combination of drugs to induce general anaesthesia during a caesarean section. Commonly, anaesthesia would be induced by an intravenous drug and then, to maintain the state, with an inhalational agent such as nitrous oxide or halothane. Muscle paralysis is obtained by the administration of a drug such as tubocurarine. Inhalation agents are time and dose dependent and may affect the fetus directly by being transported across the placenta or indirectly by altering uteroplacental blood flow.

Various factors, including the higher metabolic requirements and the presence of the fetus, make the pregnant woman more vulnerable to hypoxia should it occur during intubation. There is a rapid fall in PO_2 and hypoxia and respiratory acidosis may rapidly follow. Supine hypotensive syndrome may exaggerate the effect by reducing venous return and cardiac output so that the uteroplacental blood flow is poor; a left lateral tilt of woman on the operating table will reduce the incidence of this problem. However, with safe techniques, light to moderate anaesthesia and adequate oxygen administration, women with normal health should not have problems.

Epidural analgesia

Epidural analgesia involves the introduction of a local anaesthetic into the epidural space surrounding the spinal cord. A catheter is inserted so that further doses of local anaesthetic can be administered if needed. Epidural analgesia provides adequate pain relief in about 90% of women who are given the technique although the success rate may also depend on the experience of the anaesthetist. Most women now choose epidural analgesia, especially primigravid women. Epidural and spinal analgesia are becoming more common as a method of pain relief for caesarean section.

Anatomy of the epidural space

The epidural space is a small space about 4 mm wide situated around the dura mater and contains blood vessels and fatty tissue (Figs 38.7 and 38.8). The spinal nerves pass through it. Engorgement of the veins reduces the size of the space during pregnancy, and uterine contractions, which cause even more engorgement of the veins, reduce the epidural space even more. The aim is to surround specific fibres of the spinal nerves in order to remove the sensation of pain. The procedure is similar to a lumbar puncture but the meninges are not penetrated. Most commonly, the lumbar route is used and the alternative of caudal anaesthesia is not popular in Britain. The anaesthetic is introduced between lumbar vertebrae 3 and 4 or 2 and 3 (Fig. 38.9).

Preparation of the woman

The procedure and its risks are explained to the woman, who must give consent. Baseline readings of temperature,

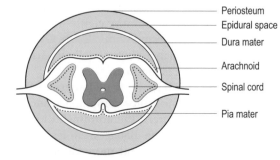

Figure 38.7   The epidural space.

pulse, blood pressure and fetal heart are recorded. The woman is encouraged to empty her bladder. An intravenous infusion of a crystalloid solution such as Hartmann's is prepared and made ready for use. The epidural can cause

sudden hypotension. If this occurs, the Hartmann's infusion is speeded up to restore normotension. Resuscitation equipment and drugs should always be available. During the siting of the epidural, the woman may be positioned on her left side or sitting up and asked to flex her back by drawing up her knees. This helps to separate the vertebrae and gives better access to the epidural space.

Procedure

Using an aseptic technique, the skin is cleaned and sterile towels are placed around the area of skin to be breached. A small amount of local anaesthetic is injected and a special epidural needle (**Tuohy needle**), which is a blunt needle with stilette, is inserted. The needle is advanced carefully until the resistance of the ligamentum flavum is reached, just before the epidural space. The stilette is removed and a syringe containing air or normal saline is attached to the needle. Further advancement of the needle brings it into the epidural space, which is recognised by a sudden loss of resistance when the plunger of the syringe is depressed. Any leakage of cerebrospinal fluid (CSF) would indicate that a dural tap has occurred.

If no blood or CSF is seen, the catheter is introduced through the epidural needle until its tip is in the epidural space. A test dose of 3–5 ml of local anaesthetic, usually

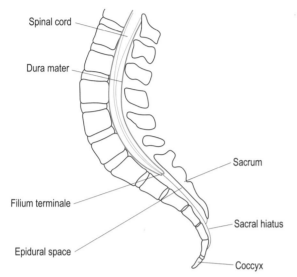

Figure 38.8   The epidural space and sacral hiatus (from Sweet B 1997, with permission).

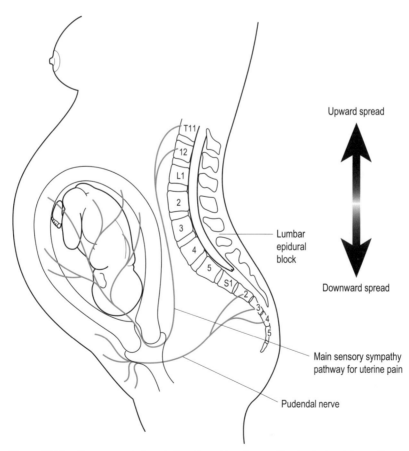

Figure 38.9   Nerve supply in relation to epidural anaesthesia during labour (from Sweet B 1997, with permission).

bupivacaine (Marcain) 0.25%, is given. A bacterial filter is attached to the end of the catheter, which is taped securely in place. Observations of maternal blood pressure and pulse and fetal heart are recorded every 5 min for 20 min and then every 30 min. This is repeated with every top-up of the epidural.

Indications for epidural analgesia

- The woman's choice of pain relief.
- Effective analgesia.
- Hypertensive conditions, to prevent the rise of blood pressure (it may even cause a small fall in BP).
- Preterm labour, to avoid the use of narcotic drugs.
- Prolonged labour, to allow rest and prevent exhaustion.
- Malpresentations such as breech, to prevent premature pushing and in case manipulations are needed in the second stage of labour.
- Malposition of occipitoposterior, to reduce pain and early pushing. However, there may be delay or no rotation of the head due to the reduced tone of the pelvic floor.
- Multiple pregnancy, to prevent the administration of narcotic drugs and in case manipulations are needed in the second stage of labour.
- Cardiac and respiratory disease.
- Operative deliveries such as caesarean section.
- Possible difficulties with intubation during administration of a general anaesthetic.

Contraindications

- Maternal reluctance for this form of pain relief.
- Sepsis near the site of the injection or systemic sepsis.
- Haemorrhagic disease or clotting disorder.
- Neurological disease.
- Hypovolaemia or hypotension.
- Spinal deformity.
- Chronic back problems.

Complications (Bevis 1999)

Hypotension   Hypotension may occur because the local anaesthetic blocks the transmission of both motor and sensory nerves and affects the sympathetic nervous system. This causes vasodilation and a fall in blood pressure may occur unless blood volume is increased by infusion (a preload) prior to the epidural block.

Dural tap   Dural tap may occur if the dura mater is punctured. It should be recognised by a few drops of CSF leaking through the Tuohy needle. If more CSF leaks, the woman may develop a severe headache, which often lasts a week. Lying flat will relieve the headache but also remove her ability to care for her baby. A blood patch of 10–20 ml of blood introduced into the epidural space usually cures the headache.

Total spinal block   Total spinal block is a rare complication and occurs if the anaesthetist fails to recognise a dural puncture and proceeds to inject the local anaesthetic. There is a profound motor and sensory block and a dramatic fall in blood pressure. The woman collapses and may have a cardiac arrest. Resuscitation and ventilatory support are needed immediately. Prevention of maternal hypoxia and restoration of normal blood pressure may allow the baby to be delivered safely as soon as feasible.

Bloody tap   A bloody tap occurs if the anaesthetist punctures an epidural vein. Blood will be seen in the epidural cannula. Resiting is necessary to avoid an intravenous injection of local anaesthetic. A patchy block with a better effect on one side of the body may occur, usually the right side. A top-up by the anaesthetist with the woman lying on the affected side may work but for a few women it may be impossible to provide total analgesia.

Other drugs

Opiates have been injected into the epidural space, including diamorphine, morphine, pethidine and fentanyl. They do not produce a block so that there is little risk of hypotension but they may reduce the amount of pain perceived, especially postoperative pain. The use of a dilute combination of opiate with local anaesthetic may give a longer, more effective analgesia with less motor blockade. The local anaesthetic blocks the A-δ fibres while the opiates remove pain transmitted by the smaller C fibres. This allows careful mobilisation of the woman and she can be more active in the second stage of labour. The drugs commonly used are **bupivacaine** and **fentanyl** and they may be given by epidural infusion as well as by bolus injection. Wild & Coyne (1992) report side-effects, including pruritus, urinary retention, postural hypotension, nausea, vomiting and respiratory depression.

Spinal anaesthesia

Spinal anaesthesia is different from epidural anaesthesia in that the local anaesthetic solution is injected into the subarachnoid space directly into the CSF rather than into the epidural space. It is quick, easy to perform and usually effective. It induces a total motor and sensory block below the anaesthetised area. There is more risk of profound hypotension occurring. It is useful for performing short procedures such as forceps delivery or manual removal of placenta. It can be used for performing a caesarean section but care must be taken that its effects do not wear off before the end of the surgery. Spinal anaesthesia may be combined with epidural anaesthesia to prevent the above risk (Bevis 1999).

Pudendal block

This is the infiltration by the obstetrician of a local anaesthetic agent via a transvaginal route into an area around the

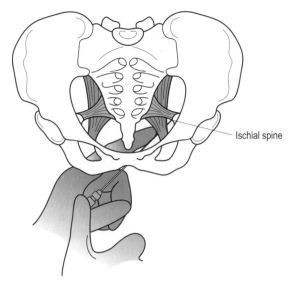

Figure 38.10   Pudendal nerve block (from Sweet B 1997, with permission).

Ischial spine

pudendal nerve (Fig. 38.10). It originates from S2–S4 and passes across the ischial spine. A special needle called a pudendal block needle, which has a guide, is used. Ten millilitres of lidocaine (lignocaine) 1% is introduced just below each ischial spine. Analgesia of the lower vagina and perineum results and is suitable for use in forceps or breech deliveries. Perineal repair may be carried out using the same analgesia although perineal infiltration would be more usual.

Perineal infiltration

This is the use of a local anaesthetic to infiltrate the perineum for either performance of an episiotomy or suturing: 10 ml of lidocaine (lignocaine) 1% solution is distributed by fan-like injections. Precautions are taken to avoid the inadvertent intravascular injection of the drug.

Complementary pain relief methods

Some women wish to avoid using pharmacological methods of pain relief or the invasive technique of epidural analgesia. Some midwives are keen to learn the techniques for complementary therapy so that they can offer a wider range of help to the women they care for but they should ensure that they are trained and that the therapy has no hidden dangers for the mother. Some women choose to be accompanied in labour by their complementary therapist. Health professionals now accept many of the complementary therapies (Tiran & Mack 2000).

Some methods that are used and have been found to benefit women in labour are massage (Kimber 2003), acupuncture (Budd 1992), hypnosis (Jenkins & Pritchard 1993), aromatherapy with oils placed in a warm bath (Burns & Blamey 1994), reflexology (Feder et al 1993) and biofeedback. Other allied therapies involve immersion in warm water, nipple stimulation to increase oxytocin production and listening to soothing music.

It is important that all practitioners of complementary therapies have received training in their use; the Midwives Rules and the Code of Practice (UKCC 1998) provide guidance for practice (Ndala unpublished work 2001, Yerby 2000).

MAIN POINTS

- The chemicals bradykinin, prostaglandin and histamine are involved in the local production of inflammation and pain. The physiological threshold for pain sensation may be similar in all people but cognitive and emotive factors alter the individual's reaction to and experience of pain. The anticipation of pain increases anxiety levels and the perceived intensity of pain.

- Somatic pain may be deep or superficial. Superficial pain tends to be brief, highly localisable and sharp or pricking in character. Deep somatic pain is described as burning or aching, is more diffuse and longer lasting. Visceral pain results from the organs of the body cavities and is often described as burning, gnawing or aching. The brain plays a large part in the modulation of pain.

- Melzack & Wall (1988) updated their gate control theory of pain. Inputs from large myelinated fibres conveying

touch and fibres conveying pain interact at the level of the spinal cord. The large-diameter sensory nerve impulses come into the spinal cord more rapidly, which inhibits the slower pain impulses presynaptically. This constitutes the gate against small-diameter fibre impulses.

- Besides the physical, emotional and cognitive factors affecting pain perception, abnormalities of labour may cause an increase in the pain perceived. Pain may be increased in labours complicated by prolongation, occipitoposterior position and borderline cephalopelvic disproportion.

- Pain may cause increased levels of catecholamine secretion, leading to increased cardiac output and heart rate, a rise in blood pressure, hyperventilation with maternal alkalosis, decreased cerebral and uterine blood flow due to vasoconstriction, decreased uterine contractions and delayed stomach and bladder emptying.

- Understanding of pain pathways and perception leads to both pharmacological and non-pharmacological methods of pain relief. The environment of the woman in labour is important and a companion of the woman's choice should stay with her throughout labour. The perception of active participation in the birth is very important. Communication of information about progress and encouragement will reduce anxiety and add to the feeling of being in control.

- Transcutaneous electrical nerve stimulation (TENS) depends on the physiology of the gate in the spinal cord. It works by interrupting the transmission of pain and is also thought to stimulate the release of endogenous opiates.

- In labour the most commonly used analgesic is pethidine. Entonox gas contains a mixture of equal parts of oxygen and nitrous oxide. It has no side-effects for the fetus and is commonly used in labour; it can be used in conjunction with other forms of analgesia.

- Epidural analgesia provides adequate pain relief in about 90% of women given the technique. There are numerous indications for epidural analgesia, including maternal choice, prolonged labour, malpresentations and malpositions, multiple pregnancy and hypertensive conditions.

- Some of the contraindications for epidural analgesia are maternal reluctance, sepsis, haemorrhagic disease or clotting disorder, and spinal deformity.

- The use of a dilute combination of opiate with local anaesthetic may give a longer, more effective analgesia with less motor blockade. This allows careful mobilisation of the woman and enables her to be more active in the second stage of labour.

- Pudendal block results in analgesia of the lower vagina and perineum and is suitable for use in forceps or breech deliveries. Perineal infiltration is used prior to performing an episiotomy or prior to suturing.

- Some women wish to use non-pharmacological methods of pain relief. Complementary therapies are now more accepted in labour. Midwives and others using these alternative therapies should be appropriately trained in their use.

References

Allan D, Nie V, Hunter M 1996 Control and co-ordination. In Hinchliff A S M, Montague S E, Watson R (eds) Physiology for Nursing Practice, 3rd edn. Baillière Tindall, London.

Barrett J W H 1983 Prenatal influences on adaptation in the newborn. In Stratton P (ed.) Psychobiology of the Human Newborn. John Wiley, New York.

Bevis R 1999 Pain relief and comfort in labour. In Bennett V R, Brown L K (eds) Myles Textbook for Midwives, 13th edn. Churchill Livingstone, Edinburgh.

Blackburn S T 2003 Maternal, Fetal and Neonatal Physiology: A Clinical Perspective, 2nd edn. W B Saunders, Philadelphia.

Budd I S 1992 Traditional Chinese medicine in Obstetrics. Midwives' Chronicle 105:140–143.

Burns E, Blamey C 1994 Using aromatherapy in childbirth. Nursing Times 9(9):54–60.

Carlson N R 1991 Physiology of Behaviour, 4th edn. Simon & Schuster, Needham Heights.

Feder E, Liisberg G B, Lenstrup C et al 1993 Zone therapy in relation to birth. In Midwives: Hear the Beat of the Future. Proceedings of the International Confederation of Midwives, 23rd International Congress, ICM, London.

Fitzgerald M J T 1992 Neuroanatomy: Basic and Clinical. Baillière Tindall, London.

Hayward J 1975 Information: a Prescription against Pain. Royal College of Nursing, London.

Hughes J, Smith T W, Kosterlitz H W et al 1975 Identification of two related pentapeptides from the brain with opiate agonist activity. Nature 258:577.

Jenkins M W, Pritchard M 1993 Practical appellations and theoretical considerations of hypnosis in normal labour. British Journal of Obstetrics and Gynaecology 100:221–226.

Kimber L 2003 How did it feel to you? An informal survey of massage techniques in labour. In Wickham S (ed.) Midwifery: Best Practice. Elsevier, London.

McCaffery M 1983 Understanding pain. In Sofaer B (ed.) The Patient in Pain. Lippincott, Philadelphia.

Marieb E N 2000 Human Anatomy and Physiology, 5th edn. Benjamin/Cummings, Philadelphia.

Melzack R, Wall P 1965 Pain mechanisms: a new theory. Science 150(3699):971–979.

Melzack R, Wall P 1988 The Challenge of Pain. Penguin, Harmondsworth.

Rang H P (ed.), Dale M M, Ritter J M 2001 Pharmacology, 4th edn. Churchill Livingstone, Edinburgh.

Telfer F M 1997 Relief of pain in labour. In Sweet B R, Tiran D (eds) Mayes Midwifery: A Textbook for Midwives, 12th edn. Baillière Tindall, London.

Tiran D, Mack S 2000 Complementary Therapies and Childbearing, 2nd edn. W B Saunders, Philadelphia.

UKCC 1998 Midwives Rules and Code of Practice. UKCC, London.

Walding M F 1991 Pain, anxiety and powerlessness. Journal of Advanced Nursing 16:338–397.

Wild L, Coyne C 1992 The basics and beyond, epidural analgesia. American Journal of Nursing April:26–30.

Yerby M 2000 Pain in Childbearing, Key Issues in Management. Baillière Tindall, London.

Annotated recommended reading

Hayward J 1975 Information: A Prescription against Pain. Royal College of Nursing, London.

The main issue in this article is the fear of the unknown in an alien environment. Hayward suggests that explanation of conditions and procedures helps people in hospital to understand and accept their condition and enables them to cope better with the pain.

McCaffery M 1983 Understanding pain. In Sofaer B (ed.) The Patient in Pain. Lippincott, Philadelphia.

In this chapter, McCaffery gives a simple definition of pain: 'Pain is what the experiencing person says it is'. This is the basis of current thinking in pain management. Pain is an individual experience and each person's pain is unique to them. This is an article worth reading.

Melzack R, Wall P 1965 Pain mechanisms: A new theory. Science 150(3699):971–979.
This publication sites the original scientific paper on the 'Gate Control Theory' which is essential reading to those interested in understanding pain or studying pain management.

Melzack R, Wall P 1988 The Challenge of Pain. Penguin Books, Harmondsworth (reprinted 1991).
A book which is easy to read and encompasses all the theories and principles of pain management. This is a reference book for those who require a deeper understanding of pain and its management.

Rang H P (ed.), Dale M M, Ritter J M 2001 Pharmacology, 4th edn. Churchill Livingstone, Edinburgh.
A very comprehensive textbook for science, medical, nursing and midwifery students. Its approach emphasises the mechanisms by which drugs act and relates these to the overall pharmacological effects and clinical issues.

Yerby M 2001 Pain in Childbearing, Key Issues in Management. Baillière Tindall, London.
A well-written book that covers key issues in pain in childbearing, facts and concepts that enable a deeper understanding of pain issues. This is an excellent reference book for pain management students.

Chapter 39

The second stage of labour

INTRODUCTION

Hillan (1999) comments that the duration of the second stage (2nd stage) is difficult to predict and in multigravidae may last for as little as 5 min whereas in primigravidae the process may take up to 2 h. Irrespective of how we analyse, divide and measure the 2nd stage of labour, much physical effort is usually provided by the mother over a comparatively short period. The physiological changes that occur in the 2nd stage are a continuation of the forces that have been occurring in the first stage of labour but there is now no impediment to descent of the fetus through the birth canal and to its birth.

The 2nd stage of labour begins when the cervix is fully dilated (Fig. 39.1) and ends when the fetus is fully expelled from the birth canal. Both midwives and their medical colleagues have used this to base the management of the delivery of the baby according to a time regime. There have been challenges to the concept that the exact timing of the 2nd stage of labour is possible and progress rather than

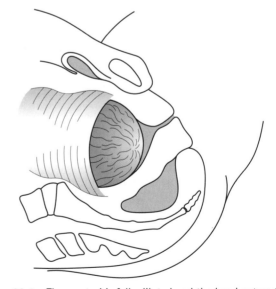

Figure 39.1   The os uteri is fully dilated and the head enters the vagina (from Sweet B 1997, with permission).

an estimated time limit is probably a more useful indicator of normality.

PHYSIOLOGY OF THE SECOND STAGE OF LABOUR

Contractions

There is often a brief lull in uterine activity at the end of the first stage (the **latent phase**) before the contractions take on their expulsive nature. The character of the contractions changes from that of the first stage. They become longer and stronger but may be less frequent so that the woman and her baby can recover between each expulsive effort. There is continued contraction and retraction of the upper uterine segment (UUS). The fetus descends the birth canal and fetal axis pressure increases flexion and reduces the size of the presenting part.

The secondary powers

As pressure is exerted on the rectum and pelvic floor, a reflex occurs which the woman feels as a compelling urge to push (the **active phase**). Normal bearing-down efforts made by a woman if left to her own devices occur for about 5–6 s several times during the contraction. Compaction of the fetus occurs during the contraction and pressure on the fetal head may evoke vagal stimuli, causing a transient fall in fetal heart rate with a rapid recovery. Reduction in oxygen supply due to compression of the placenta will add to this effect. Recent studies suggest that spontaneous pushing will prolong the 2nd stage of labour but cause fewer fetal heart rate changes, higher arterial pH and less damage to the birth canal.

Descent of the fetus

As the fetus descends the birth canal it displaces the soft tissues contained in the pelvis. Anteriorly, the bladder is pushed up into the abdominal cavity, which results in stretching and thinning of the urethra. Posteriorly, the rectum becomes flattened in the sacral curve and any faecal matter will be expelled. The levator ani muscles of the pelvic floor thin out and are displaced laterally. The perineal body is stretched and thinned.

The fetal head now becomes visible at the vulva and advances with each contraction to recede slightly between contractions until crowning of the head occurs (the **perineal phase**). The head is born and the shoulders and body of the baby are born with the next contraction, accompanied by a gush of amniotic fluid. The 2nd stage culminates as soon as the baby is completely born.

Onset of the second stage

There is often no clear demarcation between the end of the first stage and the beginning of the 2nd stage. Several signs can be taken as indicative that the 2nd stage has begun but

Table 39.1   The presumptive signs of the 2nd stage of labour

Presumptive sign	Differential diagnosis
Expulsive uterine contractions	There may be an urge to push before full cervical dilatation if the rectum is full, the head in the occipito-posterior position or the woman is highly parous
Rupture of the forewaters	This may occur at any time in labour
Dilatation and gaping of the anus	Deep engagement of the presenting part and premature maternal pushing may cause this
Appearance of the presenting part	Excessive moulding and caput succedaneum formation may protrude through the cervix prior to full dilatation as may a breech presentation.
Show	This must be distinguished from bleeding due to premature separation of the placenta
Congestion of the vulva	Pushing before full dilatation of the cervix may produce this

the midwife ought to have no difficulty in making the diagnosis. Hillan (1999) outlines the **presumptive signs** of the onset of the 2nd stage of labour and differential diagnoses (Table 39.1). The appearance of several of the signs together may indicate that the 2nd stage of labour has begun but if no progress can be seen after a few contractions, it is sometimes necessary to confirm the absence of cervix by vaginal examination.

Duration of the second stage

The duration of the 2nd stage is difficult to predict and in multigravidae may last for as little as 5 min whereas in primigravidae the process may take up to 2 h. There is no good evidence available to impose a time limit for this stage of labour and it is more relevant to base decisions on progress with evidence of adequate uterine contractions, descent and continuing good maternal and fetal wellbeing. Two phases of the 2nd stage of labour can be described as in the first stage of labour: the **latent** and **active phases**.

The latent phase begins at full dilatation of the cervix but the presenting part may not yet be visible at the pelvic outlet and the woman may not have an urge to bear down. As the fetal head descends due to the force of uterine contractions and stretches the tissues of the vagina and pelvic floor, it will become visible at the vaginal orifice. Once the fetal head is visible, pressure on the rectum will normally provide the reflex stimulus for maternal expulsive pushing and the active phase begins.

MECHANISMS OF LABOUR

The fetus is in effect a cylinder which has to negotiate the curved birth canal formed of the bony pelvis and soft tissues of the flattened and distended perineal body. There are two problems with being human and giving birth. One is the curve of the birth canal generated by the upright posture and walking on two legs (bipedalism) and the other is the large size of the baby's head due to the size of the human brain. Even so, the brain is only one-quarter of the size it will grow to in the adult. Moulding of the skull in order to reduce the presenting diameters is described elsewhere and this section will concern itself with the passive movements that the fetus makes in response to the forces exerted on it by the birth canal.

Collectively, these movements are called the mechanisms of labour and the fetus is turned slightly to take advantage of the widest part of each plane of the pelvis. The reader will remember that the plane of the inlet is widest in the transverse while the outlet is widest in the anteroposterior diameter. Knowledge of mechanisms enables the midwife to use skills in order to facilitate birth with least trauma to mother and fetus. Therefore it is important to take a fetal doll and pelvis and practise these mechanisms until they can be visualised in relation to the unseen movements during the birth of the baby. It is helpful to silently run through these when observing deliveries. It may be life-saving to understand what is occurring inside the woman's body so that external manoeuvres can be used to complete delivery.

Different mechanisms occur depending on the presentation and position of the fetus and there are principles common to all:

- descent of the fetus takes place;
- the part of the fetus that leads and meets the resistance of the pelvic floor will rotate forwards to come to lie anteriorly under the symphysis pubis;
- whatever part of the fetus emerges will pivot around the pubic bone.

The mechanism of a normal labour

There is a classical way of recalling the situation of a fetus at the commencement of the 2nd stage of labour. The terms are described in Chapter 37, p. 482. The following is for a normal labour:

- **the lie** is longitudinal;
- **the attitude** is one of good flexion;
- **the presentation** is cephalic;
- **the position** is right or left occipitoanterior;
- **the denominator** is the occiput;
- **the presenting part** is the posterior part of the anterior parietal bone.

The movements

For illustrations of the movements see Figures 39.2–39.10.

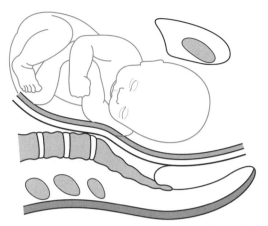

Figure 39.2   Descent of a well-flexed head into the pelvis. The sagittal suture is in the transverse diameter of the pelvis (from Sweet B 1997, with permission).

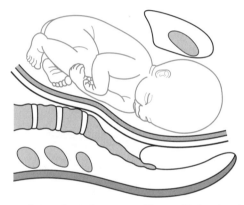

Figure 39.3   Internal rotation occurs. The sagittal suture is in the oblique diameter of the pelvis (from Sweet B 1997, with permission).

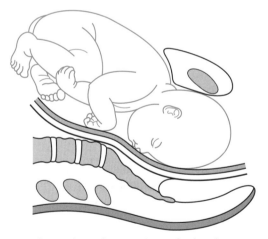

Figure 39.4   Internal rotation complete – further descent occurs. The sagittal suture is now in the anteroposterior diameter of the pelvis (from Sweet B 1997, with permission).

Descent   Descent of the fetal head into the pelvis may have occurred in the antenatal period so that the woman, especially a primigravida, begins labour with the head engaged. This usually indicates that vaginal delivery is likely.

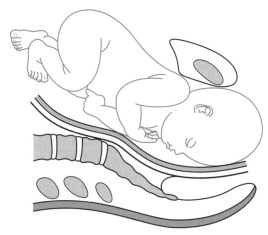

Figure 39.5   The head descended to the vulval outlet (from Sweet B 1997, with permission).

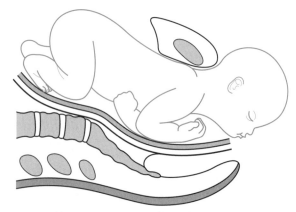

Figure 39.6   The head is crowned (from Sweet B 1997, with permission).

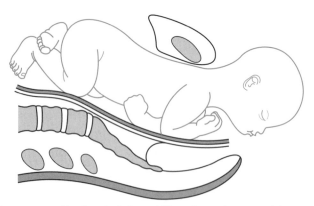

Figure 39.7   The face is delivered (from Sweet B 1997, with permission).

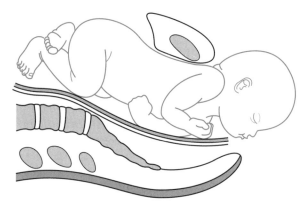

Figure 39.8   Restitution has taken place and internal rotation of the shoulders occurs (from Sweet B 1997, with permission).

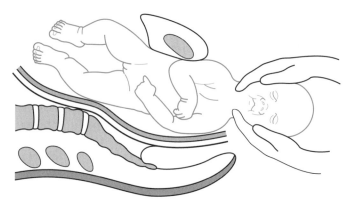

Figure 39.9   Gentle downward traction is applied to deliver the anterior shoulder (from Sweet B 1997, with permission).

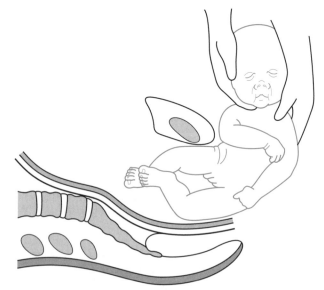

Figure 39.10   The posterior shoulder is delivered and then the trunk by lateral flexion (from Sweet B 1997, with permission).

There is continued descent during the first stage of labour and this is speeded by maternal effort during the 2nd stage of labour.

Flexion   Flexion of the fetal head on the trunk is increased during labour because the skull is attached to the fetal spine nearer the occiput than the sinciput. Pressure transmitted from the fundus of the uterus down the fetal spine will force the occiput lower than the sinciput, increasing flexion and resulting in the conversion of the suboccipitofrontal diameter of 10 cm to the favourable suboccipitobregmatic diameter of 9.5 cm.

Internal rotation of the head   As the leading part is driven onto the pelvic floor, the resistance of the muscular diaphragm and its gutter shape, sloping downwards anteriorly, cause the occiput to rotate forwards in the pelvis 1/8th of a circle to lie under the symphysis pubis and the anteroposterior diameter of the head now lies in the anteroposterior diameter of the pelvis. This causes a slight twist on the neck of the fetus so that the head is no longer aligned with the shoulders.

Extension of the head   The occiput escapes from beneath the subpubic arch and the smallest possible diameters, which are the suboccipitobregmatic diameter of 9.5 cm and the biparietal diameter of 9.5 cm, distend the vaginal orifice. The head is now born by extension as it pivots on the suboccipital region around the pubic bone. The sinciput, face and chin sweep the perineum. The widest diameter to distend the vagina is the suboccipitofrontal as the sinciput is born.

Restitution   Restitution is a movement made by the head following delivery which brings it into correct alignment with the shoulders. This will be 1/8th of a circle towards the side of the occiput.

Internal rotation of the shoulders   The anterior shoulder is the first to reach the pelvic floor and this now rotates forward to lie under the symphysis pubis. This movement is accompanied by external rotation of the head 1/8th of a circle more in the direction of restitution. The occiput now lies laterally, turned towards the woman's thigh.

Lateral flexion   The anterior shoulder is usually born first and slips under the pubic arch and the posterior shoulder passes over the perineum. The remainder of the body is born by lateral flexion as the spine bends laterally on its way through the curved birth canal.

Physiological changes

Edwards (1995) outlines the physiological principles which should underlie the management of the 2nd stage of labour. These include:

● fetal hormone secretion aimed at adaptation to independent life;
● the condition of mother and baby;
● the bearing-down reflex;
● thinning of the perineum;
● position of the mother.

MANAGEMENT

The 2nd stage of labour begins when the cervix is fully dilated and ends when the fetus is fully expelled from the birth canal. Midwives and medical colleagues have used this definition to base the management of the delivery of the baby according to a time regime. This suggests that the exact timing of the 2nd stage of labour is possible. This concept has been challenged and it is probable that progress rather than an estimated time limit is more useful as an indicator of normality (Enkin et al 2000).

At the end of the day the question must be asked about stages and phases of labour as to whether they are physiological entities or human imagination. Before describing the physiology and management of the 2nd stage, the concepts need to be examined.

The second stage of labour – two or three phases

Crawford (1983) believed that the division of labour into three stages and subdividing the stages into phases was contrary to the actual events of labour and that basing the management of labour on these concepts may lead to distress and hazard for mother and fetus. While he discussed the division of the first stage of labour into the latent and active phase, he stated that the 'distinction between the first and second stages leads to the greatest trouble in clinical practice'. He believed that the difficulty occurs because there is a lack of clear definition as to when the 2nd stage begins. If it begins with expulsive efforts by the woman, then some women wish to bear down before the cervix is fully dilated and sometimes a woman will not bear down until the presenting part is distending the perineum. Sometimes, if the woman has had epidural analgesia, she may not have an urge to bear down at all.

Aderhold & Roberts (1991) examined the concept of phases in the 2nd stage of labour with an in-depth study of four nulliparous women. They describe the above concepts of two phases to the 2nd stage as follows:

> The early phase from complete dilation until the presenting part becomes visible which lasts 10 to 30 min and generally occurs with mild or no urge to bear down. Then the period of active bearing down … follows as the fetal scalp becomes visible, and proceeds until the birth of the baby. Pushing becomes more pronounced and there is a sudden change in the woman's demeanour.

They remind readers that some authorities have gone further and described **three phases** of the 2nd stage of labour – the latent phase or lull; the descent or active phase; and the perineal phase. In their small study of four nulliparous women, they found evidence to support the three phases.

The researchers suggest that if further research verifies the phases of the 2nd stage, midwives and other obstetric care providers will be able to use this deeper understanding of spontaneous 2nd stage to inform their management. In particular, they agree with Crawford that forced expulsive efforts before the woman is ready could impose hypoxic stress on the fetus and maternal exhaustion could occur.

The length of the second stage of labour

Normal bearing-down efforts made by women if left to their own devices occur for about 5–6 s several times during the contraction (Caldeyro-Barcia 1979). Saunders et al (1992) investigated both neonatal and maternal morbidity in relation to the length of the 2nd stage of labour. They found no relation between the length of the 2nd stage of labour and the frequency of low Apgar scores or of admissions to Special Care Baby Unit (SCBU). They concluded that current management allowing spontaneous pushing, even in 2nd stages lasting up to 3h, did not carry any undue fetal risk. Recent studies suggest that spontaneous pushing will prolong the 2nd stage of labour but will cause fewer fetal heart rate changes, higher arterial pH and less damage to the birth canal.

If the three factors discussed above are considered together and applied to clinical practice, it appears that the best way to manage the 2nd stage of labour is to allow the woman to push as and when she wishes as long as maternal and fetal condition remains good and progress is occurring (Enkin et al 2000). There is a need to take to heart the modifying statement by Chamberlain & Drife (1995) that while there may be indications to change practice, further research must continue to be carried out, especially following up the infants into childhood.

Chamberlain & Drife (1995) summarised the previous decade of thinking:

> ... ideas about the length of the second stage of labour have swung from a regimented timetable to a go-as-you-please regime according to the attitudes of the mother, the midwife and possibly the fetus.

They add that the division between the first and 2nd stages cannot be timed and go on to outline a possible history of why clinicians have been so keen to establish full dilatation of the cervix, concluding it is because that is the point at which vaginal delivery can be accomplished by the use of obstetrical forceps. They finally state that no rules can be laid down about the length of the 2nd stage of labour but that research should be continued into the effects on the fetus and long-term effects on the child.

The definition at the beginning of this chapter stated that the 2nd stage begins with full cervical dilatation. At the time the woman is found to be 'fully dilated', it may be 3 or 4 hours from the previous vaginal examination (VE) and it is not possible to know exactly when full dilatation occurred. The author remembers occasions when a woman had not dilated for several hours despite having regular contractions, but by reassuring and encouraging the woman to do breathing exercises or use Entonox, within an hour, the woman felt an uncontrollable urge to push, with the vertex becoming visible shortly afterwards. It was not possible to tell when the 2nd stage of labour had begun. Another occasion is where the woman has made little or no progress and a Syntocinon (oxytocin) infusion is started as a result; very often, the cervix is fully dilated when she is next examined to check progress. The time of examination is documented as the beginning of the 2nd stage. Full dilatation of the cervix could have occurred half an hour or an hour before that time.

Medical control

Crawford (1983) stated that clinicians believe they know when the 2nd stage of labour begins and that they have an 'entrenched opinion' about how long it should last. The problem is that the woman may be asked to bear down once full cervical dilatation is established, regardless of whether she feels she wants to. This creates a situation with developing maternal exhaustion, metabolic acidosis and ending in an instrumental delivery, resulting in possible birth trauma to the woman or her baby. He believed that the woman should not be urged to bear down until she wished to or until the presenting part was distending the perineum and that if there was no maternal or fetal distress there was no need for instrumental delivery. These views were supported by Westcott (1984), who summarised them in an article looking at the wider issue of medical control of labour intended to be read by pregnant women.

In an attempt to clarify definitions, they suggested that the first part of the 2nd stage begins at full cervical dilatation and ends when the mother voluntarily bears down. She found that there were two distinguishable parts and that the second part was more likely to lead to fetal acidosis and birth asphyxia than the first part. In her last paragraph she suggests that the first part of the 2nd stage should 'really be considered as the end of the first stage of labour'. Once again, the distinction between the end of the first stage and beginning of the 2nd stage is ill defined.

Midwifery thinking

An important milestone for midwifery practice was a review of the management of women in the normal 2nd stage of labour undertaken by Thomson (1988). She described with feeling and accuracy the control exerted over the labouring woman, including position, forced expulsive efforts and the concentration on the vulva. She concluded that the available literature on managing the 2nd stage suggested an interrelationship between three factors:

1. the position of the woman;
2. the means by which the woman exerts pressure to assist the uterus to expel the baby;
3. the length of the 2nd stage of labour.

These three factors still remain valid today and will be used as a plan for discussing the physiological management of labour.

Position of the woman

In most other cultures in the world and in Europe until the 18th century, women used a variety of positions during the 2nd stage of labour. Irrespective of the position used for delivery, women have tended to deliver with abducted thighs in an upright position. In most cases women adopt upright positions so that the third lumbar vertebra is above the fifth (Thomson 1988). Upright positions include standing, kneeling, sitting on birthing chairs and squatting. The lying down dorsal position may have originated in France because of the wish of Louis XIV to witness the delivery of the baby of his mistress but has been perpetuated for the ease of the medical profession. In Britain the left lateral position may have originated as the 'London position' advocated by Smellie in 1752 (Thomson 1988).

Although the recumbent position has been until the last few decades, the most common position for delivery, it is known that it leads to supine hypotension, which may adversely affect fetal oxygenation (Enkin et al 2000). If the mother lies on her back there will be a significant reduction in maternal cardiac output and circulation of oxygenated blood through the placental tissue due to compression of the inferior vena cava and descending aorta although this does not happen if the woman lies on her side or if the uterus is tilted to the left. The upright posture has at least four beneficial effects on the progress of the 2nd stage:

1. It allows gravity to play its part in the descent of the fetus.
2. It increases the diameters of the pelvic outlet by up to 1 cm in the transverse diameter and 2 cm in the anteroposterior diameter in the squatting position. This produces a 28% increase in the area of outlet over women delivered in the supine position.
3. It increases the efficiency of uterine contractions.
4. It reduces the incidence of fetal distress and neonatal asphyxia.

Squatting   Squatting is probably the most common position for childbirth in the developing world. The mother may need the support of two people or she may support herself with her back to a wall or firm surface. The flexion and abduction of the thighs brought about by squatting has a number of advantages (Simkin & Ancheta 2000).

- provides the advantage of gravity;
- enlarges the pelvic outlet by increasing the intertuberous diameter;
- allows freedom to shift weight comfortably;
- provides mechanical advantage – upper trunk presses on fundus more than any other position;
- may enhance the urge to push;
- may hasten descent of the fetal head if it is engaged and well-aligned in an occiputoanterior position;
- may relieve backache.

However, if the fetal head is at a relatively high station and asynclitic, squatting may impede correction of the angle of the head by reducing the space available for the fetus to move into synclitism. If squatting is continued for a prolonged period, the woman should lean back or rise after every contraction to prevent compression of the blood vessels and nerves located behind the knee joints.

Hands and knees/all–fours positions   Women may often adopt a kneeling position themselves. This position also has the following advantages:

- aids fetal rotation from occipitoposterior position;
- may aid in reducing an anterior lip in the late first stage;

- allows the woman freedom to sway, crawl or rock the pelvis, which can promote rotation and increase comfort;
- reduces back pain and relieves haemorrhoids;
- may resolve fetal heart problems mainly due to cord compression.

The position allows access for vaginal examination and provides an excellent view of the fetus and perineum and causes less perineal trauma. There may be an increase in vulval trauma.

Upright positions adopted by women for labour and birth have been noted to restore normality to prolonged labour (Simkin & Ancheta 2000).

Birthing chairs   Electronically controlled birthing chairs appeared to be an alternative for supporting women in the squatting position, giving the midwife good vision and access to the fetus. However, there have been problems associated with their use. There appears to be a higher mean blood loss and an increase in postpartum haemorrhage in multigravidae. This finding may be due to the increased accuracy in measuring blood loss or there may be more actual blood loss from perineal trauma caused by obstructed venous return because of pressure on the buttocks and perineum. This pressure may also be responsible for the increase in perineal oedema and haemorrhoids in women delivered in the upright position in birthing chairs.

Review of upright positions   For centuries there has been controversy around whether being upright or lying down has advantages for women delivering their babies. In a systematic review of research studies, Gupta & Nikodem (1999) considered the benefits and risks associated with the upright or lateral positions compared with supine or lithotomy positions. They concluded that the upright or lateral positions were associated with a reduced duration of 2nd stage, a reduction in both assisted deliveries and episiotomies, a smaller increase in 2nd degree tears and an increased risk of blood loss greater than 500 ml. Women were also noted to perceive less severe pain and found bearing down to be easier. These are tentative findings and further well-controlled studies are required. In the meantime women should be encouraged to give birth in the position they find most comfortable.

Maternal effort in the second stage of labour

We may then accept that the 2nd stage of labour begins with full dilatation of the cervix but the presenting part may not yet be visible at the pelvic outlet and the woman may not have an urge to bear down. As the fetal head descends due to the force of uterine contractions and stretches the tissues of the vagina and pelvic floor, it will become visible at the vaginal orifice. Once the fetal head is visible, pressure on the rectum will normally provide the reflex stimulus for maternal expulsive pushing and the active phase begins.

Prior to the 1990s it was customary practice for birth attendants to give women formal instructions during the 2nd stage of labour (Watson 1994). The rationale for this was to reduce the length of the 2nd stage of labour and prevent too much stress for the fetus. Women were often encouraged to take a big breath at the start of each contraction and bear down as long and as hard as they can. This is known as the Valsalva manoeuvre and uses forced expiration against a closed glottis to increase intra-abdominal pressure to aid the uterus to expel the fetus. This manoeuvre causes the blood pressure to drop and rise again and women using the technique have shown alterations in heart rate and brain wave patterns. Forced pushing has been implicated as the cause of burst capillaries in the face and eyes and rarely cerebrovascular accidents (strokes) may occur.

There is no evidence to suggest that any benefits are gained from routine directed pushing and pushing from sustained bearing down, breath holding or early bearing down (Enkin et al 2000). Current practice now recommends that directed pushing should be abandoned and women should be encouraged to follow their instincts. The midwives role should be to affirm physiology, not control it or deny it, and to encourage women-centred approaches, which promote normality.

Effect on pelvic soft tissues

There are two ways of interpreting early pushing in the 2nd stage of labour: pushing in the early part of each contraction, as discussed above; and pushing in the latent phase. A paper by Beynon (1957) explains the effect that forceful pushing from the commencement of each contraction has on the soft tissues of the pelvic floor. Beynon theorised that in the early part of a contraction the vaginal muscles are drawn taut to prevent the bladder supports and transverse cervical ligaments being pushed down in front of the baby's head. Early expulsive effort may lead to incontinence and prolapsed uterus later in life. Active pushing during the latent phase of the 2nd stage of labour may strain the uterine supports and the vaginal and perineal muscle before these tissues have a chance to stretch gradually.

Perineal lacerations

During the 2nd stage of labour, **perineal lacerations** may occur. In order to control the extent of these lacerations an **episiotomy** may be performed, especially in women who have a previous history of extended tears. Depending on the depth of tissue involved in the tear, perineal lacerations can be classified as follows:

- A **first-degree** tear involves just the skin of the fourchette.
- A **second-degree** tear involves the skin of the fourchette, the perineum and perineal body. The muscles of the perineal body involved are the superficial muscles – the bulbocavernosus, transverse perinei and the ileococcygeus muscles.
- A **third-degree** tear involves all the above tissues and the anal sphincter.

- Sweet (1997) includes a **fourth-degree** tear, which includes the anal sphincter and extends into the rectal mucosa.
- An **episiotomy** includes the same structures as a second-degree tear.

Other tissues may be lacerated during delivery. **Labial lacerations** are not usually severe enough to require suturing but can be very painful, especially during micturition. **Vaginal** and **cervical lacerations** may bleed severely and need immediate pressure to control bleeding followed by suturing.

The episiotomy

An episiotomy, in a strict sense, is an incision of the pudenda. It is a deliberate incision of the perineum, through the structures involved in a second-degree tear. In common parlance, however, episiotomy is often used synonymously with perineotomy (Cunningham et al 2001). In the United Kingdom, it is an integral part of the midwife's role to perform an episiotomy and infiltrate the perineum with local anaesthetic when this procedure is required (UKCC 1998). The rationale for the incision is to enlarge the vulval outlet immediately before delivery to facilitate delivery and reduce perineal trauma. Early studies by Sleep (1984a, 1984b) demonstrated that the performance of an episiotomy was not a valid reason to prevent perineal trauma. Findings indicated that there was no reduction in trauma to the pelvic floor nor did women suffer less pain or swelling; indeed, many women felt more pain. The perineal wound, whether tear or episiotomy, healed in a similar manner. Findings from recent studies and reviews support these findings and suggest that there is no evidence to suggest that episiotomies add any protection against perineal-related problems such as sphincter tears (Carroli & Belizan 2002, Low et al 2000).

More recently, the results of a study by Goldberg et al (2002) showed a trend in the reduction of episiotomies performed over almost two decades. The overall episiotomy rates in 34 048 vaginal births showed a significant reduction from 69.6% in 1983 to 19.4% in 2000.

Recommendation for performing an episiotomy During the antenatal period women should be given a chance to discuss the possible need for the midwife to make an episiotomy to avoid confrontation situations in an emergency (Walsh 2000). It is unlikely that a woman will refuse if she is able to make an informed choice based on knowledge acquired calmly. Her wishes should be recorded on her birth plan.

Enkin et al (2000) state that there is no evidence from available studies to support the suggestion that the use of episiotomy minimises trauma to the fetal head. Recommendations for current practice should include the following:

- A reduction in the episiotomy rate for normal births to 10% or less (WHO 1996).
- Fetal indications are the only justification for performing an episiotomy: to expedite delivery if the fetal head is on

the perineum and there is evidence of fetal distress or if the fetus is preterm or is presenting by the breech to reduce the risk of intracranial trauma.

- Elective episiotomies for previous third-degree tears should be discontinued and should not be mandatory for forceps or ventouse births.
- Documented consent should be obtained from the woman.

The incision   There are two types of incision: the mediolateral and the midline. The mediolateral is most commonly used because it avoids damage to Bartholin's gland and is unlikely to extend in the midline to involve the anal sphincter (Fig. 39.11).

The perineum is infiltrated along the line of the intended episiotomy using 10 ml of lidocaine (lignocaine) 1%. The practitioner should check carefully to avoid giving the

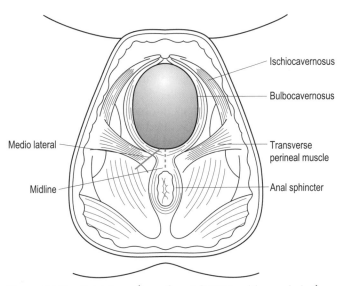

Figure 39.11   Episiotomy (from Sweet B 1997, with permission).

injection intravenously to avoid the risk of causing bradycardia or collapse. The anaesthetic takes effect very quickly and the incision can then be made using episiotomy scissors. The incision is best made during a contraction when the perineum is thinned out and should be 3–4 cm long. The practitioner should protect the fetal head during the administration of the local anaesthetic and performing the episiotomy by inserting two fingers between the head and the perineum (Fig. 39.12).

Suturing the perineum   Repair of the perineum is now an integral part of the role of the midwife in intrapartum care. This includes being able to recognise situations where it is not appropriate for the midwife to suture: for instance, if a third-degree tear has unfortunately been sustained. The advantage to the woman is that the suturing is carried out immediately and she doesn't have to wait until a doctor is available. The midwife should comply with the local policies for the use of suture materials, which should be based on up-to-date research. Aseptic technique is universal. The most important point is to explore the depth of the wound and ensure that the first suture is placed above its apex to prevent the development of a vaginal haematoma. The perineum is then sutured in layers from the inside tissues outwards (Fig. 39.13). A continuous subcuticular method of suturing is recommended using polyglycolic sutures such as Vicryl (polyglactin 910) or Dexon (polyglycolic acid), as this can result in less suturing being required and less pain (Kettle & Johanson 2002a, 2002b).

THE FETUS IN THE SECOND STAGE OF LABOUR

It is traditional to view the 2nd stage of labour as the most dangerous stage for the fetus where there is an increased risk for the occurrence of asphyxia and trauma. This has led

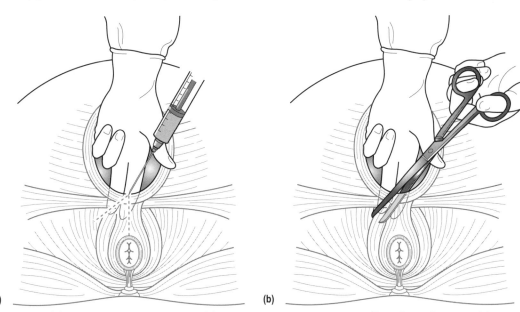

Figure 39.12   (a) Infiltration of the perineum. (b) Making a mediolateral incision (from Sweet B 1997, with permission).

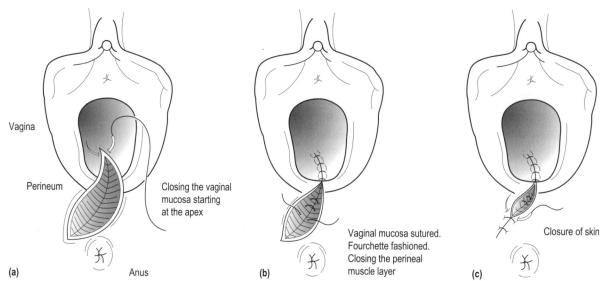

Figure 39.13 Suturing the perineum. (a) Closing the vaginal mucosa, starting at the apex. (b) Vaginal mucosa sutured, fourchette fashioned, closing the perineal muscle layer. (c) Closure of the skin (from Sweet B 1997, with permission).

to attempts to deliver the baby as quickly as possible. Although the Valsalva manoeuvre will significantly shorten the 2nd stage of labour, studies have indicated that sustained breath holding leads to abnormalities in the fetal heart (Caldeyro-Barcia 1979) and adversely affects fetal condition and neonatal outcome (Bassell et al 1980, Paine & Tinker 1992). Compaction of the fetus occurs during the contraction and pressure on the fetal head may evoke vagal stimuli, causing a transient fall in fetal heart rate with a rapid recovery.

Reduction in oxygen supply due to compression of the placenta will add to this effect. This may cause prolongation of the normal fall in fetal heart rate seen after contractions in the 2nd stage of labour. Also, if the mother lies on her back there will be a significant reduction in cardiac output and circulation of oxygenated blood through the placental tissue due to compression of the inferior vena cava and descending aorta, although this does not happen if the woman lies on her side or if the uterus is tilted to the left.

Piquard et al (1988) examined the validity of fetal heart rate monitoring in the 2nd stage of labour and whether a time limit should be placed on the 2nd stage to safeguard the fetus. They cited evidence that umbilical artery pH decreased significantly if the 2nd stage exceeded 45 min. This aspect of care in the 2nd stage will be discussed more fully in Chapter 46. In 1989 Piquard et al analysed fetal distress in relation to the concept of two biological parts to the 2nd stage of labour. They agreed with clinicians that the 2nd stage of labour is a time of risk for the fetus with distress related not only to hypoxia but also to mechanical stress.

MAIN POINTS

- At the end of the first stage of labour there is often a brief lull in uterine activity before the contractions take on their expulsive nature, becoming longer and stronger but less frequent. The fetus descends the birth canal and increasing flexion reduces the size of the presenting part.

- The 2nd stage of labour begins with full dilatation of the cervix and ends when the fetus is fully expelled from the birth canal. Progress made during this stage rather than an estimated time limit is more useful as an indicator of normality.

- The duration of the 2nd stage in multigravidae may last for as little as 5 min, whereas in primigravidae the process may take up to 2 h. Two phases of the 2nd stage of labour can be described: the latent and active phases. The latent phase begins at full dilatation of the cervix but the

woman may not have an urge to bear down. Pressure on the rectum normally provides the stimulus for maternal expulsive pushing and the active phase begins.

- The upright posture allows gravity to aid descent of the fetus, increases uterine contraction efficiency and reduces the incidence of fetal distress and neonatal asphyxia. The squatting position for labour and delivery has a number of additional advantages: it enlarges the pelvic outlet, allows freedom to shift weight comfortably, may enhance the urge to push and hasten descent of the head and may relieve backache. The hands and knees position appears to relieve backache, aids rotation and descent and causes less perineal trauma.

- Current practice recommends that directed pushing should be abandoned and women should be encouraged to follow their instincts. The midwives' role should be to affirm physiology, not control it or deny it, and to encourage women-centred approaches which promote normality.

- Perineal lacerations may occur during the 2nd stage of labour. Labial lacerations are not usually severe enough to require suturing but can be painful during micturition. Vaginal and cervical lacerations may bleed severely and may need to be sutured immediately to control bleeding.

- The rationale for the incision of an episiotomy is to enlarge the vulval outlet immediately before delivery.

Fetal reasons are the only justification for performing an episiotomy. During the antenatal period, women should be given a chance to discuss the possible need for an episiotomy.

- Perineal repair is an integral part of the midwife's role. It is most important to explore the depth of the wound and ensure that the first suture is placed above its apex to prevent the development of a vaginal haematoma. The perineum is then sutured in layers from the inside tissues outwards with a continuous subcuticular method of suturing using polyglycolic sutures such as Vicryl or Dexon.

References

Aderhold K J, Roberts J E 1991 Phases of second stage labor: four descriptive case studies. Journal of Nurse-Midwifery 36(5):267–275.

Bassell G M, Humayun S G, Marx G F 1980 Maternal bearing-down efforts – another fetal risk? Obstetrics and Gynaecology 5(1):39–47.

Beynon C 1957 The normal second stage of labour. Journal of Obstetrics and Gynaecology of the British Commonwealth 64(6):815–820.

Caldeyro-Barcia R 1979 The influence of maternal bearing-down efforts during second stage on fetal well-being. Birth Family Journal 6(1):17–21.

Carroli J, Belizan J 2002 Episiotomy for vaginal birth. Cochrane Review: In The Cochrane Library, Issue 1. Update Software, Oxford.

Chamberlain G, Drife J 1995 What is a prolonged second stage of labour? Contemporary Review of Obstetrics and Gynaecology 7:69–70.

Crawford J S 1983 The stages and phases of labour: an outworn nomenclature that invites hazard. Lancet 321:271–272.

Cunningham F G, MacDonald P C, Leveno K J et al 2001 Williams Obstetrics, 21st edn. Prentice-Hall International, New Jersey.

Edwards N P 1995 Birthing your baby the second stage. Association for Improvements in the Maternity Services (AIMS).

Enkin M, Kierse M J N C, Nielson J et al 2000 A Guide to Effective Care in Pregnancy and Childbirth, 3rd edn. Oxford University Press, Oxford.

Goldberg J, Holtz D, Hyslop J 2002 Episiotomy rates. Obstetrics and Gynaecology 99:(3).

Gupta J, Nikodem V 1999 Women's position during second stage of labour. Cochrane Review: In The Cochrane Library, Issue 1. Update Software 2003, Oxford.

Hillan E M 1999 Physiology and management of the second stage of labour. In Bennett V R, Brown L K (eds) Myles Textbook for Midwives, 13th edn. Churchill Livingstone, Edinburgh.

Kettle C, Johanson R 2001a Continuous versus interrupted sutures for perineal repair. Cochrane Review: In The Cochrane Library, Issue 3. Update Software 2002, Oxford.

Kettle C, Johanson R 2001b Absorbable synthetic versus catgut suture material for perineal repair. Cochrane Review: In The Cochrane Library, Issue 3. Update Software 2002, Oxford.

Low L, Seng J, Murtland T et al 2000 Clinical-specific episiotomy rates: impact on perineal outcomes. Journal of Midwifery and Woman's Health 45(2):87–93.

Paine L L, Tinker D D 1992 The effect of maternal bearing-down efforts on arterial umbilical cord pH and length of the second stage of labor. Journal of Nurse-Midwifery 37(1):61–63.

Piquard F, Hsiung R, Schaefer A et al 1988 The validity of fetal heart rate monitoring during the second stage of labor. Obstetrics and Gynaecology 72(5):746–751.

Piquard F, Schaefer A, Hsiung R et al 1989 Are there two biological parts in the second stage of labor? Acta Obstetrica and Gynaecologica Scandinavica 68:713–718.

Saunders N, St G, Paterson C M, Wadsworth J 1992 Neonatal and maternal morbidity in relation to the length of the second stage of labour. British Journal of Obstetrics and Gynaecology 99:381–385.

Simkin P, Ancheta R 2000 The Labour Progress Handbook. Blackwell Science, Oxford.

Sleep J 1984a Episiotomy in normal delivery 1. Nursing Times 80(47):29–30.

Sleep J 1984b Episiotomy in normal delivery 2: the management of the perineum. Nursing Times 80(48):51–54.

Sweet B R 1997 The pelvic floor and its injuries. In Sweet B R, Tiran D (eds) Mayes Midwifery: A Textbook for Midwives, 12th edn. Baillière Tindall, London.

Thomson A M 1988 Management of the woman in normal second stage of labour: a review. Midwifery 4:77–85.

UKCC 1998 Midwives Rules and Code of Practice. United Kingdom Central Council, London.

Walsh D 2000 Evidence based care series 8: perineal care should be a feminist issue. British Journal of Midwifery 8(12):731–737.

Watson V 1994 Maternal position in the second stage of labour. Modern Midwife 4(7):21–24.

Westcott V P 1984 The revolution starts here. Mother and Baby April:19–23.

WHO 1996 Care in normal birth: a practical guide. Report of a technical working group, Maternal and Newborn Health/Safe Motherhood Unit. World Health Organisation, Geneva.

Annotated recommended reading

Edwards N P 1995 Birthing your baby the second stage. Association for the Improvement in the Maternity Services (AIMS).
In this article Edwards outlines the physiological principles which should underlie the management of the second stage of labour.

Enkin M, Kierse M J N C, Nielson J et al 2000 A Guide to Effective Care in Pregnancy and Childbirth, 3rd edn. Oxford University Press, Oxford.
This is a well-written book that covers 'effective care in pregnancy and childbirth'. It provides a research-based resource.

Chapter **40**

The third stage of labour

INTRODUCTION

The third stage (3rd stage) of labour begins with the completion of delivery of the fetus and ends with the control of bleeding. During this time period vigilance is required as there are emergencies which may arise to threaten the health and life of the mother. An understanding of the normal physiology allows choice between the physiological management and active management of the 3rd stage and minimises the risk of complications by preventative treatment and rapid emergency treatment if necessary.

PHYSIOLOGY OF THE THIRD STAGE OF LABOUR

The 3rd stage of labour begins immediately following the birth of the baby. During the 3rd stage, separation and expulsion of the placenta and membranes occurs and bleeding from the placental site is minimised. This stage is most hazardous for the mother because of the risk of haemorrhage and other complications to be discussed in Chapter 45. The physiological 3rd stage normally lasts from 5 to 30 min but may take up to an hour. During the second stage of labour, the uterus is steadily emptied, accompanied by accelerated myometrial contraction and retraction.

Separation of the placenta

Separation of the placenta usually begins with the contraction that delivers the baby's body (Fig. 40.1). The placental site begins to diminish in size and the placenta is compressed so that blood in the intervillous spaces is forced back into the spongy layer of the decidua. Retraction of the oblique muscle fibres constricts the blood vessels supplying the placenta so that the blood cannot drain into the maternal vascular tree. The uterine vessels become tense and congested and burst, so that a small amount of blood collects between the spongy layer of the decidua and the maternal surface of the placenta, stripping it from its attachment.

The non-elastic placenta is detached from the uterine wall. Separation normally begins from the centre of the placenta so that no blood escapes and a retroplacental clot forms. This

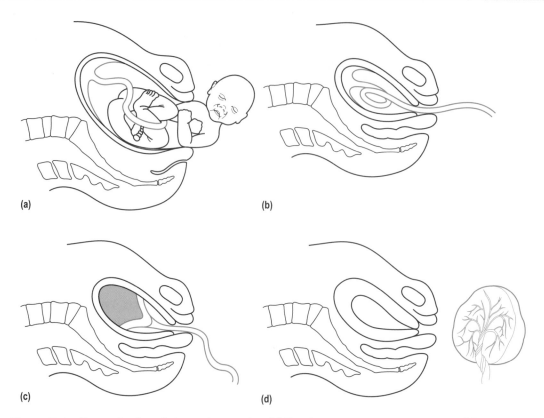

Figure 40.1 The mechanism of placental separation. (a) The placenta before the child is born. (b) The placenta partially separated immediately after the birth of the child. (c) The placenta completely separated. (d) The placenta expelled and the uterus strongly contracted and retracted (from Sweet B 1997, with permission).

probably provides a third means of separation of the placenta as the developing blood clot increases pressure and helps to strip the adherent lateral borders. The weight of the placenta strips the membranes off the uterine wall and the placenta descends fetal side first, enclosing the blood clot in a complete bag of membranes into the vagina and out of the body. **Schultze** described this method of separation and generations of midwifery students have referred to this method as 'shiny Schultze' referring to the glistening appearance of the fetal surface of the placenta.

There is an alternative mechanism of placental separation which begins unevenly at one of the lateral borders. Blood escapes from behind the placenta so that there is no formation of a retroplacental clot. The placenta folds in on itself with the maternal surface outwards and descends edge-on to appear maternal surface first. It is accompanied by a fluid blood loss which the inexperienced may perceive as the onset of a postpartum haemorrhage. This process takes longer and there is more risk of incomplete expulsion of the membranes, often referred to as ragged membranes. This process was first described by **Matthews and Duncan** and has been called 'dirty Duncan' as an *aide-mémoire*.

Control of bleeding

Once separation is complete, the uterus contracts strongly (Fig. 40.2) and the placenta and membranes fall into the

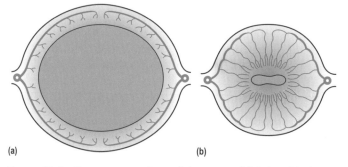

Figure 40.2 Transverse sections of the uterus. (a) Relaxed before the third stage. (b) Contracted and retracted after the third stage – blood vessels are compressed and bleeding arrested (from Sweet B 1997, with permission).

lower uterine segment and then into the vagina. It is important to remember that at least 500 ml/min of blood flows through the placental site. This flow must be stopped in seconds to prevent serious haemorrhage. Three factors are involved in the process:

- The tortuous uterine blood vessels are surrounded by the oblique muscle fibres, which retract and act as 'living ligatures' (Fig. 40.3).

- Once the placenta has left the upper segment, a vigorous contraction brings the walls of the uterus in opposition, applying pressure to the placental site.

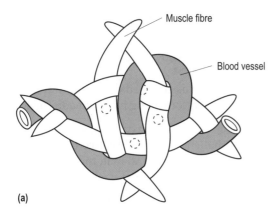

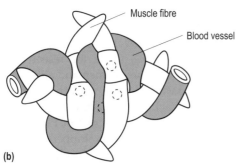

Figure 40.3   How the blood vessels run between the interlacing muscle fibres of the uterus. (a) Muscle fibres relaxed and blood vessels not compressed. (b) Muscle fibres contracted, blood vessels compressed and bleeding arrested (from Sweet B 1997, with permission).

- There is a transitory increase in the activity of the coagulation system during and immediately after placental separation so that clot formation in the torn blood vessels is maximised. The placental site is rapidly covered by a fibrin mesh.

- Putting the baby on the breast will help achieve placental separation by causing a release of oxytocin from the maternal posterior pituitary gland.

MANAGEMENT OF THE THIRD STAGE OF LABOUR

The management of the 3rd stage of labour should be based on an understanding of the physiological process: for at least the last decade there has been as much discussion on the method of management of the 3rd stage of labour. The argument centres on the benefits of **active management** versus **physiological management** (also known as expectant or conservative management) of the 3rd stage. Active management involves using a prophylactic oxytocic drug followed by controlled cord traction (CCT) (Fig. 40.4) to control the length of the 3rd stage and lessen the amount of bleeding. **Physiological management** involves letting nature take its course, as described above; it involves a 'hands off approach', waiting for signs of placental separation and allowing the placenta to deliver spontaneously (possibly aided by gravity

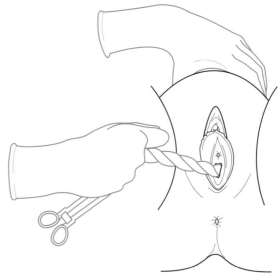

Figure 40.4   Controlled cord traction (from Sweet B 1997, with permission).

and nipple stimulation). The placenta and membranes are expelled by maternal effort but carefully grasped by the midwife to avoid retention of placental tissue or membranes.

The development and use of oxytocic drugs to manage the third stage of labour

There has been a great deal of debate over the last decade about the optimum method for the safe expulsion of the placenta after childbirth (Anderson 2003). Active versus physiological management remains a controversial issue. Begley (1990) reminded us that in the first half of this century postpartum haemorrhage (PPH) was a major cause of maternal death, with figures between 8% and 22%, depending on when and where the statistics were gathered. Increased availability of blood transfusions, the role of better antenatal care and nutrition in the prevention of anaemia and improved general health of women in Westernised countries reduced this to between 4 and 7% by 1978. However, PPH still remains the commonest cause of maternal mortality in the world (Anderson 2003).

Van Dongen & de Groot (1995) wrote an informative historical paper on the use of ergot alkaloids. The alkaloid used in the management of the 3rd stage, ergometrine, was first isolated in 1932 and was synthesised in 1938. They stated that the World Health Organisation (WHO) in 1989 estimated that of 500 000 women (half a million) who die because of pregnancy and childbirth, PPH is one of the most common causes, accounting for 13% of maternal deaths in developed countries but 33% of deaths in developing countries. Latest WHO statistics (1998) show that nearly 600 000 women die every year from complications of pregnancy and childbirth: 99% of these deaths occur in developing countries and 25% of all deaths are as a result of PPH.

The first routine use of intramuscular (i.m.) ergometrine 0.5 mg was in 1951 and it was given as the head crowned.

This shortened the 3rd stage of labour and reduced blood loss in all deliveries but, more significantly, it reduced the incidence of PPH. However van Dongen & de Groot also mention that oxytocin is as efficient as ergometrine without its dangers. The risks associated with the administration of ergometrine are severe hypertension, nausea and vomiting, and side-effects due to vasoconstriction. Maternal deaths have occurred following its administration and for these reasons the writers considered that the administration of oxytocin may be safer.

Begley (1990), cited Embrey et al (1963), who compared the use of i.m. ergometrine with i.m. Syntometrine, a product combining ergometrine and Syntocinon (oxytocin), and this rapidly became the drug of choice in Britain (Fig. 40.5). During the 1980s women were better nourished, younger, of less parity and less anaemic than their mothers had been. They were also better informed and aware of the trend towards natural childbirth. It became part of the birth plan of many women to request that these oxytocic drugs should be omitted in the 3rd stage of labour unless thought necessary in an emergency. This led to a series of trials over recent years to ascertain the safety of this practice, which was named physiological management of the 3rd stage of labour.

In 1987 Gilbert et al wrote a paper on the incidence and effect of PPH. They compared 86 women who had a PPH with 351 women whose blood loss at delivery was less than 350 ml and found risk factors of primiparity, induction of labour, forceps delivery, prolonged first and second stages of labour and the administration of oxytocin rather than Syntometrine. Epidural analgesia was an associated factor. They concluded that, 'Changes in labour ward practices over the last 20 years have resulted in the re-emergence of PPH as a significant problem'. In particular they, mentioned induction of labour, epidural analgesia and acceptance of a prolonged second stage as factors increasing the risk of PPH.

Active versus physiological management

In November 1988 Prendiville et al reported on a major trial, called the Bristol Third Stage Trial. The rationale was the challenge of routine obstetric procedures and their effects on the natural process of labour. Inch (1985) had suggested that routine management of the 3rd stage of labour led to a 'cascade of intervention', leading to controlled cord traction, because:

- women were delivered of their placentas without the aid of gravity;
- the umbilical cord is clamped early and routinely;
- a prophylactic oxytocic drug has been administered.

In particular, the use of oxytocics, usually i.m. Syntometrine, was challenged. The objective of the trial was to compare the effects on fetal and maternal morbidity of routine active management of the 3rd stage of labour and expectant (physiological) management, in particular to determine whether active management reduced the incidence of PPH. There were 1695 women of 4709 delivered between 1 January 1986 and 31 January 1997 included in the trial. They were allocated randomly to physiological management (849) and active (846) management.

After 5 months, a high level of PPH in the physiological group (16.5% versus 3.8%) made the researchers modify the protocol to exclude more women and allow those in the physiological group who needed some active management to be switched to fully active management. The physiological group continued to show a high rate of PPH and after the first 1500 deliveries the study was stopped.

Following criticism of their protocol, Prendiville et al (1998) reanalysed their results to exclude the risk categories mentioned in the Gilbert et al (1987) paper. They found that active management of the 3rd stage was preferable regardless of these first and second stage criteria. However, they also considered the effect of familiarity with the techniques of physiological management and also that midwives may find physiological management less acceptable because of their knowledge of the risks. They also considered the fact that women would have had no antenatal preparation for the maternal effort required. The main conclusion of the trial was still that active management of the 3rd stage of labour was justified.

Harding et al (1989) commented on the views of midwives and mothers participating in the trial and found that both mothers and midwives commented unfavourably about the length of the 3rd stage when it was managed physiologically. They were in favour of continuing the current practice of active management.

Following the Bristol Trial, a further study was set up, named the Dublin Trial. Begley (1990) gave the opposite point of view in a report of the findings of this randomised controlled trial of 1429 women, which compared active management of the 3rd stage of labour using i.v. ergometrine 0.5 mg with physiological management of women who had a low risk of PPH. The trial found that the use of ergometrine was associated with complications such as a greater need for manual removal of placenta, nausea, vomiting and severe afterpains, hypertension and secondary PPH. Although the incidence of PPH and postnatal Hb of less than 10 g/dl was higher in the physiologically managed group, there was no difference in the need for blood transfusion. The discussion stated that there was no need to use i.v. ergometrine in

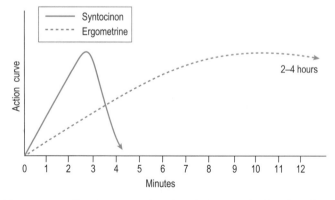

Figure 40.5   Graph representing the relative speeds of action of the drugs syntocinon and ergometrine.

women at low risk for PPH and, in fact, more complications occurred because of its administration.

Thilaganathan et al (1993) reported on a further randomised controlled trial of active versus physiological management of the 3rd stage, called the Brighton Trial. Randomisation was achieved by consecutively numbered sealed envelopes and, like the other two trials, there were some postrandomisation withdrawals due to circumstances such as retained placenta. The high-risk categories were grand multiparity, previous PPH, previous caesarean section, pregnancy-induced hypertension, antepartum haemorrhage and premature rupture of the membranes. Women who had previously consented and who presented in spontaneous labour between 37 and 42 weeks of gestation were admitted to the trial. Women who then required augmentation of labour, operative delivery, cervical laceration or 3rd-degree tear during delivery were withdrawn from the trial. It was found that active management of the third stage of labour reduces the length of the 3rd stage of labour but may not reduce blood loss when compared to physiological management in women at low risk of PPH.

Rogers et al (1998) reported on the findings from the Hinchingbrooke Randomised Controlled Trial comparing active management with physiological management of 3rd stage of labour. This trial was conducted to address those issues related to outcomes about 3rd stage that had not been answered by either the Bristol or Dublin trial. Active management included i.m. Syntometrine (or Syntocinon for women with hypertension) within 2 min of birth, immediate cord clamping and cutting of the cord and delivery of the placenta by maternal effort or CCT. Physiological management involved no administration of a prophylactic drug, the cord was left intact until pulsation ceased and the placenta was delivered by maternal effort. Women ($n = 1512$) were recruited to the trial if deemed to be low risk for PPH. Information was collected immediately after birth and up to 6 weeks postpartum and included subjective information from mothers. Midwives in this trial were already experienced in the practice of both active and physiological management.

Results indicated that women who received physiological management had a PPH rate 2.5 times greater than women who were actively managed. There was more chance of these women requiring blood transfusion and the average length of 3rd stage was 15 min compared with 8 min in the actively managed group who were also noted to have raised number of side-effects. Women in the physiological group were three times more likely to make positive comments. Positive comments related to feelings of achievement, and negative comments were related to the extra length of time.

Prendiville et al (2000) compared active versus expectant management of the 3rd stage of labour in a systematic review of the four main trials above. They conclude that routine active management of the 3rd stage is superior to expectant (physiological) management in terms of blood loss, PPH and other serious complications of the 3rd stage. However, they found that active management was associated with unpleasant side-effects such as nausea and vomiting. They

suggest that active management should be the routine management of choice for women expecting to deliver a baby by vaginal delivery in a maternity unit. The implications were found to be less clear for other birth settings, including domiciliary deliveries, developing countries and units where expectant management is the usual practice.

Syntometrine versus oxytocin

McDonald et al (1996) carried out a systematic review of six randomised controlled trials to compare the use of oxytocin and Syntometrine as prophylactic oxytocic drugs used in the active management of 3rd stage of labour. They concluded that the use of the combination preparation Syntometrine (oxytocin and ergometrine) was associated with a statistically significant reduction in the risk of PPH compared with oxytocin (5 units), but was found to be less so when 10 units were administered. No difference was found in relation to blood loss of greater than 1000 ml. Syntometrine was associated with adverse side-effects, including nausea, vomiting, raised blood pressure and a higher rate of retained placenta.

Examination of the placenta

- The placenta and membranes should be examined as soon as possible after delivery (Fig. 40.6):
  1. To see whether or not the placenta and membranes have been completely delivered.
  2. To detect abnormalities which might provide information about any intrauterine problems. This may be of help in planning neonatal care.
- Gloves should be worn to prevent the transmission of bloodborne diseases such as hepatitis or HIV. The placenta

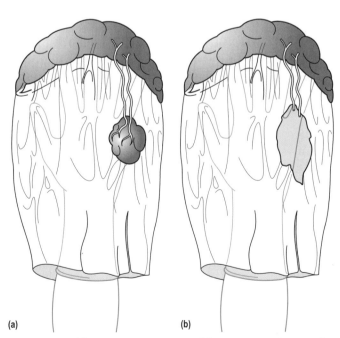

(a)   (b)

Figure 40.6   (a) Succenturiate placenta. (b) The torn membrane – the missing lobe is in the uterus (from Sweet B 1997, with permission).

should be held up by the cord top to inspect the membranes for completeness. There should be a single hole through which the fetus was delivered.

- The amnion is stripped back from the chorion to the cord insertion to ensure that both membranes are present.
- The maternal surface of the placenta should be examined to make sure all the lobes are present. Any abnormalities such as infarctions should be noted.
- The number of cord vessels should be ascertained. The absence of one of the umbilical arteries is sometimes associated with renal agenesis.
- Blood loss is measured and added to the estimated loss present in the bed linen and pads. A blood loss of more than 500 ml is considered to be a PPH and should be reported to the obstetric team.

- Cord blood should be taken when the mother's blood group is rhesus negative, where antibodies have been found in maternal blood and for haemoglobinopathy investigations.

The midwife should remain with the woman for at least 1 hour following completion of the delivery, whether this is in the maternity unit or the mother's home. The uterus should now be palpated gently to ensure that it remains well contracted. The mother's temperature, pulse and blood pressure are taken and recorded. Her lochia are inspected and she is encouraged to pass urine. An all-over wash, clean clothing and refreshment will be appreciated. Immediate care of the baby and the role of parenting will be discussed in other chapters.

MAIN POINTS

- In the 3rd stage of labour separation and expulsion of the placenta and membranes occurs and bleeding from the placental site is minimal. It begins immediately following the birth of the baby and normally lasts from 5 to 30 min but may take up to an hour.

- The placental site begins to diminish in size and the placenta is compressed so that blood in the intervillous spaces is forced back into the spongy layer of the decidua. Retraction of the oblique muscle fibres constricts the blood vessels supplying the placenta, preventing blood from draining into the maternal vascular tree. The uterine vessels become tense and congested and burst so that a small amount of blood collects between the spongy layer of the decidua and the maternal surface of the placenta, detaching it from the uterine wall.

- Separation normally begins from the centre of the placenta so that no blood escapes and a retroplacental clot forms. This probably provides a third means of separation of the placenta as the developing blood clot increases pressure and helps to strip the adherent lateral borders and the membranes.

- There is an alternative mechanism of placental separation which begins at one of the lateral borders. Blood escapes from behind the placenta so that there is no formation of a retroplacental clot. The placenta folds in on itself, with the maternal surface outwards, and descends

edge on to appear maternal surface first accompanied by blood.

- Three factors are involved in haemostasis: the action of the living ligatures; the walls of the uterus applying pressure to the placental site; and a transitory increase in the activity of the coagulation system.

- Active management involves using a prophylactic oxytocic drug followed by controlled cord traction to control the length of the 3rd stage and lessen the amount of bleeding. Physiological management involves a 'hands-off approach', waiting for signs of placental separation and allowing the placenta to deliver spontaneously (possibly aided by gravity and nipple stimulation).

- Routine active management is superior to expectant (physiological) management in terms of blood loss, postpartum haemorrhage and other serious complications of the 3rd stage. However, active management is associated with side-effects such as nausea and vomiting.

- The placenta and membranes should be examined following delivery. This is required to identify complete or incomplete delivery of the placenta and membranes and to detect abnormalities.

- The midwife should check that the uterus is well contracted and that lochia are minimal. Blood pressure, pulse and temperature are checked and recorded. An all-over wash, clean clothing and refreshment will be appreciated.

References

Anderson T 2003 Active versus expectant management of the third stage of labour – A Cochrane database review. In Wickham S (ed.) Midwifery: Best Practice. Elsevier, London.

Begley C M 1990 A comparison of active and physiological management of the third stage of labour. Midwifery 6:3–17.

Gilbert L, Porter W, Brown V A 1987 Postpartum haemorrhage – a continuing problem. British Journal of Obstetrics and Gynaecology January 94:67–71.

Harding J E, Elbourne D R, Prendiville W J 1989 Views of mothers and midwives participating in the Bristol Randomised Controlled Trial of Active Management of the Third Stage of Labor. Birth 16(1):1–6.

Inch S 1985 Management of the third stage of labour – another cascade of intervention? Midwifery 1:114–122.

McDonald S, Prendiville W, Elbourne D 2002 Prophylactic syntometrine versus oxytocin for delivery of the placenta. Cochrane Review: In The Cochrane Library, Issue 1. Update Software 2003, Oxford.

Prendiville W J, Harding J E, Elbourne D R et al 1988 The Bristol Third Stage Trial: active versus physiological management of the third stage of labour. British Medical Journal 297:1295–1230.

Prendiville W J, Elbourne D R, McDonald S 2000 Active versus expectant management of the third stage of labour. Cochrane Review: In The Cochrane Library, Issue 4. Update Software 2002, Oxford.

Rogers J, Wood J, McCandlish R et al 1998 Active versus expectant management of the third stage of labour: The Hinchingbrooke Randomised Controlled Trial. Lancet 351:693–699.

Thilaganathan B, Cutner A, Latimer J et al 1993 Management of the third stage of labour in women at low risk of postpartum haemorrhage. European Journal of Obstetrics & Gynaecology and Reproductive Biology 48:19–22.

Van Dongen P W J, de Groot A N J A 1995 History of ergot alkaloids from ergotism to ergometrine. European Journal of Obstetrics & Gynaecology and Reproductive Biology 60:109–116.

World Health Organisation (WHO) 1998 Press release WHO/33, World Health Day highlights scandal of 600 000 maternal deaths each year.

Annotated recommended reading

Prendiville W J, Elbourne D R, McDonald S 2000 Active versus expectant management of the third stage of labour. Cochrane Review: In The Cochrane Library, Issue 4. Update Software 2002, Oxford.
This is an updated review of active versus physiological management of the third stage of labour, and is essential reading for evidence-based intrapartum care.

Yuen P M, Chan N S T, Yim S F et al 1995 A randomised double blind comparison of Syntometrine and Syntocinon in the management of the third stage of labour. British Journal of Obstetrics and Gynaecology 102:277–380.
In this article Yuen et al compared the effectiveness of Syntometrine and Syntocinon and concluded that Syntometrine was the drug of choice as it was more effective than Syntocinon.

Section 3B

LABOUR PROBLEMS

SECTION CONTENTS

Although the majority of labours progress normally, problems may present at the onset or develop rapidly within labour that are life threatening to both mother and fetus. The knowledge and experience required to recognise these problems and to summon help from the obstetric team is vital to the midwife. This section is concerned with abnormal labour. Traditionally, these problems can be grouped as the effects of the 'powers, passenger and passages' on the progress of labour. Chapter 41 examines the 'powers' and presents the problems of abnormal uterine action in detail. The following two chapters discuss problems with the 'passenger', i.e. the fetus. Chapter 42 is concerned with breech presentation, while Chapter 43 discusses all other abnormal positions and presentations. Except in extreme cases, it is artificial to discuss problems with the 'passages' as these almost always relate to the size, position and presentation of that particular fetus. However, Chapter 44 is concerned with cephalopelvic disproportion. The placenta and membranes are part of the passenger and problems with their delivery are considered in Chapter 45. Chapter 46 is about perinatal fetal asphyxia and sits at the junction between labour and neonatal care. Finally, Chapter 47 looks at operative procedures such as delivery by forceps, vacuum extraction and caesarean section.

Chapter 41

Abnormalities of uterine action and onset of labour

INTRODUCTION

The length of labour is variable and is affected by the type of uterine contractions, parity, birth interval, psychological state, presentation, position, pelvic shape and size of the fetus. This chapter will discuss abnormalities of uterine action. Each of these factors must be considered in turn over the next few chapters, although in practice there may be interaction between them. This chapter on abnormal uterine action will include active management of labour. The association between the pattern of contractions and the progress of labour is highly variable and the outcome difficult to predict. Abnormal uterine action may be inefficient, resulting in prolongation of labour, or overefficient, resulting in precipitate labour.

Normal labour begins spontaneously at term, i.e. after 37 completed weeks and before 42 completed weeks of pregnancy. The contractions increase in length, strength and frequency, resulting in progressive descent of the fetus and dilatation of the cervical os until the fetus, placenta and membranes are expelled from the uterus and bleeding is controlled. Normal labour is also characterised by harmonious interaction between the two poles of the uterus: the upper uterine segment contracts and retracts and the lower uterine segment thins out and the cervix dilates. A retraction ring forms between the two.

ABNORMALITIES OF UTERINE ACTION

Prolonged labour

The first stage of labour can be described as having latent, active and deceleration phases. During the latent phase, the uterus contracts regularly and the cervix effaces and dilates. The latent phase lasts until cervical dilatation is about 3–4 cm and can take 6–8 h in a primigravida and the active phase with rapid dilatation of the cervix is at about 1 cm/h in a primigravida and 1.5 cm/h in a multigravida. Defining the term 'prolonged labour' is problematic and related to a chosen length, mainly because of a belief that the longer labour lasts, the more danger there is for mother and fetus. It is important to remember that although prolonged labour is common in primigravidae it occurs less often in multigravidae and may be due to obstruction of labour. Rupture of the uterus may follow careless use of oxytocic drugs in a multigravid labour.

There has been a trend to reduce the accepted length of labour in a primigravida over the last 40 years from 24 to 12 h. If the length of the latent phase of the first stage of labour in a primigravida is accepted as 6 h, resulting in a dilatation of 4 cm, and average progress of dilatation up to 10 cm in the active and deceleration phases is 1 cm/h, it is easy to see how 12 h has become the accepted norm. Labour may be prolonged in the latent, active or deceleration phases.

Timing of the onset of labour

A further difficulty is how to define the onset of labour. As discussed in Chapter 36, p. 471, the timing is important as it allows decisions to be made about the progress and ongoing management of labour yet it is difficult to establish with accuracy. Gibb (1988) discusses the concept of **prelabour**, meaning the changes that occur in the last few weeks of pregnancy. It is often difficult to decide when the transition from the painless uterine contractions of prelabour develops into true labour.

Latent or active phase?   There is lack of agreement about whether to count the onset of labour from the onset of the latent phase or the active phase of the first stage of labour (O'Brien 1997). The most frequently used marker for the commencement of labour is the onset of regular rhythmic painful uterine contractions. This is an arbitrary point in time rather than a biologically correct starting point (Enkin et al 2000). Vaginal examination of women at the time of admission demonstrates that the decision to present for admission in labour varies, depending on the advice the woman has been given on recognising the onset of labour and her anxieties and expectations.

Dangers of prolonged labour to the mother and fetus

Maternal risks   The physical effort, pain and anxiety of a prolonged labour result in dehydration, ketosis and tiredness. If this were to be allowed to continue:

- Maternal distress could occur: the temperature, pulse and blood pressure rise; dehydration, oliguria and ketosis develop; and the woman may vomit.
- If the membranes are ruptured, intrauterine infection is a risk.
- If undetected cephalopelvic disproportion is present, the uterus may rupture.
- Other risks include trauma to the bladder, operative interventions and postpartum haemorrhage.

Fetal risks

- Intrapartum hypoxia may cause acidosis, fetal distress, neonatal asphyxia and meconium aspiration, possibly leading to perinatal death.
- Cerebral trauma may occur due to excessive pounding of the fetal head against the bony pelvis or excessive moulding.
- Prolonged rupture of the membranes may result in neonatal infection, e.g. pneumonia.

Inefficient uterine action

Uterine contractions are inefficient if they do not result in dilatation of the cervix. Inefficient uterine action is the commonest cause of abnormal labour in primigravidae. O'Driscoll et al (1993) showed that inefficient uterine action caused delay in 65% of 9018 nulliparous women with prolonged labour. The remaining cases were caused by persistent occipitoposterior position (24%) and cephalopelvic disproportion or CPD (11%) (Malone et al 1996). There is slow progress and the length of labour is prolonged. Inefficiency may be because the contractions are too weak (**hypotonic uterine action**) or because there is loss of coordination between the upper and lower uterine segments (**incoordinate uterine action**).

Hypotonic uterine action

The uterine contractions are weak and short and there is slow dilatation or no dilatation of the cervix. The woman does not find the contractions too painful or distressing. The fetus remains in good condition. If hypotonic contractions occur from the commencement of labour, they are said to be **primary**. The cause of primary hypotonic uterine action is unknown but is more commonly seen in primigravidae. If they begin after a period of normal uterine action, they are said to be **secondary** and there may be abnormalities of labour such as CPD, malposition of the occiput, a malpresentation, maternal dehydration or ketosis. The commencement of epidural analgesia sometimes causes hypotonic uterine action (O'Brien 1997).

Incoordinate uterine action

There is loss of polarity and an increase in resting tone of the uterus. The contractions are frequent and painful and the woman feels pain between contractions. The woman feels the contraction before and after it is palpable abdominally. The cervix dilates slowly or not at all. Placental blood flow is decreased, leading to fetal distress. This type of uterine action is associated with malpositions of the occiput.

Active management of labour

In the 1960s, O'Driscoll introduced active management of labour (AML) for the management of labour in primigravidae

(O'Driscoll et al 1986). There must be accurate diagnosis of the onset of labour with painful uterine contractions and one of the following: complete effacement of the cervix, a show or spontaneous rupture of the membranes (Henderson 1996). Amniotomy is carried out shortly after admission with augmentation of labour with Syntocinon (oxytocin) if there is inadequate progress after 2 h. Some maternity units have a policy of putting up a Syntocinon infusion immediately after amniotomy. All women are given adequate emotional support and ongoing peer review to assess the efficiency and effectiveness of the protocol (Gerhardstein et al 1995, O'Brien 1997).

Augmentation of labour

A Syntocinon infusion is used to manage prolonged labour when progress is slow but otherwise normal. This is acceleration or augmentation of labour. Once delay has been diagnosed and abnormalities of presentation or CPD ruled out, the membranes are ruptured and an intravenous infusion of Syntocinon is commenced to stimulate labour contractions. Any abnormality of fluid and electrolyte balance is corrected and both mother and fetus monitored carefully. Adequate pain relief should be provided. Findings regarding the progress of labour should be recorded graphically on a partogram (Fig. 41.1) so that deviations from normal can be immediately recognised. There should be good psychological support of the woman. This should include explanation of what is happening and reassurance that everything is going as planned.

Reduction of caesarean section births   Gerhardstein et al (1995) discussed the effect of active management of labour on the reduction of caesarean section births (CS) in the USA where the rate of CS has risen dramatically. Their study found that women whose labours had been managed actively had a lower rate of CS than the control group of women who laboured spontaneously. Similarly, Henderson (1996) wrote that CS rates have escalated in all Western countries, reaching 20% of all deliveries in some units in the UK and 25% in the USA. Concern over the increased maternal morbidity and financial cost have led to attempts to reduce the CS rate to that of 5–7% of all births achieved by O'Driscoll and his colleagues in Dublin. Henderson analysed how the Dublin figures had been maintained at the low level despite the noted increase in other countries.

Other factors that could account for the low use of CS included 'an avoidance of innovations seen in most obstetric units in the 1970s and 1980s'. These innovations include low rates of induction of labour and avoidance of electronic fetal monitoring. Henderson quotes Barrett et al (1990), who concluded that 30% of CS performed for fetal distress were unnecessary. AML is a package and it is necessary to examine the individual parts of the package. Henderson concluded 'that research has failed to demonstrate that the two widely used elements of the O'Driscoll protocol, artificial rupture of the membranes and the infusion of oxytocin, reduce the rate of caesarean section'.

Amniotomy   The benefits of intact membranes throughout labour include reduced risk of intrauterine infection and of fetal hypoxia because of less placental compression and less reduction of size of the placental site. Amniotomy is the artificial rupture of the fetal membranes (ARM) that results in drainage of liquor (Shiers 1999). This procedure has been practised for several decades and is usually performed to accelerate labour. Amniotomy may also be done to examine the amniotic fluid for the presence of meconium.

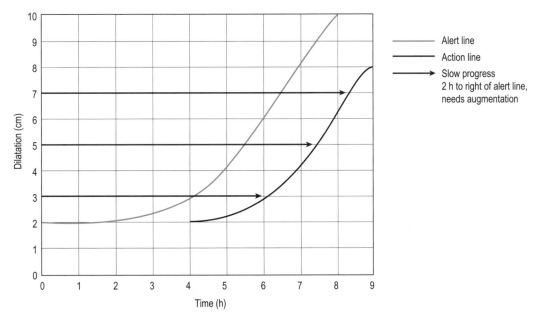

Figure 41.1   Normogram/partogram of cervimetric progress commencing at 2 cm dilatation. 'Alert', line outlines normal progress. 'Action' line indicates when augmentation should be instituted. (After Studd 1973.)

In a systematic review, Fraser et al (1999) studied the effects of amniotomy on the CS rate and other indicators of maternal and neonatal morbidity. They concluded that routine early amniotomy is associated with both benefits and risks. Amniotomy was associated with a reduction in the length of labour by 60–120 min and a possible reduction in abnormal 5-min Apgar scores. The review showed an upward trend in the number of CSs performed and evidence of an increase in fetal heart rate monitoring abnormalities in women following amniotomy. The reviewers suggest that amniotomy should be reserved for use in labours with abnormal labour progress. In similar fashion, O'Brien (1997) believes there should be a clear indication of the need for amniotomy before it is carried out.

Oxytocic infusion O'Brien (1997) reports that the use of oxytocin can be as high as that quoted by O'Driscoll et al (1993) of 45%. As described above, the benefits are correction of inefficient uterine action, a shorter labour, a reduced rate of CS with a corresponding increase in vaginal delivery. Byrne et al (1993) found no evidence that an oxytocic infusion generated excessive intrauterine pressures. However, women experience more painful contractions and are restricted in their ability to move about.

The division of the first stage of labour into latent, active and deceleration phases must be considered as being important to the use and efficacy of oxytocin. Olah et al (1993) found that cervical muscle fibres constrict in response to oxytocin in the latent phase, leading to a poor response; they also described high intrauterine pressures and the possibility of fetal distress, although O'Driscoll et al (1993) found no evidence of this.

Expectations of childbirth have developed and the medicalisation of a normal physiological process was criticised in the 1980s (Walkinshaw 1994). There is now much variation in practice between units and, until recently, maternal satisfaction with delivery has not been considered in research protocols. Enkin et al (2000) summarised the evidence and did not think there was any benefit to women and their babies of liberal use of oxytocic infusions. They concluded that although the use of an oxytocic infusion had its place in the management of women enduring a prolonged labour, other measures such as ambulation and allowing intake of appropriate nutrition should be considered before labelling a labour as abnormal and using medical intervention.

Prolonged second stage of labour

A discussion on the acceptable length of the second stage of labour is presented in Chapter 39. Delayed progress may be due to:

- inefficient uterine action (primary powers);
- inefficient maternal effort (secondary powers);
- a full bladder or rectum, a rigid perineum;
- a contracted pelvic outlet;
- a large baby;

- a fetal abnormality such as hydrocephaly or abdominal enlargement;
- persistent occipitoposterior position;
- deep transverse arrest of the head;
- malpresentation.

Management

The condition of mother and fetus should be carefully assessed and as long as progress is being made, although slowly, more time may be given. Adopting an upright position may enlarge the pelvic outlet and direct the presenting part against the posterior vaginal wall, utilising Ferguson's reflex with the release of oxytocin. If the maternal or fetal condition becomes worrying or there is no obvious progress, an assisted vaginal delivery or, more rarely, a CS may be needed.

Overefficient uterine action

Precipitate labour

A precipitate labour occurs when the uterine contractions occur frequently and are intense. There is rapid completion of the first and second stages of labour and delivery normally occurs within an hour. This condition is much commoner in the multigravid woman and is usually caused by lack of resistance of the maternal soft tissues. There may have been minimal pain in the first stage of labour and the woman becomes aware of imminent delivery when the head is about to be born.

Dangers of precipitate labour The woman may have lacerations to the cervix and perineum. Postpartum haemorrhage may follow. The baby may be hypoxic and may sustain intracranial injuries because of rapid descent through the birth canal. If the birth takes place in an inappropriate place, the baby may fall to the ground and be injured. Any woman with a history of a previous precipitate delivery should be watched very closely when in labour, i.e. should not be left alone at any time while in labour.

Tonic contraction of the uterus

This rare event, where the tone of the uterus is continuously high and there is no relaxation of the uterine muscle, is accompanied by intense pain. The fetus becomes distressed as the placental circulation is grossly restricted. Intrauterine death may occur. Causes may be obstructed labour or misuse of oxytocic drugs such as Syntocinon and prostaglandins. This is an emergency and immediate treatment may save the baby's life and prevent uterine rupture:

- if an oxytocic infusion is in progress, turn it off;
- turn the mother onto her left side to enhance uteroplacental blood flow;
- administer oxygen;
- inform the obstetrician, who will carry out a CS.

Cervical dystocia

Cervical dystocia, where the cervix dilates slowly if at all, may be congenital or acquired. Congenital problems may be fibrosis, stenosis or poor cervical development. Acquired cervical dystocia may be due to fibrosis and scarring of the cervix following surgery, cautery or irradiation. In the past when there was failure to recognise the condition, prolonged pressure would result in ischaemia and there would be annular detachment of the cervix.

If the anterior part of the cervix is trapped between the pelvic brim and the fetal head, venous return is restricted and the anterior lip may become swollen and oedematous and feel as thick as a finger during vaginal examination. The first stage of labour will be prolonged and occasionally the cervix may be seen blue and glistening between the fetal head and the symphysis pubis. The most likely cause is the woman bearing down before full cervical dilatation and it is commonly the result of a persistent occipitoposterior position. If the woman lies on her side and is encouraged to use inhalational analgesia, she will be helped to avoid pushing. Elevating the foot of her bed may also help. Epidural analgesia may occasionally be needed. It is sometimes possible to push an anterior lip of cervix up behind the fetal head but care must be taken not to tear the cervix.

PROBLEMS: TIMING OF THE ONSET OF LABOUR

Preterm onset of labour

Preterm labour is one that begins before the end of the 37th week of pregnancy. A baby born from such a labour is a preterm baby irrespective of birth weight. Not all preterm babies are of low birth weight (LBW), weighing less than 2000 g, but many babies are both preterm and of low birth weight. Babies weighing less than 1500 g are very low birth weight (VLBW), while those weighing less than 1000 g are named extremely low birth weight (ELBW). Preterm babies have different problems and needs to those babies who are of low weight because of growth retardation and the care of the babies will be discussed in the relevant chapter.

Kramer et al (1998) showed that between 1978 and 1996 the incidence of preterm delivery increased from 6.6% to 9.8% for births at less than 37 weeks' gestation, from 1.7% to 2.3% at less than 34 weeks and from 1.0% to 1.2% at less than 32 weeks. To quote Lindsay (1997), 'The incidence of preterm delivery as a proportion of all births ranges from 6 to 10% in developed countries and has changed little over the past 20 years'. Maternal mortality and morbidity is rarely affected by preterm onset of labour (Arias 1993) although women suffer feelings of inadequacy as a result of perceiving themselves to have failed. However, preterm birth is responsible for almost all neonatal deaths not due to congenital malformations and for much morbidity. As gestational age increases, so does the rate of preterm delivery. Less than a quarter of such births occur before 32 weeks.

Aetiology

Preterm births may follow a spontaneous onset of labour or be elective because of a problem for the woman or the fetus. The following conditions may lead to an elective induction of preterm delivery:

- severe pre-eclampsia;
- maternal disease such as renal disease, diabetes mellitus and maternal infection;
- severe intrauterine growth retardation;
- rhesus isoimmunisation;
- premature rupture of the membranes;
- prolapsed cord;
- placental abruption.

In about 40% of cases onset of labour occurs spontaneously with no known cause. Lindsay (1997) summarises the **risk factors** associated with preterm labour (Table 41.1). While not directly causative, they may indicate which women have an increased risk of preterm delivery. Although the above list is comprehensive, it is difficult to predict which woman will begin labour before term. A further problem is that even if the onset of preterm labour could be predicted, it is difficult to prevent the progress to delivery.

As the risk factors are so wide, attempts at reducing some of the physical or social factors have had limited success. Risk-scoring systems have been developed using the above factors but have been found to be poor predictors, especially in primigravid women. Home monitoring of uterine activity has had no effect on the rate of preterm birth. Cervical effacement can be assessed but it is not a good predictor of preterm birth and may also introduce infection.

Fetal fibrinectin   High levels of fetal fibrinectin, a component of the extracellular matrix secreted by the anchoring trophoblastic villi, have been found in cervical and vaginal secretions prior to the onset of preterm labour (Lockwood et al 1991). Separation of maternal and fetal tissue at the choriodecidual junction leads to a leakage of fibronectin and a test has been developed. The test is accurate in up to 80% of cases and can be carried out every 2 weeks after the 24th week of pregnancy. Both blood and amniotic fluid contain fibronectin and this limits the use of the test (Lindsay 1997).

Preterm rupture of the membranes

Spontaneous preterm prelabour rupture of the membranes is associated with cervical incompetence and genital tract infection. Labour may begin soon after the event, but, if delayed, bacteria may ascend the genital tract to colonise the uterus and fetus. The woman must be admitted to a hospital with a neonatal intensive care unit. No vaginal examination is performed in the absence of signs of labour and a speculum examination is carried out to visualise the cervix. A high vaginal swab is taken for culture and sensitivity testing.

Table 41.1 A summary of the risk factors given by Lindsay (1997)

Biological/medical factors	Reproductive history	Current pregnancy	Socioeconomic and psychological (Peacock et al 1995)
Age less than 15 or more than 35 Low body weight (less than 50 kg at conception) History of hypertension, renal disease or diabetes mellitus Cigarette, alcohol or drug use Short interpregnancy interval	History of previous preterm birth Bleeding in previous pregnancy Uterine abnormality Abdominal surgery	Failure to gain weight adequately Bleeding in this pregnancy Retained intrauterine contraceptive device Infections, e.g. pyelonephritis Genital tract infection e.g. bacterial vaginosis (Hillier et al 1995), *Chlamydia*, group B haemolytic streptococcus Fetal problems: multiple pregnancy, fetal malformation, rhesus disease, fetal death, polyhydramnios	Poverty and social deprivation Psychological distress Late antenatal booking and poor attendance for care

The use of drugs in preterm onset of labour and preterm rupture of the membranes

Corticosteroids The risk of hyaline membrane disease for the neonate is high and the steroid dexamethasone is given to the mother to accelerate surfactant production in the lungs. Crowley (1999) has provided an extremely detailed review of the use of corticosteroids prior to preterm delivery, analysing 18 trials and 3700 babies between 1976 and 1995. Her findings were that antenatal administration of corticosteroids to women expected to deliver preterm reduced mortality, respiratory distress syndrome and intraventricular haemorrhage in preterm infants. Crowley concluded that 'every effort should be made to treat women with corticosteroids prior to preterm delivery'. A typical regime is two doses of 12 mg given orally or by intramuscular injection 12 hours apart. The effects of the drug take 24 h and it is effective for up to 7 days.

Antibiotics Chorioamnionitis is the cause of preterm labour in up to 30% of cases. Intra-amniotic infection may exist without a rise in temperature, rise in white cell count, uterine tenderness or fetal tachycardia and the cause is poorly understood (Arias 1993). Preterm labour possibly follows infection because of an increased production of prostaglandin by the decidua and the amnion. Prophylactic use of antibiotics has resulted in the reduction of the risk of preterm delivery occurring within 1 week and the prevention of infection in the mother or baby (Enkin et al 2000).

King & Flenady (2002) completed a systematic review to assess the effects of prophylactic antibiotics administered to women in preterm labour with intact membranes. This involved 7428 women over 11 trials, including the recent large 'Oracle II 2001 trial'. The review failed to demonstrate a clear overall benefit from the use of prophylactic antibiotic treatment for preterm labour with intact membranes on neonatal outcomes. In fact, the review raised concerns about the increased neonatal mortality in those who had received antibiotics. The findings could not currently recommend prophylactic antibiotics for routine practice.

In preterm prelabour rupture of the membranes with clear evidence of infection or vaginal colonisation with pathogenic bacteria, antibiotic therapy is commenced. There is evidence to suggest that routine use of antibiotics in preterm rupture of membranes is associated with a delay in delivery and a reduction in the factors contributing to neonatal morbidity (Kenyon et al 2003).

Tocolytic drugs If preterm labour is diagnosed and the membranes are intact, β-adrenergic drugs such as ritodrine hydrochloride, salbutamol and terbutaline, which relax smooth muscle, may be administered by intravenous infusion. No effect on perinatal mortality has been found but the delay of onset of labour by 48 h gives time for the corticosteroids to be effective (BNF 2003).

These drugs affect all smooth muscle and the woman may suffer side-effects of tachycardia, cardiac dysrrhythmias, palpitations and peripheral vasodilation, resulting in hypotension and flushing (Rang et al 2001). Nausea and muscle tremors can be a problem. Pulmonary oedema may occur because of increased permeability of the alveolar–capillary barrier (Watson & Morgan 1989). There may be stimulation of the renin–aldosterone system, with increased secretion of antidiuretic hormone, leading to fluid retention. No attempt should be made to stop labour if the fetus is more than 34 weeks gestation or is estimated to be more than 2500 g (Pearce 1985).

Prostaglandin synthesis inhibitors such as indometacin may also be used; they block the production of the enzyme endoperoxide synthase, which is responsible for the conversion of arachidonic acid to prostaglandin. Maternal side-effects are nausea, vomiting, diarrhoea, dizziness and headaches. Fetal effects may be premature closing of the ductus arteriosus, right-side heart failure and death in utero. Major et al (1994) found an increased incidence of necrotising enterocolitis in neonates following exposure to indometacin in utero. Indometacin may be the best current tocolytic agent but is not the first choice because of the side-effects on the fetus (Arias 1993).

Calcium channel blockers such as nifepidine inhibit muscle contraction (Marieb 2000). There must be careful observation of mother and fetus because of the side-effects of the drugs, including blood glucose monitoring (RCOG 1994). Delivery is probably inevitable if cervical dilatation progresses to 4 cm or if the membranes rupture.

Labour and delivery

All tocolytic drugs are stopped and careful monitoring of the condition of the woman and her fetus carried out. Analgesic drugs such as pethidine and morphine should be avoided if possible and the preferred methods of pain relief are epidural anaesthesia or Entonox, neither of which affect the fetus adversely. An obstetrician and paediatrician should be present at the delivery and an elective episiotomy performed to reduce pressure on the fetal head and minimise cerebral trauma. Forceps may offer better protection. Some obstetricians prefer to deliver VLBW babies, especially if presenting by the breech, by CS. The cord should be clamped at least 10 cm away from its insertion into the abdominal wall to facilitate care in the neonatal unit. Vitamin K 0.5–1.0 mg is usually given, intramuscularly, to minimise the risk of haemorrhage.

Prolonged pregnancy

A pregnancy is considered to be post-term if the gestational age is accurate and it is prolonged beyond 42 completed weeks (294 days). The risk of prolonged pregnancy is higher in primigravidae, being about 20% higher than in women who have given birth previously. Fetal maturity can be estimated by calculation if the first day of the last menstrual period is known and the woman has a regular cycle.

Abdominal examination is not an accurate way of measuring gestational age. An early ultrasound scan will provide good assessment of fetal age and serial scans later in pregnancy can monitor continuing fetal growth. If the woman has not been seen until late in pregnancy it is possible to find ossification centres by X-ray but this is not reliable as ossification may vary up to 5 weeks between fetuses in late pregnancy. Static maternal weight, abnormal fetal

heart rate patterns and reduced fetal movements may indicate deterioration in fetal condition.

Risk factors

Post-term pregnancy is associated with a higher incidence of perinatal death and congenital malformation. After term, there may be progressive placental insufficiency and perinatal asphyxia is more common. The volume of amniotic fluid may diminish so that oxygen supply may be interrupted during contractions due to compression of the placenta. Meconium staining of the liquor is common, with the risk of meconium aspiration syndrome. Babies born after 42 weeks are more likely to weigh more than 4000 g and the increased size of the fetus may result in shoulder dystocia, accompanied by the typical trauma of brachial and facial palsy and fractured clavicle.

Management of post-term pregnancy

Conservative management of pregnancy is becoming more common if there are no complications. It is possible to monitor the wellbeing of the fetus by cardiotocography, ultrasound measurement of amniotic fluid volume and biophysical profile but there is no evidence that their use improves the outcome for the fetus. Unrestricted breast stimulation and coitus after 39 weeks may decrease the incidence of post-term pregnancy and digital separation of the membranes from the lower pole of the uterus (sweeping the membranes) may also help. Induction of labour after 41 weeks has been shown to lessen the incidence of perinatal death but there is no support for the use of induction of labour in post-term pregnancies before 41 weeks (Enkin et al 2000).

Induction of labour

Induction of labour is defined as an intervention designed to artificially initiate uterine contraction, leading to progressive dilatation and effacement of the cervix and the birth of the baby (National Institute of Clinical Excellence 2001). Induction is carried out for medical or obstetric reasons when it is thought that the health of the mother or fetus would be compromised by the continuation of pregnancy (Table 41.2).

Table 41.2   Some indications for induction of labour

Maternal indications	Fetal indications	Joint indications
Prolonged pregnancy	Placental insufficiency	Preeclampsia
Following spontaneous rupture of membranes	Rhesus isoimmunisation with haemolysis	Placental abruption
Medical conditions such as diabetes mellitus	Intrauterine death	Previous precipitate labour
Poor obstetric history such as a previous stillbirth	Severe congenital abnormalities	An unstable lie
Maternal request for social/psychological reasons		

Table 41.3 Modified Bishop's scoring system

Assessment features	0	1	2	3
Dilatation of the cervix (cm)	0	1–2	3–4	5–6
Consistency of the cervix	Firm	Medium	Soft	–
Length of cervical canal (cm)	>2	1–2	0.5–1	<0.5
Position of cervix	Posterior	Mid	Anterior	–
Station of presenting part related to ischial spines	−3	−2	−1	+1, +2

Contraindications

Contraindications include placenta praevia, CPD, oblique or transverse lie, severe fetal compromise and lack of maternal consent.

Method

Induction should be timed when the presence of favourable factors indicates readiness. The success of induction depends on the state of the cervix (Enkin et al 2000), which can be assessed by the Bishop's scoring system (Table 41.3). The prognosis for induction is good with a score of 6 or more.

Cervical ripening

Prostaglandins There are few oxytocin receptors in the cervix, making oxytocin inefficient at ripening the cervix. There is a high failure of induction, leading to long labours and an increase in the need for CS if the cervix is unfavourable at the commencement of induction. The introduction of vaginal administration of **prostaglandins** (PGE$_2$) or a smaller dose by the endocervical route for cervical ripening has increased the likelihood of a successful induction of labour, leading to spontaneous vaginal delivery within 12–24 h (Enkin et al 2000). However, uterine hypertonus occurs more often among women in whom prostaglandin ripening of the cervix has been used than in those women who received placebo or no prostaglandins. Abnormalities of fetal heart rate are also more likely to occur but neither trend appears to result in an increase in operative delivery (Enkin et al 2000).

Sweeping the membranes Sweeping or stripping of the membranes is a relatively simple technique to perform during vaginal examination. The practitioner's finger is introduced into the cervical os and the inferior pole of the membranes is detached from the lower uterine segment by a circular movement of the finger. This procedure has the potential to initiate labour by increasing local production of prostaglandins. In a randomised controlled trial of 142 nulliparous and multiparous women, membrane stripping was found to be a safe and possibly effective way of avoiding induction by promoting spontaneous onset of labour at term (Berghella et al 1996). In a systematic review of 19 clinical trials, Boulvain et al (2001) concluded that routine sweeping of the membranes from 38 weeks onwards does not seem to produce clinically proven benefits. There is agreement in the literature that a larger trial is necessary to judge the effectiveness of this procedure (Enkin et al 2000).

Amniotomy with or without oxytocin

Rupturing the membranes is a point of no return in obstetric management of labour. Once performed, the risk of intrauterine infection increases with the time interval before delivery. Amniotomy may be used on its own, accompanied by commencement of an oxytocic infusion if contractions do not commence after a few hours, or with the simultaneous commencement of an oxytocic infusion. Syntocinon infusion must be carefully regulated to avoid the complications of hyperstimulation of uterine action and water retention. Amniotic fluid embolism is a rare complication which follows hyperstimulation of uterine action.

Moldin & Sundell (1996) carried out a randomised controlled trial of amniotomy versus amniotomy with oxytocin infusion with 196 participants. All the women had a favourable Bishop's score and were at term with an indication for induction. Group A had the combined induction regime, while group B had amniotomy alone. The addition of an oxytocic drug led to a shorter induction–delivery interval due to a shorter latent phase of labour but no difference in the active phase of labour or the second stage of labour. Of the group B women who had amniotomy alone, 32% eventually received oxytocin although the length of time of oxytocin administration was nearly 5 times less than in group A where oxytocin had been commenced soon after the amniotomy. The authors concluded that the minor differences between the groups justified an individual management policy with attention paid to both the indication for induction of labour and the woman's choice.

MAIN POINTS

- The type of uterine contractions, parity, birth interval, psychological state, presentation and position, pelvic shape and size all affect the length of labour. Each factor must be considered, although there may be interaction between them.

- The first stage of labour can be described as having latent, active and deceleration phases. The term 'prolonged labour' is used because of the belief that the longer labour lasts, the more danger there is for mother and fetus.

- The dangers of prolonged labour to the mother are the physical effort, pain and anxiety, dehydration, ketosis and tiredness. Maternal distress could lead to maternal morbidity and mortality. Risks to the baby include intrapartum acidosis, fetal distress, neonatal asphyxia and meconium aspiration, perinatal death, cerebral trauma and ascending neonatal infections.

- Uterine contractions are inefficient if they do not result in dilatation of the cervix. The commonest cause of abnormal labour in primigravidae is inefficient uterine action due to hypotonic uterine action or incoordinate uterine action. Progress is slow and labour is prolonged. The administration of oxytocin corrects inefficient uterine action and shortens labour. However, women experience more painful contractions and are restricted in their ability to move about.

- Delayed progress in the second stage of labour may be due to inefficient uterine action or inefficient maternal effort, a full bladder or rectum, cephalopelvic disproportion or obstructed labour. Adopting an upright position may enlarge the pelvic outlet and directs the presenting part against the posterior vaginal wall, bringing about increased uterine action.

- In precipitate labour, uterine contractions occur frequently and are intense, delivery occurring within an hour. It is commoner in multigravid women and is usually caused by lack of resistance of the maternal soft tissues. The woman may have lacerations to the cervix or perineum and postpartum haemorrhage may follow. The baby may sustain intracranial injuries.

- Tonic uterine action is usually accompanied by intense pain. The fetus becomes distressed as the placental circulation is grossly restricted and intrauterine death may occur. Causes may be obstructed labour or misuse of oxytocic drugs such as Syntocinon or prostaglandins. Immediate treatment will prevent uterine rupture and save the baby's life.

- If preterm labour is diagnosed and the membranes are intact, tocolytic drugs may be administered. The delay of onset of labour by 48 h gives time for the corticosteroids to be effective in maturation of the fetal lungs. If delivery is inevitable, tocolytic drugs are discontinued. Analgesic drugs such as pethidine and morphine should be avoided if possible. Prophylactic antibiotic therapy is recommended for use in preterm rupture of membranes, as it is associated with a delay in delivery and benefits for neonatal morbidity.

- The introduction of vaginal or endocervical administration of prostaglandins (PGE_2) for cervical ripening has increased the likelihood of a successful induction of labour. Stripping the membranes from the lower uterine segment possibly produces increased amounts of prostaglandin and may be a safe way of avoiding induction by promoting spontaneous onset of labour at term.

References

Arias F 1993 Practical Guide to High Risk Pregnancy and Delivery, 2nd edn. Mosby Year Book, Chicago.

Barrett J F R, Jarvis G J, McDonald N H 1990 Inconsistencies in clinical decisions in obstetrics. Lancet 336:549–551.

Berghella V, Rogers R A, Lescale K 1996 Stripping of membranes as a safe method to reduce prolonged pregnancies. Obstetrics and Gynaecology 87(6):927–931.

Boulvain M, Stan C, Irion O 2001 Membrane sweeping for induction of labour. Cochrane Review: In The Cochrane Library, Issue 4. Update Software 2003, Oxford.

British National Formulary 2003 No 45, March. British Medical Association and the Royal Pharmaceutical Society of Great Britain, London.

Byrne B M, Keane D, Boylan P et al 1993 Intra-uterine pressure and the active management of labour. Journal of Obstetrics and Gynaecology 13:433–436.

Crowley P 1999 Prophylactic corticosteroids for preterm delivery. Cochrane Review: In The Cochrane Library, Issue 2. Update Software 2003, Oxford.

Enkin M, Keirse M J N C, Renfrew M et al 2000 A Guide to Effective Care in Pregnancy and Childbirth, 2nd edn. Oxford Medical Publications, Oxford.

Fraser W D, Turcot L, Krauss I et al 1999 Amniotomy for shortening spontaneous labour. Cochrane Review: In The Cochrane Library, Issue 2. Update Software 2003, Oxford.

Gerhardstein L P, Allswede M T, Sloan C T et al 1995 Reduction in caesarean birth with active management of labor and intermediate-dose oxytocin. Journal of Reproductive Medicine 40(1):4–8.

Gibb D 1988 A Practical Guide to Labour Management. Blackwell Science, Oxford.

Henderson J 1996 Active management of labour and caesarean section rates. British Journal of Midwifery 4(3):132–149.

Hillier S L, Nugent R P, Eschenbach D A 1995 Association between a bacterial vaginosis and preterm delivery of a low birth-weight infant. New England Journal of Medicine 333(26):1736–1742.

Kenyon S, Boulvain M, Neilson J 2003 Antibiotics for preterm rupture of membranes. Cochrane Review: In The Cochrane Library, Issue 2. Update Software 2003, Oxford.

King J, Flenady V 2002 Prophylactic antibiotics for inhibiting preterm labour with intact membranes. Cochrane Review: In The Cochrane Library, Issue 2. Update Software 2003, Oxford.

Kramer M S, Platt R, Yang H et al 1998 Secular trends in preterm birth: a hospital-based cohort study. Journal of the American Medical Association 280:1849–1854.

Lindsay P 1997 Preterm labour. In Sweet B R, Tiran D (eds) Mayes Midwifery: A Textbook for Midwives. Baillière Tindall, London, pp 603–609.

Lockwood C, Senyei A, Dishe M et al 1991 Fetal fibronectin in cervical and vaginal secretions as a predictor of preterm delivery. New England Medical Journal 325(10):669–674.

Major C, Lewis D, Harding J et al 1994 Tocolysis with indomethacin increases the incidence of necrotising enterocolitis in the low weight neonate. American Journal of Obstetrics and Gynaecology 170(1):102–106.

Malone F D, Geary M, Chelmow D et al 1996 Prolonged labor in nulliparas: lessons from the active management of labor. Obstetrics and Gynaecology 88(2):211–215.

Marieb E N 2000 Human Anatomy & Physiology, 5th edn. Benjamin/Cummings, New York.

Moldin P G, Sundell G 1996 Induction of labour: a randomised clinical trial of amniotomy versus amniotomy with oxytocin infusion. British Journal of Obstetrics and Gynaecology 103(4):306–312.

National Institute of Clinical Excellence (NICE) 2001 Clinical Guidelines for Induction of Labour.

O'Brien W 1997 Prolonged labour and disordered uterine action. In Sweet B R, Tiran D (eds) Mayes Midwifery: A Textbook for Midwives, 12th edn. Baillière Tindall, London.

O'Driscoll K, Meagher D, Boylan P 1986 Active Management of Labour, 2nd edn. Mosby, London.

O'Driscoll K, Meagher D, Boylan P 1993 Active Management of Labour, 3rd edn. Mosby, London.

Olah K S J, Gee A, Brown J S 1993 Cervical contractions: the response of the cervix to oxytocic stimulation in the latent phase of labour. British Journal of Obstetrics and Gynaecology 100:535–640.

Peacock J L, Bland J M, Anderson H R 1995 Preterm delivery: effects of socio-economic factors, psychological stress, smoking, alcohol and caffeine. British Medical Journal 311(7004):532–536.

Pearce M J 1985 The management of preterm labour. In Studd T (ed.) The Management of Labour. Blackwell Science, Oxford.

Rang H P (ed.), Dale M, Ritter J M 2001 Pharmacology, 4th edn. Churchill Livingstone, Edinburgh.

RCOG 1994 Guidelines No. 1 – For the Use of Ritodrine. Royal College of Obstetricians and Gynaecologists, London.

Shiers C V 1999 Prolonged pregnancy and disorders of uterine action. In Bennett V R, Brown L K (eds) Myles Textbook for Midwives, 13th edn. Churchill Livingstone, Edinburgh.

Walkinshaw S A 1994 Is routine active intervention in spontaneous labour beneficial? Contemporary Review of Obstetrics and Gynaecology 6(January):13–17.

Watson N, Morgan B 1989 Pulmonary oedema and salbutamol in preterm labour. British Journal of Obstetrics and Gynaecology 96(12):1445–1448.

Annotated recommended reading

National Institute for Clinical Excellence (NICE) 2001 Clinical Guidelines for Induction of Labour.
This document sets out research-based guidelines for induction of labour. It is essential reading for midwives and obstetricians. The reason for inducing labour remains the responsibility of the lead professional caring for the woman.

Shiers C V 1999 Prolonged pregnancy and disorders of uterine action. In Bennett V R, Brown L K (eds) Myles Textbook for Midwives, 13th edn. Churchill Livingstone, Edinburgh.
In this chapter Shiers has written comprehensively about prolonged pregnancy, disorders of uterine action and subsequent management.

Enkin M, Keirse M J N C, Renfrew M et al 2000 A Guide to Effective Care in Pregnancy and Childbirth, 3rd edn. Oxford University Press, Oxford.
This book is based on systematic reviews of care practices carried out in pregnancy and childbirth. It is invaluable to anyone caring for pregnant women and expectant parents.

Chapter **42**

Breech presentation

INTRODUCTION

Any presentation of the fetus other than a vertex is called a **malpresentation**. These include breech, face, brow and shoulder presentations. These presentations have in common an ill-fitting presenting part which may be associated with early rupture of the membranes. There is also the likelihood of poor uterine action, leading to prolongation of labour. Each malpresentation leads to a different mechanism for descent and there may be difficulties in delivery; an understanding of the movements made by the fetus in response to the maternal pelvis will help to prevent injury to the woman or her baby. The risk of morbidity and mortality for the fetus is increased and malpresentations may result in operative delivery. Breech presentation is discussed in this chapter and the other malpresentations in Chapter 43.

BREECH PRESENTATION

Breech presentation is where the lie is longitudinal but the fetal buttocks lie in the lower segment of the uterus. It is found in 3–4% of all deliveries (Enkin et al 2000). One in four fetuses will present by the breech at some stage in pregnancy but as pregnancy progresses spontaneous version to a vertex presentation is likely to occur, especially in multigravidae. Prematurity and multiple pregnancy are the main known causes. Other causes include placenta praevia and uterine or fetal abnormality (Al-Azzawi 1998).

Types of breech presentation

Depending on the relationship of the lower limb to the fetal trunk, four types of breech presentation can be described (Fig. 42.1). This can influence the diagnosis of breech presentation antenatally and the complications likely to occur at delivery:

1. **Complete or flexed breech:** the thighs and knees are flexed and the feet are close to the buttocks (tailor sitting

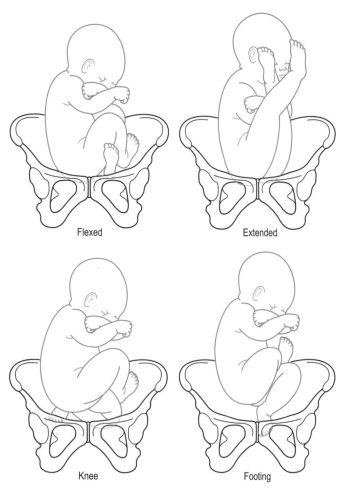

Figure 42.1   Types of breech presentations (from Sweet B 1997, with permission).

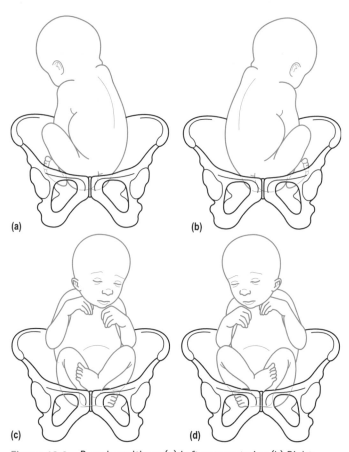

Figure 42.2   Breech positions. (a) Left sacroanterior. (b) Right sacroanterior. (c) Right sacroposterior. (d) Left sacroposterior (from Sweet B 1997, with permission).

or squatting), which occurs in 10–15% and is commonest in multigravidae.

2. **Extended or frank breech:** the fetal thighs are flexed and the legs extended at the knees. The legs lie along-side the trunk with the feet near the head. This is the most common of the four types of breech presentation, occurring in 45–50%, and is seen most commonly in primigravidae near to term. The firm uterine and abdominal muscles prevent fetal movement so that the fetus is unable to flex its knees and there is limited likelihood of a turn to cephalic presentation.

3. **Footling presentation:** one or both hips and knees are extended and the feet present below the buttocks. This rare complication is more common in preterm labour.

4. **Knee presentation:** One or both hips are extended and the knees flexed. The knee(s) present below the but-tocks. This is the least seen of the four presentations.

As in vertex presentations, the baby presenting by the breech can take up different positions (Fig. 42.2).

Aetiology

Many of the causes of persistent breech presentation are associated with conditions which either restrict the move-ment of the fetus or allow excessive movement of the fetus. Others involve the health of the fetus (see Table 42.1).

Diagnosis of breech presentation

On discussion

A past history of a previous breech presentation could sug-gest a uterine anomaly and an increased risk of repeated breech. If the woman complains of discomfort under the ribs it may be due to the presence in the fundus of the hard fetal head. The woman may also be aware of fetal kicking movements below the umbilicus.

On abdominal examination

Findings are:

● **Inspection:** usually reveals nothing unusual.
● **Palpation:** the presenting part feels firm but not hard or smooth. The head may be felt in the fundus, hard, round

Table 42.1 Possible causes of breech presentation

Restricted space	Excessive intrauterine space	Fetal causes
Primigravidae with firm uterine and abdominal muscles	Grande multiparity because of lax uterine and abdominal muscles	Fetal abnormalities
Uterine malformations such as bicornuate uterus	Polyhydramnios	Fetal death in utero
Uterine fibroids		Decreased fetal activity
Contracted pelvis preventing engagement of the presenting part		Impaired fetal growth
Multiple pregnancy		Short umbilical cord
Placenta praevia		
Oligohydramnios		

Box 42.1 Abdominal palpation of breech

Although abdominal examination is the main diagnostic tool it may be difficult to recognise in the primigravid woman with an extended breech. The breech may be deep in the pelvis and simulate an engaged head. The feet lie alongside the head and both prevent the identification by palpation and prevent movement of the head on the neck elicited by ballottment. Finally, if the breech is engaged, the fetal heart may be heard in the expected position for a vertex presentation.

and ballottable. Box 42.1 presents possible findings on abdominal palpation of breech presentation.

- **Auscultation:** fetal heart sounds may be heard above the umbilicus.

On vaginal examination

On vaginal examination, either small parts or the breech itself may be detected. It is essential to distinguish between a hand and a foot if small parts are felt. The breech itself is smooth and rounded and may feel like a vertex.

A vaginal examination will exclude a deeply engaged head either in pregnancy or labour. It is sometimes difficult to differentiate the shoulders, which lie at the level of the pelvic brim, from the breech. The author remembers numerous occasions when he was asked by colleagues to palpate the woman's abdomen as they were concerned that they may have discovered a previously undiagnosed breech presentation. On re-examination, the head was found to be deeply engaged, but in all these circumstances a vaginal examination confirmed cephalic presentation.

Ultrasound scan

Diagnosis in a suspected breech presentation can be made by ultrasound. The fetus should be examined for anomalies at the same time.

Associated risk factors

The increased risk of morbidity and mortality in breech deliveries may be four times that of cephalic presentation but is partly dependent on associated factors. These factors include prematurity, congenital abnormalities, placenta praevia and placental abruption (Enkin et al 2000). Prolapse of the umbilical cord may lead to anoxia and fetal death, as may entrapment of the fetal head behind an incompletely dilated cervix. The woman is also placed at risk because of the possible delivery by caesarean section (CS).

Congenital abnormality

The presence of a congenital abnormality occurs more frequently with a breech presentation than with a vertex. The risk of congenital abnormality may be as high as 15% in babies of less than 1500 g (Arias 1993). The most common major abnormality is a defect of the neural tube such as meningomyelocele, hydrocephaly or anencephaly. Anomalies of the internal systems such as the gastrointestinal, respiratory, cardiovascular and urinary systems are also found. Congenital dislocation of the hip is the most common problem, occurring in three times as many girls as boys.

Risks at delivery

The fetus is at risk from the following:

- **Intrauterine and extrauterine asphyxia,** because of the delay in delivery of the head after the birth of the thorax and arms. Placental separation may occur before the birth is complete and cord compression is inevitable. Hypoxia may stimulate breathing with the inhalation of blood, liquor and mucus.
- **Intracranial haemorrhage,** which used to be thought to be due to rapid compression and decompression of the brain as the head descended through the pelvis, resulting in a torn tentorium cerebelli. However, it is now thought that the main cause of cerebral haemorrhage is anoxia and congestion of the cerebral vessels.

- **Skeletal fractures and dislocations**, damage to muscles and nerves and rupture of abdominal organs due to difficulties arising during delivery or to faulty delivery technique.
- **Genital oedema and bruising**, because of the formation of a caput succedaneum.

MANAGEMENT OF PREGNANCY

Any woman found to have a breech presentation after 32 weeks should be seen by an obstetrician. With her full involvement, a decision needs to be made about the safest option for delivery. An attempt will probably be made to move the fetus to a cephalic presentation to reduce the risks mentioned above.

Cephalic version

Promotion of spontaneous cephalic version

Various exercises and positions have been tried in an attempt to turn a breech. Hofmeyr & Kulier (2001) systematically reviewed the postural techniques 'used by doctors, midwives and birth attendants to promote cephalic version.' The review cited the following five studies involving 392 women:

- **Chenia & Crowther (1987)**, who modified Elkin's procedure asking women to adopt the posture three times a day for 7 days with a full bladder.
- **Bung et al (1987)**, who used a different technique – the 'Indian' version – where women are encouraged to lie down once or twice a day in a supine head-down position with the pelvis supported on a wedge-shaped cushion.
- **Hartadottir & Thornton (1992)**, who carried out a randomised controlled trial with women with a diagnosed breech presentation after 34 weeks. One group were taught how to take up the knee–chest position for 15 min twice a day. The results were compared to a control group of normally managed women.
- **Obwegeser et al (1999)**, who asked women to adopt the supine position with the pelvis elevated by a 30–35 cm cushion for periods of 10 min twice per day.
- **Smith et al (1999)**, who asked women to assume the knee–chest position for 15 min, three times per day for 1 week.

There is insufficient evidence from well-controlled trials to support the use of postural management for breech presentation and larger trials are needed to assess the clinical value of these techniques. However, these exercises do not do any harm and there are no contraindications.

Moxibustion Moxibustion (burning herbs to stimulate acupuncture points) is a traditional Chinese method used to promote version of fetuses in a breech presentation (Enkin et al 2000). In this technique a practitioner inserts and manipulates acupuncture needles. In the heated needle method, the practitioner inserts acupuncture needles, then places small cones of moxa on the needle heads and ignites them. It is a way of applying heat locally to regulate, tone and supplement the body's flow of Qi (vital energy). This method is popular in China and Japan.

Sweet (1997) discusses the findings that 80% of breech presentations after 34 weeks can be corrected by this technique where 'the herb *Artemisia vulgaris* (mugwort) is applied to the B67 acupuncture point at the base of the little toenails twice a day for 5 days' (Budd 1992).

External cephalic version

During external cephalic version (ECV) the fetus is manipulated through the abdominal wall to turn it from a breech to a cephalic presentation (Fig. 42.3). This manual manoeuvre has always been controversial, especially if carried out before 36 weeks. There are risks attached to the procedure of bleeding from the placental site, cord entanglement, causing fetal distress, converting the lie and presentation to an undeliverable one and initiating preterm labour. To reduce these risks to a minimum, the following contraindications are described:

- a history of infertility;
- elderly primigravidae;
- hypertension;
- a rhesus-negative mother;
- cephalopelvic disproportion;
- a uterine scar;
- placenta praevia or placental abruption;
- multiple pregnancy;
- congenital malformations;
- intrauterine fetal death.

The role of ECV in three separate ways was systematically reviewed:

1. external cephalic version before term (Hofmeyr 2001a);
2. external cephalic version at term (Hofmeyr & Kulier 1999);
3. interventions to help external cephalic version at term (Hofmeyr 2001b).

External cephalic version before term does not appear to improve pregnancy outcomes in relation to the incidence of breech presentation, CS, perinatal mortality and Apgar scores below 7 at 1 min. Hofmeyr (2001a) concluded there was no place for the use of ECV before term although its use in spontaneous or induced preterm labour needs to be evaluated.

Hofmeyer & Kulier (1999) found evidence to support the use of attempting external cephalic version at term. This procedure was found to reduce the chance of non-cephalic births and CSs. In individual cases the risk of ECV needs to be weighed against the current and future risks of continued breech presentation to mother and fetus.

The interventions reviewed by Hofmeyr (2001b) for ECV included routine tocolysis, fetal acoustic stimulation, epidural or spinal analgesia and transabdominal amnio-infusion. Tocolysis involves the use of drugs that act as relaxants to the uterine musculature, such as salbutamol and ritodrine, prior to carrying out ECV. Hofmeyr found that routine tocolysis appears to reduce the failure rate of ECV at term. However, there was not enough evidence to evaluate the other types of intervention although some of the findings appeared promising. No randomised trials were found for transabdominal amnioinfusion for ECV at term.

The advantages of delaying ECV until term include:

- the delay will give more time for spontaneous version to occur;
- less reversions to breech presentation;
- a reduction in fetal mortality;
- other pregnancy complications, excluding ECV, may become apparent;
- if complications occur, the fetus is mature enough to be delivered;

- reducing the incidence of breech deliveries;
- reducing the incidence of CS.

Disadvantages are that the membranes may rupture and labour commences before version is attempted.

The procedure for ECV A skilled and experienced practitioner should carry out the procedure. A successful procedure not only depends on the practitioner but also on the position and engagement of the fetus, volume of liquor and maternal parity. The position of the breech should be confirmed by ultrasound scan and the woman should give prior consent for the procedure. The woman should be 'nil by mouth' in preparation for a potential CS after the procedure. A cardiotocography recording of the fetal heart should always be obtained prior to the procedure. The woman should be asked to empty her bladder and she then lies flat on a couch or bed. A tocolytic drug may be used although there is no firm evidence to support the use of these drugs. The obstetrician disimpacts the breech from the pelvis and then, applying pressure to both poles of the fetus, the fetus is then rotated into a cephalic presentation (Fig. 42.3). It is safer

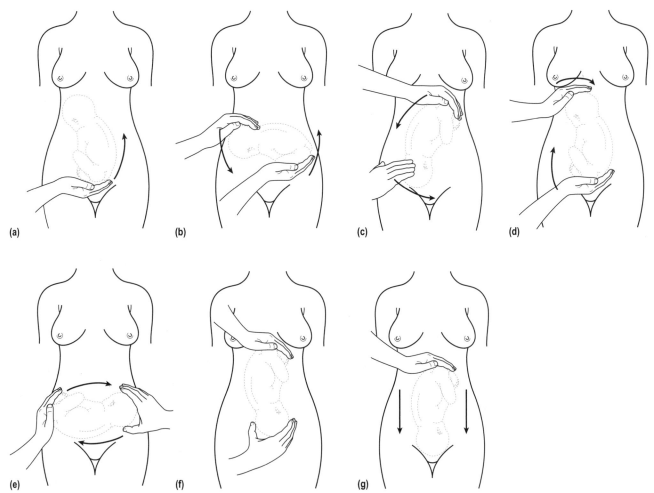

Figure 42.3   External cephalic version. (a) Palpation and mobilization of the breech. (b) Manual forward rotation using both hands, one to push the breech and the other to guide the vertex. (c) Completion of forward roll. (d) Backward flip using both hands, (e) Quarter turn accomplished. Continue to push breech upwards and vertex downward. (f) Completion of external version. (g) Gently push the breech downwards to direct vertex into pelvis (reproduced with permission from Clay et al 1993).

to achieve this by making the fetus turn a forward somersault or to 'follow its nose' as the editor's tutor used to say. A backward somersault may sometimes achieve the version easier but there is a risk of extension of the neck, resulting in a brow presentation. On completion of the manoeuvre, the fetal heart should be recorded for 30 min to ensure there is no fetal distress. Uterine contractions, signs of rupture of the membranes and any vaginal bleeding are watched for and reported to the obstetrician immediately. If the woman's blood group is rhesus negative, she should be given 500 IU of anti-D immunoglobulin after ECV.

The role of planned caesarean section at term

Over the last 25 years it has been accepted that CS should be the mode of delivery for fetuses presenting by the breech but few studies have been carried out to evaluate this use of planned CS. In a systematic review, Hofmeyr & Hannah (2000) suggest that there is not sufficient evidence to evaluate the use of a policy of planned CS for breech presentation. However, a multi-centre international, randomised controlled trial compared elective CS to vaginal delivery for selected breech presentations, including frank or complete breech, greater than 37 weeks gestation and less than 4000 g estimated fetal weight (Hannah 2000, SOGC 2000). The trial was stopped earlier than planned due to preliminary data showing a significant reduction in perinatal mortality and morbidity and no increase in serious maternal complications in the elective CS group (Hannah 2000).

In a study of long-term outcomes of children with breech presentation at term, Danelian et al (1996) reviewed data on preschool children and found that planned delivery by CS was not associated with better long-term outcomes. A handicap rate of 19.4% in 1387 children whose records were available was present in both CS and vaginal delivery groups, suggesting that planned vaginal delivery is as safe as elective CS when long-term outcome is considered. A further problem with more breech babies delivered by CS is that practitioners lose their skills, thus endangering the fetus. What appears to be more certain is the role of elective CS in the delivery of the preterm breech. A trend towards increased risk of neonatal death has been found when the baby weighs less than 1750 g (Kiely 1991) and 1600 g (Gilady & Cols 1996). Babies with birth weights over 3000 g are also at risk.

VAGINAL DELIVERY

In the event of a persistent breech presentation, the following factors are considered prior to vaginal delivery:

- **maternal age and parity** – there is an increased risk of failure with young women with low vaginal parity;
- **period of gestation** – any gestation taking into account the risk factors for the mother;
- the **history** of the present pregnancy – this should be a healthy pregnancy with no obstetric or medical problems;

- **past obstetric history**;
- **size and shape of the pelvis** – should be large enough for the particular fetus;
- the **condition of the fetus**.

There are fundamental differences in delivery between cephalic and breech presentations. With cephalic or vertex presentation, the largest part of the fetus, the head, delivers first. Moulding of the cranium can occur over several hours. In a breech delivery, the breech is first delivered followed by the shoulders and then the head. Each part of the fetus is larger and less compressible than the previous part. The aftercoming head has not had time to mould because it enters the pelvis with the base of the skull leading and this cannot mould (ALSO 2000). In a vaginal breech delivery the biggest challenge is that the head might not fit through the pelvis as it is the last and largest part to deliver.

If women are selected carefully so that the pelvis is of adequate dimensions in relation to the fetus and there are no other adverse factors, they should be able to deliver safely per vaginam. It is essential to understand the mechanism of a breech delivery so that management of the delivery can be completed without trauma. In ideal conditions vaginal breech delivery should be performed by an experienced midwife or under the supervision of a senior obstetrician. A paediatrician should be present at delivery.

Management

The mechanism of a breech delivery

There are six possible positions for a breech delivery. These are right or left sacroanterior, right or left sacroposterior, right or left sacrolateral. The mechanism of the **left sacroanterior position** will be described in full:

- the **lie** is longitudinal;
- the **presentation** is breech;
- the **denominator** is the sacrum;
- the **attitude** is one of complete flexion;
- the **presenting part** is the anterior (left) buttock;
- the **bitrochanteric diameter**, 10 cm, enters the pelvis in the left oblique diameter of the pelvic brim.

The movements

It is necessary to consider the birth of the fetus in three parts: the buttocks, the shoulders and the head.

1. Compaction and flexion Descent takes place with increasing compaction due to increased flexion of the limbs on the trunk.

2. Internal rotation of the buttocks The anterior buttock reaches the pelvic floor and rotates forwards in the pelvis 1/8th of a circle to lie under the symphysis pubis. The bitrochanteric diameter now lies in the anteroposterior diameter of the pelvis.

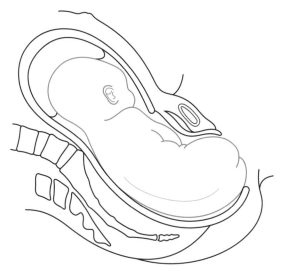

Figure 42.4   Lateral flexion and birth of the buttocks (from Sweet B 1997, with permission).

3. Lateral flexion of the trunk The anterior buttock escapes under the symphysis pubis, the posterior buttock sweeps the perineum and the buttocks are born by a movement of lateral flexion (Fig. 42.4).

4. Restitution The anterior buttock turns slightly to the mother's right side.

5. Internal rotation of the shoulders With the birth of the buttocks, the bisacromial diameter (11 cm) of the shoulders enters the pelvis in the same diameter of the pelvis as the buttocks, the left oblique. The anterior (left) shoulder reaches the pelvic floor and rotates forwards 1/8th of a circle to lie behind the symphysis pubis.

6. Birth of the shoulders The anterior shoulder and arm escape under the symphysis pubis and the posterior shoulder and arm pass over the perineum.

7. Internal rotation and delivery of the head The flexed head engages with the suboccipitobregmatic diameter of 9.5 cm or the suboccipitofrontal diameter of 10 cm lying in the right oblique or transverse diameter of the pelvic brim. Internal rotation of the head carries the occiput behind the symphysis pubis. The face lies in the hollow of the sacrum. Internal rotation of the head is accompanied by external rotation of the trunk. The chin, face, vertex and occiput are born over the perineum by a movement of flexion.

The first stage of labour

The first stage does not differ from normal labour and may be allowed to continue spontaneously if there is progressive dilatation and descent with no fetal or maternal complications. However, the risks of the delivery mean that the birth should take place in a consultant unit with an anaesthetist and paediatrician being available. Labour is normally induced at term and some obstetricians prefer to induce labour at 38 weeks when the fetus will be smaller. If the breech is flexed and not engaged, there may be early rupture of the membranes with the risk of prolapse of the umbilical cord. If the legs are extended, the breech is likely to be engaged and the risk of cord prolapse is minimal.

Epidural analgesia is the analgesia of choice from the obstetric point of view, because it prevents the desire to push too early when the buttocks slip through the incompletely dilated cervical os with a risk of entrapment of the head (Al-Azzawi 1998, Arias 1993). There is also the possibility of delivery of the head by forceps. However, Chadha et al (1992) found that the contractions in both first and second stages of labour decrease in intensity following the commencement of epidural analgesia. This appeared to increase the frequency of breech extraction (see below) or CS and its use is not advocated by all. 'Low-dose' epidurals give effective pain relief and the woman is able to push effectively when the cervix is fully dilated.

The fetus should be continuously monitored by cardiotocographic recording of the fetal heart throughout labour.

The second stage of labour

The woman must be encouraged not to push until the cervix is confirmed as fully dilated by vaginal examination. An experienced midwife or obstetrician will normally conduct the delivery. In hospital, the woman's legs are usually placed in lithotomy position for the actual delivery. All midwives should be familiar with the manoeuvres necessary to deliver the baby in case of an emergency. Simulated practice is essential. An anaesthetist and paediatrician should be present at the delivery in case of a sudden need for intervention.

Breech delivery may be spontaneous with little help needed, usually in a multigravida or with a preterm baby, or assisted where the manoeuvres are performed to assist the birth of the baby. Breech extraction may be occasionally necessary where the fetus is extracted from the birth canal by manipulation rather than by assisting the normal mechanism. This is dangerous and is not often used in developed countries.

Assisted breech delivery

The woman's bladder is emptied prior to commencement. The perineum is infiltrated with local anaesthetic and an episiotomy is performed when the posterior buttock distends the perineum. The episiotomy will not create more room in the bony pelvis but will allow the practitioner to perform various manipulations as required.

The buttocks No handling is necessary and delivery should proceed spontaneously until the fetal umbilicus appears at the introitus. When the umbilicus delivers, a loop of several inches of cord should be gently pulled down to prevent tension on the cord as the body delivers. This will also allow easy monitoring of the fetal pulse by palpation (ALSO 2000). The legs should normally deliver themselves.

The body   After the umbilicus is born, gentle downward traction may be used to deliver the body. The practitioner's fingers should be used to carefully grasp the fetal pelvis, with the thumbs placed on the sacroiliac regions to avoid injuring the abdominal organs. Traction should be in a 45° downwards direction. The body may deliver quickly with little effort.

The head   There are two alternative methods for delivering the head: the Burns–Marshall manoeuvre (Fig. 42.5) and the modified Mauriceau–Smellie–Veit manoeuvre (Fig. 42.6).

Burns–Marshall

The baby is allowed to hang by his own weight to encourage descent and flexion of the head, taking care not to let the baby's head deliver suddenly. Once the nape of the neck and hairline can be seen, the baby's ankles are grasped and with slight traction the trunk is carried in a wide arc up over the mother's abdomen. The other hand should support the perineum to prevent sudden delivery of the head. Once the mouth is clear, the baby can breathe and time should be taken to complete the delivery of the cranium.

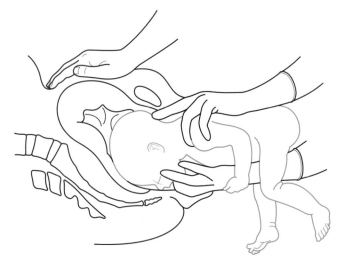

Figure 42.6   The Mauriceau–Smellie–Veit manoeuvre (from Sweet B 1997, with permission).

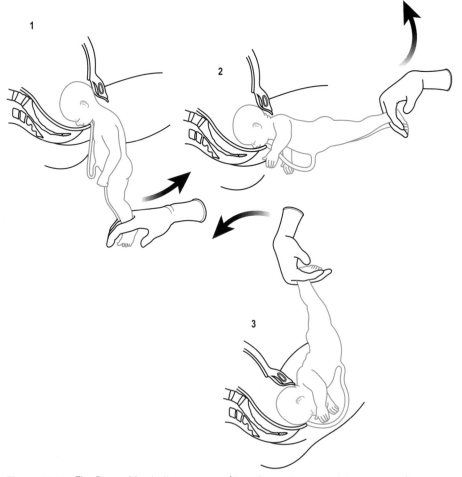

Figure 42.5   The Burns–Marshall manoeuvre (from Sweet B 1997, with permission).

Mauriceau–Smellie–Veit (modified)

This method is recommended for delivery of the head and all the movements promote head flexion. One of the practitioner's hands should be placed above the fetus, with one finger inserted into the vagina and placed on the occiput and one finger on each of the fetal shoulders. The other hand is placed beneath the fetus. The classical Mauriceau–Smellie–Veit (MSV) manoeuvre describes placing a finger in the mouth as seen in Fig. 42.6. However, traction on the lower jaw has been found to cause dislocation. As an alternative the modified manoeuvre involves placing two fingers on the maxilla instead. An assistant should follow the head abdominally and be prepared to apply suprapubic pressure to flex the head through the pelvis. The fetus may be draped on the practitioner's lower arm.

Delivery of the head commences and is flexed through the pelvis by four separate mechanisms:

1. the occipital finger applies flexing pressure on the occiput;
2. the assistant applies suprapubic pressure on the occiput as required;
3. the fingers on the maxillae apply pressure on the lower face, which tends to promote flexion;
4. some traction is also required for the delivery by downward pressure of the fingers on the shoulders.

As the mouth and nose appear over the perineum they may be suctioned. The baby's head is carefully delivered following the curve of the birth canal.

Extended legs If the legs are extended, they may splint the body and prevent lateral flexion of the trunk. The legs of a frank breech may be delivered by inserting a finger behind the knee to flex the knee and abduct the thigh. Active efforts to deliver the legs are not mandatory, as the legs will deliver spontaneously and the feet will become free eventually (ALSO 2000).

Extended arms If the baby's arms cannot be found crossed over the chest, they may be extended alongside the head, making the total diameter of the presenting part too large to descend into the pelvis. This often happens when the breech is pulled on to deliver the legs and trunk. The arms must be brought down before the head can be delivered and this is done by a beautiful manoeuvre called Lövset's manoeuvre (Fig. 42.7). The success of the manoeuvre arises from the relative positions of the two shoulders. The posterior shoulder is below the sacral promontory while the anterior shoulder is above the symphysis pubis.

The baby's thighs are grasped with thumbs placed over the sacrum. The baby is gently pulled downwards and it is

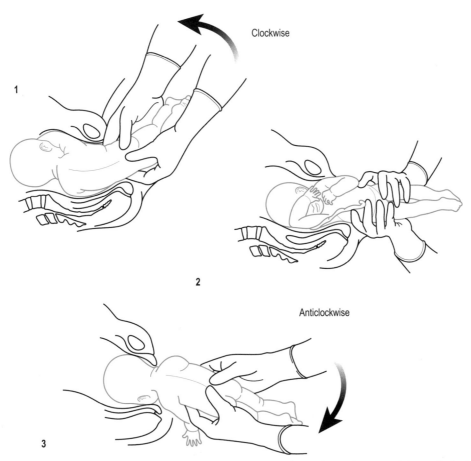

Figure 42.7 Birth of the arms using Lövset's manoeuvre (from Sweet B 1997, with permission).

critical to keep the back uppermost to allow the fetal head to enter the pelvis with the occiput anterior. The baby is rotated through 180° to bring the posterior shoulder to the anterior position but beneath the symphysis pubis. Friction of the arm against the pelvic walls will bring the arm down and it can be released. The manoeuvre is repeated in the opposite direction to release the second arm.

Extended head   If the hairline does not become visible after a few seconds of allowing the baby to hang by its weight, the head is probably extended. Forceps are usually used to deliver the head but the modified Mauriceau–Smellie–Veit manoeuvre may be used if the midwife has to conduct the delivery.

Entrapment of the fetal head   This dangerous situation arises when the fetal body slips through an incompletely dilated cervix and the head is trapped behind the cervix. In the immediate absence of medical aid it may be possible to make an airway for the baby by placing fingers or a Simm's speculum in the vagina, thus holding maternal tissues away from the baby's mouth and nose.

The obstetrician will try to release the baby's head from the cervix and one method that may help is the McRobert's manoeuvre, which is also useful in the delivery of a fetus with shoulder dystocia. The woman lies on her back, lifts her knees up to her chest and raises her buttocks off the bed. Arias (1993) stated that 'There is no adequate description in the literature of the incidence, methods of management and outcome of infants when the fetal head is entrapped during a breech delivery.' He suggested incisions into the cervix as the quickest way of freeing the head, although these are known to extend into the lower segment and cause cervical incompetence. He also suggests trying an injection of diazoxide or other drugs to relax the cervix. However, mortality and morbidity rates for the neonate are high.

Undiagnosed cephalopelvic disproportion   In an unbooked woman or where there has been failure to diagnose a degree of hydrocephaly, this dire emergency may arise as the delivery proceeds. If the breech is delivered up to the head, there is usually difficulty in performing a CS. Symphysiotomy may save the baby's life.

Posterior rotation of the occiput   This is rare complication. In this situation the back of the baby is turned towards the mothers buttocks. To deliver the head the chin and face are allowed to escape under the symphysis pubis as far as the root of the nose, and then the baby is lifted towards the mother's abdomen to allow the occiput to sweep the perineum.

MAIN POINTS

- One in four fetuses will present by the breech at some stage in pregnancy but spontaneous version to a vertex presentation is likely to occur, especially in multigravidae. Depending on the relationship of the lower limb to the trunk of the fetus, breech presentation may be complete or flexed, extended or frank, footling or knee presentation.

- There is an increased risk of morbidity and mortality in breech deliveries. Associated factors include prematurity, congenital abnormalities, placenta praevia and placental abruption, prolapse of the umbilical cord and entrapment of the fetal head behind an incompletely dilated cervix.

- At delivery, the fetus is at risk from asphyxia, intracranial haemorrhage, skeletal fractures and dislocations, damage to muscles and nerves and rupture of abdominal organs, genital oedema and bruising. Long-term problems are thought to include growth hormone deficiency.

- An obstetrician should see women with a breech presentation after 32 weeks. A decision needs to be made with her about the safest option for delivery. External cephalic version may be attempted at or after 37 weeks.

- The risks of a vaginal breech delivery mean that the birth should take place in a consultant unit. Labour is normally induced at term and some obstetricians prefer to induce labour at 38 weeks when the fetus will be smaller. If the breech is flexed and not engaged there may be early rupture of the membranes with the risk of prolapse of the umbilical cord.

- An experienced midwife or obstetrician will conduct the delivery. All midwives should be familiar with the manoeuvres necessary to deliver the baby presenting by the breech, in case of an emergency. The modified Mauriceau–Smellie–Veit manoeuvre is recommended for delivery of the head as the movements all promote flexion.

- An anaesthetist and paediatrician should be present at the delivery in case of a sudden need for intervention. Dangerous but rare complications such as entrapment of the fetal head, late diagnosis of cephalopelvic disproportion and posterior rotation of the occiput may lead to fetal death.

References

Al-Azzawi F 1998 Childbirth & Obstetric Techniques, 2nd edn. Mosby, St Louis.

ALSO 2000 Malpresentations, Malpositions, and Multiple Gestation, 4th edn. Advanced Life Support in Obstetrics, Registered Charity No 1024554, UK Office, Newcastle-upon-Tyne.

Arias F 1993 Practical Guide to High Risk Pregnancy and Delivery, 2nd edn. Mosby Year Book, Chicago.

Budd S 1992 Traditional Chinese medicine in obstetrics. Midwives' Chronicle 105(1253):140–143.

Chadha Y C, Mahmood T A, Dick M J et al 1992 Breech delivery and epidural analgesia. British Journal of Obstetrics and Gynaecology 99:96–100.

Danelian P J, Wang J, Hall M H 1996 Long-term outcome of term breech presentation by method of delivery. British Journal of Medicine 312(7044):1451–1453.

Enkin M, Keirse M J N C, Neilson J et al 2000 A Guide to Effective Care in Pregnancy and Childbirth, 3rd edn. Oxford University Press, Oxford.

Gilady Y, Cols E 1996 The delivery of very low birthweight breech. What is the best way for the baby? Israel Journal of Medical Science 32(2):116–120.

Hannah M 2000 The Term Breech Collaborative Group. What is the best way to deliver a breech baby? Lancet 356:1375–1383.

Hofmeyr G J 2001a External cephalic version before term. Cochrane Review: In The Cochrane Library, Issue 2. Update Software 2003, Oxford.

Hofmeyr G J 2001b Interventions to help external cephalic version for breech presentation at term. Cochrane Review: In The Cochrane Library, Issue 2. Update Software 2003, Oxford.

Hofmeyr G J, Hannah M E 2000 Planned elective CS for term breech presentation. Cochrane Review: In The Cochrane Library, Issue 2. Update Software 2003, Oxford.

Hofmeyr G J, Kulier R 1999 External cephalic version for breech presentation at term. Cochrane Review: In The Cochrane Library, Issue 2. Update Software 2003, Oxford.

Hofmeyr G J, Kulier R 2001 Cephalic version by postural management for breech presentation. Cochrane Review: In The Cochrane Library, Issue 2. Update Software 2003, Oxford.

Kiely J L 1991 Mode of delivery and neonatal death in 17587 infants presenting by the breech. British Journal of Obstetrics and Gynaecology 98(9):898–904.

SOGC 2000 Interim Position on Management of Term Breech. Society of Obstetricians and Gynaecologists of Canada, September 27.

Sweet B R 1997 Malpresentations. In Sweet B R, Tiran D (eds) Mayes Midwifery: A Textbook for Midwives, 12th edn. Baillière Tindall, London.

Annotated recommended reading

Al-Azzawi F 1998 Childbirth & Obstetric Techniques, 2nd edn. Mosby, St Louis.
This atlas contains superb collection of colour photographs, a pictorial demonstration of normal childbirth and its variations and a breech delivery.

Enkin M, Keirse M J N C, Neilson J et al 2000 A guide to Effective Care in Pregnancy and Childbirth, 3rd edn. Oxford University Press, Oxford.
This book is based on systematic reviews of research literature on pregnancy and childbirth and includes sections on breech delivery and external cephalic version.

Gilady Y, Cols E 1996 The delivery of very low birth weight breech. What is the best way for the baby? Israel Journal of Medical Science 32(2):116–120.
In this article, Gilady and Cols reviewed the literature on the delivery of the preterm breech. They found that babies weighing less than 1700 g were at risk of neonatal death if delivered by the breech.

Liu D T Y 2003 Labour Ward Manual, 3rd edn. Churchill Livingstone, Edinburgh.
This book is an excellent resource for a labour ward practitioner. It contains useful information on intrapartum care, including pictorial presentation of breech delivery.

Chapter 43

Malposition and cephalic malpresentations

INTRODUCTION

If the vertex is the denominator in a cephalic presentation, the term malpresentation is not used. The correct word to use for occipitoposterior position of the vertex is **malposition**. True cephalic malpresentations are face and brow. Shoulder presentation resulting from oblique or transverse lie is a rare but dangerous event. Each of these situations may affect the length and outcome of the labour and require vigilance to prevent maternal and fetal morbidity and, rarely, mortality. The more common occipitoposterior position will be discussed first as it may lead to secondary brow or face presentation.

OCCIPITOPOSTERIOR POSITION OF THE VERTEX

In occipitoposterior position of the vertex, the occiput occupies one or other of the posterior quadrants of the mother's pelvis and the sinciput points towards the opposite anterior quadrant (Fig. 43.1). Malposition is common and affects about 10% of all labours. The outcome of such labours is generally normal with rotation of the occiput to the anterior and normal vertex delivery. However, there may be prolonged labour and mechanical difficulties associated with the delivery.

Causes

There is no single satisfactory cause for occipitoposterior position. However, if the forepelvis is small, as found in android and anthropoid pelves, the head may take up a posterior position. Other possible causes include a pendulous abdomen, a flat sacrum or an anterior placenta.

Attitude

Instead of the normal well-flexed attitude with the limbs and head flexed on the trunk and the rounded back pointing towards the mother's soft abdominal wall, the fetal spine faces the forward curve of the maternal lumbar spine

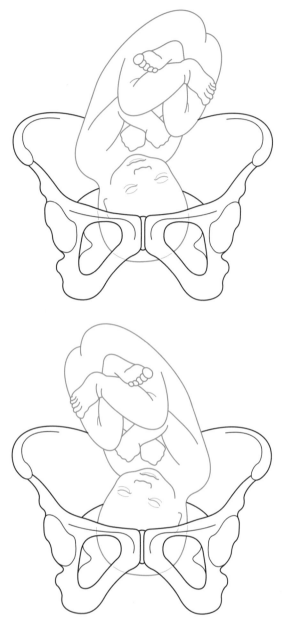

Figure 43.1 Right and left occipitoposterior positions (from Sweet B 1997, with permission).

and good flexion is not possible. The fetal spine is straightened, the head is held in a deflexed position known as the 'military position' and the anterior fontanelle is found directly over the internal os. The term bregmatic presentation is sometimes used (Sweet 1997). This position of the head brings larger diameters into relationship with the pelvic brim and engagement of the head may not occur.

Risks

- Obstructed labour if either deep transverse arrest or brow presentation result.
- Maternal perineal trauma such as a third-degree tear and bruising.

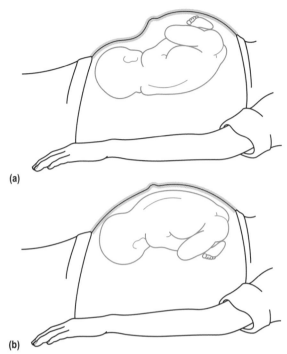

(a)

(b)

Figure 43.2 (a) Abdominal contour with occipitoposterior position, showing depression at umbilicus. (b) Rounded abdominal contour with occipitoanterior position (from Sweet B 1997, with permission).

- Cord prolapse if there is early spontaneous rupture of the membranes.
- Neonatal cerebral haemorrhage due to upward moulding of the fetal skull. The falx cerebri may be pulled away from the tentorium cerebelli, resulting in a tear of the great vein of Galen. Chronic hypoxia, if present, results in venous distension, which increases the likelihood of haemorrhage.

Diagnosis in pregnancy

Occipitoposterior position is the commonest cause of a nonengaged head in late pregnancy in primigravidae. The woman may complain that the baby has too many hands and feet and that she has to pass urine more frequently in the absence of infection (El Halta 1996). Abdominal examination will confirm the diagnosis:

- On inspection – the abdomen appears flattened. There may be a saucer-shaped depression below the umbilicus between the fetal head and limbs (Fig. 43.2).

- On palpation – the fetal head is high and deflexed. It may feel large if the occiput is more lateral but small if the occiput is quite posterior and the bitemporal diameter is palpated. Fetal limbs may be felt on both sides of the midline of the uterus and the fetal back may be felt out in the flank (Fig. 43.3).

- On auscultation – the fetal heart may be heard at or just above the umbilicus or out in one flank.

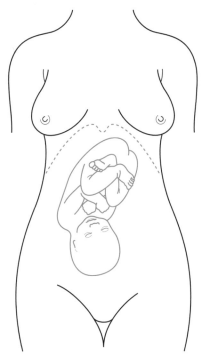

Figure 43.3   In occipitoposterior positions the anterior shoulder is well out from the midline and fetal limbs are readily palpable. This may cause a mistaken diagnosis of multiple pregnancy. (Reproduced with permission from Beischer & Mackay 1986 Obstetrics and the Newborn. Baillière Tindall, London.)

Diagnosis in labour

Abdominal examination, as described above, will indicate the presence of an occipitoposterior position although the head may be flexed and become engaged.

On vaginal examination, palpation of the anterior fontanelle is a diagnostic aid in determining occipitoposterior position (ALSO 2000). If the head is reasonably well flexed, the anterior fontanelle will be felt anteriorly and it may be possible to feel the posterior fontanelle. When the head is deflexed, the anterior fontanelle is almost central and easy to feel by its shape and size (Fig. 43.4).

The first stage of labour

The course of labour partly depends on the degree of descent and flexion that takes place (Fig. 43.5). This in turn is influenced by the strength of uterine contractions. If the head flexes, it is likely that labour will proceed normally. The engaging diameter is the suboccipitofrontal, which is 10 cm. When the occiput reaches the pelvic floor and rotates 3/8th of a circle, the baby is born with the occiput anterior.

If the head remains deflexed, problems may arise. The engaging diameter is the occipitofrontal, which measures 11.5 cm. The head may be non-engaged at the commencement of labour and early rupture of the membranes may occur. If the presenting part is high and not well applied to the cervix, there is a risk of cord prolapse.

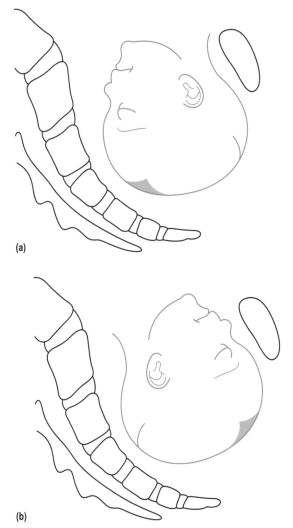

(a)

(b)

Figure 43.4   Position of the anterior and posterior fontanelles. (a) Occipitoanterior. (b) Occipitoposterior (from Sweet B 1997, with permission).

Labour is prolonged because of poor stimulation of the cervix and dilation is slow and uneven. Contractions may be excessive but uncoordinated and painful and the woman experiences severe backache. Encouraging the mother to take up a knee–chest position for 45 min may help rotation of the vertex to an anterior position (El Halta 1996). Augmentation of labour may be necessary (see Ch. 41). Care must be taken to prevent maternal loss of confidence, ketosis and dehydration and fetal distress. There may be difficulty in micturition with retention of urine and the woman needs encouragement to empty her bladder frequently. Catheterisation may be necessary if the woman is unable to pass urine.

The role of maternal position

Sutton (1996) discusses the benefits of upright and leaning-forward postures in order to encourage the fetal head to engage in the optimal occipitoanterior position. Avoidance

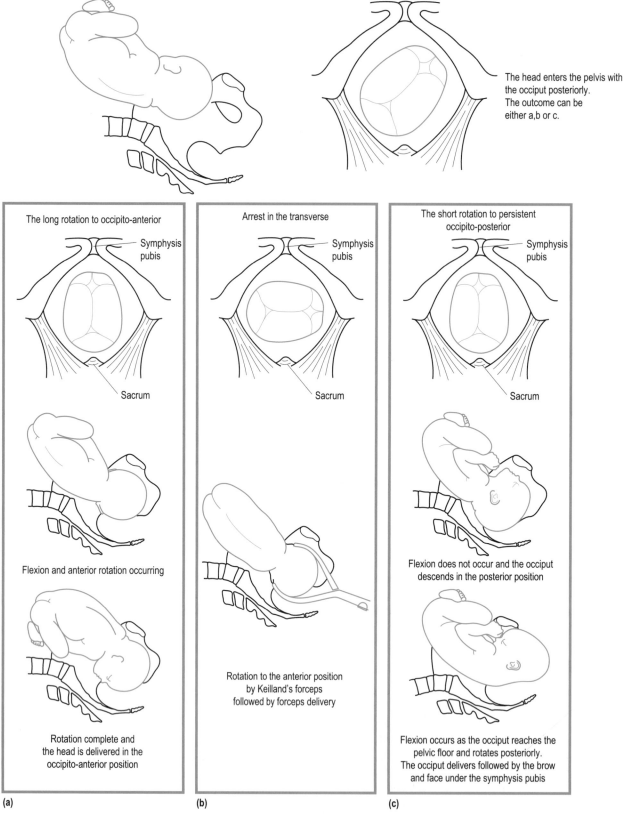

The head enters the pelvis with the occiput posteriorly. The outcome can be either a, b or c.

(a)

The long rotation to occipito-anterior

Symphysis pubis

Sacrum

Flexion and anterior rotation occurring

Rotation complete and the head is delivered in the occipito-anterior position

(b)

Arrest in the transverse

Symphysis pubis

Sacrum

Rotation to the anterior position by Keilland's forceps followed by forceps delivery

(c)

The short rotation to persistent occipito-posterior

Symphysis pubis

Sacrum

Flexion does not occur and the occiput descends in the posterior position

Flexion occurs as the occiput reaches the pelvic floor and rotates posteriorly. The occiput delivers followed by the brow and face under the symphysis pubis

Figure 43.5   Outcome of an occipitoposterior position. The head enters the pelvis with the occiput posteriorly. The outcome can be a, b or c (from Sweet B 1997, with permission).

of a reclining position with the knees higher than the hips will reduce the incidence of occipitoposterior position of the fetal head at the commencement of labour. Taking up an all-fours posture may reduce the pressure of the fetus on the maternal spine and help to reduce backache. It may also aid rotation of the fetus to an occipitoanterior position (Simkin & Ancheta 2000).

Simkin & Ancheta (2000) detail the advantages of ambulation and forward-leaning positions in labour. Freedom to move around in the first stage of labour and the maintenance of an upright position such as can be achieved by sitting astride a chair and leaning on its back have been shown to be beneficial to women with an occipitoposterior presentation. Descent of the fetal head is encouraged and good uterine contractions should follow. Progress is more likely to be normal, culminating in long internal rotation of the occiput (see below). In the second stage of labour, the squatting position increases the anteroposterior diameter of the outlet and may aid rotation, descent and delivery.

Relieving backache

To relieve the backache, many women find the kneeling position beneficial. This position may also aid rotation of the head to an occipitoanterior position. Massaging the woman's back in the lumbosacral region may also help to relieve the backache and a warm bath has been found to be helpful. Epidural analgesia is the most effective method of relieving the pain. In the second stage of labour, perineal trauma is minimised with the kneeling position.

A difficult problem to the woman in the late first stage of labour is feeling a strong urge to push before full cervical dilatation. Pushing presses the fetal head against the cervix and oedema may occur, thus lengthening the transitional stage of labour. Simkin & Ancheta (2000) suggest that the adoption of the kneeling position with the head resting on the forearms may lessen the pressure on the cervix.

The second stage of labour

The possible outcomes of an occipitoposterior position are:

1. long internal rotation of the occiput and delivery as an occipitoanterior;
2. deep transverse arrest of the head;
3. short internal rotation of the sinciput and delivery as 'face to pubes';
4. partial extension of the head to a brow presentation;
5. full extension of the head to a mentoposterior face presentation.

1. Mechanism of long internal rotation of a right occipitoposterior position

- The lie is longitudinal.
- The attitude of the head is deflexed.
- The presentation is vertex.
- The position is right occipitoposterior.
- The denominator is the occiput.
- The presenting part is the middle to anterior area of the left parietal bone.

The movements
Descent and flexion There is continued descent with flexion during the first stage of labour and the presenting diameter of occipitofrontal (11.5 cm) is converted to suboccipitofrontal (10 cm).

Internal rotation of the head The occiput reaches the pelvic floor first and rotates forwards along the right side of the pelvis 3/8th of a circle to lie under the symphysis pubis. The anteroposterior diameter of the head now lies in the anteroposterior diameter of the pelvis. The shoulders follow and rotate 2/8th of a circle. The occiput escapes from beneath the subpubic arch.

Extension of the head The head is now born by extension as it pivots on the suboccipital region around the pubic bone. The sinciput, face and chin sweep the perineum.

Restitution Restitution is a movement made by the head following delivery which brings it into correct alignment with the shoulders. This will be 1/8th of a circle towards the side of the occiput.

Internal rotation of the shoulders The anterior shoulder is the first to reach the pelvic floor and rotates forwards to lie under the symphysis pubis. This movement is accompanied by **external rotation of the head** 1/8th of a circle more in the direction of restitution. The occiput now lies laterally turned towards the woman's thigh.

Lateral flexion The anterior shoulder is usually born first and slips under the pubic arch and the posterior shoulder passes over the perineum. The remainder of the body is born by lateral flexion.

This outcome is the most common, occurring in about 65% of births.

2. Deep transverse arrest of the head

If the head remains deflexed, deep transverse arrest may occur. The fetal head has begun long internal rotation but there is insufficient flexion to complete the process. The occipitofrontal diameter is caught above the ischial spines in the bispinous diameter. Labour becomes obstructed. Weak contractions, or a straight sacrum with narrow outlet (as found in the android pelvis), may lead to this.

Diagnosis and management Diagnosis is made by finding the sagittal suture in the transverse diameter of the pelvis with a fontanelle at each end of the suture. Caput succedaneum may obscure the landmarks. It will be necessary to rotate the head to an occipitoanterior position either manually or with Kielland's forceps prior to delivery by forceps. An alternative way of rotating and delivering the fetal head is by vacuum extraction. Some obstetricians would be unwilling to do an instrumental delivery when the head has not descended below the ischial spines.

The use of the vacuum extractor is preferable to the forceps as it reduces the incidence of maternal injuries (Enkin et al 2000). Johanson & Menon (1999) found that although vacuum extraction was related to increased incidence of neonatal cephalhaematoma and retinal haemorrhage, there was less incidence of maternal trauma and caesarean section (CS). In the light of their review, they recommended the use of vacuum extraction.

3. Short internal rotation of the sinciput and delivery as 'face to pubes'

In about 5% of labours the occiput fails to rotate spontaneously to an anterior position (Arias 1993). This is known as persistent occipitoposterior position or POP. The head remains deflexed and the sinciput reaches the pelvic floor first and rotates forwards. The occiput comes to lie in the hollow of the sacrum and the head of the baby is born facing the pubic bone. Incidentally, this is the normal birth position of the great apes such as chimpanzees.

Diagnosis
- There may be delay in the second stage of labour.
- There is gaping of the vagina and dilatation of the anus due to the presence of the large occiput.
- Confirmation is by finding the anterior fontanelle directly behind the symphysis pubis. This may be masked by caput succedaneum and feeling for the pinna of the ear will aid confirmation. In a POP, the pinna will point towards the sacrum.

Management of the spontaneous delivery

The second stage is likely to be prolonged and, even when the woman wishes to push, there may be incomplete cervical dilatation (Kuo et al 1996). The squatting position may assist descent of the presenting part (Simkin & Ancheta 2000). Once the perineal phase of delivery is reached, to maintain the smallest possible diameters distending the perineum, the sinciput is allowed to emerge under the symphysis pubis as far as the root of the nose. Flexion is maintained and the occiput is allowed to sweep the perineum. The rest of the face is brought down from under the symphysis pubis. There is a high risk of perineal trauma, especially a 'buttonhole' tear in the centre of the perineum. An episiotomy may be required.

FACE PRESENTATION

The incidence of face presentation at term is about 1 in 500. In this presentation, the head and spine are fully extended and the limbs fully flexed. The fetal occiput lies against its shoulder blades and the face is directly above the internal os (Fig. 43.6).

Causes

Face presentation may be described as primary when it is present before the onset of labour. The fetus is often abnormal and anencephaly is common, while a rarer cause is due to fetal goitre which prevents the head from flexing. A secondary face presentation is one that develops as labour proceeds. In a deflexed occipitoposterior position, the biparietal diameter of the fetal head may be unable to pass through the sacrocotyloid diameter of the pelvic brim. The bitemporal diameter descends more quickly and the head extends first to a brow presentation and ultimately to a face presentation. Other causes of face presentation include a flat pelvis, a poor uterine muscle tone, prematurity, polyhydramnios or multiple pregnancy.

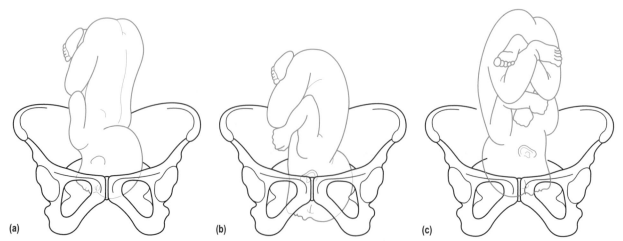

(a) (b) (c)

Figure 43.6   Face presentations. (a) Right mentoposterior. (b) Right mentolateral. (c) Left mentoanterior (from Sweet B 1997, with permission).

Risks

- Obstructed labour if either deep transverse arrest or brow presentation result.
- Maternal perineal trauma such as a third-degree tear and bruising.
- Cord prolapse if there is early spontaneous rupture of the membranes.
- Facial bruising as the caput forms over the face.
- Cerebral haemorrhage due to excessive moulding of the cranium.

Diagnosis

Per abdomen

In pregnancy, face presentation is rarely found as the majority of cases develop in labour (Coates 1999). It may be difficult to diagnose face presentation. A deep groove may be palpated between the fetal head and back. The chest wall may be pressed up against the anterior wall of the uterus and heart sounds are heard clearly on the side where limbs are palpated. However, in mentoposterior positions where the chest faces posteriorly, heart sounds may be difficult to hear. In women who have a late ultrasound, a face presentation is sometimes found.

Per vaginam

In labour, the possibility of a face presentation should be suspected if the head remains high. On vaginal examination, feeling orbital ridges and a mouth with gum margins will confirm the diagnosis. The fetus may suck the examining finger, as the author has experienced on a number of occasions. The mouth feels very different from the soft and clinging anal orifice, which would be found if the presentation was breech. Also, the examining finger may have meconium coating it if the breech was presenting. It is important to determine whether the fetus is presenting in a mentoposterior or mentoanterior position. Unless a posterior face rotates to anterior, there will be an obstructed labour. The position of the chin is the important diagnostic tool.

Progress and outcomes of labour

As in many labours where there is an irregular high presenting part, there may be early spontaneous rupture of the membranes with the risk of cord prolapse and contractions may be inefficient, leading to a prolonged labour. The face bones cannot mould and large diameters must enter the pelvis.

Mentoanterior position

If contractions are good, descent and rotation of the head occur and labour progresses to a spontaneous delivery.

Mechanism of a left mentoanterior position   There are six possible positions: right mentoanterior, mentolateral and mentoposterior; and left mentoanterior, mentolateral and mentoposterior. The mechanisms are:

- the **lie** is longitudinal;
- the **attitude** of the head and back is one of extension;
- the **presentation** is face;
- the **position** is left mentoanterior;
- the **denominator** is the mentum;
- the **presenting part** is the left malar bone.

The movements

Descent   There is continued descent with increasing extension; the mentum is the leading part.

Internal rotation of the head   The mentum reaches the pelvic floor first and rotates forwards 1/8th of a circle to lie under the symphysis pubis. The chin escapes from beneath the subpubic arch (Fig. 43.7).

Flexion of the head   The head is now born by flexion. The sinciput, vertex and occiput sweep the perineum.

Restitution   Restitution occurs as the chin turns 1/8th of a circle towards the left side of the woman.

Internal rotation of the shoulders   The anterior shoulder is the first to reach the pelvic floor and rotates forwards to lie under the symphysis pubis. This movement is accompanied by **external rotation of the head** 1/8th of a circle more in the direction of restitution.

Lateral flexion   The anterior shoulder is usually born first and slips under the pubic arch and the posterior shoulder passes over the perineum. The remainder of the body is born by lateral flexion.

Mentoposterior position

If the head is completely extended and the mentum reaches the pelvic floor first, the mentum rotates forwards into a

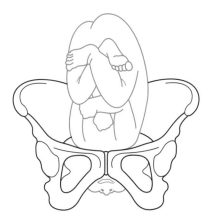

Figure 43.7   The face at the outlet, the chin passing under the pubic arch (from Sweet B 1997, with permission).

mentoanterior position and delivery is possible. If the head is incompletely extended, there is a persistent mentoposterior position and the sinciput reaches the pelvic floor first. The chin comes to lie in the hollow of the pelvis and there can be no further progress. For further progress, the head and shoulders of the fetus would have to be in the pelvic cavity together. In order to be born, the presenting fetal part must pivot round the subpubic arch either by flexion or extension. If the chin is posterior, this cannot happen as the fully extended head cannot extend further and labour is obstructed.

Management of labour   The first stage of labour is managed according to the risks. During vaginal examination, note should be taken of the descent of the mentum. If the head remains high or there is a suspicion of cephalopelvic disproportion, the fetus should normally be delivered by CS.

In the second stage, when the face appears at the vulva, the sinciput must be held back to permit extension. This allows the mentum to escape under the pubic arch before the occiput sweeps the perineum. This ensures that the smallest possible diameter, which is the submentovertical of 11.5 cm, distends the vaginal orifice rather than the large mentovertical diameter of 13.5 cm. An elective episiotomy must be made because of the large diameters distending the vaginal orifice. The chin escapes under the pubic arch and the head is born by flexion. If there is delay in descent or if the fetus remains in a persistent mentoposterior position, a forceps delivery, with rotation if necessary, may be successful. Otherwise, a CS will be needed to reduce maternal and fetal morbidity and mortality.

BROW PRESENTATION

Brow presentation occurs in about 1 in 2000 deliveries. Except for anencephaly, the causes are the same as for face presentation. The head is an attitude midway between full flexion and full extension (or face). The largest diameter of the head, the mentovertical of 13.5 cm, cannot enter the widest possible diameter of the pelvic brim, which is the transverse of 13 cm (Fig. 43.8). Unless the brow presentation extends fully to a face presentation and the mentum comes anterior, labour is obstructed.

Diagnosis

Per abdomen

The head is very high and the presenting diameter is very wide. A groove may be felt between the occiput and the back.

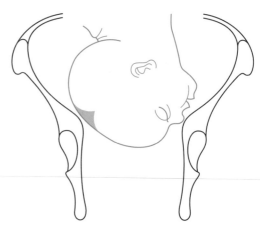

Figure 43.8   Brow presentation (from Sweet B 1997, with permission).

Per vaginam

The presenting part may be so high it cannot be reached. If the brow is within reach, the orbital ridges are felt at one side and the anterior fontanelle on the other with the frontal suture running between them. Frequently, the examination is confusing because of the oedema and unfamiliarity of the presenting features (ALSO 2000). Diagnosis can be confirmed by ultrasound.

Management

If the brow presentation is diagnosed early in labour and both maternal and fetal conditions are satisfactory, time may be allowed to see if the head will flex to a vertex or extend to a face presentation. If the brow presentation persists, a CS will be necessary.

SHOULDER PRESENTATION

Shoulder presentation in labour is the result of a non-corrected abnormal lie in pregnancy. Instead of the normal longitudinal lie, the fetus lies across the uterus either in an oblique or a transverse lie. The lie may be unstable. Shoulder presentation leads to obstructed labour and delivery should normally be by CS.

Causes

The commonest cause is grande multiparity. Grande multiparous women often have lax uterine and abdominal muscles; in this case, the fetus take the transverse lie. More than 80% of cases occur in women with three or more previous pregnancies (Arias 1993). Other causes include anything

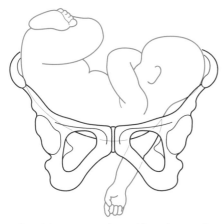

Figure 43.9   Shoulder presentation with prolapse of one arm (from Sweet B 1997, with permission).

which prevents the fetus from adopting a longitudinal lie or the fetal head from engaging. These include placenta praevia, multiple pregnancy, polyhydramnios, a uterine abnormality, a large uterine fibroid or a contracted pelvis. When the fetus dies in utero it may slump into an abnormal lie.

Diagnosis

Per abdomen

A transverse lie is easy to diagnose in pregnancy because of the abnormal shape of the uterus. The uterus is broader and the fundal height lower than normal and there may be a discernible bulge at either side of the uterus. On palpation, the fetal head will be felt on one side of the uterus and the breech on the other. The fetal back may be anterior (dorsoanterior) or posterior (dorsoposterior). There is no presenting part entering the pelvis (Fig. 43.9). In an oblique lie the shape of the uterus may be indicative and one or other pole of the fetus is found in one or other iliac fossa. Ultrasound is useful both to confirm the diagnosis and detect the cause.

Per vaginam

A vaginal examination should not be done if a transverse lie is suspected on abdominal examination in case there is a placenta praevia. Rarely, a woman will be admitted already in labour with the shoulder impacted at the brim of the pelvis. It may be mistaken for a breech presentation. The fetal cord and arm may prolapse into the vagina. On vaginal examination the shoulder is recognised by feeling the fetal ribs and the hand, which must be differentiated from a foot by the length of the digits and the presence of a heel. The safest method of delivery is by CS, even if the fetus is dead.

Management

A full examination is made during pregnancy to exclude causes such as placenta praevia. If no major pregnancy abnormality is found, the obstetrician may attempt to correct the lie to a longitudinal lie and cephalic presentation. However, reversion to the original lie is common and some doctors do not perform repeated external cephalic version (ECV) before the onset of labour, planned or otherwise. As pregnancy progresses, some lies will stabilise as longitudinal. Sweet quotes Phelan et al (1986), who found that after 37 weeks of pregnancy a transverse lie persisted in only 17% of cases.

The woman should be admitted to hospital at 37–38 weeks, when the fetus is mature for ECV and induction of labour. There is a risk of labour commencing spontaneously with early rupture of the membranes and cord prolapse. When the contractions are established and the fetal head enters the pelvis, the membranes can be ruptured. If complications arise or if the woman has a poor obstetric history, a CS is performed.

In the case of twins, if after the birth of the first twin, the second twin takes up a transverse or oblique lie, the fetus must be turned by ECV, the second set of membranes ruptured and the delivery completed.

COMPOUND PRESENTATION

This is a presentation where a hand or foot lies alongside the head. It is a rare complication and the incidence is about 0.1% of all deliveries (Arias 1993). Cord prolapse may occur in up to 20% of cases. It is more likely to happen if the fetus is small and the pelvis large or there is any condition that prevents the descent of the head such as contracted pelvis, prematurity or multiple pregnancy. The limb may recede as the head advances and the delivery proceeds normally. If the limb does not recede, it will be impossible for the head and hand to be delivered simultaneously; in this case, a CS is performed. One of the editors remembers being asked by a colleague to check and confirm compound presentation. The woman was 8 cm dilated and hand was lying alongside the head. The fingers had descended lower than the head. The obstetric registrar was immediately informed and a suggestion made that because the hand was too far advanced, it was unwise to continue with normal labour. The registrar was not happy with the suggestion as it implied making a decision for him. After he examined the woman, he said that the hand would recede and ordered that labour should continue for 3 more hours. When the woman was re-examined, the hand was found to be presenting in the vagina. The woman had an emergency CS, the baby ended up on a special care baby unit (SCBU) with very badly bruised hand and arm.

MAIN POINTS

- There is no single cause for occipitoposterior position of the vertex but if the forepelvis is small, as found in android and anthropoid pelves, the head may take up a posterior position. Other causes include a pendulous abdomen, a flat sacrum or an anterior placenta. Risks include obstructed labour, maternal perineal trauma, cord prolapse and neonatal cerebral haemorrhage.

- Antenatally, occipitoposterior position is the commonest cause of a non-engaged head in late pregnancy in primigravidae. It may be detected by a combination of maternal complaints and abdominal examination. In labour, during a vaginal examination, palpation of the anterior fontanelle confirms the diagnosis.

- The possible outcomes of an occipitoposterior position are long internal rotation of the occiput and delivery as an occipitoanterior, deep transverse arrest of the head, short internal rotation of the sinciput and delivery as 'face to pubes', partial extension of the head to a brow presentation or full extension of the head to a mentoposterior face presentation.

- If there is deep transverse arrest, the head must be rotated to an occipitoanterior position either manually or with Kielland's forceps prior to delivery by forceps.

- Face presentation may be primary when it is present before the onset of labour or secondary when it develops as labour proceeds. Risks include obstructed labour, maternal perineal trauma, cord prolapse, facial bruising and cerebral haemorrhage.

- In labour it is important to determine whether the fetus is presenting in a mentoposterior or mentoanterior position.

The position of the chin is the important diagnostic tool. In a mentoanterior position with good contractions, descent and rotation of the head occurs and labour progresses to a spontaneous delivery. In a mentoposterior position, the usual outcome is that the fully extended head cannot extend further and labour is obstructed.

- In brow presentation, the mentovertical diameter is too large to enter the transverse widest possible diameter of the pelvic brim. Unless the head extends fully to a face presentation and the mentum becomes anterior, labour is obstructed. If brow presentation is diagnosed early in labour and maternal and fetal conditions are satisfactory, time may be allowed to see if the head will flex to a vertex or extend to a face presentation. If brow presentation persists, CS is necessary.

- Shoulder presentation in labour is the result of a non-corrected abnormal lie in pregnancy. The fetus lies across the uterus either in an oblique or a transverse lie. Shoulder presentation leads to obstructed labour and must be prevented. The commonest cause is laxity of the uterine and abdominal muscles most often in multiparous women.

- In compound presentation, a hand or foot lies alongside the head. It is more likely to occur if the fetus is small and the pelvis large or there is any condition that prevents the descent of the head. The limb may recede as the head advances and the delivery proceeds normally. If the limb does not recede, it will be impossible to deliver the head and hand simultaneously; in this case, a CS is performed.

References

ALSO 2000 Malpresentations, Malpositions, and Multiple Gestation, 4th edn. Advanced Life Support in Obstetrics, Registered Charity No 1024554, UK Office, Newcastle-upon-Tyne.

Arias F 1993 Practical Guide to High Risk Pregnancy and Delivery, 2nd edn. Mosby Year Book, Chicago.

Coates T 1999 Malposition of the occiput and malpresentations. In Bennett V R, Brown L K (eds) Myles Textbook for Midwives, 13th edn. Churchill Livingstone, Edinburgh.

El Halta V 1996 Posterior labor – a pain in the back! Its prevention and cure. Clarion 11(1):12–13.

Enkin M, Keirse J N C, Renfrew M 2000 A Guide to Effective Care in Pregnancy and Childbirth, 3rd edn. Oxford University Press, Oxford.

Johanson R B, Menon V 1999 Vacuum extraction versus forceps for assisted vaginal delivery. Cochrane Review: In The Cochrane Library, Issue 2. Update Software 2003, Oxford.

Kuo Y-C, Chen C-P, Wong K-G 1996 Factors influencing the prolonged second stage and the effects on perinatal and maternal outcomes. Journal of Obstetrics and Gynaecology Research 22(3):253–257.

Phelan J P, Boucher M, Mueller M et al 1986 The non-labouring transverse lie: a management dilemma. Journal of Reproductive Medicine 31:184–186.

Simkin P, Ancheta R 2000 The Labour Progress Handbook. Blackwell Science, Oxford.

Sutton J 1996 A midwife's observations of how the birth process is influenced by the relationship of the maternal pelvis and the foetal head. Journal of the Association of Chartered Physiotherapists in Women's Health 79:31–33.

Sweet B R 1997 Malpresentations. In Sweet B R, Tiran D (eds) Mayes Midwifery: A Textbook for Midwives, 12th edn. Baillière Tindall, London.

Annotated recommended reading

Enkin M, Keirse M J N C, Neilson J et al 2000 A Guide to Effective Care in Pregnancy and Childbirth, 3rd edn. Oxford University Press, Oxford.
A well-written book based on authoritative evidence available on all aspects of care during pregnancy and childbirth. An invaluable resource for intrapartum care.

Coates T 1999 Malposition of the occiput and malpresentations. In Bennett V R, Brown L K (eds) Myles Textbook for Midwives, 13th edn. Churchill Livingstone, Edinburgh.
A chapter in an edited book in which Coates describes abnormal presentations and their management. It is an invaluable reference for those who provide intrapartum care.

Chapter **44**

Cephalopelvic disproportion, obstructed labour and other obstetric emergencies

INTRODUCTION

Two evolutionary adaptations lead to problems of fit between the female pelvis and the fetal head. Firstly the birth canal and the pathway taken by the fetus are complex as the human pelvis is adapted to a bipedal posture (Morgan 1994). Compared to other primates such as the chimpanzee:

- the anteroposterior diameter is reduced at the brim, cavity and outlet;
- there is widening of the transverse diameters;
- the sacral promontory protrudes into the pelvic inlet;
- the sacrum makes an angle with the lumbar spine – the **lumbosacral angle**;
- there is inward protrusion of the ischial spines in order to support the strong pelvic floor;
- the sacrum is curved;
- the superior ramus is thinned and elongated with widening of the subpubic angle.

Secondly the fetal head is able to negotiate the pelvis successfully because of three features:

1. spheroid shape of the vertex;
2. mobility of the head on the neck, allowing flexion or extension;
3. moulding of the bones of the vault (Abitol 1993).

CEPHALOPELVIC DISPROPORTION

Any condition leading to a misfit between the fetal head and the maternal pelvis, with failure of descent of the head into the pelvis despite good contractions, results in **cephalopelvic disproportion (CPD)**. The presenting diameters of the fetal head are larger than the diameters of the pelvis. The shape of the pelvis may be abnormal but, as long as the diameters allow passage of the fetal head, delivery should follow as there should be no problem with the rest of the fetus. Cephalopelvic disproportion is an absolute cause of obstructed labour and there are tremendous dangers for mother and fetus.

Diagnosis

In a primigravida it is expected that the fetal head should engage in the last 2–3 weeks of pregnancy. If the head does not engage, an attempt to make it engage is tried and, if unsuccessful, CPD should be suspected. The most common cause for non-engagement of the head is **occipitoposterior position**, with deflexed head and a presenting occipitofrontal diameter of 11.5 cm. However, in such cases the head flexes and descent occurs in labour. Other causes of a non-engaged head include **pelvic tumours**, **placenta praevia** and **polyhydramnios**.

A steep **angle of inclination** between the pelvic brim and the horizontal is found in some Afro-Caribbean women and may delay engagement until late in labour. The editor remembers a student midwife from the West Indies who listened intently to the session on CPD. When she had her first child a couple of years later she brought her daughter to see me and said her labour had all happened strictly according to the lecture. Those caring for her became increasingly worried during the course of labour when the head did not engage. Just as they came to take blood in case of a need for a caesarean section (CS), she wanted to push. The head engaged, descended through the pelvis and she had a normal vaginal delivery.

Maternal indications of possible CPD

These indications include:

- Bone conditions such as rickets or osteomalacia, which may have resulted in alterations in the size and shape of the pelvis.
- Spinal deformities such as scoliosis.
- Pelvic trauma and fractures which may have altered the size and shape of the pelvis.
- Previous obstetric conditions such as prolonged labour, difficult delivery or CS.
- Short stature of the woman. Mahmood et al (1988) found that the height of the woman was a better predictor of CPD than the shoe size, although 80% of women under 1.6 m still achieved vaginal delivery.

Fetal conditions leading to CPD

These conditions include:

- Size of the fetus in relation to the maternal pelvis. In a multigravida with deliveries of normal-sized infants, CPD is less likely, but in the event of a larger fetus there may be a problem. Abdominal palpation is an inaccurate method of judging fetal size, although experienced practitioners may become quite adept. Estimation of fetal size is becoming easier as ultrasound technology advances.
- Fetal abnormalities such as hydrocephalus.

Assessing the pelvis

A combination of careful history taking and clinical expertise backed up by technology should enable selection of women at risk. **Head fitting** or **pelvic assessment** examinations may be carried out. However, Enkin et al (2000) write that there is:

> reasonable correlation between clinical and radiological assessment of pelvic dimensions but neither are particularly accurate in predicting the outcome of labour and opinion varies about the value of pre-labour assessments.

Head fitting

In head fitting, the technique is to attempt to cause engagement of the non-engaged head. The woman is asked to empty her bladder and to lie flat on the examination couch. The symphysis pubis is located with the fingers of the right hand and the fetal head is held between the thumb and fingers of the left hand. The woman takes a deep breath and as she breaths out the head is pushed downwards and backwards into the brim of the pelvis. The fingers of the right hand palpate to assess whether the widest diameter of the head has entered the pelvic brim.

Pelvic assessment

Pelvic assessment of the shape and size of the pelvis is carried out by the obstetrician in the last few weeks of pregnancy if the head cannot be made to engage. The tissues will be softer, allowing ease of examination, and the fetus is large enough to relate to the size of the pelvis. The aim is to assess the brim, cavity and outlet of the pelvis. An attempt is made to measure the diagonal conjugate which runs from the lower border of the symphysis pubis to the sacral promontory and thus assess the anteroposterior diameter of the pelvic brim, also known as the **true** or **obstetric conjugate**, through which the fetus has to pass.

During a vaginal examination an attempt is made to reach the sacral promontory but in a good-sized pelvis it is unlikely to be reached as the diagonal conjugate measures 12–13 cm. If it is reached, 2 cm are subtracted to allow for the depth of the pubic bone and the obstetric conjugate is estimated. The size of the pelvic cavity is assessed by examination of the length and curve of the sacrum and by feeling the length of the sacrospinous ligament, which should accommodate two fingers.

Finally, the shape and size of the pelvic outlet can then be assessed. The ischial spines are located to see whether or not they are prominent, which may suggest a narrow transverse diameter of the outlet. The subpubic angle should be more than 90° and should accommodate the width of two fingers. One external measurement is made with the fist: the distance between the ischial tuberosities should accommodate a large fist.

X-ray pelvimetry

An erect lateral X-ray pelvimetry provides information about the size and shape of the pelvis and the relationship of the fetal head to the pelvic brim. However, there has been criticism of its use because of an association between pre-natal irradiation and childhood leukaemia. It may also be a poor predictor of CPD and the results do not appear to affect the management; therefore, an X-ray pelvimetry should seldom if ever be necessary in pregnancy (Enkin et al 2000). Details that can be seen are:

- the shape of the pelvis;
- the shape of the sacrum;
- the inclination between the sacrum and pelvic brim;
- the anteroposterior diameters of the brim, cavity and outlet;
- the width of the sacrosciatic notch;
- the depth of the pelvic cavity.

Request for pelvimetry Pelvimetry may be requested for the following factors:

- Any primigravida with the fetal head not engaged at term in whom clinical assessment suggests pelvic contraction.
- A primigravida with a breech presentation if external cephalic version has failed or is contraindicated and vaginal delivery is being considered.
- Any multipara with a history of difficult labour such as failure to progress in labour, prolonged labour and operative delivery although these women should be offered a pelvimetry in the postnatal period to avoid the risks of radiation to the fetus. A previous CS for any reason other than CPD is not a contraindication for trial of labour (Flamm et al 1994).
- Women with a history of injury or disease of the pelvis and spine or any limp or deformity.

Brock (1997) mentions a small study by Moore et al (1992) that examined the benefits of magnetic resonance imaging (MRI). More accurate measurements of the pelvic outlet without the danger of radiation may be achievable but more research is needed. Depending on the antenatal findings discussed above, there are three possibilities: disproportion is not present and vaginal delivery will be possible; there is CPD of such a degree that vaginal delivery will not be possible; and there is a degree of CPD which may be overcome in labour.

Trial of vaginal delivery

If there are no obstetric or medical complications, the woman can be admitted to hospital for a trial of labour. The aim is to allow time for the contractions of labour, aided by the abdominal and pelvic floor muscles, to cause sufficient flexion and moulding of the fetal head so that descent occurs (Abitol 1993). Engagement of the head is likely to be followed by vaginal delivery. All primigravidae with a non-engaged head are considered to be undergoing a trial of labour (Brock 1997). An old but probably useful saying is that the fetal head is the best pelvimeter.

Selection of women for trial of vaginal delivery

- The presentation must be cephalic.
- There should be no major degree of CPD.
- The woman should be healthy with a good obstetric and medical history.
- There should be no pregnancy complications such as hypertension.

Management

There must be careful monitoring of mother and fetus and facilities for the immediate carrying out of a CS if needed. All observations are plotted on a partogram and any changes in the conditions of mother, fetus or progress noted by the midwife must be reported to the obstetrician, who is the decision maker (Shiers 1999). The obstetrician may wish to conduct all vaginal examinations. Ambulation and adoption of an upright position encourages flexion and descent of the head, maintenance of good uterine action and cervical dilatation (Simkin & Ancheta 2000).

Assessment of progress Successful progression to a vaginal delivery should occur if the contractions are good, the fetal head flexes and the skull bones mould, the pelvic joints relax and maternal and fetal heart remain satisfactory. Progress is assessed by observation of descent of the fetal head by abdominal palpation. The dilatation of the cervix is assessed by vaginal examination. Progress in dilatation should follow that of 1 cm/h.

If progress is slow due to inefficient uterine action and thought to be unrelated to CPD, active management of labour can be undertaken and oxytocic drugs can be used. However, it is important to remember that the injudicious use of oxytocic drugs in the presence of more than a minor degree of CPD may lead to rupture of the uterus. If hyperstimulation occurs, the Syntocinon (oxytocin) infusion should be stopped immediately and the obstetrician informed. A CS may be necessary if:

- the progress of labour remains slow following the commencement of the oxytocin infusion;
- the head fails to descend in the presence of efficient contractions;
- fetal distress arises.

OBSTRUCTED LABOUR

Obstructed labour occurs when there is no advance of the presenting part despite strong uterine contractions (Shiers 1999). There is a large increase in maternal and fetal morbidity and mortality if labour is allowed to proceed in the presence of unrecognised obstructed labour. The situation is more common in remote areas of the world such as villages in Africa or India where women do not have access to trained personnel but it can also occur in a developed country such as in the UK if a woman fails to disclose her pregnancy or to present herself for care in labour.

Causes

- Cephalopelvic disproportion is a cause of obstructed labour that is unresolvable except by CS (in remote areas of the world, division of the symphysis pubis – symphysiotomy – or a fetal destructive operation may save the life of the mother).
- Malpositions and malpresentations of the head, such as brow, posterior face or deep transverse arrest of the head.
- Fetal abnormalities such as hydrocephalus.
- Maternal tumours.
- Fibroids.

Signs and symptoms

Early signs

- There is little progress in labour, with no descent of the head despite efficient uterine action.
- On vaginal examination, the presenting part is high.
- The cervix dilates slowly and may be felt like a curtain or empty sleeve (Brock 1997) hanging in front of the presenting part.
- The membranes have usually ruptured early and there is an ever-present risk of cord prolapse.
- In a primigravida there may be active phase arrest and the contractions stop for a while, finally restarting with increased strength. The woman may complain of severe and continuous pain.
- The multiparous woman may have tumultuous contractions that proceed rapidly to uterine rupture.

Late signs

- If nothing was done for the woman or, much more likely in the UK, if she presented herself for care late in labour, she may progress to having a raised temperature, rapid pulse and dehydration.
- On abdominal inspection, the uterus would appear to be moulded around the fetus because of tonic contraction and loss of liquor amnii.
- A Bandl's pathological retraction ring may be seen as a ridge of tissue running obliquely across the abdomen. This denotes an extremely thinned lower uterine segment and imminent rupture of the uterus.
- There will be a cutting off of the fetoplacental blood supply and fetal oxygen supply and the fetus will die.

- On examination the vagina feels hot and dry and the presenting part is high. There may be excessive moulding and a large caput succedaneum obscuring the presenting part in a cephalic presentation.
- Urinary output is reduced and a vesicovaginal fistula may occur due to sloughing off tissue due to prolonged pressure.

Management

Prevention, by achieving a high standard of antenatal care and observations in early labour, would be the best management to allow early detection of likely difficulties and treatment before obstructed labour occurs. Removal of an ovarian cyst, correction of an abnormal lie or performing a planned CS are examples of actions that minimise the chances of obstructed labour occurring. If labour is advanced when the woman is first seen, an emergency CS is carried out regardless of whether the fetus is dead or alive. Rarely, especially in developing countries, if the fetus is dead and the cervix is fully dilated destructive operations such as cleidotomy (division of the clavicles) or craniotomy (perforation of the skull) may allow vaginal delivery but there is risk of perforation of the thin lower uterine segment (Gupta & Chitra 1994).

UTERINE RUPTURE

Rupture of the uterus is an obstetric emergency and the fetus and mother may die. Rupture of the uterus may involve a previous scar, spontaneous rupture of an intact uterus or traumatic rupture. Deaths from uterine trauma have reduced to two between 1997 and 1999 compared with five deaths in the previous triennial report of the confidential enquiry into maternal deaths in the UK (Lewis 2001). The incidence of uterine rupture appears to be reducing in developed countries but may be rising in the developing countries due to vaginal delivery following a previous CS and due to inappropriate use of oxytocic infusions (Grace et al 1993).

Types of uterine rupture

Scar rupture is usually due to a previous CS. A longitudinal scar in the uterus (classical incision) is more likely to rupture than a transverse scar in the lower segment. Rupture of the classical scar occurs in about 2% of cases and is more likely to occur in late pregnancy when the upper segment is stretched to its limit. Performing a CS at 38 weeks may reduce this rate. Rupture of a transverse lower segment scar is more likely to happen in labour as the lower segment is thinned and extended. Uterine rupture following a lower segment CS is less than 1%.

Traumatic rupture of the uterus may be caused by the use of obstetric instruments such as forceps. These can cause tearing of the cervix which extends into the lower segment. Intrauterine manipulations such as internal podalic version, where the foot of the fetus is grasped at delivery to convert a transverse lie – usually of the second twin – to breech or correction of a shoulder presentation in labour, may lead to uterine rupture as may the misuse of oxytocic drugs.

Spontaneous rupture of the uterus may follow strong spontaneous uterine action such as that occurring in obstructed labour. The rupture is found most often in the lower segment. Abruptio placentae where there is extravasation of blood into the uterine muscle (Couvelaire uterus) facilitates such a rupture.

Signs and symptoms

Complete rupture

Rupture of the uterus may be complete or true, involving the full thickness of the uterine wall and the pelvic peritoneum. This is usually an acute event associated with sudden intense pain, blood loss and collapse followed by maternal and fetal death. The uterine contractions cease and there is vaginal bleeding. The fetus may pass into the abdominal cavity and be palpable outside the uterus directly under the abdominal wall.

Incomplete rupture

Incomplete or silent rupture involves the myometrium but the peritoneum remains intact. It is more frequently associated with a previous lower segment CS. Because scar tissue tends to be avascular, there are less dramatic signs. The mother's condition deteriorates slowly. Abdominal pain or scar tenderness may be present and a rise in maternal heart rate may be an indicator of impending rupture.

Management

If a ruptured uterus is diagnosed, obstetric, anaesthetic and theatre emergency teams must be alerted and the mother immediately transferred to theatre. The anaesthetist will establish venous access and start resuscitative measures while the surgeons and the theatre teams scrub up for emergency CS. A blood transfusion will be necessary. The baby is delivered and the uterus repaired if possible. A hysterectomy may be necessary if the rupture is severe and bleeding difficult to control. Postoperative treatment should include observation of severe side-effects of haemorrhage such as renal failure or, later, onset of Sheehan's syndrome. The psychological effect of the experience on the woman and her family should be anticipated and explanations and counselling made available.

SHOULDER DYSTOCIA

This term is used to describe a range of difficulties encountered with the delivering the shoulders after delivering the head.

Definition

Shoulder dystocia is a condition requiring special manoeuvres to deliver shoulders following an unsuccessful attempt to apply downward traction.

Shoulder dystocia is another obstetric emergency which may end in fetal and maternal morbidity and mortality. There is difficulty in delivering the anterior shoulder and urgent manoeuvres are necessary (Fig. 44.1). There are two causes:

1. a large baby;
2. failure of the shoulders to rotate into the anteroposterior diameter following delivery of the head.

The incidence of shoulder dystocia is about 0.2% and the risk rises as pregnancy becomes prolonged with increasing birth weight.

Discrepancies in the definition, the degree of difficulty and the manoeuvres used have resulted in variations between 0.15% and 2% of all vaginal deliveries in the reported incidence of this obstetric emergency.

Recognition

The head fails to advance and the fetus looks to be burying its chin in the perineum. This happens because the anterior shoulder is wedged firmly behind the symphysis pubis. Difficulty in delivering the face and the chin are warning signs (Shiers & Coates 1999).

Risk factors

The following factors, most of them associated with a large fetus, should be taken into consideration so that the woman can be delivered in an appropriate setting:

- if the mother is over 35 years there may be an associated increase in birth weight;
- a maternal weight of more than 90 kg is the most frequently associated factor;

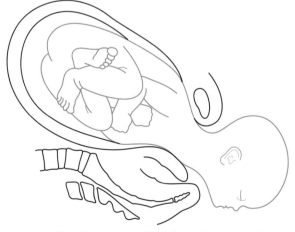

Figure 44.1   Shoulder dystocia (from Sweet B 1997, with permission).

- maternal diabetes mellitus, whether insulin dependent or gestational, is associated with fetal macrosomia and difficulty in delivering the shoulders;
- infants of increased birth weight in non-diabetic mothers have less incidence of shoulder dystocia, with a 10% risk rather than the 31% risk of the diabetic woman (Spellacy et al 1985);
- maternal high birth weight is associated with high birth weight of her own fetus;
- women with a platypelloid pelvis, where the antero posterior diameter is reduced, may develop shoulder dystocia with a normal-sized infant.

Management

Excessive force must not be applied to the fetal head or neck and fundal pressure must be avoided (ALSO 2000). These activities are unlikely to free the impaction and may cause maternal and fetal injury. If possible, the midwife should summon an obstetrician, paediatrician and anaesthetist. However, there is little time to save the life of the baby and the woman may be in her own home so the midwife must attempt to complete the delivery. It may be necessary to try more than one manoeuvre so it is necessary to keep calm and think clearly about what is happening inside the mother's pelvis.

Manoeuvres

The HELPERR mnemonic is a clinical tool that can provide practitioners with a structured framework to deal with this extremely difficult situation:

H Call for help
E Evaluate for episiotomy
L Legs (the McRoberts' manoeuvre)
P Pressure (suprapubic)
E Enter (internal manoeuvres)
R Remove the posterior arm
R Roll the woman

The manoeuvres (ALSO 2000) will be dealt with individually but this does not imply that any one technique is superior to any other; together they are a valuable tool for practitioners to take effective steps to overcome this situation. The steps should be done efficiently and appropriately as the time element is vital. An assistant can maintain relevant recordings of the events.

The three main aims of the manoeuvres are to:

1. increase the functional size of the bony pelvis;
2. decrease the bisacromial diameter;
3. change the relationship of the bisacromial diameter within the bony pelvis.

It is recommended that an episiotomy be performed, if possible. Even though the obstruction is bony, it will give

room for the manoeuvres and prevent maternal trauma. Delivery should be attempted following each manoeuvre.

The McRoberts' manoeuvre

This is a simple manoeuvre and its effectiveness makes it appropriate for the first step in the management. The woman is helped to lie on her back with her knees drawn up to her chest (Fig. 44.2), which simulates the squatting position. This manoeuvre can help to deliver the shoulders by:

- opening the pelvic inlet to its maximum possible diameter;
- flexing the fetal spine and pushing the posterior shoulder over the sacral promontory and into the hollow of the sacrum;
- rotating the symphysis pubis superiorly over the impacted shoulder;
- elevating the anterior shoulder;
- straightening any maternal lumbosacral lordosis and flattening the sacral promontory to reduce this obstruction;
- bringing the inlet perpendicular to the maximum expulsive force;
- removing the weigh-bearing forces from the sacrum;
- allowing the direction of the maternal force to be perpendicular to the plane of the inlet.

This manoeuvre can be tried twice as a first resort when shoulder dystocia has been diagnosed.

Suprapubic pressure

An assistant should attempt external manual suprapubic pressure for 30–60 s while the delivering practitioner continues gentle traction. The suprapubic hand should be placed over the fetus's anterior shoulder and pressure should be applied in a 'CPR' style in such a way as to adduct or collapse the shoulder anteriorly and pass under the pubic symphysis. Initially, the pressure should be continuous but, if not accomplished, a rocking motion is recommended to dislodge the shoulder from behind the pubic symphysis.

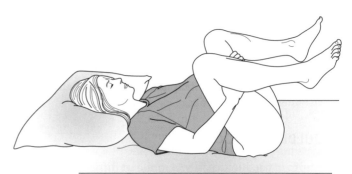

Figure 44.2   McRoberts' position (from Sweet B 1997, with permission).

Internal manoeuvres

The following two manoeuvres attempt to manipulate the fetus to rotate the anterior shoulder into an oblique plane and under the maternal symphysis pubis.

1. Rubin's manoeuvre   Rubin's manoeuvre can be described as manoeuvres I and II. The first manoeuvre is to rock the fetus's shoulders from side to side once or twice by pushing on the mother's lower abdomen (this is the **P** or **Pressure** component as previously described).

Rubin's II manoeuvre is carried out to reduce the diameter of the shoulder girdle and is the basis of the first part of the **E** or **Enter** component. The fingers of one hand are inserted into the vagina behind the anterior shoulder and pushing the shoulder towards the fetus's chest to reduce the diameter. If both shoulders are adducted, the circumference of the baby's body is greatly reduced (we use this position to squeeze through narrow spaces by bringing our shoulders forward to make ourselves smaller). This may free the shoulders from the symphysis pubis to allow delivery. The McRoberts' manoeuvre can still be applied to facilitate delivery. If unsuccessful, the practitioner should proceed to the next movement.

2. Woods' screw manoeuvre   This next manoeuvre can be combined with the Rubin II manoeuvre. The practitioner uses the opposite hand to approach the posterior shoulder from the front of the fetus, and rotate the shoulder towards the symphysis in the same direction as with the Rubin II manoeuvre. The practitioner now has two fingers behind the anterior shoulder and two fingers of the other hand in front of the posterior shoulder. The Rubin II adducts or flexes either the anterior shoulder while the Wood's screw manoeuvre abducts or extends the posterior shoulder. This is why the combination of the two manoeuvres may be more successful.

If these manoeuvres fail, then the **reverse Wood's screw** manoeuvre may be tried. The fingers of the entering hand are placed on the posterior shoulder from behind and the attempt is to rotate the fetus in the opposite direction as the Wood's screw manoeuvre. This rotates the shoulders out of the impacted position to allow delivery. This manoeuvre is identical to the Rubin II when performed on the posterior shoulder.

There remains a lot of confusion in obstetrics about performing these manoeuvres. They can occasionally be difficult to perform particularly when the anterior shoulder is partially wedged underneath the symphysis. At times it may be necessary to push the posterior shoulder, or sometimes the anterior shoulder, back up into the pelvis slightly in order to accomplish the manoeuvre (ALSO 2000). Since this is an obstetric emergency then it is important that practitioners are prepared to perform all the practical skills of the different manoeuvres. These should be practised in workgroup situations using dolls and pelvis or other similar models for simulation purposes.

Remove the posterior arm

A hand is inserted into the vagina along the sacral curve to locate the posterior arm or hand. Once located, the elbow should be flexed so that the forearm may be delivered in a sweeping motion over the anterior chest wall of the fetus, thus shortening the bisacromial diameter (Fig. 44.3). This allows the anterior shoulder to collapse as the fetus drops into the pelvic hollow, freeing the impaction anteriorly.

Roll the woman

The woman should be rolled onto the 'all fours' position. This is a safe, rapid and effective technique for the reduction of shoulder dystocia. By rotating to this position, the true obstetrical conjugate increases by as much as 10 mm and the sagittal measurement of the pelvic outlet increases up to 20 mm. The fetal shoulders often dislodge during the act of turning from supine to this position.

Other manoeuvres

Cleidotomy   This is a deliberate fracture of the clavicle but is difficult and rarely done. Spontaneous fracture may occur and facilitate delivery.

Zavanelli manoeuvre   This manoeuvre of cephalic replacement followed by CS involves returning the head to its pre-restitution position, flexing the head and pushing it back into the birth canal. Continuous upward pressure is maintained until the CS can be performed.

Outcome for mother and fetus

Maternal death is rare but can happen. Maternal morbidity is more common, with perineal, vaginal and cervical lacerations, uterine rupture, vaginal haematoma and haemorrhage possibly occurring. Postpartum haemorrhage should be anticipated and the genitalia carefully examined for lacerations.

For the baby, birth asphyxia is a complication of shoulder dystocia. Meconium aspiration may occur due to the asphyxia. Birth injury is also commonly reported with brachial plexus injury.

CORD PRESENTATION AND PROLAPSE

Campbell & Lees (2000) state that 1 in 300 births are complicated by presentation of the umbilical cord when the cord lies in front of the presenting part with the fetal membranes still intact. If a loop of cord lies alongside the fetal presenting part, it is an **occult cord presentation**. If the membranes rupture, the cord is prolapsed. Murphy & MacKenzie (1995) found an incidence of cord prolapse in 132 babies born in the John Radcliffe Hospital, Oxford, between 1984 and

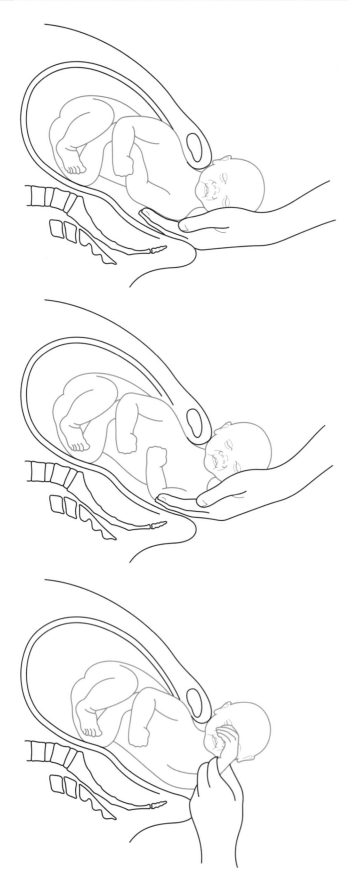

Figure 44.3 Delivery of posterior arm (from Sweet B 1997, with permission).

1992. This gave a rate of 1 in 426 total births. There were 6 stillbirths and 6 neonatal deaths, giving an uncorrected perinatal mortality rate of 91 per 1000. Of 120 survivors, only one baby was known to have developed a major neurological handicap.

Causes of cord presentation and prolapse

- A high presenting part: multiparous women, malposition of the occiput and malpresentations – brow, face, shoulder presentation (in 20%) and breech presentation (in 5%), the high assimilation pelvis found in Afro-Caribbean women, cephalopelvic disproportion, placenta praevia, fibroids.
- Preterm labour because of the increased ratio of liquor amnii to fetus and the prevalence of malpresentations.
- Multiple births, especially following the birth of the first baby.
- Polyhydramnios.
- An unusually long cord.
- Following obstetric manipulations such as external cephalic version.

Diagnosis and management

Cord presentation may be diagnosed in pregnancy by ultrasound scanning, especially in women with any of the risk factors mentioned above (Lange et al 1985). In early labour vaginal examination may occasionally find the rope-like cord between the presenting part and the membranes. It will be pulsating in time with the fetal heart rate. If cord presentation is suspected, it is essential to ensure that the membranes do not rupture. The mother is best placed in an exaggerated Simm's position with her pelvis, hips and buttocks elevated to take pressure off the cord and membranes. This is an obstetric emergency and medical assistance should be obtained immediately. If cord presentation persists, an emergency CS will be needed. If the membranes have ruptured, the cord may have prolapsed through the cervix, into the vagina or even outside of the vulva.

If the cord is prolapsed it may be felt in the vagina or seen at the vulva. The cord may be compressed, especially if the presentation is cephalic because of the hardness of the fetal head, and the fetal oxygen supply cut off. If the cord is external to the vagina, cooling, drying and handling may precipitate spasm in the umbilical vessels. If the woman is in hospital the prognosis can be good. However, if the woman is at home fetal loss may be high.

Factors to take into consideration are the stage in labour and whether or not the fetus is dead. If fetal death is confirmed, labour can be allowed to continue unless other conditions such as obstructed labour contraindicate vaginal delivery. If the fetus is thought to be alive, the treatment is immediate delivery. In the first stage of labour an emergency CS is arranged. In the meantime, pressure must be kept off the cord by positioning the woman in a knee–chest posture or exaggerated Simm's position. The cord can be replaced gently back in the vagina and oxygen therapy may be of use if there is some fetoplacental circulation remaining.

In the early part of the second stage of labour with no cephalopelvic disproportion or malpresentation, a forceps delivery is performed. If the woman is multiparous and in late second stage an episiotomy may allow early delivery.

MAIN POINTS

- Any condition leading to a misfit between the fetal head and the maternal pelvis with failure of descent of the head into the pelvis despite good contractions results in cephalopelvic disproportion (CPD). Cephalopelvic disproportion is an absolute cause of obstructed labour and there are dangers for mother and fetus.

- Maternal indications of possible CPD include bone conditions which may have resulted in alterations in the size and shape of the pelvis, spinal deformities, pelvic trauma and fractures, previous difficulties with delivery and short stature. Fetal conditions leading to CPD include size of the fetus in relation to the maternal pelvis.

- A combination of careful history taking and clinical expertise backed up by technology should enable selection of women at risk. Head fitting and clinical or radiological pelvic assessment examinations may be carried out. An erect lateral X-ray pelvimetry provides information about the size and shape of the pelvis and the relationship of the fetal head to the pelvic brim. Magnetic resonance imaging (MRI) may allow more accurate measurements of the pelvis.

- Obstructed labour occurs whenever there is an impassable barrier to the descent of the fetus through the birth canal in spite of efficient uterine action. There is a large increase in maternal and fetal morbidity and mortality if labour is allowed to proceed. Causes of obstructed labour are CPD, malpositions and malpresentations of the head, such as brow, posterior face or deep transverse arrest of the head, fetal abnormalities such as hydrocephalus and maternal tumours.

- Rupture of the uterus may involve a previous scar, spontaneous rupture of an intact uterus or traumatic rupture. Rupture of the uterus may be complete. This is usually an acute event associated with sudden intense pain, blood loss and collapse followed by maternal and fetal death. Incomplete or silent rupture is more frequently associated with a previous lower segment CS.

- Shoulder dystocia is an obstetric emergency which may end in fetal and maternal morbidity and mortality. It may be due a large baby and failure of the shoulders to rotate into the anteroposterior diameter following delivery of the head.

- Causes of cord presentation and prolapse include high presenting part, breech presentation, cephalopelvic disproportion, placenta praevia, fibroids, preterm labour, multiple births, polyhydramnios, a long cord and external cephalic version. If the membranes rupture, the cord may prolapse and may become compressed, cutting off the fetal oxygen supply. If the cord is outside the vagina, cooling, drying and handling may precipitate the umbilical vessel spasm.

References

Abitol M M 1993 Adjustment of the fetal head and adult pelvis in modern humans. Journal of Human Evolution 8(3):167–185.

ALSO 2000 Shoulder Dystocia, 4th edn. Advanced Life Support in Obstetrics, Registered Charity No 1024554, UK Office, Newcastle-upon-Tyne.

Brock M I 1997 Cephalopelvic disproportion, obstructed labour and uterine rupture. In Sweet B R, Tiran D (eds) Mayes Midwifery: A Textbook for Midwives, 12th edn. Baillière Tindall, London.

Campbell S, Lees C 2000 Obstetrics by Ten Teachers, 17th edn. Hodder, London.

Enkin M, Keirse M J N C, Renfrew M et al 2000 A Guide to Effective Care in Pregnancy and Childbirth, 3rd edn. Oxford University Press, Oxford.

Flamm B L, Goings J R, Liu Y et al 1994 Elective repeat caesarean delivery versus trial of labour: a prospective multi-centre study. Obstetrics and Gynaecology 83(6):927–932.

Grace D, Lavery G, Loughran P G 1993 Acute uterine rupture and its sequelae. International Journal of Obstetric Anaesthesia 2:41–44.

Gupta U, Chitra R 1994 Destructive operations still have a place in developing countries. International Journal of Gynaecology and Obstetrics 44(1):15–19.

Lange I R, Manning F A, Morrison I et al 1985 Cord prolapse: is antenatal diagnosis possible? American Journal of Obstetrics and Gynecology 1512:1083–1085.

Lewis G (ed.) 2001 Why mothers die, 1997–1999: the 5th Report of the Confidential Enquiries into Maternal Deaths in the United Kingdom. RCOG, London.

Mahmood T A, Campbell D M, Wilson A W 1988 Maternal height, shoe size, and outcome of labour in white primigravidas: a prospective study. British Medical Journal 297:515–517.

Moore N R, Dickenson D R M, Gillmer M D 1992 Royal College of Radiologists Annual Meeting – Abstract. Clinical Radiology 46:414.

Morgan E 1994 The Descent of the Child. Souvenir Press, London.

Murphy D J, MacKenzie I Z 1995 The mortality and morbidity associated with umbilical cord prolapse. British Journal of Obstetrics and Gynaecology 102(10):826–830.

Shiers C V 1999 Prolonged pregnancy and disorders of uterine action. In Bennett V R, Brown L K (eds) Myles Textbook for Midwives, 13th edn. Churchill Livingstone, Edinburgh.

Shiers C V, Coates T 1999 Midwifery and obstetric emergencies. In Bennett V R, Brown L K (eds) Myles Textbook for Midwives, 13th edn. Churchill Livingstone, Edinburgh.

Simkin P, Ancheta R 2000 The Labour Progress Handbook. Blackwell Science, Oxford.

Spellacy W N, Miller S, Winegar A et al 1985 Macrosomia, maternal characteristics and infant complications. Obstetrics and Gynaecology 66(2):158–161.

Annotated recommended reading

Lewis G (ed.) 2001 Why mothers die, 1997–1999: the 5th Report of the Confidential Enquiries into Maternal Deaths in the UK. RCOG, London.

This triennial report was produced for the confidential enquiries into maternal deaths in the UK. All health professionals providing care for women during pregnancy and childbirth are urged to read the full report.

Chapter **45**

Postpartum haemorrhage and other third-stage problems

INTRODUCTION

Once the baby has been born, delivery of the placenta and membranes may seem an anticlimax. However, the third (3rd) stage of labour is the most dangerous for the woman. The management of the 3rd stage should be aimed at minimising these possible serious complications but interfering as little as possible with the physiological process and the mother's enjoyment of her baby (Enkin et al 2000). A major role of the midwife is to explain the need for active interventions, such as the giving of an oxytocic drug or commencing an intravenous infusion, to the mothers, prior to labour so that women are enabled to make informed choices should the need suddenly arise.

POSTPARTUM HAEMORRHAGE

Definition

Postpartum haemorrhage (PPH) is defined as excessive bleeding from the genital tract following the birth of the child. PPH occurs in the period extending from the time of birth to the end of the puerperium. If bleeding occurs in the first 24 h, it is called **primary PPH** and complicates about 6% of labours. If the bleeding occurs after the first 24 h and before the end of the 6th week, it is called **secondary PPH**, a much less common occurrence that complicates less than 1% of deliveries.

Postpartum haemorrhage is also classified according to the site of bleeding. Most commonly, the bleeding is from the placental site and there is poor tone of the uterine muscle. This is **atonic haemorrhage**. Bleeding may also be traumatic due to a laceration of the genital tract. In primary PPH, bleeding is said to be excessive if the amount exceeds 500 ml or is sufficient to cause deterioration in the woman's condition. Because of the diuresis and haemoconcentration that follow delivery, smaller amounts of blood loss are detrimental in secondary PPH.

Primary PPH is one of the most serious complications of labour that a midwife has to deal with until medical aid arrives. At term, maternal blood is circulating to the placenta at about 500 ml/min and the blood loss may be rapid and devastating *if the bleeding is not controlled*. PPH is still a significant cause of maternal mortality, especially following a caesarean section (CS) (Lewis 2001). Measuring blood loss at delivery can be difficult. It is important to remember that blood soaks into sheets and towels and that it separates into clot and serum. Any clot placed in a jug and measured will only be 40% of the total loss so that it is easy to underestimate the total loss by up to 50%.

Primary postpartum haemorrhage from the placental site

Causes

Failure of the uterine muscle fibres to contract and retract to compress the blood vessels is the immediate cause. Risk factors are:

- a history of previous postpartum haemorrhage;
- high parity – para 3 or more;
- overdistension of the uterus in multiple pregnancy, polyhydramnios and a large fetus;
- fibroids may interfere with efficient contraction and retraction;
- antepartum haemorrhage – the bleeding that occurs into the muscle during placental abruption will reduce the fibres' ability to contract and retract and in placenta praevia there is little contractile ability in the lower uterine segment;
- prolonged labour with weak or uncoordinated contractions;
- atony caused by drugs such as antihypertensives, general anaesthesia and tocolytics;
- retained placenta;
- anaemia because even a small amount of blood loss may precipitate shock;
- inversion of the uterus;
- mismanagement of the 3rd stage of labour by fiddling with the uterus;
- coagulation defects – disseminated intravascular coagulation may complicate concealed placental abruption, amniotic fluid embolus, severe pre-eclampsia and eclampsia and intrauterine death;
- medical disorders of clotting may also lead to primary PPH.

Despite the long list of risk factors outlined above, many cases of primary PPH occur in normal labours with no explanation.

Management of primary postpartum haemorrhage

In the antenatal period Prevention is the best form of management and begins with the booking interview. If any of the risk factors described above are present, the woman should be delivered in hospital so that if bleeding does occur then treatment is immediately available. As pregnancy progresses detection and treatment of anaemia is important and it would be advantageous to raise the haemoglobin (Hb) level to at least 11 g/dl before delivery (Lindsay 1997).

In labour Women at risk of PPH must be managed carefully to minimise the likelihood of bleeding. When labour commences an intravenous cannula is inserted and blood is taken for a full blood count (FBC) and confirmation of blood group. Serum is saved for 'cross matching' blood should it become necessary to give the woman a blood transfusion. Prolonged labour, with its problems of dehydration and exhaustion, should be avoided. A Syntocinon (oxytocin) infusion should be started if labour progress is slow. The woman's bladder should be kept empty by encouraging micturition or by catheterisation, as a full bladder may inhibit uterine muscle activity and add to the risk of atony.

Management of the 3rd stage should be discussed with the woman antenatally. She should be advised that the potential for PPH is greater with physiological management of the 3rd stage than it is with 'active management'. It should be explained to her that the medical view is that it is safer to manage the 3rd stage of labour actively. In active management, an intramuscular injection of Syntometrine 1 ml, containing Syntocinon 5 units and ergometrine 500 µg, is given with the birth of the anterior shoulder. The placenta is then delivered by controlled cord traction. An intravenous or intramuscular injection of ergometrine 500 µg would be prescribed if the woman starts to bleed.

Signs of postpartum haemorrhage

It would be difficult to miss the visible bleeding and maternal collapse that can occur. Other signs may be present if blood loss is not visible. For instance, if clots were retained in an atonic uterus:

- pallor;
- a rising pulse rate and falling blood pressure;
- altered levels of consciousness;
- air hunger;
- an enlarged boggy-feeling uterus.

Management of primary postpartum haemorrhage – treatment

It is important that a midwife is familiar with the sequence of actions needed to deal with a PPH and to minimise the effects of blood loss.

If bleeding begins **before the placenta is delivered**, the following actions should be taken:

1. Ensure that medical aid is available.

2. Massage the fundus of the uterus firmly by a smooth circular motion to stimulate a uterine contraction, i.e. to

'rub up' a contraction. Bleeding indicates that the placenta has begun to separate and it is no longer necessary to await events.

3. Give an oxytocic drug. Intramuscular Syntometrine 1 ml will act to contract the uterus in 2.5 min and an intravenous injection of either Syntometrine 1 ml or ergometrine 500 μg will act in 45 s. Note that the midwife should not give more than two injections of ergometrine 500 μg as the drug may cause severe peripheral vasoconstriction and a sudden rise in blood pressure.

4. Pass a catheter into the bladder and ensure that it is completely empty.

5. Palpate to ensure the uterus is contracted, and then attempt to deliver the placenta by controlled cord traction.

6. If all else fails, the obstetrician should be asked to review. The obstetrician will try to deliver the placenta by cord traction. If this fails, the woman will need a manual removal of the placenta under spinal or epidural anaesthesia.

If the uterus is well contracted, the bleeding is likely to be from traumatic injury to the soft tissues. Locate the bleeding site and try to stem the bleeding using pressure.

If bleeding begins **after delivery of the placenta**, massage the uterus to obtain a contraction and expel any blood clots remaining in the uterus. An injection of an oxytocic drug, either intramuscular Syntometrine 1 ml or ergometrine 500 μg should then stop bleeding by achieving a sustained contraction. Ensure that the urinary bladder is empty. If bleeding continues, it is necessary to carry out bimanual compression of the uterus. Following delivery of the placenta and membranes, they should be examined for completeness. If the placenta appears incomplete, the doctor will carry out an exploration and evacuation of the uterus under spinal or epidural anaesthesia.

Bimanual compression of the uterus   Bimanual compression may be performed externally or internally. In **external bimanual compression**, one hand is dipped down as far as possible behind the uterus while the other is placed flat on the abdomen. The uterus is compressed between the two hands and pulled upwards in the abdomen. This ensures that the bleeding area of the placental site is compressed while the uterine veins are straightened out to allow free drainage, relieve congestion and decrease the bleeding (Lindsay 1997).

Internal bimanual compression is carried out if the mother is anaesthetised and still bleeding after manual removal of placenta. One hand is closed to form a fist, inserted into the anterior vaginal fornix and pushed up towards the body of the uterus. The other hand is placed on the abdominal wall behind the uterus and compresses the uterus downwards against the hand in the vagina. This applies compression to the placental site until the uterus is felt to contract (Fig. 45.1).

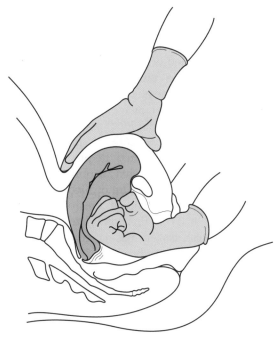

Figure 45.1   Internal bimanual compression of the uterus (from Sweet B 1997, with permission).

Once bleeding is controlled, an intravenous infusion containing Syntocinon (oxytocin) is started to maintain uterine contraction. If blood loss is excessive or if the woman had a low haemoglobin level before delivery, a blood transfusion may be necessary. It is important not to underestimate the amount of blood lost. As early as 1967 Brant found that estimates of blood loss became more inaccurate as the amount lost increased. In the case of serious PPH, the obstetrician and anaesthetist will agree on the management of fluid replacement. Each hospital will have guidelines on managing PPH; these should be followed at all times. Group O rhesus-negative blood should be available on the labour ward for use in emergencies. Where large volumes of blood are to be transfused, blood-warming coils should be used.

If the uterus fails to contract even though oxytocic drugs have been used, a deep intramuscular injection of the prostanoid carboprost, which is 15-methyl-PGF$_{2\alpha}$ (Rang et al 2001), can be given in a dose of 250 μg and repeated at intervals of 1.5 h. Carboprost is contraindicated in women with cardiac, renal, pulmonary and hepatic disease as well as in acute pelvic inflammation. It should be used with care in women who have asthma, hypertension, diabetes, epilepsy, hypotension or hypertension (BNF 2003). Different maternity units, according to their guidelines, may use different methods for controlling bleeding. In continuing haemorrhage, internal iliac artery ligation and uterine packing may be needed and, if all fails, a hysterectomy may be performed to save the woman's life. Further controlled trials are required to assess the effectiveness and safety of pharmacological and surgical interventions used for the treatment of PPH (Mousa & Alfirevic 2002).

Observations   Once blood loss is controlled, the total loss is estimated remembering how difficult this can be and that estimates become less accurate as blood loss increases. Fluid intake is recorded on a chart, as is the hourly urine output. Central venous pressure measurement may be required, depending on the blood loss and the severity of the woman's condition, which may require correct fluid replacement. Maternal pulse and blood pressure are recorded every 15 min to ensure her condition remains satisfactory. The uterine fundus is palpated frequently to ensure it remains contracted and the lochia are observed.

If the problem involves failure of blood coagulation, a haematologist should be involved. Fresh blood is usually the best treatment as it contains both platelets and coagulation factors but fresh frozen plasma, containing factors V and VIII and fibrinogen, can be used.

Traumatic postpartum haemorrhage

If the blood loss is from a laceration of the genital tract, bleeding should be stopped by direct pressure if possible and then sutured. Bleeding from a cervical or lower uterine tear should be suspected if the uterus is well contracted, no superficial bleeding can be seen and the blood loss is slow and steady. Tears of the upper part of the vagina, the cervix and lower uterine segment should be sutured under spinal or epidural anaesthesia. If severe bleeding is from the uterus and cannot be stopped, a hysterectomy may be necessary to save the woman's life.

Secondary postpartum haemorrhage

Secondary PPH is any abnormal bleeding or excessive bleeding from the birth canal occurring 24 h and 12 weeks postnatally (Alexander et al 2001). This is a complication of the puerperium and is most often seen between days 4 and 14. It is usually due to a retained piece of placenta but other causes include the presence of blood clot or a fibroid in the uterine wall. Secondary PPH is also commonly associated with infection. There may have been warning signs of heavy, red, offensive lochia and subinvolution. If infection is present, pyrexia and tachycardia may be present.

Management

If the uterus is palpable it is massaged to make it contract. Any clots are expelled and the bladder must be emptied. If bleeding is slight it may be managed at home with antibiotics and oral ergometrine tablets.

If bleeding is severe, an intravenous injection of ergometrine 500 μg or intramuscular Syntometrine 1 ml is given. If the woman is at home she should be transferred to hospital once her condition is under control. A blood transfusion may be given, depending on the blood loss and the antenatal Hb. The uterus is evacuated under spinal or epidural anaesthesia.

Complications of postpartum haemorrhage

Unless adequately treated, the woman is likely to develop **chronic iron deficiency anaemia**. Infection is more common and lactation may be poor. If shock develops, acute renal tubular necrosis may present with anuria. Anterior pituitary necrosis leading to Sheehan's syndrome may occur if the haemorrhage was severe. All women who have suffered a postpartum haemorrhage should be advised to book into hospital for any subsequent deliveries.

Haematoma formation

Postpartum haemorrhage may be concealed if progressive haematoma formation occurs in the perineum or lower vagina. A site of haematoma formation more difficult to diagnose is bleeding into the broad ligament. Up to 1 litre of blood may collect in the tissues, leading to increasing maternal pain due to pressure. The mother may collapse with signs of shock.

Management

The woman will have to be taken to theatre so that the haematoma can be drained and haemostasis achieved under spinal or general anaesthetic. Replacement of the lost blood may be necessary. Infection is a risk and antibiotics are usually prescribed.

PROLONGED THIRD STAGE

Failure of the placenta to deliver spontaneously remains an important cause of postpartum haemorrhage (Lewis 2001). If labour is managed actively, the placenta and membranes should be delivered within 10 min.

If the placenta is not delivered within 30 min, the 3rd stage is considered to be prolonged. With physiological management of the 3rd stage, up to 1 h may be allowed before considering the procedure to be prolonged. The placenta may be separated but retained, trapped behind the reforming cervix, and bleeding is likely. Alternatively, the placenta may be morbidly adherent to the uterine wall and, if there is no separation, bleeding will not occur.

Causes

- Uterine inertia.
- Full bladder.
- Mismanagement of the 3rd stage where 'fiddling' with the fundus causes irregular contractions and partial separation of the placenta.
- The formation of a constriction ring or spasm between the upper and lower uterine segments.
- A uterine abnormality such as bicornuate uterus.
- Morbid adherence of the placenta, more likely to occur in women who have had a previous CS or placenta praevia.

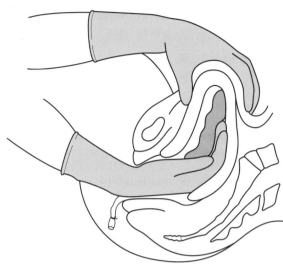

Figure 45.2   Manual removal of the placenta (from Sweet B 1997, with permission).

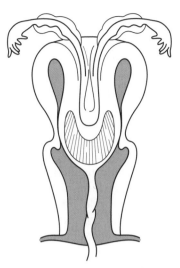

Figure 45.3   Inversion of the gravid uterus (from Sweet B 1997, with permission).

Types of adherent placenta

1. **Placenta accreta**, where the decidua basalis is deficient and the chorionic villi have attached to the myometrium.
2. **Placenta increta**, where the villi penetrate deeply into the myometrium.
3. **Placenta percreta**, where the villi have penetrated to the serous external coat of the uterus.

Management

As long as the placenta remains in the uterus, haemorrhage is a threat. If there is no success in delivering the placenta after emptying the bladder, manual removal of the placenta by the obstetrician will necessary (Fig. 45.2). The procedure may cause shock if conducted without adequate anaesthesia.

The obstetrician has two choices in deeply adherent placentae. A CS can be performed or the placenta can be left in situ to be reabsorbed. The drug methotrexate has been used to hasten the absorption of the placental tissue but is not always successful (Lindsay 1997). An intravenous oxytocic injection is given following successful manual removal followed by an intravenous infusion of Syntocinon (oxytocin). Different hospitals have different protocols for the amount of Syntocinon to be used after manual removal of placenta. Prophylactic antibiotic therapy is commenced, as manual removal of placenta may have introduced organisms into the uterus.

ACUTE INVERSION OF THE UTERUS

In this rare condition, which occurs in about 1 in 100 000 deliveries, the uterus is partly or completely turned inside out (Fig. 45.3). In **partial inversion**, the inner surface of the fundus is drawn down into the uterine cavity; in **severe inversion**, the inside of the fundus protrudes through the cervix into the vagina. If the uterus is fully turned inside out, it may appear outside the vulva. Profound neurogenic shock due to traction on the uterine supportive ligaments is likely to occur. There will be pain and possibly haemorrhage if there is partial placental separation.

Causes

- Mismanagement of the 3rd stage by applying fundal pressure or cord traction with the uterus relaxed.
- A short cord, where the fundus descends with the fetus.
- Manual removal of placenta if the operator withdraws the hand in the uterus while still applying fundal pressure.
- Spontaneous inversion, possibly due to straining, which raises intra-abdominal pressure, such as a sudden cough or sneeze.

Diagnosis and management

The woman will complain of pain and may collapse suddenly. On palpation of the uterus, it will be difficult to find the fundus of the uterus. A distinct hollow in the fundus may be felt. The woman may complain of a feeling that something is in her vagina.

The rapid replacement of the uterus will prevent the development of shock. Replacement is easier if it is carried out immediately, before uterine congestion and oedema develop. Pressure is applied first to the part of the lower segment nearest the cervix, gently proceeding upwards towards the fundus. If replacement is not possible, the uterus should be replaced in the vagina and the foot of the bed elevated to reduce traction on the uterine ligaments, fallopian tubes and ovaries. An injection of morphine 15 mg will reduce pain. If the placenta is still attached to the uterine wall, it should not be removed.

Methods of replacement

If there has been delay the woman is anaesthetised and the uterus replaced manually, as described above, by pressure in the fornices to replace the lower segment, which was last to invert, and the fundus last. If a retraction ring has developed between the upper and lower uterine segments, the replacement may be difficult. Inhalation of amyl nitrite vapour or a deep general anaesthetic may be needed to relax the uterine muscle.

O'Sullivan's hydrostatic method is preferred by some obstetricians. Two to three litres of warm normal saline are infused via a douche nozzle into the vagina while the introitus is sealed around the forearm by the other hand (Lindsay 1997). The fluid container is held about 1 m above the level of the uterus with the woman in the lithotomy position. The pressure of the liquid distends the vagina and the uterus replaces itself quite quickly. Following replacement, an intravenous injection of ergometrine 500 μg will ensure it remains in its correct position. The placenta may now be removed if necessary.

AMNIOTIC FLUID EMBOLISM

This obstetric emergency occurs when amniotic fluid is forced from the uterine venous sinuses of the placental bed into the maternal circulation. It usually follows uterine hyperactivity but may also occur near to term, before labour begins or in the 3rd stage as a result of a tear in the lower uterine segment. The embolus travels around the systemic circulation, through the heart and into the pulmonary circulation to obstruct pulmonary arterioles or alveolar capillaries.

Risk factors

Amniotic embolism is more likely to occur in women where intra-amniotic pressures are raised:

- hypertonic uterine action, spontaneous or induced by oxytocic drugs;
- older multiparous women with rapid labours;
- multiple pregnancy;
- polyhydramnios;
- uterine trauma such as CS, ruptured uterus, internal podalic version or manual removal of placenta.

Clinical signs and symptoms

The diagnosis can only be made with certainty if amniotic fluid is detected in maternal circulation and often this is postmortem when fetal desquamated skin and lanugo are also found in the lungs. There is usually sudden onset of **maternal respiratory distress** with cyanosis, chest pain, dyspnoea, blood stained frothy sputum and collapse. **Cardiovascular collapse** soon follows with tachycardia and hypotension. Amniotic fluid is rich in thromboplastins and its release

into the blood may cause **disseminated intravascular coagulation** (DIC) and coagulation failure (Davies & Harrison 1992). DIC is most likely to occur within 30 min of the initial collapse (Shiers & Coates 1999).

Management

This is an obstetric emergency. The uterus must be emptied as quickly as possible and a CS performed if necessary. Unfortunately, this rare complication often results in the death of the woman and her baby despite active treatment. Oxygen is given by face mask and cardiopulmonary resuscitation commenced if the woman collapses. Intravenous aminophylline may help relieve bronchospasm and hydrocortisone will relieve the inflammatory effect of amniotic fluid on lung tissue. An attempt is made to reverse the DIC and control haemorrhage should they occur. If the woman survives there may be **renal failure** and dialysis may be necessary if the kidneys do not respond to diuretic drugs such as mannitol.

SHOCK IN OBSTETRICS

McCance & Huether (2001) define shock as being a condition in which the cardiovascular system fails to perfuse the tissues adequately, resulting in widespread impairment of cellular metabolism. Three functions of the cardiovascular system may be altered and result in shock. If the heart is thought of as a pump, these can be summarised as:

1. **heart function** – loss of the pump;
2. **blood volume** – nothing to pump;
3. **blood pressure** – no force in the pump.

   Shock from any condition will inevitably cause progress to organ failure and death unless some compensatory mechanisms occur to reverse the situation or clinical treatments are successful.

If shock remains untreated, the body's compensatory mechanisms are overwhelmed and a downward spiral towards death will occur. The compensatory mechanisms function to maintain blood pressure and blood flow to vital organs such as the brain and the heart (Marieb 2000).

Recognition of shock

Because the body has many systems, all involving cells at the microscopic level, shock presents with many signs and symptoms. Tissue damage is diverse and subjective symptoms can be vague. A person may report nausea, weakness, feeling cold or hot, dizziness, confusion, fear and anxiety, thirst and shortage of breath with air hunger. Clinical measurements will find pulse and respiration rate increased, blood pressure and cardiac output decreased, diminished urinary output, cold, clammy skin, pallor and reduced core temperature.

Classification of shock

There are various ways of classifying shock: for example, by pathophysiological processes, by clinical manifestations or by cause. Classification by cause is the most useful as it will also indicate the likely pathophysiology underlying the shock and highlight the disorder that will need treating to reverse the shock (Tables 45.1 and 45.2). The three main cardiovascular functions that are impaired are obvious. All of the following types of shock may occur in childbearing women and will first be described in detail. Possible causes of obstetric shock will then be discussed. The danger is that the compensatory mechanisms may mask the signs of shock until maternal and fetal lives are at risk.

Cardiogenic shock

Heart failure is the cause of cardiogenic shock and most cases are due to myocardial infarction. Shock may also occur in congestive cardiac failure, myocardial ischaemia and drug toxicity. It is not very responsive to treatment and often leads to death.

Compensatory sequence of events:

- As cardiac output begins to decrease, renin produced by the kidneys stimulates aldosterone release so that sodium and water are retained.

Table 45.1 Types of shock and their immediate cause

Type	Cause
Cardiogenic	Heart failure
Hypovolaemic	Reduced blood volume
Neurogenic	Neural alterations of smooth muscle tone resulting in vasodilation
Anaphylactic	Immune system pathology resulting in vasodilation
Septic	Resulting in cardiac depression and dilatation with vasodilation

- Hypothalamic responses cause catecholamine release from the adrenal glands, resulting in vasoconstriction to maintain blood pressure.
- Cardiac performance is enhanced but there is increased demand for oxygen and nutrients.
- Tissue perfusion begins to fall and nutrient and oxygen delivery to the cells decreases.
- Cellular metabolism is impaired and signs of shock appear.

Hypovolaemic shock

Hypovolaemic shock with inadequate blood volume is the most common form. Shock begins to develop when intravascular volume is decreased by 15%. The first sign is a thready pulse as intense vasoconstriction attempts to move blood from the periphery to supply the vital organs. A sharp decline in blood pressure is a late and serious sign (Marieb 2000). It may occur because of:

1. loss of whole blood in haemorrhage;
2. loss of plasma as in burns;
3. loss of interstitial fluid;
4. diabetes mellitus;
5. excessive vomiting or diarrhoea.

Compensatory sequence of events:

- Adrenals release catecholamines, which increase heart rate and systemic vascular resistance (SVR).
- Interstitial fluid moves into the vascular compartment.
- The liver and spleen disgorge stored red blood cells and plasma into the circulation.
- Renin produced by the kidneys stimulates aldosterone release and sodium and water are retained.
- Tissue perfusion begins to fall and nutrient and oxygen delivery to the cells decreases.
- Cellular metabolism is impaired and signs of shock appear.

Table 45.2 Pathophysiological causes of shock in childbearing

Cardiogenic shock	Hypovolaemic shock	Neurogenic shock	Anaphylactic shock	Septic shock
Pulmonary embolism	Haemorrhage associated with childbearing	Acute inversion of the uterus	Adverse drug reactions	Infection in septic abortion and puerperal infection
Severe anaemia	Ruptured ectopic pregnancy	Aspiration of acid gastric contents (Mendelson's syndrome)		
Cardiac disorders such as valvular or congenital problems	Ruptured uterus	Intrauterine manipulations without adequate anaesthesia		
Severe hypertension	Coagulopathy following amniotic fluid embolism Diabetic crisis			

Neurogenic shock

Another name for neurogenic shock is **vasogenic shock**, referring to the massive vasodilation that results because of a loss of balance between the sympathetic and parasympathetic stimulation of vascular smooth muscle. Although blood volume does not change, the vascular compartment is increased drastically, resulting in relative hypovolaemia with a decrease in SVR. Vascular resistance is normally maintained by the sympathetic stimulus and if this is interrupted or inhibited for any length of time, neurogenic shock will follow. It may occur because of:

- trauma to the spinal cord;
- cerebral hypoxia;
- medullary hypoglycaemia;
- anaesthetics and other depressive drugs;
- pain and severe emotional distress.

Compensatory sequence of events:

- An increase in sympathetic activity will correct the bradycardia and very low SVR.
- Fainting ensures that the person is prevented from maintaining an upright posture so that blood pressure is equalised from head to toe and cerebral blood supply is maximised.

Anaphylactic shock

Anaphylactic shock results from a widespread hypersensitivity reaction. The pathophysiology is similar to that of neurogenic shock, with widespread vasodilation and pooling of blood in the periphery. This type of shock is very serious because it involves multiple body systems. It begins as an allergic reaction with an immune and inflammatory response to a proteinaceous substance such as insect venom, pollen, shellfish, penicillin or foreign serum. The vascular component of this response includes vasodilation and increased vascular permeability so that the relative hypovolaemia brought about by peripheral pooling is exacerbated by tissue oedema. There is bronchoconstriction so that the ability to provide oxygen to the tissues is severely compromised.

The onset of anaphylactic shock is rapid and can progress to death in minutes unless emergency treatment is available. The effects to a few people of ingesting peanuts have been widely reported in the press and illustrate the condition well. The signs are anxiety, difficulty in breathing, gastrointestinal cramps, oedema and urticaria with severe itching and burning sensations in the skin (McCance & Huether 2001). A steep fall in blood pressure follows with confusion and coma.

Emergency management   There is little time for spontaneous compensatory mechanisms and the person may die unless medical intervention is possible:

- adrenaline (epinephrine) injection will reverse airway constriction and cause vasoconstriction;

- volume expanders intravenously will reverse the relative hypovolaemia;
- steroids will end the inflammatory process.

Septic shock

Septic shock is a very complex process and the explanations for its progress are still being investigated. Gram-negative bacteria cause more than half the cases and in the non-pregnant population the most common sources of infection are the respiratory tract and the gastrointestinal tract. Infections of the genital tract are of prime importance in the childbearing woman.

Septic shock is triggered by bacteraemia and bacteria may be present in the blood for quite a long time before shock develops. It is most likely to be the elderly, critically ill or immune compromised who develop bacteraemic shock. One of the authors remembers a woman who was severely ill following insertion of an intrauterine contraceptive device. Uterine infection was followed by generalised infection and bacteraemia.

Four major body chemicals have been implicated in the development of bacteraemic shock (McCance & Huether 2001):

1. **Interleukins (ILs)** are cytokines produced by the white blood cells which cause vasodilation and increase vascular permeability. They also influence the hypothalamus to cause fever, initiate the complement cascade and stimulate the release of TNF.

2. **Tumour necrosis factor (TNF)** is a cytokine produced by macrophages, natural killer cells and mast cells. It activates both clotting and complement cascades. In addition, TNF causes vasodilation and increases vascular permeability.

3. **Platelet-activating factor (PAF)** is released from mononuclear phagocytes, platelets and some endothelial cells in response to the presence of an endotoxin. It is directly toxic to multiple organs and causes vasodilation and increased vascular permeability. PAF also mobilises white cells, activates platelets and stimulates the release of TNF.

4. **Myocardial depressant substance (MDS)** is secreted by white blood cells in response to an endotoxin. The heart responds to MDS by becoming depressed and dilated, which results in pump failure and hypotension.

As shock increases, carbohydrate metabolism is altered, with a serum increase in both insulin and glucagon. Serum glucose levels fluctuate and glucose usage by the tissues is enhanced. Glucose and glycogen stores become depleted. Depletion of glucose leads to heart failure and oxygen shortage and **multiple organ dysfunction syndrome (MODS)** may develop.

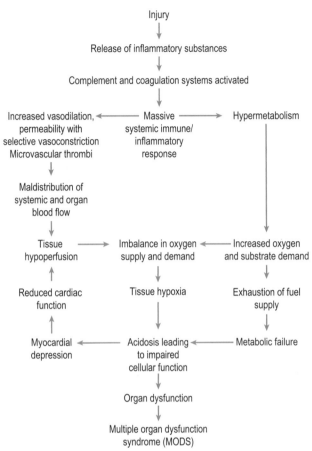

Figure 45.4 The pathogenesis of multiple organ dysfunction. (Reproduced with permission from McCance & Huether 1994.)

Multiple organ dysfunction syndrome

Multiple organ dysfunction syndrome is present if there is failure of two or more organ systems after severe illness or injury (Fig. 45.4). Sepsis and septic shock are the most common precipitating causes. Mortality is high and it is the most common cause of death following sepsis, trauma and burns. The following processes occur:

- release of the stress hormones cortisol, adrenaline (epinephrine), noradrenaline (norepinephrine) and endorphins;
- stimulation of the sympathetic nervous system;
- vascular endothelial damage by endotoxins or inflammatory substances;
- interstitial oedema;
- disseminated intravascular coagulation with microvascular thrombi and capillary obstruction;
- hyperdynamic circulation with increased venous return;
- hypermetabolism with elevated carbohydrate, lipid and protein breakdown to provide energy, leading to weight loss.

Failure of the lungs develops first with adult respiratory distress syndrome (ARDS). If this occurs, there is a mortality of over 80% (Pearlman & Tintinalli 1998). Renal and liver failure follow and there is gastrointestinal and immune system failure. Cardiovascular collapse with myocardial depression of function causes the death of the patient after about 3 weeks if treatment is unsuccessful. The normal supply of oxygen to the tissues is based on need and is met by alterations in blood flow distribution. This system fails and oxygen supply depends only on how much the circulation is able to deliver. This is known as **supply-dependent oxygen consumption**.

Outline of the management of MODS The reader is referred to McCance & Huether (2001) for a fuller description of the management of MODS. Briefly, early recognition is extremely important followed by treatment of the precipitating cause: for example, removing the source of infection. Restoration of tissue oxygenation and nutrition is very important. Individual organs such as the kidney may need supporting through the crisis.

Shock in childbearing

The above causes of shock can all be related to specific emergencies arising in childbearing and a summary is presented in Table 45.1.

MAIN POINTS

- In primary postpartum haemorrhage (PPH), the bleeding may be from the placental site but may occasionally be due to a laceration of the genital tract. Risk factors include previous PPH, high parity, overdistension of the uterus, fibroids, retained products of conception, inverted uterus, 3rd stage mismanagement and coagulation defects. If any of the risk factors are present, the woman should be delivered in hospital. Physiological management of the 3rd stage is considered unsafe.

- If bleeding commences before the placenta is delivered, the uterus is massaged to encourage contractions, an oxytocic drug is given and an attempt to deliver the placenta is made. A manual removal of placenta under anaesthesia will be necessary if the placenta cannot be delivered by controlled cord traction. If bleeding begins after delivery of the placenta, the uterus is massaged to obtain a contraction and expel any blood clots remaining in the uterus. An injection of an oxytocic drug should sustain contractions and stop bleeding.

- If the placenta is incomplete, evacuation of the uterus under spinal or general anaesthesia will be carried out. Once bleeding is controlled, an intravenous infusion containing oxytocin is commenced to maintain uterine contraction. Blood transfusion and fluid replacement may be required if bleeding is excessive. Prophylactic antibiotics will be prescribed following any operative intervention. If severe bleeding is from a tear in the uterus and bleeding cannot be controlled, a hysterectomy will save the woman's life.

- Secondary PPH is usually due to a retained piece of placenta or membrane. Other causes include the presence of blood clots, a fibroid or infection. If the uterus is palpable it is massaged until it contracts, clots are expelled and the bladder emptied. An intravenous injection of an oxytocic drug is given if bleeding is severe followed by evacuation of the uterus.

- Bleeding in the puerperium should always be reported to the obstetrician. Inadequate treatment may lead to iron deficiency anaemia, acute renal tubular necrosis or anterior pituitary necrosis and Sheehan's syndrome.

- Failure of the placenta to deliver spontaneously is one of the main causes of PPH. The placenta may be separated but retained, when bleeding is likely, or morbidly adherent to the uterine wall and bleeding will not occur. Manual removal may be necessary. In deeply adherent placentae, a CS can be performed.

- Causes of acute inversion of the uterus include mismanagement of the 3rd stage but spontaneous inversion does occur. Rapid replacement of the uterus will prevent shock.

- An amniotic fluid embolus travels into the pulmonary circulation to obstruct pulmonary arterioles or capillaries. It is more likely to occur where intra-amniotic pressures are raised and in uterine trauma. Sudden onset of maternal respiratory distress is followed by cardiovascular collapse and possibly disseminated intravasular coagulation (DIC). Oxygen is given and cardiopulmonary resuscitation commenced if needed. Intravenous fluids are administered. Mortality is high and renal failure may be a complication.

- Three functions of the cardiovascular system may be altered and result in shock: i.e. heart function, blood volume and blood pressure. Shock progresses to organ failure and death unless compensatory mechanisms or clinical treatments can reverse the pathology.

- Classification of shock by cause is the most useful as it will also indicate the likely pathophysiology and highlight the underlying disorder that will need treating. Types of shock are cardiogenic, hypovolaemic, neurogenic, anaphylactic and septic.

References

Alexander J, Thomas P, Sanghera J 2001 Treatments for secondary postpartum haemorrhage. Cochrane Review: In The Cochrane Library, Issue 1. Update Software 2003, Oxford.

BNF 2003 British National Formulary, Number 45, March. British Medical Association and Royal Pharmaceutical Society of Great Britain, London.

Brant H 1967 Precise estimation of postpartum haemorrhage: difficulties and importance. British Medical Journal 1:389–400.

Davies M, Harrison J 1992 Amniotic fluid embolism: maternal mortality revisited. British Journal of Hospital Medicine 14(10):775–776.

Enkin M, Keirse M J C, Renfrew M et al 2000 A Guide to Effective Care in Pregnancy and Childbirth, 3rd edn. Oxford University Press, Oxford.

Lewis G 2001 Why mothers die 1997–1999: The 5th Report of the Confidential Enquiries into Maternal Deaths in the United Kingdom. RCOG, London.

Lindsay P 1997 Complications of the third stage of labour. In Sweet B R, Tiran D (eds) Mayes Midwifery: A Textbook for Midwives, 12th edn. Baillière Tindall, London.

McCance K L, Huether S E (eds) 2001 Pathophysiology: The Biologic Basis for Disease in Adults and Children, 4th edn. Mosby, St Louis.

Marieb E N 2000 Human Anatomy and Physiology, 5th edn. Benjamin/Cummings, New York.

Mousa H A, Alfirevic Z 2002 Treatment for primary postpartum haemorrhage. Cochrane Review: In The Cochrane Library, Issue 1. Update Software 2003, Oxford.

Pearlman M D, Tintinalli J E (eds) 1998 Emergency Care of the Woman. McGraw-Hill, New York.

Rang H P (ed.), Dale M M, Ritter J M 2001 Pharmacology, 4th edn. Churchill Livingstone, Edinburgh.

Shiers C V, Coates T 1999 Midwifery and obstetric emergencies. In Bennett V R, Brown L K (eds) Myles Textbook for Midwives, 13th edn. Churchill Livingstone, Edinburgh.

Annotated recommended reading

Lewis G (ed.) 2001 Why mothers die, 1997–1999: the 5th Report of the Confidential Enquiries into Maternal Deaths in the UK. RCOG, London.
This report is produced from the confidential enquiries into maternal deaths and describes how midwives might affect the safe outcome of pregnancy for all women. All midwives are urged to read this report as well as the full report.

Chapter **46**

Perinatal fetal asphyxia

INTRODUCTION

Labour has been known to be dangerous for the fetus for centuries. Uterine contractions interfere with umbilical and uteroplacental blood flow and affect fetal gas exchange. The result is a normal tendency to mild metabolic acidosis in the active phase of the first stage and in the early second stage of labour. At the end of the second stage of labour there may be transient respiratory acidosis (Arias 1993).

DEFINITIONS

- **Fetal distress** is a general purpose term to indicate the fetus is in jeopardy, sometimes but not always because of hypoxia.

- **Acidosis** is an increased concentration of hydrogen ions (H^+) in blood and at the cellular level, resulting from an accumulation of acid or loss of base with a blood pH of less than 7.2.

- **Hypoxia** is a decreased concentration of oxygen in blood (hypoxaemia) and at the cellular level.

- **Hypercapnia (hypercarbia)** is an increased concentration of carbon dioxide in blood and at the cellular level.

- **Asphyxia** is a severe abnormality of gas exchange which results in hypoxia, hypercapnia and acidosis. The term **fetal asphyxia** is preferred to that of **fetal distress**, which refers to a state of fetal danger that may or may not be caused by asphyxia.

FETAL GAS EXCHANGE AND pH REGULATION

The bicarbonate buffer system which regulates fetal acid–base balance is not as efficient as in the neonate because of a decreased ability to eliminate carbon dioxide (CO_2). As carbon dioxide cannot be expelled by the fetus into the air, it must be eliminated as molecular CO_2 via the placenta to be removed by the maternal respiratory system.

Respiratory acidosis

In the placenta there is a gradient between maternal and fetal circulations down which fetal CO_2 can diffuse. Fetal scalp blood PCO_2 is about 38–44 mmHg and maternal blood PCO_2 is 18–24 mmHg. In most cases interference with fetal gas exchange involves a problem of elimination of CO_2, resulting in respiratory acidosis. An excessive rise in fetal PCO_2 causes fetal H^+ ions to be released from the unstable carbonic acid (H_2CO_3), which lowers fetal blood pH (acidosis). The buffering bicarbonate ions, which also released, are insufficient to correct the acidosis. The full equation is:

$$CO_2 + H_2O \leftrightarrow H_2CO_3 \leftrightarrow H^+ + HCO_3^- \qquad (46.1)$$

Metabolic acidosis

Decreased oxygen transfer to the fetus will also cause acidosis. Oxygen deficiency causes cells to switch to anaerobic respiration, with the release of lactic acid and H^+ ions into the blood. If hypoxia persists, the excess H^+ ions cause CO_2 and water (H_2O) to be released from the buffer bicarbonate to add respiratory acidosis to the metabolic acidosis. Water is transferred across the placenta to the maternal circulation but there is a delay in removing the CO_2. Anaerobic respiration is inefficient and utilises more energy, resulting in a decrease in glucose.

INTRAUTERINE HYPOXIA

Oxygenation of the fetus depends on maternal oxygenation, perfusion of the placental site, the fetoplacental circulation and adequate fetal haemoglobin (Michie 1999). Disruption or impairment to the flow of oxygen from the air to the fetus will result in fetal hypoxia.

Possible causes of intrauterine hypoxia

- Oxygenation of the mother may be impaired by respiratory or cardiovascular disease.
- Perfusion of the placental site may be reduced in:
  hypertension because of vasoconstriction;
  hypotension due to blood loss;
  aortocaval occlusion;
  shock;
  excessive uterine contractions.
- Prolapse, compression or a true knot in the umbilical cord may cause fetal hypoxia.
- Placental disease.
- There may be a reduction in fetal red cells caused by haemolysis.

Fetal response to hypoxia

The fetal response to hypoxia is an acceleration of heart rate to maintain oxygen supply to the brain and delivery of excess CO_2 to the placenta. As glycogen reserves become depleted, the increased supply of glucose demanded by the heart muscle because of the **tachycardia** cannot be met and the heart slows (**bradycardia**). The anal sphincter relaxes and fresh meconium is passed into the amniotic fluid. Hypoxia may stimulate the fetus to make gasping movements and meconium may be inhaled.

Physiological control of the fetal heart

The cardiac regulatory centre is situated in the medulla oblongata. Baroreceptors found in the arch of the aorta and carotid sinus are responsive to changes in blood pressure, and chemoreceptors in the same blood vessels respond to changes in blood gas tensions (Marieb 2000). These receptors send messages to the cardiac regulatory centre, which in turn sends messages via the sympathetic and parasympathetic nervous system to the heart. Sympathetic stimulation via the sinoatrial node will increase the heart rate while parasympathetic stimulation via the vagus nerve will decrease the heart rate. The continuous interaction between these two branches of the autonomic system causes small fluctuations in heart rate which lead to variability on heart rate tracings.

MONITORING THE FETUS IN LABOUR

The fetal response to labour may be monitored clinically by observing the amniotic fluid and the rate and rhythm of the fetal heart, either intermittently using a Pinard fetal stethoscope or Doppler ultrasound fetal heart rate detector or by continuous cardiotocographic monitoring. Where it is difficult to monitor the fetal heart from the mother's abdomen, for example in obese women, the fetal heart can be monitored electronically using a fetal scalp electrode, which is attached to the fetal skull and it produces a direct **fetal electrocardiogram**. Contraction length, strength and frequency can also be monitored externally by a transducer or internally by an intrauterine catheter pressure device.

Meconium

The presence of meconium in amniotic fluid is only suggestive of intrapartum asphyxia in the fetus. Meconium is a non-specific finding that may be associated with fetal problems other than asphyxia (Clark & Clark 2002, Miller et al 1975). Meconium-stained amniotic fluid is associated with cardiovascular malformations, rhesus isoimmunisation, chorioamnionitis and pre-eclampsia. However, if the pregnancy is known to be high risk and the meconium is freshly passed, as indicated by it being dark green or black, thick and tenacious, its predictive value of asphyxia is high. Old or stale meconium giving rise to lightly stained yellowish or greenish amniotic fluid does not correlate well with fetal asphyxia (Morrin 1997).

Classification of meconium-stained liquor

Meiss et al (1978) classified meconium into early light, early heavy and late meconium staining. Early staining was present from during the active phase of labour and late was newly passed in the second stage of labour. Early heavy staining and late staining were associated with a significant increase in meconium aspiration. Similarly, thick, fresh meconium at the onset of labour is associated with increased morbidity from meconium aspiration (McNiven et al 1994).

Prophylactic amnioinfusion for meconium-stained fluid

Thick, undiluted meconium reflects reduced amniotic fluid volume, which is itself a risk factor (Enkin et al 2000). Morrin (1997) summarises the arguments for and against the use of amniotomy to visualise the amniotic fluid for meconium staining. A randomised controlled trial which included nulliparous women found that routine amniotomy had little effect on the important outcomes of labour and is not to be recommended (UK Amniotomy Group 1994).

Spong et al (1994) concluded that amnioinfusion does dilute amniotic meconium but prophylactic amnioinfusion did not improve perinatal outcome and increased the risk of chorioamnionitis and endometritis. They suggested that the benefit of amnioinfusion resulted from the alleviation of variable fetal heart rate decelerations rather than meconium dilution. Hofmeyr (2001) reviewed the use of amnioinfusion for meconium-stained liquor in labour and suggested that any associated benefits seen are more likely to be due to an improvement in oligohydramnios than in dilution of meconium.

Fetal heart monitoring

Intermittent auscultation

The frequency of monitoring of the fetal heart by the midwife is decided by the frequency and strength of the uterine contractions and the effects on the fetus (Dover & Gauge 1995). Other risk factors likely to affect fetal oxygenation were also taken into account. Intermittent auscultation is usually carried out hourly in early labour, every 15 min as contractions increase and between each contraction in the late first stage and second stage of labour. The heart rate and rhythm should be listened to, commencing immediately after a contraction and counted over a full minute, to assess whether decelerations are present. The normal range is between 120 and 160 beats per minute (bpm) but in practice a better range would be between 110 and 150 bpm (RCOG 2001). The faster rate is found in preterm babies and the lower in term and post-term babies. The rhythm is regular with a coupled beat.

Electronic fetal monitoring

Continuous electronic fetal heart rate monitoring was introduced in the 1970s and adopted enthusiastically by obstetricians as 'a significant improvement in intrapartum fetal assessment' (Arias 1993). The technique was introduced before evidence of its efficacy or safety had been sought. Electronic fetal monitoring (EFM) is used in the monitoring of labour in 3 out of 4 pregnancies in the USA. EFM can be used continuously or intermittently: for instance, for 15–30 min periodically.

Concerns have been raised about the safety and efficiency of continuous EFM (Arias 1993). Thacker et al (2001) compared EFM with intermittent auscultation during labour using the results of nine randomised controlled trials (RCTs). They reviewed studies including 18 561 pregnant women and their 18 695 infants. Data from each study were used to calculate a combined risk estimate for eight outcomes:

- 1-min Apgar score below 7;
- 1-min Apgar score below 4;
- neonatal seizures;
- neonatal intensive care admissions (NICU);
- stillbirths;
- neonatal deaths;
- caesarean delivery;
- operative vaginal delivery.

When the value of EFM was compared with intermittent fetal heart rate monitoring, the results were:

- no trial showed a significant decrease in babies with a 1-min Apgar score of less than 7;
- outside of the USA there was a significant decrease in the risk of 1-min Apgar score of less than 4;
- only 1 trial showed a significant decrease in the number of babies having neonatal seizures;
- only 1 trial showed a significant decrease in perinatal mortality;
- only 1 trial showed a significant decrease in the number of admissions to NICU;
- there was a significant increase in the numbers of vaginal operative deliveries;
- there was a significant increase in the numbers of deliveries by caesarean section (CS) and the risk of CS delivery was highest in low-risk pregnancies.

Implications for practice The review found no measurable impact on morbidity or mortality, with the exception of reduced incidence of neonatal seizures, although outside the USA there was a decrease in the 1-min Apgar scores below 4. The increase of CS rates with added risk to the mother is a worrying factor. The National Institute of Clinical Excellence (NICE 2001) and expert panels in the USA and in Canada have advised against routine EFM in low-risk pregnancies and have found weak evidence for its inclusion in high-risk pregnancies. Some believe the technology was introduced before it was well developed and that more research is needed. However, despite the controversy, there seems to be no likelihood of a reduction in such monitoring occurring (Thacker et al 2001). This is because EFM is able to:

- provide reliable confirmation of fetal wellbeing;
- show the possibility of the presence of fetal problems;
- determine the presence of severe problems.

Waveform analysis

Westgate et al (1993) carried out a prospective randomised clinical trial to compare conventional cardiotocography (CTG) with waveform analysis of changes in the ST waveform of the electrocardiogram. The subjects were 2434 high-risk labouring women in Plymouth, England. The criteria used for analysis were the incidence of operative intervention and neonatal outcome. They found that ST waveform analysis discriminated between cardiotocogram changes and reduced the incidence of operative deliveries and low 5-min Apgar scores. They conclude that more research into waveform analysis is warranted. Van Wijngaarden et al (1996), in similar fashion, used PR interval analysis and found they were able to reduce the number of fetuses undergoing scalp blood sampling.

Fetal heart patterns on electronic monitoring

The following terms are used to interpret CTG readings.

Baseline fetal heart rate There is a baseline rate per minute (bpm) of 120–160, which is the rate present between periods of acceleration and deceleration. A rate over 160 is called **baseline tachycardia** and below 110 is **baseline bradycardia**. Both tachycardia and bradycardia may be associated with fetal hypoxia. Tachycardia may be seen if the woman is ketotic or pyrexial. Some fetuses normally have a bpm of 110–120. A prolonged bradycardia occurs when there is continuous compression of the umbilical cord.

Baseline variability Continuous adjustments in the autonomic nervous stimulation of the heart due to fetal response to the environment lead to minute variations in the length of each heart beat. This leads to the CTG tracing having a jagged appearance, as the baseline rate is continuously adjusting, rather than being a straight line because each beat is the same length. There should be variance in the baseline rate of at least 5 bpm. Loss of variance may be due to hypoxia. It is also seen after the administration of pethidine because of depression of the cardiac regulatory centre in the fetal brain. Fetal sleep lasting 20–30 min may also cause a reduction in variability (Gibb 1988).

Response to uterine contractions The fetal heart normally remains steady or **accelerates** during a contraction. Accelerations of 15 bpm above the baseline are associated with fetal activity and stimulation. The presence of two accelerations within a 20-min period is a sign of fetal health and the tracing is said to be reactive (Gibb 1988).

Decelerations, dips of more than 15 bpm below baseline, are more worrying.

- An **early deceleration** mirrors the pattern of the contraction. It commences at or after the onset of a contraction, reaches its lowest point at the peak of the contraction and then returns to normal by the end of the contraction. It is associated with compression of the fetal head and vagal response but may also indicate early fetal hypoxia.

- A **late deceleration** begins during or just after a contraction, reaches its lowest point after the peak of the contraction and may not recover until the onset of the next contraction. This time lag between the peak of the contraction and the low point of the deceleration is more significant than the drop in heart rate. It indicates fetal hypoxia and inadequate fetal brain oxygenation (Aldrich et al 1995) and is suggestive of cord compression. Prolapse of the cord should be excluded by vaginal examination and the obstetrician should be informed.

- **Variable decelerations**, where the heart rate varies in timing, frequency and amplitude, are associated with cord compression where there is obstruction to venous flow and a corresponding rise in fetal blood pressure. Both early and late decelerations are present. This pattern can be considered benign but if the decelerations are below 60 bpm, 60 bpm below the baseline or last for longer than 1 min the fetus may be in danger (Morrin 1997).

Two other unusual and rare patterns are observed: first, a sinusoidal pattern where there is a regular trace with a wave pattern of 3–6 per min with amplitude of 5–30 bpm (Morrin 1997) – this is associated with rhesus isoimmunisation, fetal anaemia and asphyxia; secondly, a saltatory pattern with excessive variability of more than 25 bpm this may be associated with fetal acidosis but the cause is unclear.

Fetal blood sampling

Cardiotocography can suggest the presence of fetal hypoxia but acidosis can only be confirmed by fetal blood sampling (Nickelsen 2002). The normal pH of fetal blood is 7.25–7.45 in labour. If this falls below 7.25 in the first stage of labour or below 7.2 in the second stage of labour, the fetus may be in danger and must be delivered immediately. In order to carry out a fetal blood sampling procedure, the membranes need to be ruptured and the cervix needs to be at least 3 cm dilated. An amnioscope is passed through the cervix to access the fetal scalp. The scalp is sprayed with ethyl chloride to produce a reactive hyperaemia and a thin layer of silicone gel applied to ensure blood collects in a droplet. The skin is punctured and blood is collected in a heparinised capillary tube for immediate analysis of blood pH.

MANAGEMENT OF CONFIRMED FETAL ASPHYXIA

Severe hypoxia may result in the baby being stillborn, asphyxiated at birth or suffering brain damage. If the condition of the fetus monitored by the above findings suggests a major problem, the obstetrician must be called to see the woman and her fetus. If labour is being augmented by administration of Syntocinon (oxytocin), it is sensible to reduce the force of the uterine contractions by discontinuing the infusion. Administration of oxygen to the mother may be useful if the underlying cause of the fetal hypoxia is maternal disease. Delivery will probably be either by CS in the first stage of labour or by operative delivery (forceps or ventouse extraction) in the second stage. If delivery is imminent, an episiotomy may be all that is required. A resuscitaire should be present and a paediatrician should be called to the delivery room in all cases of fetal distress as the neonate may need resuscitation.

NEONATAL ASPHYXIA AND RESUSCITATION

Initiation of respirations at birth

From about 22 weeks surfactant is produced in the fetal lung. The amount present increases until birth and there is a surge of production at about 34 weeks gestation. Surfactant has two main functions: to reduce surface tension in the alveoli so that they can expand more easily and to help prevent the alveoli collapsing at the end of each expiration. Fetal breathing movements have been identified as early as 11 weeks gestation and these increase in strength and frequency until they are present over 50% of the time. The rate varies between 30 and 70 breaths per minute.

Establishing respiration at birth

This topic is summarised below and fully explored in Chapter 48, p. 615:

- As the fetal chest is compressed by the birth canal, it is squeezed and lung and amniotic fluid are forced out of the alveoli into the upper respiratory tract. Passive recoil of the chest after delivery helps to draw air into the lungs.

- Hypoxia during the late stage of delivery occurs with the birth of the head and the beginning of placental separation. The oxygen content of the blood falls and the carbon dioxide content rises, stimulating chemoreceptors to send a message to the respiratory centre and causing onset of breathing.

- The respiratory centre is also bombarded with stimuli from handling of the baby and the temperature changes found in the nasopharynx and on the skin.

- Circulatory changes direct the blood away from the placental circulation to the pulmonary circulation and lungs for oxygenation.

- Effective oxygenation is achieved by respiratory exchange in the alveoli and by adequate circulation.

Most neonates establish respirations within 1 min of birth.

Birth asphyxia

Failure to initiate or sustain respirations at birth is called **birth asphyxia** or **asphyxia neonatorum**.

Causes

- Obstruction of the airway by mucus, blood, meconium or amniotic fluid may occur, especially if intrauterine anoxia has been present. Because of stimulation of the respiratory centre the fetus may have gasped in utero, drawing the above substances into the trachea and bronchi.

- The airways may not be patent due to congenital anomalies such as choanal atresia, hypoplastic lungs or diaphragmatic hernia.

- Lung function may be compromised by abnormalities in the cardiovascular system or central nervous system.

- Pain-relieving drugs such as pethidine and morphine and narcotic drugs such as diazepam, as well as general anaesthetics, if given in large doses, may depress the fetal respiratory centre.

- Intracranial haemorrhage may cause pressure on the cerebellum and medulla, affecting the cardiovascular and respiratory centres.

- Severe intrauterine infections following prolonged rupture of the membranes, leading to pneumonia, meningitis and septicaemia, may inhibit the efficient establishment of respiration.

- Immaturity of the neonate may lead to mechanical dysfunction because of poor lung development, lack of surfactant and a soft rib cage.

Recognition

Birth asphyxia may be classified as mild, moderate or severe, depending on scoring systems such as that devised by Virginia Apgar in 1953. Arias (1993) relates that several studies carried out in the 1980s, such as that of Sykes et al (1982), demonstrated that **Apgar scores** are poor predictors of hypoxia and acidosis. The Apgar score (Fig. 46.1) assesses the condition of the baby at birth and may be affected by all the above causes of neonatal asphyxia. It follows that babies may not always have shown pre-delivery signs of impending asphyxia, many of the causes arising suddenly after delivery. Respiratory depression by fetal hypoxia is only one factor that may cause a baby to fail to breathe at birth (Roberton 1997).

For each of the vital signs in Fig. 46.1 the neonate may be given a score of 0, 1 or 2 depending on the descriptors.

Sign	Score		
	0	1	2
Heart rate	Absent	Slow – below 100	Fast – above 100
Respiratory effort	Absent	Slow, irregular	Good, crying
Muscle tone	Limp	Some flexion of the extremities	Active
Reflex irritability	No response	Grimace	Crying, cough
Colour	Blue, pale	Body pink, extremities blue	Completely pink

Figure 46.1   The Apgar scoring system based on points being awarded for five physiological signs.

The Apgar score at 1 min is recorded and suggested parameters are:

- 7–10 – no asphyxia;
- 4–6 – mild to moderate asphyxia, response to treatment usually good;
- 3 or less – severe asphyxia, requires urgent resuscitation.

Case study

A case that illustrates how there may be no sign to predict asphyxia follows. When one of the editors was a junior sister, she and a friend had been caring for a multigravid woman in labour. Labour had commenced spontaneously, there had been no sign of fetal heart rate abnormalities and the delivery was normal.

The editor received the baby who seemed to be breathing spontaneously and, anticipating no problems, he was wrapped and given to his mother. Within 1 min he became extremely cyanosed and stopped breathing. The editor took him to the resuscitaire, gave oxygen by face mask and he recommenced breathing rapidly. This happened once more and she called the paediatric houseman. He examined the baby who was once more pink all over and breathing well. Put him in the cot was the guidance! Once more the baby collapsed. She then called the consultant who quickly diagnosed transposition of the great vessels of the heart. The baby, who is now a strapping 26-year-old man, was transferred for immediate corrective surgery.

Management of birth asphyxia

A simple way to remember the steps in resuscitation is the **ABC method** (with D added):

A = airway – ensure patency
B = breathing – ensure that oxygen enters the lungs
C = cardiac function – ensure there is an adequate heart beat and circulation
D = drugs – ensure that the resuscitation trolley with all its required components is available.

Mild to moderate asphyxia   The upper airways should be cleared gently with suction. Intermittent positive pressure ventilation (IPPV) via a face mask should be given using a T-piece or a resuscitation bag such as the Ambu-bag attached to an oxygen supply (adhere to local guidelines). This should always include a means of limiting pressure to no more than 30 cmH$_2$O to prevent pneumothorax from overinflation. The baby should become pink as oxygen supply is ensured and this should lead to an improvement in heart rate. When the baby breathes spontaneously, oxygen should be maintained until the baby's condition is judged to be satisfactory.

If the baby's temperature is allowed to fall, the demands for oxygen and glucose will increase so the baby must be kept warm throughout the procedure. If the mother has received pethidine or morphine within the last 2–3 h and the baby is unresponsive, naloxone hydrochloride (Narcan), which is a narcotic antagonist, should be given. The dose is 200 µg and it can be given intramuscularly or into the umbilical vein.

All relevant practitioners should be trained in the skills required for basic neonatal resuscitation and these skills should be maintained through practice-related activities.

Severe asphyxia   If the paediatrician is not present, he should be called as an emergency and resuscitation of the infant commenced. Endotracheal intubation will be necessary and this is normally the role of the paediatrician. However, midwives trained in this technique should become proficient so that they can carry it out in the absence of a paediatrician (Fig. 46.2). If not appropriately trained to intubate, then the midwife should ensure that the baby has a clear airway and start IPPV with bag and mask until a trained practitioner arrives. More harm can be done to the baby if an inexperienced practitioner attempts to perform intubation.

An appropriately sized laryngoscope is passed over the tongue to the posterior pharynx. It is then advanced carefully over the epiglottis until the glottis comes into view (Fig. 46.3). If the epiglottis cannot be seen, gentle pressure on the cricoid cartilage may assist. Another technique

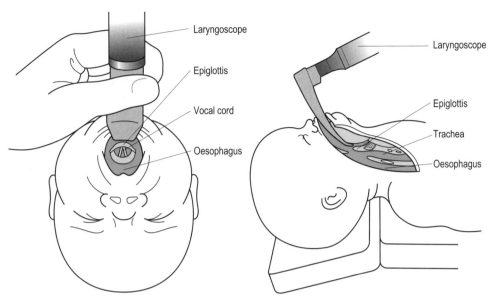

Figure 46.2   Intubation of the neonate (from Sweet B 1997, with permission).

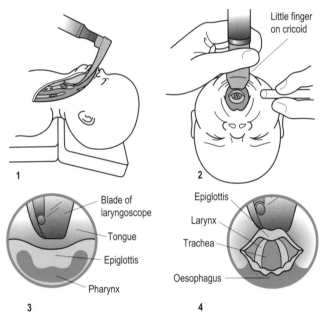

Figure 46.3   How to intubate. 1. Lie the baby on its back if possible, with the head tilted slightly downwards. Extend the neck so that the chin points upwards. 2. Take the infant laryngoscope with a straight blade and insert the blade into the infant's mouth, gently lifting the tongue. 3. The epiglottis can be seen at the base of the tongue; it hangs down obscuring the entrance to the larynx. 4. Slide the laryngoscope to the base of the epiglottis and tilt the tip of the blade upward. At the same time, press gently on the cricoid cartilage with the little finger. The entrance to the larynx will then come into view. An endotracheal tube can then be guided carefully into the trachea (from Kelnar C, Harvey D, Simpson C 1995, with permission).

is to advance the tip of the laryngoscope blade further and then slowly withdraw it. This should allow the glottis to slip into view. Aspiration of mucus can be carried out directly if necessary.

A size 2.5 for a baby weighing less than 1 kg to a size 3.5 for a baby weighing more than 3 kg endotracheal tube (ETT) is passed through the glottis into the trachea, a distance of 7–10 cm from the tip of the ETT depending on the size of the baby and the laryngoscope removed. The trachea can be cleared by passing a fine catheter through the ETT, which can then be attached to the oxygen supply connected to a water manometer. IPPV is commenced at 40–60 times per minute. The initial pressure should be 30 cmH$_2$O, reduced to 25 cmH$_2$O.

This should be continued until the baby is pink, has a heart rate of over 100 bpm and is breathing spontaneously.

External chest compression should be commenced if the baby has a heart rate of less than 60 bpm which is decreasing despite adequate ventilation. The prime purpose of chest compression in neonatal resuscitation is to deliver oxygenated blood to the coronary arteries. This is performed using two fingers to depress the sternum 1–2 cm at 120 times per min. If the heart rate is less than 60 bpm, then resuscitation should comprise 90 cardiac compressions and 30 lung ventilations per min. The Apgar should be repeated at 5 min and until the baby's condition is satisfactory. The Apgar score at 5 min has more prognostic value than the score at 1 min.

Practitioners responsible for resuscitating the newborn should read the current national literature on resuscitation of babies at birth but in practice should always follow their local hospital guidelines on resuscitation.

For midwives practising in the community it is reassuring to remember that severe neonatal asphyxia rarely occurs unannounced and warning signs identified during fetal monitoring in labour should result in the woman being transferred to a maternity unit to safeguard the fetus. A resuscitation bag such as the Ambu-bag should be sufficient. When the delivery has been an emergency and no equipment is available, mouth-to-face (over mouth and nose) resuscitation has saved lives. Just the air in the cheeks should be blown into the baby's airways.

Drugs

Drugs that may be required and should always be available on the resuscitation trolley are:

- adrenaline (epinephrine), a cardiac stimulant;
- dextrose 10%, given if hypoglycaemia is confirmed;
- dextrose 20%;
- naloxone hydrochloride, given if a narcotic antagonist is needed;
- sodium bicarbonate, to counteract acidosis;
- sodium chloride 0.9%;
- vitamin K_1, given to prevent haemorrhagic disease of the newborn;
- water for injection.

Transfer to the neonatal unit

A baby who has suffered severe asphyxia should be transferred to the neonatal unit for further observation. Complications such as cerebral oedema, hypoglycaemia, hypothermia and electrolyte disturbance should be anticipated and prevented if possible and treated if they occur. Paediatric follow-up is important to detect long-term problems such as developmental delay or cerebral palsy.

Correction of acidosis

If only one of the two types of acidosis is present, the other system can be used to compensate. The lungs are central to the control of carbon dioxide level in respiratory acidosis while the kidneys control bicarbonate level in metabolic acidosis. Acidosis in neonates tends to be mixed and the buffering systems may fail. As stated above, the administration of sodium bicarbonate is controversial and should always follow blood gas analysis. The bicarbonate combines with hydrogen ions to form carbonic acid. This then dissociates into water and carbon dioxide:

$$H^+ + HCO_3^- \leftrightarrow H_2CO_3 \leftrightarrow CO_2 + H_2O \qquad (46.2)$$

If the carbon dioxide can leave the body by the lungs, there is no problem but in respiratory difficulties it may accumulate in the body. It crosses cell membranes and the blood–brain barrier to cause intracellular acidosis, even if there seems to be a blood picture improvement in acidosis. This is because the bicarbonate buffer cannot cross cell membranes as readily as the carbon dioxide. The sodium content in sodium bicarbonate may result in an overloading of the baby's vascular system, resulting in cellular over-hydration and damage.

MAIN POINTS

- Impairment of the distribution of oxygen to the fetus will result in fetal hypoxia with acceleration of heart rate to maintain oxygen supply to the brain and deliver excess CO_2 to the placenta. As glycogen reserves become depleted, the heart muscle slows. The anal sphincter relaxes and fresh meconium is passed into the amniotic fluid. Hypoxia may stimulate the fetus to make gasping movements and meconium may be inhaled.

- The presence of meconium in amniotic fluid is only suggestive of intrapartum asphyxia in the fetus and is a non-specific finding that may be associated with other fetal problems such as cardiovascular malformations, rhesus isoimmunisation, chorioamnionitis and pre-eclampsia. Only if the meconium is fresh is asphyxia likely to occur.

- Both tachycardia and bradycardia may be associated with fetal hypoxia. Tachycardia may be seen if the woman is ketotic or pyrexial. A prolonged bradycardia suggests continuous compression of the umbilical cord.

- Fetal acidosis can be confirmed by fetal blood sampling. Severe hypoxia may result in the baby being stillborn, asphyxiated at birth and suffering brain damage. Administration of oxygen to the mother may be useful if the underlying cause of the fetal hypoxia is maternal disease.

- Birth asphyxia may be caused by obstructed airways or congenital anomalies of the respiratory, cardiovascular or central nervous systems. Pain-relieving drugs may depress the fetal respiratory centre. Intracranial haemorrhage may affect the cardiovascular and respiratory centres. Intrauterine infection or immaturity may inhibit the efficient establishment of respiration. The Apgar score assesses the condition of the baby at birth.

- In mild to moderate asphyxia the upper airways should be cleared gently with suction. Intermittent positive pressure ventilation via a face mask should be given. The baby becomes pink as oxygen supply is ensured and this leads to an improvement in heart rate. If the mother has received pethidine or morphine within the last 2–3 h and the baby is unresponsive, naloxone hydrochloride (Narcan) 200 µg, a narcotic antagonist, is given.

- If severe asphyxia is present, the paediatrician should be called. Endotracheal intubation will be necessary and all midwives specifically trained in this technique should become proficient. Cardiac massage should be commenced if the baby's heart rate is below 60 bpm or if the carotid or femoral pulses are weak or cannot be felt. The Apgar should be repeated at 5 min and until the baby's condition is satisfactory.

- A baby who has suffered severe asphyxia should be transferred to the neonatal unit for further observation. Complications such as cerebral oedema, hypoglycaemia, hypothermia and electrolyte disturbance should be anticipated, prevented if possible and treated if they occur.

References

Aldrich C J, D'Antona D, Spencer J A 1995 Late fetal heart decelerations and changes in cerebral oxygenation during the first stage of labour. British Journal of Obstetrics and Gynaecology 102(1):9–13.

Arias F 1993 Practical Guide to High Risk Pregnancy and Delivery, 2nd edn. Mosby Year Book, Chicago.

Clark D A, Clark M B 2002 Meconium aspiration syndrome. e-medicine Journal 3(1).

Dover S L, Gauge S M 1995 Fetal monitoring – midwifery attitudes. Midwifery 11(1):18–27.

Enkin M, Keirse M J N C, Renfrew M et al 2000 A Guide to Effective Care in Pregnancy and Childbirth, 3rd edn. Oxford University Press, Oxford.

Gibb D M E 1988 A Practical Guide to Labour Management. Blackwell Science, Oxford.

Hofmeyr G J 2001 Amnioinfusion for meconium-stained liquor in labour. Cochrane Review: In The Cochrane Library, Issue 2. Update Software 2003, Oxford.

McNiven P, Roch B, Wall J 1994 Meconium-stained amniotic fluid. Modern Midwife 4(7):17–20.

Marieb E N 2000 Human Anatomy and Physiology, 4th edn. Benjamin/Cummings, New York.

Meiss P J, Hall M, Marshall J R et al 1978 Meconium passage: a new classification for risk assessment during labor. American Journal of Obstetrics and Gynecology 131:509.

Michie M M 1999 The baby at birth. In Bennett V R, Brown L K (eds) Myles Textbook for Midwives, 13th edn. Churchill Livingstone, Edinburgh.

Miller F C, Sacks D A, Yeh S Y et al 1975 Significance of meconium during labor. American Journal of Obstetrics and Gynecology 122:573.

Morrin N A 1997 Midwifery care in the first stage of labour. In Sweet B R, Tiran D (eds) Mayes Midwifery: A Textbook for Midwives, 12th edn. Baillière Tindall, London.

NICE 2001 Guidelines for the Use of Electronic Fetal Monitoring. National Institute of Clinical Excellence, London.

Nickelsen C N 2002 Fetal capillary blood pH. Blood Gas News 11(1):44–46.

RCOG 2001 Electronic fetal monitoring – the use and interpretation of CTG: Evidence based clinical guideline No 8. Royal College of Obstetricians and Gynaecologists, London.

Roberton N R C 1997 Resuscitation of the newborn. In Roberton N R C (ed.) Textbook of Neonatology. Churchill Livingstone, Edinburgh.

Spong C Y, Ogundipe O A, Ross M G 1994 Prophylactic amnioinfusion for meconium-stained amniotic fluid. American Journal of Obstetrics and Gynecology 171:931–935.

Sykes G S, Johnson P, Ashworth F et al 1982 Do Apgar scores indicate asphyxia? Lancet 1:494.

Thacker S B, Stroup D F, Chang M 2001 Continuous electronic fetal heart monitoring for fetal assessment during labour. Cochrane Review: In The Cochrane Library, Issue 2. Update Software 2003, Oxford.

UK Amniotomy Group 1994 Comparing routine versus delayed amniotomy in spontaneous first labour at term. A multicentre randomised trial. Online Journal of Current Clinical Trials. Document number 122, April 1.

Van Wijngaarden W J, Sahota D S, James D K et al 1996 Improved intrapartum surveillance with PR interval analysis of the fetal electrocardiogram: a randomised trial showing a reduction in fetal blood sampling. American Journal of Obstetrics and Gynecology 174:1295–1299.

Westgate J, Harris M, Curnow J S et al 1993 Plymouth randomised trial of cardiotocogram only versus ST waveform plus cardiotocogram for intrapartum monitoring in 2400 cases. American Journal of Obstetrics and Gynecology 169:1151–1160.

Annotated recommended reading

Michie M M 1999 The baby at birth. In Bennett V R, Brown L K (eds) Myles Textbook for Midwives, 13th edn. Churchill Livingstone, Edinburgh.
This is a chapter in an edited book, in which Michie has written about the causes and management of birth asphyxia. It is an invaluable reference for intrapartum care.

NICE 2001 Guidelines for the Use of Electronic Fetal Monitoring. National Institute of Clinical Excellence, London
This publication sets out evidence-based guidelines and recommendations for the use of EFM. The guidelines recommend selective use of continuous EFM.

Nickelsen C N 2002 Fetal capillary blood pH. Blood Gas News 11(1):44–46.
In this article Nickelsen discusses the history of electronic fetal monitoring (EFM). He highlights the inadequacies of EFM that led to the introduction of fetal blood sampling as an additional method of confirming fetal hypoxia.

Thacker S B, Stroup D F, Chang M 2001 Continuous electronic fetal heart monitoring for fetal assessment during labour. Cochrane Review: In The Cochrane Library, Issue 2. Update Software 2003, Oxford.
Thacker et al compared EFM with intermittent auscultation by reviewing randomised controlled trials (RCTs). The review showed no measurable impact on fetal morbidity or mortality.

Chapter 47

Operative delivery

INTRODUCTION

Achievement of a safe vaginal delivery depends, in many cases, on the ability of the obstetrician to effect an operative delivery with forceps or vacuum (Arias 1993).

An operative delivery is performed if a spontaneous birth is judged to pose a greater risk to mother and baby. Operations are divided into vaginal assisted methods (forceps and vacuum extraction deliveries) and abdominal methods (caesarean section). Vaginal assisted deliveries should be undertaken for four basic reasons (Chamberlain & Steer 1999):

1. fetal or maternal distress in second stage of labour;
2. lack of advancement in second stage of labour;
3. control of the after-coming head in a breech delivery;
4. prophylactic shortening of second stage in, for example, heart disease.

The only absolute indications for caesarean section (CS) are cephalopelvic disproportion and major degrees of placenta praevia. Other indications demand a judgement by the obstetrician that the risk of vaginal delivery exceeds the risk of the operation or that the mother's perception is that it does (Chamberlain & Steer 1999).

FORCEPS DELIVERY

Obstetric forceps have been known and utilised in difficult deliveries since their invention by the Chamberlen family in the 17th century. Since then, there have been attempts to modify and improve their effectiveness and safety, leading to a variety of instruments available for use in different obstetric situations (Fig. 47.1). Obstetric forceps consist of two blades, each with a handle and a shank. The blades are marked 'L' left or 'R' right, according to the side of the mother's pelvis in which they lie when applied. There may be a locking or traction device incorporated into the mechanism (Bevis 1999). Whatever the variation in shape, two

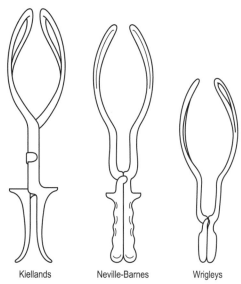

Kiellands   Neville-Barnes   Wrigleys

Figure 47.1 Obstetric forceps (from Sweet B 1997, with permission).

considerations are important leading to the addition of **pelvic** and **cephalic curves**:

- the shape and size of the fetal head;
- the curve, shape and size of the bony pelvis.

The use of forceps

The shape and size of forceps depend on its use. Forceps may be applied in midcavity or at the pelvic outlet. They may be used to *rotate* the fetal head followed by **traction** in the direction of the curve of Carus to complete the delivery or to apply traction only.

- For traction without rotation, non-rotational forceps such as those designed by **Wrigley** or **Simpson** are used for low-cavity delivery, mainly now for delivery of the after-coming head of the breech. **Neville Barnes** or **Haig Ferguson** forceps for midcavity delivery have a pelvic and cephalic curve although these are now used exclusively for low-cavity non-rotational delivery and the axis traction attachments are rarely used.

- It is important to understand that mid- and high-cavity forceps deliveries (when the fetal head is higher than +2) are no longer undertaken because of the possibility of trauma. CS is more likely to be the method of choice in those cases.

- To correct malposition from occipitolateral or occipitoposterior to occipitoanterior prior to traction, rotational forceps such as **Kielland's forceps** are the only design commonly used. These forceps have no pelvic curve (straight) so that they can be rotated in the confines of the birth canal. In malpositions there is often **asynclitism** (tilting of the fetal head). Kielland's forceps have a sliding lock so that asynclitism can be corrected prior to rotation

and traction. There is a gap between the handles when the blades are applied and there is a danger that too much pressure may be applied to the fetal head with the risk of cerebral trauma.

Applying the forceps

Positioning the forceps The blades are inserted separately on either side of the fetal head so that they are located alongside the head and over the ears (Fig. 47.2). They should be situated symmetrically between the eye orbits and the ears, reaching from the parietal eminences to the malar area and cheeks (Vacca 1999). They should come together and lock easily without the use of strength if they are applied correctly. In 1982 Myerscough described the line of application extending from the point of the chin to a point on the sagittal suture near the posterior fontanelle.

The skill of the operator The operator is a major determinant of the success or failure of instrumental delivery. Unfavourable results are almost always caused by the user's unfamiliarity with either the instrument or the rules governing its use (Enkin et al 2000). It is important that the skills of using any instrument are acquired under supervision because of the devastating consequences that could arise if mother or baby is damaged during the operation.

Prerequisites for forceps delivery (Chamberlain & Steer 1999)

No obstruction to the descent of the fetus
- The cervix must be fully dilated – attempts to apply forceps blades with an undilated cervix will lead to trauma without successful delivery.
- The membranes should be ruptured.
- The bladder must be empty – to prevent trauma.
- No obvious bar should exist such as cephalopelvic disproportion.
- Engagement of the head.

Safeguarding the mother
- Adequate anaesthesia must be available by epidural or pudendal block.
- A full explanation of the procedure should be given to the woman and her partner and consent obtained.
- An episiotomy is usually performed – to allow space for the posterior pull.

There should be as much safety, comfort and dignity for the woman as possible although the lithotomy position is essential. The procedure is carried out aseptically using sterile instruments.

Safeguarding the baby
- There should be careful and accurate identification of the presentation and position of the fetal head.

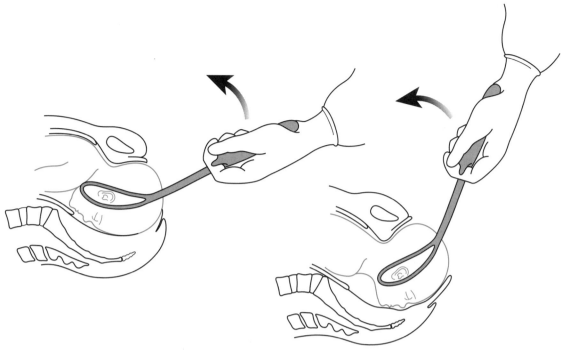

Figure 47.2   Forceps delivery (from Sweet B 1997, with permission).

- The forceps blades should be applied correctly and their position checked before rotation and/or traction is commenced.
- A paediatrician should be present at the delivery.
- Neonatal resuscitation equipment should be available.
- Some obstetricians prefer manual rotation of the head as it is thought to be less traumatic than instrumental rotation (Bevis 1999). Rotational forceps delivery may cause a significant deterioration in fetal acid–base balance (Baker & Johnson 1994).

Complications of forceps delivery

Maternal

- There may be soft tissue damage to the lower uterine segment, cervix, vagina and perineum.
- Bleeding from tissue trauma may lead to postpartum haemorrhage and shock.
- Retention of urine may occur if there is bruising and oedema of the urethra and neck of the bladder.
- Perineal pain may be present once the anaesthesia has worn off.
- Dyspareunia may occur in the long term.
- Psychological effects may lead to avoidance of future pregnancy.

Neonatal

- A cephalhaematoma may form due to friction between the fetal head and the blades or pelvic walls.

- Facial or scalp abrasions are common.
- Bruising of the scalp may lead to neonatal jaundice.
- Intracranial haemorrhage is a rare but serious problem, which may lead to convulsions.
- These problems are more often seen in rotational forceps as is failed forceps delivery resulting in emergency CS (Johanson et al 1992).

VACUUM EXTRACTION (VENTOUSE DELIVERY)

Use of the vacuum extractor

Delivery by the use of **vacuum extraction** has a history as long as that of forceps delivery and is not new. The modern version was developed by **Malmström** in the 1950s and has been modified by others (Vacca 1999). Originally, the vacuum extractor consisted of a rounded metal cup in three sizes, 40, 50 and 60 mm in diameter (Bird 1969), and this type of cup is still in use. This was attached to a **chain** and handle and a suction pump to extract air and create a vacuum. The largest cup size which can be passed through the cervix is chosen.

Cups are now available made of silastic, silicone rubber and plastic. Johanson & Menon (2000) compared soft versus rigid vacuum extractor cups. They found that soft cups were significantly more likely to fail to achieve a vaginal delivery than metal cups. They also found that soft cups were associated with less scalp injury. Metal cups appeared to be more suitable for occipitoposterior, transverse or difficult occipitoanterior position deliveries while soft cups seem to be appropriate for uncomplicated deliveries needing assistance in the second stage. Soft cups deform to follow the contours of the baby's head during application but the application is poor if there is moderate to severe caput succedaneum. The author uses the Kiwi Omnicup. The Omnicup is made of rigid plastic and can be used for malpresentations such as occipitoposterior as well as occipitoanterior positions (Vacca 1999). The omnicup forms a chignon similar to that formed by metal cups but without the associated scalp injury.

Applying the vacuum extractor

Positioning The cup is attached by suction to the fetal scalp as near to the occiput as possible and taking care to avoid the anterior fontanelle (Fig. 47.3). A **vacuum** is created with a negative pressure of 0.2 kg/cm, drawing an artificial caput (chignon) into the cup (Telfer 1997). The cup is checked for position and to ensure that no maternal soft tissue such as the cervix has been included within the rim (Fig. 47.4). The vacuum pressure is increased to 0.8 kg/cm. This can either be done in stages or in one step. One to two minutes should be allowed for the **chignon** to develop. Traction is then applied following the curve of Carus to enhance the natural forces of uterine contractions and maternal expulsive effort.

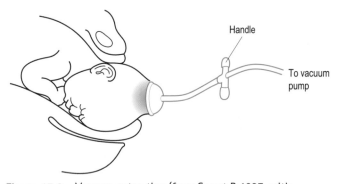

Figure 47.3 Vacuum extraction (from Sweet B 1997, with permission).

The skill of the operator Used skilfully, the advantages of the **ventouse** are that there is no increase to the presenting diameters and the instrument can be used to flex and rotate the head and to assist the mother to deliver her infant. However, some operators may be too hasty or unskilled and apply traction before suction has been achieved, resulting in the cup coming away from the scalp. Some maternity units have trained midwives to perform ventouse deliveries. The technique is also useful where midwives work alone, without obstetric colleagues, in remote areas of the world. It is important that a midwife is properly trained and is confident in the use of this device and that their employing authority approves the use of ventouse equipment by midwives.

Prerequisites
- These are as for forceps delivery.
- The vacuum extractor is not suitable for application in babies with suspected coagulability.
- It should not be used where contractions are weak or maternal effort is poor.

Complications

Maternal

There is less trauma to maternal tissues than that caused by forceps, if the cup has been applied correctly to the fetal head.

There is a tendency for more bleeding due to the abrupt distension of the lower birth canal caused by traction and friction of the fetal head.

Neonatal

- Trauma to the fetal scalp is the most common complication although this is reported as minimal if soft cups (Chenoy & Johanson 1992) or a rigid plastic cup such as the Kiwi Omnicup (Vacca 1999) are used.
- All babies will have a chignon, which is a combination of oedema and bruising.
- Abrasions of the scalp may be caused by the cup being pulled off during inexpert traction.

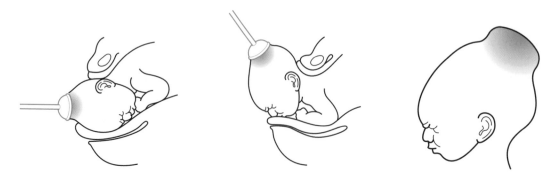

Figure 47.4 Formation of chignon and direction of traction in vacuum extraction.

- Jaundice, usually mild and responding to phototherapy, may be due to the reabsorption of the red cells which have escaped the circulatory system during bruise formation.
- Neonatal retinal haemorrhages are more common following vacuum extraction than forceps delivery but there are no long-term problems.
- Vacuum extraction has been found to be associated with umbilical cord blood acid–base changes but these changes in pH and PCO_2 were not associated with increased perinatal morbidity or mortality or acidaemia at birth. These findings suggest that vacuum extraction can be used to deliver babies with fetal distress in the second stage of labour.

Comparison of forceps and vacuum extraction

Although **assisted vaginal delivery** is performed worldwide, there is a large variation in its application, ranging from 1.5% of all deliveries in the Czech Republic to 15% in Australia and Canada (Stephenson 1992). In a systematic review of 10 studies, Johanson & Menon (1999) compared assisted vaginal delivery by obstetric forceps versus ventouse extraction. The reviewers concluded that the use of vacuum extractor appears to reduce maternal morbidity. There was a reduction in cephalhaematoma and retinal haemorrhages with forceps deliveries and this was seen to be a compensatory benefit.

This area remains controversial, although the benefits to the mother of vacuum extraction have been established. Further research using larger studies is required to provide further information about major adverse neonatal effects of both methods and improving operator skill.

CAESAREAN SECTION

Overview

Caesarean section (CS) is a surgical procedure in which the abdomen and uterus are incised to facilitate the birth of the baby. There are records of this procedure being performed prior to the discovery of anaesthetic drugs, and usually for delivery of the fetus when the mother had died. Caesarean section may be carried out as an emergency in response to adverse conditions developing in late pregnancy or in labour. Elective CS is a planned event where the timing is chosen to maximise safety for mother and fetus.

Current rates

Rates of CS worldwide have increased steadily over the last few decades (Savage 1996). In the UK they have doubled and in the USA and Canada they have tripled. The WHO (1985) said that CS rates should not need to be more than 10–15%. While Savage believes that this rate should not need to be more than 6–8%. The rate in England and Wales has been observed to increase: 11.3% in 1989–90; 15.5% in 1994–95; 18% in 1997–98; and 21.5% in 2000–01 (DOH 2001). In the early 1990s about 25–30% of births in the USA were by CS and recently there has been a drive to reduce these numbers to meet national targets.

Indications

The majority of CSs were performed for hypertensive disorders of pregnancy, antepartum haemorrhage or fetal distress (Lewis 2001). The major reasons for the increase in CS rate are for breech presentation, repeat CS or previous dystocia. The setting up of post-traumatic stress clinics for women who have had previous traumatic 'normal deliveries' may also have contributed to the rising numbers of CSs, as the women involved may opt for a CS for subsequent deliveries. Table 47.1 summarises the indications for CS.

Method

The operation of CS is a technique whereby the course of childbirth is interrupted, and delivery via the natural passage is skirted in favour of the abdominal route (Al-Azzawi 1998).

Table 47.1 Maternal and fetal indications for caesarean section

Maternal	Fetal	Maternal and fetal
Severe pregnancy-induced hypertension	Severe rhesus isoimmunisation	Cephalopelvic disproportion
Previous vaginal reconstructive surgery	Cord prolapse	Pelvic tumours
Previous third-degree tears	Multiple fetuses (3 or more)	High-risk obstetric history
A large for dates fetus (with previous shoulder dystocia)	Breech presentation	Antepartum haemorrhage
Eclampsia	Brow or shoulder presentations	Uterine rupture
Terminal illness of the mother	Severe intrauterine growth retardation (which may be complicated by maternal disease)	Failure to progress in labour
	Fetal distress in labour	Placenta praevia
	Fetal abnormality where damage may be increased by vaginal delivery	Fetal macrosomia
	Active genital herpes	Tumours

Any person called on to assist at a CS must be aware of the surgical techniques involved. Technically, there are two types of CS according to the incision in the uterus: the **lower segment** and the **classical**. There is no association with the type of abdominal wall incision although a lower segment CS is most often performed through a transverse incision, also called the **Pfannenstiel** or **bikini-line incision** (Bevis 1999). The lower segment forms from about 32 weeks of pregnancy and is less muscular than the upper segment. A transverse incision into the lower uterine segment heals more rapidly than a vertical incision into the upper uterine segment and there is less risk of rupture of the uterus in a subsequent pregnancy. For this reason, classical CS is rarely performed unless the fetus is to be delivered prior to the 32nd week of pregnancy or there is an anterior placenta praevia.

Anatomical layers incised and sutured in a caesarean section

- Skin.
- Fat.
- Rectus sheath.
- Muscle (rectus abdominis).
- Abdominal peritoneum.
- Pelvic (visceral peritoneum or perimetrium).
- Uterine muscle (sutured in two layers).

As the uterus is incised, the membranes are ruptured with the escape of amniotic fluid. There is likely to be substantial bleeding because of the increased blood supply to the uterus. Immediate postoperative care is as for any surgery but the woman will wish to see and have contact with her baby as soon as possible and to breastfeed if that is her intended method of feeding. Because of the proximity of the bladder to the lower uterine segment, urine output must be observed. A urinary catheter is inserted in the bladder for at least 24 h after the CS as there may be difficulty in micturition at first. Any presence of haematuria must be reported to the obstetrician.

Types of anaesthesia used for caesarean section

Types of anaesthesia used for CS will depend on the reason why the CS is being performed. In the case of fetal distress, where a woman already has a working epidural, the epidural will be topped-up with a stronger anaesthetic with or without an opiate drug such as morphine or fentanyl. Spinal anaesthesia is used for elective CSs or when an epidural is ineffective. In the case of severe fetal bradycardia, where the fetus has to be delivered quickly, a general anaesthetic is usually given. A general anaesthetic is also given when a patient who has had a spinal or epidural complains of pain during the operation. Women with clotting disorders will always have a general anaesthetic.

Postoperative analgesia

The anaesthetist should prescribe adequate and effective analgesia and should include:

- intramuscular analgesia, e.g. morphine sulphate injections;
- non-steroidal anti-inflammatory drugs, e.g. diclofenac 100 mg p.r. (per rectum) or oral tablets as recommended in the British National Formulary (BNF 2003);
- oral tablets, e.g. paracetamol 1 g, four times a day, or co-dydramol, two tablets taken 6 hourly;
- patient-controlled analgesia (PCA) may be prescribed, where a woman has coagulation problems, to avoid frequent intramuscular injections, and may also be necessary for women who have had a general anaesthetic for an emergency CS.

Safety

Lilford (1990) warned that any increase in the proportions of elective CS would lead to increase in the CS rate and probably in maternal mortality. Caesarean section carried out for the safety of the fetus puts the mother's life at risk (Hillan 1991). Even with the benefit of modern surgical techniques, it is still less safe for the woman than a vaginal delivery. The major hazard is **pulmonary embolism**, which is difficult to prevent (Savage 1996). **Haemorrhage** and **infection** as well as thromboembolic disorders may occur (Francome et al 1993). Long-term morbidity with **infertility**, voluntary or involuntary, may be a problem. The Confidential Enquiry into Maternal Deaths (CEMD) for the years 1994–96 reported that 48.8% of all direct deaths were following CS. However, the most recent CEMD report noted that from 1997 to 1999 there was a dramatic fall in the number of direct deaths following CS (Lewis 2001).

Neonatal behaviour

There is a profound effect on neonatal behaviour attributable to at least the following four factors (Trevathen 1987):

1. caesarean section is often carried out before term;
2. maternal medication is greater than in vaginal births;
3. in elective CS the baby is not subjected to the stress of labour;
4. hormonal influences vary depending on the time and mode of delivery.

Babies are less active if delivered by CS; they sleep more and cry less. The influence of drugs in labour on neonatal behaviour will be examined in more detail in Chapter 57.

GENERAL ANAESTHESIA IN PREGNANCY AND CHILDBIRTH

Reversible anaesthesia, which is a state of unconsciousness and muscle relaxation, is brought about by pharmacological preparations. There is a great difference in obstetric anaesthesia from general surgery as two lives have to be cared for – the mother and the fetus. The recent CEMD report recommends the need for vigilance in the care of the pregnant woman undergoing general anaesthesia (Lewis 2001).

The altered physiology of the woman increases the danger and includes raised maternal intragastric pressure, acidity of gastric contents and delayed gastric emptying, leading to the risk of acid aspiration syndrome. Aortocaval compression, the effect of drugs on the fetus, maternal hypoxia or hypotension, placental insufficiency and intrapartum fetal hypoxia also increase the risk of neonatal respiratory depression (Telfer 1997).

General anaesthetic agents

For a drug to be used as an **anaesthetic agent**, it must affect the central nervous system appropriately and be rapidly controllable so that anaesthesia can be induced rapidly, be adjusted during the operation to provide the correct level of consciousness and the effects should be quickly reversible after the operation (Rang et al 2001). Humphrey Davy suggested the use of the gas **nitrous oxide** for relieving the pain of surgery in 1800. He tested its effects on himself and a few others including the then prime minister. It was found to cause euphoria, analgesia and loss of consciousness but became famous as laughing gas until an American dentist, Horace Wells, had a tooth extracted under its influence.

Inhalational anaesthetics were used in surgery in 1846 when William Morton used ether to extract a tooth. He persuaded the chief surgeon at Massachussetts General Hospital to use it during a surgical procedure on the 16th October 1846 and it was successful; subsequently, planned protracted surgical procedures could be carried out. The famous American Oliver Wendell Holmes invented the word 'anaesthesia'. In 1847 James Simpson, professor of obstetrics in Glasgow, used the agent **chloroform** to relieve pain in childbirth, but it only became popular after Queen Victoria gave birth to her seventh child under the influence of chloroform in 1853.

The modern drugs

Although many CS are now performed under epidural anaesthesia (see Ch. 38), general anaesthesia is still used. It is now common practice to preoxygenate pregnant women prior to induction of a general anaesthetic although this may lead to stress for the woman (Bevis 1999). The choice made by the woman is important. Holdcroft et al (1995) found that one-third of the women in their small study opted to be unconscious during CS. Induction agents used to initiate anaesthesia include barbiturates such as **thiopental**, which causes loss of consciousness in 20 s if given intravenously (Rang et al 2001), or **propofol** which appears to be a good alternative to thiopental. Maternal unconsciousness follows rapidly with minimal side-effects and fetal respiratory depression can be avoided.

Anaesthesia is then maintained by inhalational anaesthetic agents such as nitrous oxide combined with a volatile agent such as **halothane** (Fluothane) or **enflurane** (Ethrane). Halothane has limited usefulness as an obstetric anaesthetic agent as it causes relaxation of the uterine muscle (Rang et al 2001). These agents deepen the anaesthesia, improve uterine blood flow by reducing circulating catecholamines and improve fetal acid–base status (Capogna & Celluno 1993).

Problems

Failed intubation

Failed intubation is an obstetric emergency requiring prompt and calm action. Most maternal deaths attributed directly to anaesthesia have been reported to be due to a misplaced endotracheal tube. It is usual to have a failed intubation drill (Bevis 1999). The anaesthetist may choose to maintain an airway with a Guedel airway and face mask, with an assistant maintaining cricoid pressure throughout the anaesthetic, or **spinal anaesthesia** may be chosen.

Effect of anaesthetics on the nervous system

The mode of action of drugs that create a state of anaesthesia is as yet unexplained. The brain has a large blood flow and the blood–brain barrier is freely permeable to anaesthetic agents (Rang et al 2001). Theories involve interaction with the lipid bilayer of the cell membrane or with hydrophobic binding sites on protein molecules. Anaesthetics inhibit the conduction of cellular action potentials and synaptic transmission.

It is probable that **anaesthetics act** on two main parts of the brain: the **reticular formation** and the **hippocampus**. Loss of consciousness is probably due to the effect of the drug on the reticular formation of the brain. Anaesthetics also cause short-term amnesia and the hippocampus is likely to be the site for this action. Many other brain functions are affected such as motor control and reflex action. It is not helpful to look for one site of action as all neurons are affected.

Muscle relaxation is achieved by drugs which **depolarise** neuromuscular messages postsynaptically such as suxamethonium (Scoline) or **non-polarising agents** which act postsynaptically such as pancuronium (Pavulon) (Rang et al 2001).

Acid aspiration syndrome (Mendelson's syndrome)

This life-threatening syndrome arises from the inhalation of acid gastric contents and was first described by Mendelson in 1946. The result of such aspiration is a chemical pneumonitis leading to **adult respiratory distress syndrome (ARDS)** with acute bronchospasm, dyspnoea, cyanosis, wheezing and tachycardia (Telfer 1997). The factors predisposing to this arise from the physiological effect of progesterone on the smooth muscle of the stomach which causes delayed emptying, decreased lower oesophageal tone, which leads to reflux, and the altered position of the stomach due to the enlarged uterus. There is also gastric hypersecretion in labour and there is still no consensus on nil-by-mouth policies. There is no firm evidence to support the policy of restricting food intake for all women in labour. Most maternity units now only restrict food intake in those women who have a higher risk of having an emergency CS.

Prevention of acid aspiration syndrome
Prevention of this syndrome is essential. The administration of drugs such as **antacid preparations** like sodium citrate 30 ml prior to anaesthetic induction and **histamine-2 (H$_2$) antagonists** such as ranitidine 150 mg are recommended. Other drugs such as **metoclopramide** act centrally in the nervous system and also locally in the gastrointestinal tract. These are antiemetic drugs, and they act as stimulants to gastric motility, accelerating emptying without stimulating gastric juice production. They increase tone in the lower oesophagus and prevent gastro-oesophageal reflux (Rang et al 2001).

During induction of the general anaesthetic and intubation, **cricoid pressure (Sellick's manoeuvre)**, part of what is referred to as '**crash induction**' along with the immediate passing of a cuffed endotracheal tube, is essential to prevent aspiration of acid stomach contents. The cricoid cartilage is compressed between the thumb and finger towards the cervical spine in order to occlude the oesophagus. Deaths have occurred due to inexperience of the practitioner and it is recommended that only an experienced anaesthetist should be involved in obstetric anaesthesia (Lewis 2001).

Aortocaval compression

The alternative name for **aortocaval compression** is supine hypotensive syndrome, which Bevis (1999) believes to be misleading as the fall in blood pressure is a late sign and placental perfusion will have occurred before the drop in maternal blood pressure. A reduction in venous return and a fall in cardiac output are produced by the weight of the gravid uterus pressing on and partly occluding the inferior vena cava. It will occur whenever the woman lies supine in late pregnancy. If fetal distress is present, the interference with placental circulation will increase the severity of hypoxia.

Prevention of aortocaval compression
If the woman has to lie supine, the sequence of events can be avoided by placing a folded blanket or a small rubber wedge under the mattress to tilt the woman's body about 15° to the left. Modern operating tables and delivery beds have this function built into their design. Wilkinson & Enkin (1997) reviewed the use of **lateral tilt** during CS but found the data to be poor. However, they stated that low Apgar scores were fewer and neonatal pH measurements and oxygen tensions appeared to be better if lateral tilt was used.

MAIN POINTS

- Forceps may be used to rotate the fetal head before traction is applied to complete the delivery or to apply traction only to complete delivery. It is necessary to confirm that there is no obstruction to the descent of the fetus before performing a forceps delivery.

- Maternal complications following forceps delivery include soft tissue damage to the lower uterine segment, cervix, vagina and perineum; bleeding from tissue trauma; retention of urine; postdelivery perineal pain; and dyspareunia in the long term. Neonatal complications are more often seen in rotational forceps and include cephalhaematoma; abrasions; neonatal jaundice; and intracranial haemorrhage.

- Equipment for vacuum extraction delivery has been modified. Cups are now available made of silastic, silicone rubber and plastic as well as the original metal. Soft cups deform to follow the contours of the baby's head during application and are less likely to be associated with scalp trauma.

- Midwives can be specially trained to perform this technique and can use the ventouse equipment for delivery if it is approved by their employing authority.

- Worldwide CS rates have risen over the last 25 years. In the UK the majority of operations are performed for hypertensive disorders of pregnancy, antepartum haemorrhage or fetal distress. Even with modern surgical techniques it is still less safe for the woman than a vaginal delivery. During CS, the altered physiology of the woman increases the danger of acid aspiration syndrome but the major hazard is pulmonary embolism.

- Although many CS are now performed under spinal or epidural anaesthesia, general anaesthesia is still used. Acid aspiration syndrome arises from the inhalation of acid gastric contents, resulting in chemical pneumonitis and adult respiratory distress syndrome. Prevention is essential and antacid preparations and histamine-2 (H$_2$) antagonists are recommended. Most maternal deaths attributed directly to anaesthesia are due to a misplaced endotracheal tube. During induction of the general anaesthetic and intubation, cricoid pressure is essential to prevent aspiration of acid stomach contents.

References

Al-Azzawi F 1998 Childbirth & Obstetric Techniques, 2nd edn. Mosby, St Louis.

Arias F 1993 Practical Guide to High Risk Pregnancy and Delivery, 2nd edn. Mosby Year Book, Chicago.

Baker N, Johnson I R 1994 A study of rotational forceps delivery on fetal acid–base balance. Acta Obstetrica et Gynecologica Scandinavica 73:787–789.

Bevis R 1999 Obstetric anaesthesia and operations. In Bennett V R, Brown L K (eds) Myles Textbook for Midwives, 13th edn. Churchill Livingstone, Edinburgh.

Bird G C 1969 Modification of Malmström's vacuum extractor. British Medical Journal 3:526.

BNF 2003 British National Formulary, Number 45 (March). British Medical Association and Royal Pharmaceutical Society of Great Britain, London.

Capogna G, Celluno D 1993 The effects of anaesthetic agents on the newborn. In Reynolds F (ed.) Effects on the Baby of Maternal Analgesia and Anaesthesia. W B Saunders, London.

Chamberlain G, Steer P 1999 ABC of labour care: operative delivery. British Medical Journal 318(May):1260–1264.

Chenoy R, Johanson R B 1992 A randomised prospective study comparing delivery with metal and silicone rubber vacuum extractor cups. British Journal of Obstetrics and Gynaecology 99:360–364.

DoH 2001 NHS Maternity Statistics, England: 1995–1996 to 1997–1998. Department of Health, London.

Enkin M, Keirse M J N C, Renfrew M et al 2000 A Guide to Effective Care in Pregnancy and Childbirth, 3rd edn. Oxford University Press, Oxford.

Francome C, Savage W, Churchill H et al 1993 Caesarean Birth in Britain. Middlesex University Press, National Childbirth Trust, London.

Hillan E 1991 Caesarean section: maternal risks. Nursing Standard 5(50):26–29.

Holdcroft A, Parshall A M, Knowles M G et al 1995 Factors associated with mothers selecting general anaesthesia for lower segment caesarean section. Journal of Psychosomatic Obstetrics and Gynaecology 16(3):167–170.

Johanson R B, Menon V 1999 Vacuum extraction versus forceps for assisted vaginal delivery. Cochrane Review: In The Cochrane Library, Issue 2. Update Software 2003, Oxford.

Johanson R B, Menon V 2000 Soft versus rigid vacuum extractor cups for assisted vaginal delivery. Cochrane Review: In The Cochrane Library, Issue 2. Update Software 2003, Oxford.

Johanson R B, Rice C, Doyle M et al 1992 A randomised prospective study comparing the new vacuum extractor policy with forceps delivery. British Journal of Obstetrics and Gynaecology 100:524–530.

Lewis G (ed.) 2001 The Confidential Enquiries into Maternal Deaths in the United Kingdom: Why Mothers Die 1997–1999. RCOG, London.

Lilford R 1990 Maternal mortality and caesarean section. British Journal of Obstetrics and Gynaecology 97:883–892.

Myerscough P R 1982 Munro Kerr's Operative Obstetrics, 10th edn. Baillière Tindall, London.

Rang H P (ed.), Dale M M, Ritter M M 2001 Pharmacology, 4th edn. Churchill Livingstone, Edinburgh.

Savage W 1996 The caesarean section epidemic: a psychological problem? Journal of the Association of Chartered Physiotherapists in Women's Health 79:13–16.

Stephenson P A 1992 International Differences in the Use of Obstetrical Interventions. World Health Organisation, Copenhagen, WHO (EUR/ICP/MCH):112.

Telfer M 1997 Anaesthesia and operative procedures in obstetrics. In Sweet B R, Tiran D (eds) Mayes Midwifery: A Textbook for Midwives, 12th edn. Baillière Tindall, London.

Trevathen W 1987 Human Birth: An Evolutionary Perspective. Aldine de Gruyter, New York.

Vacca A 1999 Handbook of Vacuum Extraction in Obstetric Practice. Vacca Research, Brisbane.

WHO (World Health Organisation) 1985 Appropriate technology for birth. Lancet ii:436–437.

Wilkinson C, Enkin M W 1997 Lateral tilt during caesarean section. Cochrane Review: In The Cochrane Library, Issue 2. Update Software 2003, Oxford.

Annotated recommended reading

Al-Azzawi F 1998 Childbirth and Obstetric Techniques, 2nd edn. Mosby, St Louis.
This book presents a pictorial demonstration of all modes of delivery, including the three main types of CS. The visual colour presentations will prove valuable to students and those learning childbirth techniques.

Chalmers B 1992 WHO, Appropriate technology for birth revisited. British Journal of Obstetrics and Gynaecology 99:709–710.
In this article, Chalmers questions the basis of the WHO's 1985 recommendations (appropriate technology for birth). Do they match up to today's research findings? The documents require critical analysis by both practitioners and decision makers.

Johanson R B, Menon V 1999 Vacuum extraction versus forceps for assisted vaginal delivery. Cochrane Review: In The Cochrane Library, Issue 2. Update Software 2003, Oxford.
This systematic review on the use of ventouse versus forceps provides useful information for those who perform instrumental deliveries and those responsible for giving advice to women and their partners.

Vacca A 1999 Handbook of Vacuum Extraction in Obstetric Practice. Vacca Research, Brisbane.
This is an excellent reference book for ventouse and forceps deliveries. Vacca is a professor of obstetrics and has been involved with the design of the Kiwi Omnicups for ventouse delivery.

World Health Organisation (WHO) 1985 Appropriate technology for birth. Lancet ii:436–437.
As a result of debates at the United Nations of increasing caesareans section in 1979, the WHO undertook research into perinatal services and developed recommendations for appropriate technology for birth. This document includes the recommendations.

Section 4A

PUERPERIUM – THE BABY

Section 4 considers the mother and her baby in the puerperium. Midwives may care for mothers and their babies for up to 28 days and it is imperative that they are able to recognise both normal appearance and behaviour and any deviations present. Section 4A is about the baby. Chapters 48 and 49 provide a detailed account of the adaptation of the fetus to independent extrauterine life. The remaining chapters provide an introduction to some commonly encountered serious disorders. These chapters cannot take the place of a specifically written textbook on neonatal care and the reader is referred to one of the many excellent books available and the papers given within the chapter reference lists. Chapter 50 is about the care of the low birthweight baby, Chapter 51 examines cardiovascular and respiratory problems, Chapter 52 is concerned with neonatal jaundice and some metabolic disorders while Chapter 53 discusses problems arising from infection or trauma.

Chapter **48**

Adaptation to extrauterine life 1 – respiration and cardiovascular functions

INTRODUCTION

Chapters 48–53 explore physiological mechanisms and pathophysiological factors affecting adaptation to extrauterine life. The neonate (from birth until 4 weeks of age) is referred to using the masculine pronoun to distinguish him from his mother. Throughout intrauterine life, the fetus is dependent on his mother for survival, yet at birth his body must make many rapid physiological and biochemical adaptations fundamental to the successful transition to extrauterine life.

Every body system contributes to the establishment and ongoing adjustment of new homeostatic values. Of immediate importance are the changes which occur in the respiratory and cardiovascular systems (Moore & Persaud 1998). The initiating biochemical and physiological factors are considerable but the fundamental feature is the significant rise in the partial pressure of carbon dioxide (CO_2) in the blood once contact with the placenta is lost. This rise is crucial to effective stimulation of the respiratory centre which induces the neonate to take the first breath. This initiates a sequence of events leading to lung expansion and inhalation of air (Coad & Dunstall 2001). The inspired oxygen stimulates the haemodynamic changes, including the augmentation of circulating blood volume, cardiac and respiratory functions. The renal system and maintenance of the acid–base balance of the body is also discussed. An understanding of physiology provides a foundation for many advances in neonatal care so it is important to assess and evaluate the changing body processes of the neonate.

THE APPEARANCE OF THE NORMAL BABY

Skin and hair

The **neonate** at term (Fig. 48.1) weighs about 3500–3750 g and is 50–55 cm long. His occipitofrontal head circumference averages 35 cm and his head is almost 25% of his total body mass (Michie 1999). He should appear plump with a

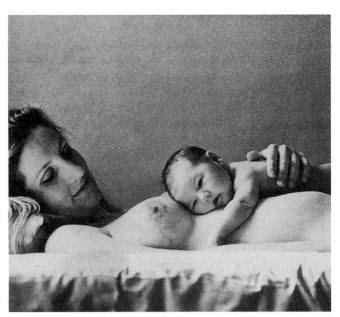

Figure 48.1   Skin-to-skin contact in a warm labour ward. (Courtesy of Professor J Hedgecoe.)

rounded abdomen, largely due to the deposition of subcutaneous fat and water. In healthy neonates the skin of the body and face should be uniformly warm and of good colour. The nails should reach the ends of the fingers and toes. The scalp should be covered with fine silky hair. Some neonates appear bald while others have luxuriant straight or curly hair. Remnants of **lanugo**, the fine hair that covers the entire body during the second and third trimester of pregnancy, may be present on the shoulders. The ears should be well developed, shaped by well-formed cartilage, and placed symmetrically on either side of head.

As long as tissue oxygenation is adequate, the neonate will have a delicate, pinkish skin and, depending on his race, may be lightly pigmented. The mucous membranes of the mouth and lips as well as the nail beds should always appear pink and show signs of good tissue perfusion and adequate oxygenation. Pigmentation of the genitalia and nipples is deeper in those with dark skins and a **linea nigra** may be present in the lower abdominal midline. Similarly, depending on racial origin, diffuse bluish-black skin colouration known as the **Mongolian blue spot** may be present, usually over the sacral area. The creases of his palms and soles are well defined (Michie 1999).

Humans are unique amongst primates in having large **sebaceous glands** which produce **sebum** over the scalp, face and upper back (Morgan 1994). Although the sebaceous glands are very active in utero, most become inactive by birth and will stay dormant until puberty when their re-established activity may lead to acne. At birth, distended sebaceous glands called **milia** may be present over the nose and cheeks. Remnants of the sebaceous gland excretion mixed with dead skin cells forms the **vernix caseosa**, covering the entire skin in later stages of fetal life. In a term infant this is usually reduced to covering the groins and axillae.

At about 5 months of gestation, the fetus develops sweat glands (**eccrine glands**) on the palms of its hands and the soles of its feet. At the same time, scent glands (**apocrine glands**), used by many mammals for sweat cooling, appear to develop throughout the body. By 7 months the apocrine glands disappear except for in the armpits, pubic area, around the nipples and lips while the eccrine glands continue to spread all over the body. In humans, but no other primates, these are the glands used for **sweat cooling** when the body temperature rises above a critical physiological point (Morgan 1994). These sweat glands are inactive for the first few days of life (Michie 1999).

Eyes

The iris colour of most babies is poorly defined, generally appearing dark blue-grey although some dark-skinned babies may have brown eyes at birth. Permanent colouring of the iris may take several years to develop. Oriental and Down syndrome babies have an **epicanthic fold** (vertical pleats of skin that overlap the medial angles of the eyes), which changes the shape of the soft tissue covering the orbital region. Epicanthic folds are common in many other infants too.

It is important to assess the structure and appearance of the eyes. Observation must include the relative size, shape and position of the eyes in their sockets. Assessing neonatal vision by an observed reaction to light is generally considered adequate unless significant structural features warrant a fuller visual assessment. However, assessing the neonate's response to light requires a relatively dark room and only a moderately bright beam of light in order to avoid stimulating reflex eye closure. Pupil size of a term infant should be within 1.8 mm (when constricted) and 5.4 mm (when dilated) diameter range. Measurements that fall outside these acceptable parameters should be considered as anomalous and investigated further (Avery et al 1999).

Neonates cannot generally shed tears, which provide a natural lubricant and antiseptic for the eyes. This may contribute to a higher incidence of eye infections such as conjunctivitis. This clinical phenomenon may be further complicated by temporary blockage of the lacrimal ducts, which under normal conditions would keep the conjunctiva clean and lubricated.

Sexual characteristics

Both boys and girls have a small nodule of breast tissue averaging 1 cm in diameter surrounding the nipple. Initially, the breast tissue may be swollen because of the high plasma oestrogen acquired from the mother and for a short time a milky fluid may be present. Traditionally, such breast milk was referred to as **witchs' milk**. No attempt should be made to remove this milk as squeezing the breast tissue may lead to bruising and abscess formation.

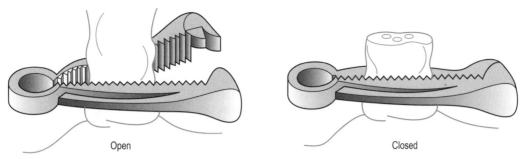

Figure 48.2   A cord clamp (from Sweet B 1997, with permission).

The testes are descended into the scrotum in boys born at term but are usually undescended in preterm infants. The foreskin adheres to the glans penis but this should not obstruct the voiding of urine. In girls the deposition of fat in the genital area ensures that the labia majora covers and conceals the labia minora. This feature is not present in preterm babies and the urethral and vaginal orifices can be seen if the labia are parted. A thick white vaginal discharge, probably a response to maternal oestrogens, may be present. The linings of the uterus and vagina consist of fairly mature epithelium and in some baby girls may have a small **pseudomenstrual bleed**. Following birth, as maternal oestrogen levels in the infant's blood fall, the genital tract returns to an infantile state.

Posture

A baby usually lies in a flexed position and resists extension of his limbs. When his arms are extended, the tendency is to move them outwards, possibly by reflex. When he is placed on his back, he will turn his head to one side, usually the right side, elevating the left shoulder. Conversely, when placed in the prone position he will draw his knees under his abdomen, elevate his buttocks and turn his head to one side. A term baby is quite active and should move his limbs spontaneously and equally on both sides of his body. Such postural phenomena may not be evident in premature infants because the neural and locomotor systems are structurally and functionally too immature.

PHYSIOLOGICAL CHARACTERISTICS OF THE NEONATE

The haematological system

Circulatory volume

The separation of the fetus from the placental circulation following birth is a major transitional event. The umbilical arteries taking deoxygenated blood from fetus to placenta for oxygenation constrict at birth but the umbilical vein remains dilated, an invaluable mechanism in limiting fetal blood loss. Fetal blood volume varies from 75 to 125 ml/kg

depending on the direction and amount of blood flow between fetus and placenta at the time of birth. Commonly, at delivery, the baby is held for 2–3 min at or below the level of the placenta and blood will flow from placenta to the neonate by the force of gravity (Coad & Dunstall 2001).

The transfer of placental blood to the fetus also depends on the timing of the clamping of the umbilical cord (Fig. 48.2). Yao & Lind (1969) found that if the baby was held at the level of the introitus until the cord was clamped, or was held 40 cm below the level of the introitus for 30 s, he generally received a transfusion of approximately 80 ml of blood from the placenta. However, if the baby was held more than 50 cm above the introitus, the transfusion of blood to the newborn infant was negligible.

Early clamping of the umbilical cord   There are advantages and disadvantages of early versus late clamping of the umbilical cord. The cord is usually clamped early (Coad & Dunstall 2001). In preterm infants, late cord clamping is associated with subsequent **hyperbilirubinaemia** due to the significant increase in erythrocytes. The concomitant increase in plasma volume may expand the vascular compartment, as well as have some effect on the extravascular space in the lungs. It is possible that the combination of these factors contributes to the development of **respiratory distress** by reducing the infant's already compromised lung compliance and functional residual capacity.

However, there is some suggestion that late clamping of the cord (after 30 s) may be beneficial to premature neonates as it increases the scope for oxygen transportation and acid–base balance. Other groups of neonates may be harmed by delayed cord clamping, particularly in neonates experiencing **hydrops fetalis**, **rhesus isoimmunisation** (Ch. 52, p. 665), those at risk of developing polycythaemia as a consequence of **cyanotic heart disease** (Ch. 51, p. 653) or **severe immaturity** due to maternal diabetes mellitus (Ch. 50, p. 637). In multiple births, the cord of the first baby should be clamped early to prevent blood loss from the unborn baby through a communicating placental circulation.

Changes in other haematologic parameters

Circulating blood volume at term averages 90 ml/kg of body weight. As in adults, each of the blood's cellular components has a finite life span and must be continually replaced. In health, haematopoiesis proceeds at a relatively fixed pace and the circulating concentrations of each cell type remain within narrow limits. Despite this relative stability, the haematopoietic system is highly responsive, with a unique capacity to up-regulate or down-regulate production of any cell type on demand. This responsiveness is essential to the ongoing adaptations in the composition of the neonate's blood. Changes continue to occur, particularly in the 1st week of life during the transitional period: for instance, the type and quantities of haemoglobin changes and mechanisms involved in fetal oxygen uptake and release are adapted to the extrauterine lifestyle.

The microanatomical and physiological processes regulating haematopoiesis are complex. This is essential to the maintenance of equilibrium between cellular production and function, and the unique demands made on the various cellular metabolic activities. For instance, in adults, mature erythrocytes circulate for approximately 120 days, platelets for about 10 days and neutrophils for 6–8 h.

Growth factors are considered to be important in haematopoeitic tissue growth and differentiation. Their molecular mass, chromosomal locations and the cell types they influence provide insight into the ongoing development and differentiation of pleuripotent stem cells into competent mature blood cells (Christensen & Schibler 1996). Several haematopoietic growth factors, including granulocyte colony-stimulating factor (**G-CSF**), granulocyte–macrophage colony-stimulating factor (**GM-CSF**), **interleukin 6** (IL-6) and **interleukin 8** (IL-8) appear to play significant roles. For example, G-CSF is involved in the stimulation of myeloid progenitor cell cycling, clonal development of neutrophils and enhancement of neutrophil function as phagocytic cells (Ch. 29).

Erythrocytes (red blood cells)

The **erythrocyte** count at birth averages 5 million/ml. Erythrocytes develop from pleuripotent stem cells found in the bone marrow. These stems cells are capable of replication and differentiation into a wide spectrum of blood cells, including erythrocytes, granulocytes, monocytes and megakaryocytes. The earliest recognizable erythrocyte comes in the form of a **normoblast**, which matures without further replication to a **reticulocyte**. This then matures, giving rise to erythrocytes.

The maturation of the precursor cells to mature erythrocytes in neonates and adults is controlled by **erythropoietin**, which is thought to bind to specific receptor sites found in the membrane of the evolving cells. The responsiveness to erythropoietin is inversely related to the ability of the progenitor cells to replicate (Wardrop et al 1996). Also, erythropoietin must be capable of binding to the specific receptor site in order to induce the process of maturation. With normal physiological and biochemical conditions at birth, the relationship between erythropoietin and red cell production should be in functional order.

The relative increase in erythrocytes due to **plasma reduction** and **haemoconcentration** in the first few hours/days of life is a transitional phenomenon, corrected by the rapid but fairly well-controlled destruction of excess erythrocytes which occurs following birth. A more acceptable physiological erythrocyte count is achieved by 6 months of life (Rudolph 2002). Nucleated, immature erythrocytes are seen during the first 24 h following birth, possibly due to the stresses of delivery, but these usually disappear within 4 days. Although erythropoietin influences cell development during intrauterine life, it disappears about 24 h after birth, to return after 2–3 months, which coincides with resumption of bone marrow activity and red cell production.

Haemoglobin Neonatal haemoglobin averages 16.5–17.5 g/dl. This may increase by a further 6 g/dl over the first 24 h due to a shift in fluid distribution leading to haemoconcentration. The decrease in circulating plasma volume results in a net increase in erythrocytes. Various physiological mechanisms contribute to the gradual reduction in haemoglobin concentration and its eventual decrease back to cord blood values by the end of the 1st week of life. By 3 months, the haemoglobin level in healthy infants has fallen to 12 g/dl (Sweet 1997).

Erythrocytes are more specialised in composition than most other cells because of the presence of their major constituent haemoglobin, which accounts for 95% of total cellular protein content. Cord blood haemoglobin content varies with gestational age but broad parameters can be detailed as follows (Sweet 1997):

- fetal haemoglobin (HbF) is 50–85%;
- adult haemoglobin (HbA) is 15–40%;
- haemoglobin A_2 (HbA$_2$) is less than 2%.

The rate of decline of HbF production after birth is considerable; at 4 months of age fetal haemoglobin will be less than 20%.

Haemoglobin combines reversibly with oxygen, permitting erythrocytes to deliver oxygen from the lungs to the tissues for use in cellular metabolic processes. This function is demonstrated by the oxygen dissociation curve, whereby the oxygen saturation of the blood is plotted against oxygen tension or partial pressure of the whole blood (Guyton & Hall 2000). The oxygen dissociation curve in the neonate is placed firmly to the left, denoting the high affinity of HbF for oxygen. This phenomenon is thought to be necessary to allow efficient extraction of oxygen from the maternal circulation but it does not allow the release of equally large proportions of oxygen to the tissues after birth.

2,3-diphosphoglycerate Mature red blood cells lack mitochondria and their glucose metabolism is anaerobic. After birth the shift in the **oxygen dissociation curve** to the right is attributable to certain organic phosphates which decrease the affinity of HbA for oxygen by competing for the same binding sites. One of these, **2,3-diphosphoglycerate** (2,3-DPG), is formed during anaerobic glycolysis and then acts as an intermediate compound, enhancing the release of oxygen from haemoglobin. An increase in 2,3-DPG production occurs when the metabolic need for oxygen is increased.

Because HbF has a lower affinity for 2,3-DPG than HbA, it is able to bind oxygen more tenaciously, and this accounts for the shift of the oxygen disassociation curve to the left in the fetus and neonate.

The postnatal shift of the oxygen disassociation curve to the right is indirectly attributable to the decreasing production of HbF and its gradual replacement by HbA, which lowers the affinity of the haemoglobin for oxygen. This makes it easier for oxygen to dissociate and so enhance oxygen release to the tissues (Marieb 2000).

White blood cells   White blood cells defend the body against undesirable cells, microorganisms and proteins (Ch. 29, p. 387). At birth most neonates show an initial increase in the number of circulating white blood cells, possibly due to their displacement from other sites provoked by the stress of birth. However, gradual reduction in these cells brings about normal cell levels by the 5th day after birth. The two main functions of white blood cells are **phagocytosis** by neutrophils and monocytes and the **competent immune response** attributed to lymphocytes and plasma cells.

Differential white cell counts in the newborn infant indicate that neutrophils account for approximately 50% and lymphocytes for about 30% of the total white blood cells. The proportion of lymphocytes then increases rapidly within the first few months to an average of 60%, a value which persists for the first 2 years of life. Monocytes are the most abundant cells in the first few weeks of extrauterine life but gradually decline to the much lower adult value.

There are numerous theories concerning neonatal susceptibility to topical and systemic infections. There may be biochemical, structural and functional differences or abnormalities in the neutrophils (Christensen & Schibler 1996). Also, there may be developmental defects in signal transduction, cell surface receptor mobility or intracellular factors such as rigidity of the cytoskeleton and microfilament contraction. Each of these factors could affect neutrophil function, undermining their responsiveness to undesirable cells or pathogens or their capacity to migrate from capillaries into the surrounding tissue.

Haemostasis   Haemostasis (Ch. 16, p. 212) depends on the interaction of blood vessel walls, **platelets** and a group of **clot-promoting factors** which make up the **coagulation system**. The neonate is considered to be at risk of spontaneous bleeding between the 3rd and 6th days of life due to a lack of **vitamin K** (Box 48.1), which contributes to the synthesis of the necessary clotting factors. However, as he begins to be milkfed, the bacteria necessary for the synthesis of vitamin K become established in the gut and this provides a natural environment for the ongoing production of vitamin K (Sweet 1997).

Platelets (Ch. 16, p. 211) are released into the circulation, as required, to support normal coagulation processes. The cell surface properties and their internal constituents play a crucial role in haemostasis. Platelet counts in adults range between 150 and $400 \times 10^9/L$ and, although term infants have similar platelet values, premature babies frequently have slightly lower values (Andrew & Massicotte 1996). This may reduce their ability to form indissolvable clots. Platelet release of substances enhancing the clotting cascade may also be reduced. For instance, reduction in **prothrombin** values occurs because of the lack of vitamin K. Similarly, clotting factors such as **factors VII, IX and X**, which are also vitamin-K dependent, are also significantly reduced. Neonatal fibrinogen levels are similar to those of an adult.

The cardiovascular system

The fetal circulation

At birth the **fetal circulation** (Fig. 48.3) changes to the configuration of the adult circulation system (Fig. 48.4). The immediate changes take place within the first 60 s but the full transformation may take up to a few weeks (Coad & Dunstall 2001). At the same time blood oxygenation changes from a placental to pulmonary source which requires the neonate to inspire sufficient oxgygenated air. The fetal circulation differs from that of the adult by several modifications, including the flow of blood bypassing the lungs and being redirected to and from the placenta for exchange of respiratory gases, nutrients and waste products via the maternal circulation. There are four temporary fetal blood vessels.

- Two sets of blood vessels transport blood between the fetus and placenta:
  1. the **ductus venosus**;
  2. two **hypogastric arteries**.
- Two right-to-left shunts allow blood flow to bypass the lungs:
  3. the **ductus arteriosus**, between the pulmonary artery and aorta;
  4. the **foramen ovale**, between right and left atria.

The ductus venosus connects the umbilical vein to the inferior vena. The hypogastric arteries branch off from the internal iliac arteries and, as they enter the umbilical cord, become the umbilical arteries. The ductus arteriosus leads from the bifurcation of the pulmonary arteries to the aortic arch, entering it just after the exit of the subclavian and carotid arteries. The foramen ovale is a temporary opening between the right and left atrium, and its role is to divert blood away from the lungs during the intrauterine life (Coad & Dunstall 2001).

The path taken by the fetal blood flow, referred to as the fetal circulation, begins at the placenta. This is best understood by reading the text and looking at the diagram:

- Oxygenated blood returns from the placenta via the umbilical vein.

- About half of this blood passes through the liver to join the inferior vena cava via the hepatic veins. The rest transfers via the ductus venosus directly to the inferior vena cava where the blood returning from the placenta mixes with the small amount of deoxygenated blood returning from the lower limbs, which reduces its oxygen content.

Box 48.1 Vitamin K and haemorrhagic disease of the newborn

The reduction of vitamin K and clotting factors results from poor placental transfer of vitamin K to the fetus and the lack of intestinal flora in the fetus. There is a further decline in these factors over the first few days following birth, particularly in breastfed babies, as breast milk contains very low levels of vitamins, including vitamin K. However, vitamin K is especially concentrated in colostrum and hind-milk (Enkin et al 2000). The content of vitamin K in cow's milk and formula milk is greater than in breast milk (Enkin et al 2000). Breastfed babies may eventually develop prolonged prothrombin deficiency. Haemorrhagic disease of the newborn occurs in 0.4–1.7% of all babies in the 1st week of life (Merenstein et al 1993). However, many early studies were carried out when breastfeeding practices were restrictive. Neonates did not receive as much colostrum and hind milk and supplementary milk feeds were frequently given.

The awareness of some of the benefits of vitamin K has resulted in its prophylactic administration (since the 1950s) to neonates at risk of spontaneous haemorrhage, in particular within the gastrointestinal tract, resulting in **haematemesis** and the passage of **melaena stools** and the umbilical cord. There is also a serious risk of **intracranial haemorrhage** in susceptible babies such as premature babies and those who experienced birth injuries.

The British Paediatric Association recommended that oral vitamin K of 0.5 mg was given with a repeat dose at 8 days. However, by 1993 there was evidence that late **haemorrhagic disease** was occurring in neonates who had been given oral vitamin K. Giving premature babies and others at risk of haemorrhage, intramuscular or intravenous vitamin K 0.5–1 mg was considered and those with haemorrhagic disease could be given Konakion (vitamin K_1 or phytomenadione) 1 mg intravenously. Most paediatricians recommended giving 0.5–1 mg vitamin K to all babies at birth, as it is difficult to predict which are likely to be at risk of haemorrhage. Enkin et al (2000) recommend giving vitamin K to all babies that are breastfed until further research is carried out. If bleeding is severe, a blood transfusion may be necessary, but normal coagulation must be re-established to limit the severity of bleeding and other undesirable pathophysiological events.

Golding et al (1990, 1992) suggested a link between the intramuscular administration of vitamin K and childhood cancer although this was not substantiated by Hull (1992) nor did the American Academy of Pediatrics find a correlation between the administration of prophylactic vitamin K and any increase in the incidence of childhood leukaemia (Merenstein et al 1993, Ekelund et al 1993, von Kries et al 1996).

Administration of vitamin K to mothers

Nishiguchi et al (1996) examined three strategies for prevention of vitamin K deficiency in neonates:

1. routine oral prophylaxis at birth;
2. additional vitamin K for breastfeeding mothers as well as routine oral prophylaxis;
3. screening and treatment of babies at greatest risk.

They found that giving babies two doses of oral vitamin K did not totally abolish the risk of haemorrhagic disease. In the group where the mothers took a 15 mg capsule of vitamin K daily for 2 weeks starting 2 weeks following delivery, no babies were found to be vitamin K deficient. However, Crowther & Henderson-Smart (2000) reviewed five trials and found no evidence that vitamin K administered to women prior to preterm birth prevented neonatal periventricular haemorrhage. Because there was no link found between vitamin K and childhood leukaemia and the inadequacy of oral administration, Puckett & Offringa (2000) recommend the use of intramuscular vitamin K.

Arguments against the policy

The need for this treatment of all neonates has been questioned. Some studies suggested that the neonate is not vitamin K deficient and that concentrations of vitamin K-dependent factors do not always increase after the administration of vitamin K. In particular, the route of administration has come under scrutiny. To assess the status of neonates against an adult norm may be inappropriate. In evolutionary terms to suggest that an entire group of a given population is disadvantaged could be misleading and yet this is what the prophylactic use of vitamin K does. Clearly, there is a need for a long-term clinical trial and review of the empirical evidence this may yield regarding the prophylactic administration of vitamin K to all neonates.

- As the inferior vena cava enters the heart, its position is aligned with the foramen ovale. The free edge of the atrial septum (the crista dividens) separates the blood flow into two streams. Most of this blood passes from the right atrium through the foramen ovale to the left atrium, creating a right-to-left shunt. From here the blood flows to the left ventricle and then to the aorta to supply oxygenated blood to the head, trunk and limbs.

- A small quantity of right atrial blood passes through the tricuspid valve into the right ventricle. About 10% of this is directed via the pulmonary artery to the lungs for

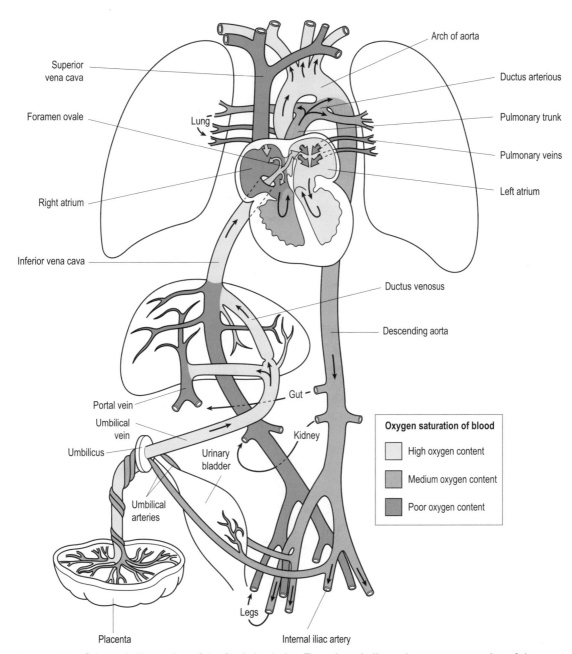

Figure 48.3   Schematic illustration of the fetal circulation. The colours indicate the oxygen saturation of the blood and the arrows show the course of the blood from the placenta to the heart. The organs are not drawn to scale. Observe that three shunts permit most of the blood to bypass the liver and lungs: (1) ductus venosus, (2) foramen ovale, and (3) ductus arteriosus. The poorly oxygenated blood returns to the placenta for oxygen and nutrients through the umbilical arteries. (Reproduced with permission from Moore 1989.)

oxygenation of the lung tissue. The remaining 90% is directed into the aorta via the second right-to-left shunt, the ductus arteriosus between the pulmonary artery and aorta. This blood mixes with the blood from the ductus venosus and is referred to as the mixed oxygenated blood.

- Deoxygenated blood from the head and neck returns to the right atrium via the superior vena cava. Here this stream of blood crosses the stream of blood coming from the inferior vena cava en route to the right ventricle, thus

reducing the oxygen content of that blood even further. The two streams in the right atrium remain separate due to the atrial shape although there is some mixing of about 25% of the blood to allow oxygen and nutrients to be taken to the lungs.

- By the time the circulating blood enters the internal iliac arteries its oxygen content is significantly reduced and so it returns to the placenta via the two umbilical arteries for reoxygenation.

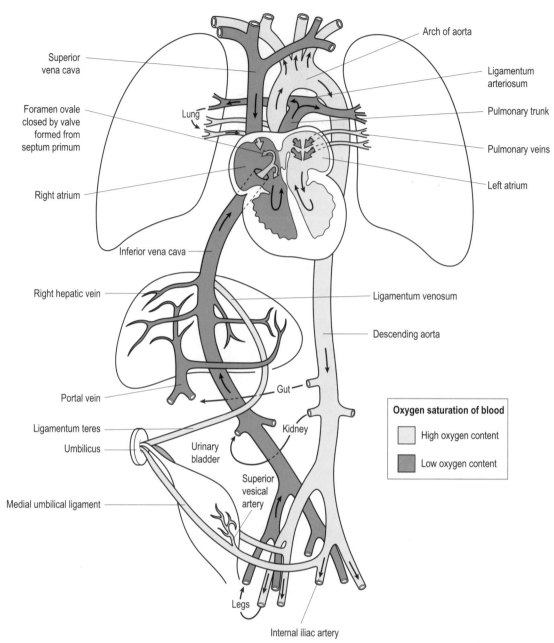

Figure 48.4   Schematic illustration of the neonatal circulation. The adult derivatives of the fetal vessels and structures that become nonfunctional at birth are also shown. The arrows indicate the course of the blood in the infant. The organs are not drawn to scale. After birth, the three shunts that short-circuited the blood during fetal life cease to function and the pulmonary and systemic circulations become separated. (Reproduced with permission from Moore 1989.)

- A small amount of blood descends to supply oxygen and nutrients to the lower limbs via the external iliac arteries and then returns to the heart via the inferior vena cava.

- The metabolic waste products of the fetus such as urea and uric acid are also transported in this manner and removed via the placental circulation for elimination by the mother.

Changes at birth

Some of the unique features of the fetal circulation must change at birth if the fetus is to survive as an independent being. The adaptation to extrauterine life is dependent to a large extent on the interplay between the cardiovascular and the respiratory systems:

- The separation of the neonate from the placental circulation results in the collapse of the umbilical vein and arteries, the ductus venosus and the hypogastric arteries. These vessels eventually fibrose and give rise to supporting ligaments.

- This results in a reduction in flow to the right atrium, causing a fall in the right atrial pressure. As blood flow through the hypogastric arteries ceases, the volume of blood is now contained in a smaller systemic compartment and this results in an increase in systemic vascular resistance (SVR), which soon increases the return of blood volume to the lungs. Larger quantities of blood are now returned from the lungs via the pulmonary veins to the left atrium, causing an increase in left atrial pressure.

- The initial equalising of pressures in the two atria closes the flap of the foramen ovale and the right-to-left intra-atrial shunt of blood ceases, although this shunt may remain patent for a few days, particularly in circumstances where the left atrial pressure falls.

- As the baby takes his first breath, the lungs expand and oxygenated air is inspired. This displaces the pulmonary fluid further and triggers the mechanisms essential to effective respiration and pulmonary gas exchange. Oxygen content of the blood increases, which brings about vasodilation of the pulmonary vascular bed. Pulmonary vascular resistance (PVR) falls by 80%, which dramatically increases pulmonary blood flow.

- At the same time the amount of blood being shunted via the ductus arteriosus is decreased. As oxygen tension in the blood rises, the oxygen-sensitive fibromuscular tissue of the ductus arteriosus constricts and eventually contributes to the successful closure of the ductus arteriosus, although it may remain patent for a few days in normal infants. In premature infants and those born with cardiovascular and respiratory anomalies, the ductus arteriosus may persist and spontaneous closure may not occur for some weeks or months.

Obsolete fetal structures remain as ligaments:

- the umbilical vein becomes the ligamentum teres;
- the ductus venosus becomes the ligamentum venosum;
- the ductus arteriosus becomes the ligamentum arteriosum;
- the foramen ovale becomes the fossa ovalis;
- the hypogastric arteries are known as the obliterated hypogastric arteries.

Persistent fetal circulation may occur in infants with respiratory or cardiac disorders (Box 48.2).

The respiratory system

At term, the acinar portion of the fetal lung is well developed and more than 25% of **true alveoli** are present (Fig. 48.5). However, as the pulmonary blood vessels are quite narrow, only a small amount of blood perfuses the lungs, although this is adequate for meeting the nutritional needs of the pulmonary tissue. As the fetus obtains oxygen and excretes carbon dioxide via the placenta and maternal circulation, its lungs are not necessary for gas exchange. At term, the lungs hold about 25 ml/kg of **pulmonary fluid**, which is partially expelled when the chest is compressed during vaginal delivery. The remaining fluid is absorbed by the lymphatic and pulmonary vascular systems. The fetus exercises its

---

Box 48.2 Persistent fetal circulation

When the neonate presents with respiratory or cardiac disorders frequently accompanied by hypoxia and acidosis, a modified form of fetal circulation may persist. The ductus arteriosus remains patent, and in some circumstances the neonate may experience a reversal of the earlier cardiovascular and pulmonary changes (Sweet 1997). This exacerbates the problem of hypoxia as deoxygenated blood from the right side of the heart is able to mix with the oxygenated blood returning from the lungs to the left side of the heart. The resulting reduction in oxygen tension relaxes the fibromuscular tissue of the ductus arteriosus and interferes with its normal closure.

Throughout fetal life the patency of the ductus arteriosus is maintained by high circulating levels of prostaglandin PGE_2 and local release of prostacyclin PGI_2. Therefore when the closure of the ductus arteriosus is compromised, prostaglandin synthetase inhibitors such as indometacin may be used to facilate its closure pharmacologically. Indometacin may reduce urinary output and it may be necessary to administer furosemide (frusemide) to ensure renal tissue perfusion and urine formation (Kelnar et al 1995). If the pharmacological method fails, mechanical or surgical intervention may eventually be necessary.

---

muscles of respiration, particularly the diaphragm, by making irregular fetal breathing movements.

Surfactant

From about 32 weeks gestation increasing amounts of **surfactant** is produced by the alveolar type II pneumocytes. Surfactant is composed of a number of **phospholipids** and specialised **protein molecules** (Fig. 48.6) which jointly reduce the **surface tension** of the alveolar fluid. The lining of the alveoli becomes thinner, increasing the surface area for eventual gas exchange. **Platelet-activating factor** (PAF) is thought to stimulate the production of the phospholipids by triggering enzymes within the endoplasmic reticulum of the **type II pneumocytes** involved in their synthesis. At term, surfactant forms a monolayer lining within the alveoli which acts as an air–liquid interface, reducing the surface tension within the terminal sacs – imagine blowing a soap bubble. This prevents the alveoli from collapsing with each expiration once respiration is established.

Onset of respirations

Most infants gasp within seconds of birth and establish regular respiration within minutes (Coad & Dunstall 2001). Respiration meets the cellular need for oxygen and removes carbon dioxide, the waste product of cellular metabolism,

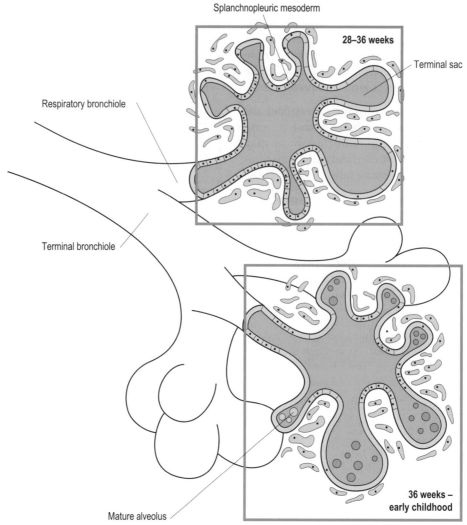

Figure 48.5 Maturation of the lung tissue. Terminal sacs (primitive alveoli) begin to form between weeks 28 and 36 and begin to mature between 36 weeks and birth. Only 5–20% of all terminal sacs produced by the age of 8, however, are formed prior to birth. (Reproduced with permission from Larsen 1993.)

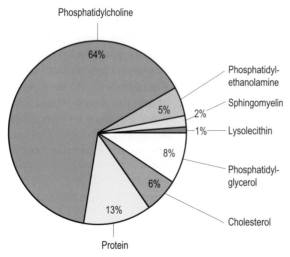

Figure 48.6 Composition of pulmonary surfactant. (Reproduced with permission from Blackburn & Loper 1992.)

so it is important that successful respiration is established without delay. The **respiratory centre** in the medulla oblongata of the brain matches respiratory effort to cellular metabolic needs. In this role the medulla is influenced by **chemoreceptors** and **stretch reflexes**; however, the neonate's response to chemoreceptor stimulus is generally weak.

During its descent through the birth canal the fetus experiences a reduction in oxygen, a period of **physiological hypoxia** and an accumulation of carbon dioxide. These biochemical changes become more profound with the cessation of the placental circulation. This hypoxia and concomitant **hypercarbia** is crucial to the establishment of a new respiratory drive within the medulla oblongata and thus contributes to more successful pulmonary ventilation.

The emptying of the pulmonary fluid from the lung combined with the expansion of the pulmonary vascular bed and pulmonary tissue creates a negative pressure of up to 9.8 kPa, which assists the first breath (Michie 1999). The elastic recoil of the rib cage at delivery increases this capacity and the infant is stimulated to inspire. At the first inspiration the diaphragm contracts strongly and the flexible ribs and sternum are pulled concave. Subsequent breaths require much less mechanical work (Coad & Dunstall 2001). The factors initiating the first breath and lung expansion are:

- compression of the chest wall during delivery and the recoil of the chest wall immediately after birth;
- chemoreceptor stimulation by the reduction in oxygen and increase in carbon dioxide in the blood;
- sensory stimuli on the skin, such as touch, pressure and cold;
- stimulation of the senses by light and noise.

Initially, the neonatal respiratory rate averages 50 breaths per minute, eventually reducing to a more acceptable parameter of 40 breaths per minute. This initially high respiratory response may result from an increase in excitatory respiratory neural synapses which increase respiratory motor activity (Avery et al 1999). Respiration is characteristically **irregular** with short periods of **apnoea** and involves the abdominal muscles but once established, the control of respiratory effort is thought to be similar to that in older children and adults.

Inflation of a normal lung in a neonate is completed within the first few breaths and most alveoli are expanded within the first few hours, establishing a fairly constant lung volume of approximately 25 ml/kg body weight. The inflation of the lungs encourages the **intra-alveolar fluid** to move into the surrounding interstitium, particularly the peribronchial and perivascular spaces. Its absorption into the vasculature and lymphatic drainage extends over a few days. Delay in the removal of this alveolar fluid will interfere with the efficiency of respiratory gas transfer and may cause cardiorespiratory distress.

The renal system

The neonatal kidney differs from that of the older child and adult in both **glomerular** and **tubular function**. Its lobular appearance too is different to the shape of a more mature kidney. By 35 weeks gestation the fetal kidney is believed to have a full complement of **nephrons**, although these may be shorter and not as functionally mature. The **cortex** is more mature than the **medulla** by the end of the 36th week of gestation and at this time **nephrogenesis** is believed to cease, with each kidney having a complement of between 850 000 and 1 000 000 nephrons (Sweet 1997). In premature babies nephrogenesis appears to continue for a variable period of time.

Postnatal development of the kidneys

At birth the kidneys must respond rapidly to functional requirements as well as to endogenous and exogeneous stresses. The kidneys must take over the control of fluid and electrolyte balance and the excretion of metabolic wastes. The clamping of the umbilical cord is the signal for a striking increase in renal function. From a value of 10 ml/min/m^2 in term neonates, **glomerular filtration rate** doubles during the first 2 weeks of life. Glomerular filtration rate is lower in very premature babies but this is gradually corrected as the glomeruli mature at a comparable rate.

Clamping the umbilical cord is a signal for the striking increase in renal function but the most likely factors which contribute to this rapid maturation in renal function are of a haemodynamic and morphological nature (Guignard 1982). Thus, a decrease in **renal vascular resistance** and the increase in **systemic blood pressure** at birth contribute to a more effective filtration pressure and an increase in glomerular permeability and filtration area. **Vasoactive substances** such as prostaglandins may also, in part, mediate the haemodynamic changes.

Renal growth in early infancy depends on hypertrophy of existing units, and kidney size correlates well with age and parameters of somatic growth. The functional maturity of neonatal kidneys has been assessed by histological appearance of the glomeruli and by the size and disposition of the different types of nephrons. The rate of glomerular growth varies and immature glomeruli may be present for many months after birth. Superimposed diseases such as inflammatory changes and urinary tract obstructions may contribute to persistence of the immature form of glomeruli.

The anatomical development of the kidneys proceeds from the corticomedullary junction out towards the periphery in a **centrifugal pattern** (Brenner & Rector 1991). This contributes to a process of budding from the ends of the collecting ducts, a mechanism that ensures that new nephrons are added to the outermost part of the kidney and allows recently formed nephrons to be fitted into the developing **cortical matrix**.

Neonatal renal physiology

In a full-term neonate tubular functions are either effective at birth or mature rapidly thereafter. They are able to lower urinary osmolality to acceptable values and contribute to the regulation of acid–base balance. Mechanisms involved in blood pressure control such as the **renin–angiotensin system** are more active at birth, possibly due to their stimulation by the excess **catecholamines** produced by the fetus in response to the stress of labour and birth. These phenomena contribute to an adequate distribution of blood to vital organs, including the kidneys.

The glomeruli In normal circumstances the relatively rapid renal growth ensures that a functional relationship is achieved between the glomeruli and the nephrons. In due course the average glomerular size of 100 μm at birth increases to 300 μm but this can be retarded or accelerated by certain pathological changes. For instance, cyanotic congenital heart disease is associated with striking glomerular enlargements.

The tubules Postnatally, tubular length increases and enhances the processing of the glomerular filtrate. The growth of the tubules appears to be relatively greater than the growth of the glomeruli, which may contribute to the ongoing maintenance of glomerulotubular balance as glomerular filtrate increases after birth. Finally, tubular growth is important in enhancing tubular capacity for transport of solutes and water during selective reabsorption, secretion and excretion.

The tubules are sensitive to **antidiuretic hormone**. The lower corticomedullary gradient may be associated with a limited rate of urea excretion and deficient transport of sodium chloride in the **loop of Henle**. Despite this, sodium balance is well maintained in neonates whose sodium fraction excretion has stabilized to 1% or less by the 3rd day of life. However, the response to sodium loading is blunted, possibly due to the high concentration of circulating aldosterone, which falls only gradually, in conjunction with similar decreases in renin and angiotensin, throughout the 1st week of life.

The bladder

The neonatal bladder is **fusiform** (cigar shaped) rather than pyramidal as in adults. It is situated almost entirely in the abdominal cavity until the pelvic cavity begins to increase as the child grows. The bladder then descends into the pelvis and the ureters lengthen. It is worth noting that distension of the bladder will increase the intra-abdominal pressure and this may exacerbate respiratory difficulties.

Renal function

The kidneys have a high rate of oxygen consumption, accounting for approximately 7% of the total oxygen used by the body. This linear relationship can be demonstrated in changes in oxygen consumption and fluctuations in sodium levels. Active transport of sodium appears to reflect the most significant energy expenditure of the kidney other than that required for basic metabolic needs.

Renal blood flow is reduced for the first few days of extrauterine life compared with that of an older baby. Glomerular filtration rate (GFR) is also lower. However, these two parameters rapidly increase after birth and double by the end of the 2nd week. This may be associated with the cessation of the placental circulation, which initiates an increase in systemic circulatory pressure, thus improving renal blood flow.

The tubular thresholds for reabsorption of solutes are lower in the neonate and they are more likely to lose sodium, glucose and other solutes in their urine. Both full-term and premature babies can excrete normal excesses of acid via the kidneys but have little reserve to cope with increased levels. The mechanism of water regulation is similar to that of the adult but ability to dilute or concentrate urine is limited because of a lower corticomedullary gradient and immature loops of Henle. This phenomenon may impact on the neonate's ability to excrete drugs efficiently.

Urine output During pregnancy the placenta acts as a **haemodialyser**, adapting to the metabolic needs of the fetus. About 25% of neonates pass urine at or shortly after delivery when the event may pass unobserved or unrecorded. Some delays can occur in those who experienced perinatal asphyxia or severe stress which may have contributed to temporary renal insufficiency. The neonate's state of hydration, cardiac output and renal perfusion must therefore always be considered in evaluating urinary output.

Urine output varies, depending on fluid and solute intake and events that occurred at the time of birth. Term neonates normally excrete between 15 and 60 ml/kg of urine daily, increasing this volume four-fold by the end of the 1st week as fluid intake increases. Dilute, straw-coloured and odourless urine is passed by reflex emptying of the bladder. It is important to observe the force and direction of the stream of urine and in boys and whether the stream leaves the tip of the penis. The use of magnesium sulphate to control eclampsia or lidocaine (lignocaine) used in epidural analgesia may delay the neonate's ability to void.

Body composition

For clinical convenience, **total body water** is divided into discrete compartments. This approach provides a basis for interpreting changes occurring in body fluids and electrolytes. **Intracellular fluid** is separated by cell walls or plasma membranes from **extracellular fluid**, which is divided into **intravascular** and **extravascular** components. Transcellular fluids formed by secretory activities within the biliary systems and the choroid plexus are referred to as **specialised fluids**.

Neonates are vulnerable to water loss because their large body surface area contributes to greater water loss by **evaporation**. There is a physiological inability of the renal tubules to concentrate urine. Neonatal high metabolic rate may also contribute to significant water loss. Water distribution between the compartments differs between infants and adults, and midwives must remember this when caring for neonates, pregnant mothers or mothers in the postdelivery stage. A healthy neonate usually exchanges approximately 50% of the total extracellular fluid over 24 h whereas an adult exchanges only 14–15% (Logan 1992).

Maintenance of normal body water content depends on the equilibrium between fluid intake and output. However, during the first few days of extrauterine life there is a significant transfer of water from the intracellular fluid compartment to the extracellular fluid compartment. This mechanism probably protects the neonate against dehydration. It also increases the already large extracellular fluid volume and could contribute to tissue oedema.

The proportion of the body consisting of water varies with age, gender and adipose tissue. Babies have the greatest total body water content although its distribution is different to that in older children. Deuterium dilution studies have shown that the total water content of the normal

Table 48.1 Total body water content of infants (3.0 kg in body weight; body surface area 0.2 m²)

Body fluid compartment	Total body water content		
	Percent of body weight	Litres	Litres/m²
Intracellular	38	1.14	5.70
Extracellular:			
● Interstitial	33	0.99	4.95
● Plasma	5	0.15	0.75
Total	76.00	2.28	11.40

Table 48.2 Total body water contents of adults (70.0 kg in body weight; body surface area 1.85 m²)

Body fluid compartment	Total body water content		
	Percent of body weight	Litres	Litres/m²
Intracellular	40	28.0	15.2
Extracellular:			
● Interstitial	16	11.2	6.0
● Plasma	4	2.8	1.5
Total	60.00	42.00	22.70

neonate averages 77%, falling to approximately 65% in babies aged 6 months (Logan 1992). A comparison of the proportions in body fluid distributions between infants (Table 48.1) and adults (Table 48.2) (Logan 1992) can be a helpful tool in the assessment and care of these two groups of patients.

In comparison to adults, neonates have considerably more interstitial fluid. The gradual translocation of intracellular fluid into the extracellular fluid compartment after birth may be attributed to withdrawal of maternal hormones or other unknown variables. They may become slightly oedematous but, as the extracellular fluid peaks at about 3 days, a **diuresis** adjusts the values of the fluid compartments. This may be partly due to a decrease in **atrial natriuretic peptide** (ANP), important in the regulation of sodium, which occurs at the same time. In neonates a loss of 5–10% of body weight in the 1st week after birth is attributed to this diuresis. The role of the cardiovascular, respiratory and renal systems as well as the fluid compartments in this physiological adaptation should not be underestimated. Fluid therapy must take into account these physiological differences to avoid fluid overload with the risk of congestive heart failure, necrotising enterocolitis and symptomatic patent ductus arteriosus.

MAIN POINTS

● A fetus is dependent on his mother for survival, using the placenta as a life-supporting unit. At birth he must adapt to an independent life. Each body system contributes towards establishing and maintaining new homeostatic values. Immediately important are adaptations that ensures oxygen uptake from the surrounding air and elimination of metabolic waste products.

● The term neonate has a rounded abdomen and varying amounts of fine silky scalp hair. Lanugo is sometimes found over the shoulders and vernix caseosa in the groins and axillae. The ear cartilage is well formed and the palm and sole creases are well defined. Both boys and girls have a small nodule of breast tissue. In boys the testes are descended into the scrotum and the foreskin still adheres to the glans penis. In girls the labia majora cover the labia minora.

● Neonatal circulating blood volume varies from 75 to 125 ml/kg depending on the direction and amount of blood flow between fetus and placenta at birth and the gestation of the infant and the time of clamping of the umbilical cord. Erythrocyte count at birth averages about 5 million/ml. The average haemoglobin is 16.5–17.5 g/dl.

● The neonate is at risk of spontaneous bleeding between the 3rd and 6th days of life due to a lack of vitamin K.

Breastfed babies may develop prolonged prothrombin deficiency. Prophylactic administration of vitamin K to prevent the risk of spontaneous haemorrhage is common. Concerns about a link between the intramuscular administration of vitamin K and childhood cancer appear to be unsubstantiated.

● The fetal circulation differs from that of the adult. Cardiovascular modifications bypass the lungs and transfer blood to and from the placenta for exchange of respiratory gases oxygenation. The changes at birth culminating in the establishment of the neonatal circulation involve the cardiovascular and respiratory systems.

● Respiratory or cardiac disorders with hypoxia and acidosis may lead to persistent fetal circulation with patent ductus arteriosus. Attempts may be made to close the ductus arteriosus using indometacin, a prostaglandin synthetase inhibitor. If this fails, methods may be used to ligate this vessel and obliterate the persistent blood flow.

● By 38–40 weeks gestation, surfactant forms a monolayer lining for the alveoli, creating an air–liquid interface and reducing surface tension in the terminal sacs. This prevents the alveoli from collapsing at the end of expiration. The respiratory centre in the medulla oblongata matches respiratory effort to the infant's metabolic needs.

- Nephrogenesis is complete by 35 weeks of gestation but in premature babies continues for a variable period of time. Renal growth depends on hypertrophy of existing units. Superimposed renal disease may contribute to persistence of immature glomeruli or cause permanent damage to the renal parenchyma.

- Clamping the umbilical cord may increase renal function but the most likely contributing factors are of a haemodynamic and morphological nature. The haemodynamic changes may be mediated by vasoactive substances such as prostaglandins.

- Neonates have larger total body water content with greater proportions in extracellular fluid. They become slightly oedematous because of a shift of intracellular fluid into the extracellular fluid compartment after birth.

- The subsequent diuresis results in a loss of 5–10% of body weight in the 1st week. Renal perfusion, glomerular filtration rate and tubular filtration adjust to neonatal metabolic demands by the end of the 2nd week.

- Tubular thresholds for solute reabsorption are lower in neonates, resulting in lose of sodium, glucose and other solutes in the urine. Infants are able to excrete normal quantities of acid via the kidneys but have little reserve to cope with increased levels that may occur in cardiorespiratory disturbances.

- The neonate's ability to dilute or concentrate urine is also limited. Most babies pass urine within 12 h of birth. It is important to observe the force and direction of the stream of urine and, in boys, whether the stream leaves the tip of the penis.

References

Andrew M, Massicotte M 1996 Haemostasis. In Gluckman P, Heyman M (eds) Paediatrics and Perinatology: The Scientific Basis. Arnold, London.

Avery G, Fletcher M, MacDonald M 1999 Neonatology – Pathophysiology and Management of the Newborn. Lippincott Williams and Wilkinson, Philadelphia.

Brenner B, Rector F 1991 The Kidney, Vol. 1. W B Saunders, Philadelphia.

Christensen R, Schibler K 1996 Haematopoiesis and the lymphoid system. In Gluckman P, Heyman M (eds) Paediatrics and Perinatology: The Scientific Basis. Arnold, London.

Coad J, Dunstall M 2001 Anatomy and Physiology for Midwives. Mosby, St Louis.

Crowther C A, Henderson-Smart D J 2000 Vitamin K prior to preterm birth for preventing neonatal periventricular haemorrhage. Cochrane Review: In The Cochrane Library, Issue 2. Update Software 2003, Oxford.

Ekelund H, Finnstrom O, Gunnarskog I, Kallen B, Larsson Y 1993 Administration of vitamin K to newborn infants and childhood cancer. British Medical Journal 301:89–91.

Enkin M, Keirse M J N C, Renfrew M et al 2000 A Guide to Effective Care in Pregnancy and Childbirth, 2nd edn. Oxford University Press, Oxford.

Golding J, Paterson M, Kinlen L J 1990 Factors associated with childhood cancer in national cohort study. British Journal of Cancer 62:304–308.

Golding J, Greenwood R, Birmingham K, Mott M 1992 Childhood cancer, intramuscular vitamin K, and pethidine given in labour. British Medical Journal 305:341–346.

Guignard J 1982 Renal function in the newborn infant. In Fine R (ed.) Paediatric Nephrology. W B Saunders, Philadelphia.

Guyton A, Hall J 2000 Textbook of Medical Physiology. W B Saunders, Philadelphia.

Hull D 1992 Vitamin K and childhood cancer: the risk of haemorrhagic disease is certain; that of cancer is not. British Medical Journal 305:326–327.

Kelnar C J H, Harvey D, Simpson C 1995 The Sick Newborn Baby, 3rd edn. Baillière Tindall, London.

Logan R 1992 Fluid electrolytes and acid–base balance. In Campbell A, McIntosh N (eds) Textbook of Paediatrics. Churchill Livingstone, Edinburgh.

Marieb E N 2000 Human Anatomy and Physiology, 5th edn. Benjamin/Cummings, New York.

Merenstein K, Hathaway W E, Miller et al 1993 Controversies concerning vitamin K and the newborn. Pediatrics 91:1001–1002.

Michie M M 1999 The baby at birth. In Bennett V R, Brown L K (eds) Myles Textbook for Midwives. Churchill Livingstone, Edinburgh.

Moore K L, Persaud T V N 1998 Before We are Born, 5th edn. W B Saunders, Philadelphia.

Morgan E 1994 The Descent of the Child. Souvenir Press, London.

Nishiguchi T, Saga K, Sumimito K et al 1996 Vitamin K prophylaxis to prevent neonatal vitamin K deficient intracranial haemorrhage in Shizuoka prefecture. British Journal of Obstetrics and Gynaecology 8(11):1078–1084.

Puckett R M, Offringa M 2000 Prophylactic vitamin K for vitamin K deficiency bleeding in neonates. Cochrane Review: In The Cochrane Library, Issue 2. Update Software 2003, Oxford.

Rudolph A, Hoffman J, Rudolph C et al 2002 Rudolph's Paediatrics. Prentice-Hall, New Jersey.

Sweet B R 1997 Physiology and care of the newborn. In Sweet B R with Tiran D (eds) Mayes Midwifery, 12th edn. Baillière Tindall, London.

Von Kries R, Gobel U, Hachmeister A et al 1996 Vitamin K and childhood cancer: a population based case-control study in Lower Saxony, Germany. British Medical Journal 313(7051):199–203.

Wardrop C, Holland B, Jones J 1996 Red cell physiology. In Gluckman P, Heyman M (eds) Paediatrics and Perinatology: The Scientific Basis. Arnold, London.

Yao A C, Lind J 1969 Distribution of blood between the infant and placenta at birth. Lancet 2:505.

Annotated recommended reading

Boxwell G 2000 Neonatal Intensive Care Nursing. Routledge, London.
This textbook outlines a range of common and challenging neonatal problems and provides helpful and directive suggestions for neonatal intensive care nursing. Critical analysis and reflection on the identified neonatal nursing concepts would reinforce best practice.

Ekelund H, Finnstrom O, Gunnarskog I, Kallen B, Larsson Y 1993 Administration of vitamin K to newborn infants and childhood cancer. British Medical Journal 301:89–91.
This article offers some empirical evidence and a critical account of some of the advantages and disadvantages of vitamin K administration to neonates

as a prophylactic measure believed to protect some neonates against intracranial bleeding.

Hull D 1992 Vitamin K and childhood cancer: the risk of haemorrhagic disease is certain; that of cancer is not. British Medical Journal 305:326–327.
This article provides a balanced consideration of the benefits of neonatal vitamin K administration, particularly in circumstances where the risk of haemorrhagic disease and intracranial bleeding is considerable.

Larsen W 2002 Human Embryology. Churchill Livingstone, Hong Kong.
This textbook offers a systematic and informative account of the current understanding of human embryology. Each chapter explores the normal developmental processes and then diversifies into the most common genetic and congenital anomalies that may evolve in the embryo or fetus.

Polin R, Fox W 1998 Fetal and Neonatal Physiology, Vols 1 and 2. W B Saunders, Philadelphia.
This textbook offers detailed accounts of important bioscientific concepts in fetal and neonatal care. A résumé of genetics underpins a more detailed exploration of normal embryonic development. The exploration of biochemical, physiological, nutritional and pathophysiological principles contributes to clinical practice and research.

Wong D 1999 Nursing Care of Infants and Children. Mosby, St Louis.
This textbook offers detailed accounts of the biophysical, psychosocial and nursing issues relevant in managing the care of infants and children. It has a range of helpful appendices, including excellent developmental screening tools and biophysical nomograms and parameters invaluable in child care.

Chapter **49**

Adaptation to extrauterine life 2 – nutritional and metabolic adjustments

CHAPTER CONTENTS

INTRODUCTION

The human placenta has evolved into a highly sophisticated interface between the mother and the fetus. It is capable of supporting the nutritional, respiratory, metabolic and excretory needs of the fetus and also offers protection against pathogenic organisms and toxins. After birth, these highly complex physiological processes are supported by the newborn infant's own systems.

THE GASTROINTESTINAL TRACT

Fetal development

The development of the gut is described in Chapter 11 and a synopsis is included here for revision. The **primitive gut** begins to form during the 4th week of pregnancy when the blind-ended **endodermal gut tube** stretches from the **pharyngeal membrane** to the **cloacal membrane**. It consists of three distinctive parts, the **foregut**, **midgut** and **hindgut**, each corresponding to important vascular territories. The neural pathways essential to digestive tract function develop from **neural crest derivatives**. During the 6th week, the endodermal epithelium proliferates until it completely occludes the gut lumen. Over the next 2 weeks **recanalization** re-establishes tubal patency. Stenosis and duplication of segments of the gastrointestinal tract (GI tract) may arise as a result of incomplete recanalization (Larsen 2001). By the 7th week, recanalization may contribute to the gradual rotation of the stomach. This ensures that the greater curvature is directed caudally and to the left, which moves the liver to the right and brings the duodenum and pancreas into contact with the posterior abdominal wall where they are fixed.

The neonate

There are significant anatomical and physiological limitations in the neonatal gastrointestinal tract. According to Polin & Fox (1998) these limitations are partly influenced by the requirement of the fetus to swallow amniotic fluid. The swallowing actions of the small bolus of amniotic fluid may play an important role in the maintenance of patency of the GI tract. There is no evidence to suggest that the gastro-intestinal system in utero serves any nutritional purposes.

The stomach at birth

The stomach has a small capacity, holding only 15–30 ml at birth, but increases rapidly within the first few weeks. Although **gastric emptying time** is both slow and inconsistent, averaging at 2–3 h, this can be influenced by nutrients: e.g. carbohydrates increase emptying time while fats decrease emptying time. The presence of mucus in the stomach during the first 24–48 h can delay gastric emptying, whereas the weakness of the **cardiac sphincter** commonly contributes to regurgitation of milk. Gastric acidity, which at birth is equal to that of an adult, rises gradually as a consequence of the significant fall in hydrochloric acid production by the 10th day, making the baby vulnerable to infection (Michie 1999).

Also, during the first 6 months the intestinal mucosal barrier remains immature so that **antigens** and other **macromolecules** can be transported across the epithelium and into the systemic circulation. However, since maternal **colostrum** is rich in antibodies, easily swallowed and helps the passage of **meconium**, the risk of systemic infection is somewhat reduced. Postnatal maturation of the gut is stimulated by increases in peptide hormones such as **gastrin** and **motilin** (Ch. 21, p. 282), which are secreted following the commencement of enteral feeding.

The neonatal intestine is long with a large surface area for absorption of nutrients and there are large numbers of secretory glands. Enteric intake stimulates the intestinal mucosa cells to divide and mature. Digestive enzymes are synthesised and released as required. However, the relative deficiency of the enzymes **amylase** and **lipase** contributes to difficulties in digesting carbohydrates and fats. The entry of food into the stomach induces a **gastrocolic reflex**, which results in opening of the **ileocaecal valve**. Consequently, as the contents of the ileum enter the colon they appear to stimulate a forceful **peristalsis**, which is in turn accompanied by a reflex emptying of the **rectum** (Michie 1999).

Meconium

Meconium is a material that collects in the intestines of the fetus from the 16th week and forms the first stools of the newborn infant. Its characteristic thick and sticky consistency and greenish-black colour is attributed to the accumulation of secretions from the intestinal glands, bile salts and components of amniotic fluid such as vernix, lanugo, fatty acids, epithelial cells, mucus and blood cells (Blackburn 2003). Initially, meconium is sterile but within 24 h of birth it begins to be colonised with bacteria largely in response to enteral feeding. Most neonates pass meconium within 24 h

of birth and failure to do so could be an early sign of intestinal malfunction, obstruction or imperforate anus.

Milk feeding induces a change in the infant's stools. As digested milk enters the colon, a gradual **transition** in the stool occurs, resulting in a stool of yellow-brownish appearance. Following this, the consistency and frequency of the stools depends on the type of feeding. For instance, breastfed babies pass loose, bright yellow, inoffensive stools on average 6–10 times in 24 h in the earlier days to once a day when feeding is established. By contrast, bottlefed babies pass paler, more formed stools with a recognisable smell and generally less frequently, with a tendency towards constipation.

THE LIVER

Fetal development

The liver is formed along with the gall bladder and their respective ducts about the 22nd day. These grow into the **septum transversum**. Subsequent hepatic growth continues linearly through the remainder of gestation. The left hepatic lobe is approximately 10% larger than the right lobe. This phenomenon is precisely opposite to the postnatal relationship in the hepatic lobes which may indicate an altered blood supply. As with most embryonic tissues, the initial growth is attributed to hepatocellular proliferation (**cell hyperplasia**), which peaks during the second trimester of pregnancy. In the third trimester a decrease in mitosis allows enlargement of individual hepatocytes, which gradually contributes to the eventual size of the whole organ.

The neonate

After birth, ongoing mitosis allows the liver to grow and mature until the end of the second decade of life. Given that the neonatal liver has less than 20% of the **hepatocytes** found in an adult liver, ongoing mitosis is critical to the ultimate construction and physiological scope of the mature organ.

The liver is a major early **haematopoietic organ**, a function later taken over by the bone marrow. At birth the liver is physiologically immature even though it accounts for 5% of the neonate's weight. The mature liver metabolises substances by utilising **oxidative** and **conjugation processes** under enzymatic control. In general, water-soluble by-products are produced. In the neonatal, however, the immature liver produces low quantities of these enzymes such as glucuronyl transferase, which is essential for bilirubin conjugation. This shortfall contributes to a rise in **unconjugated bilirubin** in the plasma, which is exacerbated by the normal higher breakdown of superfluous red cells. The binding of unconjugated bilirubin to fatty tissue contributes to a transient neonatal jaundice on the 3rd–5th days. Feeding stimulates liver function and bacterial colonisation of the gut, which in turn stimulates vitamin K production (Michie 1999).

METABOLISM

Fetal metabolic processes are directed towards **anabolism** and tissue growth. The placenta supports body temperature and functions such as respiration and nutrition. After birth, an adequate supply of essential nutrients coupled with normal enzyme and hormonal controls ensures that most newborn babies establish homeostasis and maintain an anabolic state that supports growth and development. The fetus prepares for the transition to independence by laying down a fuel store of glycogen and lipids during the last few weeks of pregnancy. This ensures that the neonate has reserves of glycogen, fat and other nutrients. Once oxygen requirements are met, the next immediate need for survival is an adequate supply of water. The relative excess of water in neonates confers no protection against dehydration since the daily turnover of water equals 15–20% of total body water.

After birth, body heat production is attributed to **brown adipose tissue** (BAT) and hepatic **tri-iodothyronine** synthesis facilitates the transition from a net anabolic to a **catabolic** state as glycogen and lipid reserves are mobilised to meet the required increase in metabolic rate (Blackburn 2003). The extent of these adaptations is strongly influenced by numerous factors such as maternal nutrition in the late stages of pregnancy and the maturity of the neonate at birth.

Glucose metabolism

Glucose is the major **substrate** for carbohydrate metabolism in newborn babies (Garrow & James 2000). At birth, the baby's plasma glucose concentration depends upon such factors as the timing of the last maternal meal, the duration of labour, the nature of delivery and the type and quantity of intravenous fluid administered to the mother during labour. After birth, as the neonate loses the maternal glucose source, falling **plasma insulin levels** and slow production of insulin prevent glucose being taken up by the cells. This is coupled with an increase in **serum glucagon levels**, which mobilises glucose from the intracellular **glycogen stores**.

Hepatic glycogen stores decrease rapidly as 90% is utilised in the first 24 h after birth. Muscle glycogen is also reduced by 50–80%. After birth, **gluconeogenesis** is regulated by changes in the serum insulin:glucose ratio, catecholamine release, fatty acid oxidation and activation of liver gluconeogenic enzymes. The concentration of these hepatic enzymes continues to increase for the next 14 days and, once milk feeding is established, additional changes in hepatic function occur.

Neonatal blood glucose levels fall to the lowest values between 2 and 6 h after delivery, become stable, then rise and equilibrate at about 3.6 mmol/L as the baby adapts to the extrauterine environment (Dodds 1996). Most paediatricians believe that the lowest safe level for neonatal blood glucose is no less than 2 mmol/L (Koh & Vong 1996). The method of feeding can influence neonatal blood glucose levels. Hawdon et al (1992) found that the average neonatal blood glucose level in 132 breastfed term babies was 3.6 mmol/L with a range of 1.5–5.3 mmol/L. These levels were significantly lower than in bottlefed babies.

Fat metabolism

Lipolysis increases rapidly after birth, reaching a maximum within a few hours. This results in a rise in plasma **free fatty acids**, which reach adult levels by 24 h after birth. During this time about two-thirds of the baby's energy is produced from oxidation of fat, the major form of stored calories in the newborn. Fat is also the preferred energy source for organs such as the heart and the adrenal cortex, which have high energy demands.

The major differences between human milk and formula milk are the absence of **long-chain unsaturated fatty acids** in the formulae compared with high concentrations of long-chain unsaturated fatty acids and cholesterol in mature human milk (see Ch. 56). The fat content in colostrum averages at 2%, but phospholipids and **cholesterol** are found in higher concentrations. Mature human milk has a fat content of 3.5–4.5% contained within membrane-enclosed fat globules, whose core consists of triglycerides, while the membrane is constructed of phospholipids, cholesterol and proteins. This **triglyceride** packaging permits dispersion of the lipids in the aqueous environment of the milk and protects them from hydrolysis by milk lipase.

Alternative fat stores and **ketone body** release are stimulated by catecholamine release commonly associated with the cooling of the body after birth. In this instance, ketone bodies are produced during fatty acid metabolism and these form important metabolites for the infant. Similarly, acetate is metabolised by the mitochondria and this contributes to further energy release. Ketone bodies may be a major energy source for the developing brain and myocardium (Polin & Fox 1998, Rudolph et al 2002).

Protein metabolism

Whereas the basic building blocks are supplied by the placenta directly to the fetus, the neonate has to digest milk proteins into **amino acids** and **oligopeptides**. This process requires **proteolytic enzymes** released into the stomach and the pancreas as well as the intestinal brush border. The relatively high concentration of free amino acids and peptides in human milk probably enhances the release of **gastrin** and **cholecystokinin**, which in turn promotes the release of the proteolytic enzymes. Neonatal ability to synthesise protein is limited, due to relative immaturity of the liver enzyme systems. As a consequence, serum amino acid levels are higher than later values in the first few weeks of life and there is a significant urinary amino acid excretion.

Calcium, phosphorus and magnesium metabolism

On comparison of the neonate's blood values with those of the mother, it becomes apparent that the neonate manifests **hypercalcaemia** and **hyperphosphataemia**.

Calcium

Calcium is the most abundant mineral in the body. Polin & Fox (1998) postulate that at term most newborn babies have accumulated between 20 and 30 g of calcium, 80% of which was accrued in the last trimester of pregnancy. Of this total body pool of calcium, 99% is located in the neonate's developing skeletal frame. Serum calcium exists in three separate fractions, which are present in dynamic equilibrium:

1. protein-bound calcium represents approximately 40% of the total serum concentration, with albumin serving as the primary binding protein;
2. calcium is also found bound to a number of other anions such as citrate, phosphate, bicarbonate and sulphate;
3. free, ionised calcium is, however, the physiologically active form of calcium.

Garrow & James (2000) postulate that the ultimate balance in plasma calcium is at least in part determined by ongoing exchange between the skeletal system, the intestine and the kidney. This significant movement of calcium is controlled by the **calciotrophic enzymes**, **parathyroid hormone**, **1,25-dihydroxycholecalciferol** and **calcitonin**. Calcium metabolism is also influenced by growth hormones, corticosteroids and a variety of locally acting hormones such as the **cytokines**.

The neonate must move from intrauterine dependence on maternal calcium sources to independent metabolism. The normal range for blood calcium in a neonate is 1.8–2.2 mmol/L (Simpson 1997). During the first 2 days of life serum calcium levels fall and there is a physiological hypocalcaemia, increasing back to normal between 5–10 days once intestinal absorption of calcium matures. Renal excretion of calcium is efficient and increases as the days pass (Pitkin 1985).

Aspects of calcium metabolism

- As serum calcium levels decrease, parathyroid hormone (PTH) levels increase. By 3–4 days the parathyroid glands are responding adequately to calcium levels.
- Calcitonin levels are normal at birth but this is followed by a surge in the next 24 h. After 36 h the calcitonin levels fall back to normal. This may act to protect the neonate from the effects of increased PTH and reabsorption of calcium from bone. Neither oral nor intravenous calcium administration seems to affect calcitonin levels.

- Term neonates can metabolise vitamin D in the liver and kidneys although absorption of exogenous vitamin D may be limited due to reduced fat absorption.

Phosphorus

As with calcium, approximately 80% of the phosphorus present in the neonate is accumulated by the fetus in the last trimester of pregnancy. Phosphorus is also divided into three component parts:

1. at least 85% of the infant's total phosphorus is contained in the skeletal system;
2. the phosphorus contained in body fluids is divided between an organic fraction composed of a number of phospholipids and phosphoesters; and
3. inorganic phosphate.

Although phosphorus levels decrease in the first 2 days after birth, they still remain higher than in the adult. Renal excretion of phosphorus is delayed with a decreased glomerular filtration rate and increased tubular reabsorption rate. Furthermore, the increased energy release with conversion of adenosine triphosphate (ATP) to adenosine diphosphate (ADP) leads to increased phosphate release. If feeding is delayed, this catabolic process is increased even further.

Magnesium

Magnesium is the second most common **intracellular cation** in the body. According to Polin & Fox (1998), the newborn term infant contains about 20 mg of magnesium/100 g fat-free weight. The infant's total body magnesium is divided between three compartments:

1. the skeletal system, which contains about 60%;
2. muscle tissue, which holds about 29%;
3. the remainder, which is distributed through soft tissue.

Plasma magnesium Only 1% of the total body magnesium appears to be located in the extracellular space. About 60% of the magnesium present in the plasma exists as **free ion** while 20% is bound to various **anions** such as phosphate and oxalate. The remaining plasma magnesium is bound to serum proteins. This binding capacity maintains magnesium within relatively tight physiological limits, which is thought to be essential in neonates, children and adults. The normal range for plasma magnesium is 0.7–1.0 mmol/L. No particular hormones have been identified as causing this fine-tuning of plasma magnesium; however, the kidneys appear to be the primary organs for regulating serum magnesium.

THE NEONATAL NERVOUS SYSTEM

In a human adult the central nervous system is thought to consist of 100 billion **neurons**. These are intricately connected with one another in a manner that makes possible consciousness, thought, learning, memory, vision and many other properties characteristic of the human nervous system. The achievement of precision of the adult neural pattern is in part dependent on environmental stimulation as children who spend most of their 1st year of life lying in their crib develop abnormally slowly (Shatz 1992).

Nervous system activity increases throughout gestation so that at term the baby is prepared to process incoming information from the environment and produce behaviour appropriate for his physical and physiological status. The transitional functions of the nervous system can be divided into in three parts, the autonomic, sensory and motor state.

Autonomic functions

At birth the newborn infant's nervous system takes over control of functions such as hunger, thirst and satiety, which are carefully balanced by specific hypothalamic centres. The centres are also thought to influence sucking and swallowing. A physiological steady state or homeostasis is achieved by the regulation of respiration, heart beat, body temperature and metabolic activity and is adjusted to ensure the body generates sufficient heat to support important enzyme activity.

Sensory functions

The neonate can detect odour, differentiate between tastes, see and observe preferential stimuli and hear and discriminate sounds, all sensory modalities that are useful in the interaction with his carers (Ch. 57, p. 727).

Motor functions

Movements in neonates, as in adults, may be reflexive or volitional. Volitional movement is under the control of the motor cortex. At first, it may appear that the neonate makes few volitional movements. However, gradual motor control becomes evident as myelination of the major central and peripheral nerve tracts progresses. It is likely that environmental stimulation contributes to the generation of new dendrites (Fig. 49.1) and interneuron connections which may ultimately contribute to the fullness and complexity of the many integrated functions of the central nervous system.

Ongoing neural development

At birth the neonate's nervous system has a considerable complement of neurons but many of these will be lost by **apoptosis** and a new complement of neurons will be generated over the next 2 years (Shaffer 2002). The significant increase in the size of the brain in the 1st year of life is attributed to the development of **neuroglia** and **myelin**. The neuroglia forms the supporting framework and protective structures for the conducting neurons. During infancy the brain and spinal cord are thought to enjoy a degree of **plasticity**, allowing ongoing modifications of the developing nervous system in response to environmental stimuli

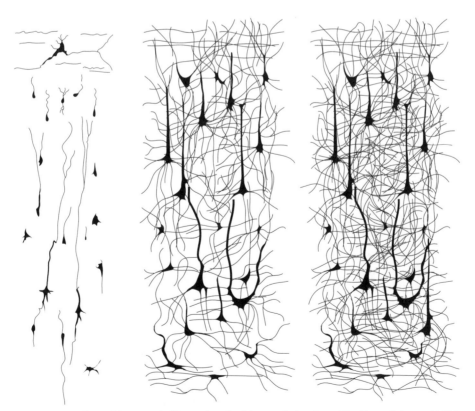

Figure 49.1   Dendritic growth. (Reproduced with permission from Blackburn & Loper 1992.)

and possibly nutrition. The infant learns through observation, auditory stimuli and perception (Greenfield 1997).

The term neonate demonstrates a typical pattern of muscle tone that changes in a predictable way as he develops. At first there is strong but passive **flexion** but as this disappears a more purposeful movement evolves, allowing greater control and accuracy. Muscle control proceeds in a **cephalocaudal** direction and amongst the first to develop are head control, turning over, reaching and grasping.

Reflexes

Reflexes are autonomic, 'built-in' motor behaviours which generally occur in the spinal cord. They are critical to the neonate's safety and survival. To some extent, these reflexes also provide carers with opportunities for assessing the infant's motor capabilities, responsiveness and needs. The absence or exaggerated state or persistence of many of these reflexes may signify brain damage:

- The **Moro (startle) reflex** involves adduction and extension of the arms with the fingers fanned out followed by abduction of the arms with flexed elbows in an '**embrace**' position. The neonate's legs initiate a similar response. This response may be accompanied by crying. Generally, this primitive reflex disappears by the 8th week of life.

- The **palmar grasp reflex** involves a neonate closing his fingers tightly around any object placed in his palm. Trevathan (1987) claims that photographs taken by Eibl-Eibesfeldt (1975) show a preterm baby suspending herself without help from a rope. Trevathan suggests that the Moro, grasp reflex, walking and crawling movements evolved to help the infant readjust to different carrying positions.

- The **tonic neck (fencing) reflex** is apparent when the neonate's head is turned to one side. He will extend the arm and leg on the side of body the head is turned to, and flex the arm and leg on the other side. This is aimed at stabilising the neonate and preventing him from rolling over.

- The **stepping reflex** is seen when the neonate is held upright with his feet touching a solid surface, in response to which alternating stepping movements are made.

- **Rooting reflex** is seen when the side of the mouth or cheek are gently stroked. The neonate will turn his head towards the source of the stimulus and open his mouth ready to suckle.

- **Sucking and swallowing reflexes** are well developed in the term neonate. Sucking and swallowing are coordinated with respiration, including gag, cough and sneeze reflexes.

- **Traction response** is observed when the neonate is held by the wrists and pulled into a sitting position. The head lags at first, then rights itself, deploying neck muscles, before falling forward.

State regulation

An excellent description of **behavioural states** is given by Prechtl & O'Brien in Stratton (1982); this term refers to the recognisable combination of behaviours seen to be repeated by the neonate over time. Such behavioural states have been investigated by observational studies, electroencephalography and polygraphy where various physiological signals such as respiration rate are studied. Prechtl defined five states using the four parameters of eyes open, respiration regular, gross movements and vocalisation. Brazelton (1984) uses similar criteria, as outlined in Michie (1999).

Sleep states

Deep sleep The eyes are closed, respirations are regular, no eye movements are present and response to stimuli is delayed. Jerky movements may be present.

Light sleep Rapid eye movements (REM) occur, respiration is irregular, sucking movements may occur, response to stimuli is rapid and may result in an alteration of state, and random movements are noticed.

Awake states

Drowsy state The eyes may be open or closed with some eyelid flutter, smiling may occur, smooth limb movements interspersed with startle responses may be present and alteration of state occurs readily following stimulation.

Quiet alert state Motor activity is minimal but the baby is alert to visual and auditory stimuli.

Active alert state The baby is active and reactive to the environment. It is in this state he will mimic facial expressions.

Active crying state The baby cries vigorously and may be difficult to console. There is considerable muscular activity.

Babies cry for different reasons such as hunger, thirst, pain, a need to change position or unsatisfactory room temperature; this is their only means of attracting attention to their needs. Although crying causes anxiety, mothers usually learn to recognise and respond to the different cries. Understanding these different behavioural states may contribute to better parenting, lessen anxiety and allow greater parental enjoyment.

THE IMMUNE SYSTEM

Lymphopoiesis (Ch. 29, p. 388) is aimed at the production of **immunocytes** capable of distinguishing between foreign and self-antigens, facilitating the elimination of foreign antigens and maintaining a memory of previous exposure to them. In order to accomplish these tasks, the development of the lymphoid tissue proceeds along the two classical pathways culminating in the formation of competent **B lymphocytes** necessary for **antibody-mediated immunity** and **T lymphocytes**, which are predominantly responsible for **cell-mediated immunity**.

Both fetus and neonate are compromised by their immature immune systems. Also, lack of exposure to common pathogens and antigens contributes to the significant delay in mounting a desirable immune response. Since cell-mediated and humoral immunity are affected, the inflammatory response and complement cascade are limited. The immaturity of the immune system may also predispose to allergy formation and, in part, be responsible for the susceptibility to gastrointestinal infections.

At birth the fetus usually leaves a sterile intrauterine environment and enters an environment containing potentially harmful pathogens. The skin, respiratory system and gastrointestinal tract must acquire normal microbe commensal populations and respond appropriately to pathogens and allergens. The initial colonisation is via the mother's genital tract during birth, then her skin organisms and finally organisms found in the environmental.

Organisms such as *Lactobacillus*, *Escherichia coli* and protective anaerobes are derived from the mother's genital tract along with pathogens such as group B streptococcus and *Chlamydia trachomatis*. As neonatal skin and mucous membranes are fragile and easily breached by pathogenic organisms, the colonisation that initially occurs on the skin, umbilical stump and genitalia followed by mucous membranes of the eyes, nose and throat can result in potentially dangerous systemic infections.

The gut

The mild acidity of the stomach secretions may afford some protection against ingested pathogens. Certainly, the colonisation of meconium, which occurs within a few hours of birth and increases rapidly over the next few days, does not always lead to infection. Breastfed babies develop a different pattern of bacterial colonisation to that observed in artificially fed babies. The acid environment in the gut in which protective organisms such as *Lactobacillus* can grow appears to prevent colonisation by pathogenic organisms. Eventually, the development of gut defence mechanisms such as 'gut closure', accompanied by the development of the mucosal barrier and other defences, renders the epithelium impermeable to pathogens.

Specific immune responses

Two specific immune responses concern immunoglobulin IgA (humoral-mediated immunity) and maturation of T cells (cell-mediated immunity).

Humoral-mediated immunity

During fetal life there is transfer of IgG via the placenta from mother to fetus, affording the fetus some degree of passive immunity. However, IgA does not cross the placenta and neonatal levels are low. Colonising IgA is transferred in the colostrum and milk, which protect it from the acidic contents and proteolytic enzymes present in the baby's gastrointestinal tract. IgM is too large a molecule to cross the placental barrier. However, the neonate is capable of producing sufficient amounts of IgM in response to a challenge by micro-organisms such as the TORCH organisms (Toxoplasmosis, Other viruses, Rubella, Cytomegalovirus and Herpes simplex).

Cell-mediated immunity

At birth, T cell numbers are similar to those found in the adult but their function is decreased. Cytotoxic activity of T cells is only 30–60% of that found in the adult. However, these T cells are naïve and require significant maturation before they can mount minimal protection.

THERMOREGULATION

Thermoregulation is the balance between heat production and heat loss.

Adult mechanisms

Humans are a **homeothermic** species, maintaining a constant body temperature independent of their environment. Skin receptors in various parts of the body send signals to the **hypothalamus**, triggering coordinated autonomic nervous system responses. The transfer of these signals to the cerebral cortex triggers learned behavioural responses. Consequently, a rise in normal body temperature in humans is accompanied by an autonomically triggered **peripheral vasodilation** and sweating and a behavioural response, culminating in the search for a cooler environment and wearing of appropriate clothing. If the body temperature falls there is usually a reflex **peripheral vasoconstriction** and shivering and the person seeks a warmer environment and more suitable clothing (Michaelides 1997).

Neonatal mechanisms

At birth the neonate passes from a thermoconstant intrauterine temperature of 37.7°C to an environment where the room temperature averages at between 21 and 25°C. This contributes to rapid and significant heat loss due to the wet, warm skin. Heat may be transferred down the internal gradient from the body core to the skin surface and to the environment. The speed with which heat passes through the internal gradient depends upon capillary blood flow and the amount of subcutaneous fat present. In contrast, the loss

Table 49.1 Sources of heat gain and heat loss in the neonate

Heat gain	Heat loss
Metabolic processes such as oxidative metabolism of glucose, fats and proteins	Evaporation – water loss from the skin and respiratory tract, most common at birth. Heat is also lost in urine and faeces
Physical activity such as crying, restlessness and hyperactivity	Convection – heat lost into the air around the baby
Non-shivering thermogenesis generated through metabolism in brown adipose tissue	Radiation – heat radiated to nearby cold solid surfaces, most common after the first week of life Conduction – heat lost by direct contact with cold surfaces touching the baby

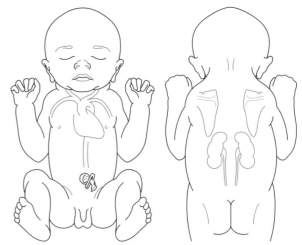

Figure 49.2 The areas where brown fat is found. (Reproduced with permission from Wallis & Harvey 1979.)

of heat down the external gradient depends on the difference between the skin temperature and the external environment and this involves the four processes of evaporation, convection, radiation and conduction. The balance between heat gain and heat loss in the neonate is shown in Table 49.1.

Thermoregulation is a common physiological problem amongst neonates largely due to the immaturity and inefficiency of the normal control mechanisms observed in adults (Michaelides 1997). For instance, in the first few days of life, neonates lose sweat only from their head region. The neonate has a much larger surface area than that of the adult. This area from which heat can be lost, of which the head makes up 25%, is relatively small when compared with the **body mass** where heat can be produced. An increase or decrease in the body surface area is achieved by the neonate's changing posture and exposure to the environment. Under normal circumstances a neonate's rectal temperature may average at 36.0–37.2°C, and skin temperature, also known as peripheral temperature, may average at 35.5–36.5°C.

As neonates are generally unable to shiver, and are limited in their ability to move about to generate heat from muscle action, they are at some disadvantage. However, they can decrease their surface area exposed to the environment by flexing their limbs and taking up the fetal position. During the first 24 h of extrauterine life, healthy term neonates will increase their body heat production by 2.5 times as a physiological response to cold. This process appears to be activated by catecholamine release, which induces **lipolysis** in the brown adipose tissue (BAT), which is also found in human adults, other animal neonates and hibernating animals.

Heat production and BAT

About 2–7% of the weight of a newborn infant is thought to consist of brown adipose tissue (BAT), which is mainly situated around the kidneys, in the mediastinum, around the nape of the neck and scapulae, along the spinal column and around the large blood vessels in the neck (Fig. 49.2). **Brown adipocytes** (fat cells) begin to proliferate at 26–30 weeks gestation and continue to increase in number for some months after birth. A small amount of brown adipose tissue persists throughout life, with greater quantities being present in slender individuals.

The adipocytes of BAT differ from those in white adipose tissue by their scope for metabolic activity and heat production. The cells contain many small fat vacuoles, numerous mitochondria and other active organelles. Brown adipose tissue has extensive capillary perfusion, which gives it the characteristically brownish colour. Activity of the sympathetic nerve fibres during cold stress causes the adrenal glands to release the necessary catecholamines, such as **noradrenaline** (norepinephrine), which stimulate the anterior pituitary gland to release **thyroid-stimulating hormone** (TSH), which in turn causes the thyroid gland to increases its production of **thyroxine** (T_4). **Adrenaline** (epinephrine) and thyroxine increase the metabolic activity within the brown fat cells and heat is produced but this process requires extra oxygen and glucose.

Care of the neonate

It is important that parents as well as professionals caring for neonates are aware of the need to keep the head and nape of the neck warm and to adjust both the environmental temperature and the amount of clothing worn in order to maximise heat regulation. It must also be remembered that at the time of birth the baby should be dried and covered and given to the mother to hold if possible. The best source of heat is from the mother's body. Implications for the care of small and sick neonates are discussed in a later chapter.

MAIN POINTS

- The nutritional, excretory and metabolic needs of the fetus and its protection against pathogenic organisms and toxins are met by the placenta. After birth these complex physiological processes function independently.

- At birth, the gastrointestinal system of the newborn infant manifests some anatomical and physiological limitations, partly influenced by fetal swallowing of amniotic fluid. The swallowing actions of the small bolus of amniotic fluid may be important in the development and maintenance of gastrointestinal patency.

- In term neonates sucking and swallowing reflexes are present at birth. The small stomach capacity increases rapidly within the first few weeks of life, allowing the infant to take larger feeds. The cardiac sphincter remains weak and milk regurgitation is common.

- The intestinal mucosal barrier remains immature so that antigens and other macromolecules can be transported across the epithelium into the systemic circulation. Colostrum is rich in antibodies and helps the elimination of meconium. The relative deficiency of the enzymes amylase and lipase means that the neonate has difficulties digesting carbohydrates and fats.

- A gastrocolic reflex ensures that feeding is often accompanied by reflex emptying of the bowel. Most neonates pass meconium within 24 h of birth. Failure to do so could be a sign of intestinal obstruction.

- The liver is physiologically immature and there is low production of enzymes such as glucuronyl transferase. Enteral feeding stimulates liver function and bacterial colonisation of the gut, which allows vitamin K to be produced.

- The fetus lays down a fuel store of glycogen and lipids during the last few weeks of pregnancy. After birth these glycogen and fat stores are used as metabolic fuel. Catecholamines released in response to body cooling stimulate the release of alternative fat stores and ketone bodies.

- Neonatal blood glucose levels fall to a lowest level between 2 and 6 h after birth, become stable and then rise as the baby adapts to his extrauterine environment. The feeding method can influence neonatal blood glucose levels.

- Lipolysis increases rapidly after birth, reaching a maximum within a few hours. In the first 24 h two-thirds of the baby's energy is derived from the oxidation of fat. The neonate's ability to synthesise protein is limited due to the relative immaturity of the liver enzyme systems. This results in higher serum amino acid levels and a significant urinary amino acid excretion.

- During the first 2 days of life serum calcium levels fall and there is physiological hypocalcaemia. Calcium then rises to normal values between 5 and 10 days of age as intestinal absorption of calcium increases. Renal excretion of calcium is efficient. Neonates metabolise vitamin D in the liver and kidneys although absorption of exogenous vitamin D may be limited because of immature fat absorption mechanisms.

- The decreased glomerular filtration rate and increased tubular reabsorption rate delay renal excretion of phosphorus. Increased energy release with conversion of ATP to ADP may contribute to increased phosphate release.

- Only 1% of the total body magnesium is located in the extracellular space. In plasma about 60% of the magnesium exists as free ion while 20% is bound to various anions. The remaining plasma magnesium is bound to serum proteins. The kidneys appear to be the primary organs for serum magnesium regulation.

- Nervous system activity increases steadily throughout gestation. At term the neonate processes incoming information from the environment and produces behaviour appropriate for its status. The relative plasticity of the brain ensures that new neural connections can be established and modified by environmental stimuli as the baby learns through observation and perception.

- The term neonate demonstrates a typical muscle tone which changes, giving rise to strong passive flexion and, eventually, purposive movement. Reflexes are critical for the baby's safety and survival. The absence of such reflexes or their unusual persistence may be indicative of brain damage.

- Neonatal behaviours include two sleep states – deep and light – and four awake states – drowsy, quiet alert, active alert and active crying. Helping parents to recognise these different behavioural states may contribute to better parenting skills and greater enjoyment of the neonate.

- Lymphoid tissue development culminates in the formation of competent B lymphocytes and T lymphocytes. Lymphopoiesis aims at producing competent immunocytes capable of distinguishing between foreign and self-antigens, processing foreign antigens and maintaining a memory of previous exposure. The fetus and neonate are immunocompromised which makes him susceptible to gastrointestinal infections.

- At birth the neonate's skin, respiratory system and gastrointestinal tract must acquire normal microbe commensal populations and respond appropriately to pathogens and allergens. The initial colonisation is via the mother's genital tract during birth, then her skin microorganisms and finally environmental organisms.

- Breastfed babies develop a different pattern of bacterial colonisation than artificially fed babies. The acid environment in the gut facilitates the growth of *Lactobacillus*, preventing colonisation by pathogenic micro-organisms. Neonates develop gut closure to render the epithelium impermeable to such micro-organisms.

- Neonatal thermoregulation can be a problem as the large body surface area contributes to greater heat loss. Shivering is limited but neonates can increase their body heat production by 2.5 times in response to cold by lipolysis of brown adipose tissue.

References

Blackburn S T 2003 Maternal, Fetal and Neonatal Physiology: A Clinical Perspective, 2nd edn. W B Saunders, Philadelphia.

Brazelton T B 1984 Neonatal Behaviour Assessment Scale, 2nd edn. Spastics International Medical Publications, Blackwell Scientific, Oxford.

Dodds R 1996 When policies collide: breastfeeding and hypoglycaemia. MIDIRS Midwifery Digest 6(4):382–386.

Eibl-Eibesfeldt I 1975 Ethology: The Biology of Behaviour. Holt, Rinehart and Winston, New York.

Garrow J, James W 2000 Human Nutrition and Dietetics. Churchill Livingstone, Edinburgh.

Greenfield S (ed.) 1997 The Human Mind Explained. Cassell, London.

Hawdon J M, Platt M P W, Aynsley-Green A 1992 Patterns of metabolic adaptation for preterm and term infants in the first neonatal week. Archives of Childhood Fetal and Neonatal Edition 67(4):357–365.

Koh T, Vong S K 1996 Definition of neonatal hypoglycaemia: is there a change? Journal of Paediatrics and Child Health 344(4):302–305.

Larsen W 2001 Human Embryology. Churchill Livingstone, Edinburgh.

Michaelides S 1997 Thermoregulation and the neonate. In Sweet B R, Tiran D (eds) Mayes Midwifery, 12th edn. Baillière Tindall, London.

Michie M M 1999 The baby at birth. In Bennett V R, Brown S (eds) Myles Textbook for Midwives, 13th edn. Churchill Livingstone, Edinburgh.

Pitkin R M 1985 Calcium metabolism in pregnancy and the perinatal period: a review. American Journal of Obstetrics and Gynaecology 151:99.

Polin R, Fox W 1992 Fetal and Neonatal Physiology. W B Saunders, Philadelphia.

Prechtl H F R, O'Brien M J 1982 Behavioural states of the full-term newborn. The emergence of concept. In Stratton P (ed.) Psychobiology of the Human Newborn. John Wiley, Chichester.

Rudolph A, Hoffman J, Rudolph C et al 2002 Rudolph's Paediatrics. Prentice-Hall, New Jersey.

Shaffer D 2002 Developmental Psychology: Childhood and Adolescence. Wadsworth, Belmont, California.

Shatz C 1992 The developing brain. Scientific American 9:35–41.

Simpson C 1997 Metabolic and endocrine disorders of the newborn. In Sweet B R, Tiran D (eds) Mayes Midwifery, 12th edn. Baillière Tindall, London.

Trevathan W R 1987 Human birth: an evolutionary perspective. Aldine de Gruyter, New York.

Annotated recommended reading

Blackburn S 2003 Maternal, Fetal and Neonatal Physiology: A Clinical Perspective, 2nd edn. W B Saunders, Philadelphia.
This textbook offers excellent accounts of bioscientific aspects of knowledge which should be taken into consideration when managing the care of an expectant mother, the fetus and the newborn infant.

Boxwell G 2000 Neonatal Intensive Care Nursing. Routledge, London.
This textbook outlines a range of common and challenging neonatal problems and then provides helpful and directive suggestions for neonatal intensive care nursing. Critical analysis and reflection on the identified neonatal nursing concepts reinforce best practice.

Dodds R 1996 When policies collide: breastfeeding and hypoglycaemia. MIDIRS Midwifery Digest 6(4):382–386.
This paper discusses why giving babies who are to be breastfed unnecessary artificial feeds is based on non-scientific physiological interpretations of blood glucose levels.

Gluckman P, Heymann M 1996 Pediatrics and Perinatology – The Scientific Basis. Arnold, London.
This textbook offers a comprehensive account of biological aspects of embryonic and fetal development and maturation. The theoretical accounts are supported by empirical evidence and conclusions are drawn about relevant biochemical, cellular, genetic, anatomical and physiological issues.

Polin R, Fox W 1998 Fetal and Neonatal Physiology, Vols 1 and 2. W B Saunders, Philadelphia.
This two-volume textbook offers detailed accounts of bioscientific concepts important in fetal and neonatal care. A résumé of genetics acts as a basis for a detailed exploration of normal embryonic development. The systematic exploration of biochemical, physiological, nutritional and pathophysiological principles makes a significant contribution to clinical practice and research.

Wong D 1999 Nursing Care of Infants and Children. Mosby, St Louis.
This textbook offers detailed accounts of the relevant biophysical, psychosocial and nursing issues in managing the care of infants and children. It contains helpful appendices, including excellent developmental screening tools and biophysical nomograms and parameters.

Chapter 50

The low birthweight baby – common problems and care

INTRODUCTION

This chapter provides an overview of some of the common problems which are encountered in low birthweight infants. The complexity and diversity of problems does not permit a detailed account of the knowledge and expertise required by those caring for neonates in neonatal intensive care units. Nevertheless, an attempt will be made to build on some of the diagnostic accounts of congenital abnormalities detailed in Chapter 15, p. 195, giving due consideration to the most relevant aspects of physiology, pathophysiology and, where appropriate, therapeutic caring interventions.

LOW BIRTHWEIGHT BABIES

The term **low birth weight** applies to all those infants who at birth weigh less than 2500 g. The improved survival of infants weighing less than 1500 g required the introduction of a new term **very low birth weight**. This term is more suited to the characteristic problems and outcomes that these very small babies experience. Given that about 70% of **perinatal mortality** (total of stillbirths and neonatal deaths) occurs in the 7% of babies whose birth weight is low or very low (Kelnar et al 1995), the problems which these infants encounter are clearly complex. The following parameters are applied regardless of the cause of the infants low birth weight (Simpson 1997a, Papageorgiou & Bardin 1999):

- low birth weight (LBW) is usually taken to include babies weighing 2500 g or less at birth;
- very low birth weight (VLBW) are babies weighing below 1500 g at birth;
- extremely low birth weight (ELBW) are babies weighing under 1000 g at birth.

Causes of low birth weight

The two factors that dominate the reasons for an infant's low birth weight are **prematurity** at birth and **intrauterine**

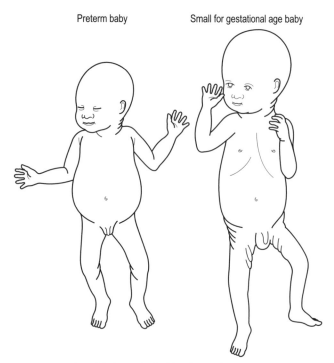

Figure 50.1   Low birthweight babies (from Sweet B 1997, with permission).

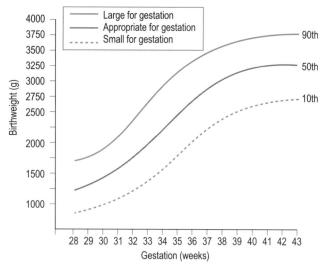

Figure 50.2   A centile chart, showing weight and gestation (from Sweet B 1997, with permission).

growth retardation (Fig. 50.1). Premature infants are born before 37 completed weeks of pregnancy, calculated from the 1st day of the last menstrual period. In this instance, the term is used regardless of birth weight.

Those infants who are **small for gestational age** (SFGA) weigh less at birth than would be predicted for the gestational age. This group usually includes those infants who are born below the 10th centile. These two major groups of newborn infants are likely to present with a range of characteristic problems which require sensitive but swift intervention. Some of these problems are present at birth while others will develop in the first few days or even weeks following birth. It is for this reason that these groups of infants must be carefully identified and their optimal care effectively managed in a proactive manner. **Centile charts**, depicting the variable birth weight parameters in conjunction with gestational age, provide a useful guide for a relatively accurate physical assessment (Fig. 50.2).

Assessment of gestational age

Small-for-gestational-age infants are defined as having a birth weight that is more than two **standard deviations** below the mean or less than the 10th percentile of a population-specific birth weight/gestational age graph plot. The terms used to define variations in fetal growth vary although reference to body weight at birth is frequently used as a constant variable. Clearly, classification by body weight alone provides little insight into fetal growth rate as

many of these infants may also be premature. Similarly, classifying neonates as premature or term on the basis of their birth weight is also misleading. A realistic assessment of fetal growth must therefore consider variations in **genetic** and **environmental factors** that could affect the expectant mother and the growth rate of her fetus.

In most instances fetal growth would be based on the length of gestation by taking into account the onset of the last menstrual period, the size and shape of the growing uterus and maternofetal hormone profile. **Ultrasound studies**, and in some instances **amniocentesis**, will provide additional information. Most fetuses fall into a **symmetric** or **asymmetric growth pattern**. Symmetric growth implies that both brain and body growths are limited, whereas asymmetric growth implies that body growth is restricted to a greater extent than head growth. The mechanisms for such asynchronous growth are not understood although Anderson & Hay (1999) suggest that increased cerebral blood flow relative to the remainder of the systemic circulation may be a contributing factor. The physical status of the neonate is often anticipated, making it necessary for a paediatric team to be present at the time of delivery.

The gestational age of such small neonates must be established soon after birth by an experienced paediatrician. Assessment of physical characteristics and neurological and neuromuscular development using **scoring systems** originally devised by Dubowitz et al (1970) is used widely within the United Kingdom (Fig. 50.3). However, as this scale awards points for neurological state as well as external criteria, it may not always be suitable for assessing the gestational age of sick and/or mechanically ventilated neonates. In these instances the Parkin score (Parkin et al 1976), which uses exclusively external criteria, is quicker, although not quite as accurate (Fig. 50.4), and may be a more appropriate assessment tool in some instances (Simpson 1997a).

External (superficial) Criteria					
EXTERNAL SIGN	SCORE 0	1	2	3	4
OEDEMA	Obvious oedema hands and feet: pitting over tibia	No obvious oedema hands and feet: pitting over tibia	No oedema		
SKIN TEXTURE	Very thin, gelatinous	Thin and smooth	Smooth: medium thickness. Rash or superficial peeling	Slight thickening. Superficial cracking and peeling esp. hand and feet	Thick and parchment-like: superficial or deep cracking
SKIN COLOUR (Infant not crying)	Dark red	Uniformly pink	Pale pink: variable over body	Pale. Only pink over ears, lips, palms or soles	
SKIN OPACITY (trunk)	Numerous veins and venules clearly seen, especially over abdomen	Veins and tributaries seen	A few large vessels clearly seen over abdomen	A few large vessels seen indistinctly over abdomen	No blood vessels seen
LANUGO (over back)	No lanugo	Abundant; long and thick over whole back	Hair thinning especially over lower back	Small amount of lanugo and bald areas	At least half of back devoid of lanugo
PLANTAR CREASES	No skin creases	Faint red marks over anterior half of sole	Definite red marks over more than anterior half; indentations over less than anterior third	Indentations over more than anterior third	Definite deep indentations over more than anterior third
NIPPLE FORMATION	Nipple barely visible; no areola	Nipple well defined; areola smooth and flat diameter <0.75 cm.	Areola stippled, edge not raised; diameter <0.75 cm.	Areola stippled, edge raised diameter >0.75 cm.	
BREAST SIZE	No breast tissue palpable	Breast tissue on one or both sides <0.5 cm. diameter	Breast tissue both sides; one or both 0.5–1.0 cm.	Breast tissue both sides; one or both >1 cm.	
EAR FORM	Pinna flat and shapeless, little or no incurving edge	Incurving of part of edge of pinna	Partial incurving whole of upper pinna	Well-defined incurving whole of upper pinna	
EAR FIRMNESS	Pinna soft, easily folded, no recoil	Pinna soft, easily folded, slow recoil	Cartilage to edge of pinna, but soft in places, ready recoil	Pinna firm, cartilage to edge, instant recoil	
GENITALIA MALE	Neither testis in scrotum	At least one testis high in scrotum	At least one testis right down		
FEMALE (With hips half abducted)	Labia majora widely separated, labia minora protruding	Labia majora almost cover labia minora	Labia majora completely cover labia minora		

Figure 50.3a Dubowitz score. (Adapted from Dubowitz L M S, Dubowitz V, Goldberg C 1970.)

THE PRETERM NEONATE

The problems of the preterm neonate can to a large extent be attributed to immaturity of the body systems (Fig. 50.5), which means that some organs and systems may not have reached the fully functional state required for adaptation to extrauterine life.

Features of the preterm neonate

- A large head in proportion to their body, with a small face.
- Brain tissue is fragile and neurological damage more likely.
- Neonates born before 24 weeks may present with fused eyelids.
- Soft skull bones with widely spaced sutures and large fontanelles.
- The skin is red and thin, subcutaneous fat is absent and surface veins are prominent.
- Lanugo may be present, depending on the gestational age.
- A small narrow chest with little breast tissue.
- A large prominent abdomen with a low-set umbilicus.

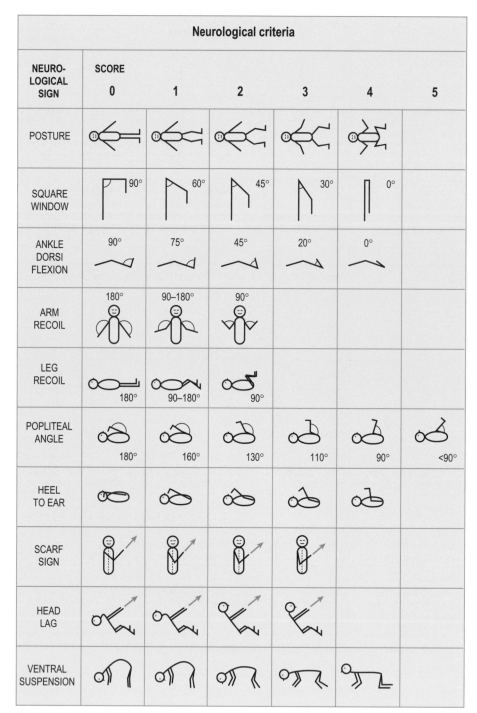

Figure 50.3b Dubowitz score. (Adapted from Dubowitz L M S, Dubowitz V, Goldberg C 1970.)

- Thin limbs with soft nails not reaching to the ends of the digits.
- Small genitalia: in girls, the labia majora do not cover the labia minora; in boys, the testes have not descended fully into the scrotum.
- Muscle tone is poor and all four limbs may be held in the extended position.
- Normal reflexes, including sucking, may be absent or feeble.

Causes of preterm birth

Premature births occur spontaneously but in many circumstances may be medically controlled for maternal or fetal safety. Although 40% of such births have no established causes, a range of contributing factors such as physical disorders in the fetus and the mother or the mother's social class may play a key role (Table 50.1). This is not surprising as many suboptimal health problems appear to be the

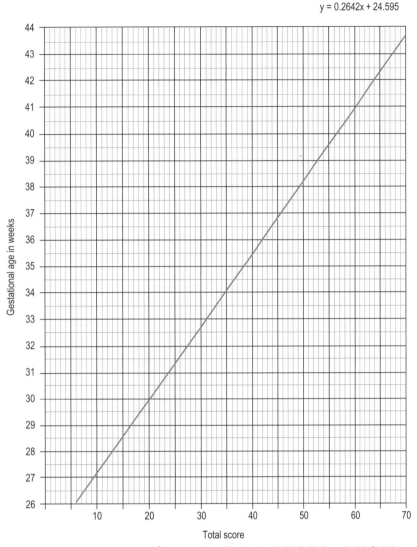

$y = 0.2642x + 24.595$

Figure 50.3c   Dubowitz score. (Adapted from Dubowitz L M S, Dubowitz V, Goldberg C 1970.)

consequence of interplays between genetic and environmental factors (Chs 8 and 15).

Immediate management

The care of the premature neonate is aimed at supporting the numerous physiological shortfalls which are apparent at birth. In most instances this care should be initiated during labour or before. Premature neonates should be delivered in maternity departments with a suitable neonatal unit as the transfer of such small neonates is fraught with problems and risks to the neonate.

In labour

Ideally, **prophylactic corticosteroids** should be administered to a mother who is in early labour and likely to give birth. Such practice is supported by Crowley (1996) and others who recommend that the administration of 24 mg

betamethasone or dexamethasone or 2 g hydrocortisone administered in divided dosages will **reduce respiratory distress syndrome** and **intraventricular haemorrhage** with no adverse effects to the fetus/neonate. The **pharmacodynamic effects** of such corticosteroids administered in these circumstances are not fully understood. Nevertheless, the positive clinical outcomes in neonates born under these conditions appear to support this practice.

The delivery of the fetus must be given careful consideration in all circumstances. Papageorgiou & Bardin (1999) advocate delivery of the fetus by elective caesarean section on the grounds that this mode of delivery improves the outcome for very low birthweight babies, weighing between 1000 g and 1600 g, particularly where the fetuses are breech presentations (Gilady et al 1996). However, Grant & Glazener (2003) conclude that there is 'not enough evidence to evaluate a policy for elective caesarean delivery for small babies'.

In cases where vaginal delivery is the elected choice, then an episiotomy is required with additional supportive

2 Parkin Hey and Clowes score

This is quicker to perform but may not be quite so accurate.

Skin texture.   Tested by picking up a fold of abdominal skin between finger and thumb, and by inspection.
0 Very thin with a gelatinous feel.
1 Thin and smooth.
2 Smooth and of medium thickness, irritation and rash and superficial peeling may be present.
3 Slight thickening and stiff feeling with superficial cracking and peeling especially evident on the hands and feet.
4 Thick and parchment-like with superficial or deep cracking.

Skin colour.   Estimated by inspection when the baby is quiet.
0 Dark red.
1 Uniformly pink.
2 Pale pink, though the colour may vary over different parts of the body, some parts may be very pale.
3 Pale, nowhere really pink except on the ears, lips, palms and soles.

Breast size.   Measured by picking up the breast tissue between finger and thumb.
0 No breast tissue palpable.
1 Breast tissue palpable on one or both sides, neither being more than 0.5 cm in diameter.
2 Breast tissue palpable on both sides, one or both being 0.5–1 cm in diameter.
3 Breast tissue palpable on both sides, one or both being more than 1 cm in diameter.

Ear firmness.   Tested by palpation and folding of the upper pinna.
0 Pinna feels soft and is easily folded into bizarre positions without springing back into position spontaneously.
1 Pinna feels soft along the edge and is easily folded but returns slowly to the correct position spontaneously.
2 Cartilage can be felt to the edge of the pinna though it is thin in places and the pinna springs back readily after being folded.
3 Pinna firm with definite cartilage extending to the periphery and springs back immediately into position after being folded.

Score each external sign in turn. Add them up. Read off the baby's gestational age on the following chart:

| | Gestational age | |
Score	days	weeks
1	190	27
2	210	30
3	230	33
4	240	34.5
5	250	36
6	260	37
7	270	38.5
8	276	39.5
9	281	40
10	285	41
11	290	41.5
12	295	42

Figure 50.4   Parkin, Hey and Clowes score. (Reproduced from Parkin et al 1976.)

intervention where forceps may be used to lessen the risk of intracranial haemorrhage. In these circumstances care must be taken not to give the mother any form of medication such as analgesia that might compromise the functional scope of the respiratory centre of the fetus and so suppress normal respiration after birth.

At birth

The delivery suite must be equipped and prepared to resuscitate the neonate. Ideally, an experienced paediatric team should be present during the delivery. Some neonates may have weak respiratory muscles and an immature respiratory centre and these may contribute to difficulties in establishing effective respiration and pulmonary gas exchange. In such circumstances, elective **endotracheal intubation** of all low birthweight babies may improve survival and later wellbeing as many of these neonates, although well at birth, may go on develop respiratory, cardiovascular and gastrointestinal problems thereafter.

Care must also be taken to ensure that the ambient temperature of the delivery suite and the neonatal unit is no less than 24°C. In order to minimise thermoregulation problems, the neonate must be dried and warmly wrapped. If the

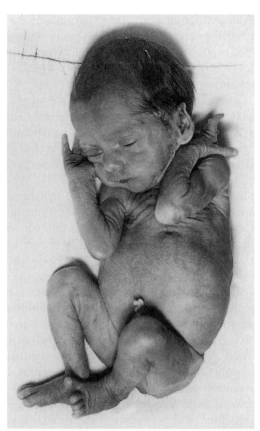

Figure 50.5   A preterm baby born in 1954 at 28 weeks gestation and weighing 1.1 kg. He was discharged in good health after 11 weeks in hospital (from Kelnar C, Harvey D, Simpson C 1995, with permission).

Table 50.1   Causes of preterm birth

Fetal causes	Maternal causes
Multiple pregnancy	Pre-eclampsia
Polyhydramnios	Antepartum haemorrhage
Congenital abnormalities	Rhesus incompatibility
	Systemic maternal disease such as diabetes mellitus
	Pyrexia associated with viral infections
	Smoking, alcohol and drug abuse
	Maternal short stature
	Cervical incompetence
	Maternal age and parity
	Inappropriate maternal nutrition

neonate's respiratory and cardiovascular functions are satisfactory, the parents may wish to hold him. However, if the mother wishes to have a more direct skin-to-skin contact with her newborn infant, then warm protective blankets (Simpson 1997a) may be required for the baby. Conversely, if the neonate needs **cardiopulmonary resuscitation**, an overhead radiant heater should be used to ensure that the immediate vicinity is warm and sensitively controlled to support the principles of thermoregulation.

Ongoing care of preterm babies

Potential problems

The preterm neonate baby may present with a potential for a range of problems and these may include:

- respiratory problems such as apnoea, respiratory distress syndrome and bronchopulmonary dysplasia;
- metabolic problems such as hypoglycaemia and hypocalcaemia;
- structural organic problems such as necrotising enterocolitis and periventricular and intraventricular haemorrhage;
- haematological problems such jaundice and anaemia;
- haemodynamic problems such as persistent fetal circulation.

Where there is evidence of such problems, the premature neonate will require supportive care to ensure survival, growth and eventually normal development. This care must include:

- maintenance of ambient and body temperature;
- supportive interventions for respiratory and cardiovascular dysfunction;
- supportive nutrition and metabolic interventions;
- prevention of infection;
- supportive intervention to maintain effective renal perfusion and function;
- monitoring of excretion;
- supportive intervention to foster the emotional relationship between the parents and their baby.

Maintenance of temperature

Compared with term infants, premature infants have a narrower thermoneutral range where heat production cannot always match the rate of heat loss. This is further aggravated by the greater heat loss due to the larger head-to-body ratio and the exaggerated body surface area which is characteristic in all premature and SFGA infants. The greater heat loss makes additional metabolic demands on the neonate, whose ability to assimilate nutrients and exchange gases will be compromised by immaturity. The administration of glucose as energy and oxygen must not be exceeded beyond the physiological norm.

To ensure that the neonate's body temperature is kept within the very narrow physiological range (Kelnar et al 1995), ambient temperatures are held between 26 and 28°C and the incubator temperature between 33 and 37°C. This generally maintains the neonate's ideal body temperature at about 37°C. By attaching a temperature-monitoring skin probe to the neonate, it is possible to control the incubator temperature, allowing it to adjust automatically in response to changes in the neonate's temperature (Simpson 1997a). Infants born before 30 weeks of gestation have porous skins through which water easily evaporates, causing an increase in heat loss. It is important to nurse them in a humid atmosphere for the 1st week. Using a heat shield when required will prevent heat loss by radiation.

Respiration

The premature infant may have a respiratory rate that averages between 40 and 60 breaths/min. This is generally considered as sufficient for adequate air intake and gas exchange. Ongoing observation and hourly monitoring will contribute to an accurate assessment of the infant's overall respiratory function and this must include:

- the shape of the chest – its symmetry, inflation and contour;
- the colour of the skin;
- the rate and rhythm and effort on respiration;
- breath sounds on auscultation.

Oxygen therapy   Oxygen therapy may be required in circumstances where respiratory distress and cyanosis develop (Ch. 51). In such instances the temperature, humidity, flow rate and concentration of inspired oxygen must be adequately controlled and monitored (Kelnar et al 1995) in order to avoid oxygen toxicity. Oxygen-enriched air may be delivered into the neonate's head box (Fig. 50.6) or in more severe circumstances by means of assisted mechanical ventilation. The amount of oxygen given must be carefully adjusted to uphold arterial oxygen tension in the normal physiological range.

Too high concentrations of oxygen can have adverse effects, particularly on the retina and the lungs, contributing to the development of **retrolental fibroplasia** (retinopathy of prematurity) and **bronchopulmonary damage**. Inadequate oxygenation or hypoxia can also be detrimental, particularly in terms of contributing to episodes of profound bradycardia and brain damage. Monitoring of oxygen administration by means of **transcutaneous oxygen monitoring** and **arterial blood sampling** is crucial, especially in very ill infants. As continuous transcutaneous monitoring has many advantages over the intermittent sampling, this is the method of choice in most neonatal (intensive) care units. Although **assisted mechanical ventilation** is an effective means of life support where reliable spontaneous ventilation is impossible, it must be curtailed as soon as the neonate's clinical condition allows.

Nutrition

The neonate's specific nutritional requirements are in part dependent upon total body stores of fat, protein and glycogen. **Hypoglycaemia** is one of the most common problems that SFGA and premature neonates develop, especially in the first 3 days of life (Anderson & Hay 1999). When planning a nutritional programme, intestinal uptake, assimilation of nutrients, energy expenditure and elimination of the by-products of digestion must be taken into consideration in conjunction with the physical maturity of such neonates.

For practical reasons, the neonate's energy requirements may be divided into two major components: the support of **physical growth** and the support of metabolic activities and energy expenditure associated with **development**. In general, the energy requirements for metabolic activities take precedence over that required for growth. This becomes evident in circumstances where compromised nutrition and energy supply fail to meet the metabolic demands and this in turn results in poor growth.

Most paediatricians and midwives recommend that term infants are breastfed where circumstances allow. Greer (1991) supports this policy by suggesting that it would be logical to establish a nutrition strategy capable of mimicking for at least a short period of time fetal intrauterine nutritional needs and growth pattern. The energy reserves and nutritional needs of preterm and LBW infants are more challenging. Ideally, appropriate nutritional support should commence within minutes of birth. However, since the initial period of the neonate's life tends to be complicated by a range of acute medical problems which require skilled intervention, nutritional support may sometimes be relegated to a secondary position. In Anderson & Hay's (1999) view, premature and SFGA neonates should receive intravenous hydration and glucose within 30 min of their birth if homeostatic problems are to be avoided.

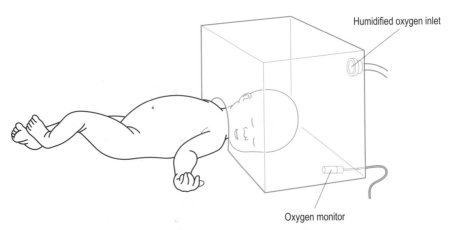

Figure 50.6   Baby being nursed in a headbox (incubator not shown) (from Sweet B 1997, with permission).

Fats Fats are the main dietary source of energy in the neonates, providing up to 50% of the total caloric needs. Yet all premature and LBW neonates have lower plasma free fatty acid levels in comparison to term neonates. Anderson & Hay (1999) reported that, once fed, these neonates appear to have a deficient oxidation of free fatty acids and utilisation of triglycerides, a phenomenon that could be partly contributing to the development of hypoglycaemia. Since fats are essential in the formation of cell membranes and make a significant contribution to the development of the nervous system, it seems logical that a balanced nutrition must contain the right kinds and quantities of fats in order to support the neonate's multifactorial needs.

Proteins Although dietary proteins supply less than 10–14% of the daily caloric needs, a daily intake of proteins is critical as a source of amino acids essential for growth, particularly in premature and LBW infants whose muscle mass is deficient. Protein intake must be adequate to replace nitrogen loss which occurs as a consequence of protein turnover. This may average 11–14% of the total body protein per day. Greer (1991) suggests that although neonates have the ability to synthesise some amino acids, **essential amino acids** such as histidine, isoleucine, leucine, lysine, methionine, phenylalanine, threonine, tryptophan and valine must be given, while VLBW infants may require additional amino acids such as cystine and taurine.

Carbohydrates Enterally fed neonates use carbohydrates, and glucose in particular, as a major source of energy (Greer 1991). The minimal 24-h glucose utilisation rate by the resting term neonate is estimated to be 4 mg/kg/min. An intake of glucose less than that rate may result in **gluconeogenesis** from non-carbohydrate sources such as amino acids. Conversely, excess glucose can be stored in the liver as glycogen and converted into glucose when required to support metabolic demands. However, in LBW neonates, glycogen stores are usually low in the early neonatal period and this is a major contributing factor to the frequent episodes of hypoglycaemia observed in these neonates. Other contributing factors may include deficient catecholamine release and decreased hepatic and muscle glycogen stores.

The best method of feeding such neonates will depend on size, maturity and physical condition. Whenever possible, the neonate's inclination to suck should be used as an indication that breast or bottle feeding could be offered with careful supervision. Premature neonates may, however, have poor sucking and swallowing abilities so that **enteral tube feeding**, which may be **nasojejunal** (Fig. 50.7) or **nasogastric**, may be necessary. Such feeding may be continuous or intermittent in circumstances where abdominal distension or severe regurgitation both become apparent.

Neonates who require assisted mechanical ventilation may run the risk of milk aspiration or the presence of milk in the stomach may embarrass respiration. In such instances **total parenteral nutrition** may be the more suitable means of providing nutritional support. It is usual to

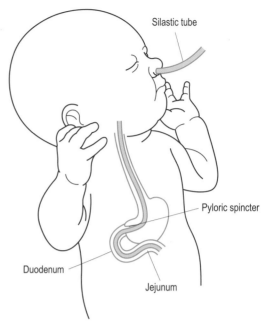

Figure 50.7 Baby with nasojejunal tube in situ (from Sweet B 1997, with permission).

commence with intravenous water and dextrose with the addition of salts such as sodium, phosphate and calcium. If parenteral feeding is to be continued, amino acids, lipids and vitamins and trace elements must be added. As the neonate's clinical condition improves, enteral feeding is introduced and gradually increased as the intravenous feeding regimen is reduced and discontinued.

Requirements Small and sick neonates will have additional nutritional requirements. Irrespective of whether enteral or parenteral feeding is chosen, the amount of fluid in which the nutrients are given must not exceed the kidney's ability to excrete the metabolic waste products. Premature neonates grow more rapidly than term babies and need therefore, on average, 600 kJ/kg/day. To achieve this level 180–200 ml/kg/day of breast milk or standard formula milk is necessary. Since this volume is excessive, the neonate's energy needs may be met by giving smaller amounts of LBW formula milk or adding calorific supplements to standard formula milk. Lucas et al (1992) reported that breast milk may be advantageous to central nervous system development and should be given whenever possible.

Nutritional supplements Growing neonates require **nutritional supplements**. These include vitamins A and D from the age of 1 month to 2 years due to the fact that premature babies have limited fat stores, which may have an impact on the neonate's ability to store and utilise fat-soluble vitamins. Vitamin C, a water-soluble vitamin, is also needed to support growth and healing and to aid iron absorption. As there is a delay in the production of erythrocytes by the bone marrow, premature infants can become very anaemic, sometimes requiring blood transfusion. In most instances, iron supplements are recommended from about the 4th week after birth until weaning.

The treatments themselves may contribute to problems. For instance, blood transfusion may suppress erythrocyte production and iron supplementation can increase the risk of infection by inhibiting the anti-infective properties of lactoferrin, allowing *Escherichia coli* to multiply. Very small babies may also require folic acid supplements. Calcium and phosphate supplementation may be required in order to increase the rate of bone mineralisation.

Excretion

Urine   As with all babies, the premature neonate should pass urine within 24h of birth and the amount should increase as fluid intake increases. All babies cared for in a neonatal unit should have their urine output measured, and the urine tested for glucose and **osmolality**. Glycosuria may indicate a lower renal threshold for glucose and this will require a review of the amount of glucose administered in order to avoid dehydration. The osmolality of the urine will indicate whether there is fluid retention or normal excretion, giving an indication of the amounts of fluids that need to be administered. Failure to produce urine or to micturate may be indicative of some haemodynamic problems such as hypotension, acute renal failure or urinary obstruction (Simpson 1997b). Each of these problems are potentially life threatening and care must be taken to monitor such developments and intervene in the earliest stages.

Faeces   The passage of meconium may be delayed in small premature infants, especially in those with respiratory distress syndrome or cystic fibrosis. Testing of the first meconium stool for the presence of abnormal constituents is important. The presence of blood and mucus in the stools may be indicative of a serious disorder such as necrotising enterocolitis and must therefore be attended to immediately.

Pain

For many years clinicians took little account of the pain suffered by newborn infants and small babies. Many believed neonates felt little pain. This view has now been largely dismissed by multiple studies showing that fetuses, neonates and small infants feel and respond to painful stimuli. From an evolutionary point of view this would seem to be an essential adaptation to extrauterine life!

Keeble & Twaddle (1995) discussed the benefits of developing an adequate tool for assessment of pain in the neonate. Response to pain stimuli may be behavioural, such as crying, grimacing and startle or withdrawing limbs; physiological, such as tachycardia, bradycardia, hypertension and increased oxygen requirements; or metabolic, manifesting as increased metabolic rate in response to decreased insulin secretion and increased corticosteroid release, leading to hyperglycaemia.

There may also be glycosuria, proteinuria, ketonuria and a raised urine pH (Simpson 1997b).

The relief of pain includes caring for the environment. Staff should develop expertise in techniques such as heel prick and intravenous line siting, procedures known to induce pain. Comfort interventions such as stroking, non-nutritive sucking, positioning and cuddling can reduce pain. Analgesia where required must be used with caution and anaesthesia should be used where invasive techniques and surgery are being carried out. Most neonates require postoperative analgesia although care must be taken not to suppress the neonate's respiratory drive and compromise respiratory function. Neonates whose respiratory function is supported by assisted mechanical ventilation may, if required, receive carefully selected sedatives and, as an adjunct to analgesia, muscle paralysing agents (Simpson 1997b).

Environmental neonatology

The premature neonate is adapted to the intrauterine environment and the effects of **noise**, **light**, **handling** and **positioning** may influence its wellbeing in the neonatal unit and beyond (Kelnar et al 1995). Such neonates require a vast amount of sleep yet neonatal units are not necessarily the most restful places for their occupants. Noise and light levels can be high and care often necessitates frequent handling disturbance. These factors are thought to contribute to apnoea and bradycardia and, in some instances, poor growth.

Noise   Noise levels are measured in logarithmic units called **decibels** (dB). The human ear is very sensitive and can hear sound over a wide range from a pin dropping to a shrieking steam whistle, a range from 0.1 dB to 120 dB. In adults, noise of 130 dB is invariably associated with inducing pain and therefore this level acts as a threshold. It must, however, be recognised that severe hearing dysfunction and loss can occur with continuous exposure to sound over 90 dB. Common sound levels include the background noise in a home (50 dB), a noisy restaurant (80 dB) and amplified rock music (over 90 dB) (Marieb 2000).

Ongoing research into the effects of noise on these babies, such as the continuous noise levels inside of an incubator, suggests that care should be taken to minimise all sounds. Kelnar et al (1995) argue in line with the British safety standard that 'the mean noise inside an incubator should not exceed 60 decibels' and yet many incubator alarms can exceed 85 dB! Sudden loud noise can cause sleep disturbance, crying, tachycardia, hypoxaemia and raised intracranial pressure in the baby (Long et al 1980). This suggests that extra care must be taken when closing portholes, cupboard doors and moving incubators.

Light   In order to observe babies adequately, the level of light in neonatal intensive care units (NICUs) has increased 5- or 10-fold in the last two decades. This, with the use of phototherapy lamps, increases the risk for the premature neonate of developing **retinopathy** (Glass et al 1985). Establishing a day/night pattern of lighting and dimming lights when not in use can reduce these harmful effects. Mann et al (1986) found that when noise and light stimuli were reduced at night the neonates slept on average 2 h/day longer and increased their weight gain more rapidly than babies who did not undergo the conventional day/night cycling. The practice of covering the neonate's eyes when undergoing **phototherapy** should be adhered to and bright sunlight must be avoided.

Handling   One significant problem in most neonatal units is the need to carry out investigations while providing invasive but comforting care. Thoughtful planning to ensure that interventions are carried out systematically and in a coordinated manner will allow for longer rest periods. Soothing and comforting interventions, including baby massage and 'kangaroo care', were evaluated by Lacy & Ohlsson (1993), who provide some insight into their benefits. **Facilitated tucking** (containment of the infant's arms and legs in a flexed position close to his trunk) was used as an intervention in mild pain and as a provision of comfort by Corff et al (1995).

Positioning   Kelnar et al (1995) cite various studies on the effects of faulty positioning in premature neonates (Fig. 50.8); for instance, Bottos & Stefani (1982) found that prolonged nursing in the **prone position** can result in externally rotated hips and everted feet, both of which may delay standing and walking. Fetters (1986) claims that a lack of careful positioning that mimics the flexed position that normal babies take up during the last few weeks in utero and extension from about 40 weeks may result in developmental delay.

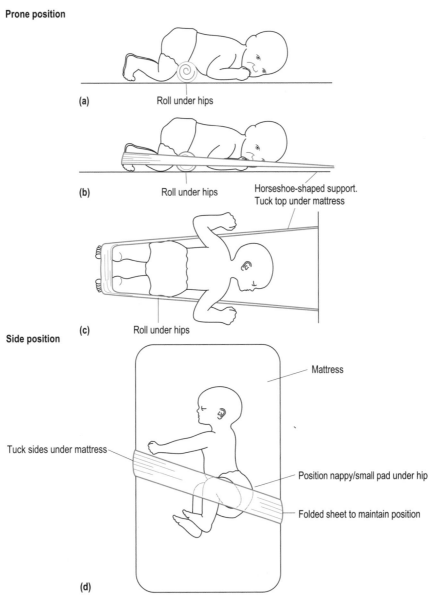

Prone position

(a)   Roll under hips

(b)   Roll under hips

Horseshoe-shaped support.
Tuck top under mattress

(c)   Roll under hips

Side position

Tuck sides under mattress

Mattress

Position nappy/small pad under hip

Folded sheet to maintain position

(d)

Figure 50.8   Prone positioning and side lying (from Kelnar C, Harvey D, Simpson C 1995, with permission).

Premature neonates often develop flattened, elongated and asymmetrically shaped heads. This can be minimised by altering the resting position of the head and taking care that the neonate's prone position is interspersed with lying in a lateral position with the hips and knees in optimal positions (Kelnar et al 1995).

Prevention of infection   Exposure to infectious pathogens is one of the most problematic experiences for the premature neonate whose immune system is not capable of mounting a full defence against infection. Therefore, the most important aspect of practice in busy neonatal units is prevention of infection by careful hand/forearm washing both before and after attending to each neonate, in conjunction with upholding the highest standards of hygiene. Appropriate liquid cleansing agents must be used and handwashing procedures must be followed. Gloves, and in some instances protective gowns, may need to be worn if body secretions are thought to be infectious.

For hygienic purposes each neonate must have a personal set of caring equipment stored in the vicinity of the incubator or cot. Care must be taken to allow sufficient space between cots or incubators to prevent cross-infection. Disposable items should be used where these are available and continuous vigilance with cleaning of equipment is essential. Staff or visitors with infections such as herpes simplex, upper respiratory tract infections, gastroenteritis or septic wounds should not enter a neonatal unit until their treatment is concluded.

THE SMALL-FOR-GESTATIONAL-AGE BABY

Neonates who are SFGA, sometimes referred to as 'light for dates', may have been affected by asymmetrical growth retardation or symmetrical growth retardation (Ch. 13). Most of these neonates are born after the 37th week of gestation and are frequently neurologically mature but lack subcutaneous fat (Fig. 50.9). As the fetal brain generally undergoes a growth spurt in the last trimester of pregnancy, there is a risk that this might have been compromised in some instances because of nutrient and oxygen deficiencies. Lack of energy stores can also compromise the fetus and its ability to cope with the process of labour and birth. The risk of **hypoxia** during labour and **hypoglycaemia** after birth is high. Other health problems which may later be attributed to the condition of these fetuses in utero are **hypertension** and **cardiovascular disease** and **mature-onset diabetes mellitus** (Barker 1992).

Asymmetrical growth retardation

According to Anderson & Hay (1999) asymmetrical growth retardation indicates that the body growth is restricted to a much greater extent than growth of the head, and thus the brain. In such cases brain growth is considered '**spared**'. Maternal conditions such as pre-eclampsia may be a

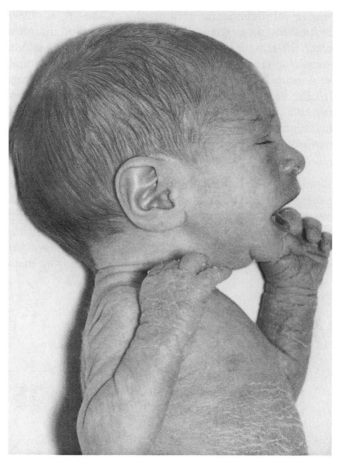

Figure 50.9   The small-for-gestational-age (SFGA or dysmature) baby (from Kelnar C, Harvey D, Simpson C 1995, with permission).

contributing factor as it frequently affects placental function to the detriment of the fetus. Fetal malnutrition may in such instances present as:

- the birth weight is low but the head circumference and length of the baby are normal for gestational age;
- there is a lack of subcutaneous fat and the body and limbs appear wasted;
- the ribs are visible and the abdomen is flat or hollow due to the small size of the liver;
- the skin is dry, loose and peeling and may be stained with meconium;
- the umbilical cord is thin and may also be stained with meconium;
- the face often looks old and wizened with large eyes and an anxious and hungry expression;
- muscle tone is generally good and the neonate is active;
- the neonate is very hungry and sucks his fist.

Symmetrical growth retardation

Symmetrical growth retardation implies that the fetal brain and body growth are limited, a phenomenon which may be apparent throughout the pregnancy (Anderson & Hay 1999). In this instance, the most common contributing factors could include intrauterine infections, maternal illness, fetal genetic or chromosomal abnormalities and maternal substance abuse. Characteristically, the neonate's head circumference is in proportion to body size and weight. These neonates may also experience greater morbidity and mortality in comparison to neonates who present with asymmetrical growth retardation.

Immediate management

Small-for-gestational-age fetuses should be delivered in a maternity hospital with a suitably equipped neonatal unit capable of providing appropriate immediate care. Complications may include perinatal asphyxia (Ch. 46), meconium aspiration syndrome, hypothermia, hypoglycaemia, **polycythaemia** and **pulmonary haemorrhage**. Most of these neonates will also present with **immunological deficiencies** such as reduction in lymphocyte number and function. As can be anticipated, some of these physical problems may extend beyond the neonatal period and therefore early specialist intervention is invaluable in limiting undesirable outcomes. Some of these problems will be discussed in Chapter 51.

Labour and delivery

Recognition of fetal growth retardation in utero offers an excellent opportunity for anticipating poor energy reserves, including limited fat, muscle and glycogen stores. It is essential, therefore, particularly during labour, to monitor fetal fitness by continuously observing fetal heart rate patterns and noting the presence of fresh meconium in the liquor. A paediatrician or midwife skilled in resuscitation should be present at the delivery and initiate appropriate therapeutic and supportive intervention when required. Since these neonates lack subcutaneous fat, loss of body heat can be rapid and the risks of hypothermia can be high. These neonates must therefore always be dried quickly and wrapped warmly as soon as practicable.

Ongoing care of small-for-gestational-age babies

The SFGA neonate has different health-related problems from the premature neonate. However, certain aspects of care such as the maintenance of body temperature, respiration, cardiac and renal function, nutrition and excretion require individual attention. Prevention of infection is a priority for both groups of babies. As these babies are usually active, vigorous, and alert and feed well, they may not require specialist care in a neonatal unit.

Transitional care

Transitional care wards have been developed in many maternity units, ideally situated near to the neonatal unit, to allow mothers to care for neonates with minor problems with supervision from experienced staff. Neonates who are small but only have minor problems, such as heat loss, benefit from being cared for by their mothers in such transitional care units. Mothers and babies are not separated and the mother is able to develop caring skills. Most of these neonates, regardless of their weight, are likely to be transferred home once they are well, providing that the home environment is suitable to their needs.

Early care in the first 48 h for such neonates is aimed at preventing complications such as hypoglycaemia, which is more likely to present following asphyxia or hypothermia. Frequent (3–4 hourly) recordings of blood glucose level are therefore important during the first 48 h or until plasma glucose values are stable. Since these neonates may develop transient neonatal diabetes mellitus, presenting with hyperglycaemia and glycosuria but no ketones in the urine, care must be taken to guard against **dehydration** and **failure to thrive** (Kelnar et al 1995). Although breastfeeding reduces the risk of infection, there is some advantage in offering such neonates LBW formula milk, which is energy dense.

All neonates require follow-up care to ensure that their growth and **developmental milestones** are monitored, especially when growth has been symmetrically retarded. Since intrauterine growth retardation may be associated with ongoing and later health problems and complications, careful monitoring of these babies may be a considerable advantage.

MAIN POINTS

- About 70% of perinatal mortality occurs in the 7% of babies whose birth weight is below the expected norm. Such neonates may be small at birth because of their prematurity or as a consequence of being small for gestational age (SFGA). Gestational age should be confirmed as soon as possible after birth using scoring systems such as the Dubowitz scale and the Parkin score.

- The woman in preterm labour must not be given drugs that could depress the fetal respiratory centre.

- An experienced paediatrician should be present at the time of delivery. As the neonate's respiratory muscles may be weak and the respiratory centre immature, difficulties may arise in establishing adequate respiration.

- Respiratory rate and effort should be adequate to keep the neonate well oxygenated. Carefully controlled oxygen therapy may be necessary to relieve cyanosis when respiratory or cardiovascular problems develop.

- Care must be taken to minimise the neonate's heat loss and body temperature maintained by providing a thermoneutral environment.

- The nutritional requirements of a neonate will depend on total body stores of fat, protein and glycogen as well as ongoing energy expenditure. Intestinal uptake and assimilation of nutrients and elimination of the by-products of digestion must therefore be carefully considered when planning any nutritional programme.

- The premature neonate is poorly equipped in terms of maintenance of metabolic and nutritional homeostasis. Fats are the main dietary source of energy and these provide up to 50% of the total caloric needs. Proteins supplies less than 14% of the daily caloric needs but are essential to ensure a steady supply of amino acids necessary to replace nitrogen lost in protein turnover.

- Enterally fed babies use carbohydrates as a major source of energy. A deficient glucose intake may result in gluconeogenesis from non-carbohydrate sources. In low birthweight (LBW) infants glycogen stores are usually lower in the early neonatal period and this may contribute to hypoglycaemia.

- The method of feeding a neonate is determined by his size, maturity and condition. If possible, breast or bottle feeds should be offered but premature neonates may have poor sucking and swallowing ability and nasogastric or jejunal tube feeding may be necessary. Ill babies may require total parenteral nutrition. Hydration is a critical component of the overall nutritional management. The neonate may also require nutritional supplements.

- All premature neonates should pass urine within 24 h of delivery and the amount should increase as fluid intake increases. Urinary output may have to be measured and the urine tested for glucose and osmolality. Glycosuria may suggest reducing the amount of glucose being administered. Urine osmolality suggests the volume of fluid required.

- The passage of meconium may be delayed in small premature neonates, especially in those with respiratory difficulties. However, the presence of blood and mucus in the stools may be indicative of necrotising enterocolitis.

- The nervous system is sufficiently developed to allow neonates to feel and react to painful stimuli. Painful responses must therefore be monitored and, where necessary, analgesia offered. Comforting interventions such as stroking can also reduce pain in some instances.

- The premature neonate gradually adapts to the extrauterine environment and the effect of noise, light, handling and positioning may influence this experience. Noise and light levels should be minimised to avoid problems such as light-induced retinopathy and noise-induced sleep problems.

- Prolonged nursing in the prone position may contribute to external rotation of hips and everted feet, which may eventually delay standing and walking. Changes in the position of the baby's head will avoid the elongated and asymmetrical head shape.

- The immune system in all premature neonates is immature and this contributes to the ongoing risk of infection. High standards of hygiene and careful handwashing and drying as well as incubator care are essential.

- Small-for-gestational-age neonates may present with asymmetrical or symmetrical growth retardation.

- Most neonates are born after the 37th week of gestation and are neurologically mature. Complications such as asphyxia, hypoglycaemia, meconium aspiration syndrome, hypothermia, polycythaemia and pulmonary haemorrhage may present after birth. They lack subcutaneous fat and lose heat rapidly but their active, alert behaviour usually poses no feeding problems.

- Small-for-gestational-age neonates may later develop long-term problems such as hypertension, cardiovascular disease and mature-onset diabetes mellitus.

- Small neonates may be cared for in transitional care wards by their mothers. It is essential to offer follow-up care to ensure that these babies meet their growth and developmental milestones.

References

Anderson M, Hay W 1999 Intrauterine growth restriction and the small for gestational age infant. In Avery G, Fletcher M, MacDonald M (eds) Neonatology – Pathophysiology and Management of the Newborn. Lippincott Williams and Wilkins, Philadelphia.

Barker D J P 1992 Fetal and Infant Origins of Adult Disease. BMJ Books, London.

Bottos M, Stefani D 1982 Postural and motor care of the premature baby. Developmental Medicine and Child Neurology 24:706–707.

Corff K E, Seideman R, Venkataraman P S et al 1995 Facilitated tucking: a non-pharmacological comfort measure for pain in preterm infants. Journal of Obstetric, Gynaecologic and Neonatal Nursing 24(2):143–147.

Crowley P 1996 Corticosteroids prior to preterm delivery. Cochrane Review: In The Cochrane Library, Issue 2. Update Software 2003, Oxford.

Dubowitz L M S, Dubowitz V, Goldberg 1970 Clinical assessment of gestational age in the newborn infant. Journal of Paediatrics 77:1–10.

Fetters L 1986 Sensory-motor management of the high risk neonate. Physical and Occupational Therapy, Pediatrics 6:217–229.

Gilady Y, Battino S, Reich D et al 1996 Delivery of the very low birth weight breech: what is the best way for the baby? Israel Journal of Medical Sciences 32(2):116–120.

Glass P, Avery G B, Subramanian K N et al 1985 Effect of bright light in the hospital nursery on the incidence of retinopathy of prematurity. New England Journal of Medicine 313:7.

Grant A, Glazener C M A 2000 Elective caesarean section versus expectant management for delivery of the small baby. Cochrane Review: In The Cochrane Library, Issue 4. Update Software 2003, Oxford.

Greer F 1991 Nutritional needs of the full-term and low-birth-weight infant. In Rudolph A (ed.) Rudolph's Paediatrics. Appleton and Lange, New York.

Keeble S, Twaddle R 1995 Assessing neonatal pain. Nursing Standard 10(1):16–17.

Kelnar C J H, Harvey D, Simpson C 1995 The Sick Newborn Baby. Baillière Tindall, London.

Lacy J B, Ohlsson A 1993 Behavioural outcomes of environmental or care-giving hospital-based interventions for preterm infants: a critical overview. Acta Paediatrica 82:408–415.

Long G J, Lucey J F, Philip A G S 1980 Noise and hypoxaemia in the intensive care unit. Pediatrics 65:143–145.

Lucas A, Morley R, Cole T J et al 1992 Breast milk and subsequent intelligence quotient in children born preterm. Lancet 339:261–264.

Mann N P, Haddow R, Stokes L et al 1986 Effect of night and day on preterm infants in a newborn nursery: randomised trial. British Medical Journal 293:1265–1267.

Marieb E N 2000 Human Anatomy and Physiology, 5th edn. Benjamin/Cummings, New York.

Papageorgiou A, Bardin C 1999 The extremely-low-birth-weight infant. In Avery G, Fletcher M, MacDonald M (eds) Neonatology – Pathophysiology and Management of the Newborn. Lippincott Williams and Wilkins, Philadelphia.

Parkin J M, Hey E N, Clowes J S 1976 Rapid assessment of gestational age at birth. Archives of Diseases in Childhood 51:259.

Simpson C 1997a The preterm baby. In Sweet B R, Tiran D (eds) Mayes Midwifery, 12th edn. Baillière Tindall, London, pp 833–851.

Simpson C 1997b Neonatal surgery and pain. In Sweet B R, Tiran D (eds) Mayes Midwifery, 12th edn. Baillière Tindall, London, pp 921–926.

Annotated recommended reading

Barker D J P 1992 Fetal and Infant Origins of Adult Disease. BMJ Books, London.
This textbook provides an invaluable account of the possible links between genetic inheritance, fetal growth and development, and the origins of disease in adults. The empirical evidence and the analytical style make a significant contribution to the practice of midwifery.

Barnes L 2000 Advances in Paediatrics, Vol. 47. Mosby, St Louis.

Barnes L 2001 Advances in Paediatrics, Vol. 48. Mosby, St Louis.
These are hugely informative textbooks that contain a considerable range of empirical evidence and some excellent critical analyses of biophysical and scientific issues of interest in clinical practice where the fetus, the neonate and the child are the focus of concern.

Blackburn S T 2003 Maternal, Fetal and Neonatal Physiology: A Clinical Perspective, 2nd edn. W B Saunders, Philadelphia.
This textbook offers excellent accounts of bioscientific aspects of knowledge which should be taken into consideration when managing the care of an expectant mother, the fetus and the newborn infant.

Boxwell G 2000 Neonatal Intensive Care Nursing. Routledge, London.
This textbook outlines a range of common and challenging neonatal problems and then provides helpful and directive suggestions for neonatal intensive care nursing. Critical analysis and reflection on the identified neonatal nursing concepts will reinforce best practice.

Grant A, Glazener C M A 2000 Elective caesarean section versus expectant management for delivery of the small baby. Cochrane Review: In The Cochrane Library, Issue 2. Update Software 2003, Oxford.
The Cochrane database offers a useful source for care in pregnancy, labour and the puerperium. Each research review is updated as necessary and the data is easily accessible in most colleges of nursing and midwifery. This update concludes that there is insufficient evidence to support elective caesarean section for small babies.

Lucas A, Morley R, Cole T J et al 1992 Breast milk and subsequent intelligence quotient in children born preterm. Lancet 339:261–264.
This is an enlightening discussion of the many advantages of breast milk feeding. Although breastfeeding offers considerable immunoprotection, its beneficial links with intelligence are not so well explored. This article exposes a new concept and invites critical analysis and possible research.

Polin R, Fox W 1998 Fetal and Neonatal Physiology, Vols 1 and 2. W B Saunders, Philadelphia.
These textbooks discuss bioscientific concepts important in fetal and neonatal care. The résumé of genetics leads to a more detailed exploration of normal and abnormal embryonic and fetal development. Overall, these books make a significant contribution to clinical practice and research.

Wong D 1999 Nursing Care of Infants and Children. Mosby, St Louis.
This textbook offers detailed accounts of the biophysical, psychosocial and nursing issues relevant in managing the care of infants and children. It concludes with a range of helpful appendices, which include excellent developmental screening tools and biophysical nomograms and parameters.

Chapter 51

Neonatal cardiovascular and respiratory disorders

INTRODUCTION

This chapter outlines common neonatal **cardiopulmonary problems** so that practitioners are aware of the need for possible intervention. Specialist textbooks should be sought where more comprehensive information is required. Avery et al (1999) and McCance & Huether (2002) provide helpful accounts of pathophysiological developments and clinical management. Neonates can become ill very quickly and practitioners' knowledge and competence may contribute to effective diagnosis and therapy to save life. All neonates causing concern should be referred to a paediatrician or a neonatal specialist.

CARDIOVASCULAR PROBLEMS

Cardiovascular abnormalities

Cardiovascular malformations make up the largest group of anomalies, accounting for about 30% of them. This averages between 7 and 8 per 1000 live births (Flanagan et al 1999). Neonates may present with **acyanotic** or **cyanotic cardiovascular anomalies**, the two categories leading to different clinical management.

Parents invariably ask why their child has a cardiac abnormality and whether it is likely to recur in future pregnancies. Although the specific cause of cardiac anomalies is unknown, links with many factors can be made, such as an association with chromosomal and genetic syndromes. For example **endocardial cushion defects** are associated with Down syndrome and **supravalvular stenosis** with Williams syndrome. The affected chromosomes/genes in many syndromes have been identified: for example, the genetic mutations encoding the **extracellular matrix proteins fibrillin-1** and **elastin** are responsible for Marfan syndrome and Williams syndrome, respectively. Genetic mutations on chromosome 22q11 may contribute to **aortic arch anomalies**, including **Fallot's tetralogy** (Flanagan et al 1999).

The cardiovascular anomalies can be differentiated into those leading to a **right-to-left shunt** in the heart, which

Table 51.1 Cardiac defects and their relative percentage occurrence

Right-to-left shunt	%	Left-to-right shunt	%	Obstructive disease	%
Transposition of the great vessels	4	Ventricular septal defect	33	Aortic stenosis	6
Tricuspid atresia	1–2	Patent ductus arteriosus	10	Pulmonary stenosis	8
Total anomalous pulmonary venous drainage	1–2	Atrial septal defect	8	Coarctation of the aorta	6

always results in **central cyanosis**, and those that contribute to a **left-to-right shunt**, which initially allows the neonate to be **acyanotic** (Table 51.1). Other cardiovascular lesions may be obstructive in nature, inhibiting either the right or the left ventricular outflow tract. Neonates that develop **heart failure** eventually present with considerable peripheral and central cyanosis (Flanagan et al 1999).

Risk factors

Contributory factors thought to play a role in the development of some cardiovascular anomalies are:

- maternal diabetes mellitus – ventricular septal defect (VSD), coarctation of the aorta and transposition of the great vessels;
- chromosomal abnormalities such as Down syndrome (40%) – atrioventricular defect (AVD), Fallot's tetralogy, VSDs and patent ductus arteriosus (PDA);
- genetic problems such as Williams syndrome;
- family history, where siblings or a parent have a cardiac defect;
- infectious agents such as those causing rubella or toxoplasmosis infection in pregnancy;
- nutritional/vitamin deficiencies;
- environmental factors and maternal drug abuse.

Presenting features in a neonate

Some of the following features may be present in neonates with cardiovascular lesions although some may also be suggestive of respiratory problems:

- tachypnoea/dyspnoea;
- grunting;
- pulmonary plethora;
- peripheral/central cyanosis;
- tachycardia;
- heart murmurs;
- poor feeding ability;
- poor weight gain;

- hepatomegaly;
- cachexia.

A paediatrician must examine all neonates presenting with any of the above symptoms. However, some cardiovascular problems may not be diagnosed for several weeks because the presenting features can at times be vague or misleading.

Investigations

Persistent tachypnoea may be the first indication of cardiovascular or pulmonary disease. Cardiovascular abnormalities with excessive pulmonary arterial blood flow or **pulmonary venous hypertension** generally contribute to pulmonary vascular engorgement and **pulmonary oedema**. These decrease the neonate's lung compliance, giving rise to increased respiratory rate and effort. In contrast, cardiovascular anomalies resulting in a decrease in pulmonary blood flow tend to contribute to intense cyanosis that elicits a tachypnoea without significant respiratory distress. A persistent respiratory rate of 60 breaths/min or greater accompanied by increased respiratory depth commonly precedes clinical deterioration.

Chest radiograph   A chest X-ray will establish the size and position of the heart in relation to the lungs and mediastinum. As some cardiovascular abnormalities change the normal size, shape and position of the heart, deviations from the normal appearance of the heart and lungs contribute significantly to the diagnosis.

Electrocardiogram   Electrocardiography is extremely valuable when the neonate presents with cardiac arrhythmia. However, ECG recordings may change rapidly in the first 72 h of life, partly reflecting the gradual transitions in right ventricular dominance normally evident in newborn infants. This must be remembered in using the ECG recordings in the overall diagnostic assessment.

Echocardiography   Exploration of the cardiovascular system by two-dimensional **echocardiography** involves ultrasound scanning (Fig. 51.1) and contributes to analysis of cardiovascular and intracardiac structures. Neonates are good candidates for echocardiographic imaging because of their thin thoracic walls. Images of the heart chambers, and valves and dimensions of the large vessels can be easily identified (Simpson 1997a). Although many abnormalities can be identified in the fetus from 16 weeks of gestation, new images are required after birth to confirm diagnosis.

Colour images help to visualise the presence and direction of blood flow in PDA, septal defects, systemic venous anomalies and arteriovenous malformations. Pulsed and continuous-wave **Doppler techniques** can estimate pressure gradients across stenotic valves, septal defects and abnormal vessel structures such as PDA and coarctation of the aorta. Surgical treatment may sometimes be initiated solely on the basis of echocardiographic findings without

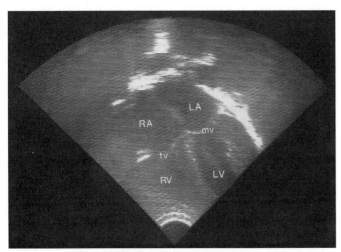

Figure 51.1   A four chamber echo of the normal heart (LA, left atrium; LV, left ventricle; RA, right atrium; RV, right ventricle; TV, tricuspid valve; MV, mitral valve) (from Kelnar C, Harvey D, Simpson C 1995, with permission).

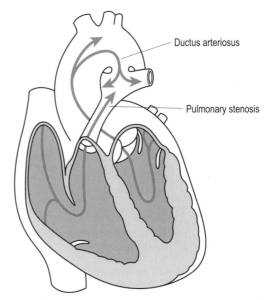

Figure 51.2   Persistent ductus arteriosus in the presence of pulmonary stenosis (from Fitzgerald M J T, Fitzgerald M 1994, with permission).

more invasive investigation such as cardiac catheterisation, but such decisions are dependent on local expertise and the nature and severity of the cardiovascular lesion.

Magnetic resonance imaging   Magnetic resonance imaging (MRI) may detect intrathoracic abnormalities of the aortic arch, the peripheral pulmonary arteries and the systematic collateral vessels which are not adequately evaluated by echocardiography.

Cardiac catheterisation and angiocardiography   These invasive investigations are required where cardiovascular defects are complex. Since such techniques are problematic, they are carried out in specialist paediatric cardiothoracic units. Cardiac catheterisation can be used to provide **palliative treatment** for neonates born with **transposition of the great arteries** or **tricuspid atresia**. Once the precise nature of the defects is established, catheterisation is used under general anaesthesia to carry out a **balloon septostomy** to enhance pulmonary blood flow. A fine catheter is inserted into the femoral vein, inferior vena cava, the right side of the heart, the pulmonary artery and its branches. If a septal defect is present, it may be possible to pass the catheter into the left side of the heart. Abnormal tracts can be identified and blood pressure and oxygen saturation within the heart and great vessels can be measured (Simpson 1997a).

Blood gases   Arterial blood gases from a baby breathing air followed by 100% oxygen can provide evidence for a differential diagnosis of a right-to-left shunt in cyanotic heart disease. PO_2 seldom exceeds 25 kPa in a baby with cyanotic heart disease breathing 100% oxygen, while a baby cyanotic because of a lung disorder will usually have a higher level of arterial oxygen. This test may provoke closure of the ductus arteriosus with disastrous consequences in neonates dependent on the ductal blood flow. In such instances prostaglandin is administered intravenously to induce the reopening of the ductus arteriosus for clinical reasons (Flanagan et al 1999).

Some common disorders – acyanotic lesions

Patent ductus arteriosus

The incidence of isolated persistent **patency of the ductus arteriosus** is about 1:2000 to 1:5000, or 10–12% of all congenital heart disease (Friedman & Silverman 2001). It is twice as common in females as in males. In a term infant the ductus arteriosus usually closes by 15 h following birth in response to increased blood oxygen saturation. Closure in premature infants may take up to 3 months when the specialised contractile tissue which enables the ductus to close develops. Under normal conditions this closure usually occurs spontaneously.

If the ductus arteriosus remains open, pulmonary resistance is reduced at birth as the blood flow is reversed and flows through the ductus from left to right, shunting oxygenated blood back into the pulmonary circulation. The ductus arteriosus may remain open when certain cardiac anomalies such as **pulmonary stenosis** are present (Fig. 51.2), providing a means of maintaining pulmonary perfusion. When spontaneous closure of this duct fails to occur, complications such as **congestive cardiac failure**, **pulmonary hypertension** and the risk of **subacute bacterial endocarditis** develop. In premature neonates the patency of the ductus contributes to the development and persistence of respiratory distress syndrome.

Symptoms of persistent PDA develop between the 3rd and 7th days following birth. The neonate develops tachypnoea, dyspnoea and lethargy. Systolic and diastolic

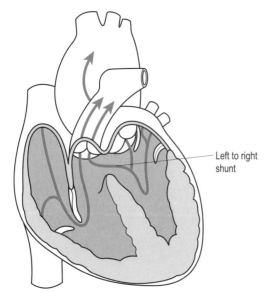

Figure 51.3 Ventricular septal defect (from Fitzgerald M J T, Fitzgerald M 1994, with permission).

murmurs are almost always present. Therapeutic intervention may include restriction of fluids, adequate oxygenation and, where necessary, treatment for congestive cardiac failure. This frequently consists of **digitalis**, **furosemide (frusemide)** and **potassium supplementation**.

Indometacin may be used to close the patent ductus in premature neonates but this is not generally effective in full-term infants (Kelnar et al 1995). Indometacin binds to plasma albumin, thus displacing bilirubin and leading to jaundice. In centres where appropriate expertise is available, transcatheter device occlusion should be the method of choice for ductal closure; however, more invasive methods of closure by means of a thoracotomy and ligation may be necessary if earlier medical management fails (Friedman & Silverman 2001).

Ventricular septal defects

Ventricular septal defects are the most common abnormality and account for approximately 20% of congenital heart malformations (Friedman & Silverman 2001). A VSD can occur as an isolated intracardiac abnormality but may also present as an adjunct to other cardiovascular lesions in about 50% of infants with congenital cardiovascular abnormalities. The defect usually occurs in the **membranous septum** but can present anywhere within the muscular part of the **interventricular septum** (Fig. 51.3).

The size and complexity of such defects varies from minute openings to almost complete absence of the interventricular septum. Knowledge of the precise size and position of the defect(s) is critical to management. The incidence of spontaneous closure is high (70%) although surgical repair is required where larger defects fail to close. Generally, infants with small defects may be asymptomatic and eventually experience spontaneous closure, resulting in normal cardiac anatomy. However, larger defects are

likely to lead to congestive cardiac failure, feeding problems and delays in normal growth.

Ventricular septal defects are commonly classified as acyanotic heart lesions with increased pulmonary blood flow because of the significant increase in left ventricular pressure which occurs after birth. The defect facilitates a left-to-right interventricular flow of blood. When there are multiple VSDs or a large VSD, the left-to-right shunt equalises the pressure in both ventricles. Thus, the rise in the right intraventricular pressure is almost entirely attributable to the ongoing shunting of oxygenated blood from the left ventricle directly into the right ventricle. As this shunting will eventually lead to right ventricular volume overload, problems such as **pulmonary plethora** and congestive cardiac failure will manifest. The persistent increase in pulmonary blood volume leads to an increased pulmonary venous return to the left side of the heart. This haemodynamic situation eventually results in left ventricular volume overload and exacerbation of the left-to-right shunt and to left ventricular hypertrophy.

For a time the enlarged left ventricle pumps more efficiently, but eventually the heart fails and pulmonary hypertension develops. If untreated, such clinical problems contribute in later childhood to the development of **Eisenmenger's syndrome** (McCance & Huether 2002). In order to avoid such difficulties, all neonates with large or problematic VSDs must be carefully managed. Congestive cardiac failure must be treated with diuretics and digitalis and potassium supplements until the defect can be closed surgically. If possible, surgery is delayed until the infant is at least 12–18 months old. All defects must ideally be closed, surgically if necessary, by the time the child enters school.

Atrial septal defect

Atrial septal defects are the most common congenital cardiac malformation. Some form of interference with atrial septal development may cause the variety of atrial septal defects (Srivastava & Olson 2000). Some may be simple, involving only the **foramen ovale**, while others may be complex, with considerable involvement of the **tricuspid** or **mitral valve**. Severe atrioventricular defects may involve the ventricular septum and mitral and tricuspid valves.

The most common of these defects are:

- **Septum primum** with endocardial cushion defects – this defect is generally associated with abnormalities of the mitral and tricuspid valves and atrioventricular canals (Fig. 51.4b). Although this defect may occur in isolation in otherwise normal infants, it most frequently occurs in infants with Down syndrome. The involvement of the endocardial cushions may contribute to the defective formation of the upper portion of the intraventricular septum.

- **Osteum secundum** – this defect is found in the central portion of the atrial septum. Because of its close anatomical association with the fossa ovalis, this defect may be appropriately known as the fossa ovalis defect (Fig. 51.4a).

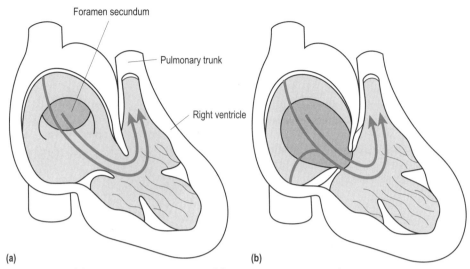

Figure 51.4 (a) Ostium secundum lesion. (b) Ostium primum lesion (from Fitzgerald M J T, Fitzgerald M 1994, with permission).

- **Sinus venosus** defect – this defect is characteristically found in the superior portion of the atrial septum and generally extends into the superior vena cava.

Simple defects cause few problems and, if spontaneous closure does not occur, surgical repairs are carried out by about 4–5 years of age. Since these defects cause a left-to-right intracardiac shunt, no cyanosis occurs. However, for babies born with atrioventricular defects (AVD), the prognosis is less favourable as they may experience conduction problems. About 30% of babies with AVD also have Down syndrome. The complex defects are usually established in the first few weeks of life as these infants present with dyspnoea, poor feeding and failure to gain weight. Mild cyanosis, abnormal heart sounds and a systolic murmur may occur (Flanagan et al 1999).

Some common disorders – cyanotic lesions

Transposition of the great arteries

Complete transposition of the great arteries (TGA) is the most common cardiovascular cause of peripheral and central cyanosis in neonates. In this anomaly, the aorta arises from the right ventricle and the pulmonary artery from the left ventricle. This complete switch of the great vessels (Fig. 51.5) leads to the formation of **two separate**, **closed circulatory systems**, whereby the blood from the pulmonary circulation cannot enter the systemic circulation and vice versa. Survival of these neonates depends on the patency of the right-to-left shunts in the ductus arteriosus and/or the foramen ovale. The presence of a concurrent VSD also permits mixing of the oxygenated and deoxygenated blood at the interventricular level. Boys appear to be affected twice as often as girls (Flanagan et al 1999).

A neonate with complete TGA and no accompanying ventricular defect will become increasingly cyanotic as

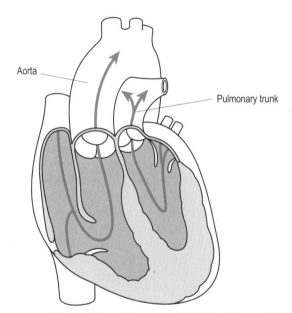

Figure 51.5 Transposition of great arteries (from Fitzgerald M J T, Fitzgerald M 1994, with permission).

the ductus arteriosus begins to close. This cyanosis is not relieved by administration of 100% oxygen and urgent life-saving intervention is needed. This is likely to consist of **prostaglandin infusion** to maintain the PDA open until palliative or corrective **surgery** can be carried out in a specialist paediatric cardiothoracic centre.

The palliative intervention may consist of a balloon septostomy (e.g. **Rashkind's**), generally carried out as an emergency to enlarge the foramen ovale and increase the interatrial mixing of blood. When it is possible, corrective surgery will be carried out some weeks later (Fig. 51.6). This consists of switching the pulmonary artery and the aorta to the appropriate ventricles and closing any remaining cardiovascular defects. Care is taken to ensure that the

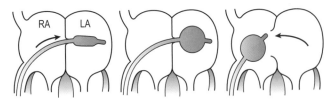

Figure 51.6   Rashkind's atrial septostomy. 1. A catheter is passed into the right atrium (RA) and pushed through the foramen ovale into the left atrium (LA). 2. A balloon at the tip of the catheter is inflated. 3. The catheter is withdrawn sharply so that the inflated balloon tears the atrial septum, allowing oxygenated blood to reach the systemic circulation. (Reproduced with permission from Wallis & Harvey 1979.)

coronary arteries can sustain **normal myocardial perfusion**. Most surgical corrections are successful with a survival rate of up to 90% (McCance & Huether 2002).

Total anomalous pulmonary venous drainage

Total anomalous pulmonary venous connection is characterised by the absence of any direct connection of the **pulmonary veins** to the **left atrium**. The pulmonary veins are connected to the right atrium, various systemic veins or the liver. Depending on these connections, oxygenated blood is returned into the right atrium, via the superior vena cava, the coronary sinus or the ductus venosus. About 30% of babies born with total anomalous pulmonary venous drainage (TAPVD) have other cardiac anomalies to consider in the management. Almost all the babies present with a right-to-left shunt of blood at atrial or ventricular level, allowing mixed arterial and venous blood to circulate to the lungs and body. Central cyanosis, dyspnoea, tachypnoea and congestive cardiac failure occur and urgent, life-saving surgical correction is necessary. Mortality can be high, averaging between 15 and 50% (Kelnar et al 1995).

Tetralogy of Fallot

The tetralogy of Fallot is the most common form of cyanotic congenital lesion in infants beyond the first year of life. Neonates can sometimes be asymptomatic. The tetralogy of Fallot classically consists of four anatomic defects (Fig. 51.7):

1. A high, large VSD.
2. An overriding aorta which straddles the VSD.
3. Pulmonary stenosis – a funnel-shaped opening at the entrance to the pulmonary artery. The pulmonary artery and valve may rarely be completely obliterated.
4. Right ventricular hypertrophy, developing because of the obstruction to blood flow.

These defects are associated with Down syndrome, first trimester rubella infection, Noonan's syndrome,

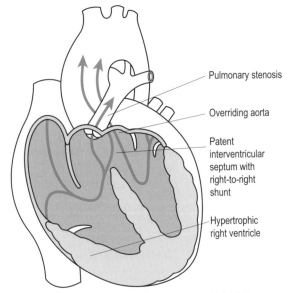

Figure 51.7   Tetralogy of Fallot (from Fitzgerald M J T, Fitzgerald M 1994, with permission).

Turner's syndrome and other undefined genetic mutations (Srivastava & Olson 2000).

The clinical features of this defect reflect the magnitude of the neonate's pulmonary blood flow, which depends on:

1. the severity of the right ventricular outflow tract obstruction;
2. the relative resistance to ventricular outflow imposed by the systemic and pulmonary circulations;
3. the presence of systemic-to-pulmonary collateral blood flow through the bronchial arteries or, rarely, a persistent ductus arteriosus.

The symptoms vary depending on the degree of pulmonary stenosis, although the size of the VSD is important. Pulmonary stenosis decreases the flow of blood to the lungs and the return of oxygenated blood to the left side of the heart. Where there is a large VSD, blood may shunt from the right ventricle to the left ventricle, causing further reduction in systemic oxygen content and an increase in central and peripheral cyanosis. However, giving oxygen in this instance may result in the closure of the PDA, further increasing cyanosis. Since hypoxia stimulates the kidneys to produce erythropoietin, most children will develop polycythaemia, which will require attention. Older children may have sudden spells of dyspnoea, cyanosis and restlessness and typically squat to alleviate these hypoxic spells.

Infants born with tetralogy of Fallot and pulmonary atresia usually require specialist surgical intervention of a corrective and/or palliative nature in the first few days or weeks of life. As most such infants will have a history of congestive cardiac failure which might impact on their growth and development, monitoring, evaluation and management in a specialist cardiac centre is advocated.

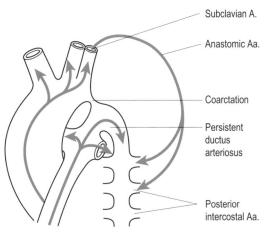

Figure 51.8   Preductal coarctation of the aorta (from Fitzgerald M J T, Fitzgerald M 1994, with permission). A., artery; Aa., arteries.

Subclavian A.
Anastomic Aa.
Coarctation
Persistent ductus arteriosus
Posterior intercostal Aa.

Some common disorders – obstructive lesions

Coarctation of the aorta

Coarctation of the aorta is characterised by an abnormal narrowing of the aorta anywhere between the origin of the aortic arch and the bifurcation of the abdominal aorta at its lower end. Commonly, it occurs at the junction with the ductus arteriosus, with 98% of cases being at this site. The narrowing may be before (**preductal**) (Fig. 51.8), at or after (**postductal**) the opening of the ductus arteriosus. In some infants **collateral arteries** develop to bypass the obstruction. Coarctation of the aorta results in obstruction to the outflow from the left ventricle and possible development of left ventricular failure. Many of these neonates eventually present with severe, life-threatening haemodynamic disturbances which can lead to acute myocardial and renal failure.

In postductal coarctation of the aorta, blood is delivered to the upper body from the ascending aorta via the subclavian arteries and the blood pressure to the upper body is increased. However, as blood flow to the lower extremities via the descending aorta is decreased, there is a significant reduction in the blood pressure of the lower limbs with decreased or absent **femoral pulses**.

Preductal coarctation is associated with a range of other anomalies. The ductus arteriosus may remain patent, creating a shunt where blood may flow in either direction depending on the pressure differences in the aorta and pulmonary artery. If blood flows from the right to the left, the right ventricle acts as a systemic pump and the blood pressure and pulse differences between the upper and lower extremities disappear. If the blood flow is directed from the left to the right, more than the normal amount of blood will be sent to the lungs, causing congestive heart failure with left ventricular hypertrophy.

Congestive heart failure may be one of the first presenting features, and must be managed accordingly. However, high oxygen levels must be avoided and prostaglandin may be given to maintain patency of the ductus arteriosus. Diuretics such as furosemide (frusemide) 1 mg/kg body weight may be given to decrease fluid overload, and the ensuing pulmonary and systemic oedema. Surgical correction and reconstruction of the defective segment of the aorta will be carried out as the infant's clinical condition is stabilised.

Pulmonary valve stenosis and aortic valve stenosis

Narrowing of the **pulmonary valve** occurs on its own in about 8% and **aortic stenosis** in about 6% of children born with congenital cardiac abnormalities. Mild cases of both valvular defects improve with age although more severe narrowing produces symptoms in neonates, most commonly pulmonary oedema and congestive cardiac failure. Surgical correction or, less commonly, valve replacement may be necessary in early infancy or childhood if cardiorespiratory function is compromising the child's growth, development and exercise tolerance.

Tricuspid atresia

Tricuspid atresia is relatively uncommon and manifests in the first few hours or days of life. The most distinctive clinical feature is extreme central cyanosis. This is caused by the entire systemic venous return entering the right atrium and exiting through the foramen ovale into the left side of the heart. As the systemic and pulmonary venous blood mix in the left atrium, the left ventricle receives only mixed oxygenated and deoxygenated blood. This is then pumped to the entire body, including the lungs. A variable, but small amount of blood will gain access to the pulmonary artery by way of the VSD. The diminutive right ventricle and pulmonary valve and pulmonary artery tend to control the pulmonary blood flow. Although the PDA will support the pulmonary blood flow initially, long-term survival will depend on the success of palliative and eventually corrective surgery.

Hypoplastic left heart syndrome

This syndrome is the consequence of a variety of specific cardiovascular malformations such as severe obstruction or atresia of the mitral valve, diminutive left ventricle, aortic atresia and malalignments of the **atrioventricular canals**. These neonates become symptomatic within the first few hours or days of life, developing congestive cardiac failure, poor cardiac output and poor peripheral perfusion. Cardiac enlargement, pulmonary plethora, hypotension and bradycardia will require supportive intervention . Most surviving neonates will require palliative surgery to enhance the quality of life. Despite advances in paediatric cardiothoracic surgery, the mortality rate for these infants is high because no successful corrective surgery is possible. **Cardiac transplantation** might be considered (Flanagan et al 1999).

Congestive cardiac failure

Congestive cardiac failure is a syndrome in which the failing heart cannot sustain a normal cardiac output and is unable to supply adequate oxygenated blood to the tissues. The major causes in the neonate are **excessive volume overload**, **excessive pressure load** and **abnormal myocardial function**.

Excessive volume overload

Large valve incompetence or left-to-right shunts are the most common causes of volume overload and in the neonate the cause is likely to be attributed to a PDA, large VSDs or endocardial cushion defects with gross valve incompetence. Less commonly, volume overload may be initiated by excessive placental transfusion at birth.

Excessive pressure load

Severe forms of aortic stenosis and coarctation of the aorta, commonly referred to as **left ventricular outflow tract obstruction**, lead to congestive cardiac failure in the first weeks of life. Infants with either of these lesions may present with very poor pulses and a large left-to-right shunt at the atrial level. The moderately severe pulmonary hypertension can be attributed to early congestive cardiac failure. Once the intra-atrial left-to-right shunt reverses or a large right-to-left shunt develops through the ductus arteriosus, the infant will present with moderately severe peripheral and central cyanosis.

Myocardial dysfunction

Hatch et al (1995) and Bristow (1996) argue that the fetal and neonatal myocardium develops much less **active tension** during **isometric contraction** than the myocardium of an adult. This may be because in the adult 60% of the myocardium is a contractile mass, whereas in the neonate or fetus the myocardium is much less compliant, resulting in a significant reduction in myocardial contractile force. The **myofibrils** are sparse, randomly organised and surrounded by considerable amounts of interstitial fluid (Larsen 2001). Therefore, the filling pressures in the heart of a newborn infant may need to be higher in comparison to the values seen in adults to optimise myofilament alignment.

Normal myocardial function in the neonate At birth the structure of the two ventricles is similar. However, as the neonate's physiological pulmonary vascular resistance falls, the right ventricle gradually adapts, losing power as it pumps to a low resistance system that doesn't require as much muscular effort. This physiological adaptation culminates in the disproportional changes and developments which characterise the two ventricles.

A characteristic feature of mature myocardium is its **sarcoplasmic reticulum**, which stores and releases calcium to support contractility. Since the neonatal myocardium has less sarcoplasmic reticulum (Bristow 1996) and reduced calcium storage facilities, it is more dependent on **trans-sarcolemmal calcium influx** than the adult myocardium. Gradual maturation of the myocardium increases the amounts of sarcoplasmic reticulum, although most neonates show a short-lived increase in ventricular performance when calcium is given to support myocardial contractility.

The neonatal myocardium is much less susceptible to hypoxia than the mature adult myocardium (Hatch et al 1995), which reflects the greater neonatal capacity for **anaerobic metabolism** and resistance to **acidosis**. This may be partly attributable to a more efficient **buffering capacity** of the immature myocytes, which allows smaller changes in intracellular pH.

Causes of neonatal myocardial dysfunction The most likely cause of neonatal myocardial dysfunction is **myocardial ischaemia** caused by an anomalous coronary artery (Freedman & Silverman 2001). However, in neonates the myocardium can also be severely depressed by **metabolic problems** such as severe postpartum asphyxia, marked hypoglycaemia, hypocalcaemia and hypomagnesaemia. **Arrhythmias** such as congenital heart block, paroxysmal tachycardia or bradycardia can cause cardiac failure in the fetus and the neonate. However, neonatal tachycardias are often intermittent and difficulties may occur in diagnosing these conditions. The causes of congestive cardiac failure must be diagnosed and successfully managed to avoid permanent damage to the heart and the entire cardiorespiratory system.

Common manifestations of congestive cardiac failure Manifestations of neonatal congestive cardiac failure include tachypnoea, pulmonary oedema, cyanosis, **diaphoresis**, feeding difficulties and, occasionally, periorbital or peripheral oedema (Rudolph et al 2002, Friedman & Silverman 2001). As the causes of congestive cardiac failure can be extensive and complex, it is essential that a specialist neonatologist establishes early diagnosis and efficient treatment. The neonate's survival and quality of life will depend on this control of the congestive cardiac failure and its primary cause.

RESPIRATORY PROBLEMS

This section is about lower respiratory tract problems in the neonate. **Breathing difficulties** are the commonest clinical problems encountered in neonates. Moreover, it is often difficult to make a clear diagnosis, even after examining a chest X-ray together with other diagnostic results. Infection is a further problem which is difficult to rule out and many neonates are given antibiotics until reliable microbiology results are available. Time of onset is important in confirming a diagnosis, as are the neonate's birth records. A major problem is the differential diagnosis of cyanosis, which may be caused by respiratory disorders or congenital heart disease (Flanagan et al 1999). A distinction must be made between these disorders if treatment is to succeed.

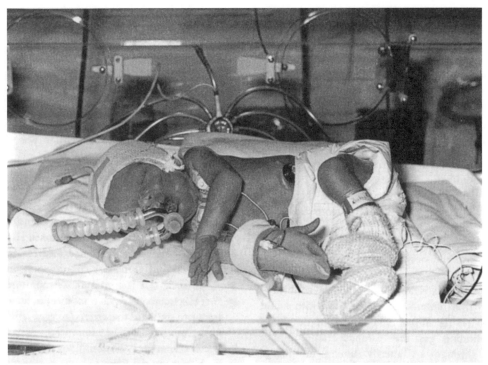

Figure 51.9   A baby having assisted ventilation (from Sweet B 1997, with permission).

Neonates with significant respiratory dysfunction accompanied by cyanosis are cared for in neonatal intensive care units by specialist practitioners (Fig. 51.9) (see Ch. 46).

Respiratory distress syndrome

The neonate initiates breathing at birth. The fluid-filled lungs inflate with air in response to inspiration. This displaces the lung fluid and contributes to enhancing pulmonary compliance and a greater pulmonary blood flow as the vascular tree expands. A 10-fold increase in pulmonary capillary blood is created, which facilitates efficient gas exchange across the alveoli walls, providing the lungs are sufficiently mature to synthesise **surfactant**.

Surfactant is a lipoprotein complex secreted by the type II pneumocytes (deMello & Reid 1995). It consists of 90% **lipids**, including **lecithin**, **sphingomyelin** and **cholesterol**; the remainder is made up of substances such as specific proteins and some carbohydrates. Surfactant originates in the intracellular lamellar bodies, from which it is extruded into the alveolar space. There, it unravels to form a complex lipid structure called **tubular myelin**, which forms the **surface monolayer**, the most functionally active form of surfactant, at the air–liquid interface in the alveolus.

The fetal lungs secrete surfactant from about the 22nd week, with considerable surges occurring at 33 weeks of gestation and at birth. Surfactant coats the inner aspect of the alveoli and reduces surface tension, ensuring that the alveoli do not collapse at the end of expiration. The ratio of lecithin to sphingomyelin (**L/S ratio**) is 1:1 at about 34 weeks of gestation, but then the amount of lecithin increases until the ratio is 2:1, comparable to a mature lung. Amniotic fluid contains both these substances and can be tested to establish fetal lung maturity.

Respiratory distress syndrome (RDS, **hyaline membrane disease**) occurs in premature neonates. This severe lung disorder causes more neonatal deaths than any other condition. The incidence is inversely proportional to gestational age. It occurs in about 70% of neonates born at 29 weeks of gestation, declines sharply to near 0% at 39 weeks (Ariagno 1995) and is rarely seen after 37 weeks of gestation. It is fairly common in term infants born to mothers suffering from diabetes mellitus. The cause is multifactorial, but insufficient active pulmonary surfactant is the major contributing factor. Predisposing factors depend on lung maturation and include:

- immature lungs, particularly in male infants;
- birth by caesarean section prior to the onset of labour;
- asphyxia neonatorum, as respiratory and metabolic acidosis interfere with surfactant synthesis;
- hypovolaemia or hypervolaemia;
- mother has a history of diabetes mellitus (this seems to delay lung maturity);
- premature/prolonged rupture of membranes;
- maternal antepartum haemorrhage;
- maternal haemodynamic instability;
- maternal substance abuse.

Pathophysiology

Respiratory distress syndrome is caused by immaturity of the type II cells and their incapacity to produce sufficient surfactant. A greater inspiratory effort is needed to keep the alveoli open. Poor alveolar stability contributes to poor lung compliance, limited lung distensibility and reduced functional residual capacity. This has a direct impact on **pulmonary perfusion** and most neonates develop a significant right-to-left shunt, which contributes to significant hypoxia with a depressing effect on myocardial function. A PDA may also contribute to existing cardiorespiratory problems. Some neonates will eventually develop hypotension and poor renal and peripheral perfusion.

Other problems such as **respiratory acidosis** and **atelectasis** (inadequate alveolar expansion and collapse of lung tissue preventing respiratory gas exchange) contribute to the ongoing events. The atelectasis is generally attributed to unequal pressures and filling capacity in some alveoli. The normal alveoli become overdistended and the smaller alveoli collapse, reducing the functional residual capacity and creating a significant **dead space** within the lungs (Blackburn 2003).

The resulting hypoxia and **hypercapnia** lead to pulmonary vasoconstriction and, sometimes, **persistent fetal circulation** with significant intracardiac right-to-left shunting of blood through the foramen ovale and ductus arteriosus. Lung ischaemia exacerbates the damage to the alveolar epithelial surfaces and capillaries. Metabolic and respiratory acidosis further suppresses the production of surfactant (Ariagno 1995, Whitsett et al 1999).

Increased alveolar surface tension combined with the low plasma protein levels present in the preterm baby leads to a shift of interstitial fluid towards the alveolar space. As the exudate is rich in **fibrinogen**, it is converted to **fibrin**, which lines the alveoli. Blood products and cellular debris present within the alveoli are bound by the fibrin and form a **hyaline membrane**, which further reduces lung surface area (Blackburn 2003) and makes the lungs less compliant.

Clinical symptoms

Affected neonates gradually develop symptoms over a few hours and, typically about 4 h after birth, they develop tachypnoea with increased respiratory effort and grunting on expiration. Characteristically, there is chest wall recession, peripheral and later central cyanosis (Fig. 51.10). A chest X-ray shows a 'ground-glass' appearance to the lungs, whereas an air bronchogram (Fig. 51.11) shows air in the larger airways against the background opaqueness (Whitsett et al 1999).

Management of respiratory distress syndrome

Prebirth maternal treatment with corticosteroids Management of RDS includes prevention and treatment. The production of surfactant in the fetal lung can be increased by treating the mother with a **corticosteroid** such as betamethasone for at least 24 h before birth. Indications for

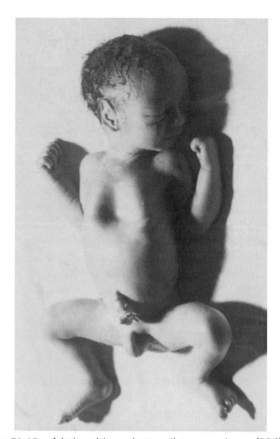

Figure 51.10 A baby with respiratory distress syndrome (RDS). Note marked sternal recession (from Kelnar C, Harvey D, Simpson C 1995, with permission).

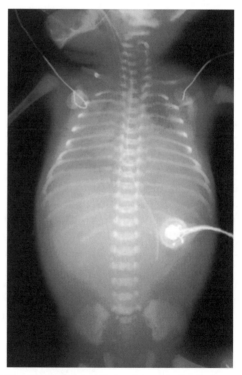

Figure 51.11 Chest X-ray showing 'ground-glass' appearance of lungs in hyaline membrane disease (from Kelnar C, Harvey D, Simpson C 1995, with permission).

commencing corticosteroid administration may be a low L/S ratio or, if this invasive test is not possible, the anticipated premature birth. Crowley's (1996) review of the research concluded that this proactive management reduces the risk of RDS in susceptible neonates and contributes to significant reduction in morbidity and mortality.

Surfactant therapy   The use of natural and artificial surfactant postdelivery has been effective in the management of affected neonates. Soll & Blanco (2001) updated earlier reviews of research into **surfactant therapy**, concerning the benefits and drawbacks of natural versus synthetic surfactant and multiple versus single dose of natural surfactant. Both natural and artificial surfactants were effective in the treatment of established RDS. There was earlier improvement in neonates who required assisted ventilatory support (Stevens et al 2002), with fewer instances of **pneumothorax** in neonates treated with natural surfactant extract. Multiple doses of natural surfactant extract resulted in greater improvements in respiratory function and oxygen levels, reducing the occurrence of pneumothoraxes. Multiple doses of natural surfactant extract appear to be the most effective treatment.

Oxygen therapy   Oxygen therapy is necessary to prevent hypoxic brain damage. Some neonates only require humidified oxygen administered into a headbox providing the necessary oxygen-rich air. Others may require **continuous positive airway pressure** (CPAP) to reduce the work of breathing by maintaining a constant alveolar end-expiratory pressure of 5–10 cmH$_2$O. However, very small babies and those with severe RDS may require mechanical ventilation by **intermittent positive pressure ventilation** (IPPV) (Simpson 1997b, Whitsett et al 1999). Complications of oxygen therapy include:

- long-term oxygen therapy and IPPV may result in pneumothorax or bronchopulmonary dysplasia;
- periventricular haemorrhages may occur where oxygen saturation is badly controlled or excessive;
- infection and secondary pneumonia may follow endotracheal intubation and periodic lavage to keep the tube patent;
- retinopathy may be caused by the administration of high oxygen concentration;
- episodes of stress may cause metabolic disturbances;
- both hypothermia and hypoglycaemia can increase oxygen requirements and energy expenditure.

Bronchopulmonary dysplasia

Bronchopulmonary dysplasia is a form of subacute or chronic **fibrosis of the lungs** associated with severe hyaline membrane disease, prolonged assisted mechanical ventilation and high oxygen requirement. This disorder affects infants weighing less than 1500 g at birth (Kelnar et al 1995). Affected infants remain oxygen dependent, have respiratory

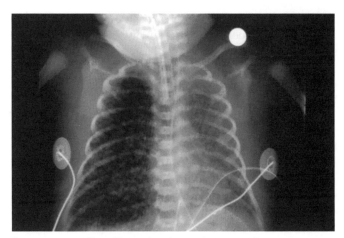

Figure 51.12   Chest X-ray showing early stages of bronchopulmonary dysplasia (from Kelnar C, Harvey D, Simpson C 1995, with permission).

Table 51.2   Some events occurring in infants with bronchopulmonary dysplasia

Pulmonary injury and barotrauma	Resolution and healing	Catch-up growth in surviving lung tissue
Pulmonary oedema	Phagocytosis and absorption of inflammatory products	Alveolar multiplication
Cell necrosis	Scarring of lung tissue	Pulmonary vascular remodelling
Hyaline membrane formation	Overinflation of the intervening lung	
Atelectasis	Increased resting volume	

symptoms such as tachypnoea and intercostal recession and abnormal lung findings on radiography (Fig. 51.12) after 28 days (McCance & Huether 2002).

Scarring of the lung tissue, **emphysema**, failure of the alveoli to multiply and inflammatory destruction of the epithelial lining of the lungs and ciliated epithelial surfaces in the bronchi are characteristic features. In addition, mucus plugs and debris clog the small-diameter airways, contributing to recurrent pulmonary infection. Many of the affected infants experience some of the events shown in Table 51.2 (deMello & Reid 1995). The clinical picture may persist for some months or years. Some babies go on to recover but others die.

Therapy involves maintenance of normal oxygen saturation, prevention of infection and adequate nutrition. Dexamethasone may be used to reduce the inflammatory changes and improve oxygenation without increasing the risk of infection (Ng 1993). Antibiotics can be used to control infection. Once the infant's condition is stabilised and the parents can manage the oxygen therapy and other supportive interventions, home care is encouraged. Ideally, a community specialist paediatric nurse and health visitor should support the family.

Meconium aspiration syndrome (MAS)

When a fetus suffers from intrapartum asphyxia, meconium is passed into the amniotic fluid and inhaled as gasping movements are made. At birth, prompt clearing of the mouth and upper airways must be carried out to avoid the consequences of such inhalation. Any meconium present must be removed.

Management

Meconium encourages growth of microorganisms and any neonate suspected of having inhaled meconium must be observed for signs of respiratory distress manifesting as tachypnoea and cyanosis for the next 24–48 h. Oxygen therapy may be required and a prophylactic course of antibiotics may be given to avert the onset of **pneumonia**. The more severely affected neonates may develop persistent fetal circulation, resulting in cardiopulmonary problems such as pulmonary hypertension, systemic hypotension and hypoxia. Pneumothoraxes are a relatively common complication (Kelnar et al 1995).

Surfactant treatment

The presence of meconium in the lung may inactivate surfactant and short-term administration of surfactant (four doses every 6 hours) commenced within 6 hours of birth improved oxygenation and reduced respiratory morbidity (Soll & Dargaville 1999). However, where persistent fetal circulation and pulmonary hypertension are severe, more drastic measures involve assisted ventilatory support using high-frequency oscillatory ventilation and nitric oxide. The relative efficacy of surfactant therapy, either alone or in conjunction with **nitric oxide** or ventilation, needs more research (Soll & Dargaville 1999).

Pneumothorax

A pneumothorax occurs as a result of injury to the pleural membranes, allowing air to leak into the pleural space. In neonates the most likely cause of pneumothorax is alveolar rupture and associated damage to the visceral layer of the **pleural membrane**. The affected lung collapses, causing a mediastinal shift and displacing the normal position of heart and greater vessels. This may in turn compromise cardiac function, initiating low cardiac output, hypotension and bradycardia. Recently, the selective use of surfactant therapy has contributed to a significant reduction in the number of neonates developing a pneumothorax and requiring additional supportive interventions.

Management

A pneumothorax does not present with the classical symptoms seen in the adult and may be difficult to diagnose. The neonate suddenly collapses and becomes cyanotic with bradycardia. There may be cardiac displacement and **transillumination**; shining a cold light against the thorax may demonstrate air around the lung (Kelnar et al 1995). Chest radiography will confirm the diagnosis (Fig. 51.13). If the neonate is otherwise in good health, draining the air may not be necessary as it will be gradually reabsorbed. However, neonates who experience respiratory distress and haemodynamic changes will require the insertion of a pleural drain connected to underwater sealed drainage that allows the air to escape and the lung to re-expand.

Transient tachypnoea of the newborn

Transient tachypnoea of the newborn (TTN) is relatively common in neonates at term who present with tachypnoea, intercostal retraction, slight grunting and possibly cyanoses. A chest X-ray will show enlarged lymph vessels, which appear as streaks, and signs of **pulmonary interstitial oedema** (Simpson 1997b). This course of events may persist from 2 to 5 days. Although the precise cause remains unknown, the most obvious factor is a mild immaturity in the surfactant system which may be responsible for surfactant deficiency or failure to absorb lung fluid following delivery (Whitsett et al 1999). Most neonates require less than 40% of oxygen to maintain systemic oxygenation.

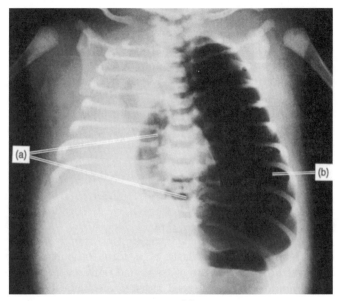

Figure 51.13 Pneumopericardium (a) with a large left pneumothorax (b) (from Kelnar C, Harvey D, Simpson C 1995, with permission).

Sudden infant death syndrome

A **sudden infant death** is the unexpected death of an otherwise healthy infant. These deaths are usually unexplained by postmortem examination. The term sudden infant death syndrome (SIDS) should only be used when it is the sole cause of death stated on the death certificate. Such deaths almost always occur during sleep and the peak incidence is from 2 to 4 months of age. Less than 1% of such deaths occur under the age of 2 months. Boys are more likely to die than girls are, and low birthweight babies are at higher risk. These deaths occur more commonly in winter. McCance & Huether (2002) suggest that SIDS is 'the greatest single cause of death amongst infants between 1 week and 1 year of age'.

The causes of sudden infant death syndrome

SIDS is a complex phenomenon (Platt & Pharaoh 2003). Although a number of key factors such as the infant's sleeping position, overheating, sudden illness and possible effects of smoking by the parents are thought to be contributory factors, further research is required.

Position of the larynx   The position of the infant's larynx and its close contact with the soft palate, which normally facilitates the infant's ability to breathe and swallow simultaneously, may be a contributing factor (Morgan 1994). From the 3rd month the **larynx** moves to a position below the back of the tongue, an arrangement necessary for speech production. Crelin (1973) first postulated that this may influence the occurrence of SIDS. The risk is highest during the transitional period and once the larynx has reached its new position at 6 months the risk of death falls. This is unlikely to be the sole cause but should be considered by researchers. Morgan also postulates that in neonates who lie in the prone position, the **uvula** may enter the larynx and block the airway. If the infant is ill, weak and cannot change the position of his head and neck, he may suffocate.

Sleeping position   The fashion for placing babies in the **prone position** for sleeping was introduced in the Netherlands in the 1970s. Babies lying in the prone position were thought to be less likely to inhale regurgitated feeds. However, this practice led to a three-fold increase in SIDS and enhanced research interest in the effects of sleeping position on the occurrence of SIDS. The studies of the 1980s concluded that death rates were lowered if infants were placed on their backs when sleeping. Fleming et al (1990) found an eight-fold increase in risk if a baby was placed prone for sleeping rather than on its side or back. Placing an infant on his side doubles the risk, possibly because babies can easily roll onto their stomachs.

Overheating   Tuffnell et al (1996) found that deep body temperature in infants who co-sleep with their parents was higher than in infants who slept alone. Parents are advised to separate their bodies from the baby by making a separate 'nest' for the baby with pillows. Mothers tend to wrap up their babies in the winter months or during illness. Fleming et al (1990) found that the occurrence of SIDS tended to coincide with infants being heavily wrapped, lain prone and allowed to sleep in an overheated room.

Smoking   Studies have shown that smoking in pregnancy increases the risk of SIDS (Schoendorf & Kiely 1992). The effects of **passive smoking** are not as easy to prove but there may be an increased risk if both parents smoke. Because of a steady rise in SIDS in England and Wales, peaking at 2.3/1000 in 1988, campaigns aimed at reducing the deaths were introduced in 1991 by the Foundation for the Study of Infant Deaths and the Department of Health. Between 1991 and 1995 the SID rate in England and Wales, which had already fallen from the high point of 1988, fell 50% from 1.4 to 0.6/1000 live births (Office for National Statistics 1996). The recommendations were that:

1. babies should not be placed upon their fronts to sleep;
2. babies should not be overheated;
3. if babies are unwell, medical help should be sought;
4. babies should not be exposed to cigarette smoke.

MAIN POINTS

- Cardiovascular anomalies, which are responsible for 30% of all congenital malformations, can be grouped into cyanotic or acyanotic heart disease. Tachypnoea, dyspnoea, cyanosis, tachycardia, bradycardia, hypo- and hypertension, heart murmurs, poor feeding, grunting and peripheral oedema may be present.

- Closure of the ductus arteriosus in the preterm infant may take up to 3 months. Therapeutic interventions include restriction of fluids, adequate oxygen administration. Indometacin and invasive ligation may be necessary if medical management fails.

- Ventricular septal defect may present with other defects in 50% of children with congenital heart lesions. Small VSDs may be asymptomatic and close spontaneously. Large defects lead to haemodynamic problems and congestive cardiac failure which must be treated prior to surgical closure.

- Simple atrial septal defects cause few problems although repair should be carried out before the child enters school. However, infants born with atrioventricular canal defects may experience conduction problems prior to and following surgical correction.

- Transposition of the great vessels leads to the formation of two separate circulatory systems which do not facilitate the transfer of oxygenated blood into the systemic circulation. The infant's survival depends on the patency of the ductus arteriosus, the foramen ovale and the existence of a VSD which must be preserved until corrective surgery is possible.

- Total anomalous pulmonary venous connection interferes with normal pulmonary venous return to the left atrium. As oxygenated blood returns to the right side of the heart, the baby rapidly develops cyanosis, tachypnoea and other haemodynamic problems requiring urgent surgical correction.

- The classical features of tetralogy of Fallot are a high, large ventricular septal defect; an overriding aorta, which straddles the VSD; pulmonary stenosis; and right ventricular hypertrophy. Surgical correction is necessary.

- Coarctation of the aorta commonly occurs at the junction with the ductus arteriosus. Collateral arteries can develop to bypass the obstruction. Abnormal blood pressure and pulses can be the first sign. Prostaglandin administration may maintain patency of the ductus arteriosus to sustain the systemic circulation until a surgical correction is possible.

- The major causes of neonatal congestive cardiac failure are excessive volume overload, excessive pressure load and abnormal myocardial function. Effective diagnosis and treatment of congestive cardiac failure is essential for survival and quality of life.

- In respiratory distress syndrome, increasing inspiratory effort and expiratory difficulties may lead to respiratory failure and atelectasis. Hypoxia and hypercapnia lead to pulmonary vasoconstriction and persistent fetal circulation. Natural/synthetic surfactant administration following birth has significantly reduced infant morbidity and mortality.

- In bronchopulmonary dysplasia infants may remain oxygen dependent. Dexamethasone may reduce pulmonary inflammation. Some infants show considerable recovery in pulmonary function whereas others experience permanent pulmonary scarring and ongoing respiratory problems.

- Inhalation of meconium may cause respiratory difficulties. Oxygen therapy and antibiotics may be needed to avoid pneumonia. Surfactant therapy commenced within 6 h of birth may improve prognosis.

- A pneumothorax may occasionally occur as a result of other primary respiratory problems. As this can influence haemodynamic stability, it will require invasive therapeutic intervention.

- Transient tachypnoea of the newborn may be caused by mild surfactant deficiency or failure to absorb lung fluid following birth. Oxygen therapy generally aids gradual recovery.

- Sudden infant death almost always occurs during sleep, with a peak incidence in the winter. Low birthweight babies are at higher risk. Causative factors include sleeping position, overheating, undetected illness and parental smoking. To date, no single common factor has been isolated. Successful campaigns aimed at reducing SIDS in England and Wales were introduced in 1991.

References

Ariagno R 1995 Respiratory problems in the preterm infant. In Reed G, Claireaux A, Cockburn F (eds) Diseases of the Fetus and Newborn – Pathology, Imaging Genetics and Management, Vol. 2. Chapman and Hall Medical, London.

Avery G, Fletcher M, MacDonald M 1999 Neonatal Pathophysiology and Management of the Newborn. Lippincott, Williams and Wilkins, Philadelphia.

Blackburn S T 2003 Maternal, Fetal and Neonatal Physiology: A Clinical Perspective, 2nd edn. W B Saunders, Philadelphia.

Bristow J 1996 Cardiac and myocardial structure and myocardial cellular and molecular function. In Gluckman P, Heyman M (eds) Paediatric Perinatology – The Scientific Basis. Arnold, London.

Crelin E 1973 Functional Anatomy of the Newborn. Yale University Press, New Haven, Connecticut.

Crowley P 1996 Prophylactic corticosteroids for preterm birth. Cochrane Review: In The Cochrane Library, Issue 1. Update Software 2003, Oxford.

DeMello D, Reid L 1995 Respiratory tract and lungs. In Reed G, Claireaux A, Cockburn F (eds) Diseases of the Fetus and Newborn – Pathology, Imaging, Genetics and Management, Vol. 2. Chapman and Hall Medical, London.

Flanagan M, Yeager S, Weidling S 1999 Cardiac disease. In Avery G, Fletcher M, MacDonald M (eds) Neonatal Pathophysiology and Management of the Newborn. Lippincott, Williams and Wilkins, Philadelphia.

Fleming P J, Gilbert R, Azaz Y et al 1990 Interaction between bedding and sleeping position in sudden infant death syndrome: a population based case-control study. British Medical Journal 301:85–89.

Friedman W, Silverman N 2001 Diseases of the heart, pericardium and pulmonary vascular beds – congenital heart disease in infancy and childhood. In Braunwald E, Zipes D, Libby P (eds) Heart Disease – A Textbook of Cardiovascular Medicine, Vol. 2. W B Saunders, Philadelphia.

Hatch D, Somner E, Hellman J et al 1995 The Surgical Neonate: Anaesthesia and Intensive Care. Edward Arnold, London.

Kelnar C J H, Harvey D, Simpson C 1995 The Sick Newborn Baby. Baillière Tindall, London.

Larsen W 2001 Human Embryology. Churchill Livingstone, New York.

McCance K L, Huether S E 2002 Pathophysiology, The Biologic Basis for Disease in Adults and Children, 3rd edn. Mosby, St Louis.

Morgan E 1994 The Descent of the Child. Souvenir Press, London.

Ng P C 1993 The effectiveness and side effects of dexamethasone in preterm infants with bronchopulmonary dysplasia. Archives of Diseases in Childhood 68:330–336.

Office for National Statistics 1996 Population and Health Monitor DH3 (Sudden Infant Deaths), 96/2. ONS, London.

Platt M, Pharaoh P 2003 The epidemiology of sudden death syndrome. Archives of Diseases in Childhood 88:27–29.

Rudolph A, Hoffman J, Rudolph C et al 2002 Rudolph's Paediatrics. Prentice-Hall, New Jersey.

Schoendorf K C, Kiely J L 1992 Relationship of sudden infant death syndrome to maternal smoking during and after pregnancy. Pediatrics 90:905–908.

Simpson C 1997a Cardiac and circulatory conditions in the newborn. In Sweet B R, Tiran D (eds) Mayes Midwifery, 12th edn. Baillière Tindall, London, pp 882–888.

Simpson C 1997b Respiratory disorders of the neonate. In Sweet B R, Tiran D (eds) Mayes Midwifery, 12th edn. Baillière Tindall, London, pp 889–895.

Soll R F, Blanco F 2001 Natural surfactant extract versus synthetic surfactant for neonatal respiratory distress syndrome. Cochrane Review: In The Cochrane Library, Issue 1. Update Software 2003, Oxford.

Soll R F, Dargaville P 1999 Surfactant for meconium aspiration syndrome in full term infants. Cochrane Review: In The Cochrane Library, Issue 1. Update Software 2003, Oxford.

Srivastava D, Olson E 2000 A genetic blueprint for cardiac development. Nature 47:221–226.

Stevens T P, Blennow M, Soll R F 2002 Early surfactant administration with brief ventilation vs. selective surfactant and continued mechanical ventilation for preterm infants with or at risk for RDS. Cochrane Review: In The Cochrane Library, Issue 1. Update Software 2003, Oxford.

Tuffnell C S, Petersen S A, Wailoo M P 1996 Higher rectal temperatures in co-sleeping infants. Archives of Diseases in Childhood 75(3):249–250.

Whitsett J, Pryhuber G, Rice W, Warner B, Wert S 1999 Acute respiratory disorders. In Avery G, Fletcher M, MacDonald M (eds) Neonatal Pathophysiology and Management of the Newborn. Lippincott Williams and Wilkins, Philadelphia.

Annotated recommended reading

Boxwell G 2000 Neonatal Intensive Care Nursing. Routledge, London.
This textbook outlines a range of common and challenging neonatal problems and then provides helpful and directive suggestions for neonatal intensive care nursing which allows critical analysis and reflection on the identified neonatal nursing concepts and reinforces best practice.

Crowley P 1996 Prophylactic corticosteroids for preterm birth. Cochrane Review: In The Cochrane Library, Issue 1. Update Software 2003, Oxford.
This article provides an invaluable review of empirical evidence concerning the use of corticosteroids as a preventative measure against respiratory distress syndrome. The overall conclusions are supportive of such prophylactic administrations of the chosen corticosteroids.

Friedman W, Silverman N 2001 Diseases of the heart, pericardium and pulmonary vascular bed – congenital heart disease in infancy and childhood. In Braunwald E, Zipes D, Libby P (eds) Heart Disease – A Textbook of Cardiovascular Medicine, Vol. 2. W B Saunders, Philadelphia.
This chapter describes congenital cardiovascular disease in infants and children. The authors distinguish between acyanotic and cyanotic lesions and detail the specific presenting features of the most common lesions that occur in infancy and childhood. They also offer a credible rationale for diagnostic and therapeutic interventions.

Hawgood S 1996 Respiratory system. In Gluckman P, Heymann M (eds) Pediatrics and Perinatology – The Scientific Basis. Arnold, London.
This section of the textbook offers an exploration of major respiratory concepts such as pulmonary structure, and the control and mechanics of breathing. By emphasising the embryonic developmental and maturational factors the text contributes to the current understanding of neonatal respiratory function.

Heymann M 1996 Cardiovascular system. In Gluckman P, Heymann M (eds) Pediatrics and Perinatology – The Scientific Basis. Arnold, London.
This section of the textbook offers an account of the fetal anatomical, physiological and biochemical principles fundamental to understanding the development and adaptation of the cardiovascular system in early childhood. The chapters provide a basis for understanding the many structural and functional problems that affect the development and maturation of the cardiovascular system.

Polin R, Fox W 1998 Fetal and Neonatal Physiology, Vols 1 and 2. W B Saunders, Philadelphia.
This textbook offers detailed accounts of most of the bioscientific concepts important in fetal and neonatal care. Genetic and chromosomal mutations, which can dominate some aspects of embryonic and fetal development, are considered. The exploration of biochemical, physiological, nutritional and pathophysiological principles contributes significantly to clinical practice and research.

Wong D 1999 Nursing Care of Infants and Children. Mosby, St Louis.
This textbook offers detailed accounts of the relevant biophysical, psychosocial and nursing issues in managing the care of infants and children. It concludes with a range of helpful appendices, which include excellent developmental screening tools and biophysical nomograms and parameters invaluable in all aspects of child care.

Chapter 52

Neonatal jaundice and some metabolic disorders

NEONATAL JAUNDICE

Morphological issues

Transition to extrauterine life ideally occurs when the fetal organs are sufficiently mature to permit independent survival. This is true of the neonatal liver and the processes of **bile synthesis**, metabolism and transport across hepatic and intestinal epithelia are relatively immature. **Hepatic disease** in neonates is not rare, and may present as a complex clinical problem.

As in adults, the neonatal **biliary apparatus** consists of primary secreting units, the bile canaliculi and a system of collecting tubules delivering the hepatocellular secretion onto epithelial-lined surfaces, the gall bladder and the duodenum. The **biliary canaliculi** are narrow tubes of about $1\,\mu m$ in diameter formed by the plasma membrane of two adjacent hepatocytes joined by occluding junctions (Bannister et al 1995). These junctions represent a barrier to the diffusion and bulk flow between plasma and bile. The lumen of bile canaliculi contains numerous **microvilli**, which increase the surface area of the canalicular membrane. Since only two hepatocytes form a canalicular lumen, most canaliculi communicate to form a complex **anastamosing network** for continuous bile drainage.

The biliary membranes are permeable to water, which ensures a continuous water exchange between plasma and bile. All hepatocytes and the bile ductal cells lining the biliary network participate in bile synthesis. Bile is **isotonic** in relation to plasma and striking concentration differences are created in these two fluids due to solutes such as bile acids. The flow of bile is an **osmotic process**. Water transport is a secondary process to the translocation of osmotically active solutes from blood to the biliary tree.

The metabolism of bilirubin

Bilirubin is a by-product of haemoglobin derived through the breakdown of haem (Fig. 52.1). Only a small proportion of bilirubin produced in the newborn infant is the

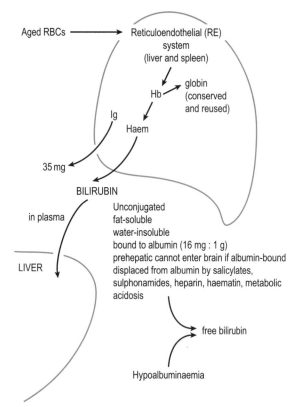

Figure 52.1   The formation of bilirubin (from Kelnar C, Harvey D, Simpson C 1995, with permission).

consequence of ineffective erythropoiesis; most of the bilirubin is synthesised from the breakdown of circulating erythrocytes.

The iron atom at the centre of the haem skeleton is reused. A molecule of carbon dioxide is removed from the haem ring and is excreted in a reaction catalysed by the enzyme hepatic **haemoxygenase**. In the bloodstream, molecules of **unconjugated** (indirect or prehepatic) bilirubin are tightly bound to serum albumin and transported to the liver for **conjugation** and excretion (Fig. 52.2). The hepatocytes easily take up unbound lipid-soluble bilirubin but need a **carrier molecule** to take up the bound complexes. The unconjugated bilirubin is conjugated (joined together) to form **bilirubin diglucuronide**, catalysed by the enzyme **bilirubin uridine diphosphate (UDP) glucuronyl transferase** (Storer 1996). Conjugation requires oxygen and glucose, and hypoxia or hypoglycaemia may slow the process down (Kelnar et al 1995).

Conjugated bilirubin is water soluble and passes into the bile. In the terminal ileum and colon some of this bilirubin is metabolised by bacterial activity to produce **urobilinogen (stercobilinogen** in the gut), which gives faeces the yellowish colour in infants and brown colour in adults. In its absence, faeces are greyish white (Marieb 2000). Small quantities of urobilinogen enter the circulation and are re-excreted by the liver and kidney as urinary urobilinogen.

Bilirubin in the neonate

Before birth, bilirubin is cleared by the placenta and maternal hepatocirculatory system. After birth, the neonate's liver takes over bilirubin metabolism, a change as complex as those in the circulatory system (Kelnar et al 1995). In term neonates, the intestines contain up to 200 g of meconium, of which 175 g may be bilirubin – about half of which is conjugated. Delays in meconium excretion, as occur in neonates with **cystic fibrosis**, may lead to the return of unconjugated bilirubin to the circulation.

Plasma bilirubin concentration   Normal neonates produce about 137–171 µmol of bilirubin per litre of plasma (Maisels 1999), which are high values compared to those of adults. This is partly explained by the higher neonatal circulating red cells which are not needed after birth and must be destroyed. There is also a shorter erythrocyte life span of about 80 days (normal 120 days) (Maisels 1999). The presence of increased numbers of immature or fragile cells may also be a contributing factor as may an increase in neonatal enteric bilirubin reabsorption compared to adults (Dennery & Stevenson 1995). Neonates produce about twice as much bilirubin as adults but plasma levels fall to normal by 6 weeks of age.

Plasma bilirubin concentration depends on the balance between production and elimination. In neonates, bilirubin conjugation and excretion are considerably less efficient than in adults, partly due to the somewhat dormant behaviour of the fetal hepatic conjugating system and bowel. Consequently, neonates usually manifest a progressive rise in plasma unconjugated bilirubin, which peaks at 180 µmol/L on the 3rd or 4th day of life, resulting in **physiological jaundice**. The increase in bilirubin sent to the liver, a decrease in hepatic uptake and a transient deficiency of hepatic bilirubin glucuronyl transferase activity culminate in reduced excretion of conjugated bilirubin. Despite its potential toxicity, bilirubin may have an important physiological role as an **antioxidant** (Maisels 1999).

Albumin binding   The transport and conjugating mechanisms for unconjugated bilirubin are not fully understood. Newly formed bilirubin is released from the **reticuloendothelial system** and is tightly bound to plasma albumin. Levels of unbound, unconjugated bilirubin are higher in neonates because of lower plasma albumin concentrations, decreasing albumin-binding capacity. There is a decreased affinity of albumin for bilirubin, possibly due to an immature albumin molecular structure (Blackburn 2003). Also, some albumin-binding sites may be **occupied by other molecules** such as **drugs**, including heparin and chloramphenicol (Sweet 1997), chloral hydrate and pancuronium (Maisels 1999). The capacity of a term neonate to excrete bilirubin is only 1/50th that of an adult, making jaundice common (Kelnar et al 1995). The delay in bilirubin conjugation leads to its deposition in fatty tissue, as unconjugated bilirubin is fat soluble and cannot be eliminated.

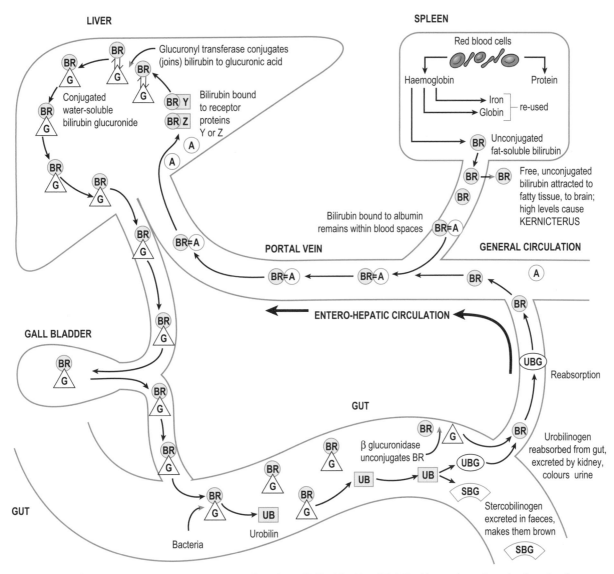

Figure 52.2 Schematic diagram showing the conjugation of bilirubin. Key: BR, bilirubin; =, bound to; A, albumin; G, glucuronic acid; UB, urobilin; UBG, urobilinogen; SBG, stercobilinogen (from Bennett VR, Brown L 1993, with permission).

Kernicterus

Unconjugated, unbound bilirubin is toxic to most cells and neural tissue and the viscera are particularly affected. The effect on **neural tissue** probably involves bilirubin deposition in the central nervous system. The brain regions most commonly affected are the **basal ganglia**, particularly the subthalamic nucleus, the globus pallidus, the hippocampus, various brainstem nuclei and the cerebellum (Maisels 1999). Unconjugated, unbound bilirubin may initiate **neural necrosis**, the dominant histopathological feature which appears around 7–10 days after birth.

Hypoxic ischaemic insults predispose the brain to bilirubin deposition in some low birthweight infants. Autopsy reports on jaundiced neonates reveal variable bilirubin staining of the aorta, pleural fluid and visceral organs (Maisels 1999). Unconjugated bilirubin has a high affinity for several plasma membrane phospholipids and forms complexes with them. The protein in membrane vesicles increases the binding of bilirubin to the plasma membranes.

Deposition of bilirubin causes irreversible tissue changes, leading to **kernicterus** (yellow kernel) characterised by yellow staining of the brain, especially the basal ganglia and cerebellum. The term **bilirubin encephalopathy** is more appropriately applied where neonates present with a mild but reversible **hyperbilirubinaemia**. The deposition of larger quantities of unconjugated bilirubin in neural tissue may cause irreversible neural damage characterised by muscular twitching, hypertonicity of the limbs and neck retraction.

There may be long-term sequelae of cerebral athetosis and mental retardation. This is most likely if the serum bilirubin level rises above 350 μmol/L although concerns should be raised when the bilirubin level rises above 250 μmol/L. Kernicterus can be prevented in all but very small, sick neonates where the blood–brain barrier may be

Table 52.1 Causes of neonatal jaundice

Prehepatic – unconjugated bilirubin	Hepatic – unconjugated bilirubin	Hepatic – mixed unconjugated and conjugated bilirubin	Posthepatic – unconjugated mixed and conjugated bilirubin	Posthepatic – unconjugated bilirubin
Physiological jaundice/jaundice of prematurity Haemolytic jaundice Bruising and haematoma Polycythaemia Postnatal infections	Breast milk jaundice	Congenital hypothyroidism Inborn errors of metabolism: galactosaemia Hepatitis, due to transplacental infections (TORCH organisms)	Congenital biliary atresia Bile plug syndrome	Paralytic ileus High intestinal obstruction such as duodenal atresia

ineffective so that quite low levels of bilirubin may damage the fragile tissues.

Causes of neonatal jaundice

Jaundice manifests as yellow discoloration of the skin and sclera caused by deposits of bilirubin. It becomes visible when the serum bilirubin rises above 85 μmol/L. Bilirubin is a normal yellowish green bile pigment which, prior to its alteration by the liver, is a weak acid, very soluble in lipid but only slightly soluble in water, making its excretion difficult. About 75% of bilirubin is released along with biliverdin when red blood cells are broken down in the liver and spleen, releasing haem and globin to the body stores. The remainder is derived from tissue **cytochromes** and other **haem** products (Storer 1996). Excessive bilirubin may enter the bloodstream in three ways (McCance & Huether 2002), all of which may affect the neonate:

1. during haemolysis of red blood cells;
2. where liver disease affects the metabolism and excretion of bile;
3. in conditions that obstruct the common bile duct, i.e. congenital biliary atresia.

Investigation and possibly therapeutic interventions are needed if:

- jaundice appears within the first 24 h after birth;
- jaundice persists for longer than 2 weeks;
- the total bilirubin level is over 250 μmol/L;
- there is conjugated hyperbilirubinaemia (above 30 μmol/L);
- jaundice appears in an ill baby irrespective of its age.

Kelnar et al (1995) divide the causes of jaundice into three groups:

1. prehepatic, originating before bilirubin arrives at the liver;
2. hepatic, with problems within the liver;
3. posthepatic, with obstruction or delay in the posthepatic pathways.

It is important to distinguish between unconjugated and conjugated. Causes of neonatal jaundice include are shown in Table 52.1 and Figure 52.3 illustrates the sites of events leading to jaundice.

Prehepatic – unconjugated bilirubin

Physiological jaundice usually appears in otherwise healthy infants around the 3rd day of life and fades gradually over the next 10 days. It is attributed to the increase in erythrocyte breakdown, which leads to greater bilirubin production and greater enteric reabsorption of bilirubin. The relatively immature liver is unable to synthesise sufficient glucuronyl transferase required to metabolise fat-soluble unconjugated bilirubin into water-soluble conjugated bilirubin. Unconjugated bilirubin cannot be excreted readily and spills over into many body tissues. The less-efficient binding of unconjugated bilirubin to plasma albumin magnifies the problem while the presence of meconium may add to the greater enteric reabsorption of unconjugated bilirubin. Late clamping of the umbilical cord increases **circulating blood volume** and **haematocrit** and may exacerbate the problem. Periodic phototherapy and increased hydration may occasionally be necessary.

Jaundice of prematurity is a more serious form of the above and is thought to be caused by the same factors. However, due to a greater immaturity of the liver, the premature neonate may manifest a more exaggerated form of jaundice, which begins earlier, lasts longer and tends to be more severe. It is essential to prevent the onset of bilirubin encephalopathy. Where **phototherapy** produces limited results, an **exchange transfusion** may be required.

In **haemolytic jaundice**, the two main causes of red cell haemolysis are **rhesus isoimmunisation**, a clinically serious problem, and **ABO incompatibility**, which is rarely severe (see Ch. 12). Jaundice generally appears in the first 24 h of life.

Bruising and haematomas such as cephalhaematoma will eventually lead to an extra breakdown of erythrocytes during the resolution of the bruise.

Polycythaemia or the presence of excess erythrocytes that must eventually be broken down will result in a greater synthesis of bilirubin. This may occur in **twin transfusion syndrome**, delayed cord clamping and infants of diabetic mothers.

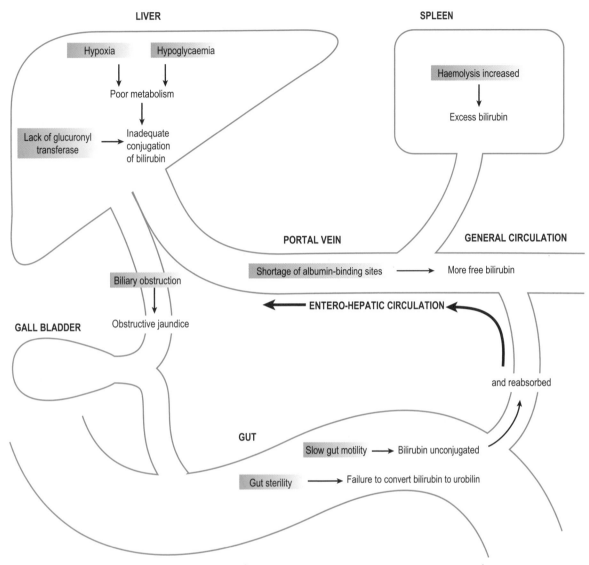

Figure 52.3   Sites of events leading to jaundice (from Bennett V R, Brown L 1993, with permission).

Following birth, **infection** such as septicaemia, urinary tract infections, meningitis and ventriculitis may also cause haemolysis of erythrocytes and consequently give rise to jaundice.

Hepatic – unconjugated bilirubin

Breast milk jaundice causes no ill effects and should not be a reason to discontinue breastfeeding but it can create anxiety for parents who see it as an illness. Breastfed babies are significantly more likely to develop hyperbilirubinaemia than bottlefed babies and it may occur early, at 3–4 days, or late, from 4 to 10 days after birth. The absolute cause of breast milk jaundice has not been established although it may involve:

- Inhibition of glucuronyl transferase by substances found in breast milk such as the maternal hormone pregnanediol and unsaturated fatty acids.

- The presence in breast milk of lipase, which releases free fatty acids into the neonate's intestines.

- The presence in breast milk of the enzyme β-glucuronidase, which will split conjugated bilirubin (Kelnar et al 1995) and increase shunting of unconjugated bilirubin from intestine back to liver.

- The delay in the passage of meconium seen in fully breastfed babies. Early breastfeeding with adequate colostrum intake will act as a laxative and prevent breast milk jaundice (Blackburn 2003, Salayira & Robertson 1993).

Hepatic – mixed unconjugated and conjugated bilirubin

Congenital hypothyroidism may contribute to jaundice. If the disorder is undetected and levothyroxine (thyroxine) supplements are not administered, it causes mental retardation. Neonatal screening using the standard Guthrie blood spot test is normally carried out on the 7th day of life and allows detection of this clinical problem. Sometimes the neonate presents early with other features of hypothyroidism as well as jaundice.

Some inborn errors of metabolism such as cystic fibrosis and galactosaemia may lead to severe jaundice. Inadequate metabolic pathways may contribute to a greater release of metabolic products which affect liver function.

Hepatitis may present as part of a syndrome accompanying transplacental infection by pathogens such as those causing rubella and toxoplasmosis, cytomegalovirus, herpes simplex or the different forms of hepatitis viruses.

Posthepatic – mixed unconjugated and conjugated bilirubin

Congenital anomalies of the biliary ducts invariably interfere with normal bile flow, leading to cholestasis. The more common biliary malformations are extrahepatic biliary atresias, intrahepatic biliary hypoplasia, cystic dilatation of the major intrahepatic bile ducts and duodenal atresia. It is important to distinguish between these dysmorphic lesions and parenchymal disorders associated with cholestasis as surgical correction of biliary malformations may be life-saving. Infants whose cholestasis is caused by inflammatory response, infections or metabolic disorders will not require surgery.

Extrahepatic biliary atresia is the commonest form of biliary malformation, with an incidence of 5–10 babies per 100 000 live births. It is more common in females. The origins of the atresia(s) are not clearly established although the prevailing histological features are associated with extrahepatic biliary obstruction, proliferation of the hepatic interlobular bile ducts and periportal fibrosis. Such babies develop a deep bronze jaundice in the 2nd week of life, the stools are putty coloured and the urine contains bilirubin (Sweet 1997). The liver becomes firm and enlarged. Because the bilirubin is conjugated, the neonate is not at risk of developing kernicterus. However, the intrahepatic accumulation of bile, if untreated, leads to progressive destruction of liver tissue, biliary cirrhosis, portal hypertension and liver failure (McCance & Huether 2002).

Depending on the extent of the obstruction, surgical intervention is usually required but the prognosis is poor because only a few babies with extrahepatic atresia are suitable for early surgery, which needs to be carried out before the liver is irreparably damaged. Liver transplantation is a long-term solution for some children but is generally carried out in older infants. When liver transplantation is not a realistic option, 80% of affected children die before the age of 3 years (McCance & Huether 2002).

Management of jaundice

Investigations

Depending on the history, signs and symptoms and gestational age, clinical investigations may include serum conjugated and unconjugated bilirubin monitoring, establishment of blood group, estimation of haemoglobin, rhesus antibodies, screening for evidence of infection, monitoring of metabolic function such as thyroxine and digestive enzyme assays.

Phototherapy

If jaundice persists, the first line of treatment to prevent the development of kernicterus is phototherapy. When a light of wavelength 400–500 nm is shone on the skin any unconjugated bilirubin is converted to a non-toxic water-soluble substance which is more easily excreted through the kidneys and the gastrointestinal tract. Phototherapy may work by inducing photo-oxidation, structural isomerisation and configurational isomerisation (Dennery & Stevenson 1995).

- Photo-oxidation is the reaction of bilirubin with singlet oxygen, leading to colourless non-reactive products that are readily excreted.
- Structural isomerisation involves the molecule lumirubin, formed by intramolecular cyclisation of the bilirubin molecule at the third carbon, leading to a polar compound.
- Configuration isomerisation involves changes in the spiral rings in the bilirubin molecules. The isomers are readily taken up by the liver and transported into the bile.

Phototherapy is not entirely risk free. Bilirubin is a photosensitiser and may sometimes act as a photodynamic agent, inducing skin blistering and bronze baby syndrome. The phototherapy light may initiate retinal damage if the neonate's eyes are not covered. According to Maisels (1999), the photodecomposition products have no known neurotoxic effects.

Clinical evidence and literature reviewed by Maisels (1999) suggest it is safe to withhold treatment in healthy term infants until the serum bilirubin reaches 320 μmol/L. However, premature neonates born around 28 weeks of gestation require phototherapy treatment when the unconjugated bilirubin level exceeds 150–180 μmol/L and neonates born about 34 weeks of gestation are likely to need phototherapy treatment at 200–240 μmol/L (Kelnar et al 1995). As phototherapy breaks down unconjugated bilirubin into the conjugated form, its excretion through the gastrointestinal tract is increased along with bile salts. This results in frequent loose stools, which may increase the risk of dehydration. Extra fluids should be given as well as normal feeding to reduce the risk of thirst and dehydration.

Exchange blood transfusion

This procedure is mainly carried out in neonates with rhesus haemolytic disease to remove excess bilirubin and antibodies from the neonate's blood. Reducing the plasma bilirubin levels lowers the risk of kernicterus and a reduction in antibodies lessens the severity of erythrocyte haemolysis which precedes the rise in bilirubin levels. Such interventions have risks, and consideration must be given to the neonate's overall state of health.

COMMON METABOLIC DISORDERS

The scope of this book does not allow exploration of the mainly recessively inherited **inborn errors of metabolism**. Detailed accounts of conditions such as **phenylketonuria**, **cystic fibrosis** and **galactosaemia** can be found in McCance & Huether (2002). Preconception, antenatal and neonatal screening tests are becoming more widely available. Disturbances in common substances such as glucose, calcium and sodium may lead to cerebral symptoms and permanent neurological damage. This is usually avoidable by prevention and prompt treatment.

Hypoglycaemia

Glucose homeostasis relies on the net balance in requirements, production and storage and regulation of glucose. A neonate's plasma glucose levels are the net result of glucose uptake, synthesis, release and utilisation. Since the neonate's **glucose homeostasis** is less than optimal due to metabolic transitions around birth, problems occur when glucose utilisation exceeds its availability or synthesis by the body leading to a fall in plasma glucose concentration. Conversely, glucose production can exceed utilisation, resulting in a constant abnormal rise in plasma glucose. Regulation of hepatic glucose production is critical to glucose homeostasis maintenance. Although the kidneys are capable of glycogen synthesis, **glycogenolysis** and **gluconeogenesis**, their glucose contribution is insufficient to maintain homeostatic balance except in prolonged starvation and metabolic acidosis. Most neonates who develop hypoglycaemia in the first 24 h after birth tend to have a history: i.e.

- a mother who suffers from diabetes mellitus;
- a mother who developed pregnancy-induced hypertension;
- stress related to neonatal asphyxia;
- being large or small for gestational age;
- may suffer from hyperinsulinism.

Most hypoglycaemic infants make a gradual but spontaneous recovery. However, recurrent or persistent hypoglycaemia may be caused by hepatic enzyme defects, endocrine deficiencies or hyperinsulinism. A plasma glucose of 2.6 mmol/L in a symptomatic baby may lead to neurological dysfunction, manifesting as tremors and seizures (Ogata 1999). Although hypoglycaemia is commoner in low birthweight babies and in babies of diabetic mothers, it can also present in neonates with a history of birth asphyxia, respiratory distress syndrome, hypothermia, cerebral damage, severe haemolytic disease or an inborn error of metabolism (Simpson 1997).

Signs

Hypoglycaemia may be asymptomatic or may be associated with other clinical problems such as lethargy, hypotonia, shallow respirations with periods of apnoea, cyanosis, muscle twitching, convulsions and coma. Prolonged hypoglycaemia may be associated with greater risks of brain damage, and associated seizures may worsen the neonate's overall prognosis Ogata (1999).

Management

Prevention is the best form of management, especially when the neonate is known to be at risk of developing hypoglycaemia. Early feeding and repeated blood monitoring is essential. In neonates whose blood glucose level is 1.7 mmol/L or more, immediate milk feed should be given. However, where the plasma glucose level is below 1.7 mmol/L a feed consisting of 10% glucose should be offered. If this is impossible, an intravenous infusion of 10% glucose solution may be necessary. If symptoms reappear, the neonate must have regular neurological and metabolic checks in order to identify or exclude more sinister problems.

Hypocalcaemia and hypomagnesaemia

During the last trimester of pregnancy, free calcium diffuses from the mother to fetus, ensuring that by term the infant's skeleton is mineralised. A manifestation of this positive calcium movement in favour of the fetus is reflected by the total and ionised calcium levels in the fetal blood, which are usually 10% higher than maternal values.

This **fetal hypercalcaemia** appears to suppress fetal **parathyroid secretion** and stimulate the release of **calcitonin**, favouring mineral deposition in the fetal skeletal system. This relative suppression of parathyroid function at birth contributes to the onset of a **transient hypoparathyroid state** with a fall in plasma calcium levels. The term neonate may show decreasing plasma calcium levels during the first 24–72 h after birth, reaching levels of 1.75–2.0 mmol/L. This physiologically induced **hypocalcaemia** may be significant, resulting in stimulation of the parathyroid glands and suppression of calcitonin secretion.

Plasma calcium levels increase to more acceptable levels within 5 days of birth. If the transition to normal calcium metabolism fails to happen, symptomatic hypocalcaemia develops. **Neonatal tetany** may occur when the plasma calcium level is less than 1.7 mmol/L. Hypocalcaemia may occur in the first 3 days of life in premature neonates where there is a history of birth asphyxia, hypothermia or respiratory distress syndrome.

Late hypocalcaemia, occurring between 5 and 6 days after birth, is usually associated with feeding the neonate unmodified cow's milk and is rare in developed countries. Cow's milk is high in **phosphorus** and the increase in serum phosphate causes the serum calcium to fall. Some immigrant mothers and mothers in lower socioeconomic groups may experience **vitamin D** and **calcium deficiencies** due to poor nutrition, leading to hypocalcaemia in pregnancy. Their babies may experience lower plasma calcium levels and higher risks of developing tetany.

Signs of tetany

Neonatal tetany results in irritability followed by **muscle twitching**, **apnoea** and **convulsions**. The neonate is generally conscious and alert between convulsions.

Management

Prevention can be aided by advising expectant mothers to increase their calcium intake. Breastfeeding is encouraged whenever possible and modified cow's milk is only given to babies when breastfeeding is unachievable. If a neonate experiences muscle twitching and convulsions, an infusion of **10% calcium gluconate** diluted in a ratio of 1:4 with sterile water or **dextrose** 10% must be considered. Regular oral calcium gluconate supplements may be continued when normal plasma calcium levels are restored. Intravenous administration of calcium gluconate must be given slowly, over 20 min (not into a peripheral vein), and with attention to cardiac function. As calcium has a direct impact on heart rate, rhythm and contractility, arrhythmias such as bradycardia may develop. If the neonate is asymptomatic, oral calcium supplements will usually be adequate (Koo & Tsang 1999).

Associated hypomagnesaemia

Failure of plasma calcium concentration to respond to administration of intravenous calcium salts should raise the suspicion of coexisting **hypomagnesaemia**. In such circumstances an intramuscular injection of 0.2 mmol/kg of **50% magnesium sulphate** will be required to correct both metabolic conditions (Simpson 1997). Hypomagnesaemia is often associated with hypocalcaemia and in such instances the serum magnesium levels may be below 0.6 mmol/L (normal = 0.6–1.0 mmol/L) and its homeostasis is thought to be controlled by the kidneys and the gastrointestinal tract. Long-term calcium and magnesium instabilities may contribute to hypoplasia of tooth enamel in the primary teeth.

Hypernatraemia

Neonatal hypernatraemia is almost always the consequence of **water depletion**. Hypernatraemia is defined by a plasma sodium level exceeding 143 mmol/L. It may be provoked by excessive fluid loss: e.g. during phototherapy or as a consequence of vomiting and diarrhoea. It may also follow excessive sodium intake, sometimes in intravenous solutions such as sodium bicarbonate. Any neonate receiving intensive care should have **plasma electrolytes** checked at least once a day.

Inappropriate infant feeding may lead to hypernatraemia. Adding extra scoops of powdered milk when mixing formula feeds will usually increase the sodium content and pose a danger to the infant. Mothers should be taught the principles of feed preparation and helped to understand the balanced hydration and nutrition that every infant requires. Where possible, breastfeeding should be encouraged. In hot weather, all infants perspire, become thirsty and cry. However, if mothers misinterpret the cry as hunger more sodium is added to the existing high plasma levels. Babies cannot excrete a high solute load by concentrating their urine. More dilute urine is produced and water is lost as it passively follows the excess sodium along the kidney tubules.

Signs of hypernatraemia

The infant may appear fretful and thirsty at first, but this is followed by dehydration, pyrexia, hypertension and a bulging pulsatile fontanelle. If the condition remains untreated, convulsions occur. Sometimes the infant may present with encephalopathy and other neurological problems which could be life threatening. The characteristic features of this clinical problem may be associated with failure to gain weight, irritability, hypertonicity and convulsions, especially when plasma sodium levels exceed 150 mmol/L. As the osmotic gradient favours maintenance of extracellular fluid at the expense of intracellular fluid, it may be difficult at times to establish the true diagnosis.

Management of hypernatraemia

Management of persistent hypernatraemia in neonates may be difficult because of its association with **cerebral haemorrhage** and **renal vein thrombosis**. Overaggressive correction may cause cellular overhydration, a problem that can affect the structural integrity of the brain tissue. Generally, the baby is slowly rehydrated with an infusion of an isotonic solution such as 0.9% saline. Sedation may be necessary to control convulsions. Any other electrolyte imbalance or hypoglycaemia must be restored. Follow-up care is necessary to observe for signs of potential neurological damage. Some mothers may require help with parenting skills, including further advice about managing the infant's nutrition.

MAIN POINTS

- Neonates produce twice as much bilirubin as adults because of the need to destroy excessive numbers of erythrocytes containing fetal haemoglobin present at birth. They also have a reduced capacity to excrete bilirubin. Although bilirubin is thought to have antioxidant properties, excessive quantities of unconjugated bilirubin can be neurotoxic.

- As the unconjugated bilirubin is fat soluble it will bind to tissue with high fat content, particularly the central nervous system. If left untreated, irreversible brain damage may occur. Kernicterus and long-term sequelae including cerebral athetosis and mental retardation will prevail. This is a preventable problem in all but the very small, sick neonates.

- Prehepatic causes of neonatal jaundice with an excess of unconjugated bilirubin include physiological jaundice/jaundice of prematurity, haemolytic jaundice, bruising and haematoma, polycythaemia and some postnatal infections.

- Hepatic unconjugated causes of jaundice include breast milk jaundice and congenital hypothyroidism. High values for mixed unconjugated and conjugated bilirubin may be attributed to such problems as inborn errors of metabolism and hepatitis due to transplacental infections. Breast milk jaundice should not be a reason to discontinue breastfeeding. However, breastfed babies are more likely to develop hyperbilirubinaemia than bottlefed babies.

- Posthepatic jaundice caused by high mixed unconjugated and conjugated bilirubin values are generally due to congenital biliary atresia, bile plug syndrome and high intestinal obstruction such as duodenal atresia.

- Phototherapy is occasionally necessary in physiological jaundice, especially in premature infants. The risk of kernicterus is minimised by using phototherapy and hydration. The need for exchange transfusion must be considered for babies at risk.

- Bruising and haematomas lead to delayed jaundice as a consequence of the breakdown of erythrocytes during the resolution of the bruise. Polycythaemia caused by twin transfusion syndrome or delayed cord clamping may induce a more extensive form of physiological jaundice.

- Neonates with biliary atresia present with a deep bronze jaundice in the 2nd week of life linked with light-coloured stools and dark urine containing bilirubin. The high concentrations of bile salts in the liver lead to progressive destruction of hepatocytes and to biliary cirrhosis, portal hypertension and liver failure. Surgical intervention is necessary but prognosis is poor.

- Disturbances in glucose, calcium, magnesium and sodium homeostasis may lead to neurological changes and permanent neural tissue damage. Plasma glucose levels of 2.6 mmol/L in babies with symptoms may lead to neurological problems.

- Hypoglycaemia is commoner in low birthweight babies and in babies of diabetic mothers. Early feeding and repeated blood screening is essential. In mild cases an immediate milk feed should be given. If the level is below 1.7 mmol/L, an intravenous infusion of 10% glucose in 0.9% saline may be required.

- Early hypocalcaemia occurs particularly in premature neonates or those with a history of birth asphyxia, hypothermia or respiratory distress syndrome. Late hypocalcaemia is usually associated with feeding neonates with unmodified cow's milk.

- Pregnant mothers with deficient intake of vitamin D and calcium may develop hypocalcaemia and their babies are at a higher risk of developing tetany. Usually, oral calcium supplements can be given. If a baby is convulsing, an infusion of 10% calcium gluconate diluted in a ratio of 1:4 with sterile water or dextrose 10% must be considered. Long-term hypoplasia of milk tooth enamel may occur.

- Hypernatraemia may be provoked by excessive fluid loss or excessive sodium intake. Since neonates cannot excrete a high solute load by concentrating urine, large quantities of water are lost in the dilute urine they normally form. The neonate is slowly rehydrated with an infusion of an isotonic solution such as 0.9% saline. Glucose and electrolyte homeostasis must be restored.

References

Bannister L, Berry M, Collins P et al 1995 Gray's Anatomy. Churchill Livingstone, Edinburgh.

Blackburn S T 2003 Maternal, Fetal and Neonatal Physiology. A Clinical Perspective, 2nd edn. W B Saunders, Philadelphia.

Dennery P, Stevenson D 1995 Management of neonatal hemolytic hyperbilirubinemia. In Reed G, Claireaux A, Cockburn C (eds) Diseases of the Fetus and Newborn: Pathology, Imaging, Genetics and Management, Vol. 2. Chapman and Hall, London.

Kelnar C J H, Harvey D, Simpson C 1995 The Sick Newborn Baby. Baillière Tindall, London.

Koo W, Tsang R 1999 Calcium and magnesium homeostasis. In Avery G, Fletcher M, MacDonald M (eds) Neonatology: Pathophysiology and Management of the Newborn. Lippincott, Williams and Wilkins, Philadelphia.

McCance K L, Huether S E 2002 Pathophysiology: The Biologic Basis for Disease in Adults and Children, 2nd edn. Mosby, St Louis.

Maisels M 1999 Jaundice. In Avery G, Fletcher M, MacDonald M (eds) Neonatology: Pathophysiology and Management of the Newborn. Lippincott, Williams and Wilkins, Philadelphia.

Marieb E N 2000 Human Anatomy and Physiology, 5th edn. Benjamin/Cummings, London.

Ogata E 1999 Carbohydrate homeostasis. In Avery G, Fletcher M, MacDonald M (eds) Neonatology: Pathophysiology and Management of the Newborn. Lippincott, Williams and Wilkins, Philadelphia.

Salayira E M, Robertson C M 1993 Relationships between baby feeding types and patterns, gut transit time of meconium and the incidence of neonatal jaundice. Midwifery 9(4):235–242.

Simpson C 1997 Metabolic and endocrine disorders of the newborn. In Sweet B R, Tiran D (eds) Mayes Midwifery, 12th edn. Baillière Tindall, London.

Storer J 1996 The liver. In Hinchliff A S M, Montague S E, Watson R (eds) Physiology for Nursing Practice, 2nd edn. Baillière Tindall, London.

Sweet B R 1997 Neonatal jaundice. In Sweet B R, Tiran D (eds) Mayes Midwifery, 12th edn. Baillière Tindall, London, pp 872–881.

Annotated recommended reading

Boxwell G 2000 Neonatal Intensive Care Nursing. Routledge, London.
This textbook outlines a range of common and challenging neonatal problems and provides helpful and directive suggestions for neonatal intensive care nursing. Critical analysis and reflection on the identified neonatal nursing concepts reinforce best practice.

Hageman J 1998 12 Neonatology Update. The Paediatric Clinics of North America 45(3). W B Saunders, Philadelphia.
This textbook offers a succinct update of a range of concepts, with emphasis on the biophysical and pathophysiological issues, central to competent neonatal care.

Polin R, Fox W 1998 Fetal and Neonatal Physiology, Vols 1 and 2. W B Saunders, Philadelphia.
This excellent textbook offers detailed accounts of the bioscientific concepts important in fetal and neonatal care. The initial résumé of genetics underpins a more detailed exploration of normal embryonic development.

Genetic and chromosomal mutations are considered. This textbook makes a significant contribution to clinical practice and research.

Wong D 1999 Nursing Care of Infants and Children. Mosby, St Louis.
This textbook offers expansive and detailed accounts of the biophysical, psychosocial and nursing issues relevant in managing the care of infants and children. It concludes with a range of helpful appendices, which include excellent developmental screening tools and biophysical nomograms and parameters invaluable in all aspects of child care.

Yau T, Stevenson D K 1995 Advances in the diagnosis and treatment of neonatal hyperbilirubinaemia. Clinics in Perinatology 22(3):741–758.
This excellent review of the diagnostic measures and therapeutic management of neonatal hyperbilirubinaemia makes a considerable contribution to the understanding of neonatal jaundice and related therapeutic factors that should be taken into consideration in the clinical context.

Chapter **53**

Infections and trauma in the neonate

INFECTIONS

Fetal and neonatal immunocompetence

Although not fully developed, the **neonatal immune system** is capable of mounting a defence against pathogens, removing worn out and damaged host cells and monitoring and destroying mutant cells. Neonates are vulnerable because of their immature and inexperienced immune system. Bellanti et al (1999) define **immaturity** as 'the genetically programmed low response or lack of response of the immune system to antigens such as bacteria, viruses and mutant cells'. The immune system is **inexperienced** because it has not undergone an immunological encounter to activate immunological mechanisms. Those wishing to review the immune system should read Chapter 29. The relative immaturity of the immune system may predispose the neonate to infection (Table 53.1).

Infections may be acquired by the fetus:

- transplacentally by the TORCH organisms (Ch. 14, p. 187);
- during invasive procedure such as amniocentesis;
- perinatally by pathogens ascending the maternal reproductive tract, especially if the fetal membranes rupture early;
- other infections acquired during pregnancy from organisms such as *Candida albicans*, *Neisseria gonorrhoeae*, *Chlamydia trachomatis*, *Listeria monocytogenes*, herpes simplex, HIV infection (Ch. 14, p. 187).

Postnatal infections

Babies become colonised by **commensal microorganisms** during labour and after birth as they are exposed to new environments. Maternal vaginal, rectal and perineal commensals and pathogens are most likely to cause neonatal **systemic** or **topical** infection. Neonatal infection is difficult to recognise as early signs may be non-specific. The infant may be lethargic, reluctant to feed, fretful and have unexplained vomiting and unusual stool pattern with weight loss. There may be poor temperature control, manifesting as either pyrexia or more commonly hypothermia, accompanied

Table 53.1 Predisposing factors to neonatal infection

Possible barriers/ mechanisms	Deficiencies in host defences
Anatomical barriers	Skin abrasions sustained during deliveries Invasive procedures: airway lavage, endotracheal intubation, umbilical artery catheterisation
Phagocytic cells	Small numbers of polymorphonuclear leucocytes Decreased polymorphonuclear cell activity Slow up-regulation in neutrophil production Poor transmission of neutrophils into the tissue
Complement mechanisms	Decreased levels of complement proteins in the blood, possibly due to immaturity of the liver
Cellular immunity	Possible defects in T-cell immunoregulation
Humoral immunity	Low levels of immunoglobulins IgA and IgM Low levels of IgG in premature infants Impaired antibody function Low levels of cytokines, e.g. interferon and tumour necrosis factor

by tachypnoea, apnoea, cyanosis and bradycardia. The neonate's skin may be mottled, jaundiced, grey or pale. Sudden collapse may occur and **differential diagnoses** include metabolic disturbances, respiratory or cardiovascular problems or intracranial haemorrhage.

Any healthy neonate who suddenly deteriorates must be examined for evidence of infection involving **microbiology screening**. Haemodynamic changes are monitored until the diagnosis is established. Early therapy may limit the severity of the infection while delays in diagnosis may contribute to spread of the pathogens and to **septicaemia**. In cases of doubt, neonates will undergo **systematic screening**, usually including nasal, throat, umbilical and skin swabs. A **full blood profile**, including white cell count, platelet count and blood culture is performed. **A lumbar puncture** will exclude **meningitis** or **ventriculitis**. Collection of **urine** and **stool samples** for culture and sensitivity may indicate the source of infection and influence management.

It is often expedient to administer **broad-spectrum antibiotics**, frequently intravenously, until the diagnosis is confirmed and the pathogens and their sensitivities identified. Most neonatal units use specific combinations of antibiotics such as **amoxicillin** and **gentamicin**, depending on which pathogens are present in that environment. The neonate will require maintenance of body temperature and adequate nutrition and hydration to avoid hypoglycaemia and acidosis. Fluid intake must be carefully managed as studies indicate that overhydration may lead to patent ductus arteriosus and **necrotising enterocolitis** (Bell & Acarregui 2001). Seriously ill neonates may require assisted mechanical ventilation.

Skin and surface infections

Neonatal skin lesions must be considered potentially abnormal, particularly if they are associated with staphylococci, which may spread from the ear, nose, mouth and skin of a carer or from another child. Due to immune system immaturity, simple lesions can rapidly lead to serious systemic infections. **Pyoderma**, the appearance of small spots or pustules on the skin, may spread rapidly in premature and ill neonates. **Paronychia** is a localised staphylococcal nail bed infection. Both infections may require antibiotics to eliminate them.

Pemphigus neonatorum is a serious skin infection caused by staphylococci entering the superficial soft tissue through a broken skin surface such as a scratch. It is highly contagious and may lead to epidemics that result in closure of maternity units. All blisters appearing on the neonate's skin should be notified to the doctor. Generally these lesions appear on the head and the trunk and, if unattended, fill with pus, break and leave raw skin surfaces open to further infection. Extensive blisters may coalesce, giving a 'scalded skin' appearance. The neonate may become seriously ill with dehydration and may develop septicaemia. Affected neonates are cared for in an isolated environment. Supportive interventions include antibiotic therapy and rehydration.

Omphalitis or infection of the umbilicus can be serious because of a possible spread of pathogens, commonly staphylococci, through the umbilical vein to the liver and kidneys (Fig. 53.1). Widespread erythema around the umbilicus or discharge of fluid or pus indicates local infection and must be treated with appropriate antibiotics and meticulous hygiene.

Ophthalmia neonatorum means the presence of a purulent discharge from the eye(s) of the neonate and develops within 21 days of birth. As it can lead to blindness, it is crucial to record any such eye infection and treat both eyes

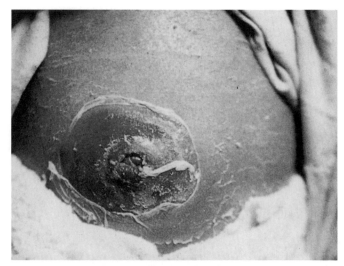

Figure 53.1 Severe periumbilical infection (from Kelnar C, Harvey D, Simpson C 1995, with permission).

with the appropriate antibiotic without delay. In severe cases, systemic antibiotics may be required. Although such severe eye infections are now rarely seen, pathogens such as the penicillin-resistant strains of *Neisseria gonorrhoeae*, staphylococci, *Escherichia coli* and *Chlamydia trachomatis* can induce them. Neonates are nursed with the affected eye in a downward position to ensure that infection does not spread to the clean eye.

Serious infections

The most serious infections are septicaemia, meningitis and pneumonia. All three present with non-specific signs such as thermoregulation problems, lethargy, apnoea and poor feeding and a differential diagnosis must be made. Group B β-haemolytic streptococcus has become an important cause of neonatal sepsis (Oddie & Embleton 2002).

Septicaemia, a serious end result of topical infection, is confirmed by blood culture. Besides the non-specific signs, abdominal distension, increased white blood cell count, hypotonia, unexplained metabolic acidosis and hyperglycaemia may occur in premature and low birthweight neonates. Occasionally, the pathogens cause disseminated intravascular coagulation (DIC). Both the systemic sepsis and the abnormal coagulation problems require swift therapeutic intervention.

Meningitis is most likely to occur in premature neonates or those born after difficult pregnancies and deliveries. Group B β-haemolytic streptococcus and *E. coli* are the most likely pathogens although *Listeria monocytogenes*, pneumococci, staphylococci and *Candida albicans* may be detected. The incidence of bacterial meningitis averages 0.4 per 1000 live births. Convulsions, bulging fontanelle and head retraction are seen in some neonates. A lumbar puncture will aid diagnosis and identify the causative pathogen. The mortality rate in neonates with meningitis averages 10–30% and frequency of complications in survivors can be high (Freij & McCracken 1999). Swift antimicrobial intervention and supportive care reduces the risk of cerebral damage, deafness, blindness and nerve palsies.

Pneumonia may follow inhalation of infected amniotic fluid and causes respiratory distress within hours of birth. Aspiration pneumonia may occur as a consequence of inhalation of milk or fluids given by nasogastric tube. This is most likely to occur in premature neonates whose swallowing and coughing reflexes are absent or weak. A range of pathogens can cause pneumonia with development of respiratory symptoms and cyanosis. All neonates require antimicrobial intervention and chest physiotherapy during the resolution phase. In milder forms of pneumonia and where the neonate is relatively strong, being nursed in an incubator with humidified oxygen may be sufficient to ensure recovery. However, premature and very small neonates may require mechanical respiratory support. Nasogastric feeding is continued if possible, but if there is severe respiratory embarrassment intravenous feeding is necessary.

Necrotising enterocolitis

Necrotising enterocolitis (NEC) is an acute inflammatory change affecting the bowel in predominantly premature neonates (Hartman et al 1999). The aetiology remains unclear (Caplan & Jilling 2001) but factors such as stress, infection, hypoxia, hypoglycaemia and inappropriate feeding may contribute. Lucas & Cole (1990) showed that NEC is up to 10 times more common in exclusively formula-fed babies than those fed with breast milk alone, and three times more prevalent in those receiving both formula and breast milk feeds. The prevention of pathogenic presence by the early colonisation of the gut by **lactobacilli** may be crucial. If the neonate is not breastfed, factors such as **IgA** and **lymphocytes** from colostrum are absent, which allows invasion of the bowel wall, portal system and bowel lymphatic glands by bacteria such as *Klebsiella*, *Clostridium* and *E. coli*.

Partial- or full-thickness intestinal **ischaemia** usually involves the terminal ileum. The sloughing of the ischaemic mucosal layer (Hartman et al 1999) contributes to gas formation within the muscular layers and the formation of **pneumatosis cystoides intestinalis**, detectable on abdominal X-ray films. Full-thickness **necrosis** leads to gut perforation and **peritonitis** and the neonate becomes critically ill. **Disseminated intravascular coagulation**, septicaemia and peritonitis may develop. An hepatic portal venous gas collection usually implies a severe or extensive form of necrosis that requires surgery.

Other clinical manifestations of NEC

- Abdominal distension.
- Acute severe abdominal pain.
- Retained gastric contents and vomiting.
- Fresh blood in stools.
- Thermal instability.
- Poor activity.
- Apnoea.
- Haemodynamic instability.

Therapeutic interventions

In mild forms of NEC diagnosed early **conservative treatment** consists of no gastric feeding, gastric decompression and intravenous antibiotics. This may avert the severe form of gut necrosis and perforation. **Intravenous fluids** are used to maintain hydration and acceptable blood glucose and electrolytes values. Regular **analgesia** such as morphine or fentanyl is administered. It is often advantageous to establish **assisted mechanical ventilation**, particularly if respiratory distress and metabolic acidosis are evident. All affected neonates will require **antibiotics** against Gram-negative and Gram-positive pathogens.

The presence of fresh blood in the stool usually confirms the diagnosis, although a stool specimen must be sent for culture and sensitivity screening. **Surgical interventions** are required if conservative medical interventions fail and the neonate shows signs of bowel perforation and peritonitis. Removal of the affected segments of the bowel with reanastomosis of the healthy segments of bowel later may have to be considered. If a functioning **ileostomy** is created, it is closed when the infant has recovered from the acute illness and surgery. Since the mortality rate averages 40% for neonates who require surgery, the onset of this acute stage of the illness must be prevented (Hartman et al 1999).

Gastroenteritis

Gastroenteritis is rare in breastfed babies and outbreaks are commonly caused by **rotavirus**, which spreads rapidly and has a high risk of mortality. Every effort must be taken to contain infection. Salmonella and certain strains of *E. coli* may also cause an outbreak. Most neonates deteriorate rapidly, and vomiting and frequent watery stools lead to severe dehydration. The gastrointestinal inflammatory changes may cause severe, spasmodic abdominal pain, requiring careful management. Segregation of the infected neonate is essential and, where more than one neonate is affected, the neonatal unit should be closed to new admissions. Affected neonates must be rehydrated and have their electrolyte imbalance and haemodynamic disturbances restored. Antimicrobial treatment is usually life-saving. An affected neonatal unit may only reopen following treatment and discharge of all neonates followed by disinfection of the clinical areas.

BIRTH TRAUMA

Uncomplicated labour rarely results in maternal or **neonatal trauma**. Severe birth trauma is now rare (Kelnar et al 1995) and should be avoidable (Greig 1999) but minor injuries may occur during difficult deliveries such as rotational forceps, ventouse extraction, shoulder dystocia or breech presentation. Neonates who are large in relation to the mother's pelvis, of low birth weight, multiple fetuses and those born by precipitate birth are also at risk. **Nerve injuries** and **fractures** of the long bones of the arm or leg may follow **shoulder dystocia** or **vaginal breech delivery**.

Head injuries

Premature neonates are at great risk of sustaining head injuries, leading to **intracranial haemorrhage** as a result of damage to protective layers around the brain (Fig. 53.2). The most severe forms of intracranial bleeding are a major cause of perinatal death. A **tentorial tear** involving the great vein of Galen, a **subaponeurotic haemorrhage** or **subdural haemorrhage** (see below) may be fatal.

Cephalhaematoma

A **cephalhaematoma** is a swelling on a baby's head caused by an effusion of blood under the periosteum of the affected skull bone (Fig. 53.3). Friction between the fetal head and the hard bone of the maternal pelvis or forceps may cause lacerations in the **periosteum**, leading to bleeding and haematoma formation. It may contribute to late onset of jaundice, as the excessive extravasated blood cells are reabsorbed. The cephalhaematoma is differentiated from the superficial oedema caused by **caput succedaneum** (Ch. 24) by characteristic features (Table 53.2).

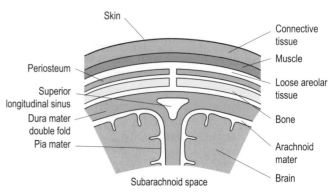

Figure 53.2 A cross-section through the skull (from Sweet B 1997, with permission).

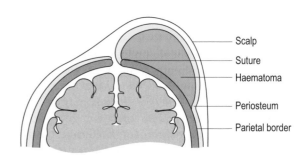

Figure 53.3 Cross-section of a cephalhaematoma (from Sweet B 1997, with permission).

Table 53.2 Differentiating between cephalhaematoma and caput succedaneum

Cephalhaematoma	Caput succedaneum
It appears in the first 12 h after birth	It is present at birth
It is clearly circumscribed and confined to one bone, never crossing a suture line	It may cross suture lines
It does not pit	As it is oedematous, pitting can occur
It tends to grow larger rather than disappear	It resolves within the first few days of life
No treatment is needed and the swelling usually disappears within 6–9 weeks, but may ossify	No treatment is necessary in normal circumstances

Subaponeurotic haemorrhage

Subaponeurotic haemorrhage is a serious birth injury commonly associated with births assisted by vacuum extraction (Greig 1999). Bleeding occurs from beneath the **epicranial aponeurosis**, giving rise to a swelling which can cross suture lines. This problem must be differentiated from caput succedaneum. A subaponeurotic haematoma is present at birth and continues to increase in size. Haemorrhage is extensive and may extend into the subcutaneous tissues of the neck or eyelids, giving rise to painful swellings. The blood loss may cause anaemia and a blood transfusion may be required. Clinical resolution is slow, extending over 2–3 weeks or longer, depending on extent and severity.

Intracranial haemorrhage

Bleeding into the **periventricular space** and other parts of brain tissue is relatively common in premature and low birthweight neonates. Ultrasound scanning, computed tomography (CT) scanning and lumbar puncture may help provide a differential diagnosis. The time of onset, duration and severity of bleeding are significant in planning a neonate's management. Intracranial haemorrhage is most likely to occur in premature neonates with a history of birth trauma, asphyxia or hypoxia. Poor autoregulation of cerebral blood flow may contribute. **Meningeal** and vessel tears occur in the **falx cerebri** or **tentorium cerebelli** (Fig. 53.4) although fragility of other cerebral blood vessels may be significant. The classical definitions of neonatal intracranial haemorrhage according to the site of bleeding are:

- subdural haemorrhage;
- subarachnoid haemorrhage;
- intraparenchymal haemorrhage;
- periventricular/intraventricular haemorrhage.

Subdural haemorrhage Subdural haemorrhage is almost exclusively associated with trauma. A tear in the tentorium cerebelli at its junction with the falx cerebri causes rupture of the **venous sinuses** and the **great vein of Galen**. Initially the neonate may appear sleepy, but becomes irritable with a high-pitched cry, vomiting and a bulging anterior fontanelle. Convulsions may occur, requiring the use of anticonvulsant drugs and dexamethasone. A subdural tap of the blood collection may be performed to alleviate rising intracranial pressure and prevent the development of meningeal adhesions, which could contribute to later development of hydrocephalus.

Subarachnoid haemorrhage In subarachnoid haemorrhage there is bleeding from small vessels into the subarachnoid space following mild trauma or asphyxia. It may be asymptomatic and undetectable on ultrasound scan and therefore more common than realised. There is often blood-stained cerebrospinal fluid (CSF). The presence of blood may initiate local inflammatory changes, which may ultimately lead to **hydrocephalus**.

Intraparenchymal haemorrhage Intraparenchymal haemorrhage is bleeding into the cerebral tissue associated with birth asphyxia or with disseminated intravascular coagulopathy. The presence of blood within the cerebral tissue will cause local irritation, possibly leading to generalised or localised convulsions. Distortion and destruction of affected cerebral tissue leads eventually to the formation of **porencephalic cysts** (Greig 1999), although these are eventually reabsorbed. Many such neonates make a slow but full recovery.

Periventricular/intraventricular haemorrhage Periventricular (PVH)/intraventricular haemorrhage (IVH) is the commonest and most serious type of intracranial haemorrhage (Fig. 53.5) in premature neonates with a history of birth asphyxia, respiratory distress syndrome and stress. It is associated with direct trauma to neurons caused by

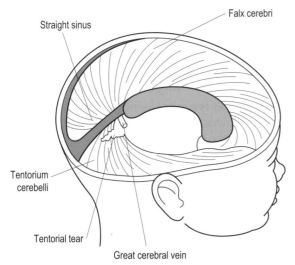

Figure 53.4   A tentorial tear (from Sweet B 1997, with permission).

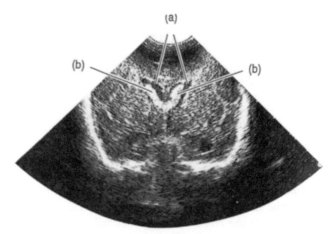

Figure 53.5   Coronal cranial ultrasound scan showing intraventricular haemorrhages (b) in dilated lateral ventricles (a) (from Kelnar C, Harvey D, Simpson C 1995, with permission).

accumulating blood, rising intracranial pressure and inflammatory changes. The accumulation of blood and inflammatory cells also interferes with normal production and circulation of cerebrospinal fluid, which may lead to hydrocephalus. Long-term outcomes may include motor and sensory disabilities and cognitive developmental delay (Blackburn 2003). This form of haemorrhage is one of the most common causes of death in neonates born before 32 weeks.

The site of bleeding is generally related to the gestation and developmental stage of the brain. The **subependymal germinal matrix** in the premature neonate is located adjacent to the lateral ventricles and contains actively dividing cells. From 24 to 32 weeks of gestation a large capillary bed supplies these cells. The large cerebral blood flow contained in relatively fragile blood vessels is incapable of autoregulation and the fragile capillary and related arteriovenous network is easily disrupted by hypoxia and hypercapnia, both capable of inducing cerebrovasodilation. This matrix almost disappears in term neonates and the risk of periventricular and intraventricular bleeding is reduced as the brain matures. In full-term neonates intracranial haemorrhage is mainly from the **choroid plexus**, contrasting sharply with the predominantly **capillary bleeding** in the subependymal germinal matrix observed in premature neonates.

The neonate with a sudden, large periventricular or intraventricular haemorrhage presents with apnoea and circulatory collapse characterised by marked bradycardia (Kelnar et al 1995). **The anterior fontanelle** may be enlarged and tense. Active resuscitation (Greig 1999) and respiratory support may be required. Balanced hydration and nutrition are administered intravenously, although fluids may have to be restricted if there is raised intracranial pressure. The prognosis for neonates with small haemorrhages is good but neonates with massive haemorrhages may suffer from convulsions, localised **cerebral atrophy** and hydrocephalus.

Periventricular leucomalacia In periventricular leucomalacia (PVL), cerebral tissue ischaemia leads to necrotic changes in the white matter surrounding the ventricles where blood flow may be interrupted due to hypotension. This area of the brain is vulnerable because it forms a boundary zone requiring blood supply from different arterial trees (Blackburn 2003). PVL destroys neural tissue of the corticospinal motor pathways, resulting in **spastic cerebral palsy** (Fig. 53.6).

Nerve palsies

Facial palsy

Facial palsy is commonly attributed to damage of the **seventh cranial nerve** by pressure applied to the facial nerve as it emerges near the angle of the jaw. The affected side of the face shows no spontaneous movement, the eye remains open and the corner of the mouth droops (Fig. 53.7). The neonate almost always recovers complete facial muscle movement.

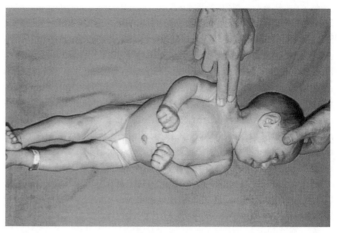

Figure 53.6 Hypertonic baby with cerebral palsy (from Kelnar C, Harvey D, Simpson C 1995, with permission).

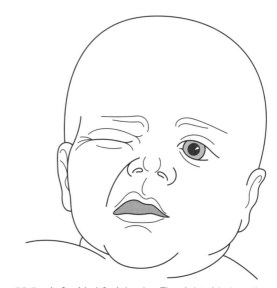

Figure 53.7 Left-sided facial palsy. The right side is active when the baby cries but the left side is relaxed (from Sweet B 1997, with permission).

Erb's palsy

Erb's palsy results from damage to the **fifth and sixth cervical nerves** caused by **compression of the upper brachial plexus** by traction or rotation applied to the neck in a breech or difficult cephalic delivery. This results in paralysis of the arm, which is inwardly rotated and hangs limply at the side, and the half closed hand is turned outwards, the characteristic 'waiter's tip position' (Fig. 53.8). As these nerves control the arm and some neck and chest muscles, any superficial or deep nerve injury will manifest in neuromuscular changes, but full recovery is often possible.

Klumpke's palsy

Klumpke's palsy is an uncommon problem caused by traction on the arm with damage to the **eighth cervical and**

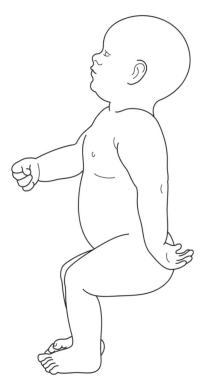

Figure 53.8   Erb's palsy (from Sweet B 1997, with permission).

first thoracic nerve roots of the lower brachial plexus. The neonate presents with paralysis of the hand and 'wrist drop' although the upper arm generally has a normal range of movement. Physical assessment and radiographic screening rule out fractures to the humerus and clavicle and identify dislocated joints. Where fractures or joint problems are present, the neonate generally cannot move his affected arm. Most neonates make a slow recovery, which may take up to 2 years. **Analgesia** will limit pain and induce local muscle relaxation to aid healing. **Physiotherapy** encourages normal muscle movement and prevents contractures. Where the neonate does not make a spontaneous recovery, **surgical intervention**, including nerve graft or repair, may be considered.

Soft tissue injuries

The most common cause of soft tissue injuries is vaginal breech delivery. Injuries include:

- superficial bruising;
- injury to liver and spleen;
- injury to the kidneys and adrenal glands;
- injury to the intestines.

Although painful superficial bruising is obvious, other more life-threatening complications may develop. This is particularly so where injury to the liver, spleen or adrenal glands results in bleeding and hypovolaemic circulatory collapse. Ultrasound scanning should establish the diagnosis. Where the neonate develops haemodynamic instability that could compromise vital organs, supportive interventions are necessary.

MAIN POINTS

- Fetal infection may be acquired transplacentally or during invasive investigations such as amniocentesis. Some infections are acquired perinatally due to pathogens ascending through the maternal reproductive tract, especially if the fetal membranes rupture early.

- Early signs of systemic infection in neonates are non-specific and include lethargy, poor feeding, jaundice, vomiting, diarrhoea and weight loss. Hypothermia, pyrexia, tachypnoea, apnoea, cyanosis, bradycardia and haemodynamic instability indicate severe infection.

- Delays in diagnosing and treating local infections may contribute to systemic infection such as meningitis and septicaemia. All infections must be treated with broad-spectrum antibiotics. Early diagnosis and treatment reduces mortality and severe complications.

- Group B β-haemolytic streptococcus and staphylococci are the commonest pathogens in septicaemia. Meningitis is frequently caused by the group B β-haemolytic streptococcus. Most neonates who develop pneumonia are very ill and require assisted mechanical ventilation, broad-spectrum antibiotics and physiotherapy.

- Gastroenteritis is rare in the breastfed baby. Outbreaks are commonly caused by rotavirus and are associated with a high mortality. *Salmonella* and some strains of *E. coli* may also cause an outbreak. Antibiotic therapy, rehydration and segregation of infectious neonates are necessary.

- Pemphigus neonatorum may lead to more serious systemic infection. Infectious neonates are isolated and treated with antibiotics. Omphalitis and ophthalmia neonatorum are potentially serious infections requiring antibiotic treatment and high standards of hygiene.

- Early diagnosis and swift medical intervention of necrotising enterocolitis may reduce its severity. Some neonates may require surgery if bowel necrosis and perforation occurs.

- Normal labour rarely results in birth injuries but minor soft tissue injuries may occur during a difficult labour. Friction between the fetal head and the maternal pelvis or forceps may cause a cephalhaematoma. No treatment is needed and the cephalhaematoma usually subsides within 6 weeks.

- Subaponeurotic haemorrhage is a serious birth injury commonly associated with vacuum extraction. Bleeding may extend into the subcutaneous tissues of the neck or eyelids, and in some instances blood will cross the suture lines.

- Intracranial haemorrhages are a major cause of perinatal death when prematurity is associated with hypoxia, asphyxia or trauma to the falx cerebri or tentorium cerebelli, resulting in subdural bleeding and subarachnoid bleeding, respectively. The time of onset, the duration and extent of the bleeding into the brain tissue are important in the overall prognosis.

- Intraparenchymal haemorrhage is frequently associated with birth asphyxia. Destruction of the affected cerebral tissue with formation of parencephalic cysts can be observed in some neonates.

- Periventricular/intraventricular haemorrhage is the most common and serious form of intracranial haemorrhage occurring in premature neonates. Some develop hydrocephalus and motor, sensory and cognitive disabilities. These neonates may develop leucomalacia. The destructive changes may result in permanent damage to the corticospinal motor pathways and cause spastic cerebral palsy.

- Nerve palsies include facial palsy, Erb's palsy and Klumpke's palsy. The most common causes of soft tissue injuries in neonates occur as a result of the fetus being in a breech position. Care must therefore be taken during such deliveries in order to avoid superficial and central organ trauma.

References

Bell E F, Acarregui M J 2001 Restricted versus liberal water intake for preventing morbidity and mortality in preterm infants. Cochrane Review: In The Cochrane Library, Issue 1. Update Software 2003, Oxford.

Bellanti J, Zeling B, Pung Y 1999 Immunology of the fetus and the newborn. In Avery G, Fletcher M, MacDonald M (eds) Neonatology: Pathophysiology and Management of the Newborn. Lippincott, Williams and Wilkins, Philadelphia, pp 1063–1122.

Blackburn S T 2003 Maternal, Fetal and Neonatal Physiology: A Clinical Perspective, 2nd edn. W B Saunders, Philadelphia.

Caplan M S, Jilling T 2001 New concepts in necrotising enterocolitis. Current Opinion in Pediatrics 13(2):111–115.

Freij B, McCracken G 1999 Acute infections. In Avery G, Fletcher M, MacDonald M (eds) Neonatology: Pathophysiology and Management of the Newborn. Lippincott, Williams and Wilkins, Philadelphia.

Hartman G, Boyajian M, Choi S et al 1999 General surgery. In Avery G, Fletcher M, MacDonald M (eds) Neonatology: Pathophysiology and Management of the Newborn. Lippincott, Williams and Wilkins, Philadelphia, pp 1005–1044.

Kelnar C J H, Harvey D, Simpson C 1995 The Sick Newborn Baby. Baillière Tindall, London.

Greig C 1999 Trauma and haemorrhage. In Bennett V R, Brown L K (eds) Myles Textbook for Midwives, 13th edn. Churchill Livingstone, Edinburgh.

Lucas A, Cole T 1990 Breast milk and necrotizing enterocolitis. Lancet 336:1519–1523.

Oddie S, Embleton N D 2002 Risk factors for early onset neonatal group B streptococcal sepsis: case control study. British Journal of Medicine 325(7359):308–311.

Annotated recommended reading

Boxwell G 2000 Neonatal Intensive Care Nursing. Routledge, London.
This textbook outlines common and challenging neonatal problems and provides helpful and directive suggestions for neonatal intensive care nursing which allow critical analysis and reflection on the identified neonatal nursing concepts and reinforce best practice.

Hill A, Volpe J 1999 Neurological and neuromuscular disorders. In Avery G, Fletcher M, MacDonald M (eds) Neonatology: Pathophysiology and Management of the Newborn. Lippincott, Williams and Wilkins, Philadelphia.
This chapter of the book offers a comprehensive account of the neurophysiology and neuropathophysiology of common neonatal problems. It enriches the existing understanding of the neuromuscular problems which may occur in neonates.

MacLean A, Regan L, Carrington D 2001 Infection and Pregnancy. RCOG Press, London.
This textbook offers excellent current reviews of microbiology. It identifies the most common pathogens that may cause maternal and fetal infection. A few chapters focus on the likelihood of transmission of infectious pathogens from the mother to the neonate.

Polin R, Fox W 1998 Fetal and Neonatal Physiology, Vols 1 and 2. W B Saunders, Philadelphia.
This textbook offers detailed accounts of bioscientific concepts important in fetal and neonatal care. A résumé of genetics underpins a more detailed exploration of normal embryonic development. The systematic exploration of relevant biochemical, physiological, nutritional and pathophysiological principles makes a significant contribution to clinical practice and research.

Tortora G, Funcke B, Case C 2001 Microbiology. Benjamin Cummings, San Francisco.
This textbook offers a balanced, reflective and well-illustrated account of the fundamentals of microbiology and how this knowledge of microorganisms can be applied in practice.

Wong D 1999 Nursing Care of Infants and Children. Mosby, St Louis.
This textbook offers detailed accounts of the biophysical, psychosocial and nursing issues relevant in managing the care of infants and children. It concludes with a range of helpful appendices, which include excellent developmental screening tools and biophysical nomograms and parameters invaluable in all aspects of child care.

Section 4B

PUERPERIUM – THE MOTHER

SECTION CONTENTS

This section examines the return to normal physiology of the woman following childbirth, the onset of lactation and the parent–baby relationship. The importance of breastfeeding cannot be overstated and breast anatomy and lactation are discussed in Chapter 54 while breastfeeding practice and problems are considered in Chapter 55. Chapter 56 is about the other physiological changes occurring in the puerperium and the pathological conditions that may affect the woman. Some pathological conditions not mentioned elsewhere in the book are discussed, including puerperal infection. The last chapter in the book considers the development of mother–baby relationships in terms of biological theories. However, the student should not lose sight of the integration of biology, psychology and sociology which underpins human behaviour.

Chapter 54

The breasts and lactation

INTRODUCTION

Lactation is the production of milk by specialised organs called **mammary glands**, named from the Latin word *mamma* for breast. Humans are classified as mammals and distinguished from other vertebrates because of their ability to produce milk for the young. Lactation was probably a key physiological feature which enabled mammals to survive the climatic changes that led to the demise of the dinosaurs about 65 million years ago (Czerkas & Czerkas 1990).

The human mammary gland, an exocrine gland, is the only organ not fully developed at birth. Dramatic changes occur in size, shape and function in the mammary glands from birth through pregnancy, lactation and ultimately involution. It is essential that all practitioners involved with women during pregnancy and childbirth have a sound knowledge and understanding of the anatomy of the human breast and the physiological mechanisms of milk production. This knowledge will help them to encourage and support women to breastfeed their babies.

THE ANATOMY OF THE BREAST

Situation, shape and size

The adult breasts are always paired and develop bilaterally on the ventral surface of the body. They possibly originate from modified apocrine sweat glands and subsequently form part of the skin. The shape of the breast varies from woman to woman but it tends to be dome shaped in adolescence, becoming more hemispheric and finally pendulous in parous females (Lawrence & Lawrence 1999). The two breasts are situated on the anterior chest wall on either side of the midline and will vary in size depending on the amount of adipose tissue present. The mature breast extends between the second rib and the sixth intercostal cartilage and lies over the pectoralis major muscle from sternum to axilla (Fig. 54.1). Mammary glandular tissue projects somewhat into the axillary region and this is known as the tail of Spence. The **nipple** is surrounded by areola and protrudes from the centre of each breast at the level of the fourth intercostal space.

Structure

The three main structures of the breast are skin, subcutaneous tissue and corpus mammae (body of the breast). The corpus mammae is the breast mass remaining after the breast is freed from the deep attachments, and the skin, subcutaneous connective tissue and adipose tissue are removed.

Corpus mammae (body of the breast)

The tissue of the mammary gland consists of two major divisions: the **parenchyma** and the **stroma**. The parenchyma or glandular tissue is the functional component of the breast tissue and the stroma comprises the connective tissue, adipose tissue, blood and lymph vessels, nerve tissue and the surrounding skin.

The parenchyma consists of the lobular, alveolar and ductular structures. It is arranged in about 15–25 **lobes** that

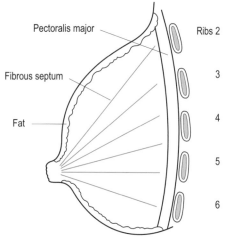

Figure 54.1   The supporting structures of the breast (from Sweet B 1997, with permission).

radiate out from the nipple like the spokes of a wheel (see Fig. 54.2). The lobes are separated from each other by fibrous connective tissue partitions so that they do not communicate with the adjoining lobes and each lobe functions independently.

The alveoli

As with all exocrine glands, the glandular tissue contains secretory and ductal tissue. Each lobe is divided into 20–40 smaller **lobules** made up of the functional milk-producing units called the alveoli and their ductules. This is known as the **lobuloalveolar system** (Fig. 54.3).

Each alveolus contains specialised milk-forming cells called acini cells, which surround a small duct. The cells are arranged in a single layer surrounding the hollow lumen. Milk is secreted into the lumen and drains via narrow ductules into the duct system. Some of the cells lining the ductules may also secrete milk.

The basal lamina   Each alveolus is surrounded by a **basement membrane** (basal lamina) made up of collagen, glycoprotein and glycosaminoglycans secreted by the epithelial cells where they are in contact with connective tissue. This provides a barrier between the epithelial and stromal components of breast tissue which cannot be crossed by cells other than leucocytes. Lymphocytes or monocytes are found wedged between the secretory cells of the alveoli and have migrated there. They play a role in local production of antibodies in the form of immunoglobulin A (IgA) for secretion into the breast milk.

The secretory cells

The secretory cells lining the alveoli are cuboidal and very polarised in structure (Fig. 54.4). The nucleus is situated at the base of the cell facing the circulation and facing the lumen is a well-developed Golgi apparatus with layers of flattened vesicles. Most of the cell is occupied by rough

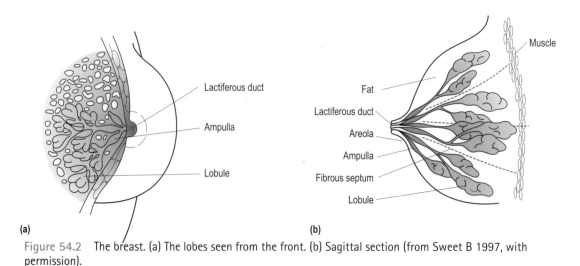

(a)   (b)

Figure 54.2   The breast. (a) The lobes seen from the front. (b) Sagittal section (from Sweet B 1997, with permission).

endoplasmic reticulum and there are a large number of mitochondria. There are large fat droplets and vesicles containing granules of protein. The basal surface of the cell has numerous infoldings for the uptake of substrate for milk production while the surface facing the lumen is covered with microvilli for secretion of milk.

The ducts

Groups of 10–100 alveoli drain into a small duct into which they pour their secretions. These small ducts join up to form larger ducts draining the lobules. The ducts from the lobules unite to form a central **lactiferous duct** for each lobe.

Each lactiferous duct expands into a dilated sac as it passes beneath the areola to form an **ampulla** (lactiferous sinus) where milk can be stored prior to suckling. It then narrows to open out onto the nipple surface. The walls of the ducts are lined by a layer of cuboidal epithelial cells resting upon a basement membrane. Surrounding the alveoli and smaller ducts are the contractile branching **myoepithelial cells**. Smooth muscle surrounds the larger ducts near the nipple.

The stroma

Connective and adipose tissue, which form the largest part of the mammary glands in the non-pregnant state, separate

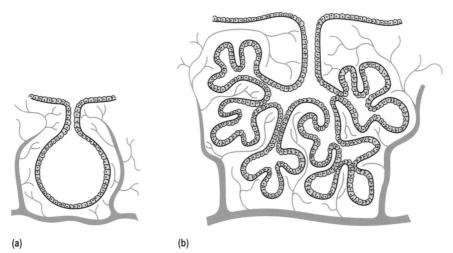

Figure 54.3   The structure of the breast. (a) Single alveolus. (b) One lobule (from Sweet B 1997, with permission).

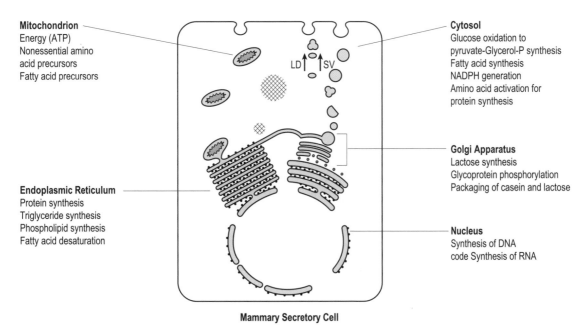

Mammary Secretory Cell

Figure 54.4   Schematic representation of cytologic and biochemical interrelationships of secretory cell of mammary gland. LD, liquid droplet; SV, secretory vesicle. (Reproduced with permission from Lawrence 1985.)

and support the radiating lobes of glandular tissue. The breasts are held in position by the suspensory ligaments of Astley Cooper which form from the interlobar connective tissue. These fibrous bands of tissue attach the breast to the underlying muscle fascia and to the overlying dermis.

The nipple and areola

The skin of the breast includes the nipple and areola which are all visible externally. The **nipple** or papilla mammae is a conic elevation located in the centre of the areola. The nipple contains about 15–25 milk ducts surrounded by a muscular fibroelastic tissue. These ducts end as small orifices near the tip of the nipple and the lactiferous ducts may merge within the nipple (Lawrence & Lawrence 1999). The milk ducts within the nipple dilate at the nipple base into the cone-shaped ampulla or lactiferous sinuses, which function as temporary milk containers during lactation. The smooth muscle fibres in the nipple represent a closing mechanism for the milk ducts and the nipple is richly innervated with sensory nerve endings. Nipple erection is induced by tactile, sensory or autonomic sympathetic stimuli. Local venostasis and hyperaemia occur to enhance the process of erection. The nipple and areola are extremely elastic due to the muscular fibroelastic system which functions to decrease the surface of the areola, produce nipple erection and empties the lactiferous sinuses during lactation. When the nipple erects, it becomes smaller, firmer and more prominent.

The **areola**, or areola mammae, is a circular pigmented area surrounding the nipple. Within the areola are about 18 sebaceous glands known as Montgomery's tubercles, which enlarge during pregnancy and appear as raised projections. These glands provide secretions to lubricate and protect the areola and nipple during pregnancy and lactation. The red pigmentation of the areola may be a visual signal for the newborn baby to find the nipple (Lawrence & Lawrence 1999).

The mammary gland, fat and connective tissue are all contained within the subcutaneous tissue. The size of the woman's breast reflects the amount of fat and connective tissue and not the glandular tissue. The size of the breast has therefore nothing to do with its function.

Blood supply The internal mammary artery and the lateral thoracic artery provide the major blood supply, with 60% of total breast tissue receiving blood from the internal mammary artery. The arterial blood supply terminates in networks of 5–12 capillaries surrounding each of the alveoli. The venous supply parallels the arterial supply and bears similar names. Veins end in the internal thoracic and axillary veins and create an anastomotic circle called the circulus venosus around the base of the papilla behind the nipple.

Lymphatic vessels There is an extensive lymphatic drainage system forming a plexus beneath the areola and between the lobes of the breast with free communication between the two breasts. The smallest of these vessels are embedded in the lobuloalveolar tissue. Lymph glands drain into the axillary nodes of both axillae, glands in the anterior mediastinum and into glands in the portal fissure of the liver.

Nerve supply The breast is innervated primarily by branches from the fourth, fifth and sixth intercostal nerves. The nerve supply to the corpus mammae is sparse and contains only sympathetic nerves accompanying blood vessels. The sensory innervation of the nipple and areola is extensive and consists of both sensory and sympathetic autonomic nerves:

- somatic sensory nerves convey impulses from skin receptors to the central nervous system;
- sympathetic (efferent) nerves innervate blood vessels and the contractile muscles of the nipple.

DEVELOPMENT OF THE BREAST

The mammary gland undergoes three major phases of growth and development before pregnancy and lactation: in utero; during the first 2 years of life; and at puberty. **Embryogenesis** refers to the embryonic development of the organ in utero. **Mammogenesis** refers to the growth and development of the mammary glands: this stage occurs in two phases as the glands respond first to the hormones of puberty and then later to the hormones of pregnancy. **Lactogenesis** refers to the initiation and production of milk.

Early development and puberty

In the 4th week of embryonic life, a primitive milk streak develops from axilla to groin on the trunk of the embryo (2.5 mm long at this stage). This streak becomes the mammary ridge or milk line by the 5th week. The ridge is actually a thickening of epithelial tissue and is accompanied by growth inward at the chest wall, which will be the region of the future gland.

Embryogenesis of the mammary glands begins in the 6-week embryo and proliferation continues until milk ducts are developed by the time of birth. During this time, processes of dividing and branching takes place, giving rise to the future lobes and lobules and much later to the alveoli. Specialised cells differentiate into breast structures such as nipple, areola, glands, hair follicles and Montgomery glands. Development is influenced by the placental sex hormones between 28 and 32 weeks to stimulate the formation of channels (canalisation). From 32–40 weeks of gestation, lobular–alveolar structures containing colostrum develop. During this time, the fetal mammary glands increase four times and the nipple and areola further develop and become pigmented. After birth, the neonate may secrete colostrum known as witch's milk.

Mammary gland development during childhood merely keeps pace with physical growth. At puberty, oestrogen becomes the major influence on female breast development. Under the influence of oestrogen, primary and secondary

GESTATION

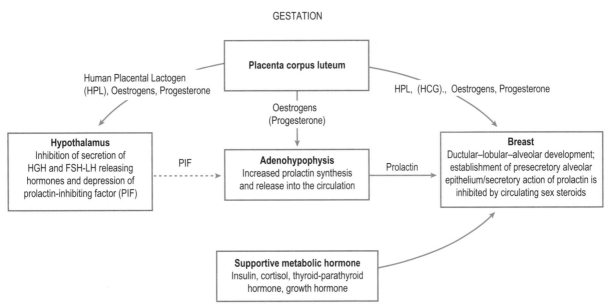

Figure 54.5   Hormonal preparation of breast during pregnancy for lactation. (Reproduced with permission from Lawrence 1985.)

ducts grow and divide and form terminal-end buds which develop into new branches and later become alveoli in the mature breast. During each menstrual cycle, proliferation and active growth of duct tissue occurs during the follicular and ovulatory phases, reaching a maximum in the late luteal phase before regressing. Complete development of mammary function occurs only in pregnancy.

Development in pregnancy

Changes in levels of circulating hormones result in profound changes in ductular–lobular–alveolar growth during pregnancy (Fig. 54.5). Breasts begin to exhibit changes at about the 6th week of pregnancy and may be useful in confirming pregnancy (Blackburn 2003).

1. Early in pregnancy, the luteal and placental hormones are responsible for a marked increase in the development of the duct system and formation of lobes. Placental lactogen, prolactin and chorionic gonadotrophin contribute to the accelerated growth. Oestrogen is responsible for development in the duct system and progesterone is responsible for lobular formation (Lawrence & Lawrence 1999). This results in the breasts feeling nodular and lumpy and the woman may feel the breasts tender and tingly. Growth continues throughout pregnancy and the breasts increase in size.

2. Prolactin is essential for the complete lobular–alveolar development. It influences the alveolar cells to initiate milk secretion and stimulates the glandular production of colostrum. By the second trimester, colostrum is secreted under the influence of placental lactogen (about 16 weeks). During pregnancy, prolactin is prevented from exerting its effect on milk excretion by the high circulating levels of progesterone.

3. Vascularity increases and the appearance of a network of subcutaneous veins is visible beneath the skin. This network increases in size and complexity throughout pregnancy.

4. By 12 weeks the nipples are now more prominent and the areola develops an increased fullness and brown pigmentation called the primary areola of pregnancy. Montgomery's tubercles further develop and become more prominent.

5. By the 24th week, there is a further pigmentation around the primary areola known as the secondary areola. This is especially noticeable in dark-haired people.

6. By term the breasts usually enlarge by 5 cm overall and increase by 1400 g in weight (Sweet 1997).

Maternal nutrition and lactation

During pregnancy, energy is stored in the form of body fat and mainly deposited on the trunk and legs. In women with adequate nutrition, this portion of the weight gain of pregnancy amounts to 4 kg, which is equivalent to an energy store of 35 000 kcal. This will provide for 4 months of lactation and 300 kcal/day for the baby, enough to ensure survival if the mother is deprived of food as may happen in famine conditions. If a woman does not breastfeed, these fat stores may be difficult to remove, leading to obesity as successive pregnancies deposit their stores. Lactating women are much more likely to regain their figures.

There are two physiological aids to the accumulation of these fat stores:

1. the effect of progesterone and other hormones on the metabolism during pregnancy;

2. the slowing down of energy usage as pregnancy proceeds.

After delivery of the baby, these extra stored calories are converted into milk. The recommendation of an additional 500 kcal/day is now considered to be the upper level for lactating women (Riordan & Auerbach 1998). The conversion of calorie intake to milk is very efficient. Women with marginal nutrition (below 1800 kcal/day), such as those in developing countries, are able to breastfeed for at least 6 months or more. This is due to the enhanced ability to store energy in pregnancy coupled with the highly efficient conversion of food energy to breast milk.

THE PHYSIOLOGY OF LACTATION

Lactation is the physiological completion of the reproductive cycle (Lawrence & Lawrence 1999). The process of lactation can be divided into three stages during which human milk varies in components, appearance and volume.

1. lactogenesis I – the initiation of milk secretion;
2. lactogenesis II – the production of colostrum and transitional milk;
3. lactogenesis III – the development of milk and the maintenance of established lactation.

Lactogenesis

There are important factors in the initiation of the cascade of events necessary to ensure that a supply of milk is readily available for the baby at birth. These include the preparation of mammary epithelium, the withdrawal of progesterone, the maintenance of prolactin levels and the removal of milk from the breast after birth (Neville et al 2001). This is achieved through the influences and control of the processes involved in lactogenesis.

Stages of lactogenesis

Lactogenesis I Lactogenesis I starts when milk components are first seen in breast tissue and colostrum can be expressed from the breast during pregnancy. A specific milk protein called α-lactalbumin can be detected in maternal blood from midpregnancy. During this stage the physical changes in the breasts are accompanied by hormonal changes resulting from the interplay between the pituitary gland, the ovary and the placenta. These will culminate in the initiation of lactation following the birth of the baby.

Lactogenesis II Lactogenesis II is initiated after birth by a fall in plasma progesterone levels and prolactin levels remaining high. There are rapid cardiovascular changes with an increase in breast blood supply, metabolic processes with the glandular tissue absorbing large amounts of milk substrates from the extra blood supply and secretory changes with the onset of milk production. Stage II begins clinically at 2–3 days after birth when 'the milk comes in'. The major changes in milk continue for 10 days when mature milk is established.

Lactogenesis III Lactogenesis III (galactopoiesis) begins around 10 days after birth once the mature milk supply is established. This involves the maintenance of established breastfeeding through milk production and removal of milk by the baby.

Hormonal control of lactogenesis

The four hormones involved in the initiation and maintenance of lactation are **oestrogen**, **progesterone**, **prolactin** and **oxytocin** (Fig. 54.6). An intact hypothalamic–pituitary axis, regulating prolactin and oxytocin levels, is essential for this process.

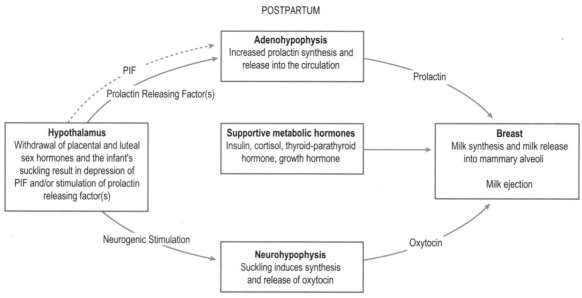

Figure 54.6 Hormonal preparation of the breast postpartum for lactation. (Reproduced with permission from Lawrence 1985.)

Oestrogen and progesterone It is highly likely that the onset and control of labour and the production of milk share the same endocrine trigger. Immediately prior to the onset of labour, during labour and following delivery of the placenta abrupt changes in the hormonal content of maternal blood occur. The pathways remain unclear in humans but it is possible for increasing fetal cortisol levels to alter the balance of the placental hormones, increasing the level of oestrogen and decreasing the level of progesterone (Lawrence & Lawrence 1999).

The fall in serum progesterone occurring just prior to the onset of labour may be the lactogenic trigger, releasing the mammary secreting cells from their inhibitory state. The secretory cells can now respond to the circulating prolactin by producing milk. Following delivery, the pituitary gland produces low levels of follicle-stimulating hormone (FSH) and luteinising hormone (LH). The ovaries respond poorly to stimulation by FSH and LH and there is a low level of oestrogen and progesterone production, enhancing the production of prolactin.

Prolactin Prolactin is a significant hormone of pregnancy and lactation. During pregnancy, concentrations of plasma prolactin rise steadily to term when they reach up to 20 times that of the non-pregnant woman. The **lactotrophs** of the anterior pituitary produce prolactin under the influence of the rising fetoplacental production of oestrogen. This stimulatory effect may be inhibited by human placental lactogen (hPL) as they are of similar activity and biological structure and compete for breast receptor sites. Prolactin is also prevented from exerting its effect on breast tissue by the high circulating levels of progesterone (Lawrence & Lawrence 1999). The inhibiting influence of progesterone is so powerful that lactation is delayed if placental fragments are retained after birth (Riordan & Auerbach 1998).

The control of prolactin secretion seems to be controlled by chemical factors, some inhibitory and some stimulatory (Fig. 54.7). The hypothalamus has a stimulating effect on the release of the majority of pituitary hormones. Prolactin is unusual among pituitary hormones because it is inhibited by a hypothalamic substance. Prolactin-inhibiting factor (PIF), which is thought to be the neuroregulatory substance dopamine, controls the secretion of prolactin from the hypothalamus (Voogt et al 2001). This factor is transported from the hypothalamus along the portal system to have its effect on the anterior pituitary.

The production of prolactin is supported by growth hormone, insulin, cortisol and thryrotrophin-releasing hormone (TRH). There is also evidence of either serotonin (5-hydroxy-tryptamine, 5-HT) release of prolactin or catecholamine–serotonin control of prolactin release. Thryrotrophin-releasing hormone is a strong stimulator of prolactin secretion but its physiologic role remains unclear, as thryrotrophin levels do not rise during normal nursing (Lawrence & Lawrence 1999).

Normally, the production of prolactin varies, following a **circadian rhythm**, with normal diurnal variation in levels in both males and females. Prolactin circadian rhythms persist throughout lactation. Prolactin levels are notably higher at night than during the day (Stern & Reichlin 1990). Increased prolactin levels are influenced by a number of factors that may be significant for lactating mothers. These include psychogenic factors, stress, exercise, nipple stimulation and sexual intercourse (Lawrence & Lawrence 1999).

After delivery of the placenta, progesterone and oestrogen levels fall abruptly and the anterior pituitary gland releases very large amounts of prolactin because it is no longer inhibited by these hormones. The decline in hPL removes any competition with prolactin for breast receptor sites. This also promotes the action of prolactin (Riordan & Auerbach 1998). Prolactin is essential for the production of milk and the amount of prolactin is proportional to the amount of nipple stimulation during the early stages of lactation. Nipple stimulation is the only factor influencing the release of prolactin. Therefore other sensory pathway are not involved in the initiation of milk production (Lawrence & Lawrence 1999).

Prolactin levels peak 30 min after a feed and return to a baseline after 3–4 h (Sweet 1997). As might be expected of a system under the influence of circadian rhythm, suckling-induced prolactin production is minimal in the morning and greatest at night. However, there is no correlation found between the amount of milk produced and the concentration of prolactin.

Oxytocin Oxytocin is essential for the removal of milk from the breast. The effective removal of milk involves two closely related aspects of breastfeeding:

- the let-down (milk ejection) reflex and the role of the posterior pituitary hormone oxytocin;

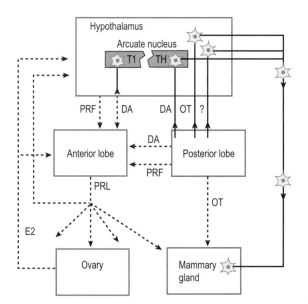

Figure 54.7 A model depicting the neuroendocrine regulation of prolactin secretion. TH, tuberohypophyseal; T1, tuberoinfundibular; OT, oxytocin; E2, oestradiol; PRF, prolactin-releasing factor; PRL, prolactin; DA, dopamine. (Reproduced with permission from Ben-Jonathan et al 1991.)

- the important role the baby has to play in suckling the breast to remove the milk.

Oxytocin is a peptide hormone produced in the hypothalamus and stored in the posterior pituitary gland. Oxytocin causes contraction of the sensitive myoepithelial cells situated around the milk-secreting glands and also dilates the ducts by acting on the smooth muscle cells lying in the duct wall (Howie 1999). Therefore, contraction of these cells has the dual effect of expelling milk from the glands and encouraging free flow of milk along the dilated ducts. This is known as the 'let down'.

The neuroendocrine mechanism or let-down reflex

Oxytocin levels in the blood often rise just before a feed, either due to the baby crying or becoming restless or the mother preparing for the feed (Lawrence & Lawrence 1999). Levels are raised within 1 min of any breast stimulation, and during stimulation the levels remain elevated and return to baseline levels within 6 min after nipple stimulation has stopped (Riordan & Auerbach 1998). Once suckling is initiated, the oxytocin response is transient and intermittent rather than sustained. The nipple and areola have a rich supply of sensory nerves. The afferent fibres terminate in the dorsal horn of the spinal cord, where they synapse on ascending fibres which transmit the messages received from the suckling of the baby to the brainstem. The messages are then relayed to the midbrain and hypothalamus, resulting in the release of oxytocin (Fig. 54.8) from the posterior lobe of the pituitary gland. This hormone contracts the myoepithelial cells and milk is propelled along the ducts. Smooth muscle contraction results in shortening and widening of the ducts to allow milk to flow into the ampullae. Some mothers may feel pressure and a tingling warm sensation during milk ejection. The baby suckling empties the breast and stimulates the release of prolactin.

The effect of higher brain centres   The **neuroendocrine regulation** of oxytocin release and the resulting milk ejection is a complex process which can be inhibited or stimulated by neural influences projected by nerves synapsing on the hypothalamus from higher centres of the brain. These include those parts of the brain involved in emotion, such as the limbic system, and the cognitive interpretation of all aspects of the activity from the prefrontal cortex. The control from higher centres can be more powerful than the nipple–hypothalamic pathway. The let-down reflex can be stimulated by other sensory pathways, such as visual, tactile, olfactory and auditory, or inhibited by emotional states. The mother can and will release milk by seeing, touching, hearing, smelling and/or just thinking about her baby. Anxiety, stress, embarrassment or emotional states can have just as powerful an effect on the inhibition of the release of milk (Wakerley et al 1994).

Suckling and removal of milk   Encouraging early and frequent breastfeeding is a simple recommendation for the initiation of breastfeeding. Following birth, there appears to be an early opportunity for the baby's suckling to stimulate prolactin receptors (Fig. 54.9), which in turn will enhance milk production. It is essential for babies to be put to the breast as early as possible after delivery, ideally in the first hour, and allow suckling as frequently as the baby demands. Milk production will be affected by factors which interfere with the process of suckling.

The baby needs to actively remove the milk by the process of suckling. This involves the baby working on the tissue of the breast with the jaw and tongue, which strips the milk from the milk ducts (Woolridge 1986). The relationship between the tongue and the lactiferous ducts is essential to good feeding and both mother and baby need to learn what constitutes good attachment and efficient removal of milk (see Ch. 55, p. 702).

Several reflexes enable the baby to play his part in breastfeeding: the rooting, suckling, swallowing and breathing reflexes. Obstetric factors such as medication, particularly pethidine, may have negative effects on the ability of the newborn baby to respond with appropriate behaviour. The reflexes are now considered.

- The **rooting reflex** is elicited when the baby's mouth is touched gently, such as by the nipple. The baby responds by turning the head towards the stimulus and opening the mouth wide. The wider the mouth opens, the easier it will be for the mother to attach the baby to the breast.

- The **suckling reflex** is complex. When the baby feels the mouth is full as far back as the hard palate and the back of the tongue, he will use jaws, tongue and cheek muscles to suckle. During suckling, breast tissue is drawn into the baby's mouth so that an elongated teat is formed from the areola and nipple and the lactiferous sinuses are within the mouth. The lips are closed around the junction of the nipple and areola. The gums are pressed against the areola and the tongue grasps the nipple and presses it against the hard palate, compressing the breast tissue beneath the areola to strip milk from the ducts (Fisher 1999). The muscles of the cheeks create suction and a negative pressure within the mouth.

- The **swallowing reflex** is well developed in the term infant and the baby swallows about 0.6 ml at each mouthful. Oesophageal function is not as developed, with irregular peristalsis.

- **Breathing** is coordinated with swallowing with an **upper airways reflex** to prevent aspiration. Under experimental conditions the introduction of water or milk from another species into the upper airway causes intermittent apnoea. Normal saline or same-species milk does not cause this apnoea. It has been observed that babies fed breast milk from a bottle suck intermittently but breathe continuously. If the baby is fed formula milk from the same bottle he sucks continuously and breathes intermittently. Breathing appears to be much more regular in babies fed breast milk. Neonates are nose breathers and cannot suckle adequately if their noses are blocked, for instance by breast tissue.

The production of milk

The consistently identifiable stages of human milk are colostrum, transitional milk and mature milk, and their relative contents are significant to nourish the newborns as they adapt to extrauterine life (Lawrence & Lawrence 1999).

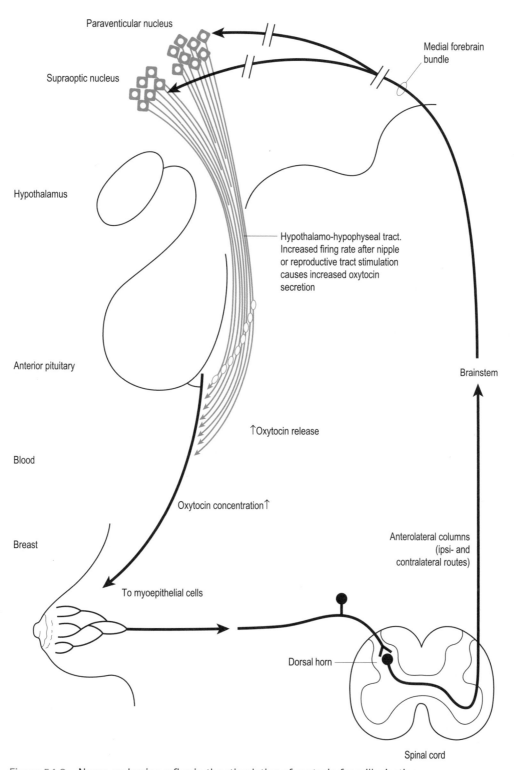

Figure 54.8 Neuro-endocrine reflex in the stimulation of oxytocin for milk ejection.

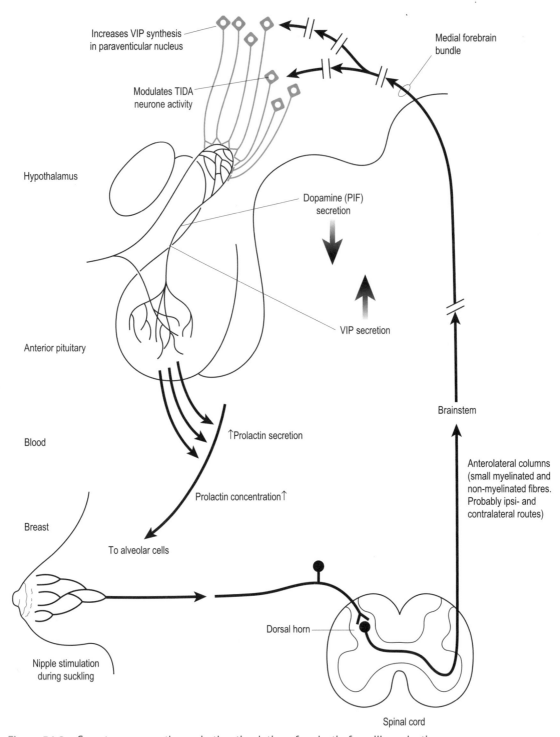

Increases VIP synthesis in paraventicular nucleus

Medial forebrain bundle

Modulates TIDA neurone activity

Hypothalamus

Dopamine (PIF) secretion

VIP secretion

Anterior pituitary

Brainstem

Blood

↑Prolactin secretion

Anterolateral columns (small myelinated and non-myelinated fibres. Probably ipsi- and contralateral routes)

Prolactin concentration↑

Breast

To alveolar cells

Dorsal horn

Nipple stimulation during suckling

Spinal cord

Figure 54.9   Somatosensory pathways in the stimulation of prolactin for milk production.

Colostrum, a thick yellow fluid, is synthesised in the breast from around the 16th week of pregnancy and gradually changes into mature breast milk between the 3rd and 14th day following delivery (Fig. 54.10). It is high in density and low in volume, containing more protein, minerals and fat-soluble vitamins (A and K) than mature milk but less lactose, fats and water-soluble vitamins. It also contains more antiinfective agents such as IgA, lactoferrin, lysozymes and leucocytes than mature milk. Colostrum facilitates the establishment of bifidus flora in the digestive tract and facilitates the passage of meconium. It is eminently suited for the newborn baby.

Transitional milk is the milk produced between colostrum and mature milk. The content gradually changes from between 7–10 days and about 2 weeks after birth. The concentration of immunoglobins and total protein decreases

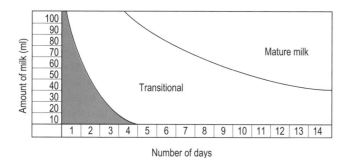

Figure 54.10   The sequence of milk production (from Lang S 1997, with permission).

and the lactose, fat and total caloric content increases. Water-soluble vitamins increase and fat-soluble vitamins decrease to the levels of mature milk.

Mature breast milk is highly variable both within and between women. Its contents change from one feed to another, over the course of a specific feed and as the baby grows and develops. The milk obtained by the baby at the beginning of a feed is called the **fore-milk** and differs from the **hind-milk** obtained towards the end of a feed.

When lactation begins, the mother's metabolism changes greatly and milk may need to be produced at the metabolic expense of other organs (Lawrence & Lawrence 1999). However, milk will continue to be produced for as long as it is removed from the breast. Recently, an autocrine regulator of milk secretion has been identified called the **feedback inhibitor of lactation** (FIH). This factor – a whey protein present in secreted milk – is able to inhibit the synthesis of milk constituents (Wilde et al 1995) and accumulates in the breast as the milk accumulates, exerting a negative control on the continued production of milk. Removing the milk also removes the regulating protein and milk continues to be produced. While breastfeeding is not a major factor for the initiation of lactation, it is essential for the continuation of lactation (Riordan & Auerbach 1998).

The contents of breast milk

The main contents of milk include proteins, carbohydrates, fats, electrolytes, minerals, vitamins, enzymes, hormones and antiinfective substances. All mammalian milks differ in the relative quantities of the above contents and have evolved specifically to maximise development of the newborn. Feeding one mammal's milk to another mammal can only be second best, although sophisticated modifications of cow's milk are achieved for human babies.

Protein

The acinar cells (milk-producing cells) are very efficient in removing breast milk precursors from maternal blood. Milk proteins are formed on the ribosomes bound to the rough endoplasmic reticulum from amino acids derived mainly from maternal blood. The protein molecules are then stored in the Golgi apparatus. Vesicles move the protein molecules to the apex of the cell where they are discharged into the lumen of the alveolus.

The main proteins of human milk are casein (40%) and whey protein (60%). These proteins are acidic in the stomach, and form soft curds, which are easily digested to provide a continuous flow of nutrients to the baby. The chief fractions of whey protein are α-lactalbumin and lactoferrin. In addition to their nutritional function, milk proteins also have specific functions. Casein is an important carrier of calcium and phosphate with which it forms micelles.

The protein in human milk is ideal for the baby and is totally different from cow's milk. Lactoferrin is an iron-binding protein which is low in bovine milk. The total protein content and the balance of amino acids present are essential for the maximum functioning of enzyme systems. The amino acids phenylalanine and tyrosine are present in much lower amounts than in cow's milk, modified or unmodified. The important amino acids glutamic acid and taurine are abundant in human milk but low in cow's milk. Taurine is necessary for the conjugation of bile salts and fat absorption in the first week of life. It is also essential for the myelination of the central nervous system (Sheridan 1997).

Carbohydrate

Lactose is the main carbohydrate in human milk and is formed from glucose or galactose in the Golgi apparatus under the influence of the enzyme lactose synthetase. The enzyme has two components – an 'A' protein called galactosyl transferase and a 'B' protein which is α-lactalbumin. Thus, the regulation of lactose is linked to the production of milk protein, in particular α-lactalbumin. Lactose in turn is linked to the water and mineral content of milk by exerting most osmotic pressure, drawing water from the cytoplasm into the Golgi apparatus. Water makes up more than 80% of milk volume. The lactose content of milk varies between a high 7 g/100 ml in human milk to 4 g/100 ml in the milk of other mammals. Cow's milk is low in lactose.

Lactose is important for brain growth. It is also necessary for the promotion of the growth of the microorganism *Lactobacillus bifidus*, the presence of which leads to increased acidity of the stool. Several important effects follow the increase in pH of the stools:

- calcium salts are easier to absorb;
- lactoferrin binds iron, making it more easily absorbed;
- the growth of pathogenic microbes is inhibited.

Fats

The fat content of human milk provides about one-half of the milk's calories and is the most important component. The lipids found in human milk are mainly globules of triglycerides (98–99%) and are easy to digest and absorb. Long-chain fatty acids are transported directly from maternal blood to the breast as chylomicrons. The acinar cells manufacture short- and medium-chain fatty acids. Although long-chain fatty acids make up most of the fat content of milks, human milk contains more long-chain fatty acids (95% against 83%) than cow's milk. In both human milk and cow's milk, 5% of the remaining fatty acids are medium-chain fatty acids and cow's milk also contains 12% short-chain fatty acids.

Arachidonic acid (AA) and docosahexaenoic acid (DHA) are two long-chain fatty acids found in human milk that are essential for the development of the brain and nervous system and for vascular tissue. The intake of biologically inappropriate fatty acids could have long-term effects on the growth of nervous tissue. The unavailability of some fatty acids with a corresponding alteration in body tissue composition may be a long-term problem for babies fed on cow's milk. In particular, the formation of the myelin sheaths may be affected permanently.

AA and another fatty acid, linoleic acid, are found in high quantities in human milk. These enable prostaglandin synthesis, which matures intestinal cells, aids digestion and adds to the antiinfective protective effect of human milk. However, the difficulty in achieving a balanced formula in modified milks was illustrated when linoleic acid was added to one infant formula to produce milk rich in polyunsaturated fats. The babies fed on this formula developed a type of haemolytic anaemia. The anaemia, caused by ingestion of large amounts of linoleic acid in the absence of vitamin E, resulted in peroxide formation and haemolysis.

Variations in fat content of milk Fats are the most variable constituent of human milk, varying in concentration over feeding, from breast to breast, over time and among individuals (Lawrence & Lawrence 1999). The fat content of the hind-milk is significantly increased, especially in late morning and early afternoon (Sheridan 1997). The fat level may reach five times the value of the initial level during the feed (Fisher 1999). The fatty acid content varies according to dietary source while the fat content varies with calorific intake. High quantities of free fatty acids and cholesterol are present in human milk and act as an important energy source for the baby, providing more than 50% of the calorific requirements. As fat contains 9 kcal/g, the calorific content will vary significantly with the fat content.

Electrolytes

Lactose secretion is directly involved in the transfer of ions across the acinar cell membrane into the milk. The total content of mineral salts is less than one-third of that present in cow's milk with only 0.2% of the sodium, potassium and chloride content. The kidney of the neonate does not cope well with an increased sodium load.

Despite modification in formula feeds, there is a risk of hypernatraemia with dehydration in formula-fed babies if the feed is reconstituted with too much milk powder over a period of time. High solute content leads to thirst and crying. Inexperienced parents may interpret this as hunger and offer more milk, which could predispose to long-term obesity. Although rare, severe hypernatraemia may result in irreversible brain damage. There may be a link between high solute loads and a predisposition to hypertension in later life. The breastfed baby is less likely to need additional fluid intake except in extreme temperatures.

Minerals

Calcium, phosphorus and magnesium are present in human milk at higher concentrations than in plasma, which suggests active transportation. Absorption in the gut of the neonate depends on the availability of fats and vitamin D. Calcium is more efficiently absorbed from human milk than from substitutes due to the human milk's high calcium: phosphorus ratio (RCM 2002). Babies fed on unmodified cow's milk are unable to absorb calcium and may suffer hypocalcaemia with tetany. Formula-fed babies tend to have lower serum calcium levels than breastfed babies even when modifications have included the replacement of the fat in cow's milk with a mixture of vegetable and animal fats and vitamin D has been added. Low levels of magnesium may exacerbate neonatal tetany.

Trace elements

The levels of iron, copper and zinc are higher in colostrum than in mature milk. More zinc is present in cow's milk but is not as readily absorbed as that present in human milk. A small amount of zinc is necessary to ensure the baby's health. Other necessary trace elements such as copper, cobalt and selenium are present in optimal quantities. These elements are associated in small amounts with the protein casein, larger amounts with whey proteins and moderate amounts with fats bound to specific carrier proteins (ligands).

Vitamins

The fat-soluble vitamins A, D, E and K are present in breast milk, with higher quantities of vitamin K than previously realised being present in colostrum and hind-milk during the early days after delivery (Fisher 1999). The need to give vitamin K to neonates is discussed in Chapter 48, p. 612. All vitamin B complex vitamins and vitamin C are also present on breast milk.

Enzymes

The function of many of the enzymes present in breast milk is unknown. The enzymes lipase, amylase and lysozyme are important. Lipase, the fat-digesting enzyme, is present in breast milk in a form which becomes active in the baby's intestine, making fat digestion easier in breastfed babies.

Also present is the starch-digesting enzyme amylase. The presence of amylase may compensate for low salivary and pancreatic amylase activity in neonates. Lysozyme is an important bacteriolytic enzyme present in many body fluids.

Hormones

Hormones present in breast milk include prolactin, oxytocin, prostaglandins, insulin, thyroid-stimulating hormone, thyroxine and growth hormones – specifically epidermal growth factor, which is important for the development of the lining of the gut. Endocrine responses are different in breastfed babies from those who are artificially fed (Sweet 1997). Growth factor concentration is maximal in the colostrum produced on the 1st day of life.

Antiinfective factors

The following breast milk factors are present (Fisher 1999):

- A high level of leucocytes are present in breast milk, especially in the first 10 days. These are mainly macrophages and neutrophils whose purpose is to surround and destroy pathogenic bacteria.

- Although immunoglobulins IgA, IgG, IgM and IgD are found in breast milk, the most important is IgA which lines the intestinal mucosal surfaces to protect against pathogenic bacteria such as *Escherichia coli*, *Salmonella* and *Shigella* spp., streptococci and staphylococci and pathogenic viruses such as poliovirus and the rotaviruses.

- Lysozyme is a protein present in breast milk in concentrations thousands of times that of cow's milk. It is bacteriolytic and helps to break down the cell walls of pathogenic organisms.

- Lactoferrin, an iron-binding protein found in human milk, increases the absorption of enteric iron. It provides protection in breastfed babies by inhibiting the growth of certain iron-dependent bacteria such as *E. coli* in the gastrointestinal tract.

- The bifidus factor present in human milk encourages the growth of the Gram-positive *Lactobacillus bifidus*, which in turn discourages the growth of Gram-negative pathogenic organisms.

The transmission of viruses in milk

In the previous decade, women infected with human immunodeficiency virus (HIV) from developed and developing countries were recommended not to breastfeed to avoid mother-to-child transmission of the infection. While feeding infants with formula milk is relatively safe in developed countries, it is very likely to increase morbidity and mortality from other infectious diseases. In light of recent studies and analysis of the situation, it is now recommended that women in developing countries should be encouraged to exclusively breastfeed to maintain the overall benefits of breastfeeding (Coutsoudis et al 1999, Morrison 1999). The World Health Organisation has shown that infants in developing countries who are not breastfed and who had received formula or other replacement feed have a six-fold increased risk of dying in the first 2 months of life (Dobson 2002).

In other viral diseases, such as cytomegalovirus, rubella and hepatitis B, the virus may be present in breast milk with no adverse effects on the baby.

Antiallergic properties

The newborn baby has an immature immune system and gut mucosa and this allows the absorption of large foreign proteins. The IgA and other factors present in breast milk encourage maturity of the gut mucosa to form a barrier against these large proteins. Sensitivity to certain allergens may be inherited, and mothers with known sensitivities may be advised to avoid eating or drinking such allergens as cow's milk for the duration of breastfeeding.

A number of reports have shown a lower incidence and severity of symptoms of atopic conditions, such as eczema and asthma, in children who were breastfed (Burr et al 1993, Oddy 2000, Saarinen & Kajosaari 1995). Findings are inconclusive at this stage as to whether the predisposing factor is breast milk or the early introduction of weaning foods. The protective effect of breastfeeding may be secondary rather than the primary factor because breastfeeding mothers tend to introduce supplements at a later stage (Howie 1999). At present, the single most effective measure against children developing allergic tendencies is probably to encourage mothers to breastfeed for at least 4 months and preferably longer (Oddy 2000).

MAIN POINTS

- Embryogenesis refers to the embryonic development of the organ in utero. Mammogenesis refers to the growth and development of the mammary glands during puberty and pregnancy. Lactogenesis refers to the initiation and production of milk (three stages).

- Mammary tissue is divided into parenchyma and stroma. The parenchyma (glandular tissue) is the functional component of the breast. The stroma comprises the other supportive tissues, including the skin.

- The parenchyma is arranged in about 15–25 lobes that radiate out from the nipple. Each lobe is divided into the lobuloalveolar system. This comprises alveoli (specialised milk-forming acini cells), ductules, ducts and an expanded central lactiferous sinus for milk storage called an ampulla.

- Alveoli and smaller ducts are surrounded by myoepithelial cells. Smooth muscle surrounds the larger ducts. The functions of the muscular fibroelastic system of the areola and nipple include decreasing the surface of the areola, producing nipple erection and emptying the lactiferous sinuses during lactation.

- Developments of the breast in pregnancy include a marked increase in the ductal system and formation of lobes; the synthesis of colostrum; increased vascularity; development of the Montgomery's tubercles; pigmentation of the areola; and an increase in size. Montgomery's tubercles lubricate and protect the areola and nipple.

- The four hormones involved in the initiation and maintenance of lactation are oestrogen, progesterone, prolactin and oxytocin. During pregnancy, progesterone inhibits the effect of prolactin on breast tissue to produce milk. Prolactin is involved in milk production (galactopoiesis) and suckling is the main stimulus for its release.

- Stimulation of the areola and nipple initiates the release of oxytocin. This causes contraction of the myoepithelial cells surrounding the milk-secreting cells and propels milk along the duct. This is known as the let-down reflex. The let-down reflex can be also be stimulated by sensory factors and inhibited by emotional states. Lactating women require an additional 500 kcal/day.

- Reflexes in the newborn that influence breastfeeding include rooting, suckling, swallowing and upper airways reflexes. Factors interfering with suckling will affect milk production. Feedback inhibitor factor (FIH) in milk inhibits the synthesis of milk constituents.

- Colostrum is high in density and low in volume and contains more antiinfective substances. Mature milk is highly variable and changes from one feed to another. The main contents of milk include proteins, carbohydrates, fats, electrolytes, minerals, vitamins, enzymes, hormones and antiinfective substances.

- Some proteins form soft curds in the stomach, providing a continuous flow of nutrients to the baby. Fats act as an important energy source for the baby, providing more than 50% of the calorific requirements. The fat-soluble vitamins A, D, E and K are present in breast milk in addition to vitamin B complex and vitamin C.

- Immunity factors present in breast milk include a high level of leucocytes and IgA. Other antiinfective agents include lysozyme, lactoferrin and the bifidus factor. Babies can be infected with HIV during breastfeeding. Exclusive breastfeeding should be encouraged in developing countries.

References

Blackburn S T 2003 Maternal, Fetal and Neonatal Physiology: A Clinical Perspective, 2nd edn. W B Saunders, Philadelphia.

Burr L, Limb E S, Maguire M J et al 1993 Infant feeding, wheezing and allergy: a prospective study. Archives of Disorders of Childhood 68:724–728.

Coutsoudis A, Kubendran P, Spooner E et al 1999 Influence of infant-feeding patterns on early mother–child transmission of HIV in Durban, South Africa: a prospective cohort study. Lancet 354:471–476.

Czerkas S J, Czerkas S A 1990 Dinosaurs, A Global View. Dragon's World, London.

Dobson R 2002 Breast is still best even when HIV prevalence is high, experts say. British Medical Journal 324(22):1474.

Fisher C 1999 Feeding. In Bennett V R, Brown L K (eds) Myles Textbook for Midwives, 13th edn. Churchill Livingstone, Edinburgh.

Howie P W 1999 The puerperium. In Edmonds K D (ed.) Dewhurst's Textbook for Obstetrics and Gynaecology for Postgraduates, 6th edn. Blackwell Science, London.

Lawrence R A, Lawrence R M 1999 Breastfeeding: A Guide for the Medical Profession, 5th edn. Mosby, St Louis.

Morrison P 1999 HIV and infant feeding: to breastfeed or not to breastfeed: the development of completing risks – Part 1. Breastfeeding Review 7(2):5–13.

Neville M C, Morton J, Umemura S 2001 Lactogenesis – the transition from pregnancy to lactation. Pediatric Clinics of North America 48(1):35–52.

Oddy W H 2000 Breastfeeding and asthma in children. Breastfeeding Review 8(1):5–11.

RCM (Royal College of Midwives) 2002 Successful Breastfeeding, 3rd edn. Churchill Livingstone, London.

Riordan J, Auerbach K G (eds) 1998 Breastfeeding and Human Lactation, 2nd edn. Jones & Bartlett, Toronto.

Saarinen U M, Kajosaari M 1995 Breast feeding as prophylaxis against atopic disease: prospective follow up study until 17 years old. Lancet 346(8982):1065–1069.

Sheridan V 1997 Breastfeeding. In Sweet B R, Tiran D (eds) Mayes Midwifery: A Textbook for Midwives, 12th edn. Baillière Tindall, London.

Stern J M, Reichlin S 1990 Prolactin circadian rhythm persists throughout lactation in women. Neuroendocrinology 51:31–36.

Sweet B R 1997 The anatomy of the breast. In Sweet B R, Tiran D (eds) Mayes Midwifery: A Textbook for Midwives, 12th edn. Baillière Tindall, London.

Voogt J L, Lee Y, Yang S et al 2001 Regulation of prolactin secretion during pregnancy and lactation. Progress in Brain Surgery 133:178–185.

Wakerley J B, Clarke G, Summerlee A J S 1994 Milk ejection and its control. In Knobil E, Neill J D, Greenwald G S et al (eds) The Physiology of Reproduction. Raven Press, New York.

Wilde C J, Addey C V P, Boddy L M et al 1995 Autocrine regulation of milk secretion by a protein in milk. Biochemical Journal 305:51–58.

Woolridge M W 1986 The 'anatomy' of infant sucking. Midwifery 2:164–171.

Annotated recommended reading

Lawrence R A, Lawrence R M 1999 Breastfeeding: A Guide for the Medical Profession, 5th edn. Mosby, St Louis.
This is an excellent reference book for health professionals involved with breastfeeding issues.

Chapter 55

Breastfeeding practice and problems

INTRODUCTION

Infant feeding affects every child for life, in many ways known and as yet unknown in other ways (Minchin 1998). Human milk nourishes the newborn, provides protection for child development in early and later life and is optimal for promoting closeness between mother and baby. In mammals, learning about breastfeeding is part of a lifelong process which begins at birth: some is instinctive but a lot is social learning and involves seeing breastfeeding as being a normal and welcome sight, involving shared experiences within the family or community. However, beliefs and attitudes about breastfeeding are very much dependent and influenced by culture, folklore and social context. For example, colostrum is accepted and encouraged as the first food for the baby in many cultures while other cultures believe colostrum to be 'old' milk and unfit for the newborn.

The majority of women are physiologically capable of breastfeeding and when this is not possible then formula milk is available for the baby as an inferior alternative. The art of breastfeeding is a specialised aspect of the science of lactation and is at risk of being lost to future generations because mothers in developed countries may choose to formula feed in favour of breastfeeding. This is concerning and makes it even more necessary to protect and support breastfeeding practices.

Although breastfeeding is partly instinctive behaviour, mothers will still need support, encouragement and good management to make breastfeeding a success. Breastfeeding is something that has to be learnt. This is true for most new mothers and it is certainly true for midwives and for other health professionals providing care and support (Inch & Fisher 1999). The information in this chapter may help to supply knowledge and information to those involved in helping mothers to successfully establish breastfeeding.

BENEFITS OF BREASTFEEDING

The benefits of breastfeeding for babies and mothers are well recognised in the current literature and it is useful to consider the benefits of breast milk and breastfeeding separately because the benefits are more than simply the advantages of feeding a baby on breast milk (UNICEF 1997). Health professionals should share information about these benefits with women when they are making a choice about feeding their baby.

Human milk is easily digested and nutritionally balanced to meet the baby's needs. In a systematic review of research studies in developed countries, Bick (2001) confirmed that breast milk has an established protection for babies against the conditions of gastrointestinal infection, otitis media and neonatal necrotising enterocolitis. Other possible benefits of breast milk for babies have been reported and include protection against lower respiratory tract infection, urinary tract infection, allergies, childhood diabetes and sudden infant death syndrome (SIDS), with neurological development of the baby being a possible advantage.

Breastfeeding may also have a positive effect for babies in relation to interpersonal relationships and sleeping patterns (Renfrew et al 2000). Babies are known to cry less if they stay close to their mothers and breastfeed from birth (Christensson et al 1995).

Increasing evidence suggests that there are long-term benefits from breastfeeding for the mother. There is a reduction in the incidence of hip fractures in women over 65 years (Cummings & Klineberg 1993) and in some types of cancer (discussed later). Breastfeeding helps the mother and baby form a close relationship and is emotionally satisfying for the mother. All of these factors can benefit the whole family emotionally and economically and improve their overall quality of life.

PHYSIOLOGY APPLIED TO PRACTICE

In Western countries it is rare for a young woman to hold a newborn baby until she bears her own and even rarer for her to closely observe breastfeeding. A primipara is therefore faced with the need to rapidly acquire these two skills without the benefit of prior experience. Midwives must be knowledgeable about the physiology of lactation and apply this to practice if they are going to help mothers to breastfeed. The baby needs adequate nourishment at the breast and the mother must be enabled to develop the necessary skills to feed the baby herself (Fisher 1999).

In recent years, a number of common breastfeeding practices have been shown to be unhelpful or detrimental to breastfeeding success. These practices were discontinued and included the separation of mothers and babies, restricted feeding and duration of breastfeeding and test weighing babies. The following practices were promoted when they were found to be beneficial in achieving breastfeeding success:

- early discharge from hospital – women who went home within 48h were more likely to be breastfeeding at 6 months postpartum (Renfrew & Lang 1999);

- provision of extra support to breastfeeding mothers – increased breastfeeding until the age of 2 months (Sikorski et al 2001).

Antenatal preparation

The decision to breastfeed by women in this society is often made before pregnancy or very early in pregnancy, while women tend to make the decision to formula feed later in pregnancy (RCM 2002). Women are unlikely to change their minds once the decision is made.

During this time, midwives should adopt a sensitive approach with women to help them make their own decision about baby feeding. Women who wish to breastfeed or are undecided should be given all the information and support they require during pregnancy. It may be a bit more difficult to give information to some women who have decided to formula feed. Women who choose to formula feed will also be given any information and support needed during pregnancy.

Preparation of the nipples is not necessary other than advising women to keep normal standards of cleanliness and wear a well-supporting bra. Women with nipple problems may find their nipples shape improves as pregnancy proceeds. Breast shells and Hoffman's exercises are ineffective in the preparation of problem nipples (Main Trial Collaborative Group 1994). Teaching pregnant women about breastfeeding physiology and skills may be more important.

The first feed

Mothers should hold their babies with skin contact at birth or within 30 min of delivery and they should be encouraged to give the first breastfeed as soon as the baby is receptive. This should be unhurried as it is important that time is taken to achieve a successful first feed. Health professionals need to know what constitutes good breast attachment to enable them to facilitate mothers appropriately with the initiation of breastfeeding. The mothers need to know how to breastfeed their baby and learn how to hold and position the baby and often they need help with this.

There are several reasons why early and frequent breastfeeding is beneficial for the mother and the baby (summarised in Riordan & Auerbach 1998):

- Suckling stimulates uterine contractions, aids expulsion of the placenta and helps to control blood loss.
- The early removal of milk creates the optimum impetus for the development and sensitivity of prolactin receptors, which ensures early milk production.
- The baby's suckling reflex is usually most intense 45 min through the second hour of labour. Initiate soon after birth to prevent any delay in gratification for the baby.
- The baby begins to get the immunological benefits of colostrums.
- The baby's digestive peristalsis is stimulated.

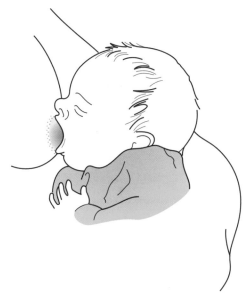

Figure 55.1   The correct position for breastfeeding (from Sweet B 1997, with permission).

- Breast engorgement is minimised or prevented by the early removal of milk from the breasts.
- Lactation is accelerated and early frequent intake of breast milk lessens neonate weight loss.
- Attachment and bonding are enhanced at a heightened state of readiness for mother and baby.

Positioning

The correct positioning of the baby at the breast is essential to the success of breastfeeding and in the prevention of potential problems for mother and baby (Fig. 55.1). The midwife needs to assess the needs and preferences of the mother and to be flexible in her approach to positioning of the baby. Special groups of mothers may need help with positioning such as new or first-time breastfeeding mothers, those with difficulties or previous difficulties with feeding and mothers with multiple births or special needs. Although the mother can adopt different positions to hold the baby, it is wise to offer the baby to the mother in a neutral position so that she can hold him on the arm she prefers for the first attempt (Fig. 55.3).

Attachment of the baby's mouth to the breast

Attachment to the breast is the most important aspect of breastfeeding and is essential for mothers to achieve success and prevent potential problems occurring (discussed later). Breastfeeding needs to be explained to the mother and she should be taught the basic skills involved. The mother should be given information:

- how to elicit the rooting reflex from the baby;
- how to offer the breast to the baby when his mouth is wide open;

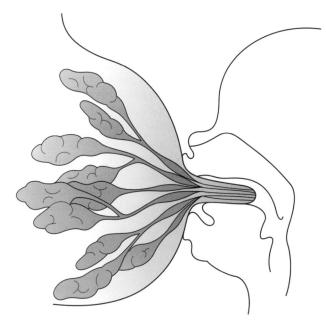

Figure 55.2   Breast tissue formed into a teat in the baby's mouth (from Sweet B 1997, with permission).

- how to recognise when the baby is properly attached;
- how the milk is released by the let-down reflex and begins to flow and how the baby uses suction to hold the breast tissue in the mouth to form a teat (Fig. 55.2) and obtain the milk by the action of the tongue pressing the milk from the sinuses into the mouth.

Four key points apply to mothers when positioning and attaching the baby to the breast:

1. the baby's head and body should be in a straight line;
2. the baby's mouth should face the breast, with the top lip opposite the nipple;
3. the mother should hold the baby close to her;
4. if the baby is newborn, then the mother should support the baby's whole body and not just the head and shoulders.

Key signs of good attachment

- More of the areola can be seen above the baby's mouth than below.
- The mouth is wide open.
- The lower lip is turned outwards.
- The chin touches the breast.

Other signs of good attachment are also found during feeding. The sucking pattern is rhythmical and changes from quick short sucks to slow deep sucks. The baby will pause from time to time and then start sucking again without coaxing. The baby can be seen or heard swallowing and is relaxed, happy and releases the breast at the end of feeding.

Nutritional aspects

The baby must be allowed to obtain both fore-milk and hind-milk from one breast before being offered the other breast. The baby should be encouraged to empty one breast before feeding from the other breast. This will ensure that the baby get the fat-laden hind-milk and will maximise calorie intake. In addition, the breast will empty of milk and will prevent protein accumulating, which exerts a negative feedback control on milk production (Wilde et al 1995). Removing milk from the breast also removes this protein and milk production is not affected. Both breasts will continue to produce milk if the next feed is commenced on the alternate breast.

Baby–led feeding

Mothers should be assured that there is no need to know how much milk has been taken (one reason for wishing to bottlefeed). The baby will be getting sufficient nourishment if satisfied and sleeping well between feeds. In particular, mothers need to understand that breast milk is not designed to last 4 full hours between each feed and that newborns do not differentiate night from day (Fisher 1999). At first, the mother may experience a few problems with tiredness due to frequent feeding but she should be reassured that this will settle down once the baby has developed his own circadian rhythms.

The role of lateral behavioural preferences

Human beings have at least three lateral preferences in behaviour that may influence the establishment of breast-feeding (Stables & Hewitt 1995):

1. the use of a dominant hand for skilled tasks, commonly the right hand;
2. the use of a dominant arm to hold the baby, usually the left arm;
3. a preference by the baby for turning his head to the right.

   Right-handed mothers may prefer to hold their baby in the left arm and if the baby prefers to turn his head to the right, there may be a preference for feeding the baby on the left breast. The mother may feel comfortable with the baby held in her left arm, leaving her dominant right hand to manipulate the breast. The baby who prefers to turn his head to the right will automatically turn to face the left breast. The mother may perceive that feeding at the right breast is more difficult. These lateral preferences occasionally cause transient problems, usually overcome by the 3rd day as the mother and baby develop skills. However, some women who are ambivalent about breastfeeding may feel unable to continue (see Ch. 57, p. 728).

   Taking note of the lateral preferences, the baby may be held across the mother's lap or tucked under her arm (see Fig. 55.3) if it is noticed that the baby consistently turns his

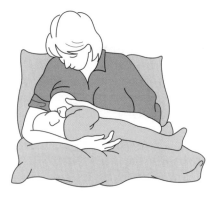

(a) The conventional hold

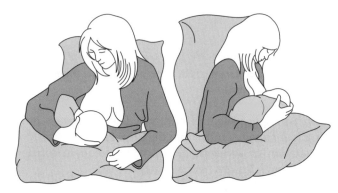

(b) Holding under one arm, dominant hand supports head **(c)** Holding across the body, dominant hand supports head

Figure 55.3   Ways of holding babies during breastfeeding.

head away from one breast (Stables & Hewitt 1995). The mother can be shown how to attach the baby to each breast using her skilful hand (Fisher 1999).

BREASTFEEDING PROBLEMS

The following common situations and conditions often cause difficulties with breastfeeding:

- insufficient milk supply;
- abnormal nipples, including flat, inverted, large or long nipple;
- sore or fissured nipples;
- full and engorged breasts;
- blocked ducts and mastitis;
- breast abscess.

Other problems include breast refusal and the mother and baby with special needs.

Insufficient milk

Almost all mothers are able to produce milk and in many cases mothers can produce more milk than is required. Although the true incidence is unknown, observations in traditional societies suggest that only 1% of women would be physiologically incapable of producing an adequate milk supply (Enkin et al 2000). However, often mothers perceive that they are not producing enough milk for their baby and this is one of the most common reasons why they start bottle feeds or stop breastfeeding.

The best means of preventing insufficient milk from occurring is unrestricted feeding by a well-positioned baby, while giving good practical and emotional support to the mother (Enkin et al 2000). Lactation is a supply-on-demand function and any formula given to top-up or replace breastfeeds will eventually diminish the mother's milk output. If the baby is not correctly positioned on the breast, there may be inadequate emptying of the breast with reduction in milk supply. Often, new mothers lack confidence and may need support and reassurance to overcome their feelings about not giving the baby enough milk. Provided there is good attachment, the most important advice is to encourage the mother to let the baby suckle often to stimulate milk production.

The only two reliable indicators that the baby is not getting sufficient milk are poor weight gain and passing small amounts of concentrated urine.

Abnormal nipples

Sometimes the size and shape of the nipple make it difficult for the baby to attach to the breast. Flat and inverted nipples commonly cause problems (Figs 55.4 and 55.5), but occasionally large and long nipples cause difficulty for small babies. If the breast tissue is soft and the baby manages to attach to the breast, this will not cause too much difficulty. However, problems can arise when the breast tissue is engorged and the baby just cannot attach to the breast. In these circumstances, it may be necessary to express milk to give to the baby until the breast texture returns to normal.

Sore or cracked nipples

Breastfeeding should be comfortable and pain free. Some mothers may feel the nipples tender for the first few days with some discomfort and even pain. During feeding, this usually occurs temporarily at the beginning of a feed only. The commonest cause of sore nipples is poor attachment to the breast caused by friction between the baby's mouth and the nipple. This is more likely to occur in women with flat or inverted nipples. Depressing the breast away from the baby's face may also alter the shape of the nipple, leading to friction and abrasion. The only factor that has been shown to both prevent and treat nipple trauma is good positioning of the baby at the breast (Enkin et al 2000). If the nipple is too sore for the mother to continue feeding, she should rest the affected breast, hand express and recommence feeding when the lesion is healed.

Full breasts and engorgement

Normal fullness of the breasts will occur a few days after delivery when the mother's milk is 'coming in'. The breasts

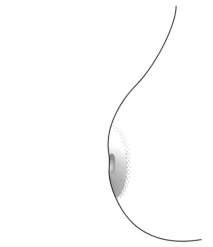

Figure 55.4   An inverted nipple (from Lang S 1997, with permission).

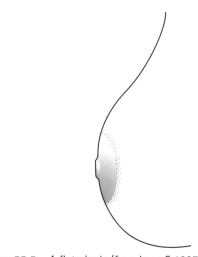

Figure 55.5   A flat nipple (from Lang S 1997, with permission).

may feel heavy, hard and hot and possibly lumpy. The milk will be flowing well and can often be seen dripping from the breasts. During this time, the mother should be encouraged to breastfeed her baby frequently to remove the milk. The breasts will feel softer and more comfortable after the feel and the breasts will adapt to suit the baby's needs within a few days.

Engorgement means that the breasts are overfull, partly with milk and partly with increased tissue fluid and blood. The breasts appear flushed, feel hard and painful and the mother may have a slight rise in pulse and temperature. This will interfere with the flow of milk, and milk production may be affected if the condition is not treated.

Allowing the baby unrestricted access to the breast while properly positioned still appears to be the most effective method of treating and preventing breast engorgement (Enkin et al 2000). The removal of milk is essential to prevent further complications such as reduced milk production, mastitis or a breast abscess. Milk can either be removed by the baby being correctly positioned and attached to the breast or by hand expressing if the baby is unable to attach.

It may help to express a little milk before the baby is put to the breast. The breasts should be well supported and analgesia may be required. The condition may be resolved more quickly if the baby is allowed to empty one breast at one feed and the other breast at the following feed.

Mastitis

Mastitis is an area of inflammation which affects part of the breast, often only one breast. It is often confused with engorgement, which affects the whole breast. Mastitis may develop in an engorged breast or it may follow a blocked duct. In these two conditions, milk stays in part of the breast, called milk stasis. If the milk is not removed, it can cause inflammation of the breast tissue, which can be infective or non-infective mastitis.

Non-infective mastitis

Non-infective mastitis occurs in a substantial proportion of women (Enkin et al 2000). It is probably due to poor drainage of milk and milk leaks into the surrounding tissue when under pressure. Milk contains substances that irritate tissue, causing an inflammatory reaction. Signs and symptoms are rarely seen before the 8th postpartum day. The affected wedge-shaped segment of breast tissue is swollen, and painful and the overlying skin is reddened. The woman complains of throbbing pain and tenderness and it is common for her to develop a raised temperature and pulse rate. Aching flu-like symptoms are often accompanied by shivering attacks and rigors.

Good breastfeeding management will help to prevent the development of mastitis. Continued breastfeeding with unlimited feeds gives the best results in milk stasis. It is important to remove milk from the breasts, as milk stasis is an ideal culture for microorganisms. Expression of breast milk alone does not have any advantage. The best outcome for women with non-infective mastitis is the continuation of breastfeeding, supplemented with expressed breast milk (Enkin et al 2000). The breast should be well-supported and warm compresses or analgesics may be necessary to alleviate any discomfort. Prophylactic antibiotics may be commenced.

Infective mastitis

Breast abscesses may develop in infective mastitis if bacteria, commonly *Staphylococcus aureus* from the baby, enter the breast through a crack in the nipple. The axillary lymph glands will be enlarged. A specimen of breast milk will confirm whether or not infection is present and antibiotics are necessary. Expressing breast milk improves the outcome for mothers with infectious mastitis (Enkin et al 2000). Pain and discomfort may be alleviated with warm compresses and analgesia.

Breast abscess

An abscess is when a collection of pus forms in part of the breast. The breast develops a painful soft swelling. Additional signs include pitting oedema of the overlying skin and a fluctuant swelling under the reddened area (Abbott 1997). Surgical incision and drainage is necessary. The baby will not be affected by the abscess and, if possible, should continue to feed from the breast. However, if the abscess is too painful or the mother is unwilling to feed, she should be advised to express her milk until the incision has healed.

Feeding after breast surgery

Nowadays it is not uncommon for women to have undergone breast surgery prior to pregnancy and lactation. Surgery may be performed for pathological conditions and include biopsy and conservative surgery for cancer or for cosmetic reasons. The latter operations include the insertion of silicone breast implants and reduction mammoplasty.

A number of factors will influence the woman's ability to lactate after surgery but success or failure will really depend on the degree to which surgery affected the internal structures involved in lactation. In general, there will be a better chance of breastfeeding if the structures are intact and functioning, but this will depend on the surgical procedure performed. For example, it is most unlikely that breastfeeding would be possible if the nipple was resited.

Women who have had silicone implants or reduction mammoplasty may be able to breastfeed successfully (RCM 2002). Breastfeeding with a silicone implant may have a higher risk of the baby developing autoimmune disease in later childhood, such as scleroderma-like oesophageal disease (Jordan & Blum 1996, Levine & Ilowite 1994). However, the benefits of breastfeeding may outweigh the slight risk of scleroderma (Williams 1994). It is possible for some women to successfully breastfeed after conservative surgery and radiation but it may interfere with milk production (Tralins 1995).

PROBLEMS ARISING WITH THE BABY

Congenital abnormalities in the baby

Structural abnormalities of the lip and palate may make a mother feel she cannot breastfeed. In practice, there should be no difficulties if the cleft is only in the lip. The baby with a cleft palate will not be able to form a teat out of the mother's breast tissue and this will prevent the baby from getting the suction necessary to withdraw the milk. Some mothers have expressed their breast milk until the defect has been repaired and then achieved successful breastfeeding (Fisher 1999). The mother of a baby with a cleft abnormality may achieve success with breastfeeding if she tries different positions to hold the baby (Fig. 55.6).

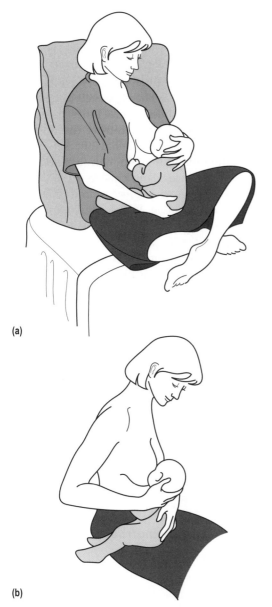

(a)

(b)

Figure 55.6   Positions for feeding a baby with a cleft abnormality (from Lang S 1997, with permission).

Prematurity in the baby

Breastfeeding will be possible with a preterm baby once the sucking and swallowing reflexes have fully developed. If the baby tires quickly at the breast, it may be necessary to use expressed milk to complement his feeding by tube. Preterm babies require a good energy source both for growth and development and to maintain an adequate body temperature. Sometimes, it is necessary to supplement human milk with a nutritional fortifier to ensure adequate growth (Jones & Spencer 2003).

CHEMICALS IN BREAST MILK

In recent years there has been much concern about the amount of environmental toxins that may be present in human breast milk (see Ch. 8). Also, most drugs are of a small enough molecular weight to pass into breast milk and can be ingested by the baby. Substances such as cocaine and nicotine taken as recreational drugs may also have adverse effects on the baby.

Medications

Careful consideration should always be given to any drugs taken by breastfeeding mothers. This is often difficult because of the many factors that can influence the potential effects of the drug for the baby such as the nature, characteristics and the route of administration of the drug and whether the drug appears in the active form or as an inactive metabolite. Other factors to be considered include whether the baby can absorb the drug from the gastrointestinal tract and, if so, whether the drug can be excreted or detoxified normally. A number of sources such as the British National Formulary (2003) or Lawrence & Lawrence (1999) can be consulted for guidance in the use of individual drugs.

Drugs taken in the first trimester may interfere with the development of the fetus while if they are taken in the later trimesters they may alter the growth and functional development of the fetus. Any drugs given to the mother during labour may affect the neonate after delivery. Insufficient evidence is available to provide guidance for breastfeeding mothers, and drugs should be avoided. If necessary, then the baby should be carefully observed for any possible adverse effects such as changing patterns in feeding and sleeping or skin rashes. Despite this information, lactating women take over-the-counter drugs, other drugs prescribed for family members and the so-called recreational drugs. All women of childbearing age should be reminded that drugs taken for minor symptoms may have adverse effects on the fetus or baby and they should be encouraged to seek advice from their family doctor for more severe illness.

Recreational drugs

Lactating women should be advised to stop or cut down their smoking. Cigarette smoking and nicotine inhalation or ingestion in breast milk can have adverse effects and may be associated with poor infant growth at 1 year (Little et al 1994) and sudden infant death (Klonoff-Cohen et al 1995). The baby may have colic and breast milk production may be reduced.

Ideally, all mothers should be free of all recreational drugs while breastfeeding. However, this is not always possible and often mothers take drugs such as marijuana, cocaine or the cheaper form called crack and various amphetamines. There is little evidence to suggest that marijuana causes serious harm to the baby and it is probably better for the occasional user to breastfeed rather than wean the baby. Cocaine and crack does harm the fetus and can seriously affect the baby who is breastfed. Cocaine in breast milk can intoxicate the baby and cause convulsions. Amphetamines readily transfer into breast milk, resulting in the baby having three times the plasma levels of the mother, although the baby does not appear to be adversely affected (Riordan & Auerbach 1998).

Environmental toxins

The type of environmental chemicals present in breast milk may include dioxin, organochlorine and methylmercury pesticides, polychlorinated biphenyls (PCBs), phthalates added to polyvinyl chloride (PVC) and heavy metals. The effects of toxins have provoked much discussion and research, especially related to the ongoing motor and mental development of the developing child.

In the meantime, the consensus suggests that women who are anxious about pollution and breastfeeding should be reassured. The advantages of breastfeeding outweigh the risks of the pollutants in breast milk and any effects present in the baby in the early months have disappeared by the age of 18 months (Koopman-Essboom et al 1996). A reduction in the duration of breastfeeding does not have any advantage either, because the milk becomes less polluted as lactation progresses (Odent 2003). Some believe the levels of such pollutants have now begun to fall following publication of popular articles and through the actions of pressure groups (DoH 1997).

Taking a wider look at infant feeding, phthalates, which act as environmental oestrogens, appear to leak out of plastics and there has recently been a huge concern about their presence in formula milks. The effect on male reproductive development and function is the possible sequel to ingestion by babies (Cadbury 1997).

SUPPRESSION OF LACTATION

The suppression of lactation is necessary in a variety of situations such as when women choose not to breastfeed, when there are absolute contraindications to breastfeeding or following the loss of a baby. As breast milk is supplied on demand, there is no need for treatment, as lactation will cease spontaneously. Women are advised to wear a well-supporting bra and although there may be discomfort for a day or two it is rare to find extreme discomfort with engorgement. There is no need to restrict fluids and the woman should not be prescribed a diuretic drug. Drugs used to inhibit milk production and suppress lactation are no longer advised because of the potential adverse effects on the cardiovascular system.

LACTATION AND FERTILITY

The natural birth-spacing effect of breastfeeding has long been recognised and the World Health Organisation has deemed it to be the most effective contraceptive worldwide.

The natural contraceptive effect of breastfeeding is not used as a reliable method of family planning in the Western world but it does play an important antifertility role in developing countries.

Natives in hunter-gather tribes have long intervals between births. These are healthy well-nourished individuals who nurse their babies several times an hour and wean them between 3 and 4 years during the next pregnancy. This intensive breastfeeding behaviour keeps the level of prolactin in their blood high enough to block the development of ovarian follicles. Four children is the average number, of which 50% may die before reproductive age and the population remains stable. In the developing world, more pregnancies are still prevented by breastfeeding than all other methods of family planning combined (Howie 1999). The current decline in breastfeeding in developing countries could cause the loss of its antifertility effect and will aggravate the increase in population.

The mechanisms of lactational amenorrhoea are complex and not fully understood. The major factor is the frequency and duration of the sucking stimulus which probably inhibits the pituitary–ovarian hormonal cycle (Howie 1999). Weight and maternal diet may be important confounding factors. Lactational amenorrhoea may last from 2 to 4 years. Breastfeeding is not absolutely reliable, especially after menstruation returns. Between 1 and 10% of women will conceive during the period of lactational amenorrhoea and most women in developed countries will need additional contraceptive protection (Howie 1999). The combined pill oral contraceptive has been shown to reduce breast milk output, an effect not seen in women who take the progestogen-only pill.

Breast cancer and amenorrhoea

There is an epidemic of breast cancer among women of developed countries in the Western world (Howie 1999). Breast cancer is a complex disease with involvement of different tissue types. About 5% of all breast cancers are familial, many involving the inheritance of the BRCA1 gene (Leutwyler 1994). Other breast cancers may be associated with environmental toxins (Davis & Bradlow 1995) and the effects of hormones on breast tissue. The relationship between breast cancer and breastfeeding remains unclear but is a question commonly asked. At present, breast cancer is uncommon in countries where breastfeeding is common (Lawrence & Lawrence 1999). Women who have breastfed also have a reduced risk of premenopausal breast cancer and some forms of ovarian cancer (Newcomb et al 1994, Rossenblatt et al 1993, Yoo et al 1999).

The incidence of breast, ovarian and uterine cancer suggests that the probability of female reproductive tract cancer at any age increases directly in relation to the number of menstrual cycles experienced. The highest risk would be an elderly woman, with an early menarche and late menopause, who had never had the reproductive cycle interrupted by pregnancy and lactation (Nesse & Williams 1995). If this is so, it will involve repeated cyclical cellular responses of breast tissue to the changing hormonal environment of the female body. Hormone manipulations may mimic the protective effects of repeated pregnancies and lactation divided by only one or two menstrual cycles. Oral contraception is protective against ovarian and uterine cancer but not breast cancer.

MODIFICATION OF COW'S MILK

Differences between human and cow's milk

All mammalian milks contain water, fat, protein, carbohydrate, minerals and vitamins. The proportions of these nutrients vary in the different milks which have evolved to maximise development of the newborn of the species. Breast milk is an incredibly complex collection of all the nutrients necessary for optimal infant development: metabolically, immunologically and neurologically (Minchin 1998). Relatively few women are physiologically unable to breastfeed but many mothers choose to formula feed their babies for a variety of reasons. Feeding one mammal's milk to another can only be second best and it is important that a safe alternative to human milk is available. There are now sophisticated modifications of cow's milk available for human babies. The main differences between human and formula milk are now discussed although the constituents of human milk were previously discussed in Chapter 54 and reference was made to some of the differences with formula milk.

Human milk contains other important factors that are absent from formula milks, including hormones, enzymes, growth factors, essential fatty acids and immunological and non-specific factors. The function of most of the hormones and growth factors in colostrum and mature breast milk is unclear. The epidermal growth factor is known to stimulate the growth and maturation of the intestinal villi, which seals the baby's intestine and helps to prevent absorption of large protein molecules without being digested. Undigested cow's milk proteins can pass through the immature gut of the baby and may cause intolerance and allergy to milk protein. The antibodies present in human milk probably help to prevent the development of allergies by coating the intestinal mucosa. Other differences are listed below:

- Lactose readily breaks down into glucose for immediate energy needs. Human milk has a high level of lactose, 7 g/100 ml, while other milks contain about 4 g/100 ml. Cow's milk is low in lactose.

- Fat is the principal source of energy for babies and is very easily digested in human milk due to the combined action of several lipases. Human milk contains essential fatty acids in different proportions to those present in cow's milk and includes some which are commonly absent in formula milk. These essential fatty acids are needed for a baby's growing brain and eyes and for healthy blood vessels.

- The levels of sodium, calcium, phosphorus and magnesium in human milk are ideal for the term baby. While human milk may contain significantly lower concentrations of minerals than formula milk, absorption may be more complete in breastfed babies because of the presence of the specific transport factors of milk. The neonatal kidney does not cope well with an increased sodium load.

- There is a high level of leucocytes in breast milk, especially in the first 10 days, mainly macrophages and neutrophils. The main immunoglobulin present is IgA, which lines the intestinal mucosal surfaces and protects against pathogenic bacteria and viruses.

- Lysozyme is present in breast milk in concentrations thousands of times that of cow's milk.

- Lactoferrin increases the absorption of enteric iron, reducing the amount of free iron. This prevents the survival of iron-dependent pathogenic organisms such as *Escherichia coli*.

- The bifidus factor present in human milk encourages the growth of the Gram-positive *Lactobacillus bifidus*, which discourages the growth of Gram-negative pathogenic organisms.

The manufacture of infant formulae

Manufacturers have achieved a high level of success in modifying cow's milk to match human milk in relation to calorific value and constituents such as electrolytes, vitamins, minerals and fluids. However, it is impossible to match the antiinfective and antiallergenic properties of human milk, and breast milk will never be totally replaced. The essential composition of infant formulae has been set down in statute and manufacturers must adhere closely to the guidelines.

Formula milk is modified from skimmed milk and whey milk and much of the casein protein is replaced by whey protein. Milks differ in the quantity of protein type: the two main groups are casein-dominant and whey-dominant milks. Although whey-dominant formulae are recommended for the early weeks and casein-dominant formulae for the older baby, there is no evidence to show that one is superior to the other. Lactose is added and some of the milk fat is replaced by vegetable fat. The solute load is reduced. Extra iron is added and the vitamin content is supplemented.

The International Code of Marketing of Breast milk Substitutes was adopted in 1981 (WHO 1981). This code aimed to protect and promote breastfeeding, to provide safe and adequate nutrition for infants, to ensure the correct use of breast milk substitutes and to control marketing of bottle milk products. The recommendations for manufactures of infant formulae include:

- no advertising of breast milk substitutes to the public;
- no free samples to pregnant women or mothers;

- no free or subsidised supplies to hospitals;
- no contact between marketing personnel and mothers;
- no free gifts such as discount coupons or special offers;
- no pictures of babies or idealising images on formula labels;
- materials for health workers should contain only factual and scientific evidence information.

A global Baby-Friendly Initiative was set up jointly by UNICEF/WHO in 1989 to protect and support breastfeeding.

In 1991, the Baby-Friendly Initiative was launched internationally to promote best practice through the implementation of the 10 steps to successful breastfeeding for maternity units and, more recently the 7 point plan for communities. The initiative was launched in the UK in 1994 and to date many health professionals have been supported in the implementation of best-practice standards in relation to infant feeding in all health care settings.

MAIN POINTS

- Human milk is specially developed to nourish the newborn and provide protection for the child in early and later life. Breastfeeding is optimal for promoting closeness between mother and baby.

- Beliefs and attitudes about breastfeeding are influenced by culture, folklore and social context. In mammals, learning to breastfeed is part of a lifelong process beginning at birth. Some parts of breastfeeding are instinctive but a lot is about social learning.

- The baby should be encouraged to breastfeed as soon as possible after birth. The position of the baby at the breast is essential to the success of breastfeeding and in the prevention of problems. Attachment to the breast is the most important aspect of breastfeeding.

- Insufficient milk is the commonest reason given by mothers for discontinuing breastfeeding. Prevention includes unrestricted feeding by a well-positioned baby. The commonest cause of sore nipples is poor attachment to the breast.

- Engorgement refers to breasts when they are overfull, partly with milk and partly with increased tissue fluid and blood. Early and unrestricted feeding helps to prevent its onset. Mastitis is an area of inflammation which affects part of the breast. If the milk is not removed, it can cause inflammation of the breast tissue.

- Environmental toxins may be present in human breast milk. Most drugs are of a small enough molecular weight to pass into breast milk. Substances such as cocaine and nicotine may have adverse effects on the baby.

- Breastfeeding has antifertility properties and prevents more pregnancies worldwide than all other forms of contraception. Lactational amenorrhoea may last from 2 to 4 years. The pattern of feeding is important, with frequent suckling being the most successful in reducing the risk of ovulation.

- About 5% of breast cancers are familial. Breast cancer risks are increased in women who have never had children. Breast cancer may be associated with environmental toxins.

- Formula milk is modified from skimmed cow's milk and whey milk. The WHO's International Code of Marketing of Breast Milk Substitutes produced recommendations to protect and promote breastfeeding on a worldwide basis.

- The UNICEF/WHO Baby Friendly Initiative is a global initiative to protect and support successful breastfeeding. It was launched in the UK in 1994 to support health professionals to implement best-practice standards.

References

Abbott H 1997 Complications of the puerperium. In Sweet B R, Tiran D (eds) Mayes Midwifery: A Textbook for Midwives, 12th edn. Baillière Tindall, London.

Bick D 2001 The benefits of breastfeeding for the infant (Structured Abstract). In the Cochrane Library, CRD Database No: DARE-20028412.

British National Formulary (BNF) 2003 No. 45 (March). British Medical Association and Royal Pharmaceutical Society of Great Britain, London.

Cadbury S D 1997 The Feminisation of Nature. Hamish Hamilton, London.

Christensson K, Cabrera T, Christensson E et al 1995 Separation distress call in the human neonate in the absence of maternal body contact. Acta Pediatrica 84:468–473.

Cummings R G, Klineberg R J 1993 Breastfeeding and other reproductive factors and the risk of hip fracture in elderly women. International Journal of Epidemiology 2(4):684–691.

Davis D L, Bradlow H L 1995 Can environmental estrogens cause breast cancer? Scientific American October:144–149.

DoH 1997 Statement Review – Toxicity of Chemicals in Food, Consumer Products and the Environment of Polychlorinated Biphenyls and Dioxins in food. Department of Health, London.

Enkin M, Keirse M J N C, Neilson J et al 2000 A Guide to Effective Care in Pregnancy, 3rd edn. Oxford University Press, Oxford.

Fisher C 1999 Feeding. In Bennett V R, Brown L K (eds) Myles Textbook for Midwives, 13th edn. Churchill Livingstone, Edinburgh.

Howie P W 1999 The puerperium. In Edmonds K D (ed.) Dewhurst's Textbook for Obstetrics and Gynaecology for Postgraduates, 6th edn. Blackwell Science, London.

Inch S, Fisher C 1999 Breastfeeding: into the 21st century, Nursing Times Clinical Monographs No 32. NT Books, London.

Jones E, Spencer A 2003 Successful preterm breastfeeding. In Wickham S (ed.) Best Midwifery Practice. Elsevier, London.

Jordan M E, Blum R W M 1996 Should breast-feeding by women with silicone implants be recommended? Archives of Pediatrics and Adolescent Medicine 150(8):880–881.

Klonoff-Cohen H S, Edelstein S L, Lefkowitz E S et al 1995 The effect of passive smoking and tobacco exposure through breast milk on sudden infant death syndrome. Journal of American Medical Association 273(10):795–798.

Koopman-Essboom C, Weisglus-Kuperus N, de Ridder M A J et al 1996 Effects of polychlorinated biphenyl/dioxin exposure and feeding type on infants' mental and psychomotor development. Pediatrics 97(5):700–706.

Lawrence R A, Lawrence R M 1999 Breastfeeding, A Guide for the Medical Profession, 5th edn. Mosby, St Louis.

Leutwyler K 1994 Deciphering the breast cancer gene. Scientific American December:18–19.

Levine J J, Ilowite N T 1994 Sclerodermal-like eosophageal disease in children breast-fed by mothers with silicone breast implants. Journal of American Medical Association 271(3):213–216.

Little R E, Lambert M D, Worthington-Roberts R et al 1994 Maternal smoking during lactation, relation to infant size at one year of age. American Journal of Epidemiology 140(6):544–554.

Main Trial Collaborative Group 1994 Preparing for breast feeding: treatment of inverted and non-protractile nipples in pregnancy. Midwifery 10:200–213.

Minchin M K 1998 Breastfeeding Matters. Alma Publications, St Kilda, Victoria, Australia.

Nesse R M, Williams G C 1995 Evolution and Healing. Weidenfield & Nicholson, London.

Newcomb P A, Storer B E, Longnecker M P et al 1994 Lactation and a reduced risk of premenopausal breast cancer. New England Journal of Medicine 330:81–87.

Odent M 2003 Intrauterine pollution and human milk pollution. In Wickham S (ed.) Best Midwifery Practice. Elsevier, London.

RCM (Royal College of Midwives) 2002 Successful Breastfeeding, 3rd edn. Churchill Livingstone, Edinburgh.

Renfrew M J, Lang S 1999 Early discharge of mothers from hospital. In Renfrew M J, Ross-McGill H, Woolridge M W (eds) Enabling Women to Breastfeed: A Structured Review of Interventions which Support or Inhibit Breastfeeding. Stationary Office, London.

Renfrew M, Fisher C, Arms S 2000 The New Bestfeeding: Getting Breastfeeding Right for You, the Illustrated Guide. Celestial Arts, California.

Riordan J, Auerbach K G 1998 Breastfeeding and Human Lactation, 2nd edn. Jones & Bartlett, Toronto.

Rossenblatt K A, Thomas D B, WHO Collaborative Study 1993 Lactation and the risk of epithelial ovarian cancer. International Journal of Epidemiology 22:192–197.

Sikorski J, Renfrew M J, Pindoria S et al 2001 Support for breastfeeding mothers. Cochrane Review: in the Cochrane Library, Issue 4. Update Software 2003, Oxford.

Stables D, Hewitt G 1995 The effect of lateral asymmetries on breast feeding skills: can midwives' holding interventions overcome unilateral breast feeding problems? Midwifery 11:28–36.

Tralins A H 1995 Lactation after conservative breast surgery combined with radiation therapy. American Journal of Clinical Oncology 18(1):40–43.

UNICEF/WHO 1997 Breastfeeding Management: A Modular Course. UNICEF UK. BFI, London (Adapted from Breastfeeding Counselling Training Course).

Wilde C J, Addey C V P, Boddy L M et al 1995 Autocrine regulation of milk secretion by a protein in milk. Biochemical Journal 305:51–58.

Williams A F 1994 Silicone, breast implants, breastfeeding and scleroderm. Lancet 343(8904):1043–1044.

World Health Organisation 1981 International Code of Marketing of Breast Milk Substitutes. WHO, Geneva.

Yoo K Y, Tajima K, Kuroisha T et al 1999 Independent protective effect of lactation against breast cancer. American Journal of Epidemiology 135:726–733.

Annotated recommended reading

Bick D 1999 The benefits of breastfeeding for the Infant. British Journal of Midwifery 7(5):312–319.
This article provides further information about original research studies on health and other benefits of breast milk for the infant.

Fisher C 1999 Feeding. In Bennett V R, Brown L K (eds) Myles Textbook for Midwives, 13th edn. Churchill Livingstone, Edinburgh.
This is an excellent well-presented and easy-to-read chapter. It describes the structure and function of the breasts, outlines the properties and components of breast milk and gives a clear account of the practical aspects of breastfeeding.

Renfrew M, Fisher C, Arms S 2000 The New Bestfeeding: Getting Breastfeeding Right for You, the Illustrated Guide. Celestial Arts, California.
This excellent book provides a detailed and clear, well-illustrated step-by-step account of how to breastfeed successfully.

Chapter 56

The puerperium

INTRODUCTION

Traditionally, the puerperium is the time after childbirth, lasting approximately 6–8 weeks, during which the maternal physiological changes, particularly in the reproductive system, resolve and return to the non-pregnant state. At the same time, the woman is going through a transition to parenthood and adapts to take on her new role and responsibilities. The puerperium commences immediately after completion of labour and is considered to be complete with the first ovulation and the return of normal menstruation.

Postpartum is a descriptive term attributed to situations and conditions following birth (parturition). The postnatal period is a social concept occurring after birth and usually involving the baby. In the Midwives Rules and Code of Practice (UKCC 1998) the postnatal period is defined as being:

a period of not less than ten days and not more than 28 days after the end of labour, during which the continued attendance of a midwife on the mother and baby is requisite.

The puerperium occurs during a time when the anticipation of pregnancy and the excitement of the birth are over. This period can be a particularly vulnerable time for women as they not only have to deal with the physiological changes to their bodies but also have to cope with any emotional, psychological and social adaptations brought about by their new role.

This chapter will address the physiology of the puerperium and the influences on emotional reactions and mental disorders associated with childbirth. Other aspects of postnatal care, which include family planning (Ch. 6) and interactive aspects of parenting (Ch. 57), are considered in other relevant sections within the book. The main maternal puerperal complications include postpartum haemorrhage, thromboembolic disorders, puerperal infections and mental health disorders. Postpartum haemorrhage can be found in Chapter 45, thromboembolic disorders, including thrombophlebitis, deep vein thrombosis and pulmonary embolism are discussed in Chapter 33 and the remaining disorders are considered in this chapter.

PHYSIOLOGICAL CHANGES

During the puerperium the physiological changes can be divided into:

- involution of the uterus and genital tract;
- secretion of breast milk and establishment of lactation;
- other physiological changes.

The major physiological event of the puerperium is lactation: therefore, Chapters 54 and 55 have been entirely devoted to this important topic. These chapters include the anatomy of the breast and the initiation and maintenance of lactation and breastfeeding.

Endocrine changes in the puerperium

Immediately following delivery of the placenta, there is a profound decrease in the serum levels of placental hormones: i.e.

human placental lactogen (hPL), human chorionic gonadotrophin (hCG), oestrogen and progesterone. The removal of the placental hormones initiates reversal of most of the pregnancy-related changes. The rate of removal of the hormones depends on their half-life. Hormones are first removed from maternal blood. Secondary removal occurs as the hormones are mobilised from the tissues. Within 24 h, plasma estradiol decreases to levels that are less than 2% of pregnancy levels. Oestrogen levels return almost to prepregnant levels by 7 days. Progesterone levels return to those found in the luteal phase of the menstrual cycle by 24–48 h and to the follicular phase by 7 days (Fig. 56.1). The enlarged thyroid gland regresses and the basal metabolic rate returns to normal.

Resumption of menstruation and ovulation

Most women are relatively infertile during the postnatal period and this may continue during the period of lactation.

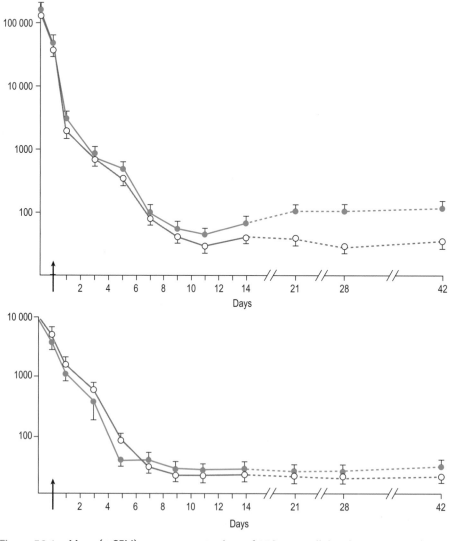

Figure 56.1   Mean (±SEM) serum concentrations of 17β-oestradiol and progesterone in lactating and non-lactating subjects. Lactating subjects (*n* = 10) ○–○; non-lactating subjects (*n* = 9) ●–● (from Sweet B 1997, with permission).

The return of ovulation is preceded by an increase in plasma progesterone. There is a wide variation in the return to ovulation, irrespective of whether the woman is breastfeeding or not. In most cases, the first menstrual cycle following delivery is anovulatory. However, ovulation may occur before menstruation in 25% of women and pregnancy may result. Anovulatory cycles are more common in lactating women (Blackburn 2003).

Two maternal hormones involved in the initiation and maintenance of lactation will be briefly mentioned here; they are discussed more fully in Chapter 55. **Prolactin** is secreted by the anterior pituitary gland in increasing amounts during pregnancy but its effects are suppressed by oestrogen. **Oxytocin** is produced in the hypothalamus and stored in the posterior pituitary gland. This hormone stimulates electrical and contractile activity in the myometrium to aid involution and is critical for milk ejection during lactation (Blackburn 2003).

Involution

The principal change in the pelvic organs is uterine involution and the uterine fundus will have disappeared below the symphysis pubis within 10 days of delivery (Howie 1999). Involution is defined as being:

a normal process characterised by a decrease in the size of an organ caused by a decrease in the size of its cells, such as is found in the involution of the uterus in the postpartum period.

During this process, the uterus returns to its normal size, tone and position and the vagina, uterine ligaments and muscles of the pelvic floor also return to their prepregnant state. The pelvic floor and subsequent problems that can arise if the ligaments and muscles are permanently weakened are discussed in Chapter 25.

Physiology

During involution there are changes to the myometrium or muscle layer and the decidua or lining of the pregnant uterus (Fig. 56.2). The muscle layer returns to normal thickness by the processes of ischaemia, autolysis and phagocytosis. The decidua is shed as **lochia** and there is regeneration of the endometrium.

Ischaemia occurs when the muscles of the uterus retract at the end of the third stage to constrict the blood vessels at the placental site, resulting in haemostasis. Blood circulating to the uterus is greatly reduced.

Autolysis is the process of removal of the redundant actin and myosin muscle fibres and cytoplasm by proteolytic enzymes and macrophages. Individual myometrial cells are reduced in size with no significant reduction in the numbers of cells.

Phagocytosis removes the excess fibrous and elastic tissue. This process is incomplete and some elastic tissue remains so that a uterus that has held a pregnancy never quite returns to the nulliparous state.

Positional changes

The most marked reduction in the size of the uterus takes place during the first 10 days. The process of involution is not complete until about six weeks and the rate at which the uterus involutes varies between women (Howie 1999).

Immediately after delivery of the placenta the whole uterus contracts down fully and the uterine walls become realigned in apposition to each other (Coad 2001). The uterus weighs about 1000 g at this time. The fundus is palpable just below or at the level of the umbilicus which is about 11–12 cm above the symphysis pubis (Howie 1999). The muscles are well contracted to aid the process of haemostasis and at this time the uterus feels globular and hard like a cricket ball. Between 1 and 12 h after delivery,

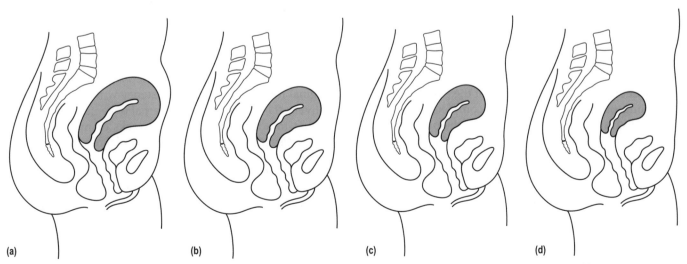

(a)   (b)   (c)   (d)

Figure 56.2   Involution of the uterus. (a) At the end of labour. (b) One week after delivery. (c) Two weeks after delivery. (d) Six weeks after delivery (from Sweet B 1997, with permission).

the myometrium relaxes slightly (Coad 2001, Howie 1999). Further active bleeding is prevented by the activation of the blood-clotting mechanisms which are altered greatly during pregnancy to facilitate a swift clotting response (Coad 2001).

On average the height of the fundus then decreases at a rate of 1 cm daily. At the end of the 1st week, the uterus has lost 50% of its bulk, weighs about 500 g and is about 5 cm above the symphysis pubis. It has returned to the true pelvis by the 10th postnatal day. By the end of the 6th week after delivery, the uterus should weigh between 60 and 80 g and has returned to its prepregnant position of anteversion and anteflexion.

This normal process of involution is slower when there has been overdistension of the uterus due to multiple pregnancy or a large baby or if the pregnancy has been complicated by polyhydramnios. Slow involution may be associated with retained placental tissue or blood clot, particularly if there is an associated infection. There is no evidence to suggest that there is any relationship between parity and the rate of involution.

Uterine contractions

During the first 24 h after delivery, oxytocin leads to uterine contractions with further retraction. The contractions can be quite strong and often result in afterpains, especially in multiparous women. Suckling stimulates oxytocin release. This gradually diminishes over the next 4–7 days and the pain is relieved by mild analgesia.

The decidua

The upper portion of the spongy endometrial layer is sloughed off when the placenta is delivered. The remaining decidua is organised into basal and superficial layers. The superficial layer consists of granulation tissue, which is invaded by leucocytes to form a barrier to prevent micro-organisms invading the remaining decidua. This layer becomes necrotic and is sloughed off as the lochia. The basal layer remains intact and is the source of regeneration of the endometrium, which begins about 10 days after delivery. The regeneration process is completed by 2–3 weeks following delivery with the exception of the placental site.

Healing of the placental site is completed by the end of 6 weeks. Immediately after delivery, the placental site is reduced to a raised roughened area about 12 cm in diameter. It contains many thrombosed sinusoids. The large blood vessels which supplied the intervillous space are invaded by fibroblasts and their lumen is obscured. Some of the blood vessels later recanalise.

Lochia

The vaginal loss during the puerperium is known as the **lochia** (a plural word). Lochia vary in amount, content and

Table 56.1 The characteristics of lochia

Type	Content	Average days
Lochia rubra	Blood, amnion and chorion, decidual cells, vernix, lanugo, meconium	1–3
Lochia serosa	Blood, wound exudate, erythrocytes, leucocytes, cervical mucus, micro-organisms, shreds of degenerating decidua from the superficial layer	4–10
Lochia alba	Leucocytes, decidual cells, mucus, bacteria, epithelial cells	11–21

colour as the excess tissue is lost. Women lose between 150 and 400 ml of lochia, averaging 225 ml. Women who breastfeed have less lochia, possibly due to more rapid involution and healing, although flow may increase temporarily during suckling. Three forms of lochia are described: **rubra** (red), **serosa** (pink) and **alba** (white).

Lochia consist of blood, leucocytes, shreds of deciduas and organisms. A summary of the characteristics of lochia is presented in Table 56.1. The lochia may remain red for up to 3 weeks or there may be a brief increase in blood content in the 2nd week. However, lochia remaining heavily blood-stained or a sudden return to profuse red lochia may suggest that placental tissue has been retained. If the lochia are offensive and the woman becomes pyrexial, uterine infection may be present, and she must be assessed by a doctor and appropriate treatment commenced.

Findings from recent research studies indicate that vaginal loss during the puerperium is considerably more varied in duration, amount and colour than classically reported and described in current textbooks (Marchant et al 1999, 2003, Sherman et al 1999).

Other parts of the genital tract

Immediately after delivery, the **cervix** is soft and highly vascular but it rapidly loses its vascularity and returns to its original form and normal consistency within a few days of delivery (Howie 1999). The external os remains sufficiently dilated to admit one finger for weeks or months (and in some cases permanently) but the internal os becomes closed during the 2nd week of the puerperium (Howie 1995). The **ovaries** and **fallopian tubes** return with the uterus to the pelvic cavity. The vagina almost always shows some evidence of parity. The **vagina**, **vulva** and **pelvic floor** respond to the reduced amount of circulating progesterone by recovering normal muscle tone. Early ambulation and postnatal exercises can enhance this return to normal. Bruising or tears to genital tissues heal rapidly and any oedema is reabsorbed within the first 3 or 4 days.

The body systems

The cardiovascular and respiratory systems

During pregnancy, the increased circulatory volume and haemodilution were needed to ensure adequate blood supply to the uterus and placental bed. Following the withdrawal of oestrogen, a diuresis occurs for the first 48 h and the plasma volume and haematocrit rapidly return to normal. The reduction in circulating progesterone leads to removal of excess tissue fluid and a return to normal vascular tone. There is an increase in atrial natriuretic peptide (ANP), which may contribute to the well-recognised diuresis that occurs during this period (de Swiet 1998). Cardiac output and blood pressure return to non-pregnant levels.

Delivery of the baby and reduction in uterine size remove the compression of the lungs. Full inflation of the lungs, including the basal lobes, is again possible. With the reduction in cardiac work and circulatory volume and the decrease in metabolism, oxygen demands now return to normal. The tendency to hyperventilation disappears, and blood carbon dioxide levels return to normal, as does the slight alkalosis.

The renal system

There is reversal of the physiological parameters of the renal system to prepregnancy levels by the end of the puerperium. During this time, the kidneys must cope with the excretion of excess fluids and an increase in the breakdown products of protein. The dilatation of the renal tract resolves with the removal of progesterone and the renal organs gradually return to their prepregnant state. During labour, the bladder is displaced into the abdomen and the urethra is stretched. There may be loss of tone in the bladder and bruising of the urethra, leading to difficulty in micturition.

Because of these features and diuresis, the bladder may become overdistended and retention of urine may occur. This may be missed if the carer fails to notice that frequent small amounts of urine are being passed with the bladder becoming ever more distended. Early ambulation with frequent encouragement to pass urine and ensuring that the bladder is emptied will help to avoid this situation. Catheterisation may occasionally be necessary.

The gastrointestinal tract

Throughout the body, smooth muscle tone gradually returns to normal due to the reduced levels of circulating progesterone. There is a rapid return to normal carbohydrate metabolism and fasting plasma insulin levels return to non-pregnant values between 48 h and the 6th week postpartum (Campbell-Brown & Hytten 1998). The minor inconveniences of pregnancy affecting the gastrointestinal tract resolve, such as constipation and heartburn. Constipation may persist as a problem, possibly due to inactivity or a fear of pain on defecation.

PUERPERAL INFECTION

At delivery, the normal protective barriers against infection are temporarily broken down, and this gives potential pathogens an opportunity to pass from the lower genital tract into the usually sterile environment of the uterus. Prior to the introduction of aseptic techniques and development of antibiotics, puerperal sepsis was an important cause of maternal mortality. Puerperal pyrexia was then a notifiable disease. Puerperal pyrexia may have several explanations but it is a clinical sign that always merits careful investigation (Howie 1999). Women are particularly at risk to infection at this time because of the presence of the placental site, the tissue trauma sustained in labour and the decidua and lochia being excellent culture mediums for the growth of bacteria.

Other sites for infection are the breasts and the epithelial linings of the veins. The possibility that the woman has developed an infection unrelated to pregnancy, such as an upper respiratory tract infection, should always be considered. Infection of surgical incisions is also a significant cause of maternal morbidity. A total of 18 maternal deaths between 1997 and 1999 were recorded as a result of sepsis, which are four more deaths than in the previous triennium report (Lewis 2001). Five of these deaths occurred in the puerperium: i.e. two deaths following vaginal delivery, one following operative delivery and two 'late' maternal deaths.

Identification of site of infection

A raised temperature and pulse rate are only indicators that infection may be present. Other signs and symptoms present on clinical examination will help to identify the site of infection. The timing of the onset of pyrexia may also indicate the source of the problem. Swabs may be taken from all possible sites, and specimens should be obtained for investigations such as organism, culture and antibiotic sensitivity. Depending on the signs and symptoms, these may include high vaginal, perineal, wound, ear, nose and throat swabs, and specimens of blood, urine, stool and breast milk. Antibiotic therapy should commence prior to the results of such investigations if the woman is ill.

Causative organisms

It takes time for invading organisms to multiply sufficiently to cause symptoms, and postnatal infection occurs after the first 24 h from delivery. As in any infection, the severity depends on two factors: the virulence of the causative organism and the resistance of the host. Infecting organisms may originate from the commensal organisms normally present in the woman's own body. These are called endogenous organisms and can cause problems if they invade susceptible sites. Such organisms may come from the vagina, bowel, skin, nose or throat of the woman and include *Escherichia coli*, *Clostridium welchii* and *Streptococcus faecalis*.

Other organisms are transmitted from sites other than the woman's body, commonly from an attendant. These are called **exogenous** organisms and are responsible for the more serious infections. The most dangerous organism is β-**haemolytic streptococcus group A** (discussed below) and it is the cause of intrauterine infection. It may be found in people with a sore throat. *Staphylococcus aureus* is a common organism which lingers in dust and can cause spots, pustules and sticky eyes in babies and breast or wound infections in mothers (Abbott 1997). A strain of this organism, called methicillin-resistant *Staphylococcus aureus* (MRSA), is resistant to most antibiotics. Overuse and misuse of antibiotics in human disease and animal husbandry has contributed to the mutations of organisms (Coughlan 1996).

Streptococci – Lancefield groups

The genus *Streptococcus* contains a wide variety of species of bacteria with many habitats. Some species are pathogenic to human beings. One group of related species are those that cause haemolysis when grown on blood agar, an action referred to as β-**haemolysis**. Streptococci are also subdivided depending on the presence of carbohydrate antigens on their surfaces and are named after Rebecca Lancefield who was a pioneer in the classification of streptococci. These are called **Lancefield groups** and are identified with letters of the alphabet such as A, B and onwards to O (Brock & Madigan 1999).

The most common organism responsible for serious and life-threatening obstetric infections is the β-haemolytic *Streptococcus pyogenes*, categorised as Lancefield group A (Lewis 2001). This organism has the ability to gain access to the circulation via the placental site, causing septicaemia and haemolysis of red cells. This strain was responsible for deaths from childbirth fever and was virulent up to the development of antibiotics, being responsible for the serious childhood illness scarlet fever, as well as for sore throats. This organism caused damage to the kidneys.

Pharmacological interventions contributed to a dramatic decrease in puerperal infections between the 1940s and the 1980s. In the late 1980s, a resurgence of infections was noted as new virulent strains of bacteria emerged, with Lancefield group B being a problem with babies (Garrett 1995). The Lancefield group B streptococcus can be found in normal vaginal flora and is most commonly associated with neonatal septicaemia and meningitis, particularly in premature infants. Serious maternal infections may also occur with this infection. The Lancefield groups C and G streptococcus may also cause serious clinical syndromes but are less common (Lewis 2001).

Group A streptococcus attack people of all ages and are lethal despite vigorous treatment. Scientists are developing new drugs to combat the ability of bacteria to resist antibiotics but it may be some years before these are readily available on the market (Chin 1996). It is imperative that vigilance in preventative measures is maintained to protect childbearing women and their babies.

Genital tract infection

Infection of the genital tract may remain localised to the perineum, vagina or cervix or may ascend the genital tract to infect the uterine cavity (**endometritis**). Infection may then spread to the fallopian tubes to cause salpingitis and to the tissues of the pelvic cavity to cause cellulitis and peritonitis.

Postpartum endometritis

Postpartum endometritis is usually caused by an ascending infection from the lower genital tract and about 2% of women experiencing vaginal births and 10–15% of those with caesarean birth are estimated to develop this condition (Walsh 2001). Other factors that may facilitate pelvic infections include prolonged labour, prolonged rupture of the membranes, multiple vaginal examinations, traumatic delivery and manual removal of placenta (Howie 1999). Antibiotic therapy is often advised for women with vaginal vaginosis.

Signs and symptoms
- Pyrexia above 38°C occurs about the 3rd postnatal day.
- Pulse rate rises by about 10 beats/min (bpm) for every degree Celsius.
- Pain is present in the lower abdomen.
- The uterus is tender on palpation.
- Headache and rigors may occur.
- Localised infection is sometimes seen in the perineum.
- Lochia may be heavy and offensive, depending on the invading organism.
- Blood cultures may be positive in up to 10% of women.

Spread of infection   The mother's condition may deteriorate rapidly if there is spread of the organism by bacteria such as *Clostridium welchii*. In the last triennium report into maternal deaths, 14 of the 18 deaths reported were directly due to genital sepsis and 4 other deaths in which it may have played a significant part (Lewis 2001).

Treatment   The woman should be isolated and examined by medical staff. In the seriously ill obstetric patient where sepsis may be implicated, it is advised that intravenous antibiotic treatment is commenced immediately (Lewis 2001). Bacteriological specimens including high vaginal and wound site swabs and urine and blood culture must be obtained prior to commencing such treatment before these results are available. The most appropriate antibiotic treatment based on the organisms currently identified as being responsible for maternal deaths would be recently introduced penicillin derivatives piperacillin/tazobactam in combination with the aminoglycoside netilmicin (Lewis 2001). Where appropriate, drugs are changed according to the sensitivity results.

Care is provided to meet the woman's needs, depending on the severity of the illness. Any dehydration should be corrected and analgesics may be required for pain relief. Haemoglobin levels will need to be assessed as anaemia may precede or follow infection. A blood transfusion is sometimes necessary. Any localised wound infections are treated. A light nourishing diet is provided if the woman is well enough to eat. The baby may also require investigation and treatment.

Urinary tract infection

Urinary tract infections are common during the puerperium, especially in women with urinary retention, indwelling catheters, operative deliveries or with a history of urinary infections (Howie 1999). Because of the delay in the return to normal in the urinary tract, there is susceptibility for infection for the first 6 weeks and this may present as cystitis or pyelonephritis. The most common organism cultured is *Escherichia coli*.

Signs and symptoms

Most infections take the form of cystitis with the usual symptoms. These include urinary frequency, urgency, dysuria and haematuria. The urine may be cloudy and offensive and there may be a slight rise in maternal temperature.

In the more serious pyelonephritis, the woman may develop:

- pain and tenderness in the renal angle which may extend along the line of the ureter;
- pyrexia and rapid pulse;
- rigors;
- nausea and vomiting.

The woman will feel ill. On urinalysis, the urine is acidic, opalescent and offensive. Pus and blood may be found on microscopic examination.

Treatment

Diagnosis can be confirmed by culturing the infecting organism on a midstream specimen of urine. A good oral intake of fluids should be encouraged and, if vomiting is present, intravenous fluids may be required to maintain adequate hydration and a good urinary output. Where necessary, drugs will be required to relieve pain, alleviate nausea and to reduce temperature. A broad-spectrum antibiotic is commenced and changed as appropriate, according to sensitivity results. Following completion of the antibiotic treatment, a repeat culture should be performed to ensure the treatment has been adequate to defeat the infection. Following the puerperium, any woman with a history of recurrent urinary tract infections should have further investigations of the urinary tract by cystoscopy and intravenous pyelography to exclude any underlying abnormality.

Other puerperal infections

In the event of puerperal pyrexia, any surgical wound should be examined for evidence of infection. This is particularly important following instrumental deliveries and surgical procedures. Wound infection will present as a reddened tender area and may be oedematous. The wound may have serous, bloodstained or purulent discharge and may be offensive in nature. There may be associated pyrexia and tachycardia with the woman being generally unwell.

Treatment will depend on the extent and severity of the infection. Bacteriology specimens required for culture and sensitivity will include swabs of the wound site for all degrees of infection and blood specimens for moderate to severe infections. Well-localised wound infections may discharge spontaneously and may only require local irrigation with an antiseptic solution. A broad-spectrum antibiotic will be required in more extensive wound infections (Howie 1999). In the majority of cases the wound will granulate from its base and heal spontaneously. In rare circumstances, the wound may need to be resutured.

If puerperal pyrexia is present, the legs should also be routinely inspected for any evidence of thrombophlebitis. Breast infections are discussed in Chapter 54.

EMOTIONAL STATES AND MENTAL DISORDERS IN THE PUERPERIUM

Behaviour is a complex function influenced by the interaction of biological factors and social, economic and cultural factors (Jessel & Moir 1995). Obstetric factors may also influence the behaviour of women during the childbearing process (Cox & Holden 1994).

Childbirth is generally recognised as being an important life event of great physiological and psychological significance. The events surrounding the birth often leave women both physically and emotionally vulnerable and they commonly experience mood changes in the postpartum period. Two classes of mental health disorders are the neuroses and the psychoses. In neuroses the individual, although likely to be depressed, remains in touch with reality. In the much more severe psychoses there is a great impairment in the perception of external reality, often with delusions and hallucinations. In most cases women with mental health disorders after childbirth will experience the neurotic disorder of postnatal depression and only a few women, many with a history of mental illness, will suffer from a puerperal psychotic episode of schizophrenia.

The spectrum of 'affective states or disorders' following childbirth is most often divided into three categories in ascending order of severity:

1. the 'baby blues' (emotional state);
2. postnatal depression (neuroses);
3. puerperal psychosis (psychoses).

'Baby blues'

The early feelings of elation in the first 3 days after birth are replaced by a normal emotional reaction to childbirth called the 'baby blues'. Over 50% of women experience this emotional reaction, which occurs from around the 3rd day after birth until about the end of the 1st week when women usually return to normal. The reaction is characterised by tearfulness, irritability, forgetfulness, fatigue and inability to concentrate and think clearly. The symptoms have a short impact on daily function and normally it is only a transient and self-limiting emotional change. However, a prolonged, serious episode may be predictive of the onset of postnatal depression (O'Hara 1997).

The cause of the 'baby blues' remains unclear. The physiological changes occurring in the puerperium are thought to be mainly responsible due to the reaction being so common at this particular time. The types of changes, which may affect behaviour, include the decrease in oestrogen and progesterone and alterations in the balance of fluids and electrolytes and neurotransmitters. These factors may interact with minor anxieties, attitudes and beliefs about the birth of the child and sociocultural stress to influence maternal mood to a greater degree. The primary treatment is to provide supportive care and to reassure the woman that the feelings that she has are normal and will subside within a few days.

Postnatal depression

Postnatal depression is regarded as any non-psychotic depressive illness of mild to moderate severity usually commencing within 2 weeks of delivery but that may develop at any time in the 1st year following childbirth. For every 1000 live births, 100–150 women will suffer from a depressive illness. This disorder is a serious condition of childbirth and should be distinguished from the brief emotional state called the 'baby blues'. The overall prevalence of postnatal depression is not significantly different from that of depression at other times but there is some evidence of an increased risk of depression occurring in the early postnatal period, being three-fold in the first 5 postnatal weeks (Cox et al 1993, Fergusson et al 1996). A significant number of these women may have developed depression in the antenatal period (Evans et al 2001).

Postnatal depression has an insidious onset, runs a chronic course and is probably the most common complication of the puerperium. Health professionals do not always detect the disorder and usually the women make a complete recovery.

Risk factors

The evidence suggests that risk factors for postnatal depression are no different to the risk factors for non-postnatal depression. Lack of social and psychological support after birth is one of the main reasons that unhappiness after childbirth is such a common problem (Enkin et al 2000).

Systematic reviews of sociological and psychological studies have identified factors with a moderate to strong association with postnatal depression (Beck 1996, Hoffbrand et al 2001). These include a past history of psychopathology and psychological disturbances during pregnancy, poor marital relationship, the 'baby blues', social factors such as poor social support and recent life events. Other factors that may also be associated with the risk of postnatal depression include a history of abuse, obstetric complications and social factors such as lower occupational status and low family income (Forman et al 2000). Stillbirth, neonatal or infant death may also affect mental health (Boyle et al 1996).

There is no persuasive evidence to support traditional explanations of postnatal depression. No biochemical explanation of women's unhappiness after childbirth has been uncovered, and psychoanalytic explanations cannot be validated empirically (Enkin et al 2000). Researchers agree that the effects of postnatal depression are detrimental and clinical efforts need to be moved towards understanding, recognising and treating antenatal depression (Evans et al 2001).

Screening and early detection

In recent years, health professionals have focused on early recognition and treatment, mainly because it occurs at such a critical time in the lives of the mother and baby and the effect on the woman and her family can be devastating. This can include maternal morbidity, neglect of the child, family breakdown, self-harm and suicide. The more common consequences for children due to maternal mental disorders include emotional and behavioural problems and cognitive delay in the children of depressed mothers (Murray et al 1999, Sinclair & Murray 1998). Overall, psychiatric disorders are known to have caused or contributed to 42 of the maternal deaths reported in the recent triennium report, which is 12% of all deaths reported between 1997 and 1999 (Oates 2001). Death by suicide was responsible for 10% of these deaths.

It is only by close contact with women, observing their behaviour and reactions to events and encouraging them to discuss their feelings and anxieties, that a midwife or doctor may recognise postnatal depression. In the neuroses the individual, although likely to be depressed, remains in touch with reality. Several of the following symptoms may be present:

- Depressed mood, manifesting as either tearfulness or social withdrawal or a change from the usual social functioning. This may include irritability and loss of libido.
- Excessive anxiety about the baby's health and no enjoyment of motherhood.
- Feelings of inadequacy and inability to cope.
- Guilt about their mothering skills and feelings towards their babies.
- Constant tiredness and sleep disturbance, with difficulty in achieving sleep and early morning waking.
- Suicidal thought or fears of harming the baby.

The most commonly used screening tool in the postnatal period is the Edinburgh Postnatal Depression Scale (EPDS). It is a simple and easy-to-use questionnaire and should always be administered by a trained health professional. The EPDS should be used approximately 6 weeks and 3 months following delivery. There is good evidence for its effectiveness as a screening tool, although diagnosis of postnatal depression does require clinical evaluation (SIGN 2002).

Management

Effective communication between all members of the multidisciplinary team is essential to ensure that the best outcome is possible for the mother and baby within the family unit. Pharmacological and psychosocial therapies are normally used in the management of mental health disorders and this includes postnatal depression. Pharmacological therapies include hormonal and homeopathic therapies and antidepressants with the additional consideration regarding the use of medication when women are pregnant or breastfeeding. These therapies have been the subject of considerable debate in recent years. The evidence relating to the role of psychosocial interventions in the treatment of postnatal depression focuses mainly on counselling, psychotherapy such as cognitive behavioural approaches in addition to a number of alternative therapies including massage, infant massage and relaxation therapies. There is evidence that women benefit from additional support and counselling, alone or in conjunction with medical therapy (Enkin et al 2000, Hoffbrand et al 2001). Women suffering a severe form of depression may need to be referred to a psychiatrist especially if suicidal.

Puerperal psychosis

Puerperal psychosis is a much less common disorder that affects one to two women per 1000 births. In general there is agreement in the literature that this rate represents a significantly increased risk for psychotic illness when compared with other times in a woman's life (SIGN 2002). The onset is quite often rapid, and typically presents in the early postpartum period, usually within the 1st month. In almost all cases of puerperal psychosis, there is a mood disorder accompanied by features such as loss of contact with reality, hallucinations, severe thought disturbances and abnormal behaviour. A key symptom is insomnia and the woman may also be confused, frightened and distressed and may be disoriented in space and time. Delusions and hallucinations often focus on the delivery or on the baby.

Risk factors

Women with a previous puerperal psychosis are at significant risk of between 25 and 57% of developing a future puerperal psychosis and an even higher risk of developing a non-puerperal relapse (Terp et al 1999). Other risk factors for women developing puerperal psychosis include a pre-existing psychotic illness (especially if it is a severe affective psychosis) and family history of affective psychosis (Schopf & Rust 1994).

Detection and management

Procedures should be put in place to ensure all women are routinely assessed during pregnancy for a history of depression. Psychosocial and biological risk factors for postnatal depression and puerperal psychosis should be routinely and systematically recorded in the antenatal period. During pregnancy, information should be available to women and their partners on the nature of postnatal mood disorders and puerperal psychosis.

Detection of the condition is more readily identified due to the nature of this disorder. Women who are at risk during pregnancy should be referred to a psychiatrist during pregnancy to ensure early detection and intervention (Cox & Holden 1994). Women who require psychiatric admission following childbirth should ideally be admitted to a specialist mother and baby unit, together with their baby (Oates 2001). Any decision taken should involve a multidisciplinary assessment, including social workers and family members. In areas where this service is not available, a transfer should be considered if the presence of the baby might hasten the mother's recovery. This should equally apply to mothers with severe postnatal depression and puerperal psychosis and those with a schizophrenic illness exacerbated by the impact of a new baby (SIGN 2002). In general, there are concerns that admission of mothers with their babies to general psychiatric wards may not adequately ensure the safety and security of the baby. Recent guidelines discourage such ad hoc arrangements and recommend the provision of mother and baby units (Oates 2000). Further research is required to review the effectiveness of mother and baby units in relation to the care of women and their families.

There is limited evidence for the effectiveness of treatment and management specifically for puerperal psychosis. As the nature of puerperal psychosis is essentially affective, treatments used for affective psychoses in general are also appropriate for puerperal psychosis. Such treatments would typically involve one or more drugs from the antidepressant, mood stabilising or neuroleptic groups. Additional considerations regarding the use of drug treatments will be required for women in pregnancy and when breastfeeding. Prognosis is good, most women recover within 6 months. However, there may be a relapse in a subsequent pregnancy (Hoffbrand et al 2001).

MAIN POINTS

- The puerperium is the 6–8 week period after childbirth during which time the maternal physiological changes resolve and return to the non-pregnant state. Women also psychologically and emotionally adapt to motherhood.

- After delivery, the subsequent removal of the placental hormones initiates the return of the body systems to its pre-pregnant state. Involution is the main change in the pelvic organs during the puerperium. The process is brought about by ischaemia, autolysis and phagocytosis. Decidua is shed and there is regeneration of the endometrium.

- Fundal height decreases at a rate of approximately 1 cm/day. Slow involution may be associated with retained products or an associated infection. Vaginal loss is termed as lochia. Three forms of lochia are described: rubra (red), serosa (pink) and alba (white). Infection may be present if lochia are offensive and the woman has a pyrexia. The cervix returns to its original form within a few days. Trauma to the genital tissues heals rapidly.

- Following the withdrawal of oestrogen, diuresis occurs and the plasma volume and haematocrit rapidly return to normal. The reduction in circulating progesterone leads to removal of excess tissue fluid and normal vascular tone returns. Cardiac output returns to non-pregnant levels.

- Delivery of the baby removes any compression on the lungs during pregnancy and ventilation returns to normal. Oxygen requirements return to normal as do carbon dioxide levels.

- A loss of bladder tone and bruising of the urethra may lead to difficulty in micturition. Retention of urine may occur. Constipation may persist as a problem.

- The main maternal puerperal complications include postpartum haemorrhage, thromboembolic disorders, puerperal infections and mental health disorders.

- Women are susceptible to invasion by pathogenic organisms in the puerperium. Puerperal pyrexia always merits medical investigation. Infection of surgical incisions is a significant cause of maternal morbidity. Treatment depends on the severity of any infection present.

- Bacteriological specimens for culture should be obtained if infection is present. In moderate to severe infections, the woman should commence antibiotics while awaiting results.

- Commensal organisms normally present in the body can invade susceptible sites and cause infection. The β-haemolytic *Streptococcus pyogenes*, Lancefield group A, is the most common organism responsible for serious and life-threatening obstetric infections.

- Predisposing factors for postpartum endometritis include prolonged labour, prolonged rupture of the membranes, multiple vaginal examinations, manual removal of placenta and traumatic delivery.

- Urinary tract infections are common during the puerperium and recurrent urinary tract infections should be further investigated for urinary tract abnormality.

- Childbearing is associated with three 'affective disorders': i.e. the 'baby blues', postnatal depression and puerperal psychosis. The 'baby blues' is a normal emotional reaction to childbirth experienced by over 50% of women. The elated emotions surrounding the birth are replaced with tearfulness, irritability, fatigue and inability to concentrate. It lasts from day 3 until the end of the 1st week after birth.

- Postnatal depression is a non-psychotic illness occurring within the 1st year of childbirth in 10–15% of women. Symptoms include depressed mood, excessive anxiety, sleep disturbances, feelings of inadequacy and guilt. The disorder responds well to counselling, cognitive therapy and antidepressant drugs. Recovery is usually complete.

- The incidence of puerperal psychosis is 2:1000 births and presents within the 1st month after birth. There is a mood disorder accompanied by feelings such as loss of contact with reality, delusions and hallucinations, and abnormal behaviour. Admission to a psychiatric mother and baby unit is usually recommended. Most women recover within 6 months.

References

Abbott H 1997 Complications of the puerperium. In Sweet B R, Tiran D (eds) Mayes Midwifery: A Textbook for Midwives, 12th edn. Baillière Tindall, London.

Beck C T 1996 A meta-analysis of predictors of postpartum depression. Nursing Research 45:297–303.

Blackburn S T 2003 Maternal, Fetal and Neonatal Physiology: A Clinical Perspective, 2nd edn. W B Saunders, Philadelphia.

Boyle F M, Vance J C, Najman J M et al 1996 The mental health impact of stillbirth, neonatal death or SIDS: prevalence and patterns of distress among mothers. Social Science Medicine 43:1273–1282.

Brock T D, Madigan M T 1999 Biology of Micro-organisms, 6th edn. Prentice-Hall, New Jersey.

Campbell-Brown, Hytten F 1998 Carbohydrate metabolism. In Chamberlain G, Broughton Pipkin F (eds) Clinical Physiology in Obstetrics, 3rd edn. Blackwell Science, Oxford.

Chin J 1996 Resistance is useless. New Scientist 12:32–35.

Coad J, Dunstall M 2001 Anatomy and Physiology for Midwives. Mosby, Edinburgh.

Coughlan A 1996 Animal antibiotics threaten hospital antibiotics. New Scientist 27:7.

Cox J, Holden J (eds) 1994 Perinatal Psychiatry. Gaskell, London.

Cox J, Murray D, Chapman G 1993 A controlled study of the onset, duration and prevalence of postnatal depression. British Journal of Psychiatry 150:27–31.

Enkin M, Keirse M J N C, Neilson J et al 2000 A Guide to Effective Care in Pregnancy, 3rd edn. Oxford University Press, Oxford.

Evans J, Heron J, Francomb H et al 2001 Cohort study of depressed mood during pregnancy and after childbirth. British Medical Journal 323:257–260.

Fergusson D, Horwood J, Thorpe K 1996 ALSPAC study team: changes in depression during and following pregnancy. Paediatric Perinatal Epidemiology 10:279–293.

Forman D N, Videbech P, Hedegaard M D 2000 Postpartum depression: identification of women at risk. British Journal of Obstetrics and Gynaecology 107:1210–1217.

Garrett L 1995 The Coming Plague. Virago Press, London.

Hoffbrand S, Howard L, Crawley H 2001 Antidepressant treatment for post-natal depression. Cochrane Review: In The Cochrane Library, Issue 2. Update Software 2003, Oxford.

Howie P W 1995 The puerperium and its complications. In Whitfield E R (ed.) Dewhurst's Textbook for Obstetrics and Gynaecology for Postgraduates, 5th edn. Blackwell Science, London.

Howie P W 1999 The puerperium. In Edmonds K D (ed.) Dewhurst's Textbook for Obstetrics and Gynaecology for Postgraduates, 6th edn. Blackwell Science, London.

Jessel D, Moir A 1995 A Mind to Crime. Signet, London.

Lewis G (ed.) 2001 Why Mothers Die 1997–1999: The Fifth Report of the Confidential Enquiries into Maternal Deaths in the United Kingdom. RCOG Press, London.

Marchant S, Alexander J, Garcia J et al 1999 A survey of women's experience of vaginal loss from 24 hours to three months after childbirth (the BliPP study). Midwifery 15(2):72–81.

Marchant S, Alexander J, Garcia J 2003 How does it feel to you? Uterine palpation and lochial loss as guides to postnatal 'recovery'. In Wickham S (ed.) Best Midwifery Practice. Elsevier, London.

Murray L, Sinclair D, Cooper P et al 1999 The socioemotional development of 5-year olds with postnatally depressed mothers. Journal of Child Psychology and Psychiatry 40:1259–1271.

Oates M 2000 Perinatal Maternal Mental Health Services – Council Report CR88. Royal College of Psychiatrists, London.

Oates M 2001 Deaths from psychiatric causes. In Lewis G (ed.) Why Mothers Die 1997–1999: The Fifth Report of the Confidential Enquiries into Maternal Deaths in the United Kingdom. RCOG Press, London.

O'Hara M W 1997 The nature of postpartum depressive disorders. In Murray L, Cooper P J (eds) Postpartum Depression and Child Development. Guilford, New York.

Schopf J, Rust B 1994 Follow-up and family study of postpartum psychoses. Part 1: overview. European Archives of Psychiatry Clinical Neuroscience 244:101–111.

Sherman D, Lurie S, Frenkle E et al 1999 Characteristics of normal lochia. American Journal of Perinatology 16(8):399–402.

SIGN (Scottish Intercollegiate Guidelines Network) 2002 Postnatal Depression and Puerperal Psychosis: A National Clinical Guideline. Royal College of Physicians, Edinburgh.

Sinclair D, Murray L 1998 Effects of postnatal depression on children's adjustment to school. British Journal of Psychiatry 172:58–63.

Terp I M, Engholm G, Moller H et al 1999 A follow-up study of postpartum psychoses: prognosis and risk factors for readmission. Acta Psychiatrica Scandinavia 100(1):40–46.

UKCC 1998 Midwives Rules and Code of Practice. UKCC, London.

Walsh L V 2001 Midwifery – Community-Based Care during the Childbearing Year. W B Saunders, Philadelphia.

Annotated recommended reading

Lewis G (ed.) 2001 Why Mothers Die 1997–1999: The Fifth Report of the Confidential Enquiries into Maternal Deaths in the United Kingdom. RCOG Press, London.

This report provides interesting and informative reading for all health professionals involved in the care of women during and following childbirth. Every case is described in detail and the reader will gain valuable and constructive information from a professional perspective.

Marchant S, Alexander J, Garcia J 2003 How does it feel to you? Uterine palpation and lochial loss as guides to postnatal 'recovery'. In Wickham S (ed.) Best Midwifery Practice. Elsevier, London.

This is an informative, well-written book providing essential reading of up-to-date midwifery practice issues. In particular, the above sections relate to the postpartum period and provide an overview of three articles about the uterus, its involution and how this is recorded by midwives and described by women.

Chapter 57

Biobehavioural aspects of parenting

APPROACHES TO THE STUDY OF BEHAVIOUR

For thousands of years the brain and mind have been seen as separate entities. The brain was the realm of scientists but the mind was studied by philosophers. In the 19th century scientists realised that sensations such as sight were the result of nerve impulses and experiments were devised to explore them. **Wilhelm Wundt** opened the first psychology laboratory at the University of Leipzig in 1879. Since then, other disciplines have been developed to study behaviour, such as:

- **ethology** – the study of natural behaviour;
- **cognitive psychology** – the way people process information;
- **physiological psychology** – the physical substance and processes in the brain;
- **behaviourism** – observed behaviour, made famous by Pavlov;
- **psychoanalysis** – people's psychological history explains their current behaviour;
- **evolutionary psychology** – the development of behaviour.

Philosophical roots

Hippocrates (460–377 BC) believed that the mind was in the brain and controlled the body. Beginning with Descartes in the 17th century, dualists considered the mind and body to be separate, with the body being constructed from matter but the mind not. The soul was thought to be located in the brain and to control the body. Later philosophers argued that Hippocrates was correct. If the soul is not part of the physical world it cannot move the physical body. If the soul can interact with the body then it must be physical. This developed into **monism**: the mind is a product of the body.

The nature of human consciousness produces a second philosophical issue; that of **determinism** versus **free will**. Most humans believe that they control their minds and choose their behaviour. This relates to **dualism**, implying that it is impossible to search for physiological causes of behaviour. There is still no agreement as to whether monists or dualists are correct in their beliefs but there is a middle course: consciousness is a process of the whole brain, not of individual brain cells.

Meanings and applications

There are two anxieties about psychosocial research findings. First they may be coloured by the biases and beliefs of the researcher's **societal norms** (Davis-Floyd & Mather 2002). Secondly, political leaders may use the theories for their own purposes. Hrdy (1999) discusses 'the politics of motherhood'. Her main concern is the role of the mother in child development. There is a typical dichotomy: should mothers stay at home or go out to work?

Human societies exhibit multiple ways of thinking, which may affect the provision of health care. Davis-Floyd & Mather (2002) describe three paradigms of health care which influence modern maternity care: the **technocratic**, **humanistic** and **holistic** models.

The technocratic model is dualistic, separating body from mind. Machinery and techniques can provide sophisticated physiological supports. This has led to the concept of the body as an unpredictable machine that is likely to need manipulation to ensure health: for example, that birth is successful. In general, the mind is not the concern of technocratic medicine.

The humanistic model developed out of a dissatisfaction of clients and many practitioners with the technological approach. It is a monistic approach that recognises the influence of the mind on the body and advocates care that considers both. Partnership between carer and client is essential. It is close to the concept of **biopsychosocial (mind–body) medicine**.

The holistic model stems from **Eastern philosophy** and was created by people dissatisfied with Western concepts of health and disease. Body and mind are fully integrated, involving the spirit or soul. The body is defined in terms of energy systems such as **chi** and its carers are often **shamans**.

Davis-Floyd & Mather (2002) visualise combining aspects of each model to provide the best system of care possible. There is evidence that the mind plays an important role in the physical state of the body. It is essential to realise the complexity of this field of research and the need for more evidence. This chapter explores two biologically based areas: ethology and physiological psychology.

Ethology

The study of animal behaviour began with Tinbergen and Lorenz in the 1950s and 1960s. Hinde (1982) wrote that:

Ethologists follow a biological tradition in attempting to start their analyses from a secure base of description … the behaviour of each species should be seen in relation to the environmental context to which it has been adapted.

Ethologists ask four types of questions about behaviour:

1. What is its immediate causation?
2. How does it develop?
3. What is its function?
4. How did it evolve?

Hinde (1982) discusses the relationship between ethology and human social sciences such as sociology, psychology and anthropology, believing that ethology alone cannot provide answers to human behaviour but that 'an amalgam of techniques, concepts and theories appropriate to the problem … is essential.' Ethology contributes towards the description and analysis of human behaviour.

Physiological psychology

Darwin's theory of natural selection suggested the concept of **functionalism**: all characteristics of a living organism perform useful functions for that organism. Structural changes between animals of a species are brought about by genetic mutations, some of which affect the way the animal is **adapted** to its **environment** and the way it behaves. Physiological psychologists ask questions about the **selective advantage** a particular behaviour may have for the species.

Recently, the new discipline of evolutionary psychology has examined the wider issue of the evolution of behaviour. Although physiological psychologists take a monistic approach to human behaviour, they remain aware that a **reductionist** process will never explain complex human behaviour.

MATERNAL–CHILD INTERACTION

Instinctive behaviour

Bowlby (1984) wrote:

Behaviour of even the simplest animals is enormously complex. It varies in systematic ways from members of one species to another and in less systematic ways from individual to individual within a species…. Yet there are many regularities of behaviour that are so striking and play so important a part in the survival of individual and species that they have earned the name instinctive.

He described four main characteristics of instinctive behaviour:

1. it follows a recognisably similar and predictive pattern in almost all members of a species (or sex);
2. it is not a simple response to a stimulus but a sequence of behaviour that runs a predictable course;
3. some of its usual consequences are of obvious value in contributing to the preservation of an individual or the continuity of a species;
4. many examples of it develop even when all the ordinary opportunities for learning are absent.

In the past there was argument over which behaviours were **innate** (inborn, genetic, natural) and which were **acquired** (learned, environmental, nurtured) but this is a meaningless division. Every biological character, physiological or behavioural, is a product of gene–environment interaction. If a biological character is little influenced by environmental variations, it is called **environmentally stable** and any characteristic that is much influenced by the environment is **environmentally labile**. Behaviour labelled instinctive is environmentally stable (Hinde 1959).

Some believe that the variability of human behaviour proves that it is culturally driven and nothing is instinctive. Bowlby (1984) disagrees. In higher species instinctive behaviour is not stereotyped but follows a recognisable pattern (characteristic 1) and runs a predictable course (characteristic 2). Mating, child care and the attachment of the young to their parents have survival value for both individual and species (characteristic 3). Despite the immense variety of childbearing cultural norms, some behaviours repeatedly emerge (characteristic 4).

Bowlby believes that behavioural attributes contribute to survival and reproduction when they operate within a prescribed environment. Environmentally stable behaviours are controlled by elements within the environment he calls 'environments of adaptedness': for instance, the range of environmental temperatures that the body can tolerate or the altitude at which the cardiovascular system can function.

The human environment of evolutionary adaptedness

Human versatility and the capacity for innovation have enabled survival in a wide range of environments (Bowlby 1984). In addition, humans have manufactured safe environments, leading to an incredible increase in world population. In the last 15 000 years a rise in **pastoralism** and **agriculture** led to the growth of cities. Unfortunately, this led to an increased risk of infection (McNeill 1979) and pollution (Colborn et al 1996).

The mother's social surroundings are part of the environment in which childbearing and childrearing take place. It is also important to consider the relationships between the sexes. The basis of sexual difference lies in investment in the gametes. Women produce fewer large ova compared to the millions of small sperms. They also provide energy to grow the fetus in utero and to supply milk during infancy (Hrdy 1999).

Lovejoy (1980) believed that pair bonding is part of human ethology, and is typical of species which produce **altricial** (needing care) infants rather than **precocial** infants (able to move about following birth). Male parenting is necessary for the support of the woman and her children during their long growth to maturity. There is no consensus on the nature of the family in human biological terms and it is risky to define evolutionary behaviour in terms of modern hunter-gatherers.

HUMAN CHILDBEARING BEHAVIOUR

Few psychologists and ethologists paid much attention to what human mothers (or fathers) did in the immediate postpartum period. Klaus & Kennel (1976) developed the concept of a **sensitive period** or **imprinting** lasting for a few minutes or hours after birth in which **maternal–infant bonding** or **attachment** (and paternal) is ensured. They define attachment as 'a unique relationship between two people that is specific and endures through time'.

Lorenz believed that if the behaviour did not occur within the **critical period** the opportunity is lost. Hinde (1982) was less restrictive and described a sensitive period as 'a given event that can be produced more readily during a certain period than earlier or later.' The presence of species-specific behaviour is important to Klaus and Kennel's theory. They were concerned about the effects of separating mothers and their babies for long periods. Rooming-in developed from their research.

Bowlby (1984) believed that the immature newborn human infant develops attachment behaviour more slowly than other species. He did not believe in a neonatal sensitive period but he did use the term imprinting, suggesting that the infant's focusing on a single figure, although slow to develop, is sufficiently like that of other mammalian species. Maternal involvement in ensuring that infants remain close to them depends on their relative helplessness. Bowlby talks of an 'evolutionary shift in balance' from the infant taking all responsibility for keeping contact to total maternal responsibility in human mothers because of infant immaturity.

Trevathan (1987) observed maternal behaviour and neonatal behaviour over the first hour after delivery. She wrote, 'Although the process may not always be perfect, behaviours of mammalian females have been selected to complement the needs and capabilities of their young'. Two categories of neonatal behaviours are described. The first is adaptation at birth and the second includes behaviours that enhance mother–infant bonding.

The neonate is described as **secondarily altricial**, requiring a **period of exterogestation** (gestation outside the uterus) with prolongation of infancy. A secondarily altricial baby has his eyes open and uses them to interpret his environment unlike a primarily altricial animal such as a kitten. Evolution has selected for onset of labour when the fetus is still immature. This is a trade-off between the size and shape of the human pelvis and the complexity and size of the human brain.

It has been suggested that the human gestation period should be about 18 months if comparisons with the maturity of infants of other species are made, but in order to be delivered safely, both for the mother and the baby, human infants are born after only 9 months and do not achieve equality of developmental status with other primates until they are 6 months old. Bowlby's observation that attachment, with purposive clinging and distress behaviour equivalent to that of a newborn gorilla, does not occur until the human infant is about 6 months old may be significant! Four important theories about childbearing behaviour are bonding, tactile behaviour, the senses and lateral preferences.

Bonding

Klaus & Kennell (1976) believed that the strong mother–infant bond formed the basis on which the infant's future attachments are formed and through which the child develops a sense of self. They suggested that there was a sensitive period when maternal and paternal attachment to their newborn took place. Although attachment is difficult if the early opportunity is missed, it still develops. Because attachment is a learning process rather than a once-only event, adoptive parents are usually able to form relationships with their children (Klaus & Klaus 1999).

Infant attachment develops over the first 6 months and Bowlby (1984) suggested that infant behaviour develops in phases from simple response to stimuli to a fully reciprocal relationship in response to parental behaviour. Parental behaviour may depend on a sensitive period and if this is disrupted, infant attachment behaviour may not develop normally. Kontos (1978) found that when mothers were allowed an hour of skin-to-skin contact following birth they demonstrated more **holding**, **encompassing** and *en face* behaviour. Their infants cried less and smiled more than those of mothers who were separated from their infants in the first hour.

Criticism of bonding theory

There has been much criticism of bonding theory. Many studies lacked scientific methodology and have been difficult to replicate. Lamb (1983) has criticised bonding theory, believing it unlikely that a species as dependent on social learning as humans would exhibit such narrow behaviour as sensitive periods. However, although early studies were flawed, events within the first few hours after birth are important.

Trevathan (1987) believes in a sensitive period in the first hour after birth which varies markedly across time and between cultures. Mothers who hold their infant close provide warmth, stimulation, eye contact and a chance to talk to the infant in the typical high-pitched voice (Kuhl et al 1997). Holding the baby on her left side near her heart beat may provide continuity from uterine to independent life for the neonate. However, Trevathen concludes that there is scant evidence that contact between mothers and their babies in the immediate postpartum period is necessary for bond formation. The observed behaviours may be 'relics from the past' and have no significant function.

Bowlby (1984) wrote: 'Almost from the first many children have more than one person towards whom they can direct attachment behaviour'. The young infant is given opportunities to form attachment to other family members, particularly the father. The mother does not usually have to accept total responsibility for childrearing. However, a child constantly surrounded by a succession of stranger carers may become withdrawn.

Tactile behaviour

Attendants present at normal births report specific maternal **tactile behaviour** when first given the infant to handle. Rubin (1963) noted an orderly progression of behaviour. Mothers took about 3 days to complete the behavioural sequence but they had limited access to their babies without clothing. Klaus et al (1970) saw the same sequence of behaviour occurring within minutes if mothers were given their naked babies to hold after birth. The mothers began with fingertip touching of their baby's extremities. Within 4–8 min they began to massage, stroke and place the palms of their hands around the baby's trunk.

Trevathan (1987) suggested that in humans stroking has taken over from the licking of young that many mammals do to stimulate breathing and defecation. Trevathan observed 66 women for the first 10 min of contact to examine tactile interaction as a possible species-specific behaviour. Touching behaviours were recorded every 10 s and grouped into seven categories:

1. holding the infant with both hands;
2. holding with one hand;
3. not holding or touching although the infant is with her;
4. holding with one arm with fingertip stroking of the infant's face;
5. holding with one arm with fingertip stroking of the infant's extremities;
6. holding with one arm with fingertip stroking of the infant's trunk;
7. holding with one arm with palmar massaging of the infants extremities and trunk.

She noted that fingertip and palmar touching behaviours reduced together over the 10 min. Fingertip touching was the most common, occurring for about 18% of the time. Palmar massage lasted for 2–6% of the time but most of the time was spent in passive holding (categories 1 and 2). Although tactile behaviours were observed in all women, they varied widely between women. Trevathan could not accept the concept of invariant behaviour and sought endogenous (from within) and exogenous (environmental) factors that might create the differences.

She analysed the behaviour in 'Hispanic' and 'Anglo' mothers and in primiparous and multiparous women. Anglo mothers spent less time holding their babies and changed state more often than Hispanic women. Primiparous women spent more time not touching their infants than multiparous women but slightly longer exploring their babies. Trevathan decided that there is a species-specific pattern of tactile interaction. Typically, mothers cradled the baby for the first few minutes after birth with occasional palmar massage. Finger exploration of face, hands and extremities followed soon.

The senses

The **motor state** of the newborn is rudimentary. However, neonates have functioning vision, hearing and olfaction and seem capable of differentiating stimuli. Studying neonatal sensory processes relies on the ability of a **stimulus** to elicit a **reflex response**. One of the best responses is that of **high-amplitude sucking** when infants are presented with visual and auditory stimuli (Siqueland & Delucia 1969). Other methods include electrical measurement of neonatal brain activity, non-invasive examination with instruments such as an ophthalmoscope and observation of responses to stimuli such as head turning.

Babies left to lie on their mothers' abdomens for an hour after birth retain their body temperature (Christensson et al 1992), crawl up the abdomen and find a nipple (Klaus & Klaus 1999) and begin to suckle unaided. They may use their senses of smell (Varendi et al 1994) and sight as well as the stepping reflex to achieve this. However, many mothers and babies are not given time for such behaviour to occur.

Vision

Newborn babies do not focus very well and **visual acuity** (what detail can be resolved) is about 20–30 times lower than in the adult. Infants focus best at a distance of between 30 and 50 cm (Slater & Findlay 1975), which is approximately the distance between them and the adult face when cradled in adult arms (*en face* position). Infants prefer some visual stimuli rather than others. They prefer to look at moving objects and follow them with their eyes and head (Brazelton et al 1966). They prefer three-dimensional objects over two-dimensional, high-contrast to low-contrast patterns, curved contours rather than straight contours (Fantz & Miranda 1975) and novel objects more than familiar ones.

The *en face* position is part of attachment behaviour between mothers and fathers and their infants. Klaus et al (1975) noted that a mother's interest in her baby's eyes increased during the first 10 min following birth. It is the distance that a mother holds her baby when she is breastfeeding, a time of optimal contact for the mother and her baby (Fig. 57.1).

Trevathan (1987) found that all her mothers spent time in the first hour after birth looking at their infants *en face*. Neonates recognise their mothers' faces from very early in life and will suck faster to see an image of their mother preferentially to other faces as early as 4 h after delivery. **Women cradle their newborn babies on their left arms, regardless of their own handedness** (Salk 1960, Hope 2002). This **holding preference** is linked with monitoring the emotional state of the baby (Manning & Chamberlain 1991).

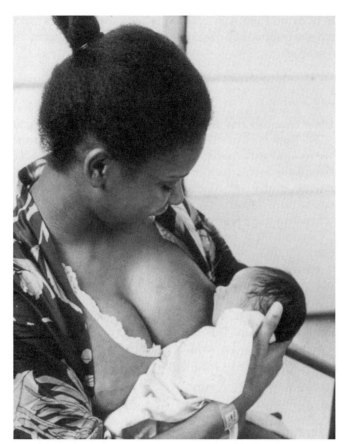

Figure 57.1   Eye contact during breastfeeding (from Kelnar C, Harvey D, Simpson C 1995, with permission).

Imitation of facial expressions (Kaitz et al 1987) suggests that the newborn recognises expressions and can copy them. This is amazing as facial expressions utilise many muscles. If you stick out your tongue, a baby may poke out his tongue in imitation. Babies also imitate an open mouth expression. As early as 14 days after delivery some babies smile in response to social interaction.

Hearing

Neonates orient to sound by turning their heads. They show interest in human speech and suck more vigorously in response to the mother's voice as early as 3 days after birth (DeCasper & Fifer 1980). Researchers have recorded that women (and men) speak to babies in a **high-pitched voice** (Lang 1972). The neonatal auditory system responds more readily to higher frequencies of the human voice.

Speech is not one-sided. **Entrainment** is the rhythmic movement made by a baby in response to the mother's voice, or indeed any human in response to speech. Condon & Sander (1974) demonstrated this **interactional synchrony** as early as 12 h after birth. Besides altering the pitch of their voices, adults tend to use repetitive, simplistic language when talking to infants (and pet animals). The baby moves its body and limbs in synchrony with the mother's voice and she responds by continuing to talk, thus prolonging the synchrony.

Olfaction

Babies recognise and distinguish different smells (Macfarlane 1975). They may use the smell and taste of amniotic fluid and its similarity to the smell and taste of the oil produced around the areola to locate the nipple (Schaal et al 1995, Varendi et al 1994). Macfarlane demonstrated that young babies turn towards breast pads worn by their mother rather than those worn by other lactating mothers.

Fleming et al (1995) confirmed that mothers quickly learned to recognise their babies' odour, especially if given an early opportunity to hold and feed their babies. They recognised T-shirts worn by their babies when allowed to choose between them and T-shirts worn by other babies. Vernix provides a source for bacterial colonisation and odour production. This recognition may be important for bonding and the importance of human olfaction is supported by studies of people recognising the smell of their partners.

Lateral preferences

Maternal holding preference

Salk (1960) discovered that women prefer to hold their babies on the left side of their bodies irrespective of handedness. This observation has been confirmed by many studies over the last 30 years. Various hypotheses have been put forward to explain this preference, all derived from a belief that **the baby elicits the behaviour**. Salk thought that when the baby was held on the left side of the thorax the maternal heart beat sounds soothed the infant. Ginsburg et al (1979) found mothers' holding side preference was related to their baby's head-turning preference; infants who preferred to turn their heads to the right (more than 80% of them) were carried on the left side of the body and vice versa. Mothers carrying their babies on their left may be monitoring their infants' emotions with the right side of their brain (Manning & Chamberlain 1991, Hope 2002).

Neonatal head-turning preferences

More than 80% of newborn babies prefer to turn their heads to the right when lying supine (Gesell 1945, Turkewitz et al 1965). This may be linked to eventual handedness developing out of continued attention to the hand most often in their visual field (Michel 1981). Liederman & Kinsbourne (1980) found evidence that head-turning behaviour is genetically programmed. They believed the asymmetrical

behaviour was linked to asymmetry in the motor development of the brain hemispheres. Cornwell et al (1985) found that the strong right-sided preference at birth had disappeared by 3 months.

Implications for practice

Attachment theory

If the sensitive period is present in humans, how should the professional interpret the first hour after birth? Sweet (1997) advises midwives that they have a duty to ensure that all mothers have the opportunity to be with their new babies during this hour. Absence of this time may adversely affect the way mothers perceive the birth and this is still evident 6 weeks after the delivery (Ball 1994). Although maternal–infant attachment may not suffer if this behaviour is omitted, the mother may find birth less fulfilling. Those helping the mother at birth should help to create the relationship between mother and baby. Klaus & Klaus (1999) are adamant that at least an hour should be set aside for this interaction.

Lateral behavioural preferences

Mothers often report more difficulty feeding their babies on one breast than the other (Stables & Hewitt 1995). The problem often arose when the woman was right-handed, preferred to carry the baby on her left and the baby preferred to turn its head to the right. This made the left breast much easier to feed from as the woman held the baby on her left arm and had her right dominant hand free to offer the baby the nipple. When the baby turned his head to the right he turned towards the breast. When she tried to feed with her right breast she was uncomfortable with the baby on her right arm, clumsy with her left hand and the baby turned away from the breast. Unfortunately, this group included most mothers!

Although most mothers adapted after a few feeds, some women gave up feeding because of the initial difficulty. Midwives can use their skills by varying the way the mother holds the baby to ensure that early feeding is successful. In women with the above problem, the following should be tried:

1. the baby is tucked under the right arm with his head cradled on her left hand;
2. he can then suckle with his head turned towards the right;
3. the mother can use her right hand to offer him the nipple.

This is not a new strategy. Midwives have used it for decades, but may not have known why. That is why research-based practice is so important to decide what care is of value.

MAIN POINTS

- Hippocrates believed that the mind was in the brain and controlled the body, a monistic theory. Based on Descartes' ideas, dualists consider the mind and body to be separate. There is still no agreement as to whether monists or dualists are correct in their beliefs. There is a second major philosophical issue: determinism versus free will.

- Psychosocial research findings may be coloured by the biases and beliefs of the researcher's societal norms. Three paradigms of health care which influence modern maternity care have been described: the technocratic, humanistic and holistic models.

- Ethologists ask four types of questions about behaviour: What is its immediate causation? How does it develop? What is its function? How did it evolve? Physiological psychologists ask questions about the selective advantage a particular behaviour may have for the species but are aware that human behaviour is complex and reductionism cannot predict it.

- Biological characters are products of the interaction between genes and the environment. A character little influenced by environmental variations is environmentally stable and any characteristic that is much influenced by the environment is environmentally labile.

- Humans have manufactured safe environments within which environmentally stable components of behaviour are found. The social surroundings of the woman are part of the environment in which childbearing and child-rearing take place.

- Some believe that pair bonding is part of human ethology. Male parenting is necessary for the support of the woman and her children during the long growth to maturity of the human child. There is no consensus on the nature of the family in human biological terms and it is risky to define evolutionary behaviour in terms of modern hunter-gatherers.

- Klaus and Kennel developed the concept of a species-specific sensitive period lasting for a few minutes or hours after birth in which maternal–infant attachment is ensured. Rooming-in developed from their research. Bowlby suggested that the infant's focusing on a single figure, although slow to develop, is like that of other mammalian species.

- The baby can be described as secondarily altricial at birth requiring a period of exterogestation to complete maturation. The onset of human labour at 40 weeks means that the neonate is still immature compared to most mammals. This is a trade-off between the size and shape of the human pelvis and the complexity and size of the human brain.

- It is possible that human gestation should last about 18 months and babies do not achieve equality of developmental status with other primates until they are 6 months old.

- There is little evidence that early contact between mothers and their babies is necessary for bond formation but when mothers are allowed an hour of skin-to-skin contact following birth they demonstrated more holding, encompassing and *en face* behaviour.

- Most infants are given an early opportunity to form attachment to other family members, particularly the father. Feminists objected to bonding studies because they believed that the theory was an attempt to keep mothers tied to their babies and in the home.

- When first given the infant to handle, mothers began with fingertip touching of their baby's extremities. Within 4–8 min they began to massage, stroke and place the palms of their hands around the baby's trunk.

- The motor state of the newborn is rudimentary but neonates have functioning vision, hearing and olfaction and seem capable of differentiating stimuli. One of the best-used stimuli for eliciting neonatal responses is that of high-amplitude sucking.

- Babies left to lie on their mothers' abdomens for an hour after birth retain their body temperature, crawl up the abdomen and find a nipple and begin to suckle unaided. They may use their senses of smell and sight as well as the stepping reflex to achieve this.

- Newborn babies do not focus very well but prefer to look at moving objects. They prefer three-dimensional objects over two-dimensional and high-contrast to low-contrast patterns, curved contours to straight contours and novel objects more than familiar ones. Women hold their babies in the *en face* position and neonates can recognise their mothers' faces from very early in their life. They can also imitate facial expressions.

- Women speak to babies in a high-pitched voice and the neonatal auditory system responds more readily to the higher frequencies. Babies move their bodies and limbs in synchrony with the mother's voice. She responds by continuing to talk, prolonging the synchrony.

- Babies can recognise and distinguish different smells and may use their sense of smell to locate the nipple. Mothers quickly learn to recognise their babies' odour, especially if they have been given an early opportunity to hold and feed their babies.

- Women prefer to hold their babies on the left side of their bodies irrespective of handedness. Various hypotheses have been put forward to explain this, all derived from a belief that the baby elicits the behaviour. About 90% of newborn babies prefer to turn their heads to the right when lying supine. The right-sided preference disappears by 3 months.

- Mothers report more difficulty feeding their babies on one breast than the other. The problem arises when a right-handed woman prefers to carry the baby on her left and the baby prefers to turn his head to the right. The left breast is much easier to feed from. After a few feeds most mothers and babies soon adapt, but some women give up feeding because of the initial difficulty.

- Midwives could vary the way the mother holds the baby to ensure that the early feeding efforts are successful. In the women with the above problem, if the baby is tucked under the right arm so that he can suckle with his head turned towards the right, the mother is more likely to be successful.

References

Ball J A (ed.) 1994 Reactions to Motherhood. Hale: Books for Midwives Press, London.

Bowlby J 1984 Attachment and Loss: Vol. 1 Attachment. Penguin Books, Harmondsworth.

Brazelton T B, Scholl M L, Robey J S 1966 Visual responses in the newborn. Pediatrics 37:284–290.

Christensson K, Siles C, Moreno L et al 1992 Temperature, metabolic adaptation and crying in healthy, full term babies cared for skin-to-skin or in a cot. Acta Paediatrica 81:488–493.

Colborn T, Myers J P, Dumanoski D 1996 Our Stolen Future. Little, Brown and Company, Philadelphia.

Condon W S, Sander L W 1974 Neonate movement is synchronised with adult speech: interactional participation and language acquisition. Science 183:99–101.

Cornwell K S, Barnes C L, Fitzgerald H E, Harris L J 1985 Neurobehavioral reorganisation in early infancy: patterns of head orientation following lateral and midline holds. Infant Mental Health Journal 6(3):126–136.

Davis-Floyd R, Mather F S 2002 The technocratic, humanistic and holistic paradigms of childbirth. MIDIRS Midwifery Digest 4(12):500–506.

DeCasper A J, Fifer W P 1980 Of human bonding: newborns prefer their mothers' voices. Science 208:1174–1176.

De Swiet 1998 The cardiovascular system. In Chamberlain G, Broughton Pipkin F (eds) Clinical Physiology in Obstetrics, 3rd edn. Blackwell Science, Oxford.

Fantz R L, Miranda S 1975 Newborn infant attention to form and contour. Child Development 46:224–228.

Fleming A, Corter C, Surbey M, Franks P, Steiner M 1995 Postpartum factors related to mothers' recognition of newborn infant odours. Journal of Reproductive and Infant Psychology 13(3–4):197–210.

Gesell A 1945 The Embryology of Behaviour. Harpes, New York.

Ginsburg H J, Fling S, Hope M L, Musgrove D, Andrews C 1979 Maternal holding preferences: a consequence of newborn head turning behaviour. Child Development 50:280–281.

Hinde R A 1959 Some recent trends in ethology. In Koch S (ed.) Psychology: a Study of a Science. McGraw-Hill, New York.

Hinde R A 1982 Ethology. Fontana, London.

Hope J 2002 Why women cradle babies on their left. Daily Mail, Saturday September 7:41.

Hrdy S B 1999 Mother Nature. Pantheon, London.

Kaitz M, Good A, Rokem A M, Eidelman A I 1987 Mothers' recognition of their newborns by olfactory cues. Developmental Psychology 20:587–591.

Klaus M H, Kennell J H 1976 Maternal–Infant Bonding. C V Mosby, St Louis.

Klaus M H, Klaus P H 1999 Your Amazing Newborn. Perseus Books, Cambridge, Massachusetts.

Klaus M H, Kennell J H, Plumb N, Zuehlke S 1970 Human maternal behaviour at first contact with her young. Pediatrics 46:187–192.

Klaus M H, Trause M A, Kennell J H 1975 Does human maternal behaviour after birth show a characteristic pattern? Parent–Infant Interaction. Ciba Foundation Symposium 33, Elsevier, Amsterdam. In Trevathan W R 1987 Human Birth: An Evolutionary Perspective. Aldine de Grutyer, New York.

Kontos D 1978 A study of the effects of extended mother–infant contact on maternal behaviour at one and three months. Birth and the Family Journal 5:133–140.

Kuhl K, Andruski J E, Chistovich I A et al 1997 Cross-language analysis of phonetic units in language addressed to infants. Science 277:684–686.

Lamb M E 1983 Early mother–neonate contact and the mother–child relationship. Journal of Child Psychology and Psychiatry 24:487–494.

Lang R 1972 Birth Book. Genesis Press, Ben Lomond, California. In Klaus M H, Kennell J H 1976 Maternal–Infant Bonding. Mosby, St Louis.

Liederman J, Kinsbourne M 1980 Rightward turning bases in neonates reflect a single neural asymmetry in motor planning. Infant Behaviour and Development 3:245–251.

Lovejoy O 1980 Hominid origins: the role of bipedalism. American Journal of Physical Anthropology 52:250, cited in Johanson D C, Edey M A Lucy 1981. The Beginnings of Mankind. William Clowes (Beccles) Ltd, Beccles and London.

Macfarlane A 1975 Olfaction in the development of social preferences in the human neonate. In Parent–Infant Interaction, CIBA Foundation Symposium, 33:103–113. Elsevier, Amsterdam.

McNeill W H 1979 Plagues and Peoples. Penguin Books, Harmondsworth.

Manning J T, Chamberlain A T 1991 Left-sided cradling and brain lateralisation. Ethology and Sociobiology 12:237–244.

Michel G 1981 Right-handedness: a consequence of infant supine head-orientation preference? Science 212:685–687.

Rubin R 1963 Maternal touch. Nursing Outlook 22:828–831.

Salk L 1960 The effects of the normal heart beat sound on the behaviour of the newborn infant: implications for mental health. World Mental Health 12:168–175.

Schaal B, Marlier L, Soussignon R 1995 Responsiveness to the odour of amniotic fluid in the human neonate. Biology of the Neonate 67:397–406.

Siqueland E R, Delucia C A 1969 Visual reinforcement of non-nutritive sucking in human infants. Science 165:1144–1146.

Slater A, Findlay J 1975 Binocular fixation in the newborn baby. Journal of Experimental Child Psychology 20:248–273.

Stables D, Hewitt G 1995 The effect of lateral asymmetries on breast feeding skills: can midwives' holding interventions overcome unilateral breast feeding problems? Midwifery 11:28–36.

Sweet B R 1997 The psychology of childbirth. In Sweet B R, Tiran D (eds) Mayes Midwifery, 12th edn. Baillière Tindall, London, pp 151–158.

Trevathan W R 1987 Human Birth: An Evolutionary Perspective. Aldine de Grutyer, New York.

Turkewitz G, Gordon E W, Birch H G 1965 Head turning in the human neonate: spontaneous patterns. Journal of Comparative and Physiological Psychology 59:189–192.

Varendi H, Porter R H, Winberg J 1994 Does the newborn find the nipple by smell? Lancet 344:989–990.

Annotated recommended reading

Bowlby J 1984 Attachment and Loss: Vol. 1 Attachment. Penguin Books, Harmondsworth.
This book is grounded in ethology and lays the foundations for much ongoing discussion and styles of care provided for mothers, fathers and their babies.

Davis-Floyd R, Mather F S 2002 The technocratic, humanistic and holistic paradigms of childbirth. MIDIRS Midwifery Digest 4(12):500–506.
The descriptions of three paradigms of health care that influence contemporary childbirth in industrialised nations are clear, highly significant for midwives and provide a basis for understanding of the many theories that complicate care provision.

Hrdy S B 1999 Mother Nature. Pantheon, London.
Sarah Hrdy is qualified in anthropology, primatology and evolutionary theory and has combined motherhood with an academic career. This book reassesses key assumptions about human evolution and reproduction in the light of human social organisation.

Human Nature Part 1 2003 New Scientist 178(2395):33–48.
Human Nature Part 2 2003 New Scientist 178(2396):37–57.
These two multi-authored supplements bring the sciences mentioned in this chapter up to date as of May 2003. The articles by internationally known scientists such as Sarah Hrdy include infant behaviour, gender and women's issues and recent thinking on the nature of mind.

Klaus M H, Klaus P H 1999 Your Amazing Newborn. Perseus Books, Cambridge, Massachusetts.
This is a book full of knowledge about the neonate backed up by excellent photographs. It is suitable for both parents and care providers as there is a reference section at the end full of original research.

Index

Note: page numbers in *italics* refer to boxes, figures and tables.

diabetes mellitus 462
effectiveness 60–61
emergency 65
failure rate per hundred woman years 61
fertilisation prevention 64–66
natural methods 68
physiological application 61–64
preconception counselling 85
vaccines 70
see also combined oral contraception
(COC); oral contraceptives
contraceptive sponge 66
contractions 476
fetal heart response 491–492
first stage 479–480
monitoring 586
second stage 510
stress testing 181
controlled cord traction (CCT) 523, 524
conus medullaris 359
convulsions
hypernatraemia 672
tonic–clonic 428
Coombes' test, direct 183
copper in breast milk 696
cord blood banks 34
cordocentesis procedure 196
cornea 127
coronary arteries 221
myocardial perfusion 654
coronary artery disease 459
coronary circulation 221
corpora atretica 46
corpora cavernosa 55
corpus albicans 45
corpus luteum 45, 46
maintenance in pregnancy 403
menstrual cycle 48
regression 46
corpus mammae 686
corpus spongeosum 55
cortical reaction *100*
corticospinal tract 367–368
corticosteroids
labour preterm onset 536
preterm rupture of membranes 536
prophylactic in preterm labour 637
respiratory distress syndrome 658–659
surfactant production 536
corticosterone 381
corticotropin-releasing hormone 381
cortisol 376, 381
biosynthesis block 465
changes in pregnancy 383
functions 381
prolactin production 691
cortisone 381
coughing 241
countercurrent exchange 259
countercurrent multiplier 259
coupled transporters 18
covalent bonds 4, 6
Cowper's glands 55
cows' milk modification 707–708
see also infant formula
coxsackie virus 458

crack cocaine 705
cradling 727
cranial nerves 359
palsy 680
crash induction 602
cremaster muscle 52
Crick, Francis HC 24
cricoid pressure 601
cristae 15–16
critical period 725
crown–heel length 101
crown–rump length 101, 145, 166, *168*
gestational age 170
crying 628
crypts of Lieberkühn 283, 284
Cushing's syndrome 271, 465
cyanide 86
cyanocobalamin *310*
cyanosis
central 650
oxygen therapy 640
cystic fibrosis 28, 30, *31*, 198–199, 671
gene therapy 34, 199
jaundice 670
meconium passage 642, 666
mutations 198–199
stem cell therapy 34
cystic fibrosis transmembrane receptor
(CFTR) 198, 199
cystic hygroma 196
cytochromes 668
cytokines 396, 404
inhibition 397
neonatal 626
cytokinesis 20
cytomegalovirus (CMV) 188
cytoplasm 10, 11, 13–16
cytosines 15
cytoskeleton 13, 16–17
cytotoxic T lymphocytes (CTLs) 187, 395, 397
cytotrophoblast 147
migratory 147–148
cytotrophoblastic shell 148–149

D

D cells 282
dairy products 87
dartos muscle 52
D-dimer estimation 440
DDT 86, 88
death
fetal demise
early 411
single 173
fetal in hyperthyroidism 464
neonatal 535
in utero fetal 537
see also perinatal death
decidua 104, 149, *150*, 151, 344
labour onset 473
puerperium 714
decidual cells 344
deep vein thrombosis 439–440
defecation 289

defensins 389
deglutition 280
dehydration 271, 457, 696
dehydroepiandrosterone sulphate (DHEAS)
383, 472
7-dehydroxycholesterol 320
delivery
breech presentation 546–550, 678
risks 543–544
cardiac disorders 424
diabetes mellitus 462
face to pubes 558
fibrinogen degradation products 475
herpes simplex infection 188
hypertension 429
IUGR infant 182
multiple pregnancy 176, 609
occipitoposterior position of vertex 557–558
operative 595–602
placenta praevia 417
placental abruption 419
premature 637–638
small for gestational age baby 645
traumatic 461
see also forceps delivery; vaginal delivery
delusions 718
dementia, Huntington's disease 198
dendrites 350, 496
dental lamina 121
dentine 121
deoxyhaemoglobin 208
deoxyribonucleic acid *see* DNA
depolarisation 339, 352
Depo-Provera 65
depression, postnatal 718
Derbyshire neck 465
dermatomes 120, 360, *361*
pain perception 498
dermis 120
Descartes, Renée 723
desferrioxamine 439
desmosomes 222
desogestrel 64–65
desynchronised sleep *357*
detergents 87
determinism 723
detrusor muscle 261
developing world, breastfeeding 706
dexamethasone 659
dextrose 672
diabetes mellitus
control 461
gestational 458–459, 462–463
juvenile onset 458
low birth weight 311
maternal 609, 650
metabolic changes *460*
obesity 83
pathological effects 459
pathophysiology 457–458
physiological effects *460*
pregnancy 457–463
care 461–462
prepregnancy care 82
type 1 458
type 2 458